Advanced Yoga Practices

—

Support Forum Posts of Yogani

—

2005-2010

Yogani

Cover image of radiating *OM* symbol drawn by the author.

Advanced Yoga Practices (AYP)

For ordering information go to:

www.advancedyogapractices.com

NOTE: For a free download of the original eBook version of this volume, containing live links to the underlined internet links herein, go to the Contact link on the above website to submit a request. The ebook comes in several popular formats covering most eBook reading devices. Please include verification of purchase with your request.

ISBN 978-1-4793887-4-5 (Paperback)
ISBN 978-0-9819255-0-9 (eBook)

Also by the Author

Yogani is an American spiritual scientist who, for nearly forty years, has been integrating ancient techniques from around the world which cultivate human spiritual transformation. The approach is non-sectarian, and open to all. His books include:

Advanced Yoga Practices – Easy Lessons for Ecstatic Living (Two Volumes)

Two large user-friendly textbooks providing over 400 detailed lessons on the AYP integrated system of practices.

The Secrets of Wilder – A Story of Inner Silence, Ecstasy and Enlightenment

This modern novel was written before AYP, helping inspire the extensive practical writings on self-directed spiritual practice that became the AYP system.

The AYP Enlightenment Series

Easy-to-read instruction books on yoga practices, including:

- *Deep Meditation – Pathway to Personal Freedom*
- *Spinal Breathing Pranayama – Journey to Inner Space*
- *Tantra – Discovering the Power of Pre-Orgasmic Sex*
- *Asanas, Mudras and Bandhas – Awakening Ecstatic Kundalini*
- *Samyama – Cultivating Stillness in Action, Siddhis and Miracles*
- *Diet, Shatkarmas and Amaroli – Yogic Nutrition and Cleansing for Health and Spirit*
- *Self-Inquiry – Dawn of the Witness and the End of Suffering*
- *Bhakti and Karma Yoga – The Science of Devotion and Liberation Through Action*
- *Eight Limbs of Yoga – The Structure and Pacing of Self-Directed Spiritual Practice*
- *Retreats – Fast Track to Freedom – A Guide for Leaders and Practitioners*
- *Liberation – The Fruition of Yoga*

For up-to-date information on the writings of Yogani, and the free *AYP Support Forums*, please visit:

www.advancedyogapractices.com

We who practice and share are
Candles lighting candles
Until all candles are lit…

Introduction

When the Advanced Yoga Practices (AYP) online lessons began on <u>Yahoo Groups</u> in 2003, there was an immediate flow of email coming here with questions on practices and experiences. The resulting email correspondences with hundreds of people became a mainstay in the development of the lessons, and in the evolution of the way the implementation of the integrated system of practices was adapted to accommodate a worldwide community of practitioners. The email interactions and online lessons led to publication of the first <u>AYP Easy Lessons for Ecstatic Living book</u>, and all the books that followed.

From the beginning, readers of the lessons were asking for a forum community so practitioners could communicate with each other. It was not undertaken immediately because the amount of administration that would be required to set up and operate such an online community was daunting. Later on, as people stepped forward to assist with moderation and other aspects of setting up and running a forum, an AYP forum was <u>launched on Yahoo Groups</u> in February of 2005. It soon had over 1,000 members, communicating on many aspects of spiritual practice and experience. As you will see in the last chapter of this book, my participation in that first AYP forum on Yahoo was limited, because extensive email communications were continuing here, and new lessons and books were being written. It was only later that practitioners began relying less on my email and more on the support forum community as the primary place for communicating on their practices and experiences.

While the first AYP forum was a good start, it soon became apparent that a more fully-featured forum environment would be necessary, with capabilities for managing multiple public forum categories for the growing online community, plus backrooms for administration and projects. So in July of 2005, the forum was moved to its current location at <u>www.aypsite.org/forum</u>. Since then, the AYP community has steadily grown in size and scope, covering every aspect of spiritual practice in a well-moderated environment. As of this writing, forum membership is approaching 4,000, which is but the tip of the iceberg in terms of overall readership. The AYP support forums and free website lessons saw over <u>130,000 unique visitors in 2010</u>, coming from nearly every country in the world.

Since the forum moved to <u>www.aypsite.org/forum</u>, my participation has been much more, with the majority of email support shifting to the public forums, and with many other experienced practitioners participating in the support function as well. In this way, support for spiritual practices and experiences has become much more efficient, and beneficial for many with the ongoing public discussions. The forums are also serving as a launching platform for many "real world" activities, like local meditation groups, training, retreats, and research on practices. All of these activities are on the rise worldwide.

To date, the public AYP forums have received over 65,000 posts, with about 2,000 of those coming from me. This book contains the 2,000 posts. They are organized by 23 public forum categories, with posts in ascending order by date in each forum category (oldest first). At the beginning of each forum "chapter" (see table of contents), a link to the category in the actual forum is provided, and a link is provided to the actual post for every post in this book. All links in the text of the posts are "live" in the original eBook edition, whether they go to other posts in the forums, to AYP online lessons, or anywhere else on the internet.

This paperback edition has been published in 2012 to provide a physical record of the forum posts for those who may wish to have them. This is a volume that can be placed on the shelf along with the other AYP books. While physical books offer advantages, this one is lacking in its ability to provide quick access to internet links that are included in the original forum posts and the original 2011 eBook edition. Also, in order to keep the number of pages in this paperback edition at a level that would be physically manageable and affordable for the reader, the formatting and fonts have been modified from the original eBook edition.

NOTE: <u>For a free download of the original eBook edition</u> of this volume containing live links to the underlined internet links herein, go to the Contact link at <u>www.advancedyogapractices.com</u> to submit a request. The eBook comes in several popular formats covering most eBook reading devices. Please include verification of purchase of the paperback edition with your request. The full benefits of the eBook will be most accessible on reading devices that have browser and internet capability.

In many cases, a post here can stand on its own, providing useful information on the AYP practices. In other cases, links in the post text will provide the full context of the discussion in the actual forum topics, AYP lessons, or elsewhere on the internet.

This book has been published to create a permanent archive for all posts from me in the 2005-2010 period. It is also to provide better access to the writings. In the eBook edition, it will be easier to search 2,000 posts than to search 65,000 posts in the live forums. The latter is actually a topic search and does not zero in on specific posts the way it can be done in the eBook. In this way, much more targeted searches can be accomplished. So the free eBook edition can be a useful companion to this paperback edition.

The posts in this book have not been edited for content. Nearly everything is just as it appears in the actual forum. So what you see is what you get. Hence, in some posts there may not be much information on practices, where a simple "thank you" is being expressed, input on a forum operations discussion, AYP promotion discussion, or whatever. In many other posts, there is a lot of information on practices, supplementing the AYP lessons and books. That is the real value of the forums and this book – to supplement the baseline AYP writings. As we have often said, the forums should not be used as a primary instructional tool for practices. For that, they are not complete. Better to go to the AYP lessons and books first, and then use the forums to supplement that, as needed.

Because the same questions keep coming up from many practitioners, you will find redundancy in many of the forum posts here. That is just how human interactions on spiritual matters occur. It is like touching an elephant from many different angles. It is the same elephant, whether we are feeling the tail, the leg, the tusk, or the trunk. It can seem redundant when we keep touching the same parts, but we will notice differences also. In time, the redundancies and the differences add up to the whole. It is not a bad thing. The forums are especially that way, where everyone is touching the elephant again and again. We keep answering the same questions coming from many angles. If we are engaged in daily practices, our level of consciousness will be continually expanding, so reading the same things every few weeks or months will bring new perspectives. This book can be handy for that, as can reading any of the AYP lessons or books more than once.

You may also find a few posts from me here challenging certain members who are pressing an agenda, proselytizing, attacking a teaching or a guru, etc. While the AYP community is very tolerant of all spiritual paths, there is a limited tolerance for attempts to force an agenda on others. If such attempts are borderline and make it past moderation into the forum discussions, they will likely be challenged, and there is some of that in here. All of my posts are here. As they say, it is "the good, the bad, and the ugly." Hopefully not too much bad and ugly. :-)

On translating the 2,000 forum posts to the published book environment, some technical compromises were necessary to make it work. Images in large quantities are difficult to translate to the several book formats, so the various kinds of "smilies" in the live forum have either been converted to a text equivalent, like the one immediately above, or eliminated.

Finally, it should be emphasized that my posts represent a small fraction of the vast online resource the AYP support forums have become for assisting many to navigate the path of self-directed spiritual practice. My deepest thanks go to all who have contributed to the support forums, whether it be with their experience in spiritual practices, administration or technical skills. Without the help of many, the AYP forums and this book would not have been possible.

It is hoped you will find this book helpful as you continue on your chosen path. Practice wisely, and enjoy!

The guru is in you.

Yogani
January 2011
(Edited September 2012 for the paperback edition)

Table of Contents

Forum 1 – Overview and Announcements

AYP Forums instructions, guidelines and news.
http://www.aypsite.org/forum/forum.asp?FORUM_ID=26

2005/07/10 10:42:17
Overview and Announcements
http://www.aypsite.org/forum/topic.asp?TOPIC_ID=273
Press Release - History of AYP

FOR IMMEDIATE RELEASE

Contact:
Yogani at AYP Publishing
yogani99@yahoo.com
www.aypsite.org

Advanced Meditation Techniques in Everyone's Reach with New Books and Website

Jacksonville, FL -- July 1, 2005 -- What can a new offbeat novel called "The Secrets of Wilder" do for you? Maybe a lot if you resonate with its solid grounding in actual secret spiritual practices.

About two years ago, a Florida man took the name "Yogani" and started putting lessons on the Internet intimately describing advanced deep meditation, spinal breathing methods and tantric sexual techniques. He did not expect that he would end up with thousands of readers worldwide and two books published. But that is what happened, and now Yogani has emerged as one of the leading exponents of public teaching of formerly secret ancient spiritual practices which cultivate lasting inner peace, happiness and an unmistakable ecstatic radiance.

Such breaks with tradition are typically American, and Yogani is definitely that. Born in New York, he grew up Christian in the 1950s and 60s, securing an education in science followed by career, marriage and children. All the while he was steadily expanding from his Christian roots, systematically integrating esoteric methods from the Far East into his daily spiritual practice routine. Over thirty years later and retired, he decided to write it all down so there would be a record of his research left behind for other seekers of truth. The Internet writing has evolved to become a vast non-sectarian website with hundreds of free lessons on spiritual techniques, as well as numerous other resources for avid seekers. Along with its huge following has come a mountain of reader testimonials. You can find it at http://www.aypsite.org

Just published, "The Secrets of Wilder" is Yogani's second book. It is a fast-paced tale that begins with a young athlete's commitment to "spiritual transformation" made on a wind-swept Florida beach. After a hair-raising journey of change lasting some ten years, John Wilder and his devoted beautiful love-mate, Devi Duran, end up bringing a generous dose of enlightenment to the world. But at what cost? It is a story of unwavering personal resolve, the discovery of powerful spiritual practices and their far-reaching effects, simmering romance, adventure, humor, miracles and ultimate sacrifices. Interestingly, "The Secrets of Wilder" takes place in the setting of mainstream American Christian culture, expanding the view of what a journey to enlightenment can be from a Christian perspective.

The first book, published last December, is called "Advanced Yoga Practices - Easy Lessons for Ecstatic Living." It is a large, user-friendly textbook on spiritual practices that goes well beyond the website lessons. It is a blend of East and West, with a down home writing style, all woven together into an open system of daily practices that is as pragmatic as it is profound in its results. Readers are calling it one of the clearest and most comprehensive books ever written on spiritual techniques. From the standpoint of practices, it serves as an optional in-depth reference book for those who read "The Secrets of Wilder."

Yogani has several more books in preparation and will continue adding to the free Internet lessons as long as his typing fingers are able. He treasures the relative peace and quiet of anonymity, and adamantly rejects the "guru" label. In fact, every lesson he puts on the Internet ends with, "The guru is in you."

For more information:
Website – http://www.aypsite.org
Books Page - http://www.aypsite.org/books.html
Book Flyer - http://www.aypsite.org/11-AYP-Flyer-ivory.pdf

For all the AYP Press Releases, see:
http://www.aypsite.org/pressrelease.html

2005/07/13 14:09:57
Overview and Announcements
http://www.aypsite.org/forum/topic.asp?TOPIC_ID=292
Navigation and Posting Guidelines

Please register for the AYP Forums whether you plan on posting messages or not. It is free and only takes a minute. It will open up many AYP forums features to you, and will be helpful for monitoring reader interest. Your email address is revealed only to those you write to directly. Select "**Register**" on the top menu.

The structure of the AYP forums is simple, and most actions are easy to intuit from the forum icons. There are two main categories of forums:

The aypsite.org forums - These were created specifically for this site and there are more than 20 of them, most with a lead-in posting from Yogani. An unlimited number of new topics may be created in these forums. Replies are automatically appended to each topic in a string, or thread.

The Yahoo AYP Forum Archive - These are from the old Yahoo forum, with over 1,000 postings in over 200 topic threads, preserved here on this site. These can still be replied to. It is requested that new topics be started in the aypsite.org forums.

Search: Any or all of the forum and archive topics can be searched for words and phrases. Select "**Search**" on the top menu. "Subject Only" searches will yield more targeted results.

New Postings: To find new activity since your last visit, or for any prior period desired, select "**Active Topics**" on the top menu.

Bug Note: Direct links in postings will not work if followed immediately by a punctuation mark like a period, comma or semicolon. Parentheses and brackets are okay, and will not disable the link.

Moderating: All forums are moderated to assure the appropriateness of the discussions, correct topic placement, and no spam. Inappropriate material (abusive conduct, off-topic posts, proselytizing, ad nauseum arguing, guru-bashing, spam, etc.) will not be posted. If a topic is placed in a mismatched forum, it may be moved by a moderator, so please do your best to post in a forum appropriate to your subject matter. The IDs of those who come to the forums to post spam will be locked.

The focus of the AYP forums is on spiritual practices and experiences. Posts focusing on political, cultural, social, environmental, etc. issues and causes will not be approved by the moderators. This is not to say such matters are not important, but they are not appropriate for the AYP forums. If such discussions were permitted, it would distract from the purpose of the forums.

Copyrighted Material: It is recommended to use good judgment ("fair use") in quoting copyrighted material, so as not to infringe upon the owner's rights. This would include listing the title and author of material quoted (and a link if available), so interested readers may obtain the book or article being referred to. Members are responsible for all content they post in the forums.

Please make sure to clearly identify material you are quoting by using quotation marks, the quote icon function, or a different color than the rest of your post.

Also be aware that AYP does not condone posting of links to websites that enable illegal downloading of copyrighted material. Whenever we become aware of such links, they will be removed. If you are aware of any such links in the AYP Forums, please notify the moderators by email at aypforum99@aypsite.org.

AYP Website and Lessons: The AYP Forums are part of the AYP website and are closely related to the hundreds of free lessons on advanced yoga practices available here. Select "**Home**" on the top menu to go to the AYP home page. The home page address is http://www.aypsite.org From there, it is easy to find the Main and Tantra Lesson Directories, Links Section, Testimonials, Topic Index, etc.

AYP Books: The **AYP Easy Lessons** books, the **Secrets of Wilder** novel and the **AYP Enlightenment Series** books are available via links throughout the website, or directly at http://www.aypsite.org/books.html

Questions: If you have questions about navigating the AYP Forums or Lessons, please post them in the **Satsang Cafe**. Also review the the Forum FAQ.

May you find useful information here, and good friends. Practice wisely, and enjoy!

The guru is in you.

2005/07/15 12:30:53
Overview and Announcements
http://www.aypsite.org/forum/topic.asp?TOPIC_ID=297
Registration Problems

The Snitz Forum software utilizes cookies in your browser. If cookies are turned off, membership functions will not work.

Firewalls can sometimes prevent cookies from functioning. See this support forum for further discussion:
http://forum.snitz.com/forum/topic.asp?TOPIC_ID=56465&SearchTerms=cookies

From that help link:

"Over the course of the past year, we have had a number of people who could not register, with the forums behaving as if they were not allowed to make cookies.

One of my forum members figured out what was going on. Apparently, some firewalls will not allow the creation of the cookie for getting past the acceptance screen. The solution to this is for the person to turn off their firewall, subscribe and turn it back on immediately. This has worked for about a half dozen folks on my forums so far who have had this problem.

Just thought I would share the information."

2005/07/22 07:46:08
Overview and Announcements
http://www.aypsite.org/forum/topic.asp?TOPIC_ID=347
How to Find New Postings Easily

It is very easy to find and view new postings if you go to "Active Topics" on the top menu of the forum. You can select any time frame you wish. As default, Active Topics will tell you what is new since your last visit. Try it and see.

In Active Topics, the entire list can be "marked as read" with the little two-tone folder icon in the upper left corner. This resets your last visit to the current date and time.

In addition, forums and topics with new postings since your last visit will be marked with a purple/pink folder on the left side in the forum and topic listings.

You can find other tips on viewing and posting in "Navigating the AYP Forums" here in the Overview and Announcements Forum.

For several reasons, the subscription feature (email notification of new postings) has not been activated for the AYP Forums at this time, so it is necessary to check "Active Topics" here on the website to see what is new.

Wishing you the best on your chosen path. Practice wisely, and enjoy!

The guru is in you.

2005/08/01 17:56:29
Overview and Announcements
http://www.aypsite.org/forum/topic.asp?TOPIC_ID=375
"Previous & Next" Links added to AYP Lessons

All of the lessons on http://www.aypsite.org now have "**Previous & Next**" links at the top and bottom of the page for better navigation.

This means you can "page through" the lessons forward or backward, if you wish, instead of going back to the lesson directory for every page change.

The **Main and Tantra Lesson Directories** will continue to be useful for surveying the overall list of lessons and for going to specific lessons. The **Topic Index** and **Site Search** will also continue to be useful means for finding and going directly to lessons of interest.

Keep in mind that there are some unused lesson numbers in the early stages of the lessons due to editing that was done in the original Yahoo Group lessons. The **Previous & Next** links skip over these unused lesson numbers, so you will notice a few skipped numbers in the sequence as you are paging through. If you spot any errors in the **Previous & Next** links, please let me know.

Wishing you smooth and speedy progress on your chosen path. Enjoy!

The guru is in you.

2005/08/23 14:10:32
Overview and Announcements
http://www.aypsite.org/forum/topic.asp?TOPIC_ID=430
Google Site Search added to aypsite.org

Google Site Search has been added to aypsite.org. Searches done here will pull up results from the AYP lessons, Forums, Links Section and every other nook and cranny of the AYP website. You can also expand your searches to the entire web here as well. Pretty handy. See: http://www.aypsite.org/SiteSearch.html

For easy access, this link has been been added to the "Overview and Announcements" forum header text. It can also be reached from the top menu of all the AYP lesson pages.

The Snitz Forum search (on top menu here) is still the way to go for specific searches in the AYP Forums, because it will shade search terms in yellow in the results -- much easier to find. Google does not provide the "cached" pages with shading of search terms for their site search feature like they do for their standard web searches.

If you want to search all the AYP lessons and also see where your search terms show up site-wide, Google Site Search is the way to do it.

"Seek and ye shall find!"

The guru is in you.

2005/08/27 00:29:41
Overview and Announcements
http://www.aypsite.org/forum/topic.asp?TOPIC_ID=437
Moved Topics -- Why? And How to Find Them

Hello All:

From time to time new topic postings may be moved to a forum that is a better fit for the subject being written about. This will happen either before a moderator approves the posting, or sometimes shortly after. In either case the author of the posting will receive an automatic email notification of the move.

If a topic is moved after posting the author will still be notified, but the rest of the forum readers will not. So, if you notice a new topic is not where you last saw it, chances are it has been moved. It is easy to re-find these simply by going to "Active Topics" on the top menu and selecting a time frame of one or two days back. This will bring up everything posted in that period, including any moved topics. Postings can also be located by search words, date or author in the Search feature on the top menu. If you are a forum member, you can also look up recent postings of any member in the Member list.

The author of a moved topic (or any forum member) can flag the moved topic by posting a reply to it. This will bring it up to the minute in the Active Topics list, so everyone will see it in their "Since Last Visit" listing.

To minimize the number of moved topics, please try and place new topic postings in a forum that matches the subject matter as closely as possible. After checking the list of forums, if you can't see anyplace where your topic fits, then just put it in the "Satsang Cafe" -- that is the catch-all.

Also keep in mind that we'd like to provide useful information across the board in the AYP Forums. That will sometimes weigh into a moderator decision to move a topic. For example, a topic on "Christian Meditation" posted in "Deep Meditation and Samyama" will likely be moved to "Other Systems of Spiritual Practice" because we'd like to provide a separate resource for those who are interested in Christian systems of spiritual practice. It is hoped that the "Other Systems" forum will eventually blossom into a wide array of discussions providing useful information on spiritual practices from many traditions around the world. This would be in addition to the many discussions on yoga practices going on in the yoga-related forums.

Apologies for the moved topics, but it is necessary in order to build up the forums in an organized and balanced way over the long term. Sounds analogous to good spiritual practice, doesn't it? :-)

The guru is in you.

2005/09/02 12:51:51
Overview and Announcements
http://www.aypsite.org/forum/topic.asp?TOPIC_ID=458
Glossary of Sanskrit Terms added to aypsite.org

Hello All:

A **Glossary of Sanskrit Terms** has been added to aypsite.org and can be found at http://www.aypsite.org/glossary.html

There are also links to it on the Home Page, Topic Index, Site Search page and Links Section (under "Sanskrit").

This glossary is tailored to the AYP lessons, providing additional perspectives relating to our practices and experiences. Enjoy!

The guru is in you.

2005/09/08 17:46:32
Overview and Announcements
http://www.aypsite.org/forum/topic.asp?TOPIC_ID=471
"Wide Page" Problem - How to Fix

Hello:

We have a newly discovered forum software glitch.

If you draw a continuous line wider than the page in a posting, it will cause all the text in the whole topic to run off the right side of the page.

_____ ...a line like this only much wider >>>

This problem is easily avoided by keeping any continuous lines (or characters) narrower than the page. If you have any postings that are triggering this "wide page" software glitch, it will be appreciated if you go back and shorten any wide continuous lines you have in there so we can see the text within the width of the page. Thanks!

The guru is in you.

PS -- This situation applies to any string of characters with no space in it that is wider than the page. The longer the unbroken string of characters, the wider the software will make the page for the whole topic.
2005/10/10 12:29:46
Overview and Announcements
http://www.aypsite.org/forum/topic.asp?TOPIC_ID=512
Bookmark new forum address http://www.aypsite.org/forum

Hi All:

As of 10/9/05 we are on a new hosting server with the AYP forums, which should serve our expansion needs for some time.

In doing the move, we started a new domain and website for AYP -- http://www.aypsite.org
That's ".org" as opposed to the old extension, ".com"

The new AYP forums address is http://www.aypsite.org/forum
   Make sure to bookmark it.

The old forum address http://www.aypsite.com/forum is being forwarded to the new address, so the move is transparent as far as using your current bookmarks goes. **However, the forwarding may not always be there, so that is why it is important to bookmark the new address**. It is as simple as changing the ".com" to ".org"

The intention is to keep both websites active indefinitely. These are with separate hosting services, so we now have some extra security for the AYP online lessons.

All online AYP sites will be kept current as new lessons and resources are added.

The guru is in you.

2005/12/31 09:14:59
Overview and Announcements
http://www.aypsite.org/forum/topic.asp?TOPIC_ID=680
How to Support the Work of AYP

Hi All:

Donations for helping make the AYP writings available to everyone around the world are accepted, and may be made to AYP on Paypal.com.

Also see the AYP Book Quantity Discount Program for obtaining copies of the AYP books for handing out or reselling.

If you would like to participate directly in promoting, translating, publishing, or selling the AYP books, please write to Yogani. All assistance is greatly appreciated.

The guru is in you.

2006/06/30 17:06:49
Overview and Announcements
http://www.aypsite.org/forum/topic.asp?TOPIC_ID=1265
No Links in Signatures Please

Hi All:

Some members here are in the habit of advertising their website either as part of an automatic signature or as a manual addition to all of their postings. There have been some complaints about this, so we are instituting a rule that homepage and favorite links are no longer allowed to be included routinely in postings.

Such links can be placed in your member profile by clicking on "Profile" in the top menu. The link placed in the "Homepage" box in the profile is accessible directly to everyone via the "little house" icon found at the top of every post. The profile containing all information supplied by a member is also easily accessible from several sources, beginning with clicking on the member's name.

Those who have links in their signature are requested to remove them -- this can be done in the member profile. Future postings containing homepage or favorite page links will be subject to rejection.

We'd like to keep the AYP forums as focused as possible on the topics being discussed, with minimal promotional distractions.

For the same reason, signatures that are excessively promotional in terms of font size or number of lines may be subject to rejection as well.

Thank you for your cooperation in this matter.

The guru is in you.

2006/07/13 11:30:19
Overview and Announcements
http://www.aypsite.org/forum/topic.asp?TOPIC_ID=1265&REPLY_ID=9324&whichpage=-1
No Links in Signatures Please

Hi All:

After a number of ups and downs on various issues related to automatic signatures, it has been decided to turn off the automatic signature feature.

This will not affect signatures in existing posts, but will prevent them from now on.

I have never used the automatic signature feature, and have not found it to be a hardship. Not having automatic signatures makes for much cleaner and more readable forums.

If you want to manually add a sign-off to your posts, please keep it to a line or two and do not include promotional links.

Many thanks, and all the best!

The guru is in you.

2006/09/25 16:29:27
Overview and Announcements
http://www.aypsite.org/forum/topic.asp?TOPIC_ID=1542
Press Releases on New AYP Books

Hi All:

For the latest press releases on AYP Books, see:

http://www.aypsite.org/pressrelease.html

Practice wisely, and enjoy!

The guru is in you.

2008/03/16 17:38:24
Overview and Announcements
http://www.aypsite.org/forum/topic.asp?TOPIC_ID=3623
Live RSS Feed Added for the Forums

Hi All:

A "**Live RSS Feed**" for the AYP Support Forums has been added as a link in the left side border of all AYP forum and website pages. (RSS means "Really Simple Syndication.")

This enables anyone with a live feed reader to see the last post in the last 15 forum topics updated, and link directly to the actual forum topics. The posts in the RSS feed are listed from the most recent to the oldest.

Note: If your browser is not RSS capable, you will see computer code or an error message when you click on the RSS link.

To see the feed, you will need an RSS feed reader, such as:

Mozilla Thunderbird (Free -- see download and setup instructions here)

Microsoft Outlook (v2007 or later -- see setup instructions here)

Firefox (v2.0 or later -- Free download. RSS can be viewed as an up-to-date web page or via subscription.)

Google Reader (Infrequent updates. New posts in topics previously listed are not highlighted.)

My Yahoo! RSS Module (Infrequent updates. Incomplete listings.)

...or other RSS feed reader. If you find a better one, be sure to let us know in the RSS discussion topic. Frequent updates and chronological listing of new and edited posts are desirable features.

For more information on RSS, see:

Video: RSS in Plain English: http://www.commoncraft.com/rss_plain_english

In-depth article on Wikipedia: http://en.wikipedia.org/wiki/RSS

If you have questions or suggestions on improving live RSS feed access, or on sharing live feeds with others to help spread the word about AYP (through social networks, directories, etc.), please post your comments here:
http://www.aypsite.org/forum/topic.asp?whichpage=3&TOPIC_ID=1786

All the best!

The guru is in you.

2008/08/27 16:26:05
Overview and Announcements
http://www.aypsite.org/forum/topic.asp?TOPIC_ID=3623&REPLY_ID=36864&whichpage=-1
Live RSS Feed Added for the Forums

Mozilla Thunderbird can do several functions, but one of the most interesting is how it reads RSS feeds. Here is a simple how to on Thunderbird configuration to use the RSS feed from AYP.

1. Thunderbird can be downloaded from http://www.mozilla.com/en-US/products/thunderbird/. There are versions for Windows, Mac and Linux.

2. Once you download it, install it as you would do with any other application.

3. Once installed, you will need to add a new account. To do that, choose Tools->Account Settings. You will get to the screen shown on the image below. Click the Add Account button.

[img]RSS/img1.jpg[/img]

4. You will need to choose the account type. Choose RSS News & Blogs and click Next

[img]RSS/img2.jpg[/img]

5. Choose a name for the account. AYP sounds about right. Click Next.

[img]RSS/img3.jpg[/img]

6. Once you do that, you can specify some configuration values for the account. I recommend that you check the 3 options below. Set the interval used by Thunderbird to refresh the feed to your liking

[img]RSS/img4.jpg[/img]

7. You will then need to specify where the feed should get its data. Click the button Manage Subscriptions, in the previous screen. You will get to the screen below. Click Add.

[img]RSS/img5.jpg[/img]

8. Specify the URL for the feed as seen below and set the messages to be stored in the account named before.

[img]RSS/img6.jpg[/img]

Once you're done, click OK and then click OK several times to close the open windows, so that you get to the screen below

[img]RSS/img7.jpg[/img]

9. That's it. The previous image will show you the look of Thunderbird with several posts. You can see that the posts look a bot like regular email messages. This will allow you read access to the forum posts without visiting the forum.

2008/08/28 04:45:43
Overview and Announcements
http://www.aypsite.org/forum/topic.asp?TOPIC_ID=3623&REPLY_ID=36888&whichpage=-1
Live RSS Feed Added for the Forums

1. Adding a RSS feed to Microsoft Outlook 2007 is really simple. Outlook 2007 has a RSS Feeds folder right from the beginning, so adding a new feed can be achieved simply by right clicking it and choosing Add a New RSS Feed from the menu.

[img]RSS/img8.jpg[/img]

2. Once prompted for it, just insert the URL for the AYP RSS Feed

[img]RSS/img9.jpg[/img]

3. Outlook will ask for your confirmation

[img]RSS/img10.jpg[/img]

4. And that's basically, you will be able to access AYP Forum's posts in a very easy and straghtforward way.

The feed will be updated periodically, according to the time settings you have Outlook configured for.

[img]RSS/img11.jpg[/img]

2008/11/24 23:01:11
Overview and Announcements
http://www.aypsite.org/forum/topic.asp?TOPIC_ID=4796
Latest AYP Online Lessons

Note: This listing will be flagged in "Active Topics" for the AYP Support Forums when new lessons are published. For all of the AYP online lessons, see the **website directories** for the Main and Tantra lessons. For email delivery of new online lessons, sign up at the **AYP Yahoo Groups** for the Main Lessons and Tantra Lessons.

Latest AYP Online Lessons:

8/25/10 - Main Lesson 430 - **Freedom**
http://www.aypsite.org/430.html

8/24/10 - Main Lesson 429 - **We Can Do This**
http://www.aypsite.org/429.html

8/19/10 - Main Lesson 428 - **The Transformation of Ego**
http://www.aypsite.org/428.html

8/18/10 - Main Lesson 427 - **Taking the Leap to Direct Experience**
http://www.aypsite.org/427.html

8/13/10 - Main Lesson 426 - **Enlightenment Time Line**
http://www.aypsite.org/426.html

8/12/10 - Main Lesson 425 - **Urgent Bhakti and Overdoing**
http://www.aypsite.org/425.html

8/6/10 - Main Lesson 424 - **After the Ecstasy**
http://www.aypsite.org/424.html

7/22/10 - Tantra Lesson T80 - **Tantra – Much More Than Better Sex**
http://www.aypsite.org/T80.html

7/19/10 - Main Lesson 423 - **Why So Much Fuss about What is So Simple?**
http://www.aypsite.org/423.html

7/15/10 - Main Lesson 422 - **Curing Kundalini Excesses**
http://www.aypsite.org/422.html

7/14/10 - Main Lesson 421 - **Spirits?**
http://www.aypsite.org/421.html

7/11/10 - Main Lesson 420 - **The Doctor Is In**
http://www.aypsite.org/420.html

7/9/10 - Main Lesson 419 - **Where's the Shaktipat Coming From?**
http://www.aypsite.org/419.html

7/8/10 - Main Lesson 418 - **Gurus, Teachers and Self-Sufficiency**
http://www.aypsite.org/418.html

7/7/10 - Main Lesson 417 - **Automatic Yoga Revisited**
http://www.aypsite.org/417.html

7/5/10 - Main Lesson 416 - **From Third Eye to Sixth Sense, and Beyond**
http://www.aypsite.org/416.html

6/21/10 - Main Lesson 415 - **Samyama and Prayer for Dissolving Global Problems**
http://www.aypsite.org/415.html

6/17/10 - Tantra Lesson T79 - **Celibacy, Sexual Obsession and Self-Pacing**
http://www.aypsite.org/T79.html

6/16/10 - Main Lesson 414 - **Off to a Good Start with Meditation, but...**
http://www.aypsite.org/414.html

6/14/10 - Main Lesson 413 - **Is Enlightenment No-Thing or All-Things?**
http://www.aypsite.org/413.html

6/10/10 - Main Lesson 412 - **Will Kechari Mudra Practice Deform the Soft Palate?**
http://www.aypsite.org/412.html

6/9/10 - Main Lesson 411 - **Less is More**
http://www.aypsite.org/411.html

6/7/10 - Main Lesson 410 - **Early Signs of Kundalini Awakening**
http://www.aypsite.org/410.html

6/4/10 - Main Lesson 409 - **Asanas (Postures) and Premature Kundalini Awakening**
http://www.aypsite.org/409.html

6/3/10 - Main Lesson 408 - **Samyama, Elbow Grease and Non-Duality**
http://www.aypsite.org/408.html

6/1/10 - Main Lesson 407 - **Pranayama for Relaxation or for Kundalini Awakening?**
http://www.aypsite.org/407.html

5/28/10 - Main Lesson 406 - **Kundalini Conundrum**
http://www.aypsite.org/406.html

5/27/10 - Main Lesson 405 - **The Uncertainty of Life**
http://www.aypsite.org/405.html

5/26/10 - Main Lesson 404 - **On Jumping to the Third Mantra Enhancement**
http://www.aypsite.org/404.html

5/19/10 - Main Lesson 403 - **The Question with No Answer**
http://www.aypsite.org/403.html

5/18/10 - Tantra Lesson T78 - **Tantra and Erectile Dysfunction**
http://www.aypsite.org/T78.html

5/17/10 - Tantra Lesson T77 - **Amaroli, Fertility and Pregnancy**
http://www.aypsite.org/T77.html

5/14/10 - Tantra Lesson T76 - **Tantric Sex and Birth Control**
http://www.aypsite.org/T76.html

5/14/10 - Main Lesson 402 - **About that word "Advanced"**
http://www.aypsite.org/402.html

5/13/10 - Main Lesson 401 - **Mulabandha and Full Yogic (belly) Breathing**
http://www.aypsite.org/401.html

5/11/10 - Main Lesson 400 - **Theory and Practice**
http://www.aypsite.org/400.html

5/6/10 - Main Lesson 399 - **Mind - Faster than the Speed of Light**
http://www.aypsite.org/399.html

5/4/10 - Main Lesson 398 - **Is Self-Inquiry Necessary for Enlightenment?**
http://www.aypsite.org/398.html

5/3/10 - Main Lesson 397 - **Deep Meditation and Analysis Paralysis**
http://www.aypsite.org/397.html

4/29/10 - Main Lesson 396 - **Do Online Forums Inhibit Spiritual Progress?**
http://www.aypsite.org/396.html

4/27/10 - Main Lesson 395 - **The Power of the Pen, and the Keyboard**
http://www.aypsite.org/395.html

4/23/10 - Main Lesson 394 - **Satsang - The Importance of Spiritual Community**
http://www.aypsite.org/394.html

4/21/10 - Tantra Lesson T75 - **Tantra After Prostate Surgery**
http://www.aypsite.org/T75.html

4/20/10 - Tantra Lesson T74 - **Breast Stimulation and Ecstatic Conductivity**
http://www.aypsite.org/T74.html

4/16/10 - Main Lesson 393 - **On Self-Defense and Forgiveness**
http://www.aypsite.org/393.html

3/31/10 - Main Lesson 392 - **The Aloneness of Enlightenment**
http://www.aypsite.org/392.html

3/22/10 - Main Lesson 391 - **Changes in Bhakti from Dual to Non-Dual**
http://www.aypsite.org/391.html

3/16/10 - Main Lesson 390 - **When Will I be Enlightened?**
http://www.aypsite.org/390.html

3/7/10 - Main Lesson 389 - **Why Won't You be My Guru?**
http://www.aypsite.org/389.html

2/27/10 - Main Lesson 388 - **Our Role as Teachers**
http://www.aypsite.org/388.html

2/26/10 - Main Lesson 387 - **Retreats**
http://www.aypsite.org/387.html

2/25/10 - Main Lesson 386 - **Group Practice**
http://www.aypsite.org/386.html

2/24/10 - Main Lesson 385 - **Review on Building a Baseline Practice Routine**
http://www.aypsite.org/385.html

2/19/10 - Main Lesson 384 - **Baseline Systems of Practice and Research on Modifications**
http://www.aypsite.org/384.html

2/16/10 - Main Lesson 383 - **Yoga Asanas (postures) - Traditional or Modern?**
http://www.aypsite.org/383.html

2/5/10 - Main Lesson 382 - **Is Ecstasy a Prerequisite for Enlightenment?**
http://www.aypsite.org/382.html

2/4/10 - Main Lesson 381 - **Ida, Pingala and Kundalini Awakening**
http://www.aypsite.org/381.html

2/3/10 - Main Lesson 380 - **Catching the Attaching**
http://www.aypsite.org/380.html

1/28/10 - Tantra Lesson T73 - **Possession and Sexual Exploitation**
http://www.aypsite.org/T73.html

1/27/10 - Main Lesson 379 - **Swallowing Air**
http://www.aypsite.org/379.html

1/13/10 - Main Lesson 378 - **How Does Pranayama Awaken Kundalini?**
http://www.aypsite.org/378.html

1/12/10 - Main Lesson 377 - **Inner Sound During Meditation**
http://www.aypsite.org/377.html

1/9/10 - Tantra Lesson T72 - **Tantra and Self-Pacing**
http://www.aypsite.org/T72.html

1/8/10 - Main Lesson 376 - **Beyond Death**
http://www.aypsite.org/376.html

For previous lessons, see the AYP website Main and Tantra lesson directories.

2010/08/25 18:40:18
Overview and Announcements
http://www.aypsite.org/forum/topic.asp?TOPIC_ID=4796&REPLY_ID=72370&whichpage=-1
Latest AYP Online Lessons

Hi All:

The above list of **Latest AYP Online Lessons** has been updated with new lesson(s).

Practice wisely, and enjoy!

The guru is in you.

2008/12/21 10:14:58
Overview and Announcements
http://www.aypsite.org/forum/topic.asp?TOPIC_ID=4924&REPLY_ID=42684&whichpage=-1
Profile & Email Address Update Reminder

Hi All:

A key reason for keeping your email address up to date in your profile is so you can receive moderator notices if and when any posts of yours are put on hold or rejected. Explanations and suggestions for how to fix an on-hold or rejected post are usually sent.

If you prefer not to be contacted by other forum members through the forum email service, that can be turned off in your profile (moderator notes will still come). Your email address is never revealed to others, unless you reply to an email received through the forum email service.

Broadcast emails are never sent through the forum email service. If you ever receive spam or any annoying email through the forum email service, do let me know and it will be addressed. We are very happy to be a spam-free community, and will do what is necessary to keep it that way.

Thank you for your participation in the forums, and all the best! :-)

The guru is in you.

PS: Also, for a variety of reasons, it is good to make sure to have your country designated in your profile.

Forum 2 – Satsang Cafe – General Questions on AYP

Put your feet up and relax with fellow spirit travelers. Newcomer questions are welcome!
http://www.aypsite.org/forum/forum.asp?FORUM_ID=19

2005/07/10 10:08:25
Satsang Cafe - General Questions on AYP
http://www.aypsite.org/forum/topic.asp?TOPIC_ID=272
Newcomer Questions Welcome!

No one is an expert in yoga, and at the same time everyone is.

This is because we all have the same divine source, and the same evolutionary potential for enlightenment. Yet, none of us knows "everything" there is to know about the means for cultivating the greatness within us. It is only a matter of degree, you know. Some of us have been doing the yoga and spiritual practices thing a very long time. Some of us may be just coming on to practices for the first time. It does not matter. We all can pick up and go from right where we are.

What matters most is how we feel about it -- about the journey. Are we ready to "give it a go?" If so, that feeling alone (your feeling) will make all the difference.

If you have that feeling, you are in a place where a lot of helpful information and support can be found. Do take advantage.

If you are new to yoga or AYP, the best place to start is at the beginning of the AYP lessons. You can find the main lessons here:
http://www.aypsite.org/MainDirectory.html

Here you will find easy-to-follow instructions on deep meditation and many other yoga practices. In these forums all of these practices are discussed from the point of view of many practitioners. That can be very helpful to develop perspective on the particulars of practice, and on where yoga can lead us.

While the title of the lessons and these forums is "Advanced Yoga Practices," the progression is such that someone brand new to yoga can learn the essentials and gradually build up over time to a powerful routine of daily spiritual practices. This is true for all who come to AYP, even some who have been doing practices for many years. There is an openly available integration of practices in AYP that is unheard of anywhere else. So, there is something here for just about everyone.

If you'd like a helping hand here in the forum -- a few pointers and some encouragement -- just put your reflections, questions or concerns right there in the Satsang Cafe. Someone who knows something about yoga and AYP will be happy to help you out in a jiffy.

Whatever your chosen path may be, I wish you all success as you continue forward. May your life be filled with divine light and joy!

The guru is in you.

2005/07/17 22:01:29
Satsang Cafe - General Questions on AYP
http://www.aypsite.org/forum/topic.asp?TOPIC_ID=305&REPLY_ID=73&whichpage=-1
duh - AYP Forums navigation

Hi Meg:

Sorry, no email message delivery. Just click "Active Topics" on the top menu for what's new since your last visit, or pick any past time frame you want there. Also, forums with new messages should have a purple folder on the left side. See also:
http://www.aypsite.org/forum/topic.asp?TOPIC_ID=292

The guru is in you.

2005/07/22 12:29:10
Satsang Cafe - General Questions on AYP
http://www.aypsite.org/forum/topic.asp?TOPIC_ID=348
Welcome to the Satsang Cafe
Satsang means "spiritual company." When we gather for the purpose of our mutual spiritual growth, something extra gets created - a positive influence that can be felt working within and around us.

Jesus said, "Where two or three are gathered in my name, I am there among them."

It is satsang, where, in this case, Jesus represents the divine spirit in all of us. It can just as easily be Krishna, Buddha, Allah, God the Father, pure bliss consciousness, or any other representation of the Truth within us. It is the same dynamic. When people gather for a spiritual purpose, for Truth, something extra is going on. We have all felt this at some time or other. If we are blessed, we feel it all the time, for it is certainly possible to be in a "spiritual gathering" even when sitting alone somewhere. That is what long-term daily practice of yoga can do for us. When we are established in the inner silence of the divine through deep meditation, we are never alone.

Here in the AYP forums, it was felt that a home base forum would be helpful. Someplace where there is no set topic. A place to just "hang out" and be with others of like mind and purpose. So here it is, the Satsang Cafe. Enjoy the expanding good vibes here. In your gathering, the divine is among you.

The guru is in you.

2005/08/25 14:39:54
Satsang Cafe - General Questions on AYP

Hello Paul:

Thank you for your heart-felt perspective and excellent points.

It is important for everyone reading here to know that all of us are ordinary folks, and that all ordinary folks have extraordinary capabilities. That means everyone. No exceptions. It is what our status as human beings guarantees. Our nervous systems are wired for enlightenment. This is the truth. All we have to do is step up and claim it.

No one has to take that proclamation on faith. Just sit down and begin deep meditation, and see for yourself. Then, a little later on, when you feel ready, add spinal breathing pranayama and you will be well on your way to unfolding the extraordinary you. No one has a monopoly on this. Anyone can learn the methods to accelerate the rise of peace and joy that are already stirring within us, longing to express in full bloom. Contrary to what many of us have been taught since childhood, this is not an exclusive gift reserved for the few. It is something everyone can do, once the means are known. These discussions are about the practical utilization of those means by everyone.

As for posting here in the AYP Forums, that is the best way we have come up with so far for folks to both give and receive help via the ever-expanding network of practitioners. The more who come on line, the more benefits there will be for everyone, because there is great power for uncovering truth in a networked approach, especially in matters of human spiritual transformation, where each of us is a living laboratory of the enlightenment process and its many nuances. So, no matter what level of experience we happen to be at, there is much to discuss and much that can be done to improve our progress. Beginning and advanced practitioners have a lot in common -- all want to move to the next stage of development. That is what these discussions are for -- helping everyone move to the next stage, no matter what it may be. Believe it or not, beginners can contribute tremendously to the progress of advanced practitioners simply by sharing experiences and asking questions. All interactions are a two-way street, with everyone gaining according to their participation.

For those who have been posting here, you will be interested to know that, while the registered membership of the AYP Forums is modest, the unregistered readership has been in the thousands of page visits every day. As a matter of fact, about two-thirds of all page visits to aypsite.org are to the forums. There are lots of readers here from all around the world, and that is wonderful. So, if you are posting here, know that many are reading. And if you have not posted here yet, that is perfectly okay. It is a joy to know so many are finding the AYP writings to be helpful, especially now that so many others are involved in sharing their experiences along the path. It has added a whole new dimension to AYP.

So, please do carry on, everyone. These are your forums. Everyone has experiences to reveal on so many different levels. All are welcome to share. What you may feel is mundane or somehow not worthy of discussion will be absolutely profound to others. Your openings will be everyone's openings. Share your journey ... learn, practice, grow and enjoy!

The guru is in you.

Hi Jim:

For what it might be worth, my resting heart rate lurks somewhere between 50 and 60 these days. That is significantly lower than in years and decades past. Blood pressure, which has tended to be high in the past, is medium to low now also. I attribute these health benefits to long-time yoga practices, a low fat low salt diet, and the yoga-friendly toning and aerobic exercise program described in the AYP book.

The guru is in you.

Hi Milissa:

Are you saying that the conventional wisdom about high salt/sodium consumption being a factor in high blood pressure is not the salt/sodium, but the impurities in processed salt? If so, can you point to any studies on this? I'm not a doctor, but I believe there have been a lot of studies pointing to a relationship between high salt/sodium intake and high blood pressure.

The relationship of high fat intake and high blood pressure is another well-researched aspect. Particularly the "DASH" diet research done in Boston some years back, which demonstrated in a large group study that a low fat diet with fresh foods leads to reduced blood pressure. I believe the DASH diet also includes reduced salt/sodium intake. See http://www.bu.edu/bridge/archive/2002/02-08/dash.htm

Cardiovascular "aerobic" conditioning is yet another important factor in reducing blood pressure, not to mention its other health benefits.

On the yoga side, I think it is much more simple. Yoga reduces metabolism (reflected in reduced breath and heart rate), as well as tension in the nervous system, which one might logically expect to relax the veins and arteries (and BP) on the inner-most level. As we know, the effects of meditation and other yoga practices eventually become a 24 hour experience in the nervous system, and this is how we feel the benefits rising in everyday life. That is a layman's point of view on the medical aspects, of course. There have been a lot of stress reduction studies on meditation and other yoga practices that would seem to bear this out. Of course, the proof of the pudding is in the eating, and most yoga practitioners are not complaining.

We have much bigger fish to fry anyway, yes? :-)

The guru is in you.

2005/10/06 13:52:14
Satsang Cafe - General Questions on AYP
http://www.aypsite.org/forum/topic.asp?TOPIC_ID=502&REPLY_ID=856&whichpage=-1
Concept of "better" path

Hi Meg:

Just to clarify, a belief in reincarnation, or, in fact, whether it exists or not, is not a prerequisite for the AYP approach. It is used as a talking point that many are familiar with to explain the diverse tendencies we are born with, even in the same genetic family. Maybe these tendencies come from somewhere else. It doesn't really matter, as long as we have the means to unwind them in a way that leads to a higher quality of life here and now. "Then" and "when" don't matter much. What we are doing now is everything.

What is important is that we find the motivation to practice, and that is the manifestation our bhakti, which is entirely personal and does not require a specific belief system -- not here anyway.

It has been said that "reincarnation is for the ignorant." That is a clever play on words that carries several meanings, pro and con.

As for making the case for reincarnation, there is a ton of literature out there, pertaining to all religions, or no religion at all. The death and dying (life before and after death) movement is an entity unto itself these days. The AYP book list has a section on it too:
http://www.aypsite.org/booklist14.html

The guru is in you.

2005/10/16 10:25:40
Satsang Cafe - General Questions on AYP
http://www.aypsite.org/forum/topic.asp?TOPIC_ID=525&REPLY_ID=987&whichpage=-1
AYP and pregnancy

Hi Lili:

If a pregnant woman is already practicing, I'd suggest continuing with only light meditation and very light spinal breathing, with little or no mudras, bandhas or kumbhaka. Very gentle... If she is not practicing already and not really hankering to, then waiting until after the pregnancy is a reasonable course... It is really a function of the person's desire.

There are also hatha yoga classes available specifically for pregnant women. Presumably these are very gentle also, which would be fine.

Obviously, practices should be discontinued at the first sign of any excessive energy flow. How that goes is a function of the individual nervous system. "Self-pacing" emphasized yet again. :-)

The guru is in you.

2005/10/22 16:28:50
Satsang Cafe - General Questions on AYP
http://www.aypsite.org/forum/topic.asp?TOPIC_ID=542&REPLY_ID=1099&whichpage=-1
Help on the Heart

Hi Frank:

Is this the topic you are looking for?
http://www.aypsite.org/forum/topic.asp?TOPIC_ID=340&SearchTerms=heart,breathing

The heart has been discussed from several angles so far. There are so many ways to approach it. Let's face it, the heart is involved in everything we do, whether we are thinking about it or not. The spiritual condition of our heart determines how we express on this earth plane.

In AYP, the heart is discussed a lot from the standpoint of following our yearnings in the bhakti sense in relation to doing our practices, and in our activities in daily life also. We have the greatest respect for the whispers of the heart. It is the divine in us,

There is also the heart breathing technique covered in the AYP lessons at http://www.aypsite.org/220.html and http://www.aypsite.org/221.html which is an effective combination of bhakti and inverse direction spinal breathing pranayama between the third eye and heart.

There is always room for different points of view on practice, especially on the heart, which has unlimited dimensions, so feel free to explore. The tiniest place in the heart is as large as the cosmos inside.

May divine love reverberate endlessly in your infinite ecstatic heart space!

The guru is in you.

2005/11/27 22:48:19
Satsang Cafe - General Questions on AYP
http://www.aypsite.org/forum/topic.asp?TOPIC_ID=554&REPLY_ID=1676&whichpage=-1
Where's the Enlightened?

Hi Meg:

Oh, now I see better where you are coming from on the Secrets of Wilder story. It appears you have raised the bar higher for the mythic hero than Joseph Campbell did. He recognized all heroes in all stories of all cultures, real or imagined, as being on the hero's journey -- including such luminaries as Luke Skywalker of Star Wars fame.

Indeed, Campbell's first book, written in the 1940s, was called "The Hero with a Thousand Faces." This is not necessarily the returning enlightened egoless hero, but anyone who makes personal sacrifices to help advance the society he or she lives in.

Campbell also pointed out that the hero's journey is ultimately a spiritual one, and Jesus certainly fills the bill for that role. But remember, Jesus had his doubts in the Garden of Gesthemane, or so it has been written.

Heroes do what they do because they can, and because they must. Where it falls on a scale of perfection is not nearly as important as the fact that they gave all that they had and made a difference. Real heroes are ordinary people making extraordinary contributions. That is what makes them so inspiring, because they demonstrate that any of us can do the same.

And they are all around us...

That is what I was aiming for with the novel. I understand that it may not be the "enlightenment story" everyone would prefer, and that is okay. It was the truest hero's journey I could come up with in this time and place. And, of course, it is loaded with instructions on spiritual practices too.

The guru is in you.

2005/12/02 10:39:03
Satsang Cafe - General Questions on AYP
http://www.aypsite.org/forum/topic.asp?TOPIC_ID=554&REPLY_ID=1745&whichpage=-1
Where's the Enlightened?

Hi All:

This Jesus/perfection discussion is touching on yama and niyama, and whether "conduct" can rise to perfection via inner silence and the connectivity of yoga. In fact, it raises the question of the interconnectivity of yoga in general, which is the conductivity that rises in our nervous system with a range of practices, connecting all the limbs of yoga within us.

So the question really is, how efficient a spiritual vehicle is the human nervous system? Can it be brought to the high states of spiritual interconnectivity (and conscious spiritual conduct) that we would call enlightenment? That is the whole point of the sages, avatars, spiritual teachers, spiritual practices, and even organized religion.

Obviously, something is going on in there. How far can we take it? We can speculate about the condition of "the enlightened," and it is a worthy examination of our possibilities. That is what we are really after, yes? Our possibilities. Ultimately, the answer sits waiting right here within us. With practices we will find out day by day.

So, "Where's the enlightened?"

Meditate every day, and then go take a look in the mirror. You will see it coming, or maybe not. Just keep your sunglasses handy... :-)

Frank, this is a terrific topic you started! Obviously one of great importance to many people. Thank you.

Keep it goin' folks.

The guru is in you.

2005/11/02 12:39:09
Satsang Cafe - General Questions on AYP
http://www.aypsite.org/forum/topic.asp?TOPIC_ID=561&REPLY_ID=1334&whichpage=-1
Hello fellow Yogis

quote:
_____
http://www.thetaobums.com/forum/index.php?showtopic=933
_____

Hi Sean:

Welcome aboard! I hope you will find AYP to be a useful resource as you travel along your chosen path.

Forums are a great way to explore and expand on spiritual knowledge and methods. You have a nice one going there in "Tao Bums." Glad we can have some cross pollination going on.

I saw over there that a discussion on AYP tantra has come up, with particular focus on the idea of semen entering the bladder, and how this can lead to spiritual developments higher up in the body. A question about the physical plumbing aspect came up -- How can vital essences get from the bladder to the brain?

I wanted to point out that it is not only physical plumbing that is involved in this. It is quite complex, really, involving physical, biological and neurological processes in the body, all of which are connected as human spiritual transformation advances. Not only the bladder is involved. There are other pathways through the sacrum to the spinal cord and up. And it also reaches up into the digestive system where a lot of activity can be observed related to the awakening of an ecstatic radiance throughout the whole body. All of this depends on our rising inner silence gained in deep meditation. The rest of the methods in AYP build on inner silence ("moving stillness") to bring up the ecstatic aspects of our development. The union of inner silence (shiva) and ecstatic conductivity (kundalini/shakti) results in the complete unfoldment in the human being. In the end, what we have is unshakable inner silence, ecstatic bliss and outpouring divine love.

So it is a complex process going on there in the pelvic region that is part of a much greater whole. Fortunately we do not have to understand it all to move forward through the transformation, any more than we have to understand how our inner biology works for our normal functioning every day. All we have to know is how to stimulate this natural process that leads us to higher functioning. That is what yoga is about, of course. Someday the scientists will unravel the inner workings of human spiritual transformation. In the meantime, we can intelligently apply and enjoy the fruits of the wonderful practices that have been handed down to us by the many great ones who have come before.

Btw, the processes of spiritual transformation discussed above are the same in women as in men, including the entry of vital essences into the bladder, etc. There is more on all of this in the AYP lessons. So read on, share your thoughts here if you like, and enjoy!

The guru is in you.

2005/11/02 16:13:39
Satsang Cafe - General Questions on AYP
http://www.aypsite.org/forum/topic.asp?TOPIC_ID=566&REPLY_ID=1345&whichpage=-1
*** Happy AYP Birthday !! *** -- and THANKS

Hi All:

Thank you so much for your kind notes. When David wrote me about this yesterday, asking if there was anything we could celebrate, this was my reply:

"I am not for celebrating 'Yogani,' but am for celebrating the anniversary of the AYP lessons. November 2, 2003 is special for me too, because that is when the divine flow started going out to the world. I am a witness to it as much as anyone, and have benefited from it as much as anyone. So I celebrate that, and everyone involved is to be celebrated equally. We have all come a long way together. Bravo for that!"

So, my hat is off to all of you. I am only the person writing the lessons. You are the ones putting them into practice. Yoga is only yoga when people are doing it and benefiting. Knowledge is only useful when it is applied. That is what AYP is about. That is what I am celebrating today, and every day! :-)

The guru is in you.

2005/11/04 14:41:52
Satsang Cafe - General Questions on AYP
http://www.aypsite.org/forum/topic.asp?TOPIC_ID=566&REPLY_ID=1380&whichpage=-1
*** Happy AYP Birthday !! *** -- and THANKS

Hi Folks:

The "helping" discussion here is much appreciated. I'm not very comfortable engaging directly in the pubic money raising discussion, so pardon my silence. Individual inquiries about it can be sent to my email. That goes for both donations and "deep discount" quantity book purchases. On the latter, there is some good news. It looks like we will be able to ship direct from London, UK, as well as Tennessee, USA, so that bodes well for the shipping costs to the UK and Europe. More on that soon in the Quantity Discount Topic.

At this point I am not in a position to set up for automatic money transfers on a regular basis on this end. Maybe Paypal can do it from the sender's end, though I have not spotted that option in there so far.

For those who are interested, here is the direct AYP/Paypal Donation Link. Any donations should only be for the perception of value received already. I am most comfortable with that.

The guru is in you.

2005/12/13 14:52:30
Satsang Cafe - General Questions on AYP
http://www.aypsite.org/forum/topic.asp?TOPIC_ID=641
Spammer Banned

Hi All:

Several have reported spam coming through the AYP Forums mail server today. I have responded with the following message, which I hope will serve to explain actions taken on this end.

Re: Michela Doujey spam letter

Hi:

It is spam. The member (nana01) has been banned. Apologies on that.

The good news is that no one has your email address. This was sent by individual transmissions one by one via the AYP forum email server where email addresses are not revealed.

If it happens again, we will tighten up the sign-up process for the forum, and take whatever further measures are necessary to stop the offending conduct.

The guru is in you.

Yogani

2006/02/11 09:51:09
Satsang Cafe - General Questions on AYP
http://www.aypsite.org/forum/topic.asp?TOPIC_ID=641&REPLY_ID=3247&whichpage=-1

Spammer Banned

Hi All:

The forum has been hit by another round of spam from this source.

Sincere apologies to all who have received it. The ID, adoujey01, has been disabled.

This is a well known nuisance spammer who has a knack for invading all sorts of Internet communities with his/her sob story scams. It has been going on for years. Whoever is doing it is not doing Africa a favor.

Email addresses are not revealed in the AYP forums. However, if someone of low character sneaks in through the registration process, emails can be sent one at a time via the email link on each person's profile page. This has happened only twice -- both cases are covered in this topic.

If you want to block all mail coming through your AYP forums email link, just go to your "profile" on the top menu and turn off email. Then you will not be bothered with these occasional nuisance spams, but you will not be able to be reached directly by legitimate forum members either. It's up to you.

Again, apologies for the intrusion. We are doing all we can to minimize this sort of thing.

The guru is in you.

2005/12/16 10:14:51
Satsang Cafe - General Questions on AYP
http://www.aypsite.org/forum/topic.asp?TOPIC_ID=651&REPLY_ID=1984&whichpage=-1
Endings

Hi Jim:

Enjoy the scenery, but then easily go back to the practice. You are right -- it never ends. Stillness in action goes on forever.

The minute we stop on the outside the gears will grind on the inside. I once had a similar watershed career event like you mentioned. I stopped to reflect for a few weeks and got sick. It was only when I moved on into the next phase that I felt better. The next phase of work is the break.

On the other hand, taking a break in an active way can be good too -- a change in scenery before the change in scenery. But somehow that works better when we are going back to the same job, not a new one. Too much anticipation, you know. As for a meditative retreat, same deal -- too much anticipation. Maybe better to just move on into it. Breaks work best when there is sameness on both ends -- then we are renewing something that was getting old. Nothing to renew in your case. The change is the renewal, yes?

I go through this with every new book out these days. It is like, "Oh, that's done, now for a break." But it doesn't feel right to pause for long -- I mean, one day's pause is almost too much. What feels right is the work, as long as there are practices and a balanced routine.

We are stillness longing to be in action. Action is what we do best. We are the rider in the ever-moving chariot of life. What physicists are now calling "the ghost in the machine." Even they know ... we are That.

The guru is in you.

2005/12/27 07:40:43
Satsang Cafe - General Questions on AYP
http://www.aypsite.org/forum/topic.asp?TOPIC_ID=670&REPLY_ID=2193&whichpage=-1
If You Could Ask One Question...

Hi Frank:

I think the answer to your first question is, yes, God can eliminate ignorance, but it must be through the questioner. And who is the questioner? Why, he/she is God. Only if God is presumed to be separate from self is there the dilemma. Recognition of God being within increases the flow of bhakti leading to practices and the elimination of ignorance -- in the questioner and in everyone.

On your second question, who is it that decides that someone is suffering? Suffering is identification with pain, and how can we impose that on others, least of all babies? Certainly no one wishes for there to be starving babies. Yet, the fact that they are there provides the opportunity to move beyond judgments on suffering, and simply act with divine love. Again, the question is a call for the questioner to act.

The American spiritual teacher, Ram Das, said that in all of his travelling around the world over the years to help disadvantaged people, the greatest suffering he ever saw was in the corporate board rooms of America. Why? Because these were the people most identified with their personal self-interest and least aware of the wholeness of life. Net result -- acute separation and great suffering...

Of course, we can say that the corporate executives picked their own fate. But can we be absolutely sure that the starving babies did not? One thing is certain. There are opportunities to dissolve ignorance everywhere, beginning right where we are sitting. We can be sure God is in the details of that. :-)

My one question is: How can we provide everyone on earth the means to live the reality of God within full time, if they choose to?

The guru is in you.

2005/12/27 13:06:37
Satsang Cafe - General Questions on AYP
http://www.aypsite.org/forum/topic.asp?TOPIC_ID=670&REPLY_ID=2209&whichpage=-1
If You Could Ask One Question...

quote:
_____
Originally posted by nearoanoke

I feel Yogani's question was more like...what if everyone choses and wants to meditate "full time"? Who will take care of the other material things in the world?

I might be wrong.
_____

Hi Near:

Jim got it mostly right. It was actually a practical question. How do we reach everyone around the world with the knowledge of open source self-directed practices, so they will be free to choose them when they wish? You can see where my head and heart are these days. In the trenches of applied yoga science... :-)

The guru is in you.

2005/12/31 21:34:15
Satsang Cafe - General Questions on AYP
http://www.aypsite.org/forum/topic.asp?TOPIC_ID=673&REPLY_ID=2304&whichpage=-1
Holosync

Hi All:

There are ayurvedic diet suggestions from several sources provided in the AYP web pages here: http://www.aypsite.org/ayurveda.html

One of the links there is to a food chart I have used for many years, supporting vata, pitta and kapha pacifying diets. Here is the pitta recommendation from there on spices:

Yes – coriander, cinnamon, cardamom, fennel, turmeric, black pepper (small amount)

No – all other spices

The guru is in you.

PS -- I just noticed that the Maharis
Hi Ayurveda free resource site pages (under http://www.ayurveda-ayurvedic.com) listed on the above AYP resource list are no longer operating. Only their product sales site is working (http://www.mapi.com).
2006/01/05 22:12:49
Satsang Cafe - General Questions on AYP
http://www.aypsite.org/forum/topic.asp?TOPIC_ID=693
The Evolving Forums

Hi All:

This was posted in a kundalini topic and I thought to repost it here for general information and further discussion on where we can go with these forums:

David wrote:
Quite some time ago you expressed a wish to be asked questions by email rather than on the forum. I am quite sure many people (many of whom are newcomers since you expressed your wishes) simply missed that . (Or if you told us of a change of mind on that issue, I missed that myself!)

Has that changed though? Have you adjusted happily to answering questions directly?

Yogani wrote:
Good question about where I am answering questions. Everywhere they come it seems! :-)

Originally, I was concerned that I would be bombarded with so many questions in the forum that the forum would become about me, which I do not want. I want it to be a community where everyone is helping each other at increasingly higher levels. I think this is a healthy path of evolution for the AYP community -- and we all know it will go higher and higher as everyone advances. This will open the door for many more seekers to find assistance, with less reliance on me for the answers. Many of you are answering questions on a very high level already, based on your own experiences. Bravo for that!

So here is the deal. Anyone can ask anything they want here of me or the community. If others can cover the questions, I will not say much (even if it is addressed to me). If there seems to be a gap, I'll jump in. Whatever makes sense. But let's make it a community, not a Yogani Q&A. I think we are doing so, and I hope it will continue to grow like that. The theory is that by the time there are too many questions for me to answer here, there will be many others who can answer them. Let's see if it works.

Given the above community-building plan and my commitment to writing more books and online lessons, I have shifted my position on emails to encouraging everyone to bring their questions here to the forums. That way many of you can help with answering questions and more people will benefit immediately from the public discussion. In other words, the quantity of private emails I will be doing will go down as most of it shifts here to the forums. This is how it should be for all the reasons mentioned. It also adds diversity and more opportunities for exploration of ways to optimize the practices.

Neither AYP nor I have all the answers. AYP is a suggested baseline from which many things can be explored and tested. I believe Jim called it a "safe harbor." That is exactly the function AYP should serve, and yoga should move on to increasingly optimized levels of application as research and practical results warrant. As long as we are working with the underlying principles of human spiritual transformation and a basic set of guidelines like AYP, then we have set the stage for tremendous progress both short term and long term. We are giving birth to a new applied science here...

The language in the forum introductions was modified several weeks ago to cover the shift to encouraging everyone to bring their questions to the forums, and it was also covered in the latest lesson #279 -- http://www.aypsite.org/279.html

The guru is in you.

2006/01/08 09:21:24
Satsang Cafe - General Questions on AYP
http://www.aypsite.org/forum/topic.asp?TOPIC_ID=693&REPLY_ID=2389&whichpage=-1
The Evolving Forums

Hi Jim:

Thank you. Excellent perspectives on using AYP. You are doing it! And thanks also for your insightful suggestions on keeping the forums grounded and heading in the right direction, which will lead to more for everyone.

While the practices of AYP are effective and well-integrated in their own right, the methodology of application itself (safe harbor/level ground approach, cause and effect testing, self-pacing, etc.) allows practitioners to reach far beyond a "cookbook" approach to spiritual development. That is what I had in mind when writing the original lessons, the Wilder novel, and now the AYP Enlightenment Series of short books -- all tools that enable independent practitioners to fly while relying increasingly on their internal compass rather than an external one.

Once people become convinced of the fact that spiritual transformation is something centered within them, not coming from an external source, then the door opens for huge progress.

It is like the revelation that the earth is round instead of flat. With the new understanding, the paradigm quickly shifts to a new level of progress. Same thing here. With a shift to recognition of the center being in every person, the efficiency of the overall process of human spiritual transformation will increase dramatically.

With this, people don't need to be told where to look to find the divine. They only need an easy-to-use and adaptable methodology that can aid them in unfolding the vast potential that they already know is present within them. It is much easier...

The guru is in you.

2006/01/14 10:44:15
Satsang Cafe - General Questions on AYP
http://www.aypsite.org/forum/topic.asp?TOPIC_ID=725&REPLY_ID=2536&whichpage=-1
Pausing to Reflect VS Sheer Escapism

Hi Jim:

If you have not already, you may wish to review Lesson #209 on fitting practices into a busy schedule, particularly the part about "honoring the habit." There are lots of ways to compress things down. But most important is to not lose the habit during extended periods of intense activity. It takes a few minutes twice per day to sustain it, and then it (the habit) is there when we are ready to resume full practices again. If we do not honor the habit, over time we will be in increasing danger of losing the whole practice. I have seen it happen many times.

Having spent decades in the corporate world, I learned about this by trial and error. It is not something we find in the yoga books. It is a modern yogi/yogini survival technique. Very necessary in this day and age ... guerrilla yoga!

The guru is in you.

2006/01/17 14:23:18
Satsang Cafe - General Questions on AYP
http://www.aypsite.org/forum/topic.asp?TOPIC_ID=739&REPLY_ID=2599&whichpage=-1
Prayers for a friend....
Melissa, you have my deepest prayers, coming on waves of inner silence.

The guru is in you.

Yogani
2006/01/22 07:55:23
Satsang Cafe - General Questions on AYP
http://www.aypsite.org/forum/topic.asp?TOPIC_ID=759
Saturday Night (1/21/06) Posting Outage

Hi All:

You may have noticed that the forum was not accepting new postings on Saturday night (USA time). This was due to a glitch that occurred while a software upgrade was being done. The problem has been corrected and all is back to normal now.

Sincere apologies for the disruption.

The guru is in you.

2006/01/22 16:51:57

Hi Guy:

I think it has been said in here somewhere before: The "tapping" of the breastbone in the *Secrets of Wilder* is a literary metaphor for the passing of the knowledge. Which is not to say there is no energy transfer involved -- a boost of sorts. But it comes mainly from the inside. In fact, I sometimes tell people that the first time one sits to meditate with "I AM" they are tapped from the inside. There is an inspiring Rumi quote along those lines: http://www.aypsite.org/forum/topic.asp?TOPIC_ID=606

There are all sorts of energy "jump starts." The most important one comes from our ongoing bhakti (desire for God or Truth). With that occurring, all other stimuli will appear to do wonders. Whatever else may seem to be going on, it is an inside job from start to finish.

Wishing you the best on your path. Enjoy!

The guru is in you.

2006/02/03 10:18:45

Hi All:

One of the moderators can lift the appropriate replies on the gap here and make a new topic out of them.

The guru is in you.

2006/02/10 13:23:51

Hi All:

For anyone wondering what happened to the fledgling "gap" discussion, it was split off from from the coffee topic where it started, and here it is.

We will try and announce such topic splits in the future in this way, so the new topic thread can be found in the active topics list.

Gap connoisseurs rejoice. It is all gap! :-)

The guru is in you.

2006/02/09 09:56:13

Hi Katrine and welcome!

I have been enjoying your beautiful poetry the past few days. When experiences reach a certain depth and intensity, poetry is about the only way to capture the feelings. I don't know why exactly, but fewer words can say more in describing such experiences. Perhaps it is the inner silence that shines through between the lines. Rumi is one of the masters of this, and so is St. John of the Cross. Leaping through traditions there. The tradition does not matter. It is the divine expression surging through the human nervous system that does. We are the doorway.

Speaking of surging, your experiences described above are also beautiful. Your journey verifies that there is certainly more than one way to go through the process of human spiritual transformation. At the same time, you are running into some of the same opportunities and limits we all find as we move ahead with practices and find ourselves in the resulting experiences. We want to let it happen fully, yet we must self-pace or face a bit of chaos. It is a matter of managing the process of purification that is occurring within us. I am very happy you are finding spinal breathing and some of the other methods in AYP to be helpful. As for the crown, well, I think you are finding what we have been discussing in the AYP lessons. It can be approached directly, but only with great care in later stages. That too is self-pacing.

As for the psychological component -- how we lose our center, how we get it back, and how we make our choices in daily activity. Of course, it will be much better to focus on how to cultivate our center than to be laboring over how we may have lost it. In the AYP approach, we focus on developing inner silence, and later on, ecstatic conductivity, and when we are not in sitting practices we just go out and live our life. Then we become naturally radiated from within in much the same way you have described the natural illumination that came to you during the powerful events that happened in your life. The more we go out and walk through our desires, challenges and fears, the more the inner divine will express and become stabilized in us. Sitting practices set the stage for this in a big way. But we still have to go out and actualize the inner transformation in our daily life. For that, all we must do is engage in what is before us. To pick up on another topic, it is hardly a sanyasin's (renunciate's) life.

There is a very good discussion on making our choices in daily living over here: http://www.aypsite.org/forum/topic.asp?TOPIC_ID=790

AYP does not pretend to know how everyone ought to be choosing in daily living. It is such an organic process, and unique to each person. Yet, we can lay an inner foundation that will illuminate the process of choosing from the inside. Then we are empowered in our individual lives to fulfill a divine purpose, each in our own way. That is a surrender, of course. First a surrender to the means that can transform us inwardly, and, ultimately, to the infinite power of God that seeks to express out through us. It is through this surrender that both we and the world can be illuminated.

Thank you for joining in and sharing, Katrine. Wishing you the best on your path. Enjoy!

The guru is in you.

2006/02/19 13:05:39
Satsang Cafe - General Questions on AYP
http://www.aypsite.org/forum/topic.asp?TOPIC_ID=803&REPLY_ID=3579&whichpage=-1
Integrating Psychology and Spirituality

Hi Katrine:

I agree with you 100%. Inner silence is our starting point and ending point. Cultivating it is essential. But to do so without engaging in life (our own process) in some way is like building a foundation with no house on it.

Many years ago I knew a man who had spent decades meditating in a secluded environment. The radiance of silence around him was palpable. Yet, if anything in his physical environment became displaced, he would throw a hissy fit.

It was then that I knew there is more to this game than cultivating stillness.

Enlightenment = Stillness in Action!
...and that is ecstatic divine love expressing in the world.

The guru is in you.

2006/02/17 16:13:17
Satsang Cafe - General Questions on AYP
http://www.aypsite.org/forum/topic.asp?TOPIC_ID=838&REPLY_ID=3489&whichpage=-1
Shabd, Nada & the end game

Hi Trueadept, and welcome also!

You can find the low-down on kechari in lesson 108 (complete with illustrations) here: http://www.aypsite.org/108.html

Like Victor, I am not familiar with Shabda.

I am moving this topic from Deep Meditation into the Satsang Cafe where a more general discussion on your thoughts can happen. You can find a wealth of information on spiritual practices and experiences around here. Kick the tires all you like. Whatever you feel might be missing, feel free to add on ... that is how we do it here.

Wishing you all the best on your path. Enjoy!

The guru is in you.

2006/02/20 10:44:38
Satsang Cafe - General Questions on AYP
http://www.aypsite.org/forum/topic.asp?TOPIC_ID=843&REPLY_ID=3620&whichpage=-1
my own post is new (purple) topic?

Hi Etherfish:

I have found the active topics link on top of the page to be the most reliable place to manage new postings, including my own. That includes checking back as many hours as necessary there to catch any posts that slip through the active listings. It can happen.

The active topics list (and all pink folders) can be cleared by clicking on the two-tone folder icon in the upper left corner of the active topics window.

The guru is in you.

2006/02/25 17:22:08
Satsang Cafe - General Questions on AYP
http://www.aypsite.org/forum/topic.asp?TOPIC_ID=846&REPLY_ID=3855&whichpage=-1
psychedelic Yoga?

Hi Trueadept:

The presence of sound and other inner sensory elements is familiar, but the path mentioned is not. In AYP, inner sensory experiences are regarded as effect rather than cause in practices -- part of the scenery as we travel along on our journey home.

In some systems, nada (inner sound) is used. In AYP, mantra is used. The mantra is always available on whatever level we are. With nada, sometimes it is there, sometimes it is not -- then we are waiting... For this reason, mantra-based deep meditation with the right procedure is more efficient and effective for long term practice. That is why we use it, and regard all the comings and goings of inner experience as scenery we encounter as we cruise along the highway to increasing inner silence. Our practice remains the same no matter what the sights and sounds may be.

As for taking psychedelics, not recommended in AYP. We already have all that is necessary within us. Additives are not necessary -- more likely to be counter-productive, especially if the aim is to cultivate advanced stages of purification and opening in the nervous system.

All the best!

The guru is in you.

2006/03/01 12:42:29
Satsang Cafe - General Questions on AYP
http://www.aypsite.org/forum/topic.asp?TOPIC_ID=859
Avoiding Forum Confusion

Hi All:

The forums have been a real boon for collectively exploring the AYP practices, associated experiences, and a lot of other things.

Yet, some have come to the forums looking for a primary teaching and have been confused. No wonder. Everything in the realm of spiritual practices is being discussed here, and we are only getting started!

Below is an email interchange in part on the subject of the forums and how they relate to the AYP lessons. I think it is important for everyone to understand this relationship to avoid confusion.

Q: I just want to let you know that my energy difficulties have subsided considerably ever since I took your advice and started a routine of daily physical exercise. But I will still go slow on pranayama for a month more till I get back to normal levels of silence in meditation as you have advised.

To tell you the truth, I am still finding the Forum a little difficult to understand. I mean, it's hard to see which topic is related to my question sometimes. Where can I start in the forum, since it is quite huge?

A: Glad to hear you are finding some stability. From there you can build up in an orderly step-by-step way.

Keep in mind that the forums are not intended to be the primary teaching tool. The AYP lessons and books are, and do answer many questions in a logical sequence. If we are grounded in the lessons as a foundation, then the forums will make much more sense and can add a lot of perspective to our path. Going into the forums to learn AYP or any particular practice from scratch is difficult, if not impossible. But as an interactive expansion on the AYP lessons that everyone can use, the forums are terrific.

Once you have been through the AYP lessons, if you are looking for an answer to a specific question, I suggest you search both the AYP lessons and the forums. Each has its own search function. The main website Topic Index is also a handy tool for finding information in the lessons. The AYP books are good for research too -- they go well beyond the online lessons and can be scribbled in and dog-eared to the n-th degree. :-)

All the best!

The guru is in you.

PS -- Perhaps in a couple of years the best of the forums can be included as part of *AYP Easy Lessons, Volume 2*, for a permanent record and easier access to the information. Or maybe by then the forums will be worthy of their own volume. Of course, the copyrights of all contributors would be honored. Time will tell...

2006/03/01 15:00:20
Satsang Cafe - General Questions on AYP
http://www.aypsite.org/forum/topic.asp?TOPIC_ID=859&REPLY_ID=3980&whichpage=-1
Avoiding Forum Confusion
PPS -- The thought occurred, if others write books that are within the realm of what we are doing here, it could be possible to publish them through AYP Publishing, which has distribution from the USA and UK.

But please don't send any manuscripts today. I have four books to finish this year!

Just some food for thought for those who feel they may have something of value to share along the lines of spiritual practice and experience -- cause and effect, you know. That is what we are into here.
Katrine? :-)

The guru is in you.

2006/03/01 16:24:02
Satsang Cafe - General Questions on AYP
http://www.aypsite.org/forum/topic.asp?TOPIC_ID=860&REPLY_ID=3984&whichpage=-1
Symbols

Hi Katrine:

Looks like a vivid radiation from the ajna (third eye), which is the area extending from the point between the eyebrows back to the center of the brain and down the medulla oblongata (brain stem). While traditional depictions of the ajna do not include the yoni symbol (inverted triangle), no one disagrees on OM being the sound. The Sri Yantra is the geometric manifestation of OM and it is based on the inverted triangle -- made out of them, as a matter of fact. Well, it is a bit more involved than that. See here for more, including links to some diagrams of the Sri Yantra:
http://www.aypsite.org/T25.html

It should be mentioned that this lesson was spruced up quite a bit in the AYP Easy Lessons book.

On your question elsewhere about what to do with OM, I have always found it better to go back to mantra meditation than to become nada-bound.

If mantra meditation is done correctly, it will never seem coarse without good reason -- some purification going on, which, along with spinal breathing and other means, leads to more and more nada (inner sound) and the full range of inner openings including all the senses, whole body, heart, mind ... the works...

I am not very familiar with nada yoga, so cannot go very far in describing its practice and effects. I do know that it is not a very good place to start, as few of us start out with nada, and fewer still have it all the time. If we do have it all the time (I do too) I suppose it can become the focus, but to me it still looks more like effect than cause, definitely an enjoyable thing to become absorbed in during spare moments. It's more like a self-indulgent hobby for me -- overwhelming ecstatic bliss. Ahhh...

This is not to say it cannot become in-the-trenches spiritual practice with a solid cause and effect dynamic. It just has not been the route I traveled all these years, so I cannot say. But, to the question, "Does AYP bring nada?" I can answer a resounding, "Yes!" In the AYP terminology, nada (OM) is associated with the rise of whole body ecstatic conductivity and radiance.

When OM comes, what each of us does with it is up to us ... hopefully not at the expense of our effective yoga practice. Nada folks might see that statement as blasphemy. Sorry. I just don't know if I could have gotten here with nada alone, with or without the help of spinal breathing. It does not offer what deep meditation does -- reliable twice-daily merging with inner silence.

To get back to the inverted triangle, it is the symbol of the feminine aspect of existence, the creative power, the word -- OM. So this discussion of inverted triangle and OM fits together, doesn't it?

We are like babies waking up to what we are. If we are a baby noticing our toes for the first time, does that mean we should meditate on our toes for the rest of our life? They are just our wonderful wiggly toes. I see OM as being like that. The wonderful ecstatic aspect of what we are, and of what everything is. So will we be infatuated with OM all the time like our baby toes? We can move beyond both. Inner silence is not so concerned about it. In time, stillness and ecstasy (OM) merge to become something much more. The outpouring of divine love into the world -- that is the big transformation for each of us, and for everyone. It is stillness and OM merged and in action.

Maybe just regard the inverted triangle as part of the OM experience, and carry on as you see fit ... if it grows to become a full blown Sri Yantra on your forehead, you will become a pilgrimage destination. It could be worse. :-)

The guru is in you.

2006/03/05 18:24:38
Satsang Cafe - General Questions on AYP
http://www.aypsite.org/forum/topic.asp?TOPIC_ID=878
Yoga - Then and Now
Picking up on a private conversation here...

Hi Jim:

Theosophy was really huge around 1900, before and after -- the only real Eastern wisdom game in town in the West until Vivekananda, Sir John Woodroffe and a few others began promoting, writing about and teaching practices. Then came Yogananda...

See lesson 253 for more history on Yoga coming to the West.

Theosophy and its off-springs (Steiner, Bailey, etc.) have Western 19th century spiritualism, intellectual mysticism and Pagan leanings mixed in, as there were no real practices to speak of coming West from India much before 1910-20 or so, so the Europeans and Americans did the best they could with all that Eastern philosophy.

Aren't you thrilled to know all this, Jim? Ah, but you'd rather just "point an click" in practices. Me too! :-)

The guru is in you.

2006/03/06 12:21:39
Satsang Cafe - General Questions on AYP
http://www.aypsite.org/forum/topic.asp?TOPIC_ID=878&REPLY_ID=4163&whichpage=-1
Yoga - Then and Now

Hi Jim:

Newton's laws of motion have been around for a long time too, and look how far we have come in applying them. I think yoga is like that. As we move from rigid past-based applications and evolve toward results-oriented real time application of yoga practices, I think we will see a great acceleration in both the understanding and the utilization of the principles that are involved. Yoga is only reflecting what is within us already, just as Newton's laws reflect how physical motion has always occurred. The refinement of application in both cases is a process, not an absolute. This has been a mistaken notion about yoga over the centuries. Yoga is not a monolith. It is an evolving interpretation of human capabilities, and manifesting them in the most efficient ways. Will that process ever end? I think not.

Over the past 100 years there has been huge progress, but it is only the beginning of far greater things. We can do this!

The guru is in you.

2006/03/06 12:42:30
Satsang Cafe - General Questions on AYP
http://www.aypsite.org/forum/topic.asp?TOPIC_ID=878&REPLY_ID=4166&whichpage=-1
Yoga - Then and Now
PS - This private conversation was just posted here in the satsang cafe. An exciting topic for sure, at the heart of all we are doing in AYP. Enjoy! :-)
2006/03/13 13:24:53
Satsang Cafe - General Questions on AYP

http://www.aypsite.org/forum/topic.asp?TOPIC_ID=897&REPLY_ID=4445&whichpage=-1
Breakdown of inner silence...

Hi Shanti:

Often tmes, symptoms of purification can mimic feelings we have had at an earlier time when we were much more stuck in a particular blockage. That can be a little unnerving for sure. Over the past few years, I have seen quite a few situations like this, with things clearing up and a happy ending. Well, no ending -- just a new opening and on to more purification, beginning from a much better place than we were before.

Of course, we can't say what exactly is happening in your case. The unwinding is as unfathomable as karma itself. You are wise to self-pace and be patient. You are doing just right. Something tells me that you will be through this sooner rather than later.

Don't forget to do some daily exercise. If you treat this like an energy excess (hitting the emotions in this case) and do a good amount of grounding activity, it will help.

The guru is in you.

2006/03/22 16:27:17
Satsang Cafe - General Questions on AYP
http://www.aypsite.org/forum/topic.asp?TOPIC_ID=933&REPLY_ID=4894&whichpage=-1
Symptoms

Hi All:

OM can be in one ear also. It can move around during various stages of purification. The symptoms of purification can be asymmetrical according to the pattern of inner obstructions that is unwinding. It is quite common and is discussed in the lessons here --
http://www.aypsite.org/207.html

However, if there are health concerns, it is better to check them out than continue to be distracted by them, especially if there is some medical history along the same lines.

The guru is in you.

2006/03/23 09:33:03
Satsang Cafe - General Questions on AYP
http://www.aypsite.org/forum/topic.asp?TOPIC_ID=933&REPLY_ID=4931&whichpage=-1
Symptoms

Hi Vicki:

The thing to do is slow down a bit on practices, and do some grounding activity -- a long walk or some physical exercise is a good place to start right away. It would be good to have grounding activity like that in the daily routine. Also, other activities that take your mind off the energy are good -- like helping others in some way that you enjoy. Check lesson 69 for additional remedies for too much energy running around --
http://www.aypsite.org/69.html

If you are not doing spinal breathing see if 5 minutes of it twice a day before meditation helps. If not, back off accordingly.

Good things are happening. The key now is stable practice, avoiding overdoing it, and bringing the energy into your daily life in productive ways. Self-pacing, grounding and service activities are some of the tools to apply. The less preoccupied we are with the energy, the smoother it will be. It wants to flow through us into the environment, and that is why becoming more external in our view can be helpful. In the end, it becomes an infinite flow of divine love pouring out of us.

The guru is in you.

2006/03/20 21:41:58
Satsang Cafe - General Questions on AYP
http://www.aypsite.org/forum/topic.asp?TOPIC_ID=947&REPLY_ID=4798&whichpage=-1
Degrees of Consciousness Evolution?

Hi Kathy:

You can find a slimmed down version of what Frank is talking about by looking at the lessons under "Enlightenment Milestones" in the Topic Index here: http://www.aypsite.org/TopicIndex.html

This model is experience-based -- observer and observed, whereas the other model mentioned by George is energy based -- the opening of particular chakras. As Melissa pointed out above, we don't do much with the chakra model in AYP. In fact, we don't dwell much on the AYP model either. Better to have the experience itself, and then we can describe it in any way we choose. There is nothing sacred, or even that useful about enlightenment models for their own sake, except as they can inspire us to practice. Ultimately, we are the model!

The guru is in you.

2006/03/23 15:06:35
Satsang Cafe - General Questions on AYP
http://www.aypsite.org/forum/topic.asp?TOPIC_ID=962&REPLY_ID=4968&whichpage=-1
Satire as a means to counter destructive myth

Hi David:

The bottom line is we are always responsible for how our actions affect others, regardless of our intentions.

Like intent, "style" has never been a good excuse for harming anyone. I'm not sure there ever is a good excuse, though we all do it, and we all have our excuses.

That is why Patanjali put a yama (restraint) in his Yoga Sutras called "ahimsa." It means "non-harming," and it is there for a reason. To do otherwise increases bondage. What we do to others, we do to ourselves.

In stillness we know the truth.

The guru is in you.

PS -- As for "destructive myth," it undoes itself in due course. In any case, it is not AYP's mission to confront all the destructive myths out there. The focus here is on utilizing the tools of yoga for promoting spiritual progress by those who have the desire to make the journey.

2006/03/23 17:09:24
Satsang Cafe - General Questions on AYP
http://www.aypsite.org/forum/topic.asp?TOPIC_ID=962&REPLY_ID=4979&whichpage=-1
Satire as a means to counter destructive myth

Thanks, Jim.

I am glad you shared that. Wow, it is downright beautiful.

Yes, everything matters. It is a shock to find out -- hard to face. Inner silence (the witness) delivers the realization. Once we become more attuned to it and learn to operate on true cause and effect instead of on our often misguided "best intentions," it is a huge breakthrough -- the unraveling of karma. We shift from being careless to caring. It makes all the difference. Then we seek to inspire instead of criticize. "Do unto others..." comes alive. A big shift in energy flow to divine love comes with that. Then we really know what ahimsa is. It is part of our essential nature.

The guru is in you.

2006/03/24 01:34:35
Satsang Cafe - General Questions on AYP
http://www.aypsite.org/forum/topic.asp?TOPIC_ID=962&REPLY_ID=5018&whichpage=-1
Satire as a means to counter destructive myth
David: You quoted me out of context. Here is the rest of what I said, which was intended to be a balanced statement in reply to Richard's concerns about how the Maharis
Hi treated the UK:

"As for the Maharishi, he has had his own agenda, and unfortunately the spiritual aspirations of people everywhere have gradually slipped into a distant second place from his point of view. It is no reflection on the UK or any other nation that has seen the teaching of Transcendental Meditation whither away. It has happened in the USA too, and I think we have been similarly blasted. When someone blames others for their own problems, it is pretty much over, isn't it?

"The unstoppable force of spiritual evolution goes on at an ever-increasing rate. Interestingly, and very much to his credit, the Maharis
Hi played an important role in fostering the shift of human consciousness during the 20th century. But now we are in the 21st century and the rules of the game are changing fast. We are moving into powerful integrated systems of self-directed practice. The age of wide open yoga science is dawning!

"We owe much to the people and nations, warts and all, who have played a role in getting us to this point. Hopefully we, warts and all, can do as good a job as they did in passing something useful on to our successors."

Yes, I do believe it is over as far as the Maharishi's role on the world stage is concerned. Few today would argue that, given his actions in recent years. Hey, he is well up in his 90s, and has made remarkable contributions over his lifetime. But something has gone wrong and everyone knows it. So the world moves on. This is not an ongoing program of trying to undo anything or anyone. It is what it is, and that is my opinion. No satire. No games. No tricks. And most of all, no ongoing program of character assassination.

As I wrote in lesson 260, contrary to popular belief, enlightened people do make mistakes. They do not know everything. When someone like the Maharis
Hi makes mistakes (and he has made plenty), it does not mean that everything he has ever done ought to be flushed down the toilet. A wise course is to take the good and let the bad go. The right thing to do is give credit for the good even while acting to avoid the bad. We had the discussion about throwing the baby out with the bathwater a month or two ago, and it seemed that everyone got it. Well, maybe not.

If there is an agenda to destroy the work and reputation of this sage because he has made mistakes, I am not for it. It becomes especially offensive when it is veiled behind satire, wittiness, or any other mask that assumes self-evident truth. The end does not justify the means if the end is wrong. I believe it is wrong to try and entirely discredit anyone by any means. In fact, we have a rule here in AYP that no teacher or tradition is to be disrespected. If I did so by expressing my opinion about the shortcomings of a great teacher, then I do apologize.

Let us have no ongoing programs of discrediting teachers or traditions going on here. It is an unnecessary distraction from the important work of AYP, which is the effective application of spiritual practices.

And if you want to use satire, David, make sure you use it for something that is not a foregone personal conclusion that may be biased and unfair. In that case, satire is only a gimmick, a ruse. Better to come out and give a straightforward opinion, so we can see what is really on your mind. In either case, if it is about systematically discrediting a spiritual teacher or tradition, it does not belong here.

The guru is in you.

2006/03/25 08:30:21
Satsang Cafe - General Questions on AYP
http://www.aypsite.org/forum/topic.asp?TOPIC_ID=962&REPLY_ID=5066&whichpage=-1
Satire as a means to counter destructive myth

Hi David:

To be honest, I really could not think of a spiritual use for satire. The word reminds me of the proverbial heartless theater critic, running roughshod over the hard work of dedicated artists with his/her twisted wit.

Then it occurred to me, an excellent spiritual application for satire would be to do it on ourselves! Turn it into a mirror and then we will have something useful. Can you do that?

I am not trying to be a smart Alec here. It is a time-tested principle that when we examine ourselves with as much intensity as we examine others, much bigger positive changes can be accomplished.

Maybe that is why the wisest people are self-deprecating to the point of satirizing themselves, while the rest of us idiots are out skewering each other to no avail.

The importance of focusing on fixing ourselves instead of others has already been said by several in this thread. The only suggestion I am adding is to take the satire itself and use it for self-examination.

As Jesus said, "You see the speck in your brother's eye; but you do not look at the plank in your own eye."

The guru is in you.

The anonymous, humble, and not nearly as holy and smart as everyone thinks,
Yogani :-)

PS -- The biggest "destructive myths" are the ones within us.

2006/03/25 17:15:53
Satsang Cafe - General Questions on AYP
http://www.aypsite.org/forum/topic.asp?TOPIC_ID=962&REPLY_ID=5101&whichpage=-1
Satire as a means to counter destructive myth

Hi All:

I never studied Franz Barton, though it sounds like one of those analyze-yourself-to-death systems. That is certainly not what I had in mind for turning satire around. It is just the concept of turning a tendency to criticize back in toward the criticizer for spiritual benefit. It is a form of bhakti. If we can redirect our emotions, whatever they may be, toward spiritual practice, then that is the thing.

I suppose if someone is prone to criticize all the time, it could turn into non-stop self-criticism when turned around, which is not a good thing. On the other hand, it can also be morphed into a stronger desire to do yoga practices, which would be a good thing. The point is, all emotions can be transformed to a higher purpose -- it is the essential principle of bhakti. Those who are dedicated to doing that are on a high path of yoga, because every thought and feeling is transformed into spiritual practice and progress. See lesson 67 for more on this -- http://www.aypsite.org/67.html

Now, did someone say there are some money changers around here somewhere? Harrumph! :-)

The guru is in you.

2006/03/26 13:23:44
Satsang Cafe - General Questions on AYP
http://www.aypsite.org/forum/topic.asp?TOPIC_ID=962&REPLY_ID=5163&whichpage=-1
Satire as a means to counter destructive myth

Hi LittleDragon:

In the fray, I neglected to welcome you into our midst. Welcome!

There is also the story of Jesus cursing the barren fruit tree -- a "Do something or get off the pot!" scenario. I can relate to that in my own spiritual career. Do you think I have a sense of urgency about all of this? You bet. The clock is ticking...

The guru is in you.

2006/03/31 09:07:41
Satsang Cafe - General Questions on AYP
http://www.aypsite.org/forum/topic.asp?TOPIC_ID=962&REPLY_ID=5434&whichpage=-1
Satire as a means to counter destructive myth

Hi David:

If you told me we have 1,000 gallons of bathwater with one ounce of baby hidden in it, I would say, let's concentrate on finding the baby and forget about the bathwater. AYP has been about that since the beginning, and I hope it always will be. Nothing bland about it, assuming we are into finding babies instead of processing bathwater.

The guru is in you.

2006/04/05 08:52:55
Satsang Cafe - General Questions on AYP
http://www.aypsite.org/forum/topic.asp?TOPIC_ID=1016&REPLY_ID=5636&whichpage=-1
drugs, depression, and yoga
Welcome Tros!

I get asked about this from time to time in private email, sometimes by someone who has used drugs as a stepping stone to yoga or other spiritual practices, and other times by someone who regards drugs themselves as the path. Invariably, the former is much better off in terms of clarity and progress than the latter.

Here is a recent interchange with an aspirant who used drugs for spiritual purposes and then moved beyond them:

Q: ...I am genuinely curious if you know about how and why marijuana affects kundalini. I know that some sadhus and yogis smoke marijuana or hashish to aid in their meditation, and I think its affect on kundalini is probably why. For a while I experimented with that but deemed it a crutch and hated how it polluted my body, so I quit for good. I do not put strange foreign substances into my body anymore.

A: Drugs can provide an initial (and artificial) introduction to the inner dimensions. This may inspire one to take up practices. Once spiritual practices are underway, then the drugs quickly become counter-productive to purification and opening to higher states, and improved inner seeing from practices reveals this. This scenario of drugs leading to spiritual practices has been fairly common over the past 50 years at least -- drugs as a stepping stone to something more.

For others, the spiritual momentum of past lives (or from somewhere) is more than enough to launch one on a path of practices in this life. In that case, drugs will not be a factor at all, and will be seen as an impediment right from the start. It all depends on the inner condition of the person.

Whichever way it happens, as our natural inner light emerges via effective practices, drugs will be a hindrance rather than a help. Why use a facsimile when we can have the real thing? No additional imprints are needed. We'd like to remove all imprints. Then we can live full time the truth that is inherent within us. :-)

See also lesson 29 -- http://www.aypsite.org/29.html

All the best on your path. Practice wisely, and enjoy!

The guru is in you.

2006/04/10 19:06:04
Satsang Cafe - General Questions on AYP
http://www.aypsite.org/forum/topic.asp?TOPIC_ID=1025&REPLY_ID=5832&whichpage=-1
Down-and-Out Yoga and Flying High Yoga

Hi Shanti:

In time, people will question what is different about you less and come to rely on your rising inner strength more. You will have more to give and will be feisty again, because that is you. You will be reborn in spiritual feistiness. We are all being reborn as our spiritual selves. Nothing is lost except the darkness, and everything is gained. That is how it goes.

Yogis and yoginis are ugly ducklings that turn into stunningly beautiful swans.

So, ugly ducklings everywhere, take heart! :-)

The guru is in you.

2006/04/14 16:09:58
Satsang Cafe - General Questions on AYP
http://www.aypsite.org/forum/topic.asp?TOPIC_ID=1043&REPLY_ID=5970&whichpage=-1
the "plank" in our own eye

Hi Anthem:

Thanks for the Jesus quote, and the stimulating plank ponderings.

It is an interesting question on whether to expend effort to solve the "puzzle of life," or just do our practices and let it solve itself.

I think it takes both. We all know the old saying, "God helps those who help themselves." Of course, that could apply to meditating only, but I think there is more to it. That is why we meditate and then go out and do. The blending of inner silence and outer puzzle-solving is essential to bring the process of transformation to fruition.

It reminds me of a lesson I wrote way back in 2003 (#36) called, "Meditation and the Fifth Dimension."

The implication there is that it is much easier to solve a puzzle when we can see in five dimensions, instead of only in four. Deep meditation is what gives us the fifth dimension. We still solve the puzzle, only it is easier to do with the extra seeing that inner silence brings us in every moment.

Of course, this is making the case for "self-inquiry," once inner silence is coming up. Certain practices are fifth dimension oriented and we cannot be very productive with them until we have that extra dimension. Sort of like trying to solve a three dimensional puzzle in two dimensions. I think to solve this one, ya gotta have five. :-)

The guru is in you.

26 –   Advanced Yoga Practices

2006/04/21 16:36:44
Satsang Cafe - General Questions on AYP
http://www.aypsite.org/forum/topic.asp?TOPIC_ID=1063&REPLY_ID=6243&whichpage=-1
Can the path to enlightenment change ppl bad?

quote:
_____
http://www.energygrid.com/spirit/ap-falsegurutest.html
_____

Thanks Near, there are a few really good ideas in there.

Let's see, "His Holiness The La Dee Da Yogani"

Only kidding! Dying laughing here. Sorry... :-)

Btw, I think you all have done a wonderful job with this topic. Not kidding on that.

The guru is in you.

2006/04/27 22:46:19
Satsang Cafe - General Questions on AYP
http://www.aypsite.org/forum/topic.asp?TOPIC_ID=1080&REPLY_ID=6446&whichpage=-1
Electricity in right palm
Welcome, Nsantoo!

I'm happy to see you got signed up in the forum okay. The answers given already are the same I would have given. It will be all for the good as you move into practices for purifying and opening from within. Then you will become even more a channel for the divine flow.

AYP is an open source integration of the world's most effective spiritual practices and can be useful for self-directed practitioners. Just follow the lessons from the beginning as the others have suggested.

It should also be added that sensations of energy moving, of which there are many kinds, are the "friction" of energy passing through still not fully purified parts of our spiritual neurobiology. As inner purification advances over time, then the energy sensations will become less, even as the energy flows become much greater.

This growth is dependent primarily on the cultivation of unbounded inner silence via deep meditation and related methods, and also the cultivation of body-wide ecstatic conductivity through spinal breathing pranayama and related methods. These two, inner silence and ecstatic conductivity, join to become the full flowering of divine love flowing through us. What you are experiencing now is a small taste of this.

It is also possible for devotion/bhakti (in the temple environment you mentioned in your previous email) to bring on the kind of symptoms you are experiencing.

And, of course, the gifts we have in this life have been cultivated in times long before our current recollection. You are picking up where you left off.

I wish you all the best on your chosen path. Practice wisely, and enjoy!

The guru is in you.

2006/05/11 15:57:51
Satsang Cafe - General Questions on AYP
http://www.aypsite.org/forum/topic.asp?TOPIC_ID=1130&REPLY_ID=6820&whichpage=-1
Turn the other cheek - Injustice ?

Hi Wolfgang:

I could be wrong, but I believe all completed auctions on eBay are binding contracts, with payment due before shipping by the seller (unfortunate about paypal not working, but the contract is still there). Which is no excuse for rudeness, of course...

It seems the simple way out of this is to pay the money, get the power supply (maybe it will be your spare by then - so sell it on eBay!), place a bad report on the seller if need be (ASAP - as *short* as possible), and move on.

They say that yogis have the ability to stay out of the mud and the thorns. That's one way to do it. Nothing to prove here, except that you can extricate yourself quickly and let go of it. Just a suggestion.

Inner silence has an amazing ability to cut through these kinds of muddy, thorny situations. Very practical. All the more reason to keep meditating. The best cheek to turn is the one that is like infinite inner space. Everything passes right through it. Then nothing sticks and it is easy to be a good Christian. :-)

All the best!

The guru is in you.

2006/05/14 19:47:11
Satsang Cafe - General Questions on AYP
http://www.aypsite.org/forum/topic.asp?TOPIC_ID=1145&REPLY_ID=6962&whichpage=-1

Mama's Day

Hi Shanti:

Will do. Thank you. We had a celebration for both mothers here today, as I am sure many of you did.

Happy Mother's Day to all divine mothers here and everywhere!

The guru is in you.

2006/05/16 13:12:23
Satsang Cafe - General Questions on AYP
http://www.aypsite.org/forum/topic.asp?TOPIC_ID=1153&REPLY_ID=7057&whichpage=-1
Global Rapture

Hi Wolfgang:

Apologies for the rearrangement. It was a random event that you ended up on top of the list of posters in this topic. If it is not okay, I will see what we can do to change it.

The reason for the rearrangement is because the AYP forums do not host political discussions, and this entire topic was going to be deleted for that reason. The moderators felt that there was useful spiritual (non-political) discussion in the topic (including your fine posts), so a salvage effort was undertaken (the first time such a thing has been done here). And you ended up on top. What luck! :-)

If this is not okay with you, let me know.

By the way, I share the belief of many that we are in the midst of an accelerating global spiritual transformation. AYP is doing its part to try and help the process along by offering an open source of effective integrated spiritual practices to everyone. Why not? It is time for human evolution to move on ... the "rapture" can be seen in that way as a positive event.

Thank you for your valuable contributions to the discussion, and all the best!

The guru is in you.

2006/05/16 14:07:55
Satsang Cafe - General Questions on AYP
http://www.aypsite.org/forum/topic.asp?TOPIC_ID=1153&REPLY_ID=7063&whichpage=-1
Global Rapture

Hi Wolfgang:

Thank you for your understanding.

Incidently, your randomly placed starting post was a good answer to Etherfish's initial question and turned out to be the perfect beginning for this renamed topic.

So, was any of this random? :-)

The guru is in you.

2006/07/20 10:09:38
Satsang Cafe - General Questions on AYP
http://www.aypsite.org/forum/topic.asp?TOPIC_ID=1196&REPLY_ID=9715&whichpage=-1
Secret of Siddhi

quote:
_____
Maatsuah said: I have to wonder, like Meg, whether this so called desire for God above else is any different from other desires. God is not an entity or idea that has been clearly defined because this entity is above the human condition (language, logic, emotions,even polarity). I have heard conflicting definitions of who or what God is from people of all backgrounds and intellectual/spiritual levels.
_____

Hi Maatsuah:

The eastern concept of "Ishta" goes a long way toward answering this question. It means "chosen ideal" (for each person) and it can be whatever one's concept of the highest ideal is -- God (specific or non-specific), truth, peace, knowledge, need to evolve, whatever turns the person on ... an emotional connection is the key.

If one's ishta is used to channel desire, it has great spiritual power. When it becomes continuous, it is called devotion, or bhakti. Desire/bhakti is the primary engine of all spiritual practice, as discussed in the AYP lessons here:
http://www.aypsite.org/12.html
http://www.aypsite.org/67.html
...and in many more lessons.

The idea that everyone must be devoted to the same ishta (ideal) has been a primary cause of strife and suffering throughout the ages. A key aspect of ishta is also to accept the beliefs of others. We call it tolerance, and it is a natural part of our evolution -- an innate divine quality in us all.

There is no one answer to the question, Who or what is God? We each have our own answer within us, and that is our ishta. It will evolve over time as we do, as our perception expands. All the while, our desire for our ideal will drive us to practices, and that is how evolution is accelerated. Bhakti and practices go hand-in-hand like that. So desire has an essential role to play on the spiritual path. With desire, things happen. With desire raised to devotion/bhakti, spiritual progress is assured.

As for siddhis, they are a by-product of purification and opening in the nervous system -- nothing more, nothing less. "Seek first the kingdom of heaven..."

On the other hand, if a desire for siddhis drives us to practices, it is better than no desire to do practices. Once in daily practices, our ishta will gradually evolve as we see more, and we will aim higher -- expanding ishta! :-)

Interestingly, as our ishta expands, so does our surrender to the process of spiritual transformation occurring within us. Then we have desire and surrender mixed -- active surrender to the divine expanding within and around us. In the end, it is all surrender ... with desire transformed to a constant outpouring of divine love, and that is how we carry on in the world.

All the best!

The guru is in you.

2006/06/13 09:07:54
Satsang Cafe - General Questions on AYP
http://www.aypsite.org/forum/topic.asp?TOPIC_ID=1212&REPLY_ID=8019&whichpage=-1
Changes in faith

Hi All:

It raises the question: Are teachings like AYP an aberration, small windows of opportunity for the few, or the wave of the future for the many?

I believe it is we who will choose, more so than the stars.

It is said that those with handicaps grow the most because they have the most to overcome. The human spirit is at its best when facing adversity. If that is the case, there is great hope for humanity.

We can do it, and it is all right.

Pssst, pass it on...

The guru is in you.

2008/11/03 10:22:18
Satsang Cafe - General Questions on AYP
http://www.aypsite.org/forum/topic.asp?TOPIC_ID=1309&REPLY_ID=39857&whichpage=-1
visualization

Hi Newpov:

Localized sensations, light, and other symptoms in deep meditation are effect rather than cause, and the instruction is to easily favor the mantra, which is the underlying cause of symptoms of purification and opening, and of the rise of abiding inner silence.

This is not to say that energy centers, light, sound and other inner phenomena cannot be used as objects of meditation, but that is a departure from the method of AYP deep meditation, and will be the practitioner's experiment, or perhaps following the guidance of another teaching. It is best to continue with one approach, and not be jumping around too much.

Remember, if we are digging a well to find water, one deep well will usually be better than many shallow ones. :-)

The guru is in you.

2006/08/10 12:30:37
Satsang Cafe - General Questions on AYP
http://www.aypsite.org/forum/topic.asp?TOPIC_ID=1400&REPLY_ID=10374&whichpage=-1
Some questions about AYP

Hi Mystic:

I try not to get fixed on labels, focusing more on the thing itself, and the audience it is being conveyed to. For example, the Secrets of Wilder uses common English terms for just about everything we talk about here, because it was written primarily for western Judeo/Christian readers.

The AYP lessons and books use Sanskrit, but it is simplified as much as possible to reach a wider audience.

As they say, "A rose is still a rose by any other name."

Keeping that in mind, here are responses to your questions:

1. In AYP, "advanced" does not necessarily refer to the people using it, but to the integrated open source system that AYP is, which can be used by anyone at beginning, intermediate or advanced levels. I think most would agree that the system itself is pretty advanced in ultimate capabilities, not only because of the full-scope integration of techniques, but for its easy access, the simplicity of the practices, and, of course, self-pacing at every level.

These days, we know that "advanced" technology in the public domain is technology that is powerful and easily accessible to people at all levels of expertise.

Oops, my cell phone is ringing. Someday I will learn to operate all the features on this thing. I'm glad it is so easy to use as a basic telephone ... very advanced!

That is the concept in AYP too.

2. "Amaroli" was used because the term was already in common use in the west. The term "Shivambu Kalpa" was considered, but in the end I decided to use amaroli as the key word -- less esoteric connotation and easier to remember. It was as simple as that. Amaroli is one of the few AYP practices not covered in the Secrets of Wilder. If it were, you can be sure it would have a simple English name. But not Pee Drinking!

3. On "spinal breathing pranayama," I don't believe this wonderful practice has had a common usage name, only many sectarian names. So I made up a descriptive non-sectarian name that everyone could easily understand and relate to. That is where it came from. East meets west!

If this is all wrong, please forgive me. I know terminology is very important, and you should feel free to use whatever terms you are comfortable with. Just make sure we can understand what you are talking about. :-)

Ease of understanding and implementation have been the main criteria used in the development of AYP. It is a blending of the ancient and the contemporary.

It is the practices themselves, and the results, that count. That is always first and foremost here. A rose is still a rose...

The guru is in you.

2006/08/11 11:30:10
Satsang Cafe - General Questions on AYP
http://www.aypsite.org/forum/topic.asp?TOPIC_ID=1400&REPLY_ID=10401&whichpage=-1
Some questions about AYP

Hi Mystic:

You got me curious, because I have not heard of amaroli referred to as anything but taking urine -- the same as shivambu kalpa. In the Hatha Yoga Pradipika, the word amaroli is used in that way. In the Damar Tantra, shivambu kalpa is used. Both are describing the same action of urine ingestion (Damar Tantra in much more detail). The Hatha Yoga Pradipika is the better known of the two scriptures, so perhaps that is why Amaroli is the term in common usage in the west.

Below are excerpts from both. I see the tie-in with vajroli in the Hatha Yoga Pradipika, but these still are two distinct practices, though they certainly impact one another through the natural interconnectedness of all yoga practices in the nervous system. Both are the "taking back in of bodily substances," so that is the similarity I suppose.

In AYP, we take a more natural and refined approach to vajroli than is described in the Hatha Yoga Pradipika. See http://www.aypsite.org/130.html and http://www.aypsite.org/T40.html.

While it may sound sacrilegious, I consider vajroli as described in the Hatha Yoga Pradipika to be a distortion of the natural processes of preservation and cultivation of sexual energy that occur in us with the rise of ecstatic conductivity in the nervous system. Even if vajroli in the HYP is not intended to be macho and chauvinistic, that will be the outcome for most eager male practitioners anyway, and have little to do with real yoga. There are much better ways to get there, while honoring and promoting the divine unfoldment in both sexes.

We should always keep in mind that ancient scriptures, while extremely valuable, were written by people too, in their own cultural climate, and are sometimes edited over the centuries. They offer much important knowledge to us, but must stand the test of real-time experience, the final arbiter of truth. The quest for truth in scripture is noble. Yet, it is to be finally transcended as the truth unfolds within each of us.

The guru (and final scripture) is in you.

From Hatha Yoga Pradipika:
http://www.santosha.com/philosophy/hathayoga-pradipika-chapter3.html

The Amaroli.

94. In the doctrine of the sect of the Kapalikas, the Amaroli is the drinking of the mid stream; leaving the 1st, as it is a mixture of too much bile and the last, which is useless.

95. He who drinks Amari (urine), snuff it daily, and practices Vajroli, is called practicing Amaroli.

From Damar Tantra:
http://www.audarya-fellowship.com/forums/health-wellbeing/29086-shivambu-damar-tantra.html

O Parvati! I shall expound to you the recommended actions and rituals of Shivambu Kalpa that confers numerous benefits. Those well versed in the scriptures have carefully specified certain vessels for the purpose. (1)

Utensils made from the following materials are recommended: Gold, Silver, Copper, Bronze, Brass, Iron, Clay, Ivory, Glass, Wood from sacred trees, Bones, Leather and Leaves. (2, 3)

The Shivambu (one's own urine) should be collected in a utensil made of any of these materials. Among them, clay utensils are better, copper are by far the best. (4)

The intending practitioner of the therapy should abjure salty or bitter foods, should not over-exert himself, should take a light meal in the evening, should sleep on the ground, and should control and master his senses. (5)

The sagacious practitioner should get up when three quarters of the night have elapsed, and should pass urine while facing the east. (6)

The wise one should leave out the first and the last portions of the urine, and collect only the middle portion. This is considered the best procedure. (7)

Just as there is poison in the mouth and the tail of the serpent, O Parvati, it is even so in the case of the flow of Shivambu. (8)

Shivambu (auto- urine) is heavenly nectar, which is capable of destroying senility and diseases. The practitioner of Yoga should take it before proceeding with his other rituals. (9)

After cleansing the mouth, and performing the other essential morning functions, one should drink one's own clear urine, which is the annihilator of senility and diseases. (10)

etc...
2006/08/14 13:27:41
Satsang Cafe - General Questions on AYP
http://www.aypsite.org/forum/topic.asp?TOPIC_ID=1426&REPLY_ID=10499&whichpage=-1
Ancient Dance during jaap?

Hi Nsantoo:

I concur with Dave. It is energy moving with inner purification, which can produce movements of various kinds -- mudras, bandhas, dancing, jerking motions, hopping on the meditation/samyama seat, etc. In AYP we favor the practice we are doing over these energy surges, combined with self-pacing in practices (in bhakti too) as necessary to regulate the underlying cause for good progress with comfort and safety. There is much more in the lessons on this. See "Automatic Yoga (and movements)" in the topic index -- http://www.aypsite.org/TopicIndex.html

The guru is in you.

2006/08/16 12:23:52
Satsang Cafe - General Questions on AYP
http://www.aypsite.org/forum/topic.asp?TOPIC_ID=1433&REPLY_ID=10588&whichpage=-1
Lonliness

Hi Alvin and all:

After a long, arduous and not always happy journey, the meaning of life as I have come to understand it is to help others as best we can, without expecting a particular outcome or payback.

That comes in a thousand forms and degrees. We will know we are heading into the right form for us if we feel good about what we are doing. It is a process of optimizing cause and effect. It is also called coming into our *dharma*.

For each of us it is about identifying what we are really good at (everyone is good at something) and finding ways to bring benefit to others with our gift, whatever it may be. If we do that with all our heart, the rest will take care of itself.

Spiritual practices will naturally take us in the direction of our dharma. It may not be what we were expecting or planning on, so there can be plenty of grinding of the gears along the way -- it can feel like loneliness as our illusions about life are dissolving. Becoming empty can be unnerving, for sure. But somewhere along the line the impulse to move will come from within, and we can choose to go with it.

In the end, surrendering to what is within us will yield lasting happiness. That is because the flow of life comes first from within. As we learn to let it animate our actions in a creative expression of helping others, loneliness and troubles will gradually give way to an inherent joy. It can happen in the same surroundings we have always been in.

Inner stillness is the foundation of the entire process.

The guru is in you.

2006/08/27 09:08:50
Satsang Cafe - General Questions on AYP
http://www.aypsite.org/forum/topic.asp?TOPIC_ID=1469&REPLY_ID=10936&whichpage=-1
Patanjali's Yoga Sutras Lessons

Hi Bipinjoshi:

Yes, the AYP online writings may be quoted and linked. This is covered in the copyright statement at the bottom of the website homepage. As many lessons as desired can be linked directly.

Thanks much for your contributions here, and for your interest in alerting others of our presence. :-)

The guru is in you.

2006/09/07 11:36:06
Satsang Cafe - General Questions on AYP
http://www.aypsite.org/forum/topic.asp?TOPIC_ID=1494&REPLY_ID=11152&whichpage=-1
Giving up the soul

Hi All:

Reminds me of the old saying:

"Oh God! if there is a God,
Please save my soul! if I have a soul."

:-)

What you are bringing up here relates to the vedanta/advaita (non-dual) branch of Indian philosophy, which technically is not the system of yoga -- well, jnana yoga crosses over, not to mention actual experiences that arise from yoga practices.

Advaita is similar to the Buddhist view of everything being spun as illusion from one thing, or no-thing. On the other hand, yoga-style practices (and even tantra) exist in Buddhism (though maybe not in Zen). It is not only intellectual in any particular system, yet the intellect has an important role to play. By a variety of means it is doing leading to non-doing in doing, if that makes sense. And the more non-doing there is, the more doing there may be -- divine doing, which is the ultimate non-doing!

So, among friends, an integration of methods can't hurt. In fact, it is essential. Each practice leads to the others, and vise versa, and eventually to the final result. That is the beauty of it all. Then we know the answers to the questions raised in the two-liner above. The reality is within us, everywhere and nowhere, in stillness.

The guru is in you.

2006/09/08 11:41:59
Satsang Cafe - General Questions on AYP
http://www.aypsite.org/forum/topic.asp?TOPIC_ID=1494&REPLY_ID=11174&whichpage=-1
Giving up the soul

quote:
_____
Originally posted by Anthem11

quote:
_____
yogani said: So, among friends, an integration of methods can't hurt. In fact, it is essential. Each practice leads to the others, and vise versa, and eventually to the final result.

Andrew said: Is there a "final result" as in an ending of the process of expansion in body and awareness? To elaborate, I could see how just "being" could be a final result, but isn't there an endless unfolding of the energies in the body as it opens up to the divine or is there a final culmination of this process of some kind? Do you perceive there to be an infinite process of increasing awareness too or does it end with perceiving the "oneness" of it all?

_____

Hi Andrew:

The "final result" is beyond human reckoning, and beyond anyone's ability to explain. As long as we are in human form, who knows where it ends? Yet, so many make the attempt to both reckon and explain. And why not? It is our nature. It is also our nature to be going somewhere. So let's go wherever "That" is...

Obviously, something profound is happening inside us. By "final result," I mean the unknowable end of the process, which is "being." Oddly enough, knowing isn't being, and being isn't knowing. It is like deep meditation, which most of us here can easily relate to. Who can say, "Now I am immersed in inner silence." No one. We can only say it after, in past tense. Yet, we can live stillness in action, becoming consciously "That" in this world -- a paradox. We can observe and explain what it is like. Yet, being does not see itself, just as the eye cannot see itself -- not without a mirror, that is. And therein lies a clue. We can see being in the actions of being, as reflecting in the mirror of the world. We are That -- an unending becoming expressed in the unending evolution of all that is manifest. We can also know That as being -- with nothing happening in the midst of it all. Everything is both.

Btw, Andrew, all of this is just a longer way of saying what you already said above. :-)

How are we doing here with the Zen, Louis?

The guru is in you.

2006/09/29 12:44:08
Satsang Cafe - General Questions on AYP
http://www.aypsite.org/forum/topic.asp?TOPIC_ID=1552&REPLY_ID=11708&whichpage=-1
Thanking God for evil

Hi All:

For some related thoughts, see my post here today on conduct, ahimsa (non-harming) and sin:
http://www.aypsite.org/forum/topic.asp?whichpage=1&TOPIC_ID=1553#11706

The guru is in you.

2006/10/05 10:17:52
Satsang Cafe - General Questions on AYP
http://www.aypsite.org/forum/topic.asp?TOPIC_ID=1572&REPLY_ID=11931&whichpage=-1
Problems with my AYP practice

Hi Andy:

Glad to see you chiming in for some input -- you have got plenty of good perspectives coming here.

As we have discussed in emails, if AYP helps you find your path, whatever that may be, then I am happy.

Of course, the path is in us already, and it is only a matter of finding resonance with that in the sources of spiritual knowledge and training we explore. No one body of knowledge is complete (including AYP), but inside you are, waiting to be revealed. Develop confidence in that and just keep going, and you cannot not miss.

Enjoy the journey. It is where all the fun is, in the now... :-)

The guru is in you.

2006/10/28 16:32:39
Satsang Cafe - General Questions on AYP
http://www.aypsite.org/forum/topic.asp?TOPIC_ID=1589&REPLY_ID=12653&whichpage=-1
Situation...

Hi Shweta:

Would anyone notice if you had been this way all along? No. They would just take your strength for granted. It is the period of change that raises the questions, for you and for those around you. Once it has progressed, your loved ones will count on your rising inner strength, and you will be glad to have it to give. Take it from someone who has traveled a similar path.

Nothing is being subtracted. Something important is being added, and that will become more apparent to all concerned as time goes on.

While no one is particularly comfortable with change, it is a fact that you will become even more the rock of your family than ever in the past.

Dispassion is profoundly passionate on the deepest level in us, and it will not be lost on anyone as it continues to manifest in your daily life in practical ways. Weakness and fear are being replaced with unshakable inner strength, compassion, and the power to stir many to choose their own freedom, no matter what the circumstances of life may bring. What a wonderful gift to give your children. Someday they will thank you for it, even though the changes might seem strange to them now.

It is not always easy to let go into our destiny, even with assurances that we will be all right. This is the very destiny that the scriptures have promised us, yes? Yet, we get nervous when we see it coming up. It is a natural reaction to an evolutionary transformation in us that we might not have considered to be within our reach. Well, it is ... and something inside us has known it all along.

The guru is in you.

2006/11/02 12:12:35
Satsang Cafe - General Questions on AYP
http://www.aypsite.org/forum/topic.asp?TOPIC_ID=1662&REPLY_ID=12835&whichpage=-1
Happy Birthday Yogani and AYP!!!

Thank you very much, All.

I am celebrating too. It is three years of wonderful sharing by so many dedicated practitioners, and lots of spiritual growth all the way around, including here.

So, today I am celebrating you, and all you have accomplished. Many thanks!

It is only the beginning... :-)

The guru is in you.

2006/11/02 17:30:02
Satsang Cafe - General Questions on AYP
http://www.aypsite.org/forum/topic.asp?TOPIC_ID=1662&REPLY_ID=12848&whichpage=-1
Happy Birthday Yogani and AYP!!!

quote:

Originally posted by Yogini

Question for David and many happy returns of this anniversary of the birth of this awesome series of lessons indeed Yogani! (in reverse order, i.e. first the congratulations, then the question for David:-)

David: you speak of exactly 3 years ago when the first lesson was posted - Would you happen to have the exact time? As an astrologer I'm curious...
Thanks in advance!

Hi Yogini:

The Main AYP Yahoo group was started on November 2, 2003 (no time available). There was a false start with nine lessons, which were deleted (don't remember why -- no dates or times available). The first lesson (#10) is time stamped "Sun Nov 16, 2003 11:45 am" eastern USA. Hey, we can celebrate again in a couple of weeks! :-)

Not sure if you can do anything with that astrologically, but that is what it is. Oh, and I should also mention that the first draft of the Secrets of Wilder was written much earlier in 2003, so the writing started before the writing started, so to speak. As is so often the case, we just pick a date to remember and celebrate, and the stars will accept it. Or did the stars do the picking in the first place? Will we ever know?

Well, here we are anyway ... in the NOW. We have always been in it. :-)

Thank you again, All, for your kind wishes. It has been and will continue to be an exciting joint effort!

The guru is in you.

2006/11/04 11:15:07
Satsang Cafe - General Questions on AYP
http://www.aypsite.org/forum/topic.asp?TOPIC_ID=1662&REPLY_ID=12919&whichpage=-1
Happy Birthday Yogani and AYP!!!

quote:
_____
Originally posted by Yogini

...AYP is likely to grow and grow over time, at least for the next 14 years...
_____

Hi Yogini:

With prognostications like that you are in danger of being elected official AYP astrologer. :-)

Clearly we are in some kind of a window of opportunity, with a convergence of knowledge and experience for all of us. The stars are doing their part, I'm sure.

You know what they say about a window of opportunity -- jump through!
No telling how long it will be open.

From this end, an ambitious writing plan has been laid out, and many have come to help by sharing their knowledge, experiences and passing the word. It has made a huge difference. AYP is a collaboration for sure.

Looking ahead over the next year or two, there will be significant refinements and additions to the overall AYP offering, for both inside and outside sitting practices. It is like the evolution of electronics. First we had big devices that got the job done (like the old family record player). Later on, the devices got much smaller and much more efficient (iPod). From the point of view here, the AYP-style approach will travel a similar route. Many will continue to take it forward, far beyond the next few years of my little window...

I believe a much bigger window is opening for efficient and safe cultivation of human spiritual transformation worldwide, and it is going to stay open for a long time.

Let's not waste a minute of it.

The guru is in you.

2006/11/04 10:39:24
Satsang Cafe - General Questions on AYP
http://www.aypsite.org/forum/topic.asp?TOPIC_ID=1672&REPLY_ID=12915&whichpage=-1
Yoga schools in Tamil Nadu region
Welcome, Prana608!

You may wish to contact Nandhi, a spiritual teacher who is from that area. He is currently living in Los Angeles.

http://www.nandhi.com/home.htm

All the best on your chosen path. Enjoy!

The guru is in you.

2006/11/17 13:22:12
Satsang Cafe - General Questions on AYP
http://www.aypsite.org/forum/topic.asp?TOPIC_ID=1715&REPLY_ID=13397&whichpage=-1
Mozart's Requiem

Hi All:

Interesting perspectives all the way around.

Just to add a few more cents, here is an AYP lesson on intelligence, bhakti and genius: http://www.aypsite.org/246.html

The meeting of heart, mind and the infinite intelligence behind it all...

All the best!

The guru is in you.

2006/11/18 17:15:02
Satsang Cafe - General Questions on AYP
http://www.aypsite.org/forum/topic.asp?TOPIC_ID=1728&REPLY_ID=13447&whichpage=-1
What are the obstructions?

quote:
_____
Originally posted by Chiron
Couldn't find anything about "Grathi".. Christi, do you have any more info/links about the term?
_____

Hi Chiron:

It is also spelled granthi(s). Here is an AYP lesson on it: http://www.aypsite.org/276.html

All the best!

The guru is in you.

2006/11/19 08:40:22
Satsang Cafe - General Questions on AYP
http://www.aypsite.org/forum/topic.asp?TOPIC_ID=1728&REPLY_ID=13465&whichpage=-1
What are the obstructions?

Hi All:

Can a coin be regarded as legal tender without both of its sides? :-)

The guru is in you.

2006/11/20 16:38:15
Satsang Cafe - General Questions on AYP
http://www.aypsite.org/forum/topic.asp?TOPIC_ID=1728&REPLY_ID=13537&whichpage=-1
What are the obstructions?

Hi All:

Ahem, read all about the spectacular miracles here: http://www.aypsite.org/76.html

Those are the ones we all are cultivating. :-)

It happens to be the subject of the next book being worked on here -- Samyama. It is about clearing out the inner obstructions more than about making miracles, though one naturally leads to the other in its own way and time. Not by our will -- by the divine will flowing out through us with fewer impediments.

The greatest miracle is that we (every one of us) can become infinite channels of divine love like that. It is a non-doing, and the outcome does not belong to us. At the same time, it is us.

The guru is in you.

2006/11/21 10:55:25
Satsang Cafe - General Questions on AYP
http://www.aypsite.org/forum/topic.asp?TOPIC_ID=1728&REPLY_ID=13569&whichpage=-1
What are the obstructions?

quote:
_____
Originally posted by david_obsidian

Hi Yogani, It might be a good time to spell out to Christi that you cannot (as of yet anyway) levitate in any true sense of the word, meaning remain suspended in the air in defiance of the laws of gravity, in such a way as to be able to prove levitation to Randi in the lab. Just in case he thinks that you are just being modest, since your post above and the lesson you link to don't constitute a direct, unambigous denial. :-)

If you leave any room at all for being mythologized on this matter, you will be. Trust me.
_____

Hi David:

I am not, but believe that I can. Therefore, I will not say that I cannot, and neither should anyone else.

This line of relationship within ourselves is important for everyone, as it is an essential constituent of bhakti. As we all know, bhakti is the primary engine of yoga. It is the part of us that believes, and belief is essential for us to take that next step on our path, however small or large it may be.

At the same time, as we engage in the practices of deep meditation, spinal breathing, samyama, etc., this line of internal relationship (bhakti) arises naturally, and we will no longer doubt our potential, regardless of the externals. Anything becomes possible, and the externals become all but irrelevant in the face of the steadily increasing divine outpouring. Our good intentions will manifest one way or another. How is not for us to judge...

To favor the external over the internal is a kind of mytholization that will hold us back. Isn't it obvious? Thank goodness practices will take care of it in time, so we don't have to be endlessly wrestling with our beliefs and thought patterns. Of course, we will anyway, for a while anyway. Eventually it all goes to stillness, and then we know...

Believe!

Miracles do happen (constantly) for those who believe. With respect to what we can accomplish, the word "cannot" is completely irrelevant.

The only problem with mythologizing in my opinion is that it is most often pointed in the wrong direction, externally toward others, which saps our ability to fully express our innate potential. We should be pointing it inward, and using it as inspiration for our practice.

This is the essential point in the great myths -- not to mythologize the hero as an external phenomenon, but to inspire the hero within us all. So often this point is missed. It is also a failing in the guru system. No one is to blame. It is our inner obstructions. Now we are catching on as inner silence and the light of knowledge are rising.

We ordinary folks are full with extraordinary possibilities. Let's never forget that. :-)

The guru is in you.

2006/11/26 11:44:49
Satsang Cafe - General Questions on AYP
http://www.aypsite.org/forum/topic.asp?TOPIC_ID=1728&REPLY_ID=13800&whichpage=-1
What are the obstructions?

Hi All:

The "truth" of the scriptures is only real if it can be verified in human experience, because human experience is what the scriptures are recording in the first place. The scriptures were written (or orally transmitted) by human beings! They are "absolute" only when mythologized to be so, and this has both pros and cons. The best scriptures are those which can also provide practical means for cultivating the spiritual potential which their authors professed to be resident in all human beings.

Scriptures can be useful when taken on blind faith over the short term, aiding in promoting bhakti and direct spiritual experience, and thus helping dissolve blind faith. But, if taken as absolute truth on blind faith indefinitely, without ongoing spiritual growth via effective practices, scriptures can become the foundation (or excuse) for grossly aberrant conduct in human beings. Any knowledge reduced to the level of an "ideology" and taken on blind faith on an ongoing basis will lead to conflict with other ideologies also taken on blind faith. When a scripture has been reduced to an ideology, beware!

Like any knowledge, scriptures can be well-used or terribly misused.

The real test of any scripture is in whether its highest ideals can be actualized in human experience. That is where the rubber meets the road. For thousands of years many dedicated practitioners have recorded their experiences on the path of human spiritual transformation, and, in some cases, recorded practical means to cultivate the divine outpouring in everyone. We owe them a great deal. How we use the information is up to us -- hopefully for the betterment of all humankind.

Just one person's opinion. :-)

The guru is in you.

2006/11/19 09:27:04
Satsang Cafe - General Questions on AYP
http://www.aypsite.org/forum/topic.asp?TOPIC_ID=1735&REPLY_ID=13466&whichpage=-1
A curiosity?

Hi Andrew:

I agree with Doc. We pick up here where we left off previously.

The ecstatic currents we experience with developing kundalini are, for the most part, a transitional stage involving the friction of the inner energies passing through the purifying subtle neurobiology. As this happens a more refined awareness develops, characterized by conscious living in pure/eternal bliss consciousness (sat chit ananda). It is our constant innate potential.

This is not to say your friend will not experience further ecstatic energy currents (purification) at some point along the way. But clearly she has done a lot of work previously and is manifesting the fruit of that. "Old souls" have that vibration about them.

Karma yoga (being there for others) is an important aspect of the path also, especially as our sense of self merges with moving inner silence. Your friend continues to evolve as she uplifts everyone around her. That is a stage expanding beyond the inner fireworks we tend to focus on while they are happening.

Every step along the way is sacred. Sometimes there is overlap, and sometimes we might appear to be mainly in one stage or the other. The common constituent in all stages of rising enlightenment is joy. When there is abiding joy, we are inclined to let go into that. Joy has its own agenda, and we can trust it.

The guru is in you.

2006/12/01 10:22:10
Satsang Cafe - General Questions on AYP
http://www.aypsite.org/forum/topic.asp?TOPIC_ID=1775&REPLY_ID=13936&whichpage=-1
SYMBOLS

Hi Vil:

Deep meditation mantras (like I AM, plus enhancements) are taken for their inner sound quality only (not meaning), and are therefore no more visually specific than, say, musical tones. The more content (visual or other) we try and attach to a mantra during practice, the less well it will work. Whether a mantra used in deep meditation is a symbol or not will depend on one's interpretation, I suppose, but the more interpreting one does, the less useful the mantra will be for deep meditation.

Interesting topic, but not with much overlap into the simple practice of deep meditation. As has been said by the great sages of lore: "KISS" (Keep it simple, stupid!) :-)

All the best!

The guru is in you.

2006/12/01 16:49:22
Satsang Cafe - General Questions on AYP
http://www.aypsite.org/forum/topic.asp?TOPIC_ID=1775&REPLY_ID=13948&whichpage=-1
SYMBOLS

Hi Vil:

Have you been through the lessons? Particularly those having to do with deep meditation and mantras (see topic index). I think everything you are asking is pretty well covered in there. If I missed anything, let me know. :-)

The guru is in you.

2006/12/10 10:08:46
Satsang Cafe - General Questions on AYP
http://www.aypsite.org/forum/topic.asp?TOPIC_ID=1775&REPLY_ID=14361&whichpage=-1
SYMBOLS

Hi All:

It has been said that "Man is God playing the fool."

That covers a multitude of sins, doesn't it? While offering great hope...

So the order of the day (and every day) is purification and opening, because we are all emerging channels of the infinite, however impure we might seem in the moment, or at any time in the past. We are symbols of the divine, and much more -- we are the reality itself, however limited the expression is or has been.

Put another way: "If God is omnipresent, in what is God not present?" This is conceptual, of course. All concepts of God are human inventions.

Reality is what it is, and we can find out through direct experience by going within. That is where the rubber meets the road. All the rest is, well, you know -- yak yak yak... :-)

The guru is in you.

2006/12/03 07:09:05
Satsang Cafe - General Questions on AYP
http://www.aypsite.org/forum/topic.asp?TOPIC_ID=1781&REPLY_ID=13995&whichpage=-1
Night shift/ yoga nidra

Hi Bewell:

That "someday" on yoga nidra is getting closer. The samyama book coming out in a month or so will address it in an additional practical way -- a new practice.

As for shift work, it has been said that all days or all nights is better than mixing and matching. The latter can produce the equivalent of "jet lag," though some can handle it without difficulty. It really depends on your own tendencies/inner energy dynamics, and you will be the best judge of it.

All the best!

The guru is in you.

2006/12/05 09:28:56
Satsang Cafe - General Questions on AYP
http://www.aypsite.org/forum/topic.asp?TOPIC_ID=1789&REPLY_ID=14100&whichpage=-1
Mind transformation

Hi EMC:

The initial difference is in having more choice on the thoughts we entertain from the position of rising inner silence (pure bliss consciousness). Thoughts gradually become like objects we can move around at will, and subconscious mental structures have less and less sway in our life. Over time, all thinking becomes illuminated from within with love, strength, creativity and bliss, and we can choose even better. :-)

The guru is in you.

2006/12/05 11:17:44
Satsang Cafe - General Questions on AYP
http://www.aypsite.org/forum/topic.asp?TOPIC_ID=1789&REPLY_ID=14105&whichpage=-1
Mind transformation

Hi EMC:

You would still have the thought, but would have less tendency to choose it. In not choosing the thought, it will become weaker over time, until it is hardly noticed at all. This is the dissolving of samskara to the so-called "burnt seed" level, where pure bliss consciousness does the burning via divine outpouring and the subsequent changes in the choices we make. Those seeds can sprout a little anytime down the road due to the karmic currents constantly flowing in us. But with abiding inner silence present and the corresponding habit of choosing, they are burnt again.

The work of Byron Katie (Book: "Loving what Is") is a good application of the choosing principle, though it takes inner silence for it, or any choosing, to go consistently higher.

The reason 12 step programs work so well is because they involve surrender to a higher power/ideal, which is bhakti. Bhakti all by itself will cultivate inner silence. We can also go on to deep meditation and samyama to get the inner silence engine really humming and manifesting in our life.

There is little chance of thinking our way through it without another aspect of practice brought in that cultivates inner silence. Any jnana/intellect-based system that works will have the element of inner silence brought in somehow. Without that, intellectual methods alone are like pushing on a string, or building castles in the air, or both! :-)

The guru is in you.

2006/12/20 10:07:45
Satsang Cafe - General Questions on AYP
http://www.aypsite.org/forum/topic.asp?TOPIC_ID=1789&REPLY_ID=14646&whichpage=-1
Mind transformation

Hi EMC:

Your mind is not you. It is a machine running on old subconscious baggage, and the attention you invest in it, which reinforces it. If you can observe your mind and thoughts as objects, without investing in what does not serve your wellbeing, those old kneejerk patterns will gradually fade (that's Katie and all of self-inquiry in a nutshell). This is not active rejection of particular thought patterns, which is more mental projection. It is favoring what nurtures us, and letting go of what does not. Abiding inner silence (witness/self) helps a lot in this. It is what nurtures us. It is us. Hence, daily deep meditation, samyama, etc.

There will be ups and downs on our sea of stillness. Yet, we remain unchanged...

The guru is in you.

2006/12/20 16:02:49
Satsang Cafe - General Questions on AYP
http://www.aypsite.org/forum/topic.asp?TOPIC_ID=1789&REPLY_ID=14660&whichpage=-1
Mind transformation

Hi Yoda:

I don't necessarily buy the "reality is a projection of our mind" idea; as in, nothing exists except through our projection of it. Sometimes "serious" jnana (discrimination) can lead to the nonsensical in this respect - "That truck that just ran over me doesn't exist, and neither do I, anymore!" :-)

However, our interpretation of reality and thinking about what it is (and acting/karma-ing that out) is just as you say, building layers and layers of "knee-jerks" (samskaras/baggage) in the subconscious mind/nervous system, and then we find ourselves living within our own illusions, often not even knowing we are in that mode. And so it goes.

Of course, the full scope of yoga is for unwinding all of this, and the whole thing can be taken back to the original "happy" of stillness/self in action.

It takes a while... With effective methods, progress is noticeable. Watching illusions dissolve is one of the most fun things there is, though it can be a bit scary in the beginning: "Pleeeease, don't take my illusions away! They are all that I think I have!"
What's that about?

The guru is in you.

PS: Reminds me of the once well-known bumper sticker -- "My karma ran over my dogma."

2006/12/20 16:28:57
Satsang Cafe - General Questions on AYP
http://www.aypsite.org/forum/topic.asp?TOPIC_ID=1789&REPLY_ID=14662&whichpage=-1
Mind transformation

Hi EMC:

Do what you have to do to keep your life on a steady keel. No point standing in the middle of the highway during rush hour.

As for all the kundalini stuff (that's what it is), there have been some who have arrived here in that condition. It has its pluses and minuses. The trick is to get smart about self-pacing and grounding, and embrace the process. Katrine can offer plenty of pointers on that, I'm sure.

The guru is in you.
    :-)

2006/12/10 09:52:44
Satsang Cafe - General Questions on AYP
http://www.aypsite.org/forum/topic.asp?TOPIC_ID=1809&REPLY_ID=14359&whichpage=-1
Vishudd
Hi Chakra

Hi Aditya:

Chin pump (dynamic jalandhara) is also very good for throat opening (and much more), preferably taken in order in relation to the rest of the practices presented in the AYP lessons. All things in good time.

Wishing you all the best! :-)

The guru is in you.

2006/12/28 17:43:12
Satsang Cafe - General Questions on AYP
http://www.aypsite.org/forum/topic.asp?TOPIC_ID=1858&REPLY_ID=14982&whichpage=-1
Physical Exercise and AYP Practice

Hi Billeejak:

Exercise in relation to yoga is like exercise in relation to anything else. Overdoing it in exercise will compromise our life. Likewise it can compromise our spiritual progress. So can overdoing it in spiritual practices.

Which is not to say long distance running or other intense physical activities are anti-yoga. It is only a matter of prudent conditioning and balancing our exercise in relation to everything else, including yoga. It can be done. Look at our fearless friend, John Wilder -- cross-country runner and wunderkid sage, all at the same time. :-)

There is no doubt that a moderate and stable exercise program will help our spiritual progress, and just about everything else in our life. This is touched on in the lessons here http://www.aypsite.org/80.html ...and in more detail in the Asanas, Mudras & Bandhas book, and AYP Easy Lessons book, where a yoga-friendly exercise program is offered.

All the best!

The guru is in you.

PS: Also see http://www.aypsite.org/69.html for the energy grounding aspect.

2007/02/23 23:41:06
Satsang Cafe - General Questions on AYP
http://www.aypsite.org/forum/topic.asp?TOPIC_ID=1864&REPLY_ID=17996&whichpage=-1
Power of the sub-conscious mind

quote:
_____
Originally posted by Jim and His Karma

It's a question of attitude. The spiritual path is about LESS YOU. Thy will be done...not MY will be done. When the construct of "you" drops away, what's left is pure love and power. But if you go for the power before that all-essential drop-away, it ain't ever gonna drop. Because that which needs to drop clings to the desire for power and glory. And it rationalizes its grasping for power by saying "I can use it to do good." Through the ages, that's been one of the great traps. I'll grow to be a superstar...and then I can HELP!
_____

Hi Jim:

But isn't "attitude" a doing also? This is one of the gripes we can have about advaita teachers who encourage us to walk around developing "an attitude" about the non-duality of existence, while ignoring the rest of the yoga tools that are available to us. Non-duality is inspiring. Yet, it will not take us far without bringing other elements of yoga in, like bhakti, deep meditation, pranayama, samyama, and the rest.

Letting go isn't going to be letting go until we are doing something else to enable it. :-)

Taking advaita to be a magic bullet is as flawed an approach as taking any other single aspect of yoga to be a magic bullet. I know that is not what you are advocating, Jim. It was felt the point ought to be emphasized though, because so many get the idea that spiritual practice is a non-doing. Well, it is, and it isn't. When we find ourselves in that paradox, even in our daily practices, we will know we are on to something. Like in that AYP lesson, "The Art of Doing Nothing."

Stumping for "letting go" can be like three day old fish, if nothing else is added into the mix. No two people are in exactly the same place consciousness-wise, and "letting go" is a "place" thing, not something we "do." It depends almost entirely on our experience of inner silence. In the vast majority of cases where real spiritual practices and progress are occurring, the habit of letting go in daily living is an effect rather than a cause. Yet, as soon as it (non-duality) appears it is often granted primacy in the over all scheme of practices, like a holy grail that anyone can grab instantly. The irony is that non-duality is nothing but an illusion for all but the anointed few, and those few do not help us much by offering it as a magic bullet. Personally, I think everyone will be anointed, but it won't happen by beating on the illusion of non-duality, no matter how real it ultimately will become for all of us.

So why do we keep telling people that "letting go" in everyday activity is a primary practice and cause of enlightenment? It is one of the the hardest ways there is to approach spiritual development. Hard because it sounds so good, makes so much sense, produces wonderful fantasies, and rarely delivers except to those who have significant exposure to other spiritual practices. It is very difficult (dare I say impossible?) to use an effect as a primary cause, because the effect must come to us from a deeper cause, something that will transcend our mind, and our attitudes.

It takes an integration of practices to get the job done. If we have found out one thing here in AYP, it is that an integration of effective yoga practices produces far more results than any magic bullet practice can, including the self-inquiry of advaita. All of these methods are meant to work together over time, and none stands alone. If we have to pick one practice, better make it deep meditation, as it is the one most likely to lead to all the rest, because it is the direct cultivation of inner silence within us.

Of course, even deep meditation must be preceded by desire, which we call bhaki. Bhakti (our desire for higher truth) is the primary engine of the entire process. All endeavors in yoga need desire, including advaita and its tools of self-inquiry. Oddly enough, self-inquiry is closer to bhakti and relies on it more than nearly every other branch of yoga, even as it denies it!

With an integrated approach to practices, we can bring fruition to self-inquiry, to non-duality, and to stillness (non-duality) in action as outpouring divine love. When we have found ourselves in the middle of that wonderful paradox, we will know we are on to something beyond the imaginings of the mind. The world is both non-dual and dual. This is a fact that neither side of the argument finds easy to accept. Until we find ourselves in the paradox, we will not see the whole picture. It is what it is, in us, not what anyone else says it is. We will find out what it is by our own direct experience, assuming we practice wisely and avoid getting shot with one of those magic bullets.

Well, just some food for thought. And then for letting go, of course. :-)

The guru is in you.

2007/02/24 08:45:40
Satsang Cafe - General Questions on AYP
http://www.aypsite.org/forum/topic.asp?TOPIC_ID=1864&REPLY_ID=18013&whichpage=-1
Power of the sub-conscious mind

quote:
_____
Originally posted by ajna

This discussion is getting interesting. As Yogani pointed out the world is both dual and non-dual simultaneously. We can only experience either of the states, not both at the same time (as told by Ramana Maharishi). When we are at the door-step of the metaphorical door separating the dual and non-dual states, we have a choice to look one way or the other, not both. But to get the ability to reach the door-step at will, practices are essential . After that there is a choice to drop practices.
_____

Hi Ajna:

But "stillness in action" is both, and therein lies the paradox of both the world and human enlightenment.

It is time for us to cross this bridge in our understanding of the nature of yoga practices and spiritual experience, mainly so we can practice with confidence and quit being a yoga house divided. The practical (and self-paced) integration of all yoga methods is the key to getting everyone anointed -- self-anointed, that is. :-)

The guru is in you.

2007/02/25 11:44:10
Satsang Cafe - General Questions on AYP
http://www.aypsite.org/forum/topic.asp?TOPIC_ID=1864&REPLY_ID=18085&whichpage=-1
Power of the sub-conscious mind

Hi Jim:

An attitude can be either a doing or a non-doing, depending on whether it is projected desire or desire released into inner silence. In the latter case, the attitude will arise as stillness in action.

In other words, we have to learn to let go into inner silence before we can let go. :-)

Obviously, for this, the cultivation of inner silence as a priori is necessary, via deep meditation, and also learning to let go into That, which is samyama. When the released/surrendered impulses of our mind surge out from inner silence, it is something else besides personal projection. It is stillness in action, or outpouring divine love. No need to worry about that running amuck, or tempting us in any way. By the act of real samyama, we have gone beyond all such personal trifles.

If we have some fear about personal corruption, or whatever, that's okay. We can just keep meditating and the fear will go sooner or later, along with the possibility for egoic mishaps.

Of course, no one will ever be absolutely perfect, but there is no need to get in a tangle over it. The more advanced we become in yoga, the easier it is to compensate for our shortcomings. That too is an inner silence thing. :-)

The guru is in you.

2007/01/05 15:10:23
Satsang Cafe - General Questions on AYP
http://www.aypsite.org/forum/topic.asp?TOPIC_ID=1886&REPLY_ID=15426&whichpage=-1
We are the truth

Hi Andrew, Katrine and All:

Beautiful descriptions of the indescribable. :-)

Grace is our joining with the divine process, and the divine process joining with us, which is knowingness, oneness and outpouring divine love. It is what we find on the other side of purification, in bits at first, and eventually full time. The clouds are clearing.

It doesn't burn because the burning is done, at least for now. :-)

As our sphere of stillness expands in the environment, there will be more purification -- no one will be left behind.

The guru is in you.

2007/01/14 16:20:56
Satsang Cafe - General Questions on AYP
http://www.aypsite.org/forum/topic.asp?TOPIC_ID=1949&REPLY_ID=16065&whichpage=-1
AYP for the Blind and Visually Impaired

Hi All:

Yes, the ebooks are enabled for audio generators (every AYP book is available in ebook format), plus we have audiobooks for the E-Series books read by guess-who coming, starting sometime this year with Deep Meditation -- downloadable MP3s.

There is sensitivity to the needs of the visually impaired here. Have been in touch with several folks in that mode since early on, and doing what I can to help.

The guru is in you.

2007/01/15 22:31:47
Satsang Cafe - General Questions on AYP
http://www.aypsite.org/forum/topic.asp?TOPIC_ID=1949&REPLY_ID=16147&whichpage=-1
AYP for the Blind and Visually Impaired
Actually, I was thinking of Groucho glasses, with a cigar, of course. :-)

http://en.wikipedia.org/wiki/Groucho_glasses

The guru is in you.

2007/02/07 09:04:55
Satsang Cafe - General Questions on AYP
http://www.aypsite.org/forum/topic.asp?TOPIC_ID=2034
Those Moving Topics

Hi All:

You may have noticed that a lot of topics have been moved from the Satsang Cafe to other forums lately. These have been accompanied by a moderator note: "Topic moved for better placement."

This is a one-time housekeeping function that has been undertaken to better organize topics by subject, going all the way back to the beginning of the AYP forums. It is nearly done now, and apologies for any inconvenience this activity may have caused anyone.

All the best!

The guru is in you.

2007/02/24 09:04:18
Satsang Cafe - General Questions on AYP
http://www.aypsite.org/forum/topic.asp?TOPIC_ID=2107&REPLY_ID=18015&whichpage=-1
New and have a question...

Hi Mattimo, and welcome!

Samad
Hi means absorption in silent Self, or pure bliss consciousness. Deep meditation leads directly to this, and the many other methods we employ add a substantial boost, including the judicious voluntary use of kumbhaka (breath suspension) in certain techniques.

Automatic breath suspension may also occur naturally in samadhi. Anyone who has practiced daily deep meditation for a while can attest to this. But stopping the breath is not the object. Cultivating inner silence is. If we have abiding inner silence, do we really care whether we are breathing or not? It can be a distraction in deep meditation, so we just easily favor the mantra over all that.

An even better condition than samad

Hi with no breath is samad

Hi while breathing and being active in the world. Then we are bringing stillness into the world in everything we do. Better not to keep our light under a bushel, or in suspended animation. Divine stillness likes to move, breathing sweetly out on everyone. :-)

All the best!

The guru is in you.

2007/03/08 11:53:47
Satsang Cafe - General Questions on AYP
http://www.aypsite.org/forum/topic.asp?TOPIC_ID=2195&REPLY_ID=18510&whichpage=-1
Non dual duality?

Hi All:

"Stillness in action."

Can we have one without the other?

Must we have one without the other?

Can advaita (non-dualism) be upheld as "stillness in action?" Perhaps not logically or philosophically. But experientially it certainly can.

Where there is such a paradox, the divine is surely interpenetrating, while doing nothing at all. :-)

The guru is in you.

2007/03/08 12:39:44
Satsang Cafe - General Questions on AYP
http://www.aypsite.org/forum/topic.asp?TOPIC_ID=2195&REPLY_ID=18514&whichpage=-1
Non dual duality?

quote:
_____
Originally posted by Doc
Accept no substitutes, there simply is no short-cut around a well established Sadhana.
_____

Amen to that.
2007/03/20 09:47:34
Satsang Cafe - General Questions on AYP
http://www.aypsite.org/forum/topic.asp?TOPIC_ID=2250&REPLY_ID=19046&whichpage=-1
I.Q.

Hi All:

Here is an AYP lesson on "Intelligence, Bhakti and Genius":
http://www.aypsite.org/246.html

Enjoy!

The guru is in you.

2007/03/29 10:46:08
Satsang Cafe - General Questions on AYP
http://www.aypsite.org/forum/topic.asp?TOPIC_ID=2353
New Yoga FAQ!

Hi All:

You will notice a new forum category has been added just above the Satsang Cafe, called **"Yoga FAQ"**.

This new feature of the AYP Forums was conceived by Etherfish, and developed with Shanti and other forum member volunteers. It is a job very well done. Thank you, Etherfish, Shanti and all who have been involved!

The FAQ covers many of the "frequently asked questions" that have come up and been discussed on numerous aspects the AYP integrated system of practices. A concise answer is provided for each topic question, as well as links to pertinent lessons and forum postings. The FAQ will be gradually improved as the discussions continue to evolve in the AYP Forums.

The Yoga FAQ itself is not a discussion area, and the reply function for the FAQ topics is not enabled there. Discussions on the FAQ topics are welcome, and can be conducted in the public forums (including in this Satsang Cafe topic), with links back to FAQ topics of interest, as desired.

Suggestions on improving the Yoga FAQ are welcome!

The FAQ can be searched using the top menu search link, which will default to search the Yoga FAQ if clicked from any page within the FAQ.

For in-depth research on specific topics, also see the Topic Index for the AYP Lessons and the site search features for the AYP Website and the AYP Forums.

We hope you will find the Yoga FAQ to be a useful resource as you travel along your chosen path. Practice wisely, and enjoy!

The guru is in you.

2007/04/13 16:11:29
Satsang Cafe - General Questions on AYP
http://www.aypsite.org/forum/topic.asp?TOPIC_ID=2422&REPLY_ID=20345&whichpage=-1
frustration on progress

Hi Guy:

When I think back to my early days of meditation, we had three young boys (we called them "the wrecking crew"), and I was working long hours and going to graduate school at night, with occasional meditation retreats -- way too occasional. It was nuts. All I knew was that there was something important going on underneath my daily meditation sittings and that it was a long term gig. So I kept on with it, and expanded over the years into the range of practices that now make up AYP.

I had some experiences in the early days, but it wasn't anything dramatic like the idyllic scenarios we see being described here almost daily. Well, maybe not so idyllic -- a lot of what are seeing today is spiritually challenging. The one thing that is the same is that, like then, the trick now is to just keep going and measure progress over the long term. Admittedly, "decades" may seen daunting to those starting much later in life. But every bit helps, and if there is such a thing as reincarnation, we will take what we have accomplished with us and move forward from there at the next opportunity. And even if there is no reincarnation, it can be gratifying in the present to be pursuing a worthy cause -- our enlightenment and the enlightenment of those around us. We should do what brings us the most happiness, whatever that is. That is all that matters.

Regarding what is the best approach for you, you should always follow your heart on that. For most of us, it will be a combination of things that move us forward. Typically, the point where we find the most resistance will usually be the place we need to walk through, sooner or later. Not always easy to do. It is discussed here from many points of view -- whether it is an energy experience we seem to be stuck in, a time of life, a personal situation, health issue, or some other thing that seems to be buried in us. The nice thing about deep meditation is that it chips away at all the subterranean stuff whether we are noticing it or not. Then, one day, the clouds part a bit, and there is the sunshine.

To be honest, I did not know for sure when AYP started if it would work for anyone. I just had to put what I knew out there, and hope for the best. It was, and is, an experiement. It is the best I can do. It is not my dharma to become a traditional teacher. If it were, it would have happened long ago. I am a researcher in spiritual practices and a writer, a pretty private person really. Nothing more than that. I don't think that me becoming a visible personality would change anything for anyone. Well, it would change things for me, in ways that do not favor the writing I have left to do. I sense that time is short for that, so every minute has to count. It is a relatively small window I am jumping through -- trying to squeeze as much of it through as possible in a usable form before the window closes.

If more direct contact with others on spirituality is what you feel you need, I suggest plugging into resources you have in your area -- a yoga class (asanas can help get our nervous system off the dime), spiritual gatherings of various types, teachers who are passing through, whatever draws your interest. Also, more can be done with AYP by starting a meditation group. That is one way to bring AYP into "up close and personal" mode, greatly increasing the inner silence and energy through the group effect. Well, these are just some ideas. Do what you feel drawn to do.

That is terrific news about your senior Hollywood friend reading a couple of the books. Thanks very much for making that connection. You can be sure that you did not exaggerate in saying a friend of yours wrote Wilder. I am a friend to you and everyone here. Just not a friend of the ordinary kind. Maybe these kinds of friendships are extraordinary? :-)

Someday I hope John Wilder will make it to Hollywood. It was his destiny in the story, and perhaps it will be in real life too. Well, thanks to you he is being pondered a bit. I think he has visited Hollywood through a few other channels too. The more the better. If AYP becomes more widely known, maybe the movie industry will stand up and take notice.

All the best!

The guru is in you.

PS: Come to think of it, we have spoken, on the radio! :-)

2007/05/25 09:08:04
Satsang Cafe - General Questions on AYP
http://www.aypsite.org/forum/topic.asp?TOPIC_ID=2592&REPLY_ID=22313&whichpage=-1
Breath and heart pondering

quote:
_____
Originally posted by Etherfish

The breathless state is caused by the use of prana instead of air to nourish blood cells. It is not caused by spinal breathing.
_____

Hi All:

Right, awakened inner vitality can reduce the need for oxygen as ecstatic conductivity expands. All practices that contribute to the rise of ecstatic conductivity play a role in this, including spinal breathing pranayama.

Breath suspension is also caused by a natural reduction in metabolism, particularly during deep meditation. This is a common experience for those who practice deep meditation.

So, both inner silence and ecstatic conductivity contribute to the phenomenon of respiration slowing down.

And, yes, we do not make a goal of breath suspension in AYP. It is a natural result of inner purification and opening.

Prudent voluntary regulation of breathing can be utilized in practical ways during certain practices -- comfortable slowing of the breath during spinal breathing pranayama, and short periods of kumbhaka during yoni mudra and chin pump.

The best way to find the answers is to practice daily, building a routine gradually over time, with self-pacing applied as needed. Then the questions will eventually be forgotten in a sea of abiding inner silence and ecstatic bliss. :-)

And, as has been said many times before, the cessation of substance abuse is a necessary prerequisite for inner purification. There is no getting around it.

The guru is in you.

2008/01/09 09:21:44
Satsang Cafe - General Questions on AYP
http://www.aypsite.org/forum/topic.asp?TOPIC_ID=2592&REPLY_ID=28652&whichpage=-1
Breath and heart pondering

Hi Paw:

Your journey is beautiful, going to show we each will find our own way. If AYP can help a little in that, it is serving its purpose. It's a great way to be spending our evening years, yes?

Remember to look beyond the thing of the moment. As we are called to serve by the outpouring of divine love, we will breathe again. Self-pace as necessary. :-)

The guru is in you.

2007/06/13 08:01:52
Satsang Cafe - General Questions on AYP
http://www.aypsite.org/forum/topic.asp?TOPIC_ID=2664&REPLY_ID=23108&whichpage=-1
can't let go of breath

Hi Mikael:

A preoccupation with the breath, or anything else, is a thought, or a pattern of thought. The body knows how to breathe without our supervision. Obsessive thoughts about breath we might have during meditation are a symptom of the process of release of inner obstructions. It is a good thing...

In deep meditation, when we realize we are off the mantra and into thoughts (no matter what kind), we just easily favor the mantra again. If the thoughts continue even as we pick the mantra back up, that is okay. There can be multiple things going on with the mantra present. Our job is not to analyze. We don't hang on to things (including the mantra) and we don't try and push things out (including attention on the breath). We just favor the mantra and let it go how it will. Every time we realize we have lost the mantra, this is a dip into inner silence, whether we have noticed or not. Purification is happening!

We just keep up the simple procedure for the time of our practice, and then make sure to take some rest (5-10 min) before getting up. The measure of our meditation is not in the sitting itself, which can be anything. It is in how we feel later on when we are active during the day.

Over time of twice-daily practice of deep meditation, thoughts that have preoccupied us will tend to become less binding. This is the dissolving of obstructions in our nervous system and the rise of abiding inner silence. It is a gradual shift that takes some time.

If we can't easily pick up the mantra due to an overwhelming sensation or feeling, then we can just be easy with it for a few minutes, letting the attention be drawn to the physical location of the discomfort. This will help dissolve it. Then, after a while (maybe only a few minutes), the sensation will fade and we will be able to easily pick the mantra back up again, continuing with our session. We count the time of easily being with a strong sensation as part of our meditation time.

All the best!

The guru is in you.

2007/06/12 11:35:20
Satsang Cafe - General Questions on AYP
http://www.aypsite.org/forum/topic.asp?TOPIC_ID=2665&REPLY_ID=23079&whichpage=-1
Heat on the Heel

quote:
_____
Originally posted by Srinivas_Mallya

Hi,
I am Srinivas, practicing AYP since last 5 months. I am doing spinal breathing and deep meditation. Recently added Sidhasana during the sitting. But I feel intense heat on the heel at the point of Contact with the root(perineum), particularly at the end of meditation. Is it OK to Continue with Sidhasana during meditation at this stage.
I am enjoying AYP and practicing twice daily.

Thank You
_____

Hi Srinivas:

It is okay to continue in siddhasana if there is not distracting discomfort. If there is, then back off with the heel as necessary to assure smooth practice and results. You also have the option to use siddhasana only in spinal breathing (or only part) until the energy symptom runs its course and stabilizes. Make whatever adjustment that is necessary to keep on a stable path of practice. This is self-pacing.

Also make sure to take adequate rest (5-10 minutes or more) when coming out of sitting practices, and keep active during the day to stablize all the good things that are happening inside. :-)

All the best!

The guru is in you.

2007/06/15 21:59:32
Satsang Cafe - General Questions on AYP
http://www.aypsite.org/forum/topic.asp?TOPIC_ID=2671&REPLY_ID=23195&whichpage=-1
Bodybuilding & Enlightenment

Hi theglock:

You might find this AYP lesson on physical fitness helpful: http://www.aypsite.org/80.html

Fitness is also discussed, with yoga-friendly exercise recommendations, in both the AYP Easy Lessons and Asanas/Mudras/Bandhas books. And, yes, the Secrets of Wilder has it too. Our hero is a champion high school cross country runner, who parlays his intense spiritual desire and dogged determination into full-blown enlightenment.

Go for it. And don't forget to self-pace as needed. :-)

All the best!

The guru is in you.

2007/06/16 10:33:23
Satsang Cafe - General Questions on AYP
http://www.aypsite.org/forum/topic.asp?TOPIC_ID=2671&REPLY_ID=23214&whichpage=-1
Bodybuilding & Enlightenment

quote:
_____
Originally posted by karmamechanic

quote:
_____
Originally posted by theglock
This leads me to believe that since my protein intake is probably nowhere near 1g/lb, maybe not even 0.2g/lb, I won't get "big" which isn't my goal, rather to have toned muscles and body strength.
_____

You can achieve this goal without lifting weights. If I recall correctly, Bruce Lee injured his back while lifting weights and switched to isometrics, which can be done without equipment. Isometrics and other forms of self-resistance exercise are much safer than lifting weights (no danger to the spine and connective tissue). I lifted weights for nearly thirty years but gave it up because I find self-resistance much more satisfying. To learn more, visit http://www.transformetrics.com. Here's another excellent site: http://www.angelfire.com/ny5/shenandoah/OBB/OBB.html. Good luck and have fun.
_____

Hi karmamechanic:

Thanks for that input. The AYP yoga-friendly exercise program covered in the books mentioned above is based on isometrics also. No trips to the gym necessary. :-)

The guru is in you.

2007/06/18 10:21:44
Satsang Cafe - General Questions on AYP
http://www.aypsite.org/forum/topic.asp?TOPIC_ID=2685
Finding our Dharma?
Q & A from a recent email exchange, posted with permission:
----

quote:
_____
From: http://www.aypsite.org/forum/topic.asp?TOPIC_ID=1433#10588

Hi Alvin and all:

After a long, arduous and not always happy journey, the meaning of life as I have come to understand it is to help others as best we can, without expecting a particular outcome or payback.

That comes in a thousand forms and degrees. We will know we are heading into the right form for us if we feel good about what we are doing. It is a process of optimizing cause and effect. It is also called coming into our dharma.

For each of us it is about identifying what we are really good at (everyone is good at something) and finding ways to bring benefit to others with our gift, whatever it may be. If we do that with all our heart, the rest will take care of itself.

Spiritual practices will naturally take us in the direction of our dharma. It may not be what we were expecting or planning on, so there can be plenty of grinding of the gears along the way -- it can feel like loneliness as our illusions about life are dissolving. Becoming empty can be unnerving, for sure. But somewhere along the line the impulse to move will come from within, and we can choose to go with it.

In the end, surrendering to what is within us will yield lasting happiness. That is because the flow of life comes first from within. As we learn to let it animate our actions in a creative expression of helping others, loneliness and troubles will gradually give way to an inherent joy. It can happen in the same surroundings we have always been in.

Inner stillness is the foundation of the entire process.

The guru is in you.

Q: Dear Yogani,

When I was reading AYP forums I came across the above post yesterday. I wanted to let you know that I was deeply moved by your words on the quote above. It made me realize how deep your understanding of the spirituality and human nature is. I should admit that the absolute humility with which the above quote was written brought certain humbleness in me. I could feel inside me that your words are true. I was filled with a strange emotion for a while after reading the post.

I want to share some things that were going on with me in the past few years. I work as a software consultant. In the past few years (5 to 10 years), I realized that I lost interest in what I was doing. I do not get satisfaction after I do my work as I used to get. I used to get depressed often (still do at times). I did not know the reason for a long time. I took some pills for a while. After I turned to yoga and meditation I did get some relief and was able to stay out of medications. But I still do get depressed at times for no reason at all. I feel that it is the loneliness inside me that is causing these feelings. You have mentioned that the meaning of life is to help others as best as we can without expecting outcome of payback. I feel that this is the only way I can stay out of the grueling depression cycles that I go through. I feel deep inside a longing to do something else than what I am doing right now which could help others. But I have a family to take care of and I continue on my profession right now. But inside me I feel that this is not really what I want to do. While I keep doing what I am doing, I am not deriving the satisfaction from what I am doing. I become lethargic at times because it does not interest me and fall into the depressive cycles. You were talking about "coming into our dharma", I feel that I do not have an option but to come back to my dharma since the life is kind of forcing me to get there with the depressive cycles if I do not follow my dharma.

But to get to my dharma, I should know what it is. At this point I only have a vague feeling in my heart (some kind of yearning). Scriptures point out that all work is equal and we just have to do it 100% sincerity. On the other hand the sanatana dharma prescribes duties based on the caste on which one is born. Between all these, how is one to find his dharma? Right now I feel that I have to continue in the profession that I am in to support the life style of my family. But I feel in my heart that this is not my dharma. The yearning inside me to do something different (I do not know what this something different is. May be my dharma?) is very powerful. As long as I do not obey this inner intuition, it is merciless and forces me back into the depressive cycles. The path I am on right now does not seem to be a healthy one. I keep telling myself that all work is equal. Whatever I do is also helping people. So I should do it 100%. But I am not doing it 100%, I just couldn't. My mind is not in it.

So my question is how can I find my dharma fast? The reason I say fast is because I feel if don't at least make a move towards my dharma starting right now; I am going to continue to feel depressed. You have also pointed out that it may not be what we are expecting or planning. This exactly seems to be my case. My plan is to stay on my profession and continue to provide the same kind of lifestyle that my family is accustomed to. So, there is obviously some conflict. I can see that the answers to my questions are also given on your post above. You have mentioned that the spiritual practices will naturally take us to our dharma. But I am writing this mail in the hope to get some more information or help from you on this regard. I feel that in order to even do my spiritual practices regularly I should be aligned with my dharma or at least moving in that direction.

I am not sure whether I have communicated my problem well on this email. But I am hoping that you will understand the issue. I just felt like sending this on an email to you rather than posting this question in the forum. But if you want to, you can use this email in the forum in any way that you see fit.

I know how busy you can be with all the books and running the AYP. So, please reply whenever you get a chance. No hurry! I unable to express in words, the gratitude that I feel towards you and AYP for providing these lessons and forum which has helped me tremendously in the past months.

PS: Just wanted to add to my mail that I felt that your words, "the meaning of life as I have come to understand it is to help others as best we can, without expecting a particular outcome or payback" and the subsequent sentences in the quote sounded like the essence of all the lessons in AYP to me. I felt that this is all everything in this life boils to.

A: Hello:

My suggestion would be to be patient while continuing your work and spiritual practices, while taking additional opportunities that come along to advance your spiritual progress, like spiritual gatherings, meditation group, study, retreats, developing an attitude of service, etc. If you don't have access to the spiritual group activities mentioned, consider starting them yourself, to the degree practical. In that way you can help yourself and others at the same time.

I spent many years in jobs that seemed not to be my dharma, while spending my spare time on practices, study, spiritual groups and retreats, when able. In the end, I realized that the jobs were my dharma after all, because they played an essential role in bringing me to where I am now, while enabling me to fulfill my responsibilities to my family (we have three grown children, and are now going to be grandparents!). This is why I say our dharma can be right under our nose in our present life and activities. The change is an inner one, not an outer one, and that will happen right where we are, wherever that may be. The important thing is for us to choose our spiritual course within our present circumstances. As we do that each day, all the doors open in time.

So, my suggestion is to count your blessings, face each day prepared to give your best, and always keep an eye out for ways to improve your role as a husband, father, provider, and spiritual practitioner. They are all part of the same thing. That's what I found out.

It will work out through dedication to what is right in front of you. Focusing on excelling in the present (right now, today) is the best way to secure the future, and be in dharma. It is the only way, because the only thing that exists is right now.

All the best on your path. Enjoy the ride!

The guru is in you.

Response: Dear Yogani,

Advanced congratulations on becoming grandparents! I guess that might be really exciting. Thanks for your immediate reply. You can use my email in any way as you see fit to post in the forum or otherwise.

Your reply was re-assuring. My plan was also to continue on my work and spiritual practices. But there was just a powerful yearning for release from, inside when I read your quote on loneliness. That was what prompted the email. At the same time, I also felt that if I change anything in terms of profession etc, I might end up with the same feeling in whatever new that I do after a while. So, I wonder at times if it is just some escapism from my current environment that the mind wants. At any cost, your mail is pretty clear, especially the part where you say "I realized that the jobs were my dharma after all…" and "The change is an inner one, not an outer one". I realize now that this is what the scriptures and the sanatana dharma mean when they state that all work are equal and none is better than other. I guess I need to get to that stage. I don't know how far it is from where I am. But I will continue on the present work and spiritual practices and hope that I will reach there some day.

2007/06/19 12:08:27
Satsang Cafe - General Questions on AYP
http://www.aypsite.org/forum/topic.asp?TOPIC_ID=2685&REPLY_ID=23329&whichpage=-1
Finding our Dharma?

quote:
_____

My plan was also to continue on my work and spiritual practices. But there was just a powerful yearning for release from, inside when I read your quote on loneliness. That was what prompted the email. At the same time, I also felt that if I change anything in terms of profession etc, I might end up with the same feeling in whatever new that I do after a while. So, I wonder at times if it is just some escapism from my current environment that the mind wants.

_____

Just to clarify, if there is a deep desire to make a change to a more fulfilling job, start a business, etc., there is nothing wrong with pursuing our desires. Denying our deepest impulses can be counter-productive. Dharma also means the outer expression of our inner unfoldment.

Other times, change may be thrust upon us, and this is always an opportunity to improve our circumstances, though it may not seem like it at the outset.

When engaged in changes, attend to the necessary details using good common sense, while making best use of time, talent and training. If we are doing our best each day, there is nothing more to labor over. Our spiritual unfoldment is found in our doing, and in our letting go. Stillness in action...

Engagement in effective daily spiritual practices over the long term, while maintaining an active and purposeful lifestyle, assures the outcome in each moment. And that is all we ever have -- this moment. Let's make the most of it. :-)

The guru is in you.

2007/06/26 16:01:21
Satsang Cafe - General Questions on AYP
http://www.aypsite.org/forum/topic.asp?TOPIC_ID=2701&REPLY_ID=23560&whichpage=-1
Which realized teachers don't endorse meditation?

quote:
_____

Originally posted by david_obsidian

The logic of it goes something like this:

"I was chronically sick, so someone suggested I try healthy eating and living and it might help eventually. But in my third year of healthy living and eating, I just got better all by myself. So obviously, all that healthy eating and living was a complete waste of time, and I wouldn't recommend it to anyone."

_____

Forgetful mountain climbers. :-)

On the art of doing nothing: http://www.aypsite.org/84.html

The guru is in you.

2007/07/01 10:28:10
Satsang Cafe - General Questions on AYP
http://www.aypsite.org/forum/topic.asp?TOPIC_ID=2718&REPLY_ID=23688&whichpage=-1
Delicate Subject; require advice

quote:
_____
Originally posted by Mattimo

I have adhered to the meditation practice, for 10 days or so now, and for the last 2 days extended my practice time considerably. I am aware this isn't necessarily advised but I cannot even begin to describe the relief I felt from meditating longer and more frequently. I could immediately feel bodily tension just sinking away (as best I can explain it).

_____

Hi Mattimo:

It is suggested to focus on developing a steady routine that you can stay with for the long term. The approach you are taking with deep meditation will not do that for you, because you are almost certain to run into large releases by greatly increasing meditation time and frequency. Keep in mind that there is often a time delay in the effects, so you are heading for an overdose, and I suggest scaling back immediately.

Much better to become stable with two times 15-20 minutes. If that proves to be good for you over a month or two, then consider light spinal breathing (a few minutes before meditation), which provides for balanced energy cultivation.

As for asanas, these are very good too, in moderation, and well integrated with other practices. As Jim says, asanas can be a good place to start in yoga, but not everyone is inclined to do that. Follow your inner inclination, but use good common sense also. The AYP writings attempt to provide reasonable guidance for a full range yoga practices.

People come to AYP from many different backgrounds (asanas, breathing, kundalini, tantra, self inquiry, drugs*, etc.), and it always boils down to each person finding their own balance while integrating new and powerful methods of yoga into a progressive, stable and safe daily routine. It takes time, with prudent self-pacing being necessary every step along the way.

Wishing you all the best on your path. Practice wisely, and enjoy!

The guru is in you.

*PS: On the drug angle, see my recent post here: http://www.aypsite.org/forum/topic.asp?TOPIC_ID=2702#23513

The spiritual inspiration sometimes provided by drugs is often offset by the obstacles that are introduced, as you well know. Yoga practices will help you dissolve the obstructions, but be very careful not engage in yoga practices in excessive ways, for this can lead to additional difficulties. In yoga, as with many things, more can be less, and less can be more. Keep it in mind. :-)

2007/07/03 11:34:41
Satsang Cafe - General Questions on AYP
http://www.aypsite.org/forum/topic.asp?TOPIC_ID=2718&REPLY_ID=23743&whichpage=-1
Delicate Subject; require advice

quote:
_____
Originally posted by karmamechanic

Sadhak, you make an excellent point about how asanas without breathwork are just stretching exercises. I've never practiced yoga asanas consistently, but it seems to me that qigong moves integrated with breathwork may accomplish the same purpose as asanas. Yogani, what do you think about this? You write in AYP that you've practiced tai c
Hi (a form of qigong) for decades. Do the benefits of qigong/tai c
Hi differ from those of asanas? If so, how?

_____

Hi Karmamechanic:

There is overlap in effects between asanas and tai chi, but there is a distinction. Tai c
Hi is mostly grounding with some inner opening, while asanas are mostly inner opening with some grounding. This is why tai c
Hi is good for helping to stabilize energy difficulties, and asanas are a good preparation for sitting practices, including spinal breathing pranayama and deep meditation.

As for breathwork during asanas, it is not specifically recommended in AYP, due to the possible "doubling up" effect with spinal breathing and other pranayamas used in sitting practices. Too much pranayama (with possible delayed effect) can lead to excessive purification and its associated physical and emotional discomforts. In AYP we suggest gentle awareness of natural breathing and body positions during asanas. We also have a samyama method that can be used as an alternative during asanas with good results -- it is provided in the AYP Samyama book.

All the best! :-)

The guru is in you.

2007/07/03 12:17:26
Satsang Cafe - General Questions on AYP
http://www.aypsite.org/forum/topic.asp?TOPIC_ID=2718&REPLY_ID=23746&whichpage=-1
Delicate Subject; require advice
PS: It can also be said that tai c
Hi (and Taoist methods in general) finds its origin in martial arts, while yoga postures have their origin in being aimed at relaxing and opening the sushumna (spinal nerve). The difference in origin may account for the variations in both practice and effects between these two systems. The overlaps are apparent, as are the differences.

2007/07/04 10:03:34
Satsang Cafe - General Questions on AYP
http://www.aypsite.org/forum/topic.asp?TOPIC_ID=2718&REPLY_ID=23782&whichpage=-1
Delicate Subject; require advice

quote:
_____
Originally posted by Jim and His Karma

quote:
_____
Originally posted by yogani

[quote]

As for breathwork during asanas, it is not specifically recommended in AYP, due to the possible "doubling up" effect with spinal breathing and other pranayamas used in sitting practices.
_____

Oh no! Yogani, I just realized...I'm following an exercise protocal from the book Mind, Body, Sport (I posted about it a few weeks ago). It recommends doing all exercise (aerobic, weight lifting, etc) with slow, calm, very deep inhale and ujiya exhale, and with mouth closed. It's real smart and very helpful (I can get up lots of stairs without getting winded, weight training's more intense, I don't get as "anguished" while running). But I'm doing this 45 mins day or more every single day....so, yes, "doubling up" has to be an issue!

And now....I'm not sure what to do! Any suggestions?
_____

Hi Jim:

It is important to recognize that similar practices, derived from different sources, done in the same day, have cumulative effects. The effects may be delayed...

If adverse symptoms arise, self pace accordingly. Better yet, anticipate possible effects beforehand, and tread carefully.

More can be less, and less can be more. :-)

The guru is in you.

2007/07/11 16:16:14
Satsang Cafe - General Questions on AYP
http://www.aypsite.org/forum/topic.asp?TOPIC_ID=2742&REPLY_ID=24109&whichpage=-1
Exercise to speed your path to self-realization

quote:
_____
Originally posted by Sparkle

When recently at a Byron Katie workshop in Dublin, at which emc also attended, I was fortunate to have a little chat with Katie during a book signing.

Part of the chat went something along the lines:

L: I have been reading your latest book "A Thousand Names for Joy". I didn't realise you were so enlightened untill I read it.
BK: Well therein lies the question of what is enlightenment.
L: Yes, eventually its probably to do with "service".
BK: Yes, service to "me"
L: And that service doesn't stop untill everything everywhere is enlightened.
BK: Yes, that's correct.

This reflects what has been said on the forum here about enlightenment, so it was nice to hear BK with the same slant.

It appears to me then that a combination of this view of enlightenment and what Christi said above would mean that your art as "art in service" "in the constant state of amazement at the miracle and beauty of God's creation" might not produce too bad a canvas.
_____

Hi Louis and All:

Very well put.

You don't have to worry about losing your motivation, Meg. As a matter of fact, as we advance, our personal motivation gradually gets multiplied by at least 6.5 billion as it expands beyond our body-mind to encompass everyone else on the planet, and beyond. We will not necessarily see it in terms that large, of course, but that is what it is, because we will be doing for others in every moment, and there is no limit to what divine love can do. You can be sure you will have the motivation to go along with the divine love. Can't have one without the other.

The good news is that we can actually handle the vast dimensions of this without falling over, assuming we have learned to self-pace along the way. Then it is just chopping wood and carrying water. Or, as another Buddhist saying goes:

"Don't sweat the small stuff.
It's all small stuff." :-)

I am also reminded of a scene in the Secrets of Wilder where Devi asks John why he is taking on the spiritual destiny of the entire planet. His answer is simple enough: "Because I can."

And that is it, you know. We are all doing what we can. As we purify and open from inside, we can do more. We can accomplish the infinite, because we are that. Whether it is through our art, our hands-on teaching, building a service organization, supporting our family, or helping an ill loved one or friend make it through the day, we do it because it is there to do, and because we can.

The image of enlightened people hanging around with no motivation to do anything, basking in their inner silence and spouting platitudes is completely false. It is a fantasy, and not a very appealing one at that, as you have rightly noted. It isn't real.

Real enlightened people are out there in the trenches of life working in their own way for the betterment of all humankind. They are working for themselves -- the "me," the oneness of "i am."

That is unity doing what unity does.

The nature of enlightenment is stillness in action, and the primary characteristics of that are unending ecstatic bliss and outpouring divine love.

It also means facing challenges, meeting deadlines, and paying the bills. So chop wood and carry water as you see fit, and enjoy the ride! :-)

The guru is in you.

2007/07/12 10:05:49
Satsang Cafe - General Questions on AYP
http://www.aypsite.org/forum/topic.asp?TOPIC_ID=2742&REPLY_ID=24134&whichpage=-1
Exercise to speed your path to self-realization

quote:
_____
Originally posted by meg

So if what's being said above is true, we should be able to reassemble our world view from where we sit, simply by shifting our awareness. If I'm experiencing lack, I should be able to shift to abundance simply by looking for it. If I'm experiencing fear, I should be able to dispel it by looking for love and beauty. Whatever we look for will be there in great abundance. Seek and ye shall find. Can it really be so simple?
_____

Hi Meg:

In theory that is true, and we should always follow our instincts for more joy. The "instant enlightenment" teachers would like us believing it is this simple. However, the instant approach is a path fraught with tangents and disappointments, because the process of human spiritual transformation is <u>not</u> instant. Blame is often placed on the aspirant for this, either self-blame or coming directly from the teacher, which leads to spiritual "performance anxiety." Not helpful.

The truth is that the neurobiology has to make the transition, and this takes some time. This is what practices are for. Our experiences and attitudes shift along with the purifying and opening neurobiology. It is all fueled by our bhakti, of course, our desire for awakening, which is the stirring seed of the awakening itself. It is a <u>gradual</u> transition from contraction and fear to expansion and love. Our motivations in life shift accordingly.

It is more like cultivating a garden than flipping a switch, though we'd all prefer the switch, I'm sure. The problem is the switch rarely will work as advertised, so better keep tending the garden. :-)

The guru is in you.

2007/07/12 19:14:00
Satsang Cafe - General Questions on AYP
http://www.aypsite.org/forum/topic.asp?TOPIC_ID=2742&REPLY_ID=24161&whichpage=-1
Exercise to speed your path to self-realization

quote:
_____
Originally posted by Etherfish

Usually people can't find love and beauty just by looking because they need to clean the windshield first.
Then that switch can be made faster, and ultimately even pain can be experienced in a non-suffering way.
Then it's easier to help other people do that.

Yes, if the voltage (inner silence) is limited, flipping the switch (self inquiry) will not do much. As the voltage is gradually increased (through daily deep meditation, etc.), the switch will work much better. :-)

This is where the non-dual and dual approaches to spiritual realization meet.

The guru is in you.

2007/07/15 11:23:28
Satsang Cafe - General Questions on AYP
http://www.aypsite.org/forum/topic.asp?TOPIC_ID=2770&REPLY_ID=24208&whichpage=-1
"The Work" and Deep Meditation

Hi Louis:

It is not recommended to introduce any new mental procedure into our deep meditation session, as this would take away from our systematic cultivation of abiding inner silence.

It is great to hear that Katie endorses the benefits of meditation. However, the real benefit is not the meditation itself, but the inner silence we gain from it in daily living. This provides the fuel for effective self inquiry anytime. Katie's "the work" is one of the most practical and useful self inquiry methods available. With the addition of more and more abiding inner silence in our daily activity (the witness), "the work" will become more and more effective. So it is not necessary to blend "the work" into our AYP sitting routine to gain the combined benefits of AYP and "the work." With rising inner silence, "the work" will increase in effectiveness naturally as we apply it in the way Katie instructs.

If we are inclined to focus directly on "the work" in sitting practices, as Katie suggested to you, this is possible utilizing specific sutras in samyama. Good suggestion, Riptiz. :-) There is guidance in the AYP Samyama book on adding sutras to our regular routine of samyama, and there can be opportunities for incorporating "the work" into sitting practices in that way. It will be "research," as any sutra addition in samyama practice is, including adding sutras from Patanjali listed in the appendix. It is suggested that such research be undertaken in systematic steps as discussed in the Samyama book. The most important aspect of samyama practice (and any yoga practice) is a stable routine maintained over the long term, so switching things around often in our daily samyama routine is not recommended.

"The work" can also be incorporated into samyama-based prayer, which may be less structured, and is also covered in the Samyama book.

Keep in mind that as inner silence cultivated in deep meditation becomes a constant feature in our daily living, samyama will be occurring automatically in all of our mental activity and actions at all times, especially if we are using the basic routine of samyama sutras in our daily sitting practices, which cultivate this tendency -- no special additions to our sutras required to achieve this global effect. Basic samyama, practiced daily after deep meditation, gradually enables all of our thinking to manifest consciously from within stillness, and this is why all of our actions become more centered, harmonious and powerful ... Stillness in action.

Inner silence will inevitably lead to effective self inquiry, by virtue of the rise of the witness. Hence the rise in effectiveness in doing "the work." However, it does not work so well going in the other direction -- self inquiry alone does not easily lead to abiding inner silence. So it is a matter of keeping the cart in front of the horse -- inner silence cultivated in front of self inquiry, not the other way around. This is the most effective role for meditation in relation to self inquiry, not necessarily a blending of the two techniques in the same sitting, which is counterproductive -- like trying to do pranayama and deep meditation at the same time. That doesn't work very well either. Each practice in its own time -- then the benefits will be crossing over via the natural connectedness of all yoga within us.

The guru is in you.

PS: I am hoping to have the AYP Self Inquiry book out in the Autumn. It is aptly called: "Self Inquiry - Dawn of the Witness and the End of Suffering."
The Samyama book is available now here:
http://www.aypsite.org/books.html#sam
(in a couple of weeks it will be out in audio download too)

2007/07/17 09:22:27
Satsang Cafe - General Questions on AYP
http://www.aypsite.org/forum/topic.asp?TOPIC_ID=2770&REPLY_ID=24252&whichpage=-1
"The Work" and Deep Meditation

quote:
_____
Originally posted by Sparkle

Yogani said:
quote:
_____
PS: I am hoping to have the AYP Self Inquiry book out in the Autumn. It is aptly called: "Self Inquiry - Dawn of the Witness and the End of Suffering."
_____
I will need to order another batch of books from you soon Yogani. When you say Autumn, is this September or later?
_____

Hi Louis:

September would be the earliest on Self Inquiry, and unlikely at this point. There are more simultaneous AYP projects going on these days, so whipping out new books is taking longer than before. Diet, Shatkarmas and Amaroli is just about done (finally), and I am very much looking forward to Self Inquiry. The practical integration of inner silence and self inquiry is coming together nicely, as is well evidenced in this topic discussion. :-)

The guru is in you.

2007/07/19 09:00:35
Satsang Cafe - General Questions on AYP
http://www.aypsite.org/forum/topic.asp?TOPIC_ID=2778&REPLY_ID=24276&whichpage=-1
parenting

Hi Glow:

There are lots of parents (and some grandparents) here in the forums, myself included.

Many are on summer vacation now, with their kids of course. :-)
I am sure you will have more feedback when everyone returns.

Yoga practices and parenting are very compatible. The challenge of scheduling practices in a busy family life are more than made up for by the balance, inner wisdom and creative energy that are brought into the equation. The entire family benefits over the long term.

During pregnancy, it will be good to go lightly with yoga, particularly with physical practices, including pranayama. Prenatal yoga classes (very gentle) are popular these days and can be beneficial.

Enjoy!

The guru is in you.

2007/07/28 10:36:26
Satsang Cafe - General Questions on AYP
http://www.aypsite.org/forum/topic.asp?TOPIC_ID=2796&REPLY_ID=24418&whichpage=-1
We and our decisions

Hi All:

There are a variety of ways to go about self inquiry, all based on the concept that thoughts are objects we can choose to identify with or not. But who is choosing? It is a relationship between the intellect (that which discriminates, or chooses) and our awareness behind that.

If our awareness has not risen to know thoughts as objects, then it will not be so simple with any system of inquiry, and the choosing will be much more encumbered with the perception, "I am these thoughts."

We are not the thoughts, of course, but try and tell that to someone who has little inner silence -- the witness. And therein lies the key point in all self inquiry, the cultivation of inner silence. Without it, doing self inquiry will be like trying to bake a cake with no flour -- not much of a cake.

That's why, in AYP, deep meditation is regarded to be the primary prerequisite for self inquiry. That hasn't been mentioned much in the several self inquiry topics going on in the forums at the moment, so thought to take the opportunity to remind. It is especially important for newcomers who may not be familiar with where all this budding self inquiry is coming from. It is bubbling out from stillness, like everything else. :-)

The guru is in you.

2007/09/06 11:16:37
Satsang Cafe - General Questions on AYP
http://www.aypsite.org/forum/topic.asp?TOPIC_ID=2861&REPLY_ID=25333&whichpage=-1
The Passing of Time

Hi All:

The cultivation of abiding inner silence goes a long way toward resolving issues of aging, fear, death, and the role of service in our life. In fact, inner silence goes all the way.

The role of the mind is elevated as inner silence comes up underneath, where our thoughts and reactions to life become objects we can accept as being "true" or not. This is the subject matter of the upcoming book:

"Self-Inquiry - Dawn of the Witness and the End of Suffering"

It is what this discussion is really about -- inquiring about finding peace with the inevitabilities of life, which we must face every day. The answer is in inner silence and our doing, allowing our actions to come from stillness. Under the right circumstances the mind can be an aid in this. The rest of the time, the mind is mostly a pitfall. It is not possible to analyze our way out of fear. Fortunately, there is a vastly bigger dimension within us, which we call inner silence -- pure bliss consciousness. :-)

The greatest asset the mind brings to the table is not in its ability to analyze, but in its ability enabling us to choose.

What is it we are choosing today? Are we choosing with intensity what will uplift us? This is how we pull ourselves up by our bootstraps. And as we become committed, all of nature will run to help us. Understanding that, we will understand everything, and fear no more.

The guru is in you.

2007/09/06 18:24:41
Satsang Cafe - General Questions on AYP
http://www.aypsite.org/forum/topic.asp?TOPIC_ID=2861&REPLY_ID=25341&whichpage=-1

The Passing of Time

Hi EMC:

By "true" I mean perceptions that lead to expansion rather than contraction -- to abiding peace, joy and boundless creativity.

We make a choice about everything that occurs in our life, consciously or not, and these choices are what determine our life experience.

Life is 100% an interpretation by us, no matter what our circumstances may be.

Of particular significance are the choices we make about daily spiritual practices, which can leverage our desire for expansion tremendously.

Seeing what is true is much easier with a foundation of inner silence arising within us. There is a snowball effect -- more clarity in stillness leads to more of the same. Then contractive perceptions tend to roll off us like water off a duck's back. In time, we lose the habit of contractive perception, because it has no traction in stillness, and becomes insignificant. The illusion of negative thinking is then continuously dissolved before it can arise to the point of dictating our mood or our actions. What remains is a constant flow of divine love.

This has many practical consequences in daily living.

We cannot think our way to this condition. It is an inner transformation that is beyond thinking. This, by definition, is meditation -- the movement of our attention from objects to reside in inner silence. This residing in inner silence, whether for an instant, or a lifetime, is samadhi. There are many grades of it.

To the extent self-inquiry promotes inner silence/samadhi, it is meditation. Sincere self-inquiry is also an effect of rising inner silence. All the limbs of yoga are connected within us like that.

And, of course, this is a journey beyond the constraints of time and space. Waves on the infinite ocean... :-)

The guru is in you.

2007/09/20 11:12:16
Satsang Cafe - General Questions on AYP
http://www.aypsite.org/forum/topic.asp?TOPIC_ID=2931&REPLY_ID=25601&whichpage=-1
Surrender - kind of important

quote:
_____
Originally posted by Christi

I don't know if you have read the Secrets of Wilder novel by Yogani, but towards the end of the novel there is a chart which clearly outlines which practice to add when, and which practices to combine with which as we progress. It also shows which order to do the practices in. I find it very useful as it can get confusing without this chart. I am surprised that Yogani has not put it on the main website.
_____

Hi Christi:

Glad you have found the Secrets of Wilder practice chart useful. The plan is to expand on it and include it in the upcoming Eight Limbs of Yoga E-Series book. Then it will appear, probably enhanced further, in the AYP Easy Lessons Vol 2 textbook (another big one), along with a lot of other new information. For now, the only place to find the chart is in the Wilder novel.

The reason why the practice chart hasn't shown up on the website is because AYP isn't financially solvent yet. So the emphasis these days is on writing, publishing and distributing books, ebooks and audiobooks, and keeping in touch with everyone here in the forums. Interestingly, this approach, brought about by necessity, has been opening many new doors to the public that would not have been opened as quickly otherwise. So there is a method in the madness of having to expand AYP into multiple publishing and media channels simultaneously. I am just along for the ride.

In the writing, my first love is sharing online, and I look forward to getting back to that when AYP is finally self-supporting with a larger body of published work in the marketplace. That will mean more free online lessons and information, including charts. It is a matter of finding a balance between the publications which will support AYP and the free website. We'll get there. :-)

These forums are an important part of it, and I greatly appreciate the ongoing contributions by everyone to each other and the growing public knowledge base. There are a lot of gems here -- both people and knowledge.

All the best!

The guru is in you.

2007/09/18 15:28:42
Satsang Cafe - General Questions on AYP
http://www.aypsite.org/forum/topic.asp?TOPIC_ID=2932&REPLY_ID=25568&whichpage=-1
self inquiry book?????

Hi Eitherway:

The Self-Inquiry book is at least month away, likely more. There was a death in the family here in August, so everything has been delayed. Your interest is much appreciated, and I am still hoping to have it out in the autumn.

In the meantime, you may like to take a look at the work of Byron Katie. Her flagship book is, "Loving What Is". While the AYP Self-Inquiry book will take a broader "yogic" view, what Katie offers is a practical "nuts and bolts" form of self-inquiry that can have an immediate positive impact on navigating the challenges of daily living. It is a good complement for those already engaged in deep meditation and other yoga practices.

In fact, just about any truth-based system of self-inquiry can shine if there is daily deep meditation going on to provide a solid foundation of inner silence -- the witness. Maybe that is why there is so much posting on self-inquiry and advaita (non-duality) here in the forums these days. The witness is with us, and is us. When we see the truth these days, it is recognized much more easily than in times past. It is a good thing. :-)

This rising recognition of truth hereabouts could be viewed as an indication that inner silence leads to self-inquiry, and the reconciliation of the non-duality/duality paradox. It is the increasing direct perception of everything we see and do as "Stillness in action."

What is less certain is whether self-inquiry by itself leads to inner silence. It has something to do with carts and horses being put in the right order. :-)

All the best!

The guru is in you.

2007/09/25 10:37:33
Satsang Cafe - General Questions on AYP
http://www.aypsite.org/forum/topic.asp?TOPIC_ID=2939&REPLY_ID=25665&whichpage=-1
Why Is Shakti Female and Shiva Male?

Hi Jim:

As mentioned in a recent Samad
Hi topic, it is what it is and our naming of it won't change the reality of what is happening within us. Maybe there is no language or metaphor that can get it completely, because human spiritual transformation is a unique stage of evolution with its own dynamics.

Yet, we humans will always be trying to correlate and name things to suit our curiosity. The mind is a thought machine. :-)

The obvious sexual nature of an awakening kundalini leads us to metaphors of gender and procreation. But how long does the 'kundalini as male' metaphor hold up after the sex act is complete and the birthing is underway? In other words, what is the longer view of the process?

Perhaps the reason why traditional models view the energetic life force as feminine is because it is the creative aspect of our nature, while inner silence remains unmanifest as pure potential (seed), even as all of creation is expressing outward from an energetic source (womb). This is where the phrase "mother nature" comes from, and this is apparently what is being mirrored metaphorically in our inner processes as well. "Father" is generally not considered to be part of external nature (creation), but hidden behind in seed form. This parallels our experience of inner silence.

The Sri Yantra offers a clear representation of this, with the male principle represented as a bindu dot at the center of an ever-expanding array of feminine yoni triangles. The paradox in this is that inner silence (tiny bindu dot) is eternal unbounded pure bliss consciousness, while the vastness of the ecstatic energetic creation (all those expanding yonis) is an ephemeral play of waves upon the infinite ocean of consciousness. So there are several ways to look at it, even within the Shiva/Shakti model.

On the other hand, I believe it is correct that the Taoist system views masculine (yang) as active, and feminine (yin) as passive/receptive. Perhaps that has to do with the stage you are describing, Jim -- more about the sex act itself than what comes later. What is the Taoist view of the subsequent birthing stage? Surely the feminine is not passive/receptive then. Is there an equivalent for dynamic "mother nature" in the Chinese system?

Well, there are no right or wrong answers in this. We can call it whatever we wish. It is the experience that counts -- the full range of human spiritual transformation. Carry on! :-)

The guru is in you.

2007/10/14 13:26:40
Satsang Cafe - General Questions on AYP
http://www.aypsite.org/forum/topic.asp?TOPIC_ID=2969&REPLY_ID=26035&whichpage=-1
Phases of the Moon

Hi EMA:

If you check "astrology/jyotish" in the topic index, you will find a few lessons that touch on this subject.

While "macro astrology" has some value for inspiring daily practices, either to go with the flow or to oppose it (like a salmon swimming upstream :-)), I have found the utilization of "micro astrology" to present unnecessary obstacles to the natural flow of bhakti, practices, divine energy and spiritual progress, which are largely beyond celestial influences and are best not over-regulated.

By "micro astrology," I mean any sort of prediction or direction that will impose on our natural tendency to evolve in our daily practices and activities -- like what time of day to practice, which way to face, which door to use in our house, whether we ought to go out at all today, etc. It is very easy to get loaded down with such things to the point of distraction in practices, and in life.

Just some food for thought.

The guru is in you.

2007/10/14 13:33:57
Satsang Cafe - General Questions on AYP
http://www.aypsite.org/forum/topic.asp?TOPIC_ID=2989&REPLY_ID=26036&whichpage=-1
Any word on when the new books drop?

Hi EMA:

More or less on schedule, if we consider autumn to end in December.

The dates have been pushed back a bit on the books page. Lot's of delaying factors here over the past few months.

A new reader just put a review up on Amazon USA for the AYP Easy Lessons book. Reviewing the existing books while waiting for the new ones is always appreciated. :-)

The guru is in you.

2007/10/27 12:30:29
Satsang Cafe - General Questions on AYP
http://www.aypsite.org/forum/topic.asp?TOPIC_ID=3035&REPLY_ID=26404&whichpage=-1
New intro for me

Hi Scott, and welcome!

Well, now that you have confessed to being the radio guy, let me offer a big thank you for those interviews, which can be found linked in the upper right corner of this page. A big thank you also to Will Brashear of the Cincinnati Yoga School, who conceived and sponsored the radio show, **"Yoga - The Other Ninety-Eight Percent."** An apt title for sure. :-)

I hope the show comes back someday. It was a lot of fun. On this end, it also led directly to the AYP Enlightenment Series AudioBooks, so the audio lives on!

Regarding being up in the head after practices, if asanas (postures) are not your thing (some are encouraged as preparation for sitting practices), there are other ways to deal with energy blockage in the head. We call it "grounding" around here. It is about getting involved in physical and external activities, whether it be a regular exercise program, digging in the garden, volunteering for your favorite cause, whatever you enjoy that is not internal activity. Such activities help stabilize what we gain in our daily practices. Yoga isn't just about inner purification and opening. It is also about getting out there and giving it all away in daily activity. Very important. This is how the results of practices become stabilized in daily life, so we see steadily increasing "stillness in action" as we go about our daily business.

Chin pump (dynamic jalandhara) is also very good for bringing energy down from the head, though there can be more stimulation of energy with that also. It is for those well-established in deep meditation and spinal breathing pranayama, preferably with some ecstatic conductivity coming up. Chin pump really shines in that situation, literally.

If there is some inertia in the body that seems to be causing a separation, it could be a "kapha" imbalance, and it is suggested to check the ayurveda diet guidelines here, or for more detail, check the appendix in the Diet, Shatkarmas and Amaroli book.

If nothing seems to be working to bring the energy down (getting the whole body involved) and there is ongoing discomfort or strain, it may be time to self-pace, scale back on practices a bit until balance returns, and then creep back up with practices as comfortable. And, of course, always take adequate rest before getting up from spinal breathing pranayama and deep meditation. This is the first, and most important, step in transitioning from practice sessions to activity.

There are additional methods for grounding that come from the Taoist system. A daily routine of Tai C
Hi or QiGong can help a lot. "Jim and his Karma" is our resident expert on integrating more focused Taoist methods with AYP for aiding with the kind of blockage you are describing. Maybe he will add a few words. You can find some of his thoughts on this here:
http://www.aypsite.org/forum/topic.asp?TOPIC_ID=2395#25244

Sooner or later, all the answers will be there for you. Keep knocking, and the doors will open. :-)

All the best!

The guru is in you.

2007/11/02 15:31:48
Satsang Cafe - General Questions on AYP
http://www.aypsite.org/forum/topic.asp?TOPIC_ID=3082&REPLY_ID=26642&whichpage=-1
****** Happy Birthday AYP******

Thank you very much, All.

The time has flown by. Eternity in an instant. And how everyone has grown! :-)

The guru is in you.

2009/11/06 08:00:59
Satsang Cafe - General Questions on AYP
http://www.aypsite.org/forum/topic.asp?TOPIC_ID=3082&REPLY_ID=59382&whichpage=-1
****** Happy Birthday AYP******

Hi All:

Thank you, not only for your kind anniversary wishes, but for your dedication on your path. Without you, AYP would be meaningless. I celebrate you. Bravo! :-)

The guru is in you.

2007/11/04 12:03:13
Satsang Cafe - General Questions on AYP
http://www.aypsite.org/forum/topic.asp?TOPIC_ID=3087&REPLY_ID=26703&whichpage=-1
Guru/Not Guru?

quote:

_____
Originally posted by Jim and His Karma

...the faux-messiah shouts to the crowd "You must think for YOURSELVES!" and they all chant back, in perfect unison "We will think for OURSELVES!".

It's a sticky wicket!

_____

Hi Jim and All:

Yes, it certainly is. Do hash it out. These forums are a good place for that.

The forums were originally set up for support, wide-ranging discussions, exploration of all spiritual practices, productive debate, and hopefully revelations leading to advancements in the field from the practical perspective of each individual's practices.

It's really got little to do with me. My role has been to put something out there based on my experience that is hopefully a reasonable starting point, and it is up to everyone to carry it forward from there in whatever form that works best. That means the *ongoing evolution of applied knowledge*. So, while I may be the guy who set the ball in motion hereabouts, it is up to everyone else to keep it in motion -- the never-ending process of separating wheat from chaff, which is the optimization of applied knowledge.

On the other hand, it is useful to keep a systematic approach preserved, particulalry for those who are starting from scratch -- the "state of the art" as it were, if there is such a thing in the spiritual arena. The forums are structured for that also. We can't really progress much in any applied science unless we launch from what has gone before. The wheel does not have to be reinvented by everyone who is starting out. That does not work very well in any field, including yoga. Progress will be assured if we take what has been found to work, and improve upon it. That has always been what it is about at AYP, and it has barely begun.

Well, so far, this post has been deliberately off topic. AYP has never been about guru/not guru, though it lurks in many minds. This will be transcended as we get on with the real task, which is the optimization of applied spiritual knowledge. So effective practices are what ought to be focused on.

I have a theory that the whole guru fixation thing is the product of inadequately applied spiritual knowledge. Find an entrenched guru, and there you will likely also find a group of followers who are not developing very fast. Effective applied knowledge on the individual level will eliminate this problem, making the entire situation much more fluid, because the principles of human spiritual transformation are readily available within everyone. They only need be activated by effective means.

It has been said that in the land of the blind, the person with one eye will be king. But what if everyone had one eye? Or, better yet, a surefire ability to grow two eyes? Where would the king (guru) be then? Sprouting up everywhere!

The guru is in you.
 :-)

PS: Oh, and if anyone wants to disagree with anything I say, or any aspect of the AYP approach, feel free to do so. It happens just about every day somewhere in the forums, and I welcome it. If something better can be offered that can bring practical results to many people, I will be one of the first to come along. But do keep in mind that it is hard to cross a river with each foot in a different boat. That may be one reason why folks tend to hush up when alternatives are presented. No one likes to have their boat rocked. But a certain amount of rocking is necessary for progress. AYP itself is a boat-rocker. So carry on, with prudence. :-)

2007/11/23 12:07:27
Satsang Cafe - General Questions on AYP
http://www.aypsite.org/forum/topic.asp?TOPIC_ID=3162&REPLY_ID=27209&whichpage=-1
For ex-SRFers

Hi All:

There can be no doubt that there have always been people who wished to openly share the knowledge of spiritual practices. The more we study our ancestors, the more we find they were very much like us. So why didn't they?

The times were different then, and this limited the kind of knowledge sharing and progress we are able to achieve today. We tend to take for granted the basic freedoms and technology we now enjoy. In those days there was limited freedom of speech, no free press, and no broad communication networks for sharing knowledge like we have today. War (often clothed in religious superstition) was the rule rather than the exception. So the sharing of spiritual methods (and all kinds of knowledge) was limited. The traditions grew up in that environment.

We still have traces of those past limitations, but it is getting better. The fact that advanced yogis were able to come to the west over the past century, planting the precious seeds of knowledge they did, is a good sign. The fact that a fledgling open resource like AYP on the integration of best-in-class practices has not been quickly stamped out is a measure of our times.

The emergence of the scientific method a few centuries ago (optimization of causes and effects via open source networking) has changed much about the way we live. It has taken a while for it to come to the knowledge of human spiritual transformation, but it finally has. It is my hope that applied spiritual science will keep marching forward. It will be a great support to what is true in every tradition.

Aside from the enabling freedoms and technologies we now have, it has also been a matter of real spiritual experience rising increasingly in the people, providing the basis for ongoing exploration and progress in optimizing causes and effects in spiritual practice. Without the rise of experience (effects), there would be little basis for proceeding with the widespread investigation and application of spiritual methods.

It is in your hands.

The guru is in you.

2007/11/24 14:19:37
Satsang Cafe - General Questions on AYP
http://www.aypsite.org/forum/topic.asp?TOPIC_ID=3179&REPLY_ID=27242&whichpage=-1
Enlightened = know everything?

Hi Near:

Here is a lesson that touches on this subject:
http://www.aypsite.org/260.html

In this case, the word "perfection" could be equated with knowing everything, which enlightened people do not. But they keep smiling anyway, due to the inner illumination radiating from beyond worldly knowledge, and their obvious limitations. :-)

All the best!

The guru is in you.

2007/11/25 12:13:19
Satsang Cafe - General Questions on AYP
http://www.aypsite.org/forum/topic.asp?TOPIC_ID=3179&REPLY_ID=27270&whichpage=-1
Enlightened = know everything?

quote:
_____
Originally posted by nearoanoke

Enlightenment seems less and less powerful the more and more I know about it. :-)
_____

Hi Near:

Actually, it is just the opposite, where less can be more. One of those divine paradoxes.

Which is more powerful, that which is manifest, or that which is the inner source of all that is manifest?

Which is more powerful, worldly knowledge, or all peace, creativity and divine love? Can worldly knowledge add anything to divine love? Not really. Can divine love add anything to worldly knowledge? Everything. Without the flow of divine love, worldly knowledge has no meaning whatsoever. What is life on this earth without love? Nothing.

The story of the destination of loveless (unenlightened) knowledge has been told a thousand times -- always a dark tale. And when the happy ending comes, it is always brought by love. The only happy ending there can be for worldly knowledge is enlightenment producing outpouring divine love. The story always leads to that outcome, sooner or later.

Knowledge can be found when needed. Divine love is the need itself. Enlightenment is not about getting something. It is about learning to release the unifying flow of divine love within us, which is the greatest joy that can be known in human life, and the fulfillment of all knowledge. It is our destiny.

The guru is in you.

2007/11/28 11:28:28
Satsang Cafe - General Questions on AYP
http://www.aypsite.org/forum/topic.asp?TOPIC_ID=3194&REPLY_ID=27404&whichpage=-1
beginner questions

Hi Growant, and welcome!

Christi and Bewell covered your questions pretty well. Maybe more folks will chime in.

Everyone will follow their own inclinations in practice, and that is how it should be. It is suggested to take the lessons in order, without trying to look too far ahead, and see what happens.

Wishing you all the best on your chosen path. Enjoy!

The guru is in you.

2007/12/22 10:01:06
Satsang Cafe - General Questions on AYP
http://www.aypsite.org/forum/topic.asp?TOPIC_ID=3292&REPLY_ID=28145&whichpage=-1
Seasons Greetings Everyone
Happy holidays All! :-)

May outpouring divine love overflow from within ever-abiding stillness in our hearts.

The guru is in you.

2008/01/29 16:10:50
Satsang Cafe - General Questions on AYP
http://www.aypsite.org/forum/topic.asp?TOPIC_ID=3325&REPLY_ID=29438&whichpage=-1
Interpretation of right palm thing happening

Hi EMC:

Another day at the office. :-)

Carry on!

The guru is in you.

2008/01/17 15:20:35
Satsang Cafe - General Questions on AYP
http://www.aypsite.org/forum/topic.asp?TOPIC_ID=3382&REPLY_ID=29030&whichpage=-1
Knot of Brahma

Hi John:

Here is an AYP lesson on the three granthis (knots): http://www.aypsite.org/276.html
A clinical approach. :-)

Yes, we yogis and yoginis still grieve, but a part of us remains untouched, even as we melt in tears. Our Silent Self. It is pain without suffering. But certainly not indifferent -- feeling much deeper than we could before -- surrendering to the opening -- and somehow finding wholeness in the tragedies of life. Perhaps it is because love is never destroyed. No matter who or what we lose, we will always have the precious eternal love that has been shared. That goes on forever.

The guru is in you.

2008/01/17 17:58:55
Satsang Cafe - General Questions on AYP
http://www.aypsite.org/forum/topic.asp?TOPIC_ID=3382&REPLY_ID=29038&whichpage=-1
Knot of Brahma

Hi John:

No doubt the two approaches are compatible. We can only smell the flower if the nose is clear. :-)

That is why optimizing integrations of the most effective methods is the main focus in AYP. As soon as we fixate on one particular aspect of practice or experience, something is lost. If we open the whole, even as we are releasing it, then we will know what it is. Knowing it is becoming it -- *That*.

The guru is in you.

2008/02/19 10:33:07
Satsang Cafe - General Questions on AYP
http://www.aypsite.org/forum/topic.asp?TOPIC_ID=3390&REPLY_ID=30259&whichpage=-1
Picking up other's emotions

quote:

Originally posted by Jim and His Karma

In more poetic terms, you watch the dance, you may even choose to join the dance from time to time, but you exist beyond dancing.

Hi Jim and All:

Great discussion. I might add that we will know stillness is moving beyond the initial stage of witnessing when it joins the dance in earnest. And the dance is called "Service."

Then we are no longer only in expanding empathy, which is still a reaction in the field of duality.

Rising unity is becoming the other, and engaging for the benefit of the other in ways that are non-dual and non-reactionary. Then, no longer do we feel invaded, nor wondering why people are reacting to us in the ways they do. They can sense the rising unity, the dissolving separateness, and are attracted to it within themselves, even as we are becoming it. It is the resonant entrainment of stillness in action.

The step from witness to stillness in action is a conscious choice each person will make along the path. It involves acting from the level of witness (not retreating into witness), walking straight through duality and the reactions structured in it (fear - ours and others). It is a walk into true relationship in service, rather than the mode of, "I'm okay, and what on earth is everyone else doing?"

That must give way to something much greater, something much more courageous. That something is service, the outpouring of divine love, which is anything but passive observation, even while it is occurring in our absolute stillness.

So, don't analyze -- Act!

The guru is in you.

2008/02/19 18:04:54
Satsang Cafe - General Questions on AYP
http://www.aypsite.org/forum/topic.asp?TOPIC_ID=3390&REPLY_ID=30275&whichpage=-1
Picking up other's emotions

quote:
_____
Originally posted by Lila

[quote]*Originally posted by yogani*

Yogani - would you be able to give any more specifics on how one is able to move into rising unit? How does one find the place of stillness in action?

If there is something you would suggest reading that explains this more I would appreciate that as well.

Namaste,
Lila
_____

Hi Lila, and welcome!

It begins with two short daily sessions of deep meditation. This is how we cultivate abiding inner silence in our daily life. Everything else proceeds from there.

Reading-wise, the best place to start is at the beginning of the main lessons (see link at the top of this page). It goes pretty much in order step-by-step, and you will see the progression. There is also a series of books that expands on the online lessons.

The Samyama and Self-Inquiry books focus more on cultivating stillness in action, as will the next book on Bhakti and Karma Yoga. The prerequisite for all of these is daily deep meditation.

There is also an "energetic" side to the process of human spiritual transformation, with associated practices covered in sequence in the lessons -- spinal breathing pranayama, asanas, mudras, bandhas, etc. The awakening of ecstatic conductivity in the nervous system plays a key role in the rise of stillness in action and unity. It can be said that our inner silence radiates outward from us on the wings of ecstasy. That is the connection. Enlightenment is a blend of abiding inner silence and natural ecstatic radiance. Together they yield endless outpouring divine love leading to unity.

Wishing you all the best on your chosen path. Enjoy!

The guru is in you.

2008/02/21 09:50:17
Satsang Cafe - General Questions on AYP
http://www.aypsite.org/forum/topic.asp?TOPIC_ID=3390&REPLY_ID=30357&whichpage=-1
Picking up other's emotions

Hi YB:

The witness never does anything, even while it is doing everything. As we become established in the witness, our ability to consciously act as divine outflow increases. It is the epitome of less becoming more -- the divine paradox.

The role of self-inquiry in this is to let it go and allow it to proceed. The faculties of mind become illuminated by the witness. The witness is that which is behind and within all objects, including all thoughts, feelings and the outer world. In letting go, the outer expression of the witness (while doing nothing) will increase as radiance. This is why I regard self-inquiry as a technique of unity, along with samyama and karma yoga (service). These are outpourings of the divine which illuminate and unify everyday living.

This view of self-inquiry is contrary to the convential wisdom that less is less and more in the world is illusion. But the conventional wisdom proves to be untrue when the self-inquiry is "relational" -- with the witness increasingly present. Then less becomes more in the world, and the so-called illusion of duality dissolves.

Stillness in action!

It cannot be understood by the intellect, but the intellect can make the necessary choices along the way. If we engage in the practices and let it happen, then we will know it for what it is. No need to take my word for it. :-)

The guru is in you.

2008/01/21 08:28:48
Satsang Cafe - General Questions on AYP
http://www.aypsite.org/forum/topic.asp?TOPIC_ID=3395&REPLY_ID=29120&whichpage=-1
Third eye opening

Hi Tibetan Ice:

Please keep in mind that the key to progress on the path is stable practice over the long term. If we keep adding on and modifying our practice every time we have an experience, there will be no stability and little chance for manageable progress.

The suggestion is to work with one practice and build a good foundation with a steady twice-daily routine for some time before considering adding anything on. Deep meditation is where we start in AYP. And we favor the procedure of the practice as given over the all the experiences. If you simplify what you are doing in that way, it will be much easier to proceed, and to address questions that come up. At the moment your practice is too spread out to facilitate much in the way of meaningful progress or support.

It is much more about building a foundation of inner silence than all the rest of the stuff.

Wishing you all the best on your path. Practice wisely, and enjoy!

The guru is in you.

2008/01/23 09:12:22
Satsang Cafe - General Questions on AYP
http://www.aypsite.org/forum/topic.asp?TOPIC_ID=3395&REPLY_ID=29204&whichpage=-1
Third eye opening

Hi Tibetan Ice:

Inner silence is the beginning and the end. It is the beginning as the witness, and the end as stillness in action, outpouring divine love and unity. Energy (kundalini/shakti) plays a supporting role in this evolution, with a thousand by-ways which can be traveled. If there is inner silence, the by-ways will be illuminated and stabilized as part of the enlightenment process. And if inner silence is limited, the by-ways will become personal tangents leading to who-knows-where. "Gifts" will not be enlightenment in that case. That's why we suggest favoring the procedure of practice over the experiences, with deep meditation being the primary practice.

It is good that you are moving into samyama. Systematic practice over time will yield the best results -- stillness in action. Yes, systematic may seem rather clinical. Yet, that is how a progressive journey is conducted -- by steady driving. All the rest is the scenery along the way. :-)

Likewise, kundalini can be addressed systematically with some more of those clinical practices, nurturing the ecstatic wings upon which inner silence flies. If the kingdom of inner silence is cultivated first, and then ecstatic energy from the center, then the gifts will flourish as part of the natural divine outflow, and everyone will benefit. That is enlightenment.

Carry on!

The guru is in you

2008/02/03 23:26:29
Satsang Cafe - General Questions on AYP
http://www.aypsite.org/forum/topic.asp?TOPIC_ID=3428&REPLY_ID=29663&whichpage=-1
Insight

Hi VIL:

Yes, EMC had quite a ride through the Self-Inquiry book, and her humorous account had me falling off the chair in laughter. I did not know the book could be such a dramatic trip -- mental rags to mental riches and back to mental rags again, and somehow illuminating from within along the way. It is in the reader for sure. :-)

http://www.aypsite.org/forum/topic.asp?whichpage=1&TOPIC_ID=3427

As far as the word "insight" is concerned, I think she was quoting her own mind in that post, her mind ever eager for more.

The word "insight" appears in only one place in the Self-Inquiry book, in a way that lends itself more to interpretation than to direct experience, as in: "...there are spontaneously awakened souls who dazzle us with their insight, and who are often idolized and imitated."

What it means in that context is in the eye of the beholder, yes? That is the only place the word is used. However, the word "inspiration" is used in many places in the book.

I would agree that true insight and inspiration are rooted in a knowingness that is eternal and always in the present, always in stillness. This is also where true self-inquiry is -- abiding in the witness. In the book this is called "relational self-inquiry."

All the best!

The guru is in you.

2008/02/08 09:55:02
Satsang Cafe - General Questions on AYP
http://www.aypsite.org/forum/topic.asp?TOPIC_ID=3440&REPLY_ID=29811&whichpage=-1
Dear Yogibear

Hi Cyberboy, and welcome!

I'm not YB either, but would like to mention that Ajita visited the AYP forums briefly a couple of years ago. You can find his posts with associated discussion here: http://www.aypsite.org/forum/pop_profile.asp?mode=display&id=342

As I recall, we did not mesh very well, due mainly to what you are discussing above -- control for control's sake, versus control for the sake of release into pure bliss consciousness, or, as Katrine loves to call it, "the shine." No control in that. We sometimes call it "active surrender." Doing something to be doing nothing, which is doing everything. :-)

The other thing I recall is that with all that structure and control, it was not clear at the time what Ajita's recommended daily routine of practice was. Perhaps he has refined and simplified (or made more public) his approach since then. Hopefully...

And in the immortal words of Joe Walsh (from his opus magnum -- Life's been good to me so far):
"People tell me I'm lazy, but it takes all my time..."

If it isn't relaxed, or leading to relaxed, it isn't IT. :-)

All the best on your chosen path. Practice wisely, and enjoy!

The guru is in you.

2008/02/11 11:38:09
Satsang Cafe - General Questions on AYP
http://www.aypsite.org/forum/topic.asp?TOPIC_ID=3440&REPLY_ID=29953&whichpage=-1
Dear Yogibear

quote:

Originally posted by yogibear

Yogani, can you explain what **you** mean by "control for release into pure bliss consciousness? "

Hi YB:

Did I say that?

In deep meditation, it is an easy procedure that favors some activity in the mind without a direction specified. The mantra is only a vibration, not a direction. When brought back to this condition repeatedly, the attention naturally goes beyond mind to underlying inner silence, also called pure bliss consciousness. So we do not "control" the process of meditation. We only create the condition in the mind for it to happen naturally. "Meditation" (dhyana) is the natural process of attention dissolving when placed on an object (dharana) to absorption in inner silence (samadhi). It is this natural process we are facilitating in deep meditation.

Then, in daily activity, we begin to find an increasing degree of resident inner silence, and gradually all objects become associated with that stillness, which is becoming our sense of self. This is when self-inquiry methods become most useful, or "relational," when there is a relationship developing between inner silence (the witness) and our thoughts, feelings and the external environment. Then life is becoming filled with peace, energy, creativity and happiness, with more and more outpouring divine love leading to unity.

So, if this control, it is only of the efficient levers of letting go. To try and control all this with the mind is a much tougher slog. Nature knows how to do it much better. It always boils down to surrender to *That*.

It is only a matter of doing something that leads us systematically to doing nothing, even while we are doing everything. :-)

The guru is in you.

2008/02/12 11:55:57
Satsang Cafe - General Questions on AYP
http://www.aypsite.org/forum/topic.asp?TOPIC_ID=3440&REPLY_ID=29993&whichpage=-1
Dear Yogibear

Hi YB:

It is fair to say that there is no attention in samadhi, which is the absorption of attention, or the transcendence of attention to it's native state -- pure awareness. In order for there to be attention, there must be an object, and there are no objects in samadhi, at least not in nirvikalpa samadhi. There are various grades of samad
Hi where objects can be present, but I am not much for making all those distinctions -- it gets to be too much of a measuring thing, and this is not what yoga is about. A fairly prominent yoga teacher once stomped off in disgust from AYP because I refused to get into grading people according to their level of samad
Hi (needing to do this measuring is a sign of slow meditation methods, btw). I prefer to avoid putting people in pigeon holes as much as possible. And we don't have to, because deep meditation is zip zip and gone to nirikalpa.

Much better to be using very efficient techniques and just enjoy wherever we happen to be at the moment. We do the practices, and find out the next things as naturally as possible. Well, it is impossible not to anticipate, but we do our best. :-)

Anyway, the grades of samad
Hi are one thing on the way out to establishing samad
Hi with no attention (no objects = nirvikalpa), and something else on the way back in to the rise of abiding inner silence during our daily activities. This is samad
Hi with attention present, relating to objects while operating in the world. In this case the objects of perception are becoming effused with inner silence, our sense of Self, and this is the unity process underway. Samyama, self-inquiry and karma yoga (service) are for accelerating the rise of inner silence in daily living. Samad
Hi coexisting with activity in the world is the next step after nirvikalpa -- the outpouring of divine love leading to the unified condition of awareness -- *"I am That." "You are That." "All this is That."*

It has been called sahaj samadhi, which means "with eyes open." Well, it is much more than with eyes open. It means with heart, mind and all the faculties of action open and fully engaged. It is stillness in action.

So there is a going out to establishment of abiding inner silence (witness), and then a coming back into full action with inner silence. That is the journey of yoga. That is why daily activity is an important part of the over all practice, to stabilize stillness in action. We are not leaving forever into samad
Hi without objects. It is not a one way trip. We are systematically going out and bringing samad
Hi back into daily living. So it is very practical.

Both aspects of going out and coming back can be occurring at the same time. We don't have to be measuring it all. It can become a distraction. Having a general idea about what is happening will be good enough to help us stay on track. We just keep favoring the practice over the experience and everything will work out just fine. :-)

The ideal amount of control in this is for activating the non-invasive levers that promote the over all process.

The guru is in you.

2008/02/14 11:49:09
Satsang Cafe - General Questions on AYP
http://www.aypsite.org/forum/topic.asp?TOPIC_ID=3440&REPLY_ID=30055&whichpage=-1
Dear Yogibear

quote:
_____
Originally posted by Suryakant

Mildred Lisette Norman Ryder, more widely known as Peace Pilgrim, personified the process you describe, yogani.

In her own words (http://www.peacepilgrim.com/book/chapt2.htm), Peace Pilgrim described what she called her "spiritual growing up period", which consisted of gradually developing samyama through self-inquiry, selfless service, and self-discipline.
_____

Thank you, Suryakant.

Beautiful. A sage worth studying.

The guru is in you.

2008/02/24 10:24:40
Satsang Cafe - General Questions on AYP
http://www.aypsite.org/forum/topic.asp?TOPIC_ID=3498&REPLY_ID=30499&whichpage=-1
Help: yoga school after kundalini ?

Hi Pascal, and welcome!

You might try contacting the translator of the AYP lessons in France, by replying to any post at the forum here:
http://fr.groups.yahoo.com/group/Pratiquesavanceesdeyoga

Your inquiry will not post publicly, but will go directly to his email. His name is Bernard. Perhaps he or someone he knows can point you to schools nearby.

If you are looking for a prominent school in India, the Bihar School of Yoga is very well-known and highly regarded. It was founded by Swami Satyananda, a leading disciple of Swami Sivananda. The school offers many fine books on yoga also, which are available worldwide.
http://www.yogavision.net/home.htm

Also, if you check the AYP Links Section, you will find schools and retreat centers of many kinds all over the world.
http://www.aypsite.org/Links.html

While I believe that AYP is a more fully integrated, non-sectarian and flexible path than most, we don't have physical schools or facilities, except for your computer of course. :-)

So be sure to check in here with questions and sharings that may come up along the way. There is a lot of information and help available here, and no one will tell you what you must do. That is up to you. Whatever is best for everyone's spiritual progress according to personal choice is what I want.

Wishing you all the best on your path. Practice wisely, and enjoy!

The guru is in you.

2008/03/26 11:22:44
Satsang Cafe - General Questions on AYP
http://www.aypsite.org/forum/topic.asp?TOPIC_ID=3650&REPLY_ID=31784&whichpage=-1
deeper samad
Hi - sakshatkara

quote:
_____
Originally posted by Tibetan_Ice

The general message on this site is that Jesus is just another vision and surely must be a premature crown opening. They will tell you to back off, reduce practice or simply ignore Him.

Hi TI:

For the record, in AYP, relationship with our divine beloved, whomever or whatever that may be, is not discouraged. It is the relationship with our chosen ideal (ongoing devotion - bhakti) that leads us along our path, including to practices.

When we are in practices, we follow the procedure of the practice, which means favoring the practice over visions and other experiences that may come up during that brief structured time in our day. Then our experience during everyday living will be all the more infused with stillness and divine energy, including our divine beloved. If purification and opening occurring within us crosses over into excess, then we self-pace as necessary -- in our practices, and also tempering the intensity of our relationship with our divine beloved if our stability and health are at risk.

Balance in all things ... we each know what we can accommodate. It is a matter of understanding and applying the underlying principles of human spiritual transformation, and proceeding with reasonable prudence over the long term. Then there will be steadily rising joy and outpouring divine love in all aspects of our life, and our divine beloved will be with us always.

The guru is in you.

2008/04/11 13:46:17
Satsang Cafe - General Questions on AYP
http://www.aypsite.org/forum/topic.asp?TOPIC_ID=3770
On creating change in the world...
Excerpt from an email interchange:

Q: ...How do I move in the world to help create positive change without fueling the very thing I am trying to help change? I am thinking that there must be a subtle change in the energy with which I act and think about it, but I can't put my finger on it.

A: Stand up for what you believe in, while cultivating inner silence each day. And consider the lives and works of people like Gand
Hi and Martin Luther King.

Move as stillness moves, not as fear would have you move.

The guru is in you.

2008/05/16 14:18:42
Satsang Cafe - General Questions on AYP
http://www.aypsite.org/forum/topic.asp?TOPIC_ID=3913&REPLY_ID=33829&whichpage=-1
Froth/foam

quote:
_____
Originally posted by emc

And hey, if they joke about it in relation to kundalini blockages... it MUST be a well-known phenomena, right??? Is it familiar to anyone?
_____

Hi emc:

It is likely a symptom of inner energy moving, associated with purification -- not only your purification, but also of whomever you may be interacting with.

There are many stories about gurus undergoing symptoms associated with the purification of others. I am thinking of a woman guru of South India (now gone) who used to spit stuff out whenever her disciples were close by.

Like all symptoms of purification, this too will pass. Hopefully you will not have to wait for the entire planet to be purified. If so, you are on a great mission there -- to spit out all impurities everywhere!

We are all doing what we can to help out.

Don't forget to self-pace. :-)

The guru is in you.

2008/07/12 12:21:10
Satsang Cafe - General Questions on AYP
http://www.aypsite.org/forum/topic.asp?TOPIC_ID=4136&REPLY_ID=35418&whichpage=-1
Question about emails

Hi Coleslaaw:

It is 5. Sorry for the inconvenience. It is a spam measure.

Welcome to the forums, and all the best on your path!

The guru is in you.

2008/08/04 18:43:36
Satsang Cafe - General Questions on AYP
http://www.aypsite.org/forum/topic.asp?TOPIC_ID=4240&REPLY_ID=36036&whichpage=-1
Yogani just one last question....

Hi Maha:

The further we go along the path, the more obvious it becomes that the methods of yoga have been derived from observed natural capabilities contained within the human nervous system. The development of practices has been done by dedicated people working at it over many centuries. We could say such people have been devoted to a chosen ideal that propelled them forward on their journey of spiritual discovery. In that sense, a belief in *something more* is important, as it is in every far-reaching endeavor in life. This is the element of spiritual desire (bhakti), which is the engine of yoga. Then all we must do is *act*.

Yoga is like any other knowledge, gradually developed through the examination of causes and effects over time, with the accumulated knowledge of each generation being passed along to be further built upon by the next generation. Of course, this evolution has at times been retarded by rigid thinking, and the superstition that it breeds. We are working on moving beyond those limitations in this modern information age, and finding some pretty good results as we continue to pull many powerful methods of yoga together into an effective integration. That has perhaps never been done before in an "open source" way. So, here we are...

While something deep within us finds comfort in the belief that all this knowledge is being handed down from benevolent celestial beings, it is not quite that glamorous. It is much more a case of God helping those who are helping themselves. Calling it a *partnership* is a much healthier and progressive approach than waiting for the manna to fall from heaven.

Happily, the result of effectively applied spiritual practices is <u>much</u> more glamorous than any mysterious celestial hand-me-down we could imagine, because we become the thing itself -- abiding inner silence, ecstatic bliss, outpouring divine love, and unity. We come to experience ourselves as *That*. It is both glamorous and ordinary -- our natural condition.

So, there is a celestial being watching out for us after all -- our own divine *Self*. :-)

Wishing you all the best as you move forward with your practices. If you need help with anything, you can find it here. Enjoy!

The guru is in you.

2008/08/14 16:43:08
Satsang Cafe - General Questions on AYP
http://www.aypsite.org/forum/topic.asp?TOPIC_ID=4293
Forum Outage

Hi All:

We had an unscheduled forum outage today from about 1:00-4:30pm USA eastern time.

Apologies to all for any inconvenience.

The guru is in you.

2008/09/08 17:15:08
Satsang Cafe - General Questions on AYP
http://www.aypsite.org/forum/topic.asp?TOPIC_ID=4293&REPLY_ID=37395&whichpage=-1
Forum Outage

Hi All:

We had another unscheduled forum outage today lasting from about 12:00 noon until 5:00 pm USA eastern time.

Apologies again for the inconvenience. Hopefully we can avoid this in the future.

The guru is in you.

2008/08/18 13:09:39
Satsang Cafe - General Questions on AYP
http://www.aypsite.org/forum/topic.asp?TOPIC_ID=4307&REPLY_ID=36506&whichpage=-1
the state of witness and pain

quote:

Originally posted by Ananda

...and i would like to hear your opinions and the rest of the forum members on pain and the state of witness and why does if it's something natural for it to come when very vibrant activities do occur in our lifes.

Hi Ananda:

My deepest prayers are with you and your family during this difficult time.

Yes, it is natural for inner silence (the witness) to be noticed during times of extreme activity. It is common for nearly everyone to experience "time seeming to stand still" during accidents and other sudden life-changing events. But true witnessing goes far beyond that.

For those who are engaged in daily deep meditation, the ability to witness is close to the surface and more prevalent at all times. In fact, the witness condition does not change at all during a traumatic event. It is only more revealed by the greater contrast of events. It is not our inner silence that is coming up more at these times -- it is the extremes of the event that reveal how well-established our witness truly is. It is during chaotic events that we find out what our spiritual practices have been cultivating. During the ongoing pain of loss or injury we will see our spiritual condition more clearly also.

There is a difference between pain and suffering. Pain is pain, a sensation we can all feel, and it will be with us to greater or lesser degrees as long as we are here on this earth. Suffering is the identification of consciousness (our sense of self) with pain through limited perceptual interpretations of the mind. By cultivating inner silence, we are able to break the grip of suffering, because we no longer see ourself as the one who is in pain. Then it is just pain uncolored by self-identification. In this condition as witness we also are in a much better position to perceive and understand what is happening within and around us, and act in ways that are most beneficial for the present situation. The natural rise of relational self-inquiry (in stillness) plays a part in this. It is the mind operating within stillness, as stillness in action, rather than separating us from what is happening.

It is a paradox, because as we move from within the witness state we become the thing that is happening and there is no more fear or suffering, while when the mind is identified as the thing that is happening there is great fear and suffering. The event may be the same, but we are not the same in our relationship to it. This also explains how the same karma can produce entirely different outcomes, depending on the spiritual condition of those who are involved. So there is a lot we can do to reduce suffering and the perceived effects of karma within and around us.

Like we always say, the results of our practices are best measured outside practices during our life activities. During a crisis, we will see the truth of our spiritual condition more clearly than at any other time.

But none of this removes the profound loss you are feeling during this time and the suffering around you, dear Ananda, and for that we continue to send our love and prayers.

The guru is in you.

PS: Such a beautiful post and Gibran quote from Anthem...

2008/08/19 16:38:28
Satsang Cafe - General Questions on AYP
http://www.aypsite.org/forum/topic.asp?TOPIC_ID=4315&REPLY_ID=36552&whichpage=-1
Exercise to Try- Nothing Exists but Now

Hi Folks:

When there is inner silence present, it is a breeze, isn't it? We can make hay with someone else's self-inquiry system, or invent our own. It all becomes relational -- occurring in stillness. And, yes, samyama is a close cousin in this.

No problemo... :-)

The guru is in you.

2008/08/24 11:03:46
Satsang Cafe - General Questions on AYP
http://www.aypsite.org/forum/topic.asp?TOPIC_ID=4346
Using quotes in your posts

Hi All:

We sometimes quote the writings of others in our posts. This is fine as long as it relates to our discussions on spiritual practices and experiences, and we follow the posting guidelines for copyrighted material.

Sometimes quotes are being formatted in ways that make it difficult to tell what is quoted material and what is written by the person posting.

Please make sure to clearly identify material you are quoting by using quotation marks, the quote icon function, or a different color than the rest of your post. These edit functions can be found at the top of the "reply to topic" window and the "edit topic" window.

If quoted material is not clearly identified, such posts may not be approved.

Thank you for your consideration in this matter.

All the best!

The guru is in you.

2008/08/26 13:41:55
Satsang Cafe - General Questions on AYP
http://www.aypsite.org/forum/topic.asp?TOPIC_ID=4352&REPLY_ID=36803&whichpage=-1
A shameful dream confronts me with life's choice

Hi newpov, and welcome!

Nothing can change the fact that ultimately we are not our thoughts and emotions, or even our actions. We are the pure consciousness behind all that. What is shame but an attachment to a perception? It is identification.

This is why we meditate daily, to cultivate pure consciousness, that abiding inner silence -- the witness. Then, as we observe all that is going on, we can allow it and let it go. When we do, the compulsive conduct and self-judgment begin to relax. That is how it is done.

All emotions, including shame and regret, can be converted with the methods of bhakti. See the Bhakti and Karma Yoga book. All attachments can be be released in the mind by systematic means. See the Self-Inquiry book.

If there is a stubborn addiction, then additional help from a 12 step program can be very good. The 12 step support program is a systematic way to step out of a destructive attachment by surrendering to a "higher power," which is also our inner silence.

There are many tools available. All we have to do is use them as best we can and keep going.

Btw, sexual lifestyle is not an obstacle to spiritual development. The underlying principle of preservation and cultivation of sexual energy can be applied within any lifestyle. This is what the Tantra lessons, book and forum discussions are about. Even pornography can be used by bhakti, leading to sound application of tantric principles: http://www.aypsite.org/T38.html

So don't be too hard on yourself. What you seek you will find, and you are obviously aiming higher. Good things are happening. :-)

The guru is in you.

2008/08/26 17:14:22
Satsang Cafe - General Questions on AYP
http://www.aypsite.org/forum/topic.asp?TOPIC_ID=4352&REPLY_ID=36817&whichpage=-1
A shameful dream confronts me with life's choice

Hi newpov:

Well, call me dull and uninteresting, but I do not place much stock in dreams. :-)

The aiming higher I was talking about is from waking state, and you are doing fine in that department. As long as we have a higher ideal for ourselves, and a willingness to act, we will move ahead. This is the essence of bhakti. As mentioned above, negative emotions can be used in this process also.

As long as we wait for someone or something other than ourselves to do the choosing and acting, we will be ... waiting.

It is suggested to review the AYP lessons from the beginning. There are many things to act on there that can leverage our desire into action and real results. In this way our point of view can be steadily changed to one with much more freedom -- the rise of inner silence, the witness, our true *Self*. Once we choose to move steadily toward *That*, then we are chosen.

The guru is in you.

2009/03/20 11:47:19
Satsang Cafe - General Questions on AYP
http://www.aypsite.org/forum/topic.asp?TOPIC_ID=5359&REPLY_ID=47669&whichpage=-1
Surrender

Hi All:

Surrender is reaching the point (again and again) of being able to admit that we do not know, and can never know. That is when all knowing comes pouring through!

It becomes much easier with rising inner silence, because we are in the habit of residing in *That* which is both unknowable and alive with all knowledge.

The guru is in you.

2009/03/27 16:48:38
Satsang Cafe - General Questions on AYP
http://www.aypsite.org/forum/topic.asp?TOPIC_ID=5400&REPLY_ID=48054&whichpage=-1
Are the lessons on this site complete?

Hi Non:

Carson is correct, except the AYP Easy Lessons book goes to Main Lesson 235 and Tantra Lesson 35. There is about 20% additional material in the book related to those lessons, which is listed here: http://www.aypsite.org/book-additions.html

Some of the extra material has found its way onto the website over time, like the Sanskrit Glossary and Asana Illustrations.

Can you build an AYP practice routine without the books? Absolutely, the website is designed for that. However, the books provide significantly more clarity and depth.

Also, the books provide financial support for the free AYP online resources. AYP has a dual personality -- one that wants provide everything for free, and the other that wants to support itself. :-)

All the best on your path!

The guru is in you.

2009/04/18 08:46:33
Satsang Cafe - General Questions on AYP
http://www.aypsite.org/forum/topic.asp?TOPIC_ID=5468
From Anandatandava

Hi All:

I have had a request from a lady whose brother, Roy, is in prison, has read some of the AYP books, and is looking for contact with other practitioners. He has no internet access, and I have been asked to post this for possible responses:

"Sorry for any redundancy, but I'm speaking blindly from prison through my sister. Is the experience of "flame-forms" from hand mudras, a common occurrence? Has anyone else explored the influence of the vagus and other cranial nerves on the autonomic nervous system as pertains to AYP yoga? I'm thinking specifically of the parasympathetic, the primary driver in experiences of profound love.

Anandatanbada"

I sent the below reply back via email. Further thoughts on Roy's inquiry will be appreciated. I will make sure his sister has the link for this topic, so she can print any further insights and send them to him.

Thanks!

The guru is in you.

My emailed reply (excerpt):

"...Energy experiences like you mentioned are common, and the suggestion is to easily favor the practice we are doing over any experiences that come up. If experiences come up during daily activity between our practice sessions, then we can enjoy them and carry on with our activity, whatever it is. Too much mental analysis can get in the way of practices and our spiritual growth. For those who are intellectual by nature, and want to pursue that line, then the AYP Self-Inquiry book is suggested.

There is no question that much more research on the neurobiology of human spiritual transformation is coming down the road, so your interest in that area will no doubt be addressed by modern science increasingly as time goes on. We are in the beginning stages of it now. I am very much in favor of this. See some of my thoughts on "applied spiritual science" here: http://www.aypsite.org/forum/topic.asp?TOPIC_ID=3267 (print and send posts of interest).

The guru is in you.

2009/05/03 20:05:19
Satsang Cafe - General Questions on AYP
http://www.aypsite.org/forum/topic.asp?TOPIC_ID=5468&REPLY_ID=49943&whichpage=-1
From Anandatandava

Hi All:

For those who are new to this discussion, the previous post is from Roy.

Welcome, Anandatandava! :-)

The guru is in you.

2010/01/23 14:10:26
Satsang Cafe - General Questions on AYP
http://www.aypsite.org/forum/topic.asp?TOPIC_ID=5468&REPLY_ID=63636&whichpage=-1
From Anandatandava

Hi Anandatandava:

"Knitted brow" is an aspect of Sambhavi Mudra (Lesson 56, plus others in the Topic Index), which is ancient and found under various names in many traditions, including in the Bible. It came to me from several sources and was integrated into the overall mix of the AYP system of practices on the basis of results.

As we know, no practice stands alone. It is so much about how practices are integrated together and optimized for good progress with comfort and safety. The AYP system is a baseline for this, and "self-pacing" is the means by which anyone can customize a daily routine of practice for best results on the individual level, as you are doing.

All the best!

The guru is in you.

2010/04/17 14:31:17
Satsang Cafe - General Questions on AYP
http://www.aypsite.org/forum/topic.asp?TOPIC_ID=5468&REPLY_ID=67380&whichpage=-1
From Anandatandava

quote:
_____
Originally posted by anandatandava

NEW LESSONS

Since I don't have the ability to determine which new lessons are pertinent to myh interests, looks like I'm going to have to try to get them all printed out and sent to me. Anyone willing to tackle a piece of this? It seems like it might be an unreasonably large task. Is it? The tiniest legible font would be fine, even preferred.

————

Hi All:

This has been taken care of, so Anandatandava will be as caught up as possible with the online lessons. Later this year, all of the online lessons since the first AYP book will be published (with additions) in AYP Vol 2. It is already in the right hand border here -- click the light blue book cover for a description.

All the best to Anandatandava, and everyone. Practice wisely, and enjoy!

The guru is in you.

2010/05/28 11:46:16
Satsang Cafe - General Questions on AYP
http://www.aypsite.org/forum/topic.asp?TOPIC_ID=5468&REPLY_ID=69322&whichpage=-1
From Anandatandava

Hi Anandatandava:

Many thanks for your ongoing chronicle. Helpful to many I am sure, and often deeply touching. If you don't see a lot of response here, it is only because we are speechless. Don't stop. You are sharing a glimpse of something that is rarely seen in the great record book in the sky we call the internet. Many will benefit.

If hardships are stimuli on the spiritual path, then you are in the fast lane for sure. Most of us grumble when our car won't start or our internet connection is busted. When we don't know better, we tend to wear our woes like a badge. The temptation is always there, no matter how great or small the obstacles in our life. But badges don't carry us forward. Walking through them does. When we know how to do that in stillness, then every hardship becomes a doorway to new openings. Not always easy, especially in cases like yours. The payoff is proportional to our letting go of judgment, surrendering to what is, and walking through, no matter what may be happening. The walking through is the most important part -- acting in the flow. Spiritual surrender is not a passive thing. We have called it "active surrender" here. In its advanced stages, we have called it "stillness in action." We become a channel for *That*.

Not that we should court trouble and hardship. Surely more than enough will come our way that we did not plan on. When it does come, there is that door, as you have amply described again and again for the benefit of the many here who live in relative comfort. We need to hear about it. Life is not so different on the outside. Admitting it or not, we are all in the prison of mortality, until we open on the inside. Outer circumstances will lead us there sooner or later. It does not matter where we are. Our inner nature (the divine) will find us, and prevail. The anvil of experience transforms us to eternal silent joy amidst the ups and downs of life. As we know, effective spiritual practices can greatly accelerate the process.

Regarding the AYP writings, for someone at your level of experience, the lessons in book or online form (printed by your sister) are the most complete coverage. The small Enlightenment Series books are more organized in terms of presenting the essential practices in easily accessible compartments. The lessons are an ongoing discussion, somewhat less organized than the E-Series, but covering more techniques and nuances of practice. Therefore the lessons are more complete, if not as easily accessible as the E-Series. So maybe you will want both sets of writing. The Secrets of Wilder novel is instructive also. It is where AYP sprang from originally, and covers more than any of the AYP writings on the stages of spiritual intensity (tapas) and hardship that can be encountered on the path, especially when an established baseline system of practice is not available (lots of trial and error in the novel). Since 2003, AYP has been an endeavor to fill in what was lacking by design in the Secrets of Wilder story, and also lacking in the real world.

I am sure we can work something out with your sister for reducing the size of fonts, pages, etc., for all the writings to meet your space limitations. Have her contact me.

Wishing you all the best on your continuing path.

The guru is in you.

2009/05/01 12:10:44
Satsang Cafe - General Questions on AYP
http://www.aypsite.org/forum/topic.asp?TOPIC_ID=5526&REPLY_ID=49788&whichpage=-1
The Times They are A-Changing'

quote:
————
Originally posted by miguel

Where can i learn more about active surrender Carson?Its related to bhakti?some yoganis lesson?im interested!:-)
I need Gods hand now!:-)

————

Hi Miguel:

The reason the "stop seeking" thing is so confusing is because for everyone it is different. We may stop seeking in the end, and some may make an ideal out of that. On the other hand, everyone is seeking according to their own situation, even (especially) the one who says, "Stop seeking!" That person is seeking your non-seeking. :-)

The key is to go with your own highest ideal (ishta) and forget about what anyone else tells you your ideal should be. The Bhakti and Karma

Yoga book goes into this in some detail, including the phenomenon/practice of active surrender.

Youth is the time to be going for it. The energy of youth, well applied, blossoms into the direct experience of divine presence. Later on, the body will slow down and there will be more work going on inside. So wherever we are in life, let's not waste a minute.

In the latest lesson (#326), seeking is noted to be a form of self-inquiry, and like all self-inquiry, the more relational (in stillness) it is, the less it will be seeking, and the more effective it will be. We know we are getting closer when we are becoming comfortable with such paradoxes, and not worrying about whether it is one thing or the other. It is all One.

In the Bible, Jesus says, "Seek and you will find. Knock and the door will open."

The answer is to keep seeking until you don't feel the need to any more. It will not hold you back. Seeking is the source of your unfoldment, until it dissolves in stillness and isn't personal seeking anymore. Then it is "stillness in action," which is a divine seeking. You know what it is for you today, and that is how it should be. No one else can tell you what it must be for you in this moment.

Just to stay with the topic, yes, the times they are changing. The lesson (#93) I wrote on this 5 years ago seems ancient compared to what is happening in the world now. Is it all going too fast? Boy, that is music to my ears. It's about time. Much better to be learning how to self-pace rapid openings (individually and globally) than to be "seeking" for centuries more for the key levers of human spiritual transformation. It's time to move on. :-)

All the best!

The guru is in you.

PS: Many well-known non-duality (advaita) teachers preach that everyone should stop seeking. It is bad advice for most people.

2009/05/01 13:57:29
Satsang Cafe - General Questions on AYP
http://www.aypsite.org/forum/topic.asp?TOPIC_ID=5526&REPLY_ID=49798&whichpage=-1
The Times They are A-Changing'

quote:
_____
Originally posted by CarsonZi

Hi Miguel...Yogani...

quote:
_____
Originally posted by yogani

Many well-known non-duality (advaita) teachers preach that everyone should stop seeking. It is bad advice for most people.
_____

Sorry if I was giving "bad" advice or speaking out of turn here. It wasn't intended (is anything ever intended to be "bad"?). I was only speaking from my heart. Hope I didn't confuse you Miguel. You should just forget what I said and go with Yogani's advice. Obviously.

Love,
Carson

Hi Carson:

"Active surrender" (you mentioned) is very good advice, which is doing (seeking) even as we are letting go. It is something we become familiar with in daily samyama sitting practice, and it creeps out into our normal activities during the day, making life much easier ... relational ... doing in stillness ... stillness in action. :-)

Bhakti, deep meditation, samyama, self inquiry, kundalini, etc ... all of these things are interwoven, in practice, and ultimately in the wholeness of our daily living. The lessons will discuss more on these integrations in results as we move along.

Ether, I was not responding to your mention of "stopping seeking" as much as to some reading I have been doing lately. Just yesterday, I was reading a famous non-duality author who suggests that everyone should stop seeking. That is a very relative statement, applying only in certain circumstances, like in one who is experiencing "active surrender," which is not something everyone can jump into overnight. Likewise, relational self-inquiry does not happen overnight, but it does happen for those who are willing to do the groundwork.

Without the groundwork, "stop seeking" and "be here now," are mere platitudes, no matter how much gorgeous language these may be wrapped in. If taken too seriously at the wrong time they can cause confusion and delay, as Miguel and others here have experienced.

For those who have done the groundwork, and then some, the platitudes become common experience, not needing much of a recommendation. It is a matter of putting the horse in front of the cart. Doing that will keep the times a-changing. :-)

The guru is in you.

2009/05/02 00:51:07
Satsang Cafe - General Questions on AYP
http://www.aypsite.org/forum/topic.asp?TOPIC_ID=5526&REPLY_ID=49818&whichpage=-1
The Times They are A-Changing'

quote:

Yogani wrote:

quote:

Without the groundwork, "stop seeking" and "be here now," are mere platitudes, no matter how much gorgeous language these may be wrapped in. If taken too seriously at the wrong time they can cause confusion and delay, as Miguel and others here have experienced.

_____

Thank you Yogani:
But don't you think "stop seeking" and "be here now" can be at least partially easily implemented by curtailing habitual thinking of the future? Some people are stuck in the past, and some in the future.
If you make at least some effort to think in the present, I think it can be of great benefit during your non-practice time of the day.

_____

Hi Ether:

As general philosophical concepts, sure, there is nothing wrong with discussing these, or any expressions of ultimate truth. They can inspire. But if the concepts are imposed thereafter as a rule for practice (or non-practice), either in opposition to one's natural bhakti to practice in other ways, or as a stand-alone approach that blocks other options altogether, then there is a problem. It can add more layers of mind-stuff.

This is the hazard of trying to carry such concepts beyond initial inspiration by themselves. They are only mental concepts, after all. In and of themselves they are not practice. Only when they become relational in stillness do they have the ability to promote the later stages of human spiritual transformation.

We have seen people get hung up in this so often, sometimes for years. It is particularly problematic when coming from an influential teacher. How could someone so great be wrong? If it isn't working for the student, if there is ongoing doubt and confusion occurring in the student (mind running in circles), then there must be something wrong with the student, right?

Wrong.

This is a scenario we should guard against for the sake of all practitioners. For the same reason, when people come to me in private with budding non-duality experiences, saying they want to share that with everyone, I remind them not to forget to tell others how they got there. The destination is not the path. The concept of the destination isn't the path either. "Stop seeking" and "be here now" are the destination. Not the path. Something more is required before these can be experienced authentically -- groundwork!

Once our inquiry becomes relational in stillness, all concepts become fair game for practice between our sittings. :-)

This was also discussed in a recent lesson called "self-inquiry - from inspiration to realization" -- http://www.aypsite.org/324.html ...and in the lessons before and after too.

The guru is in you.

2009/06/21 12:01:14
Satsang Cafe - General Questions on AYP
http://www.aypsite.org/forum/topic.asp?TOPIC_ID=5820&REPLY_ID=52616&whichpage=-1
A question for Yogani

quote:

I wondered if Yogani still does the twice daily regime or passed beyond this. Seems to me that once self realised then the circuit is complete as far as any further regular practise is concerned as it should just become a part of daily life 24/7. Bit like riding a bike, no need for regular practise and stabilisers once you realise you can ride thats all that is needed ??

_____

Hi Karl:

Yes, twice daily here, with self-pacing as needed. The rest of the day takes care of itself.

I concur with Ether that there is no end point. If there is such a thing as self-realization, it too is a stepping stone on the never-ending path of universal awakening. I will no longer need to practice when everyone no longer needs to practice. We are all in it together, as _One_. :-)

The guru is in you.

2009/07/18 12:02:57
Satsang Cafe - General Questions on AYP
http://www.aypsite.org/forum/topic.asp?TOPIC_ID=5820&REPLY_ID=53669&whichpage=-1
A question for Yogani

quote:

_____

I'm not sure why I was a little surprised that self-pacing was still needed at your stage of the game...I imagine that your not suffering from the more pedestrian kundalini symptoms like energy headaches, insomnia, etc, etc...is it more trying to avoid a premature John Wilder event like at the end of S.O.W.?

Bowing to the guru in all of us...

_____

Hi Parallax:

It should be pointed out that no practice is an end in itself, and therefore not deserving of excess, even if the excess can be handled by advanced practitioners. Overdoing time spent in one practice will be at the expense of downstream practices and the compounding of positive effects. There are only so many hours in the day, and it is important to use them wisely, for all practitioners at any stage.

The "downstream" we are talking about here could be viewed generally as spinal breathing enhancing deep meditation, deep meditation enhancing samyama, samyama enhancing self-inquiry, self-inquiry enhancing divine outpouring and service, and so on. This is a simplification, but you get the idea. Other practices that may be woven in provide similar strengthening of downstream effects, according to their known characteristics.

So, self-pacing is not only a good defense on the path. It is also the essence of a good offense. This has implications reaching far beyond our local concerns.

On the "John Wilder event," what you suggest is not too far-fetched. As we advance, while our personal energy issues may become much reduced, or irrelevant, there is also the matter of keeping cause and effect in balance covering a much wider range of influence. In that sense, you could say that stabilizing a John Wilder-like event on a global scale is part of the program. That event is not only about the individual. It is about everyone.

We are, in fact, currently in the midst of such an event, with many "John Wilders" involved. It is occurring in slow motion, rather than as a sudden spiritual energy explosion, as it was dramatized in the novel. This does not mean bodies are going to vaporize into thin air. But body/mind self-identification will. The Secrets of Wilder novel is a metaphor (Campbell-esque myth) for something equally (or more) dramatic that is currently playing out in the world.

The guru is in you.

2009/07/17 10:30:42
Satsang Cafe - General Questions on AYP
http://www.aypsite.org/forum/topic.asp?TOPIC_ID=5959&REPLY_ID=53627&whichpage=-1
A request to GURU YOGANI.
Welcome Phoenix!

Not much to tell about me really. What little there is was put in a press release several years ago: http://www.aypsite.org/pressrelease1.html

The real story is about what all of you are doing -- the fantastic global opening that is occurring. All I can say to that is, Wow!

Phoenix is rising from the ashes. :-)

I am honored to play a small part in it, along with everyone else.

The guru is in you.

2009/07/17 12:05:28
Satsang Cafe - General Questions on AYP
http://www.aypsite.org/forum/topic.asp?TOPIC_ID=5959&REPLY_ID=53632&whichpage=-1
A request to GURU YOGANI.

Hi Carson:

Some plans are being put in place to provide for continuity of the AYP writings and these forums. When the writing stops here, for whatever reason, it will continue with everyone else. My family and a few others have the necessary administrative access.

My view of AYP is as a shared resource. It has never been about me. The further along the writing gets, the less significant my role. We are pretty far along now, with still some more to go. I honestly don't know where the writing will end up, but do feel there is enough out there now to be a useful resource for any sincere aspirant on the path. These forums are an important part of that -- the shift in focus from one person's journey to the journey of many.

I'm like a guy who marked a trail on the trees as he found his way through the forest. Sooner or later the guy will leave the forest. What will matter in the long run is the marked trees, and what others choose to do with them.

The guru is in you.

2009/07/17 14:04:04
Satsang Cafe - General Questions on AYP
http://www.aypsite.org/forum/topic.asp?TOPIC_ID=5959&REPLY_ID=53640&whichpage=-1
A request to GURU YOGANI.

Hi Parallax:

I can't really say exactly where the writing is going. The key AYP practices are out there already. It is now a matter of clarifying, optimizing, observing how emerging inner silence is moving, and suggesting ways to carry it forward to benefit the most people. There could be some useful revelations in that. Time will tell.

The evolving trends among practitioners at all stages here in the online community, and everywhere, give a feel for where it is heading, and what may need further attention.

The funny thing about stillness is that it is never standing still, at least not for we who have a toe in the forest. :-)

Thanks all for being part of it!

The guru is in you.

2009/07/19 10:28:46
Satsang Cafe - General Questions on AYP
http://www.aypsite.org/forum/topic.asp?TOPIC_ID=5959&REPLY_ID=53712&whichpage=-1
A request to GURU YOGANI.

Thanks much, All.

For Christi, my age: older than Ether. :-)

For Akasha, on the Secrets of Wilder: It is a symbolic story, a novel, not an autobiography. Like all novels, it is assembled with a mixture of real and fictional events to tell the story. A relevant aspect of Wilder was discussed recently here:
http://www.aypsite.org/forum/topic.asp?TOPIC_ID=5820#53669

There is more on Wilder elsewhere in the forums, but I can't locate it right now. Try a search. The important things to know about the Wilder novel are that it is "fiction with teeth" -- the practices in it are real. And that it was written before AYP was started in late 2003. So AYP is an ongoing expansion and refinement, based on the real life experiences of many. The novel stands as a pretty good metaphor for what is happening in the world today -- global human spiritual transformation! Not without its tribulations (some are graphically depicted in the novel), so we self-pace and carry on.

For Harmony: I have previous connections with many teachings (nothing formal with SRF or Sivananda, though am familiar). Not connected with anything now except stillness in action. :-)
For some history and reading, see the AYP extended booklist discussion here: http://www.aypsite.org/253.html
The booklist is in need of updating -- I have moved on. And so should we, from me...

The guru is in you.

2009/07/19 11:07:50
Satsang Cafe - General Questions on AYP
http://www.aypsite.org/forum/topic.asp?TOPIC_ID=5959&REPLY_ID=53714&whichpage=-1
A request to GURU YOGANI.

quote:
─────────
Originally posted by gumpi

Yogani, if you have no connections with SRF where did you come across the spinal breathing technique?
─────────

Hi Gumpi:

Numerous places. Spinal breathing dates back more than 4000 years to the Vigyan Bhairava, and probably beyond. No teaching is an edifice, except unto itself. AYP is always looking beyond fixed structures, to the truth, which is found within every human nervous system.

AYP spinal breathing pranayama is an optimization derived from many sources, most importantly from actual results in practice. This is true of all the AYP practices. That is why we keep monitoring results, and are constantly looking for improvements on the level of the individual practitioner. This is science. We only look back so we can go forward! :-)

The guru is in you.

2009/07/20 12:00:09
Satsang Cafe - General Questions on AYP
http://www.aypsite.org/forum/topic.asp?TOPIC_ID=5959&REPLY_ID=53751&whichpage=-1
A request to GURU YOGANI.

quote:
─────────
Originally posted by gumpi

Yogani,

Thanks for clarification. I was interested in where you yourself first found the spinal breathing technique. For example, did you find it online? The Bihar School of Yoga didn't teach kriya yoga until about the 80s i think. previous to that it wasn't written in book form and unavailable everywhere.

Also, the path the imagination takes to trace the spinal nerve seems odd to me because is it based on actual energy flows? People seem to have many different types of experiences of energy. I wonder why spinal breathing takes the route it does.

_____

Hi Gumpi:

Too much analysis can lead to paralysis. It is suggested to have a little faith and do the practice twice-daily, followed by deep meditation for best results. If there are doubts on practice, see the AYP Spinal Breathing Pranayama book.

If someone gives us a bicycle, we can either take it apart or ride it. Can't do both at the same time. Riding is preferred, since this is what the bicycle has been designed for.

Relax and enjoy the ride!

The guru is in you.

2009/07/21 11:57:16
Satsang Cafe - General Questions on AYP
http://www.aypsite.org/forum/topic.asp?TOPIC_ID=5959&REPLY_ID=53825&whichpage=-1
A request to GURU YOGANI.

quote:
_____
Originally posted by mimirom

I think what we are experiencing is at least as big as the Copernican revolution in the 16th century, where the Earth was suddenly displaced from the center of the Universe, and the astronomical universe itself revealed it's true vastness to human comprehension.

_____

Hi Roman:

I agree. A huge pardigm shift is occurring. We are witnessing the end of body/mind self-identified awareness and the birth of spiritual Self-awareness. The truth is setting us free.

Let's get on with it! :-)

The guru is in you.

2009/07/21 13:18:23
Satsang Cafe - General Questions on AYP
http://www.aypsite.org/forum/topic.asp?TOPIC_ID=5959&REPLY_ID=53838&whichpage=-1
A request to GURU YOGANI.

quote:
_____
Originally posted by gumpi

Yogani,

I understand that analysis is sometimes overdone and practice is perhaps neglected. However, i would really just like to know where you got spinal breathing from.

Also, what are your thoughts on the amount of time spent in meditation - that is, are longer times unhealthy?

_____

Hi Gumpi:

We are not going to further dissect my background. There are good reasons why AYP is presented the way it is. It will be much better to practice and go out and live a full life.

If you are really interested in the effects of longer deep meditation sessions, try it and see what happens. It is suggested to read the AYP Deep Meditation book first.

The guru is in you.

2009/07/21 14:07:42
Satsang Cafe - General Questions on AYP
http://www.aypsite.org/forum/topic.asp?TOPIC_ID=5959&REPLY_ID=53841&whichpage=-1
A request to GURU YOGANI.

quote:
_____
Originally posted by gumpi

I have read your deep meditation book. I don't recall anywhere where you say that long meditations can be bad for health. I have done long meditations in the past but not regularly. So i don't know the potential bad effects.

Hi Gumpi:

See page 50 in the Deep Meditaton book on "*Fine-Tuning Our Meditaton Time.*" Also see the numerous discussions on overdoing and self-pacing in the lessons and forums.

While uncomfortable, short term overdoing in deep meditation will not be unhealthy for most. Self-pacing and grounding will resolve short term imbalances. As with anything, deliberate long term overdoing can be be unhealthy, and the road to recovery will be longer. In this case the problem is not with the practice, but with the obsessive or misguided overdoing. Less will very often be more, and that is an important lesson for many of us to learn. A moderate routine practiced twice-daily and balanced with normal activity in the world over the long term has been found to produce good results, i.e., steadily rising enlightenment.

The guru is in you.

2009/07/25 00:20:46
Satsang Cafe - General Questions on AYP
http://www.aypsite.org/forum/topic.asp?TOPIC_ID=6012&REPLY_ID=54020&whichpage=-1
Masters and Paths
Welcome Uma!

No special claims here. If the writings are helpful to you on your path, that is all that matters.

Regarding what teaching to follow, you might find this lesson helpful: http://www.aypsite.org/19.html

As far as the AYP approach is concerned, it is step by step, a little bit at a time, not all at once. It is suggested to review the lessons in order from the beginning and see what resonates. Take what works for you, and leave the rest.

You can find a lot of help from many skilled practitioners here in the support forums.

Wishing you all the best on your path. Enjoy!

The guru is in you.

2009/08/04 17:11:33
Satsang Cafe - General Questions on AYP
http://www.aypsite.org/forum/topic.asp?TOPIC_ID=6079&REPLY_ID=54655&whichpage=-1
Radio Shows of Yogani

Thank you, Uvavilala.

Happy to hear you are enjoying the interviews, and happy to commute with you. :-)

No direct representation here of any of those you mentioned, or anyone else. Just a deep appreciation for the journeys they undertook on our behalf.

We are standing on the shoulders of many giants. Let's make the most of it. Yes, we are all connected. We are all *One*.

The guru is in you.

2009/08/04 17:15:04
Satsang Cafe - General Questions on AYP
http://www.aypsite.org/forum/topic.asp?TOPIC_ID=6081&REPLY_ID=54657&whichpage=-1
Request for samyama.

Hi Miguel:

Glad to have you still with us in this precious life. :-)

These things do happen. Who can say why? In the long run we may see such events as turning points in our lives.

I had one too, in 1995, and it was definitely a turning point.

Rest, recover, and carry on!

The guru is in you.

2009/09/16 11:07:31
Satsang Cafe - General Questions on AYP
http://www.aypsite.org/forum/topic.asp?TOPIC_ID=6352&REPLY_ID=57022&whichpage=-1
Private Questions?

Hi lucilledweck, and welcome! :-)

See this contact link from the top menu on the main website: http://www.aypsite.org/contact.html

All the best!

The guru is in you.

2009/09/22 13:16:35
Satsang Cafe - General Questions on AYP
http://www.aypsite.org/forum/topic.asp?TOPIC_ID=6394&REPLY_ID=57379&whichpage=-1
just curiosity...

Hi Miguel:

"The blues" have been wrapping themselves around the globe a bit lately. There have been several forum topics started about this. Personally, I think it is the dark before the dawn. Well, maybe not "The Dawn," but yet another dawn in the endless flow of dawns along the way. We are talking planetary here, and each of us can feel it in our own way.

Yes, I feel what you are feeling. Put on your sun glasses everyone. :-)

The guru is in you.

2009/09/22 13:26:33
Satsang Cafe - General Questions on AYP
http://www.aypsite.org/forum/topic.asp?TOPIC_ID=6395&REPLY_ID=57381&whichpage=-1
A sugestion

Hi Lucilledweck:

All of the AYP Enlightenment Series books are available in MP3 audiobook format. See the AYP books page, and also here: http://www.aypsite.org/books-xdirdownload.html
The Enlightenment Series covers the essential practices from the AYP lessons in a focused and organized manner.

There is also a list of radio interviews that can be listened to online, or downloaded in MP3, here: http://www.aypsite.org/audio.html

Speaking of which, the latest radio interview was pre-recorded last week on "Self-Inquiry," scheduled for broadcast and website posting October 4th. More on that when we get closer to the date.

There is also a lot of audio, some with creative video added, on the AYP Youtube channel, here: http://www.youtube.com/user/yogani99

After all of that, you will surely be sick of listening to me! :-)

All the best!

The guru is in you.

2009/09/29 12:43:10
Satsang Cafe - General Questions on AYP
http://www.aypsite.org/forum/topic.asp?TOPIC_ID=6443&REPLY_ID=57799&whichpage=-1
Where do the practices come from

Hi Lucilledweck:

As with all human knowledge, practical spiritual methods have evolved over the centuries, and they continue to evolve.

This lesson was just posted, which might add some perspective:
http://www.aypsite.org/364.html

How's that for timing? :-)

The guru is in you.

2009/09/29 13:34:44
Satsang Cafe - General Questions on AYP
http://www.aypsite.org/forum/topic.asp?TOPIC_ID=6443&REPLY_ID=57802&whichpage=-1
Where do the practices come from

quote:
_____
Originally posted by Christi

Hi Yogani,

We cross posted. :-)
_____

Excellent reply. :-)

2009/10/25 14:54:29
Satsang Cafe - General Questions on AYP

http://www.aypsite.org/forum/topic.asp?TOPIC_ID=6586&REPLY_ID=58963&whichpage=-1
The increasingly "subtle" projecting mind.

Hi Anthem:

Once we have loosened identification with thoughts through cultivation of silent witness, we can enjoy the nice dreams, and "turn around" the nightmares through inquiry so they will be nice dreams too. :-)

The guru is in you.

2009/12/07 12:56:27
Satsang Cafe - General Questions on AYP
http://www.aypsite.org/forum/topic.asp?TOPIC_ID=6690&REPLY_ID=60844&whichpage=-1
Have you had direct contact with God?

quote:
_____
Originally posted by chinna

Upasani Maharaj used to throw bricks at visitors, which was an even more effective a way of turning away those who were not ready for this teaching.

The Maharis
Hi Mahesh Yogi invested huge resources in applying science to yoga and meditation and got nowhere. It's a category error.

chinna
_____

Hi Chinna:

It seems you are suggesting the traditional esoteric approach for the transmission of spiritual knowledge: "Favor the gifted and drive everyone else away."

Given that we all have inherent spiritual capability and have the right to an education in modern times, do you think you are espousing a practical point of view?

If so, we should only be teaching reading, writing and math to those who are gifted, and drive everyone else away. Then it is back to the dark ages, which is what we are just beginning to creep out of in the field of spiritual education.

There were reasons why spiritual teachings (and also literacy and math) were held esoteric in the past, but those reasons no longer exist. Yet we keep hearing how only the few are qualified for spiritual knowledge and advancement. Balony!

Open science and education are the ways forward for the unfoldment of human spirituality on a mass scale. By "science," I mean verifiable cause and effect in methodology. With that becoming increasingly developed, no one will be without the means to awaken according to their own desire. There is no difference between this and the democratization of any other kind of knowledge. Yes, it is messy at times, but that is no excuse to shrink from the task. It is the only way that the whole of humanity will be uplifted.

And Gumpi, may I remind you that these are the "AYP Support Forums." If the practices are not working for you, this is not the place to be making a blanket case to convince others that practices will not work for them. We are interested in what works. If you have something to contribute on that front, we'd love to hear it. And if you need help with practices, we will be happy to do what we can.

All the best!

The guru is in you.

PS: Chinna, millions would take issue with your belief that yoga science is going nowhere. After all, you are posting in a yoga science forum!

PPS: Nothing I have said here need be at issue with a non-dual point of view, unless of course that view is really duality in disguise, producing endless posturing and debate. Much better to focus on means than ends. If we take care of business, no need to worry about contacting God. S/He will contact us. :-)

2009/12/07 17:22:55
Satsang Cafe - General Questions on AYP
http://www.aypsite.org/forum/topic.asp?TOPIC_ID=6690&REPLY_ID=60868&whichpage=-1
Have you had direct contact with God?

Hi Chinna:

Contrary to the stereotype image of scholarly PhDs with their lab coats and equipment, science is the search for ever more reliable causes and effects by any and all means possible.

That is what the AYP Support Forums are about. Admittedly, there is a lot of noise here, and an underlying resistance to change (awakening). Neither of those things have much to do with science, but are always present in any collective search for truth. Ultimately, all obstructions are overcome and the truth prevails. Evolution flows like water running downhill, steadily wearing away obstacles. With more and more people engaged in effective spiritual practices around the world, the hill is getting steeper and the water is running faster all the time. Stillness in action!

In the early stages of a new paradigm, "ragtag" science can be the best science, because it does not stand on ceremony. It only wants results. Once results are occurring that can no longer be ignored, the "white coats" come in to verify, codify and expand on what has been discovered. That is when everyone gets on board. We can look forward to it.

On a related subject, the differences you and I have had seem to relate mainly to the spiritual assistance needs of the few versus the many. We are really talking about two different things. Perhaps you are interested in the few who can go straight into non-duality school. Looking for some company? I am always looking for how to make room in a school for everyone at every grade. I like lots of company.

Certainly the few can thrive in a school for the many, but the many will not thrive in a school for the few. That seems to be the rub we have had. Perhaps we can minimize misunderstandings by clarifying when we are talking about the few or the many. Both have their place and appropriate means in the overall scheme of spiritual evolution.

The guru is in you.

2009/12/07 20:59:10
Satsang Cafe - General Questions on AYP
http://www.aypsite.org/forum/topic.asp?TOPIC_ID=6690&REPLY_ID=60885&whichpage=-1
Have you had direct contact with God?

Hi Chinna:

Of course you are welcome, and I hope you will continue contributing. The advaita (non-dual) perspective is very valuable for those who are ready to hear it, even while posing an intellectual diversion for many others. So bear with me when I jump in from time to time to add context for the broad AYP community. A little balance never hurts. The result will be more people consciously living non-duality. :-)

The guru is in you.

2010/01/05 11:36:12
Satsang Cafe - General Questions on AYP
http://www.aypsite.org/forum/topic.asp?TOPIC_ID=6940&REPLY_ID=62169&whichpage=-1
Very Complex Inner Situation...HELP!

Hi All:

Ida and pingala balance in relation to sushumna opening is discussed here from the AYP perspective:
http://www.aypsite.org/forum/topic.asp?TOPIC_ID=6661#59564
(and in previous posts in that topic)

That discussion is from the point of view of awakening ecstatic conductivity (kundalini). It is also relevant in discussing AYP deep meditation, which does not produce the kind of imbalance being suggested here. The utilization of nadi shodana (alternate nostril pranayama) is discussed elsewhere in these forums and in the AYP lessons.

This is not to say that Omarkaya's advice is not valid within the context of Satyananda's system of practice. If Satyananda's system is working over there and the AYP system is working over here, then that is fine. But it is not fine for one to be imposing on the other. That will only bring confusion, because no one can practice two systems at the same time.

Omarkaya, it is suggested to please keep that in mind when dispensing advice in the AYP Support Forums. The place to be presenting alternate approaches is in the "Other Systems" forum category, where it will be clear to everyone that alternate approaches are being considered, rather than proselytizing one system over another one in a support discussion. All approaches are welcome to be discussed in the forums, as long as each respects the other, and practitioners are free to make their own choices.

Thanks!

The guru is in you.

2010/01/05 12:38:59
Satsang Cafe - General Questions on AYP
http://www.aypsite.org/forum/topic.asp?TOPIC_ID=6940&REPLY_ID=62176&whichpage=-1
Very Complex Inner Situation...HELP!

Hi Juan, and a belated welcome! :-)

You will find that there is plenty of room here in the forums to express your opinions, advice, and even your frustrations. You will find many approaches to spiritual practice (and non-practice) discussed here, more or less in ways that enable serious seekers to make their own choices. The AYP system is offered as a baseline, and practitioners can take it wherever they wish from there.

We try and minimize confusion for those getting started on the path, while at the same time pointing out options and alternates along the way. It is a bit of a tight-wire act, but worth the effort, I think.

So, have a good time here, practice wisely, and enjoy!

The guru is in you.

PS: Here is a note I posted a few weeks ago on Satyananda's passing: http://www.aypsite.org/forum/topic.asp?TOPIC_ID=6811#60934

2010/01/07 09:22:36
Satsang Cafe - General Questions on AYP
http://www.aypsite.org/forum/topic.asp?TOPIC_ID=6940&REPLY_ID=62319&whichpage=-1

Very Complex Inner Situation...HELP!

quote:
_____
Originally posted by Rael

Dear Yogani

Might you have any comments on Omarkaya's approach?........I am reading the Samayama book now, which, so far has explained a little , but not to a great extent yet.

This seems like a core issue material, so, if you have a minute?.....

_____

Hi Rael:

It is not recommended to try and follow multiple approaches at once, especially beginners.

There are at least 108 ways to do everything in yoga, and we can only do one thing at a time. Those who advise complicating practice without regard for the practices you are already learning ought not be heeded. As mentioned earlier, such advice belongs in the "other systems" forum category where it is not being imposed on people seeking support.

It is very easy to find (or give) endless advice on spiritual practices, but not so easy to stay focused on one approach that will bring us steady progress with stability over time of consistent daily practice. A competent teacher knows this, and will respect the journey of the aspirant, rather than try and bend it to personal will.

I suggest using the "KISS" method, which means "Keep it simple stupid!" That goes for beginning mantras too. :-)

It is up to you.

The guru is in you.

PS: Also see this lesson: http://www.aypsite.org/19.html

2010/01/07 12:01:12
Satsang Cafe - General Questions on AYP
http://www.aypsite.org/forum/topic.asp?TOPIC_ID=6940&REPLY_ID=62329&whichpage=-1
Very Complex Inner Situation...HELP!

Hi Omarkaya:

I am not so concerned about kirtans, or anything else the practitioner may be drawn to on their path. I am concerned with imposing one thing over another, because there are unlimited ways that can happen from many sources, and that helps no one.

So the practitioner has to be careful what they are considering to do when, and how much distraction it may cause to core practices. This is especially important for beginners who do not have a solid foundation of daily practice.

Of all the things we discuss in AYP, and nearly all other systems, the most important by far is the consistency of daily practice over the long term.

So the practitioner should always be asking themselves about that when considering anything that is offered. It begins with asking, "What is my daily practice?"

There may or may not be additional things the practitioner is drawn to after the core practice routine is established. Whatever the case may be, it is easy to get lost in the details and lose our core practice (if we ever had one), because the options for additional practice are unlimited.

There are thousands of kirtans. We could list hundreds here from many sources. Which one should the practitioner choose? Only they can know. And many can get lost in endless detail trying to find out. That is why I say "KISS! (keep it simple stupid)" :-)

That is also why we have the "other systems" forum category, where many methods can be considered, without being imposed on anyone.

Please keep it in mind when offering add-ons. Offering the add-on is the easy part. It is the practitioner who then has the burden of sorting out the 108 add-ons that are being promoted. Is this fair to beginners? I think not. Which is why I am giving you a hard time about this, for their sake, and yours.

Ultimately, we all make our own choices. That is what AYP is about. Part of that is developing a clear understanding about what is essential and what is overload. It will be a little different for everyone. This is why nothing in AYP is imposed. All is suggested for the practitioner to make their own choice. So the suggestion is to **suggest rather than direct**, keeping in mind that there are many factors in play. Then the practitioner will decide based on inputs available, their bhakti and personal inclinations.

We have found this to be a workable approach for many different kinds of practitioners. The reported results speak for themselves.

The guru is in the practitioner.

2010/01/14 11:37:48
Satsang Cafe - General Questions on AYP
http://www.aypsite.org/forum/topic.asp?TOPIC_ID=6940&REPLY_ID=62797&whichpage=-1
Very Complex Inner Situation...HELP!

Hi Akasha:

If you feel you should be doing alternate nostril breathing, then do it. It is your choice. That is more concession than you will find from those who approach yoga through ida, pingala and chakras, who will find it hard to admit that all of these things can be balanced by purifying and opening the sushumna directly, which is what spinal breathing pranayama is about.

So, it is a question of the angle of approach, not whether the AYP system has missed something. I can assure you that the choice of spinal breathing as core practice, and not alternate nostril breathing, was a conscious one. Not an omission, oversight or error. The approach in AYP is entirely different, going for the highest first in all areas of practice -- the master principles and controllers of human spiritual transformation. With the main controls well in hand, the rest is automatically taken care of, and regarded to be "under the hood."

For those who are attracted to alternate nostril breathing, an addition to Lesson 41 is provided in the big AYP Easy Lessons book.

From the AYP point of view, alternate nostril breathing is a relaxation technique. If and when AYP is taught in yoga studio settings, alternate nostril breathing will probably be introduced as such, and then it will be on to spinal breathing pranayama without delay. The baseline system of AYP is not going to change. And I expect the variations that people wish to bring to it will continue to be unlimited. It has been like that since AYP started in 2003. These are the two constants in yoga: The baselines that advanced practitioners took the time to put together, and the unending barrage of variations that are thrown at them by the crowd. It is the nature of open source. :-)

The least we can do is keep baselines of practice from barraging each other, which is why in these forums AYP support discussions are best carried out in one place, and evaluations of other systems of practice carried out in another place. The two cannot be done in one place without seriously compromising AYP support.

So it is not a question of whether Omarkaya, or Tibetan Ice, or anyone else, is working from a better baseline, or has a better approach. It is a matter of respecting all approaches and allowing them to maintain their integrity and consistency, while at the same time looking across traditional lines for logical improvements that will benefit practitioners. It is a tightwire act that requires careful discrimination, and above all, mutual respect for the established baselines of practice.

These forums were established first and foremost for practitioner support for the AYP baseline system as described in the AYP lessons and books. From the beginning it has been felt that discussions on other systems of practice would be healthy and provide useful cross-fertilization going in both directions. But what has happened is that the AYP system has found itself being constantly battered and overrun by other approaches in the forums, which has been an ongoing disappointment and constant source of confusion to beginning practitioners.

So steps are gradually being implemented to reclaim part of the forums for AYP support only, while retaining the other systems and alternatives categories of discussion.

The first step was to designate the Deep Meditation/Samyama and Spinal Breathing Pranayama/Mudras/Bandhas forums to be for AYP support only. We are now doing the same with Satsang, because this is where many beginners come with questions on AYP. You will note that the title of "Satsang Cafe" has been changed to be "Satsang Cafe - General Questions on AYP." In addition, two new forum categories will be added within a couple of months that will be exclusively for discussion of the AYP Main and Tantra lessons.

All of these actions are for the purpose of restoring these forums to their original purpose -- AYP practitioner support. Other systems and alternative practice discussions will continue to be welcome in their respective categories.

Those who are not able to respect the integrity of these categories of discussion, who continually bring confusion to practitioners seeking AYP support, are going to find themselves not welcome to participate in the forums anymore.

That is how it is going to be. It is hoped that everyone will take note of it, and respect it.

Thanks!

The guru is in you.

2010/01/15 12:16:06
Satsang Cafe - General Questions on AYP
http://www.aypsite.org/forum/topic.asp?TOPIC_ID=6940&REPLY_ID=62902&whichpage=-1
Very Complex Inner Situation...HELP!

quote:
_____
Originally posted by Akasha

quote:
_____

From the AYP point of view, alternate nostril breathing is a relaxation technique.
_____

I don't know where you got this from. But i disagree here. It serves to balance ida & pingala, and both brain hemispheres.
_____

Hi Akasha:

= relaxation ... :-)

From the AYP point of view, that is what it is. It may be something more from other points of view (under the hood), but that is not for discussion in this AYP support topic. Kindly take it up in other systems. Pursuing it here will only confuse the issue.

Thanks!

The guru is in you.

PS: For context, please <u>review this</u>.

quote:

From the AYP point of view, alternate nostril breathing is a relaxation technique. If and when AYP is taught in yoga studio settings, alternate nostril breathing will probably be introduced as such, and then it will be on to spinal breathing pranayama without delay.

<hr>

2010/01/17 12:30:43
Satsang Cafe - General Questions on AYP
http://www.aypsite.org/forum/topic.asp?TOPIC_ID=7008&REPLY_ID=63050&whichpage=-1
Scenery

quote:

<hr>

Originally posted by SeySorciere

Yogani calls what we experience during meditation i.e. the strange lights, smells, God, lower beings, higher beings, hallucinations, whatever else... "scenery". Question: What is this scenery really?? Delusions of the mind?? Real??

<hr>

Hi SeySorciere:

Symptoms of purification and opening. That is why we always easily favor the practice over the experiences that come up. Practices produce spiritual progress. Experiences do not.

All the best!

The guru is in you.

<hr>

2010/01/16 10:37:24
Satsang Cafe - General Questions on AYP
http://www.aypsite.org/forum/topic.asp?TOPIC_ID=7037&REPLY_ID=62992&whichpage=-1
Is prana/kundalini biochemical?

Hi TI:

Prana certainly has a biochemical (neurobiological) component. The tools of hatha yoga are for addressing that (pranayama, asana, mudra, bandha). <u>But prana is not only that.</u> It (the life force) covers a continuum from physical to pure consciousness, including the full spectrum of emotion, mind, and sensory experience. We have bhakti, meditation, samyama, self-inquiry, etc. operating across that spectrum. In AYP we work toward cultivating the opening on all levels in a consistent and balanced way that can be helpful to many. Openings on any level affect all other levels. Everything is interconnected, and this is well recognized in the integrative approaches of yoga.

The One is the many and the many are the One.

The guru is in you.

<hr>

2010/01/13 21:20:39
Satsang Cafe - General Questions on AYP
http://www.aypsite.org/forum/topic.asp?TOPIC_ID=7116&REPLY_ID=62748&whichpage=-1
Credentials?

quote:

<hr>

Originally posted by Kitten

Yogani,

What types of counseling degrees do you have to provide counseling advice to troubled, needy people? Do you have a PHD in Psychiatry? Or at least a Master's degree in something counseling related?
Your Tantra site is about sex, are you a licensed sex therapist? Have you graduated from any college, with what degree?

Please let me know.

kitten

<hr>

Hi Kitten and welcome.

This particular discussion is about the yogic aspects of diet and nothing else. For that, or anything in AYP, I claim no special credentials. Only the decades spent on the path, and a desire to give something back.

All are free to take what helps here, or leave it alone. We are not focused mainly on troubled, needy people here. Rather, the focus is primarily on those who are very interested in spiritual growth, and in doing something about it. A range of optional yogic tools are offered to assist with that. Those in need of professional counseling or medical attention are advised to seek professional assistance as appropriate. We are not here for that.

If you take a closer look at the AYP writings and these forums, you will gain a better understanding of what this open resource on spiritual practices is about, and what people are doing with it. And if it is not your cup of tea, that is okay.

Wishing you all the best on your path.

The guru is in you.

2010/01/28 00:09:14
Satsang Cafe - General Questions on AYP
http://www.aypsite.org/forum/topic.asp?TOPIC_ID=7170&REPLY_ID=63985&whichpage=-1
Any suggestions?

Hi BellaMente:

"Yoga" is one of the six primary systems of Indian philosophy (you can Wikipedia the rest), expounded in the Yoga Sutras of Patanjali, which is all of 25 pages long. Commentaries are many and much longer.

Can't get much more quantum than yoga.

The One is the many and the many are the One. :-)

The guru is in you.

2010/02/03 09:47:41
Satsang Cafe - General Questions on AYP
http://www.aypsite.org/forum/topic.asp?TOPIC_ID=7219&REPLY_ID=64427&whichpage=-1
Reincarnation

Hi Ashwathama, and welcome!

We don't make too much of reincarnation in AYP. It is a matter of personal belief, and yoga will work either way.

Here are some references from the lessons and forums: http://www.aypsite.org/forum/topic.asp?TOPIC_ID=2313

Wishing you all the best on your path. Enjoy!

The guru is in you.

2010/03/10 11:53:42
Satsang Cafe - General Questions on AYP
http://www.aypsite.org/forum/topic.asp?TOPIC_ID=7407&REPLY_ID=65922&whichpage=-1
The Crow

Hi Mani:

Keep practicing. :-)

There has been movement in the direction you desire, right? And, therefore, with continuation of practices, the movement will continue.

The mind will not go. It will still be there. It is the center of gravity of "self" that shifts from mind toward abiding inner silence, until the mind no longer rules. Then the mind continues as servant, not master.

Our relationship with the "crow" is a barometer of our condition. It will change as our sense of self gradually stabilizes in stillness.

As for "when," I can't tell you for sure. Each of our journeys is unique, with underlying principles, methods and experiences that we share in common. The "when" is the subject of an upcoming lesson.

The guru is in you.

2010/03/25 18:44:12
Satsang Cafe - General Questions on AYP
http://www.aypsite.org/forum/topic.asp?TOPIC_ID=7489&REPLY_ID=66517&whichpage=-1
A question for Yogani

Hi arzkiyahai:

Obviously, for each of them, it was where they experienced it. And for you, it will be where you experience it. One place it will never be, and that is where another tells you it is that is contrary to your own experience. This is assuming you continue with practices for as long as it takes to find out for yourself. :-)

The guru is in you.

2010/05/07 18:37:40
Satsang Cafe - General Questions on AYP
http://www.aypsite.org/forum/topic.asp?TOPIC_ID=7719&REPLY_ID=68412&whichpage=-1
It's ok to think right?

Hi tonightsthenight:

Ultimate answers about spirituality cannot be found in the mind, or in any conceptual knowledge, though we all love to try. They can only be found in the cultivation of abiding inner silence. Then the paradoxes of spirituality make perfect sense. It is a knowing that happens as we become the unknown. The mind can never get this conceptually, but it can be fulfilled. The mind finds fulfillment by experiencing its source, by merging with it, and moving in it. That's why deep meditation is the first practice in AYP.

And this is not to say we should not be out in the world using our gifts and enjoying the journey as we may like. Everyone has their own life to live. Absolutely! It's just better to operate from the infinite source that is our essential nature than from a patchwork of mental structures. Way better. :-)

So make sure you have a solid meditation practice, and all the rest will come. "Seek first the kingdom..."

The guru is in you.

2010/05/11 15:10:56
Satsang Cafe - General Questions on AYP
http://www.aypsite.org/forum/topic.asp?TOPIC_ID=7764
Scientific Research Project on AYP - Input Needed!
Reply Requested

Hi All:

Dr. Kavitha Chinnaiyan ("kami" here in the forums) is a cardiologist in Detroit, Michigan, USA, and is interested in performing scientific research on the AYP practices for health and quality of life effects, as related to the heart. This will include development of a state-of-the-art research program supported by grant funds and ongoing networking with the scientific community.
Her website is: http://www.healyourheartfreeyoursoul.com

This can be a big step forward for AYP in supporting scientific research on spiritual practices, as discussed here:
http://www.aypsite.org/forum/topic.asp?TOPIC_ID=3267
I am very appreciative of Dr. Chinnaiyan's efforts, and hope we can help by providing useful information from the AYP community.

Below, you will find a questionnaire developed by Dr. Chinnaiyan covering specific areas of health and quality of life. We'd like to obtain current feedback from as many of you as possible. Please reply in this topic with personal experiences in these areas, or other health and quality of life effects you would like to report:

quote:

The specific measures we would initially look for are:
1. High blood pressure - if someone has reported lowering and numbers before and after.
2. Diabetes - lowered blood sugars as a result of AYP
3. Chest pain or angina - resolution of symptoms or lowered frequency/intensity of pain/pressure/discomfort
4. High cholesterol - lowered numbers
5. Overall health rating (perception of overall health) before and after AYP practices
6. Response to stress - as a result of increasing inner silence and bliss, have people noticed that they are less affected by life stressors and events? This will be where we might get the most data on (albeit subjective). This is fine, since it has a direct effect on the heart.
7. Others' perception of the practitioner's changed personality/mood/temperament/response to stress.
8. Depression - change in medications since start of practice
9. Anxiety/Panic - change in meds since starting practice
10. Addictions - smoking, alcohol, drugs and coming off these with the aid of practices.
11. Heart failure symptoms - shortness of breath, swelling in the legs and change since AYP.
12. Palpitations (or heart rhythm problems) - alleviation in symptoms
13. Respiratory symptoms - asthma, COPD and alleviation in symptoms (pranayama has shown improved respiratory parameters in COPD patients)

For each of these, we'd like to know specifically what the practice routine was, how long practicing with which techniques, and background in practices (if any) before coming to AYP.

This information can be posted anonymously. It will be used to help develop criteria and biomarkers for the research program. If you prefer to report your information privately, you can email directly to Dr. Chinnaiyan by clicking on her forum member name.

If anyone would like to participate directly in the research program, as either researcher or subject, please contact Dr. Chinnaiyan or me.

All information is greatly appreciated. Many thanks!

The guru is in you.

PS: We are also supporting this effort by "data mining" the AYP support forums for health and quality of life testimonials and data posted here over the past five years. There is a huge amount of health-related information here, and we are doing what we can to retrieve whatever might be useful in the research arena. Current experiences are preferred, so please review the questionnaire list above and comment on effects you have noticed in any of those areas. Thanks!

2010/05/24 10:21:29
Satsang Cafe - General Questions on AYP
http://www.aypsite.org/forum/topic.asp?TOPIC_ID=7838&REPLY_ID=69131&whichpage=-1
The Arrival

Hi Carson:

Just arrived back after 4 days without internet.

Bravo! Wishing your growing family eternal joy!

The guru is in you.

2010/05/25 16:46:53
Satsang Cafe - General Questions on AYP
http://www.aypsite.org/forum/topic.asp?TOPIC_ID=7841&REPLY_ID=69195&whichpage=-1
How to mend a hardened heart?

quote:
_____
Originally posted by brunoloff

Once again, I refer you to the site of http://www.actualfreedom.com.au
It seems to signify that not only you can realize no-self, but you could just as well, by extension, realize the no-Self. It seems to imply that the "I am THAT" sentence that yogani so often repeats, just means that HE didn't get rid of this process...

People who underwent this kind of transformation clearly state that "there is no sense of being whatsoever."

It was this possibility which scared me, and still does, irrespective of me being able to see that scare as "not me," i.e., not "the subject".

I wonder what yogani has to say about this...
_____

Hi Brunoloff:

Well, at least I didn't write a book called "I am THAT." Nisargadatta beat me to it. :-)

Anyway, I generally don't say "I am THAT." I say "We are *That*." There is a difference. One separates us, and the other brings us together.

What else do I have to say about it? Not much. Better to meditate daily and find out for yourself what *THAT* is. You will see there is nothing to fear. Who fears freedom anymore, having tasted even a little of it?

Until there is abiding inner silence, these kinds of discussions are mostly mind games -- building castles in the air. Not that we should not have them. But we should know them for what they are -- scenery that cannot enlighten us. Only effective practices can do that.

So practice wisely, and enjoy!

The guru is in you.

2010/05/25 21:31:42
Satsang Cafe - General Questions on AYP
http://www.aypsite.org/forum/topic.asp?TOPIC_ID=7841&REPLY_ID=69202&whichpage=-1
How to mend a hardened heart?

Hi Brunoloff:

Yes, it does all end up in the same place. And where is that? Is it a place of non-doing, or a place of outpouring divine love? Or both at the same time? And if it is a doing, is it personal, or absolutely impersonal? A non-doing that is doing? What we have many times called "stillness in action." It is a paradox.

There is only one way you will find out what this is about. Practice.
Don't take anyone's word for it. Practice.

This cannot be resolved in thinking. Only in going beyond thinking. This recent lesson addresses it: http://www.aypsite.org/403.html

There is no answer. Only a becoming, which is an undoing.

The guru is in you.

PS: It is also the undoing of a hardened heart. It may begin with tears of sorrow, which in time transform to tears of joy. In stillness we will know both deeply, while remaining untouched.

2010/08/13 10:27:27
Satsang Cafe - General Questions on AYP
http://www.aypsite.org/forum/topic.asp?TOPIC_ID=8257&REPLY_ID=71894&whichpage=-1

Does anyone keep an AYP diary?

Hi All:

Writing, in whatever form, can be a useful aid on our path -- a mirror of our journey, and a tool for awakening.

See this lesson on "The power of the pen, and the keyboard" : http://www.aypsite.org/395.html

The lessons immediately before and after that one add further perspective on the spiritual role written communications can play in online forums.

All the best!

The guru is in you.

2010/08/26 08:20:52
Satsang Cafe - General Questions on AYP
http://www.aypsite.org/forum/topic.asp?TOPIC_ID=8320&REPLY_ID=72380&whichpage=-1
Latest Lesson 430

Hi Anthem:

On the "going out" from identification with objects of perception and then "coming back" into relationship with objects in unity, it is a function of self-inquiry, and that does not lend itself to a reliable formula approach as much the core practices in AYP do. It is largely personal choice. Either way, identification and suffering have been alleviated. Who is to say how one will choose to engage with objects -- as witness separate from objects, or as witness merged with objects?

There has been so much emphasis on non-duality and the "illusion" of the world (a duality!), that I felt it might be good to point out that there is a broad continuum on the enlightenment scale that can be called "freedom," where duality is still operating to greater or lesser degree.

So how long will it take to dissolve into non-dual unity? It depends on the person, the nature of their bhakti, and the exercise of self-inquiry after the "going out" from identification with objects has occurred (or as it is occurring). It could be instant, or it could not happen for a long time. Your choice. :-)

One thing is for sure, the "coming back" cannot happen until the "going out" has at least begun to happen, i.e., relational (in stillness) self-inquiry leading to unity relies on the rise of witness.

It should be mentioned that unidentified awareness without full unity with objects is not a sterile condition of non-engagement in the world. Whenever we see that sort of dry aloof dispassion, the condition will be suspect. Real spiritual dispassion is very passionate about the well-being of others. This gets to your next question.

Whether we call it "unconditional love" or "outpouring divine love," it is the same flow that emerges as abiding inner silence and ecstatic conductivity/radiance are merging in daily activity. It can also be known as an unmoving flow, which is a deep acceptance and the ability to absorb in loving stillness (and illuminate from within) whatever may be happening. This is unconditional love for Self and all. This too leads to unity, for the lover wants nothing but to merge with the beloved, which is ultimately seen everywhere. It is the fruition of bhakti and karma yoga. It too is a matter of personal choice.

So much of this is automatic, except in cases where it is beaten to death with the intellect, as advaita teachers (and their students) are so inclined to do, or with endless ritual, as is so common on bhakti paths. With a systematic approach involving daily yoga practices, it is all going to happen anyway, and the practitioner can finish it off in any way desired. That is the advantage of systematically putting in a solid foundation of abiding inner silence and cultivating it outward in ecstatic divine flow. Once that is taken care of, the rest is easy. Ripe fruit will fall off the tree sooner or later. It's as easy as one, two, three... :-)

The guru is in you.

2010/09/16 11:15:58
Satsang Cafe - General Questions on AYP
http://www.aypsite.org/forum/topic.asp?TOPIC_ID=8320&REPLY_ID=72927&whichpage=-1
Latest Lesson 430

quote:
_____
Originally posted by Anthem11

I don't quite understand your perspective here, in the AYP lessons you say that first comes witness separate from objects and then there is the merging between witness and object for ongoing 24/7 unity experience. Sounds like you are saying above that it is a choice and the person may elect not to experience the unity perspective and still not suffer 24/7?
_____

Hi Anthem:

The milestones/stages in AYP are the mechanical aspect of rising inner silence, ecstatic conductivity, and their merging in unity. It is a map that can be helpful, and we have practices that address these aspects of development quite clearly.

But then what? It boils down to how we choose to see the world in everyday living, and that is still a function of personal choice (in stillness), with personality still present in our actions. If someone is in unity (subject and objects merged), interactions will still be happening with this and that. The view from the doer's perspective can be of this and that, or of no this and that. It is a choice whether the world is viewed as a sandy beach with attributes, or as an endless sea of sand with no attributes. Which do you prefer? Those who choose to see the undifferentiated sand only may not be doing much practical work. But they do radiate divine love and giggle a lot. :-)

With unity, there is the ability to view it either way, and both ways. How it is viewed in the moment is a choice. There is no requirement that an enlightened person see things in a particular way. "Freedom" means seeing and doing freely in stillness, beyond definitions and the psychosomatic condition of identification and suffering (I, me & mine out in front all the time).

This is better to be lived than to be understood. It can be lived by everyone, but it cannot be understood by anyone. What can be understood is that it is a paradox, a liberated and happy one, with mind operating in the background instead of out in front. Effective practices combined with an active life bring us there in due course.

The guru is in you.

2010/10/02 10:55:40
Satsang Cafe - General Questions on AYP
http://www.aypsite.org/forum/topic.asp?TOPIC_ID=8509&REPLY_ID=73431&whichpage=-1
It's been a while

quote:
_____
Now, what I really wanted to share is that I've stopped practicing AYP about a month and a half ago. I started in March and was doing it every day, sometimes even three or four times a day.
_____

Hi CE:

Good to see you again.

It should be pointed out that practicing an AYP routine "three or four times a day" is certain to lead to difficulties, and so it did.

It is suggested to take a more measured approach to daily practice as you move ahead. The AYP system is a baseline, and variations (like excessive practice) can lead to unpredictable results. In cases like that, it is no longer AYP, but the practitioner's research.

Live and learn... :-)

The guru is in you.

2010/10/16 12:37:47
Satsang Cafe - General Questions on AYP
http://www.aypsite.org/forum/topic.asp?TOPIC_ID=8570&REPLY_ID=73882&whichpage=-1
Meeting other AYP practitioners

quote:
_____
Originally posted by Assorted Vibrations

I'm in Oregon. Nice to make your acquaintance faileforever. I looked through the list (http://www.aypsite.org/events.html) and I am surprised that there are no groups on the west coast. I would have guessed there would at least be something in California. I would love to start a group in Oregon but I am not in a place where I have the ability to do so right now. As soon as I can however, I would love to get on that.
_____

Hi Assorted Vibrations and faileforever:

It is not necessary to be starting a meditation group or anything specific to become a local AYP contact. Many of the people on the contacts/events list are "planning contacts," meaning they can be emailed to begin forming local networks of practitioners, which can lead eventually to meditation groups, training, retreats, etc. It does not necessarily mean taking the lead in doing any of these things.

If you would like to become a "planning contact" for your area, let me know via email and we can add you to the list. The experience has been that being on the list does not produce a flood of email, so not to worry about that. It does provide a means for a few people in each area to get in touch, and see where it might go from there. Being on the list as a planning contact involves no commitment beyond that -- pretty much what you have been looking for here in the forums, but with some better ongoing AYP visibility for your area.

Yes, it is surprising that we don't have any contacts listed for the west coast USA, particularly since a large portion of the AYP readership is there. Perhaps it is time to remedy the situation? :-)

The guru is in you.

2010/10/15 10:22:37
Satsang Cafe - General Questions on AYP
http://www.aypsite.org/forum/topic.asp?TOPIC_ID=8579&REPLY_ID=73842&whichpage=-1
Yogani - AYP for kids??

Hi njethwa:

See this lesson: http://www.aypsite.org/256.html

Wonderful to be spontaneously sharing your divine openings with your children.

The guru is in you.

2010/10/22 11:28:29
Satsang Cafe - General Questions on AYP
http://www.aypsite.org/forum/topic.asp?TOPIC_ID=8613&REPLY_ID=74091&whichpage=-1
Yogani ji's Guru?

Hi manigma:

My teachers were quite a few over the years, across a variety of traditions that I prefer not to name, so as to avoid unnecessary distractions. AYP does not rely on any lineage to project credibility, and must stand on its own, based on the direct experiences of those who use it -- it is about cause and effect.

And no, I have no relationship with Swami J. He was actually following AYP for a while in the early days, but departed the scene when I refused to get into identifying (labeling) particular levels of samad
Hi in practitioners for the application of particular practices. It is apparently what he does in his approach.

His way is respected, of course, but that is not the AYP way. Over time, I think we have gotten a pretty good handle on the overall process of human spiritual transformation via "self-directed" practice, which has been the objective since the beginning.

So, while AYP stands on the shoulders of many who have gone before, it is also an original approach that aims to empower the individual practitioner.

The guru is in you.

2010/10/27 10:43:56
Satsang Cafe - General Questions on AYP
http://www.aypsite.org/forum/topic.asp?TOPIC_ID=8625&REPLY_ID=74290&whichpage=-1
AYP Retreat Experience, Mensch Mill, PA - Oct 2010

Hi All:

Very happy to hear that the Pennsylvania retreat proved beneficial for so many of you.

On the subject of additional retreats, it will be good to do annual events -- everywhere. But this will not be enough. The ideal for many practitioners will be attending retreats 2-4 times per year. They don't have to all be in the same place, though it would be nice to have places where retreats are occurring quarterly like clockwork. Eventually it will get to that stage of development. It will evolve organically. Now that the "cat is out of the bag" that retreats really do work, there will likely be increasing demand for them. Bravo!

Speaking of which, we are now a "go" for the Kripalu March 20-25, 2011 retreat. So we have a world class facility lined up in Massachusetts, USA for a larger AYP retreat 5 months from now. Here we are on the Kripalu schedule. This information will be linked from the top left border of the AYP website and forums soon. Sign-ups will be through Kripalu.

You may have noticed me dropping a few hints in the forum recently that anyone anywhere can arrange for a facility, and we can provide the retreat leadership and help find attendees for it. Let me know if you are interested, and we can provide support.

In the course of doing more retreats here and there, it is expected that others will learn the ropes for leadership (encouraged), so we can be increasing our team of AYP retreat leaders, and keep expanding the number of retreats occurring around the world. It can grow organically like that.

Onward!

The guru is in you.

2010/11/02 07:08:09
Satsang Cafe - General Questions on AYP
http://www.aypsite.org/forum/topic.asp?TOPIC_ID=8625&REPLY_ID=74623&whichpage=-1
AYP Retreat Experience, Mensch Mill, PA - Oct 2010

quote:
_____
Originally posted by Victor

I would have loved to have been there and if ever a retreat is held on the west coast please count me in!
Pa is not out of the question for me as I have family in Philadelphia but it does take time to plan a trip out there. I would love to meet all of you face to face sometime!
_____

Hi Victor:

Sooner or later we will be having AYP retreats on the west coast USA. We finally have planning contacts in SF, LA and Seattle, and someone just volunteered for Oregon. See the "Meditation Groups, Training & Retreats" link in the top left column of this page.

The Kripalu retreat in western Massachusetts next March will be a 5 day one (the biggest one yet), and would be worth the trip from the west coast. There is a link for it in the top left border here.

If you'd like to get involved in planning a retreat for the west coast USA, let me know via email. We now have the ability to provide leadership for AYP retreats (small or large) anywhere.

All the best!

The guru is in you.

2010/10/27 06:19:37
Satsang Cafe - General Questions on AYP
http://www.aypsite.org/forum/topic.asp?TOPIC_ID=8633&REPLY_ID=74269&whichpage=-1
Energy drains to help others?

Hi Phil:

When coming off a retreat, it is common to feel somewhat invincible with all that inner silence, and we might be tempted to jump back into activity with both feet, including doing some things we might have hesitated to do before. Nothing wrong with this. We can do more. But it is suggested to allow a few days for the results of a retreat to settle in, easing back into activity gradually, if possible. There can be a bit of tenderness there, and it will stabilize as we integrate new levels of inner silence into our daily activity.

In other words, always self-pace. :-)

The guru is in you.

2010/10/27 10:07:08
Satsang Cafe - General Questions on AYP
http://www.aypsite.org/forum/topic.asp?TOPIC_ID=8633&REPLY_ID=74288&whichpage=-1
Energy drains to help others?

Hi Sage:

I don't recall anyone raising this issue in your case, though you are obviously sensitive about it. That's a good thing. "Awareness" will solve everything for us in time. As we know, meditation increases awareness.

Which brings me to ask, what are you doing here if you are not meditating? This is a forum about practices and experiences.

You are welcome to hang around, but what is the point if you are not into what is going on here? An ounce of real practice is worth ten pounds of talk. Try and see. :-)

All the best!

The guru is in you.

2010/11/13 11:52:22
Satsang Cafe - General Questions on AYP
http://www.aypsite.org/forum/topic.asp?TOPIC_ID=8644&REPLY_ID=75209&whichpage=-1
Deal with post-retreat purification

Hi Carson and Phil:

Along with self-pacing, more grounding activity and a heavier diet leaning toward pita pacifying can help. Basically all the measures discussed in Lesson 69.

More importantly, if this sort of overload and sensitivity is occurring for people coming off a retreat, then we will go back and look at the retreat structure and fine tune it for a smoother transition back into daily activity. Being the first in the USA, the Allentown retreat was rather gung-ho in a variety of practice areas, and now we are seeing the results of that. It's okay. These are matters that can be addressed with the retreat leaders for implementing a less aggressive retreat structure, leading to smoother transitions back into activity. It is yet another aspect of self-pacing.

We keep learning as we go along. :-)

The guru is in you.

2010/12/18 19:31:14
Satsang Cafe - General Questions on AYP
http://www.aypsite.org/forum/topic.asp?TOPIC_ID=8823&REPLY_ID=77097&whichpage=-1
Happy Holidays

Thank you All and happy holidays!

The guru is in you.

2010/12/17 08:08:28
Satsang Cafe - General Questions on AYP
http://www.aypsite.org/forum/topic.asp?TOPIC_ID=8908&REPLY_ID=76993&whichpage=-1
Derivation of "Yogani"?

Hi tamasaburo:

Yes, just something I picked up somewhere. No special meaning or connection intended other than the obvious yoga aspect.

From antiquity, Yogani is a female goddess, but there is no connection with that here. I only heard about it after.

And I only heard about "Yogani Studios" (in Tampa, Florida) later also. No connection there either.

All the best!

The guru is in you.

Forum 3 – Support for AYP Deep Meditation and Samyama

Entering and moving in stillness. The heart of yoga.
http://www.aypsite.org/forum/forum.asp?FORUM_ID=14

2005/07/10 11:26:40
Support for AYP Deep Meditation and Samyama
http://www.aypsite.org/forum/topic.asp?TOPIC_ID=275
Deep Meditation and Samyama

In the Psalms of the Old Testament of the Bible it says, "Be still and know I am God."

In the Bhagavad Gita it says, "If one can see stillness in action, and action in stillness, one is the wise one among men."

For a long time, wise people around the globe have been agreeing on this one point -- Inner stillness is the essence of enlightenment.

How do we cultivate this in ourselves? -- Deep Meditation!

This is why in the AYP lessons, deep meditation is the first practice covered, as soon we establish some clarity about our desire to undertake practices. Once we are established in a twice-daily meditation routine, all the rest of the practices tend to fall into place quite naturally. A little bit of inner stillness goes a very long way toward putting us on an even keel in yoga, and in everything else we undertake in life.

Meditation is the primary means for cultivating the inner peace and happiness that we all have been longing for. The longing is natural, for inner peace and happiness are found to be resident aspects of our inner nature when the obstructions in our nervous system begin to dissolve from the purifying influences of yoga practices.

In the AYP lessons, instructions on deep meditation begin at Lesson #13, and continue in many more lessons. See http://www.aypsite.org/13.html

Samyama is a practice that takes advantage of resident inner stillness (silence) we have cultivated in our nervous system through our daily meditation sessions over a period of time. Once we are able to introduce a faint intention in silence, then we can "move in stillness." This is samyama. The practice of samyama develops in us that sense of "seeing stillness in action and action in stillness." In that state, our desires become expressions of our inner silence and find fulfillment in ways we could not have anticipated before. For instructions on samyama, see http://www.aypsite.org/150.html

Samyama expands our daily life from the ordinary to become a constant stream of small miracles -- and sometimes big miracles. Such occurrences moving from within stillness are called "siddhis."

That is the beauty of yoga. We can begin to find some immediate practical benefits with deep meditation today, and, later on, we can find our experience still expanding. The possibilities in all of us are truly profound.

In this forum we hope the discussion will center on the thing that deep meditation and samyama have in common, stillness -- what it is and how to cultivate it in and around us. Keep in mind that we should be meditating for some time before we undertake samyama. That is covered in detail in the lessons. There is a logical progression in all of this. Rome was not built in a day...

In the many cultures and religions, the inherent ability in human beings to experience inner stillness has been called many things: inner silence, pure bliss consciousness, sat-chit-ananda, the void, tao, god the father, the silent seed, and so on. All these names mean the same thing.

As they say, "A rose is still a rose by any other name."

Begin deep meditation and find out for yourself what the rose is. You will find many here doing the same thing, and there will be much you can share.

The guru is in you.

2005/07/16 16:20:27
Support for AYP Deep Meditation and Samyama
http://www.aypsite.org/forum/topic.asp?TOPIC_ID=301&REPLY_ID=65&whichpage=-1
Lightening the karmic load

Hi Kathy:

When we talk about "releasing" karma in meditation, what we really mean is "transforming" it to a higher manifestation than would have happened otherwise. As the nervous system purifies, the shadowy elements of our karma become illuminated by pure bliss consciousness. The seeds of the karma remain, but with the light blooming through them from within we are inspired to act differently. So, if we wronged someone in the past (we all have), and the light is coming up, the seeds of that will inspire us to some kind of service that will not only illuminate others, but further illuminate us as well. In this way, karma is transformed to higher purpose.

As you know, when content comes up in meditation (all related to purification), we just easily go back to the mantra. In the process of purification we don't have to be analyzing the exhaust of it, which is what all thoughts, feelings and physical sensations are in meditation. We just keep letting go with the mantra into the infinite. Over time, that changes our relationship with our karma, and with everyone else's too. What we end up with is outpouring divine love sprouting out of those illuminated karmic seeds. That's why enlightenment comes in so many flavors -- so many flavors of pure love!

The guru is in you.

2005/07/20 13:35:59
Support for AYP Deep Meditation and Samyama
http://www.aypsite.org/forum/topic.asp?TOPIC_ID=306&REPLY_ID=103&whichpage=-1

First Time at Samyama

It only takes a little inner silence to begin to gain some benefit from samyama practice. In the AYP lessons we can leap-frog to samyama as soon as we feel we are ready. See the recent lesson on this at http://www.aypsite.org/269.html

Leap-frogging is not recommended for any other practice in AYP. But for samyama, it can serve us well if we have some inner silence coming up.

How do we know if we have some inner silence? If we find the mantra fading naturally and we are picking it up at very refined and fuzzy levels when we go back to it, then that is inner silence. That is also where we do samyama, at that fuzzy level on the edge of no thoughts at all. It is very simple. It is usually easy to notice if we are picking up the mantra at a refined level. We cannot force this to happen. It happens according to ongoing purification. It will not be refined like that all the time either. It depends on what purification is going on in our nervous system at the moment. If it is refined like that from time to time, then we can benefit from samyama. In fact, samyama will improve our ability to pick up the mantra deep in the mind.

So, if we are having that experience of fuzzy mantra fading away, then samyama will not be a waste of time. If we start too early with samyama, we will not do ourselves any harm either. As always, it is up to you. Here it is: http://www.aypsite.org/150.html Make sure to read the lessons before and after too, so you will get the whole picture.

The guru is in you.

2005/07/20 19:51:39
Support for AYP Deep Meditation and Samyama
http://www.aypsite.org/forum/topic.asp?TOPIC_ID=306&REPLY_ID=109&whichpage=-1
First Time at Samyama

Thanks, Jim.

Yes, it takes time to undertake all these practices, and jumping the gun on next steps will give us symptomatic feedback from within pretty soon. We will be wise to pace ourselves accordingly, allowing weeks, months or longer between forays into new practices, giving adequate time to acclimate to the one we last took on, like samyama in this case.

With all these powerful practices lined up in a row in the AYP lessons, we have all but eliminated the age-old problem of finding them. Now we are limited only by our capacity to absorb them smoothly and safely with the accelerated purification in the nervous system they cultivate. We are all different in this, so it becomes a matter of personal management, which we call "self-pacing" in the lessons.

With the practices readily available, self-pacing becomes a huge deal. As important as any practice -- maybe more important, because, if we can't build our daily routine in an orderly fashion we will not be able to continue steadily toward our enlightenment. Given the crucial role of self-pacing in AYP, a whole forum is devoted to it here. See http://www.aypsite.org/forum/forum.asp?FORUM_ID=18

In that forum, we can look at self-pacing from many angles with lots of feedback from practitioners. It is in the Q&As of the AYP lessons quite a lot already. See "self-pacing" in the topic index at http://www.aypsite.org/TopicIndex.html for links to many case study lessons on self-pacing. There is much more we can discuss on this.

The guru is in you.

2005/10/06 10:42:31
Support for AYP Deep Meditation and Samyama
http://www.aypsite.org/forum/topic.asp?TOPIC_ID=505&REPLY_ID=850&whichpage=-1
Meditation and Hypnosis

Hi Jim:

There's no doubt that auto-suggestion is real. It is what most self-improvement systems rely upon, and most popular approaches to spiritual development as well (including fads).

I do not regard deep meditation to be auto-suggestion, as it is not involved with meaning. Rather it is setting the mind up to be active without a particular meaning or direction. In this situation it naturally goes to its source, which is pure bliss consciousness. As you know, we easily favor the mantra when we realize that thoughts or sensations have come up. The result of this process over time is abiding inner silence -- not by auto-suggestion, but by natural exposure to that quality of stillness within us.

I believe there are people who use auto-suggestion to induce transcendence to inner silence, which is a far cry from ordinary behavior modification oriented hypnosis. I know little of it, except that it exists, and seems to have ancient origins.

In samyama, which is a special form of auto-suggestion, the suggestions are manifested from within pure bliss consciousness for spiritual purification and opening, and this process is morally self-regulating. Our inner silence (inner guru) is the source of all truth and love.

As for abuses by third parties, well, it can happen. That's why I always say...

The guru is in you.

2005/10/18 13:37:56
Support for AYP Deep Meditation and Samyama
http://www.aypsite.org/forum/topic.asp?TOPIC_ID=529&REPLY_ID=1011&whichpage=-1
Mantra Enhancement

Hi All:

Glad to hear some are finding the mantra enhancements to be effective for broadening the swath of the purification process going in and coming out through the mind and nervous system in deep meditation. That is just what the enhancements are for.

Keep in mind that the measure of our meditation is not in our subjective experience while doing it. That can be anything, from the sublime to the ridiculous, according to the purification that is occurring at any point in time. If we are observing the easy procedure of meditation, it will be right and the results will be there. <u>The true measure of meditation is in how we feel afterward in daily activity.</u>

Anthem is right in mentioning the potential hazards of using the mono-pole OM syllable alone in deep meditation. While it may feel great for a while, it will more than likely lead to some imbalance somewhere along the line. OM is the natural vibration of our nervous system when awakened to ecstatic conductivity and radiance. Then OM emanates naturally from the medulla oblongata (brain stem) and reverberates throughout the nervous system, and beyond. But OM is not the ideal vehicle to use alone in deep meditation to achieve that awakening. We are all attracted to it, and would like to see OM in there at some point, and that is what we do down the road in the second enhancement of the mantra -- incorporate OM in a balanced dual-pole way once we reach an adequate level of purification in our nervous system.

Modifying our mantra based on how it "feels" during meditation is not a sound approach. This week it will feel great. Next week it will not feel so great. Then what will we do? Change it again? That's not a practical formula for achieving effective long term results. It is like following the ever-changing scenery instead of the road. Where will we end up? Who knows?

Much better to stick with our mantra and regard all the ups and downs equally -- using thought streams as signals to easily come back to the mantra. It takes many months for a mantra to settle in. Deep meditation is a marathon based on steady practice, not a sprint based on the local scenery -- sort of a tortoise and hare thing, you know.

On pronunciation, "I AM" is like the English. Or "AYAM," if you'd like to drop the English spelling -- same pronunciation. The quality of the mantra is not determined by how it feels at its gross level of pronunciation in the mind. In fact, pronunciation will rarely be clear as we go deep during our meditation. At the deepest levels in the mind, there will be no discernable pronunciation at all -- just a faint impulse. A vague vibration deep inside us, even as we open to the vastness of pure bliss consciousness within. So, no one is asking you to be hollering "AYAM!" in the depths of your being. The mantra is a vehicle that dissolves into the pure bliss consciousness that is the essential fabric within us. The mantra vehicle is designed to resonate throughout a particular subtle neurological range within our nervous system (the sushumna), thus purifying it. That is true of the enhancements as well, as discussed in lesson #188, which goes into the design principles of the AYP mantras: http://www.aypsite.org/188.html

For the reasons given in the lesson, it is suggested that changes in mantra be based on sound principles and good self-pacing, rather than on the subjective experiences of the day. You will know you are on the right track with your practice if you feel more steadiness and joy in daily activity, no matter what the subjective experience in meditation may be.

Some other lessons on mantra and enhancements are:

First instructions on deep meditation - http://www.aypsite.org/13.html
On OM and the dual pole principle - http://www.aypsite.org/59.html
On changes in mantra during meditation - http://www.aypsite.org/79.html
On mantra mixed with thoughts - http://www.aypsite.org/195.html
On first enhancement of mantra - http://www.aypsite.org/116.html
On second enhancement of mantra - http://www.aypsite.org/186.html

There is a third enhancement of the mantra in the AYP Book.

The guru is in you.

2005/10/18 14:12:13
Support for AYP Deep Meditation and Samyama
http://www.aypsite.org/forum/topic.asp?TOPIC_ID=529&REPLY_ID=1013&whichpage=-1
Mantra Enhancement

David & Meg:

Yes, ahhh versus ehhh is okay, though the original is as in Sam, ham, bam, ram, etc. Then the OM syllable opens it up much further with the second enhancement. As mentioned, OM is not the best place to start.

On ayOM, you may be jumping the gun on that one for reasons mentioned above, Meg. It is up to you. Do let us know how it goes.

Actually, the same goes for Rob with the inclusion of OM instead of I AM after SHREE in the first enhancement.

This is the OM freelancer topic!

Better to follow the prescription for all the reasons mentioned.

The guru is in you.

REVISED WITH CLARIFICATIONS
2005/10/18 17:24:32
Support for AYP Deep Meditation and Samyama
http://www.aypsite.org/forum/topic.asp?TOPIC_ID=529&REPLY_ID=1021&whichpage=-1
Mantra Enhancement

quote:
_____

Rob wrote: So from everything i have gathered (and again thanks to all) i should consciously go back to the i am vibration/sound.
_____

Yes, right, Rob. That is normal meditation. Other mantras that may come up are to be treated like any other thought in meditation, and we just ease back to the mantra we have been using.

If we are deep, and the mantra is faint, we do not have to come back to a clear pronunciation of the mantra. If I AM (or whatever enhanced version we are using) becomes very faint and then we realize we are off into something else that is also faint, then we can easily come back to the faint version of our mantra, like that. If we come out into a clear (surface level) thought stream, then we can pick up the mantra clearly at that level and let it refine again. In other words, whatever level we are at in the mind when we realize we are off the mantra, that is the level where we can pick up the mantra again. In this way we take maximum advantage of the mind's natural ability to go to stillness.

The guru is in you.

2005/10/19 12:22:32
Support for AYP Deep Meditation and Samyama
http://www.aypsite.org/forum/topic.asp?TOPIC_ID=529&REPLY_ID=1038&whichpage=-1
Mantra Enhancement

Hi All:

I have some reservations about trying to peg the pronunciation of the mantra exactly. It is fine to offer some suggestions, written or oral, but you should keep in mind that the mantra is <u>yours</u> and best kept internal to your process of deep meditation. This is part of why traditional mantra initiations are often kept secret. The personal internal aspect of it is pretty important. Otherwise, we can be digging things up too much.

Consider this: There have been cases where secret mantras have been compared between people after many years of successful practice, only to find that the pronunciations of the very same mantra have been different. And, in fact, different oral traditons do use different pronounciations. So then you get into the argument on who is right. Endless nonsense! The one who is right is the one who is meditating and not arguing. :-)

The mantra is a vibrational frequency in thought that we use to go beyond thought. Whether we start a few hertz this way or that way is not going to make a difference. We want to be comfortable with the process of using our mantra. That is most important, and it takes some time to settle in with that. Spending a lot of time and effort trying to peg the frequency exactly can become a distraction that can undermine our confidence and our process of meditation. There is no such thing as an exactly right mantra pronunciation. There are many degrees, and that is okay. If your meditation is bringing good results in daily activity, then continue without unnecessary second-guessing. If it is bringing some roughness in activity, it will very unlikely be the mantra. 99.9% of the time it will be straining or overdoing in some way. So the best place to put our attention is on keeping the innocence of the deep meditation process, and on self-pacing of our practices as necessary. Taking it easy is the key. Less fuss will bring better results. We have all experienced that, yes?

As mentioned, some temporary roughness or other experiences within our meditation itself will not be mantra pronunciation related either. Experiences in meditation are due to our cycles of purification. From the lessons we know the procedures for dealing with that.

So carry on with your practice, and enjoy!

The guru is in you.

2005/10/20 12:14:35
Support for AYP Deep Meditation and Samyama
http://www.aypsite.org/forum/topic.asp?TOPIC_ID=529&REPLY_ID=1056&whichpage=-1
Mantra Enhancement

Thank you, David. Your sharings are always valuable insights.

One thing I would like to avoid is: "This is IT and you are damned if you are doing anything else."

I know you are not thinking like that, and the pronunciation suggestions are much welcome.

At the same time, we'd like to avoid absolutes in implementation, allowing everyone to find their own comfort level with their personal practice. That is essential. If we are each applying the underlying principles on the basis of cause and effect, we will be doing just right. That is the scientific approach.

Being an "open source," AYP is different from the established traditions. We do not want to create another one of those! Instead, we would like to help everyone find their way into the "ball park" of effective yoga practices. From there, it is a matter of each practitioner developing self-sufficiency. That is the key to traveling this, or any, road to enlightenment. Hopefully, AYP provides everyone enough solid information and "wiggle room" to do just that. Each person can use the teachings as they like, and not be condemned for being creative, or simply going with what resonates. As mentioned in the past, I do not consider AYP to be the last word on yoga, and I hope others will carry this exciting field of applied yoga science forward into the future. The AYP writings are intended to be a point of reference to aid in the ongoing process of self-discovery, which is the process of human spiritual transformation.

The real goal here is to develop a sound, flexible open source methodology that will stimulate the evolution and horizontal (person to person) transmission of practical yogic knowledge indefinitely. There is room for many points of view along the way to unfolding the truth within us.

So keep on sharing, everyone, and all the best!

The guru is in you.

2005/11/06 00:20:36
Support for AYP Deep Meditation and Samyama
http://www.aypsite.org/forum/topic.asp?TOPIC_ID=529&REPLY_ID=1397&whichpage=-1
Mantra Enhancement

Hello Farooq, and welcome!

Of course, I cannot confirm every sound that new meditators may wish to consider trying for mantra. There are sacred names in all the traditions that may or may not make suitable mantras. It is the sound vibration, not the meaning, that matters when we go deep into the nervous system. The underlying principles are reviewed in the AYP lessons -- see my first October 18th post in this topic for links to some lessons on this.

Of particular importance is the pairing of linear and circular components in the mantra that will enliven and open the spinal nerve in a balanced way. This is the nature of the I AM mantra, as well as the enhancements which come later. This theme of cultivating and balancing our inner polarities runs through all of the other AYP practices, as well.

I certainly do not disparage you your urge to honor your traditional roots in Islam. Cultivating inner silence in your nervous system through deep meditation will definitely aid in this. This is the magic of inner silence. It enlivens our perception of the truth in all the religions, especially our own. But engaging in deep meditation on syllables that are dear to us in meaning is not always the most efficient way to do this. If we do so, we will be engaging in our own research, and that is not something that can be measured in a few days or weeks, and definitely not known subjectively within meditation itself. Our experience in daily activity over time is the truest measure of the success of our practice. Also, keep in mind that when we begin to consider mantra enhancements later on, it will be more complicated if we are using a different mantra on the front end.

Of course, the choice is yours. Certainly there are many ways to conduct the process of human spiritual transformation. I am just not in a position to vouch for the efficiency of all of them at this time. Keep in mind that mixing approaches can sometimes lead us to less instead of more, as has been discussed here in the AYP forums from time to time. If we keep at the discussion long enough, I am sure we will come to know much more about variations that will work, and about ones that will not. That is the mission of open spiritual science. The important thing is that we keep moving forward with the sincere intention to find and optimize means that will bring us the best results on our path, and the most useful knowledge we can record for the benefit those who come after us.

As Rumi, the great Sufi master said:
"Keep walking, though there's no place to get to.
Don't try to see through the distances.
That's not for human beings.
Move within,
But don't move the way fear makes you move."

All the best!

The guru is in you.

2005/11/06 13:00:54
Support for AYP Deep Meditation and Samyama
http://www.aypsite.org/forum/topic.asp?TOPIC_ID=529&REPLY_ID=1404&whichpage=-1
Mantra Enhancement

Hi again:

Great topic links, Jim.

Farooq, it can also be mentioned that "allah" is phonetically similar to "namah," which is in the 2nd and 3rd AYP mantra enhancements. As discussed in lesson #188, "namah" is added "for its syllables (lengthening), and as a traditional transition in mantra repetitions. It resonates ecstatically in the heart, cultivating bhakti, and has a purifying effect throughout the nervous system."

We do not start with "namah" as a beginning mantra because it is necessary to prepare the nervous system for the additional heart opening it brings, as well as for the additional syllables. From the AYP perspective, perhaps "allah" would fit as a replacement for "namah" at that stage. It is just a possibility -- not tested for longevity here. But perhaps a reasonable approach that is in the direction of the AYP style of mantra progression.

It is not recommended to jump straight to mantra enhancements in AYP. Better to follow the guidelines in the lessons. If we go too soon, it can be unsettling, like shifting gears in a manual transmission car prematurely.

Food for thought... :-)

The guru is in you.

2008/05/09 16:04:52
Support for AYP Deep Meditation and Samyama
http://www.aypsite.org/forum/topic.asp?TOPIC_ID=529&REPLY_ID=33568&whichpage=-1
Mantra Enhancement

Hi Thomas:

It can be either, according to your choice. Some go for the ooo..., and others go for the aaww...

It was discussed in some detail beginning here: http://www.aypsite.org/forum/topic.asp?TOPIC_ID=3473&whichpage=2#30249

Pronunciation is less important than the systematic refinement of the mantra to stillness in deep meditation. If pronunciation is focused on too much, the refinement can be disrupted as the mind keeps grasping for the object near the surface. Meditation is the dissolving of the mantra to stillness/samad
Hi over and over again. So pick your starting point and go. It will be faint and fuzzy soon enough, and that is good.

If I offer a particular starting pronunciation, someone is sure to get overly concerned about this, and no one should. So the advice is to make it your own ... it will be very good. :-)

Enjoy!

The guru is in you.

2005/10/27 11:56:20
Support for AYP Deep Meditation and Samyama
http://www.aypsite.org/forum/topic.asp?TOPIC_ID=546&REPLY_ID=1220&whichpage=-1
cotton, earplugs

Hi All:

Interesting discussion.

A reminder: When we are meditating, we easily come back to the mantra when we realize we are off into thoughts or sensations. That applies to sensory inputs too, like noise. We don't hang on to sensory inputs, or try and push them out either. We just easily favor the mantra. That is the procedure. This makes it possible to meditate effortlessly on planes, in buses, or right next to road construction if we have to. I think you have touched on these points already, so pardon me for repeating.

There is also another dimension to this...

As we gain more experience in meditation, there is a certain charm that develops in it -- we become more connected with inner silence and naturally go there, barely favoring the mantra. We still use the procedure of meditation, of course, but the attractiveness of inner silence finds an increasing role. Then it is like listening to our favorite music. Outside inputs, like noise, are barely noticed. And if they are, they do not hold our attention for long. Our "intention" automatically goes to the joy of inner silence. So what begins as a mechanical procedure (meditation), eventually becomes a natural absorption of the mind in blissful silence (samadhi). We never give up the easy mental procedure we are in the habit of using during meditation. It refines and blends to become part of our increasingly-present inner silence.

We become inner silence. Inner silence becomes us. Then, even noise is heard in silence, and we don't mind. Daily life in activity gradually becomes like that too. It is a great way to live!

This is not to guide either way on the ear plugs. Do what is comfortable for you, and know that it will all work out fine over time. And do favor keeping the eyes closed while meditating. That is part of creating the best condition we can under the circumstances. If we were fish, we'd have to meditate with eyes open. But since we are not fish, we don't have to. There is plenty of time to see the world colored with our blissful inner silence during our daily activity. :-)

The guru is in you.

2005/11/06 13:22:16
Support for AYP Deep Meditation and Samyama
http://www.aypsite.org/forum/topic.asp?TOPIC_ID=572&REPLY_ID=1406&whichpage=-1
Shutting off the senses

Hi Etherfish:

How about cultivating inner silence naturally in deep meditation and samyama, awakening prana (ecstatic conductivity) in the spine and nervous system with spinal breathing, mudras, bandhas, etc., and then let the senses fall where they may?

With all of that, the senses are naturally drawn inward to ever-increasing levels of ecstatic bliss in stillness, which is what pratyahara is experientially. It is effect in this case. Very easy and enjoyable effect -- with zero extended concentration involved.

It is attraction toward something (adding) rather than pushing away from something (subtracting)...

The guru is in you.

2005/11/06 17:51:35
Support for AYP Deep Meditation and Samyama
http://www.aypsite.org/forum/topic.asp?TOPIC_ID=572&REPLY_ID=1412&whichpage=-1
Shutting off the senses

Hi again:

Other ways of looking at it from the AYP perspective are:

1. We do not deny the senses. We expand them to divine experience, so we are naturally drawn to endlessly more refined inner enjoyment.

2. We do not deny sexuality. We expand it inward to higher expression in the nervous system where levels of divine enjoyment far exceed the carnal.

3. We do not try and stop the mind. We lure it inward to its own endless bliss of inner stillness.

So, you see, we are following the same principle of attraction in all the AYP practices. In this way all of our external experiences are eventually purged with outpouring joy and love.

If we are lost in the revery of Mozart, will we hear the cricket chirping outside our window? For us, the cricket will be playing Mozart too!

The guru is in you.

2005/11/20 11:40:14
Support for AYP Deep Meditation and Samyama
http://www.aypsite.org/forum/topic.asp?TOPIC_ID=598&REPLY_ID=1578&whichpage=-1

losing control/ witnessing thoughts in meditation

Hi Alvin:

Going back to the mantra is not imperative under all circumstances. We only do it when it is easy -- never forcing or laboring over it. You will become more familiar with this with more experience, and be less concerned when you get into those occasional fuzzy sleep-like states. Just keep in mind, if we are remembering to pick up the mantra but it is not easy, then we just passively witness whatever is happening until things clear up enough for us to easily come back to the mantra. So you are right on that.

However, we do not deliberately try and do both things at the same time -- mantra and witnessing. That is giving attention to two procedures at once, which divides the mind, weakening the meditation. If we have the ability to choose, we always choose the mantra, because that procedure will take us deep over and over again. The witnessing procedure is okay to use separately for expediting a dominant process of purification (that is the prescription in AYP), but is not as progressive for taking us deep as effective mantra use is. That is why passive witnessing-style meditation systems take much longer to produce the same results that proactive mantra-style meditation does. Passive witnessing by itself works, but yields slower purification and requires longer sittings. That is why in AYP meditation we always favor the mantra when we have the choice to easily do that. The result is much more progress in much shorter sittings. Efficiency!

As a result of deep meditation over time, the witness will rise and be there naturally without any conscious effort. That is different. Then we will be witnessing the mantra and everything else inside and outside meditation. That does not change the procedure of meditation, which is the cause of the rising witness and all that springs from it later on.

This is covered from several angles in the lessons, and even more so in the new book coming out soon -- "Deep Meditation."

All the best!

The guru is in you.

2006/02/07 14:08:13
Support for AYP Deep Meditation and Samyama
http://www.aypsite.org/forum/topic.asp?TOPIC_ID=598&REPLY_ID=3138&whichpage=-1
losing control/ witnessing thoughts in meditation
That's right, Anthem.

When we are riding a bike, do we think, "Now I will lean this way and then that way to stay up."

No. We just ride the bike without thinking about how we are doing it. Only in the very beginning while we were learning did we think about how to do it.

It is the same with deep meditation. We think about the procedure while we are learning. Once we know how, have the habit, it has become automatic. Then we just easily come back to the most comfortable level of the mantra when we find ourselves somewhere else, anywhere else. Nothing to wait for or think about. We just do it. The practice becomes transparent to the thinking process, just as riding a bike is.

The simple habit of this procedure in deep meditation has huge implications in our daily life, not the least of which is a rising ability to easily walk past all the obstacles that stand between us and our destiny.

The guru is in you.

2005/11/28 14:54:01
Support for AYP Deep Meditation and Samyama
http://www.aypsite.org/forum/topic.asp?TOPIC_ID=609&REPLY_ID=1682&whichpage=-1
The ..I AM.. meditation and astral music

Hi Chiron:

No, music is not recommended to be intentionally used during deep meditation. It can divide the mind and impede the process of attention going beyond the mind to inner silence. Here are a couple of lessons that discuss it further -- covering all sensory inputs introduced intentionally in deep meditation that can divide our attention in practice:

http://www.aypsite.org/37.html
http://www.aypsite.org/31.html

This does not mean we can't meditate with inner or outer stimuli present. The procedure of easily favoring the mantra when we realize we are off into thoughts, feelings or sensations takes care of this. But we do not intentionally introduce stimuli into our awareness.

With good deep meditation, according to the simple procedures of practice, we will benefit even more when listening to the music afterward, as discussed in the second question here:

http://www.aypsite.org/161.html

The guru is in you.

2005/11/29 10:24:35
Support for AYP Deep Meditation and Samyama
http://www.aypsite.org/forum/topic.asp?TOPIC_ID=609&REPLY_ID=1690&whichpage=-1
The ..I AM.. meditation and astral music

Hi Chiron:

Yes, do follow David's advice and go through the lessons in order. Then if there are further questions, fire away.

One additional point on noise in your environment: There is a topic here on using earplugs, white noise, etc. to deal with a noisy meditation place. See http://www.aypsite.org/forum/topic.asp?TOPIC_ID=546

Such measures are not going to block "inner" sensory experiences, so I am more inclined to encourage everyone to develop the habit of easily favoring the mantra over whatever is going on inside or outside. But if you are in a "rough patch," getting started in a noisy place, then do what is necessary to develop a comfortable routine of practice.

I suggest you stick with 20 minutes meditation. This is discussed in the lessons. And try and resist going off in too many directions at once. Save your time and energy for a smooth logical build-up. Believe me, there is plenty more to do in AYP, in due course. You will read all about it ... the most important thing is to develop a stable routine that you can stay with for the long term. The path of yoga is a marathon, not a sprint.

The guru is in you.

2005/12/01 09:45:22
Support for AYP Deep Meditation and Samyama
http://www.aypsite.org/forum/topic.asp?TOPIC_ID=609&REPLY_ID=1730&whichpage=-1
The ..I AM.. meditation and astral music

Hi Chiron:

The main difference in effect between padmasana and siddhasana is in the degree of direct tantric stimulation. This is discussed in an AYP lesson here: http://www.aypsite.org/127.html

All the best!

The guru is in you.

2005/12/12 23:08:24
Support for AYP Deep Meditation and Samyama
http://www.aypsite.org/forum/topic.asp?TOPIC_ID=639&REPLY_ID=1927&whichpage=-1
Meditating with the 'I am' mantra

Hi Matthew, and welcome!

It is good that you are making the separation between mantra and breathing now, as it will enable you to go much deeper.

Whenever we add a new practice or make a change, there will be that "clunky stage" in the beginning. After a while things smooth out. You will find it to be the case with this also. If you just treat the breath like any other thought, emotion or sensation, and easily favor the mantra when you realize you are off it, that will be correct practice and things will smooth out soon enough.

A rhythm with the mantra can be there, but it will change according to whatever is going on in our nervous system. Also, it can be quite clear in pronunciation or very fuzzy and indistinct, or practically nothing at all. We just easily go with it at whatever level it is, not forcing it to go one way or the other. We do not decide the mantra's journey with any exterior bias. If we follow the procedure, the mantra will take us much deeper than any particular enforced rhythm, visualization or following the breath can.

At times there will be little to no breath when using the mantra in this easy way. We will be free of breath, and still going deeper far beyond breath, without even noticing it. Breathing stopping is not intentional (not a goal). It happens by itself without us doing anything with breath. It is the metabolism we are automatically slowing down in deep meditation, and the breath naturally follows.

Breath is a good follower in deep meditation like that. It is not a good leader in meditation. When breath is leading we are doing pranayama, and that has a different purpose than meditation. Pranayama can be very pleasant, ecstatic even, but we do not want to confuse that with meditation. We also do plenty with pranayama in AYP in other parts of our sitting practice. It is an important practice. But meditation and pranayama are separate practices with separate purposes. Pranayama is for cultivating ecstatic conductivity in the nervous system. It also paves the way, preparing the ground for deep meditation which goes much deeper, cultivating our inner silence. So there are two purposes which have profound long term results if developed in that way. That is why Patanjali has these two elements as separate limbs in the eight limbs of yoga.

Wishing you all the best on your path. Practice wisely, and enjoy!

The guru is in you.

2005/12/14 15:08:52
Support for AYP Deep Meditation and Samyama
http://www.aypsite.org/forum/topic.asp?TOPIC_ID=639&REPLY_ID=1955&whichpage=-1
Meditating with the 'I am' mantra

Hi Matthew and Ute:

The listening is okay if there is something stirring in the mantra department. However, if nothing is stirring, the procedure is to easily pick it up. Deep meditation with mantra is proactive, while passive listening and waiting for something to emerge is a different practice. The latter is a common meditation technique used in some of the traditions, particularly with OM -- listening, waiting for it to come. In our AYP deep meditation sessions we do not wait.

As it has been said, "If the mountain will not come to Mohammed, then Mohammed will go to the mountain."

The guru is in you.

2005/12/15 08:22:16

Hi Matthew:

The next thing to let go of is the analysis of what the mantra is doing during meditation. When you find yourself thinking in meditation, "Oh, the mantra is doing this or that," just treat it like any other thought and easily go back to the mantra at whatever level it is comfortable.

You will be an expert at this in no time. Less is more. :-)

The guru is in you.

2005/12/15 10:37:15

Hi Alvin:

We treat physical sensations, including muscular movements that might happen with mantra, the same as thoughts and feelings, and just easily come back to the mantra. The more we "work" on these other things coming to our attention, the more of an impediment they become, and we will be off the practice. The idea is to develop the habit of easily favoring the mantra over everything that comes up in body, mind or feelings. There is nothing to work on or solve. We just go with the procedure. Very simple...

Except, of course, unless someone yells, "Fire!" Then we do whatever is necessary to save life and limb. :-)

The guru is in you.

2005/12/18 10:59:35

quote:
_____
Originally posted by rabar

I have been concentrating on "pronouncing" (silently) I AM
with the true 'flat' A. When I focus on the actual pronunciation
of the 'A,' the mantra seems to merge with another ongoing sound
that I describe as around the notes 'g' and 'a' three octaves above
middle 'C'. Technically known as 'tinnitus,' this sound increases
for me during meditation. Someone recently mentioned that in his practice it increases during the headstand. I also remember back in 'head stand' days that was true for me as well. But thinking the 'AM' with the correct 'A' - if sounded aloud you have to smile to say it - is quite interesting.
_____

Hi Rabar:

While all of these experiments sound interesting, I hope you are not doing them during your regular deep meditation sessions. It is so much simpler than that. In fact, the success of the practice depends on maintaining the simplicity of the procedure. Correct practice involves no analysis whatsoever, and no concentration. We are just easily picking up the mantra when we realize we are off with our attention into anything else. Anything else. And the pronunciation is as simple as how they say "I AM" on the English-speaking evening news. Spell it "AYAM" if you like -- this removes the meaning, which is not part of deep meditation. There is wiggle room on pronunciation, as has been discussed in detail in this topic: http://www.aypsite.org/forum/topic.asp?TOPIC_ID=529

It is not necessary to peg the pronunciation or frequency of the sound, or anything like that. It is going to be changing during deep meditation anyway, according to purification going on in the nervous system. We let it change however it will. We just begin, and then follow the procedure for coming back to the mantra at whatever level we find ourselves inside when we realize we are not on it. That is all there is to it ... all the rest we are inclined to put into the process is baggage that will only hamper our natural merging with pure bliss consciousness -- our inner silence.

All the best!

The guru is in you.

2005/12/21 13:38:40
Welcome Robert!

We do not deliberately synchronize mantra and breath. And we only sit to meditate twice per day for 20 minutes. Below is a section from the new book, *Deep Meditation*, on breath in AYP deep meditation. You can find useful information in this small book on the key aspects of beginning and maintaining your meditation practice.

Note: See also my posting of Dec 12th in this topic on mantra and breath.

The guru is in you.

From the Deep Meditation book:

Breath Slowing Down

When our mind settles down during deep meditation, the body naturally goes with it. This can be measured directly in a variety of our biological functions. One of these is the breath, which is tied to our rate of metabolism. So, mind slows down, energy consumption in the body slows down, metabolism in our cells slows down, and breath slows down.

In fact, sometimes, breath can practically stop during our deep meditation. This is nothing to worry about. It means that our body is going to profound levels of quietness during meditation, and this is the catalyst for deep purification within our nervous system. So, the breath slowing down in deep meditation is a precursor of purification in the nervous system, a natural manifestation of the presence of inner silence.

It is very revealing that the breath slows down automatically as the mind goes to stillness. It is direct proof of the intimate mind/body connection that exists in us. We don't need a laboratory experiment to verify this. All we have to do is sit and meditate, and we will see for ourselves soon enough.

We do not make an effort to slow the breath while we are meditating. Neither do we deliberately synchronize the mantra with the breath. If it happens inadvertently, it is okay, but we do not favor it. We just leave the breath to do naturally what it will in deep meditation.

This is how we will achieve the best results. Deep meditation is just a simple procedure of easily favoring the mantra, no matter what else may come to our attention – breath, thoughts, feelings, physical sensations, and so on. In our practice of deep meditation, less will be more and more will be less. While other systems of practice may use the breath as an object of attention, we do not in deep meditation.

It is by following the procedure of deep meditation that the process of purification will be conducted automatically in our nervous system. Sometimes the mind will go very still, and usually the breath along with it. Other times we will be filled with thoughts and sensations inside, and the breath will be normal. It is even possible for the breath to speed up for short periods if the body is undergoing strong purification. But the more common experience will be a slowing down of the breath. It is normal, and part of the beneficial effects of deep meditation.

2005/12/22 12:07:12
Support for AYP Deep Meditation and Samyama
http://www.aypsite.org/forum/topic.asp?TOPIC_ID=661&REPLY_ID=2082&whichpage=-1
Meditation, Detachment and Daily Activity

Hi Y:

As the witness comes up, there can be that sense of separateness. It can be misinterpreted as an aloofness, but that is only a temporary situation or stage that we can easily let go of in favor of so much more. Inner silence wants to move out from us into the environment in many ways. That is its (our) nature. In fact, the expression of concern you have given here is a symptom of silence wanting to move outward!

It is a normal evolution of consciousness you are going through.

In the new book, **Deep Meditation**, the progression is covered from inner silence to witness stage, to rising ecstasy, and to the unity of outpouring divine love. It just keeps evolving like that.

Good experience ... it is freedom on the rise ... your freedom, and everyone's. Carry on! :-)

The guru is in you.

2005/12/26 11:10:25
Support for AYP Deep Meditation and Samyama
http://www.aypsite.org/forum/topic.asp?TOPIC_ID=667&REPLY_ID=2168&whichpage=-1
samadhi

Hi All:

I view the various symptoms being discussed here as manifestations of inner silence and its first child, pranic energy flow which is where the dramatic experiences come from. The manifestations can be called "grades of samadhi," but I think it is not important to be categorizing these, especially since they have no bearing on our practices themselves (AYP style, that is). Some teachers attempt to categorize levels of samad Hi among their adherents and then assign different kinds of practices for each. I think this is a fruitless task -- not to mention that having "adherents" is not part of the new paradigm of knowledge transmission anyway. Last year I was chastised by a well-known guru for taking the view that categorizing levels of samad Hi is not relevant, and for refusing to impose a "samad Hi ranking system" on the AYP readers.

As you know, my point of view is that the relevance is in the practices themselves that will lead inevitably to all the rest, and we do not have to be measuring results except for the purpose of regulating our bhakti and practices for speed and comfort. In other words, we don't get hung up in the "scenery."

Having said all that, let me throw something into the samad Hi discussion...

First off, samad Hi has no edges. If we are feeling any drama or excitement, we are having an energy experience, not a samad Hi experience. Of course, we can feel the edge after the samad Hi experience, but that is energy too. We can have inner silence and energy mixed, and to the extent it has an edge, that is the energy moving. Inner silence has no edges. Energy is very edgy, and that edginess is due to "friction" of the energy moving through the obstructions in our purifying nerves. Ecstasy is that also, until it has been refined and joined back with inner silence. With the refinement and joining of the edgy energy experiences with inner silence, a new dynamic is begun which ends up being anything but flat and boring. Inner silence (the witness) alone can be flat and unedgy, but it is a step on the way to a new dynamism that makes our original peak experiences pale by comparison.

Inner silence wants to move. The more of it we are experiencing (or becoming), the more we want to move. That movement is something different from our old energy experiences, and it is not ego-based. It is along the lines of samyama, which is inner silence expressing out into the world on waves of ecstatic bliss, or divine love. Then we are a channel, rather than a purifying vehicle sputtering on the energy boiling out from our newly cultivated inner silence trying to get free to flow into the world in huge endless waves of divine love.

So we go from inner silence, to energy experiences born of the friction of neurological purification, to the flat witness, to energy becoming ecstatic conductivity, to the merging of ecstasy and inner silence and becoming ecstatic bliss, to the unity experience of outpouring divine love.

Maybe there are samad
Hi labels corresponding with all of that, but I think not nearly as descriptive of what is happening. It is a neurobiological progression, after all.

So, we just keep doing our practices and take the rest in stride. What was dramatic will become flat, will become ecstatic, will become quiet again (ecstatically blissful), and then the avalanche of divine love will be pouring out constantly as thundering silence.

Not to worry, it will all be there. It is already written in our nervous systems.

And yes, we do get used to each new stage quickly and the contrasts fade accordingly. Going home is like that...

The guru is in you.

2005/12/26 11:57:47
Support for AYP Deep Meditation and Samyama
http://www.aypsite.org/forum/topic.asp?TOPIC_ID=667&REPLY_ID=2172&whichpage=-1
samadhi
Great Meg:

I made a point of covering this in the new book, "Deep Meditation" too, because invariably when people find themselves becoming "the witness," they ask, "Is that all there is?"

There is much more. 24 hour witness is stage one enlightenment.

The guru is in you.

2005/12/29 10:26:36
Support for AYP Deep Meditation and Samyama
http://www.aypsite.org/forum/topic.asp?TOPIC_ID=678
Procedure with Mantra

Hi all:

From my email today:

Q:
I have been doing meditation in the AYP method for the last 8 months. I still cannot keep my mind on the mantra. My mind wanders a lot and these days I cannot seem to meditate for than 10 mins.. my mind just wont co-cooperate. At the most I can keep the mantra for 6 or 7 secs...and then I am lost... come back..and maybe another 6 or 7 secs. Am I doing something wrong? How will I ever progress at this rate. Is this common... after 8 months to be meditating like a beginner. I have never been able to keep my mind on the mantra for more than 10 sec. and that had not improved in the least bit over the 8 months. However I could easily sit for 20 mins before but now after 10 my mind just wont go back to the mantra... my eyes open and my mind almost refuses to co-operate. I must be doing something wrong....How do I keep my mind on the mantra for more than 10 secs and how do I go back to my 20 mins?

A:
The object of meditation is not to stay on the mantra. It is to easily favor it when we realize we are off it. Big difference. Losing the mantra is the name of the game. With that, the mind goes to stillness. It might be for an infinitesimal second and then back into thoughts and feelings. The thoughts and feelings are the signal that it has happened, so they are a good sign. Then when we realize we are in thoughts, we just pick up the mantra again wherever we left off. We do not hang onto the mantra. It will go away and that is perfect. Neither do we hang onto thoughts and feelings. We do not hang on to anything. We do not analyze during our meditation. We just do the procedure.

I think the new *Deep Meditation* book is pretty clear on this. Maybe review it again. It is always good to have confirmation on what the practice is. The mind can make it complicated in 1000 ways. It always comes back to the simplicity of the procedure -- picking the mantra up when we realize we are off it. It may happen only once in a session. Or it may happen 100 times in a session. It doesn't matter. That is the procedure no matter what happens. And that is what will give us the result -- growing inner silence in our life.

If there is restlessness that makes if difficult to effortlessly pick up the mantra, we can stop and just be with the sensations for a few minutes. Just being with the strong sensations will help the purification that is going on to complete itself. Then when things settle down, we can go back to the mantra.

Make sure to take adequate rest before getting up after meditation. That is important. No matter how the purification goes in our meditation session, the test will be in how we feel afterward in activity. If there is some roughness in activity, then we may need to self-pace our practice a bit until things smooth out. It is all about purification and opening -- a process we are managing. It is not about sticking on the mantra or anything else except the easy procedure, and then going out and living our life normally in-between meditation sessions.

The number of months, years or decades we are meditating does not translate into more time with the mantra. The procedure will not change. Over time, the experience will change inside and outside meditation as our nervous system becomes more pure inside. Then we will lose the mantra even quicker! We will close our eyes and be gone into inner silence. It is not something we can judge or regulate. It will be what it will be. What we do have control over is how we meditate each day, and that is very simple, yes?

You are doing just fine. You will know when to inch your session time back up as the process of purification smooths out. You are wise to keep the time tempered to suit the situation.

All of this is in the little blue book. Just let the process do its thing. Good things are happening. :-)

The guru is in you.

2005/12/30 11:54:31
Support for AYP Deep Meditation and Samyama
http://www.aypsite.org/forum/topic.asp?TOPIC_ID=678&REPLY_ID=2269&whichpage=-1
Procedure with Mantra

Hi Weaver:

It sounds like you are having good results with the mantra without interrupting the process to introduce the thought "let the mind be relaxed." So I do not recommend adding that extra thought, which is a move to less inner silence not more. It is not necessary to keep picking the mantra up over and over if you are absorbed in it. It is okay to be absorbed like that. It is not concentration. It is samadhi, which is absorption in inner silence.

In Patanjali's yoga sutra's it is a three stage process comprising the last three of the eight limbs of yoga:

1. Concentration - attention on an object (dharana)
2. Meditation - dissolving of the object (dhyana)
3. Absorption - pure bliss consciousness with no object (samadhi)

All of these are included in our easy deep meditation procedure. First we pick up the mantra (1). We don't try and keep it as a rock solid clear pronunciation -- we just easily repeat it inside, letting it go how it will to less and less distinctiveness (2). At some point we will lose the mantra completely (3). Then we will be out again on some thoughts or feelings and pick it up again (1). Or, if we stay in (3) for the entire session, that is fine. We don't have to deliberately pick up a thought to come out so we can pick up the mantra again. In fact, if we do that, we have had a thought already, and that is the time to pick up the mantra instead (1). We can do this in a very fuzzy way, with the mantra barely touched as a faint impulse. Wherever we left off in clarity of pronunciation is where we pick up the mantra again. That is the easiest, most natural and effective way to be going inward. It is highly efficient. As soon as we become passive in the process (like "observing" or "relaxing"), we are losing the natural inward momentum set up by the mantra procedure. It is not a plus to diverge in this way.

In the end, concentration, meditation and samad
Hi are all happening in virtually the same place in the mind/body, blended with inner silence. That is where you appear to be in the process you described. It is the same mantra procedure going forward from there. No change is necessary.

Keep in mind that your meditations will not likely stay in this mode all the time. As purification advances, the experience will change. You may find yourself back out in surface thoughts at any time, like the original inquirer above. It is not a bad thing. And she can find herself in absorption at any time too. It is all part of the process of purification going forward. The experience will change over time. Guaranteed!

It is very important that the procedure with the mantra not change through all this. If we keep adjusting the procedure to what we think fits our experience in the moment, we will not have a stable and effective long term practice. And that is a big "uh oh."

Interestingly, samyama utilizes the same three limbs of yoga going in the reverse direction -- from inside outward. When we have developed to the point where we can have 1, 2 and 3 happening more or less in the same place (translation: some degree of resident inner silence), then we can initiate and release thoughts in inner silence and they will boomerang out, greatly amplified, through our nervous system and into the world. This is how stillness moves into action. It is a morally self-regulating process because neither ego nor negative intentions exist in our infinite field of pure bliss consciousness. As time goes on, this process of intentions flying out from inner silence becomes an avalanche of divine love flowing out from us into the world. And here we are! :-)

All the best!

The guru is in you.

2005/12/30 22:45:43
Support for AYP Deep Meditation and Samyama
http://www.aypsite.org/forum/topic.asp?TOPIC_ID=678&REPLY_ID=2281&whichpage=-1
Procedure with Mantra

Hi Darvish and Anthem:

There is no set rhythm for repetition. Whatever is comfortable, and it can change according to purification going on. No set location for the mantra either. It can locate or not for the same reason. We do not favor any particular rhythm or location. If one happens, fine, but we do not hang on to it. We don't hang on to anything, not even the mantra at any particular level. We let the attention slide ever deeper into inner silence with the ever disappearing mantra. This is covered from quite a few angles in the Deep Meditation book.

On mechanical repetition of the mantra in silence, yes, letting it go to less is the way, and picking it up as less when we realize we have gone off it. We don't stop and watch when we know we can continue with the mantra. Btw, noticing characteristics such as these (and the knee-jerk analyses of the mind) are signs of the re-emergence of thoughts and, hence, the signal to go back to the you-know-what. :-)

The guru is in you.

2006/02/02 17:30:25
Support for AYP Deep Meditation and Samyama
http://www.aypsite.org/forum/topic.asp?TOPIC_ID=678&REPLY_ID=2999&whichpage=-1
Procedure with Mantra

quote:

...a realisation that we are within the silence?

Hi WhiteCrane, and welcome!

...a realization that we <u>are</u> the silence. Not an intellectual realization, but a permanent experience of that. It first comes as an experience of "witnessing," and expands from there.

The guru is in you.

2006/01/10 09:47:34
Support for AYP Deep Meditation and Samyama
http://www.aypsite.org/forum/topic.asp?TOPIC_ID=713&REPLY_ID=2432&whichpage=-1
Question on mantras for Yogani

Hi Snake:

Sorry, but I am not a position to comment on the TM system of mantras.

There are books full of mantras, though rarely an effective method for using them. I am asked about different mantras all the time, and I usually beg off. It is impossible to explain what everyone else is trying to do with mantras.

The goal in AYP has been to come up with a simple "universal" approach to mantra utilization that is effective for both immediate and long term purification and opening. I'd like to stick with that as a baseline.

Of course, anyone is free to explore anything else. I would only caution not to try and do too many things at once with mantra. The results can get diluted very quickly. Remember, the purpose in mantra yoga is to ride (refine) the mantra inward to where there is no mantra at all -- Only pure bliss consciousness. Less is more in deep meditation. So, the less mental baggage we are carrying, the better.

Also, when digging a well, success is most likely if we keep digging in one place. In other words, switching mantras around often is not necessarily the best strategy for maximizing our progress. In the end, is not about the mantra(s). It is about how well we have become stabilized in pure bliss consciousness, which is beyond all mantras. For achieving that, the correct use of a single mantra will be most effective.

The guru is in you.

2006/01/11 10:28:12
Support for AYP Deep Meditation and Samyama
http://www.aypsite.org/forum/topic.asp?TOPIC_ID=719&REPLY_ID=2466&whichpage=-1
"negative energy"

Hi Nicole:

Thanks for bringing this question to the forum after we covered it in email. As you can see, those who have been meditating for some time have had a similar experience.

To add to the mix, here is my original email reply to the question:

"Possession" has no bearing in deep meditation, which operates far beyond the realm of such things.

The new AYP book, **Deep Meditation**, clears up most questions that can come up on deep meditation, including the "negative energy" thing. You may wish to review it.

I would add that the only power that entities have is the power we give them. By practicing deep meditation we are not even in the same neighborhood, so the question of empowering negative energies is mute. This is also covered in the AYP lessons on Samyama.

There are other mental techniques (not AYP) that work on the level of entities, and there can certainly be problems there. Those methods can not rightly be called "meditation." Meditation is the journey of attention from an object (mantra) to pure bliss consciousness with no objects (samadhi). In AYP-style deep meditation it is one step and gone -- express car right past all the other planes of existence to inner silence. Swoosh! And that is what we are stabilizing more and more each time we meditate -- inner silence, which is impervious to the energies you ask about. So if we have had problems with entities in the past, we will be much less inclined to once we are established in a stable routine of twice-daily deep meditation. Entities cannot latch on to inner silence. They can only latch on to the obsessive fears that feed them. There is no fear in pure bliss consciousness.

Interestingly, those who are constantly ranting about possession are fostering it. Those who are always warning about the devil are, in fact, empowering the negative forces. Better to meditate, live your life with naturally increasing purity, and you will find yourself letting go of those who engage in fear mongering. In fact, by your mere presence you can reduce their fear via your own progress. Even just a little light can dispel the darkness.

I suggest you bring your questions to the AYP forums for additional points of view. Then many can benefit from the discussion.

The guru is in you.

2006/01/12 07:21:16
Support for AYP Deep Meditation and Samyama
http://www.aypsite.org/forum/topic.asp?TOPIC_ID=720&REPLY_ID=2497&whichpage=-1
Some thoughts on meditation

Hi Alvin:

Mantra with thoughts is a common experience, and not a barrier to effective meditation. No need to make a drama of it. Just follow the procedure for effortless meditation. It is covered in the new Deep Meditation book.

The guru is in you.

2006/01/12 07:31:14
Support for AYP Deep Meditation and Samyama
http://www.aypsite.org/forum/topic.asp?TOPIC_ID=723&REPLY_ID=2498&whichpage=-1
Question on allowing

Hi Chris:

If we realize we have a choice of where to put our attention, we are on the way out already, even if there is a mixture of inner silence, thoughts and mantra. We always favor the mantra in these situations. This can be favoring very refined and fuzzy values of the mantra -- going ever deeper. If we choose to stand pat in "peace," we will be short of samadhi, and deep meditation stops right there. That's why we always follow the procedure.

The guru is in you.

2006/01/20 10:41:39
Support for AYP Deep Meditation and Samyama
http://www.aypsite.org/forum/topic.asp?TOPIC_ID=748&REPLY_ID=2675&whichpage=-1
what to do?

Hi Anthem and all:

Good perspectives on the experience here. It is purification to a degree more noticeable than has happened before. So we can get used to that. It can be with light or darkness, joy and sometimes a little fear. Hopefully not too much of the latter, especially not overflowing into daily activity. If so, then we know that extra attention on self-pacing of practices will be in order.

A theme in the replies that is clear is the gradual rise of surrender. By this, we do not intend to let the energy go to excess, and surrender to the resulting chaos. No. What we want is a stable unfoldment, and then gradually increasing levels of surrender within that platform of stability. Eventually, the platform of regulated practices will become completely transparent, just as our nervous system becomes a pure channel of divine love flowing into the world. Then our surrender becomes unconditional, and the world around us is transformed by the infinite divine flowing through us.

I remember for quite a few years I was chasing spiritual transformation. That chase is what drove my path. Then, when things started to break loose, I soon came to realize that spiritual transformation was chasing me. That changed the whole dynamic. That was when I had to get serious about self-pacing, and also about letting go, surrendering into what was happening. There is really no other choice, because the process itself comes to be in charge at a certain point (it always was) and the best we can do is learn to navigate skillfully like we are in a kayak going down the rapids. Sometimes we are in total surrender. Other times we are holding back so as not to overdo.

We could call this process navigating the awakening of kundalini, but that is sort of a cliche. I prefer to call it navigating the process human spiritual transformation, which includes so many more nuances than the cliche.

The John Wilder story is about this transformation from seeking to self-pacing and surrendering, and the ultimate consequences of that. In the end, it is no longer about our individual self, but the common good (universal Self). The metaphor of the caterpillar transforming into a butterfly captures it. Total sacrifice leading to radiant new life that uplifts all of nature. We are that...

In any case, it is what it is. All paths are determined by the natural processes of evolution occurring within the human nervous system. All we are doing here is awakening them in the most progressive and safest ways we know. The final destination is not determined by us. It is determined by our letting go -- our surrender by degrees to what will be. In doing so, we open the door to our illumination and to the illumination of the world.

The guru is in you.

2006/02/07 10:12:25
Support for AYP Deep Meditation and Samyama
http://www.aypsite.org/forum/topic.asp?TOPIC_ID=796&REPLY_ID=3134&whichpage=-1
Meditation

Hi Whitecrane:

This lesson can shed some light on that: http://www.aypsite.org/92.html with a followup here: http://www.aypsite.org/179.html

The experience can have many variations according to the course of individual purification, but the inner neurobiology involved is the same.

The guru is in you.

2006/02/16 10:59:18
Support for AYP Deep Meditation and Samyama
http://www.aypsite.org/forum/topic.asp?TOPIC_ID=831&REPLY_ID=3410&whichpage=-1
How to be easy/let go in meditation

Hi Alvin:

As you gradually reprogram youself, you will not only learn easy deep meditation -- you will learn how to live more easily too.

It is worth the letting go (not the effort).

There is no escaping this. No matter what real spiritual path you follow, it will always be about learning to let go. Deep meditation is a way to do it without so much fuss and fanfare. It is a simple procedure. A mechanical habit we develop that leads to not thinking about the doing of it anymore. Then it creeps out into every aspect of our life as inner silence. Very simple.

Interestingly, we gain much greater power of concentration and analysis from this simple process. Very relaxed infinite concentration, and very relaxed infinite analysis. This simple procedure awakens the genius in us.

You are in a clunky stage. It will get better if you stick with the easy procedure. Regard all the analysis coming up as any other thoughts in meditation. You know what to do then, yes? -- Easily back to the mantra. No one is asking you to invest your attention in all that analysis during meditation. If you save it for later, it will make for better meditation and much better analysis when out of meditation.

The guru is in you.

2006/02/16 22:37:58
Support for AYP Deep Meditation and Samyama
http://www.aypsite.org/forum/topic.asp?TOPIC_ID=831&REPLY_ID=3440&whichpage=-1
How to be easy/let go in meditation

Hi Meg:

This generic discussion on switching mantras is from lesson 186 (second enhancement of mantra), and might help with your question:

"If we have shifted to an enhanced mantra too early, we will know it soon enough. We will feel like we are slogging through mud. We will be bogging down and not having good results in daily activity. It is not the end of the world. If we find ourselves in this situation ongoing, the solution is simple. We just shift back down to our previous mantra and go with that for a few more months, or however long it takes us to reach the point when we are ready to shift up. Self-pacing, remember?

"A false start with a mantra enhancement can happen, but we should avoid it if we can. The reason is it takes time for a new mantra to settle in. If we have shifted too early and are trying to settle in with the new mantra, and then decide to go back to the previous one, it will take time again to change the pattern of the mantra deep in the mind. For this reason we do not change mantras often, up or down. We want to be going deep with our mantra in one place. These enhancements are for facilitating that process. Beyond these basic shifts we do not switch our mantra around. Neither do we try and use multiple mantras, not with the approach in these lessons. We want to cultivate the ability to go deep in every sitting. To do this, we will be best served by using a single vehicle, our mantra."

The guru is in you.

2006/02/25 11:42:18
Support for AYP Deep Meditation and Samyama
http://www.aypsite.org/forum/topic.asp?TOPIC_ID=854&REPLY_ID=3846&whichpage=-1
Samyama, picking up word or not?

Hi Weaver:

When we pick up a sutra in samyama the meaning is implicit in the faint feeling of the sound of it deep in the mind. We do not contemplate it during our practice, as that pulls us to the surface of the mind. The idea is to pick up the impulse of the sound of the sutra and let it go in inner silence. That is where the power comes from in samyama -- inner silence. That is where the power comes from in all we do. We just have not been accessing it directly until now. Inner silence is also where all divine love and moral conduct come from, so this practice is morally self-regulating.

"Akasha - Lightness of Air" has two components, and they should be preserved in use of the sutra. One is akasha, which actualizes the body as empty space (it is, yes?). The other is lightness which moves the body -- or at least creates the inner impulse for that, which has great inner purifying effect. It is like blowing up a balloon (step one) and then giving it a push to float through the air (step two). The sutra becomes easy with some practice -- we do it without undue delay between the two parts. It is one sutra. Like every other practice we begin in AYP, there is a clunky stage with samyama too. It will pass.

Abundance is best used in the genral sense of, well, abundance. It applies to many things, not just material wealth, though you may get that pile of gold too. :-) But more important is the purification in the nervous system that promotes abundance of divine flow in all that is manifest everywhere. Samyama practice is both individual and cosmic, promoting the divine flow from within us -- from inner cosmic to outer cosmic. How important are levitation and piles of gold compared to that? Not very ... we treat them like scenery if and when they occur, favoring the far greater opening of outpouring divine love into the world, which comes from letting go of the sutras into inner silence, and letting go of their results too. A channel does not concern itself with the before and the after. The ecstatic bliss of becoming the channel itself is more than enough.

As for selection and order of sutras, what you see is my best list based on covering the full range of body, heart, mind and all within and around us. Obviously, sutras can be selected and arranged many ways. Whatever one is using for samyama, I encourage that a steady twice-daily routine of samyama after deep meditation with the same list be adhered to. Otherwise we will not be going deep. Remember the well-digging analogy? Better to dig deep in one place to find water than to dig many small dry holes all over the place. The list of sutras, all together, is one digging in one place. We'd like to go deep there, and take all of those avenues of purification and opening into inner silence with us. If we do, we will find all of our desires coming to fruition more smoothly in daily life and an increasing divine quality naturally coming up within them.

The guru is in you.

2006/02/25 18:02:06
Support for AYP Deep Meditation and Samyama
http://www.aypsite.org/forum/topic.asp?TOPIC_ID=854&REPLY_ID=3856&whichpage=-1
Samyama, picking up word or not?

Hi Jim:

Yes, that is a good way to look at it, as long as we don't become obsessed with letting go, which is a hanging on. :-)

Some inner silence (the witness) cultivated in deep meditation takes care of it automatically. That is why having some resident (abiding) inner silence is the main prerequisite for samyama. Then there is no intentional letting go. We just pick up the sutra (faint or fuzzy), and our resident inner silence swallows it. After weeks, months and years of practice (digging the well in one place) we have the habit of samyama and all of our thoughts, feelings and actions spring from inner silence. Then we are living from the source, so to speak. Nothing to hang on to, nothing to let go of. Just a divine flow and endless merging of inner and outer.

For those who are jumping in here, take a look at <u>lesson 150</u> and the lessons that follow it for details on samyama practice. <u>Lesson 149</u> ties samyama in with the rest of what we are doing in AYP

The guru is in you.

2006/03/05 09:17:41
Support for AYP Deep Meditation and Samyama
http://www.aypsite.org/forum/topic.asp?TOPIC_ID=854&REPLY_ID=4114&whichpage=-1
Samyama, picking up word or not?

Hello Ajita:

Yes, your sharing is very welcome. However, if the method of samyama you teach is substantially different from the approach we use in AYP, it would be good to put it under "other systems of practice" so as not to confuse readers (and newcomers especially) between different methods. Perhaps call it "Ajita's Method of Samyama," or something like that. Same with meditation or any other teachings you would like to share that involve a different method. In that way, there is room for all approaches here.

The guru is in in you.

2006/03/05 11:13:43
Support for AYP Deep Meditation and Samyama
http://www.aypsite.org/forum/topic.asp?TOPIC_ID=854&REPLY_ID=4124&whichpage=-1
Samyama, picking up word or not?

Hi Jim:

Yes, the witness is first noticed naturally in relation to activity, especially with some intense activity going on, which increases the contrast between inner and outer. Even those who are not doing practices will clearly "witness" an accident or other traumatic event, noticing the part inside that is untouched. The truth is we are always the witness. It is our very consciousness, after all. As we are cultivating inner silence in deep meditation, a greater contrast comes into our awareness where we notice the increasing inner part of us that is not moving, is untouched, in relation to outer activities, and eventually in relation to all of our thoughts and feelings too. It is our own consciousness, cultivated to a greater presence, and it gradually becomes the center of our self-awareness instead of all the stuff that is happening around us and inside us. This centeredness, and natural access to our native creativity, energy, compassion and other divine qualities, provides a great advantage in many things, of course.

The interesting thing, and this is where samyama comes in, is that inner stillness "moves" outward into our daily life over time, eventually permeating every aspect of our thinking, feeling and doing. That is the "outflow" I mention pretty often. Samyama cultivates this, as does being active in the world in-between our practice sessions.

So, yes, first we notice a contrast between activity and witness. Sometime after, we come to see that we are primarily the witness itself -- the only thing in our life that is constant, unchanging, the essence of our being. Then, as this quality flows out, we come to know that everything is That.

That's where the Vedic proclamation comes from:
"I am That,
You are That,
All this is That."

It is also where the Biblical phrase comes from:
"Do unto others have you would have them do unto you."
We and they are woven of the same cloth -- brothers and sisters in oneness all.

And another way of saying it:
The One is the many,
And the many are the One.

It looks great philosophically, but it is far more that that. It becomes known by direct perception on the path of yoga. Anyone who is engaged in effective sitting practices finds out for themselves.

The guru is in you.

2006/03/05 11:56:20
Support for AYP Deep Meditation and Samyama
http://www.aypsite.org/forum/topic.asp?TOPIC_ID=854&REPLY_ID=4128&whichpage=-1
Samyama, picking up word or not?

quote:
_____
Originally posted by Shanti

Is it something like being in the middle of a conversation and suddenly feeling like you are outside watching? Is that what you mean by the witness?
_____

Hi Shanti:

Yes, or inside watching. Everywhere watching. :-)

There is nothing we have to do with this when it happens. We'll just notice from time to time. It is an experience that comes to us gradually from our practices. So the best way to cultivate it is to continue with our normal practice routine. Gradually and automatically, the habits we develop in practices become part of daily life. Stillness, love, joy, energy and much more natural purity and effectiveness of our intentions (samyama).

The guru is in you.

2006/03/10 13:17:06
Support for AYP Deep Meditation and Samyama
http://www.aypsite.org/forum/topic.asp?TOPIC_ID=854&REPLY_ID=4355&whichpage=-1
Samyama, picking up word or not?

Hi Melissa & Shanti:

If we have some symptoms in samyama that are erotic, that is how it goes. It is a common occurrence with just about any of the AYP practices -- it's even covered in the Deep Meditation book. The symptoms will pass as our purification progresses in that area, and then it all goes higher. Good things are happening!

If it gets to be too much, then some self-pacing of our practice will be in order. That could consist of taking a break from siddhasana, if using. If it is only the samyama, then you can at your option reduce the number of repetitions, or take a break from samyama for a few sessions until things settle down in your practice routine.

Grounding activity like regular physical exercise between sittings can also help smooth out the obstructions causing erotic friction.

This is not a permanent aspect of your practice -- only a phase of purification. It will pass and expand to become something much more in the realm of ecstatic bliss. Then you will be favoring your practice over that "scenery" too. So it goes, onward up the scale... :-)

The guru is in you.

2006/03/05 10:02:40
Support for AYP Deep Meditation and Samyama
http://www.aypsite.org/forum/topic.asp?TOPIC_ID=873&REPLY_ID=4117&whichpage=-1
questions on samyama

Hi Alvin:

1. No, not invented by me. It has been around for thousands of years. Nothing in AYP is new except the simplification and integration of effective methods across the limbs of yoga , open source approach, and development of self-pacing. Samyama is documented very little anywhere (except regurgitating theory) beyond the Yoga Sutras of Patanjali, and what little it is taught can be very divergent in method. As usual, I go for the easiest, most effective method encountered.

2. It is okay to start samyama as long as you have some inner silence and are stable in all you have taken on already. Make sure to take plenty of rest at the end of your session. If you are premature in taking up samyama, it is not hazardous, there will just not be much effect.

3. Yes, samyama will both cultivate and stabilize inner silence in our nervous system, in addition to increasing its presence in our daily activity -- improving both the purity and power of our intentions.

The guru is in you.

2006/03/05 11:27:05
Support for AYP Deep Meditation and Samyama
http://www.aypsite.org/forum/topic.asp?TOPIC_ID=873&REPLY_ID=4125&whichpage=-1
questions on samyama
Yes, that's right. The seed of meaning in samyama is language-related, so translations are appropriate in this case. Also remember that it is a feeling. Fuzzy feeling is the code that disappears into inner silence with each repetition. The effectiveness of samyama is in the letting go ... as is the case with so many things in yoga, and in life. All of this is the cultivation and expression of inner silence in our daily life.

The guru is in you.

2006/03/08 09:49:59
Support for AYP Deep Meditation and Samyama

questions on samyama

Hi Alvin:

Some resident inner silence present from deep meditation primes the pump of samyama. In order for samyama to cultivate more inner silence and move it outward, there must be some to begin with. That is why we do samyama right after meditation -- best time for stillness. In order for this to be, deep meditation is best well stabilized -- at least a few months from starting. Otherwise samyama will be kind of like pumping an unprimed pump. Not the end of the world, but not very efficient either. Once we do get started with samyama, regular practice is the key to good progress. This is true of all the practices, subject to the regulation of self-pacing, of course.

The guru is in you.

2006/04/03 11:32:31
Support for AYP Deep Meditation and Samyama
questions on samyama

Hi All:

Yes, that is it, Weaver and Jim. The meaning is implicit in the word(s) and the "faint feeling" is for the word(s), not the meaning. Then we let it go. So, it is not that some sutras are more feeling oriented than others. The picking up of the sutra is not about the nature of the content. That is implicit. It is exactly the same procedure for all sutras. In time, operating more in inner silence becomes a habit in all of our thinking, and our thoughts in daily activity naturally become more evolutionary and powerful.

I hope that answers your question, Frank.

Kathy, wonderful experience with samyama. And you are right -- by "having some inner silence present," it is not meant we should practice samyama only when we feel that we have some inner silence. Once we decide to practice samyama, it should become a part of our regular sitting practices. Like with all the practices, regularity over time is the key to success with samyama, and it will not always be the kind of experience we'd like to write home about, due to purification going on. It is the same with samyama as with all the practices -- a long and winding road that leads home, with the scenery always changing, gradually getting better and better. :-)

The guru is in you.

2006/04/04 08:35:12
Support for AYP Deep Meditation and Samyama
questions on samyama

Hi Ether:

Yes, we humans have a gift for making the simplest things so complicated. It must be why Jesus said, "You must become as little children to enter the kingdom..."

We could talk about it forever here in ten-thousand ways, and not one word would be wasted. So great are the benefits of simplicity.

And ... there are some new perspectives coming. Always new perspectives. :-)

The guru is in you.

2006/03/18 11:30:48
Support for AYP Deep Meditation and Samyama
Evolving Style of Meditation
Secret Wisdom:

The road to enlightenment is paved with pillows.
2006/03/26 23:45:55
Support for AYP Deep Meditation and Samyama
involuntary movement during meditation

Hi Bill:

It is something we call "automatic yoga." It can happen along the path and is not something to be overly concerned about. If you look it up in the topic index, you will find a number of lessons on this phenomenon. Here is one that covers your situation: http://www.aypsite.org/183.html

The guru is in you.

2006/04/28 09:40:54
Support for AYP Deep Meditation and Samyama
involuntary movement during meditation

quote:
————

Bill said: My question now is that I become distracted from the mantra by the movement and try to stay focused despite it, should I try to sit still and focus on the mantra or should I go with the flow and let the movements clear things up? When I find I'm off the mantra and moving around then I stop, straighten up, and go back to the mantra (and movement soon after).

Hi Bill:

This sounds like a reasonable procedure, given the circumstances, except don't force your way back to the mantra, of course. Just easily favor it when you realize you are off into thoughts, feelings, or movements. That process of going back to the mantra will naturally attenuate the movements, at least for a while. If the movements become too much in a given session, discontinue favoring the mantra for a while and just let attention easily be with the energy sensations, and that can help unwind them. This counts as meditation time, and should only be used if the sensations become excessive to the point that getting back to the mantra is not easy. One thing we never do in deep meditation is force.

In time, this should all settle down. It is obstructions in the neurobiology that are causing the movements as energy lurches through there. When the pathways become more clear, the movements will become less, even as more energy is flowing.

If it is all too much, then self-pacing the time of practices until you find a reasonable balance will be the thing to do. That is covered in the lessons, as you know. If spinal breathing seems to be causing more movement, then self-pace it more as necessary. Usually spinal breathing has a strong influence in balancing energy flows, but there are exceptions, so each application has to be judged on its results. We do not stand on fixed formulas around here. Experiences and self-pacing are the key factors to consider in gauging the measure of our practices.

Yes, asanas before sitting can help, as can more physical exercise (of the aerobic variety) during the day on a regular basis. A grounding practice like a daily Tai C
Hi routine can also help a lot. It is all about working the obstructions out. This can be promoted from both outside (physical activity) and inside (sitting practices).

Keep us posted. And all the best on your unique journey through purification and opening!

The guru is in you.

2006/04/14 11:17:22
Support for AYP Deep Meditation and Samyama
http://www.aypsite.org/forum/topic.asp?TOPIC_ID=1033&REPLY_ID=5948&whichpage=-1
Numbness on tongue + lips

Hi WhiteCrane:

At the risk of sounding like a cliche, I'll say it is purification. By now it may be past and moving on to some other manifestation of opening in the nervous systems. Has it?

Typically, symptoms around the tongue and mouth are precursers of increased kechari-related activity -- it can be soon, or much later. Just take it one day at a time.

Of course, sometimes symptoms can be medically related, so we do not turn a blind eye to that. If a symptom becomes chronic, it is a good idea to get it checked out medically, though this one you are mentioning seems pretty benign.

The guru is in you.

2006/04/14 13:07:14
Support for AYP Deep Meditation and Samyama
http://www.aypsite.org/forum/topic.asp?TOPIC_ID=1033&REPLY_ID=5959&whichpage=-1
Numbness on tongue + lips

Hi WC and Meg:

Ah, the rise of ecstatic conductivity. Sometimes it is noticed going down before it goes up and everywhere.

Walking is the prescription for spreading the energy sensations in the legs and feet out to the rest of the body and beyond. Remember, the ecstatic sensations are the friction of energy passing through purifying nerves, and gradually they will spread out and become the outpouring flow of divine love, which is even better than orgasms in the feet. :-)

The guru is in you.

2006/04/11 11:54:36
Support for AYP Deep Meditation and Samyama
http://www.aypsite.org/forum/topic.asp?TOPIC_ID=1034
Weird Bouncing

Hi All:

Here is an interesting one from my email. Comments welcome.

Q1: I have been reading your website for about six months and have been actively meditating for over a year now.

In the last few weeks, things have intensified and strange things have been happening. The pleasure that starts in my root has become very intense, as soon as I get into siddhasana... it fires right up and begins to move upward.

Lately though after only a few minutes I feel my head and neck straighten on their own, and then my head snaps down to my chest. I feel a vibration coming up, and my head begins to shake forward and backward. My mulabhanda gets tighter on it's own, and then I start to bounce. Literally bounce. Weird. I thought it was just a subjective feeling, but when my knee ran into the coffee table, about a foot and a half from the blanket I was sitting on, I knew it was real.

I tried to concentrate on the bouncing, but it didn't stop. When I went back to my mantra, the bouncing got stronger and stronger. This has only happened twice in the past couple of weeks. I thought about what you said in several postings about backing off, but my body didn't want to. I rode it out, and afterwards was totally worn out but elated. What is that?

A1: It is energy moving, yielding purification and opening. In this case you are finding some lurching that comes with energy passing through remaining inner obstructions. You also have some "automatic yoga" going on, which are yogic maneuvers like mudras, bandhas and asanas occurring automatically due to energy flow in the body.

The guideline on experiences like this is to favor the practice we are doing over the experience. If the experience becomes too intense for that, then we just let our attention relax with what is happening, not concentrating or focusing intently on it. Just easily being with whatever is happening. That will usually draw our attention to a physical location and aid in dissolving the obstruction, wherever it may be. Then, when things settle down, we can return to our practice. We count all the time spent as practice time, not starting over after an intense energy/automatic yoga episode. Make sure to take some extra rest before getting up after sessions with that much energy movement going on.

By the way, the energy surges, automatic yogas and hopping, similar to what you describe, are symptoms that more commonly occur during samyama practice, especially when doing the "akasha - lightness of air" sutra. It is all purification and opening stimulated by the outward movement of our inner stillness -- what I call "stillness in action." So, even though you are apparently not doing samyama yet, you are having some similar effects in your meditations. It can happen...

Later on, this phenomenon of the outflow of stillness into energy manifestion becomes much smoother and more organized, leading to a multitude of positive expressions in our daily life. It is an outpouring of divine love from us. It may not seem like it now, but that is where it is heading. It becomes much less physically dramatic, even as it becomes far more influential as invisible positive energy radiating out from us into the surrounding environment. Our actions are colored by the endless outflow of divine love as well, which changes our relationships for the better in a thousand subtle and not-so-subtle ways.

On the purification and opening energy management side, check these lessons:
On automatic yoga and siddhis: http://www.aypsite.org/210.html
On energy surges and hopping in samyama: http://www.aypsite.org/155.html
Also see the topic index for more lessons on "automatic yoga" and "samyama."

Q2: I appreciate your timeliness and your wisdom. In your opinion should I start to take a look at starting a samyama practice in my daily routine? It is interesting to note that this did not start to happen until I made a concerted effort to increase my bhakti, my desire to get closer to God, to allow God to get closer to me...when my desire grew, the intensity of meditation grew, the inner space in my head has grown bigger, and the there is more of a feeling of "becoming" the mantra.

A2: Obviously, you have enough inner silence for samyama practice. You can take it up at any time. It is a matter of preference and self-pacing, meaning, keeping your practice stable while being progressive at the same time. There are a lot of ways covered in the lessons to stabilize excess energy movements. My last note only touched the subject. A lot of the discussions in the forums are on this too.

Yes, bhakti will do that. It does everything, really. :-)
Sometimes we end up having to "self-pace" our bhakti to keep things from flying too fast.

All the best on your path. Enjoy!

The guru is in you.

2006/04/11 17:30:40
Support for AYP Deep Meditation and Samyama
http://www.aypsite.org/forum/topic.asp?TOPIC_ID=1034&REPLY_ID=5869&whichpage=-1
Weird Bouncing

Hi Jim:

Physical movements within safe limits (with adequate padding underneath) do not necessarily imply instability. In fact, they can be common and occur off and on for years, especially in samyama where inner silence is being stirred from many angles. If we rest adequately at the end of a session with physical movements in it, get up feeling refreshed, and go out into our day feeling clear with good energy, then it is good practice. We do not normally favor movements with attention, favoring the procedure of our practice instead, which may bring more movments or not. The movements are not a prerequisite for progress, and neither do they have to hold us back from advancing in our practices and on our path. They are a symptom of purification and can be a normal part of the scenery.

Now, let's not all go out and be deliberately jumping all over the meditation room. It's not necessary. Just be easy and natural about practice and the resulting symptoms of purification, whatever they may be. And self-pace as necessary, being sure to maintain an even tempered about all of this -- that preserves our bhakti and our motivation to carry on.

The main source of instability in practices is usually psychological rather than physical. If we become irritable or upset due to too much purification going on, and movements are there also, then this is a clear signal for self-pacing. In fact, if there are no movements and we find ourselves drifting emotionally off center, then this alone is a signal for self-pacing. On the other hand, if we feel steady inside and are having some movements, then this can be good practice, as mentioned above.

This is why I said that the questioner may consider taking on samyama if he wishes. His movements have been occasional so far, and for the most part emotionally uplifting. If he starts samyama, the movements may or may not increase. Either way, the purification will continue. In the end, the movements will subside as the nervous system becomes pure and offers less resistance to the flow of inner energy. As mentioned, this over all process could take a long time. So, in the meantime, we just go with it, following the procedures of practice and the principles of self-pacing --

optimizing always for speed and comfort. And maybe that means hopping around a bit. It would not be the first time, and it is certainly not the end of the world. Actually, it can be a beginning. A step along the way from duckling to swan. :-)

On "becoming the mantra," while we'd all like to "Be here now," the becoming-ness of it is impossible to avoid. It is a matter of point of view. If I am out here in ego and go in on the mantra, I may appear to become the mantra as it and my egoic sense dissolve into stillness, which is my self. If I am in there already (as inner silence - witness), looking from the inside out, then there is no self-becoming as the mantra makes the same journey. The process is the same. Only the point of view is different. In the case of our questioner, he saw his ego self dissolve to become the mantra refining into expanding stillness. Nothing wrong with that, as long as it is only an observation of scenery and not an imposition on the procedure of deep meditation itself.

Of course, we cannot intellectually locate ourselves in one point of view or the other -- not organically anyway. Our point of view from ego or stillness is where it is depending on the condition of our neurobiology, and we will describe the experience from that angle accordingly. Over time, the point of view gradually shifts as our sense of self changes from external to internal. Then we can say, "Hey everyone, I'm really here now!"

In truth, we probably won't say much, and just go do the dishes and take out the trash. Nothing changes, even as everything does. We are becoming "That" even though we already are "That." I guess that is why they call it "realization." Realizing something that is already. It is a becoming ... a journey from here to here...

The guru is in you.

2006/04/11 23:19:45
Support for AYP Deep Meditation and Samyama
http://www.aypsite.org/forum/topic.asp?TOPIC_ID=1034&REPLY_ID=5876&whichpage=-1
Weird Bouncing

Hi Shanti:

What surprises me is that anyone wants to read it. :-)

It is amazing that we can have so many subjective discussions going on here and find so much common ground. Surely the end result is an objective exploration of practices and experiences.

That is a statistical statement, of course. If we toss a coin 100 times and it comes up heads 75 times, it is a significant outcome that says something about the coin. If it happens with 1000 throws (750 heads), it becomes down right scientific.

Like that, the discussions here keep touching on the same themes of purification, inner openings, witnessing, ecstasy, self-pacing, etc. With enough of that it moves from subjective (internally observed) to objective (externally observed). That is very significant, assuming we are not engaged in "group think" here, and relate our experiences as honestly and subjectively as we can. Oddly enough, the more subjective we each are in sharing, the more objective the long term outcome will be, because there will be a high degree of independence in the information inputs.

The emails received here, like the one above, are especially revealing in that way, because they often come from people I have had little or no prior contact with. Many times the experiences are significantly outside what is in the AYP lessons. Yet, they usually have some sort of overlap with the lessons or with previous discussions here and can be incorporated into the over all picture, enriching the entire body of knowledge. In that way we find both confirmations of experience and expansions of knowledge occurring at the same time. It is a remarkable process.

So, I think these forums are much more than a bunch of discussions. They are shaping up to be a pretty accurate picture of the process of human spiritual transformation. Just think what that picture will look like in a few years with thousands more discussions added.

That isn't about my writing. It is about all of yours. And it does not surprise me.

You see, I knew it all along ... The guru is in you.

2006/04/11 23:45:16
Support for AYP Deep Meditation and Samyama
http://www.aypsite.org/forum/topic.asp?TOPIC_ID=1034&REPLY_ID=5877&whichpage=-1
Weird Bouncing

Hi Anthem:

Which one are you referring to? I'll see what can be done.

In the old days, I would have posted both the Q&A and follow-ups in the lessons. Of course, there would not be the follow-ups like we have here. That is the beauty of the forums. They stimulate more discussion. The disadvantage is that things gradually fade into the woodwork in the forums. Maybe I'll make a big book of goodies from the forums a few years from now. Now there's a project!

Posting website lessons is not as easy as it used to be. Updating four web locations is a chore, especially with so much else on the plate these days. Nevertheless, for certain things it is well worth the effort, especially for new practices. :-)

The guru is in you.

2006/04/12 14:44:46
Support for AYP Deep Meditation and Samyama
http://www.aypsite.org/forum/topic.asp?TOPIC_ID=1038&REPLY_ID=5898&whichpage=-1
Overcoming Pushiness in Meditation

quote:

David wrote: It does not stop with Yogani, yes?

Hi All:

Hopefully it doesn't stop with me. If it does, we are all in trouble. I didn't have a clue about Shanti's perspiration, other than the possibility of purification continuing outside practices (maybe). It took another woman to expand the perspective on that one (menopause -- thank you, Meg). See, Shanti, I don't know everything. Seems I can only prove the worth of AYP as a self-sustaining and growing knowledge-base by proving myself to be ordinary. I like it that way. The smaller they are, the softer they fall, you know. Therefore, perfectly flat is good. :-)

I do have a few practical thoughts on the latest interchange above.

I think we are talking about "ritual," at least in part -- personal ritual in particular. What does it take for any given person to sit down and relax and be set up to practice deep meditation? Well, who knows? It is personal to a large degree. For whatever reason, maybe someone can't sit down and relax until they have walked around the kitchen table three times. That is a personal thing. It is not opposed to good practice. As long as rituals do not invade the conduct of the practice itself, it will be all right. That is the key point. The procedure itself, once underway, is non-negotiable. We are either doing it or we are not. There is no in-between on that. If someone wants to do a hula dance before meditation, be my guest. Just don't get too winded. :-)

The ancient yogis offer some advice on this that is less about ritual and more about neurobiology. I tend to favor that. The progression of a short routine of asanas to pranayama, and then into meditation has been known for centuries to provide a consistent pathway for settling the nervous system into deep meditation. I recommend it because of its time-tested consistency. If something else is needed to settle down, then that is up to each individual, and I honor it. Just keep the practice of deep meditation itself in its simplest form, and everything will be fine.

Also keep in mind that the experience in meditation will be up and down and sideways from day to day and week to week. That is the ever-changing process of purification going on within us. Whatever we are doing before meditation will have minimal effect on that, so let's not knock ourselves out trying to set up for a particular experience in deep meditation. Our nervous system knows what it needs, and all we have to do is go along for the ride in our practices -- self-pacing as necessary, of course.

We cannot know what each meditation will be clearing out. But we do know the simple procedure for optimizing the process, and the recommendation is to always favor that. If the preparation beforehand involves a personal ritual or something else conducive, that is okay too. Enjoy!

The guru is in you.

2006/04/14 11:27:12
Support for AYP Deep Meditation and Samyama
http://www.aypsite.org/forum/topic.asp?TOPIC_ID=1040&REPLY_ID=5951&whichpage=-1
Adding Mantra enhancements

Hi Richard:

Sounds like a good start with the mantra enhancement. Of course, all experiences in deep meditation are transient due to the ever-changing patterns of purification going on within us. So, this too shall pass and you will be back to normal session durations soon enough. It is okay to go over on time innocently. We just don't do it deliberately, always favoring the procedure, including our predetermined session length, as our awareness in the moment allows.

Make sure to take adequate rest before getting up, especially if the session runs over like that. This will assure a smooth transition into daily activity.

The benefit of all this, deep meditation, enhancments of mantra, and so on, is increasing depth and stabilization of inner silence in daily activty. That is the payoff. How we get there is a long and winding road with all sorts of scenery -- much of it quite lovely. Enjoy! :-)

The guru is in you.

2006/04/18 09:37:36
Support for AYP Deep Meditation and Samyama
http://www.aypsite.org/forum/topic.asp?TOPIC_ID=1047&REPLY_ID=6101&whichpage=-1
Vacation Day

Hi Jim and Katrine:

My feeling about it is that the ecstatic process is what it is, or not, and we don't have to label it. Of course, we do. It goes all the way back to Adam and Eve -- the labeling.

Interestingly, our quest for this kind of pleasure leads to its own fulfillment. It is God's snare, so to speak.

In any case, I think you have put a wonderful description to it, Katrine, the ero/ecstatic roar refining to a vapor, and this is what gives our inner silence the wings it needs to pour out in every direction. A very delicate and subtle process of marrying these two sacred qualities that live in us -- stillness and ecstasy. Once it has happened, it is not so subtle. It is stillness in action, divine love relentlessly penetrating every cell of our being, every cell of the cosmos within and all around us.

I tried to put words to this in the new book "Spinal Breathing" with more clarity than perhaps in the past. Please let me know at some point if I succeeded.

Thank you for shedding more light on the sacred marriage. It is very significant that we can be having these open conversations. Collectively, we are making good progress. It is an unending celebration! :-)

The guru is in you.

2006/04/19 11:02:08
Support for AYP Deep Meditation and Samyama
http://www.aypsite.org/forum/topic.asp?TOPIC_ID=1047&REPLY_ID=6152&whichpage=-1
Vacation Day

quote:
────────
Bewell wrote: I do a double take and some redefining when you take jabs (perhaps friendly jabs) at orthodox Christian theology.
────────

Hi Bewell:

My formative religious inspiration is Christian, and I am also a strong believer in the maxim: "God helps those who help themselves." I am not opposed to saviors and especially not to surrender to our chosen ideal, whoever or whatever that may be. Practices play a key role in this process of opening and surrendering to what is ultimately real for us, and that is the focus of AYP.

If some of my writing seems reactionary in relation to traditional religious themes, it is only because the institutions have distorted religion so badly, and we will be wise not to go along with that. Not if we expect to achieve real spiritual progress in this life. This by no means takes anything away from our heartfelt surrender to Jesus, Mary, or any Beloved One in any of the traditions of the world. That is personal, and certainly valid. For many of us, it is the wellspring of our spiritual desire (bhakti), and I highly respect and encourage that in whatever way one is most inclined. My main advice on religion is, let's make the connection that is natural for us and not sell out to the institution itself, whose goals are likely not in full alignment with our own spiritual longings. In other words, the institution cannot do for us what we can do for ourselves -- commune directly with God within ourselves, and in that way bring the divine out into full expression in the world.

There are some, maybe many by now, who believe that organized religion, with all of its terrible history of manipulation, murder and mayhem, ought to be done away with, and are making a big effort in that direction. I do not believe in that. It is just more fighting over nothing. I think that all the people within the religions should do what is necessary to bring about a rapid expansion of divine consciousness from within themselves, and then transform the institutions accordingly. I believe this is what will happen as millions rise into enlightenment in the decades to come. The religious institutions are not going to go away. They are going to be transformed, because the people within them are rising rapidly in divine consciousness. And all of this is about practices...

The guru is in you.

2006/04/21 14:05:33
Support for AYP Deep Meditation and Samyama
http://www.aypsite.org/forum/topic.asp?TOPIC_ID=1066&REPLY_ID=6238&whichpage=-1
Vibration in throat

Hi Brett:

Most inner vibration like that is energy passing through some obstruction -- friction. With practices, accompanied by good self-pacing, it will clear up in time. If it is taking more time than we expected, then we can be sure it is something pretty deep unwinding in there. So much the better once it is finally unraveled. We will know it has when we can still sense the energy flowing through there, and it is smooth and pleasant (or ecstatic!). There are all sorts of positive implications in this for our daily life, of course.

If you are not into chin pump yet, doing a comfortable daily session of chin pump lite (starting out very short) can help with throat energy obstructions. Make sure to cycle the attention between root and brow with breathing when doing it, just as we do in spinal breathing. This will help balance the energy.

Any other safe activity we can do to exercise the affected region can help also -- asanas, verbal expression, like Meg suggests, and just generally letting the energy work itself through, rather than holding it back, when we are not in sitting practices. You might find that as you do that, some sensations can happen in other areas, especially the heart/emotions. So, we don't overdo too much in specific areas, knowing that the energy will always be shifting elsewhere and making some friction at the point of most resistance.

That's why we keep up the "global" program of purification and opening that deep meditation and spinal breathing provide. This way, we will not be running from trouble spot to trouble spot all the time, but cleaning out the whole nervous system simultaneously instead.

Finally, if the symptom is coming up in meditation with intensity, we can always let the attention rest innocently on the sensation for a while, and this will usually aid in dissolving it. Never underestimate the healing power of pure bliss consciousness -- the witness! :-)

All the best!

The guru is in you.

2006/05/06 09:48:02
Support for AYP Deep Meditation and Samyama
http://www.aypsite.org/forum/topic.asp?TOPIC_ID=1109&REPLY_ID=6640&whichpage=-1
Samyama - Effects of each sutra?

Hi Cosmic:

Sounds like you are having good results with samyama. The practice is not so much about individual effects as it is about the over all effect of the full range of sutras combined -- a broad expansion of inner silence from within producing profound purification and opening in and around us. Also, the full range of sutras greatly strengthens the power of our desires and thoughts in general in everyday living. This is in tandem with the expansion of inner silence, so there is a moral quality that comes up with all of this as well. Aren't we glad? :-)

I suggest you keep going, and not be too concerned about meanings of sutras. Your inner silence knows and that is where it is orginating, not out here...

If you would like to read a saga of samyama, expanded to Biblical proportions in modern times (why not?), check out the Secrets of Wilder novel.

The guru is in you.

2006/05/12 09:41:06
Support for AYP Deep Meditation and Samyama
http://www.aypsite.org/forum/topic.asp?TOPIC_ID=1109&REPLY_ID=6833&whichpage=-1
Samyama - Effects of each sutra?

quote:
_____
Cosmic wrote: Do our desires and thoughts become more intense and "louder"? Or do they become more causative (or maybe both/neither)?
_____

Hi Cosmic:

Causative, but not necessarily in ways we can predict from our individual egoic level. And, likewise, the more power there is as we advance with samyama practice and our over all purification and opening, the more corresponding divine morality will be there. That is why I call the whole process "morally self-regulating." We do not have to worry about it. Samyama is a means to become a channel for divine outflow into the world -- stillness in action. This is contrary to the common belief that we are developing "personal power" with this technique. Well, it is true that it is our power, but it is about us becoming a channel for the divine need rather than the divine becoming a channel for our personal needs. That is the distinction. It is not a coincidence that surrender of each sutra to the infinite within us is the essence of the technique. It will be the ultimate outcome in all that we do -- surrender of all intentions to the divine flow. And it will flow! :-)

The guru is in you.

2006/07/02 13:50:31
Support for AYP Deep Meditation and Samyama
http://www.aypsite.org/forum/topic.asp?TOPIC_ID=1270&REPLY_ID=8774&whichpage=-1
Arent we meditating all our life?

Hi Near and All:

The difference between meditation and what we do when concentrating in daily activity is in the absence of content (meaning) in the mantra. In deep meditation we are systematically picking up the thought of a particular sound with no meaning, and this leaves the mind/attention free to expand to its native inner silence -- infinite pure bliss consciousness. The vibrational characteristics of the mantra (not any meaning) have an influence on how this expansion of attention takes place, and its subsequent effects in the nervous system.

Of course, there is some similarity in concentrating on meaning in our daily activity -- the mind can let go of meaning and go to quieter states in that way also, though it is not nearly as efficient as systematic deep meditation using mantra with no meaning involved. Nevertheless, the letting go after concentrating on meaning can and does bring the silent inspiration of genius that lies within all of us, proportional to the degree that inner silence is available in us at a point in time. This is also the principle of samyama, which is a systematic way of letting go of specific meanings (sutras) into inner silence to achieve global purification in our nervous system and beyond. Samyama is the means by which inner silence is brought into more active manifestation in our daily living.

In time, rising inner silence becomes a dynamic in everything we do -- which brings us back to the significance our daily activity. So, when we are doing something, fading off from it, and returning to it, we are returning to it with our attention established increasingly in inner silence. This makes all of daily life more purposeful and powerful -- a kind of automatic ongoing samyama, an outer expression of the divine within us. Then, indeed, all of life becomes meditation/samyama. But to get to that stage, it is necessary to cultivate our inner silence efficiently via deep meditation. Cultivating inner silence only by concentrating on meaning, losing it, and coming back again, is not nearly as efficient as deep meditation. If it were, we'd be making much more progress without deep meditation in the picture.

With systematic deep meditation (using mantra with no meaning), everything becomes much more powerful.

As for the role of bhakti, real bhakti is inner silence stirred to activity by our desire. If we are actively surrendered to our most cherished ideal, then this stimulates us deep inside similar to the way samyama does. Of course, we do not actively engage in devotional activity while doing our other practices (we always favor the practice we are doing over all other experiences). If we have strong bhakti (desire/surrender to grow) in our life it will be there as an inner habit all the time. Then, whatever practice we are doing will be amplified in its effects. It all works together like that...

The guru is in you.

2006/07/10 10:00:53
Support for AYP Deep Meditation and Samyama
http://www.aypsite.org/forum/topic.asp?TOPIC_ID=1287&REPLY_ID=9203&whichpage=-1
comparing different forms of meditations

Hi All:

Just a reminder that the procedure of deep meditation is very simple -- favoring the mantra when we realize we are off it. The exact same principle applies to tracing the spinal nerve in spinal breathing pranayama -- gently favoring the route of the spine when we realize we are off it. We do not have to hammer either of these into concreteness. Both are allowed to refine and fade to subtleness. The AYP Enlightenment Series books are pretty clear on these points.

Another thing: Modifying any procedure of practice "in flight," as it were, is not the procedure. These things are very simple. The input of the mind has no relevance during the practices, other than to follow the simple instructions.

As they say: "KISS" -- Keep it simple stupid! :-)

Regarding other forms of meditation -- whatever turns you on over the long haul is what matters. Make your decisions on that before or after practice, and never during. Tinker at your own risk. The mind is not always our friend in these things ... that is why the procedures of practice are what they are...

All the best!

The guru is in you.

2006/07/30 12:04:26
Support for AYP Deep Meditation and Samyama
http://www.aypsite.org/forum/topic.asp?TOPIC_ID=1296&REPLY_ID=10043&whichpage=-1
Chakra question

Hi Yogaguy:

Chakras are not considered useless in AYP. It is only that they are not considered to be major control levers to promote the enlightenment process. Certainly the car will not go without the engine and transmission under the hood, but to make the car go we use the gas pedal, gear shift, and steering wheel. We don't hold the engine in our arms to make the car go. :-)

Chakras are profoundly affected by deep meditation, spinal breathing, asanas, mudras, bandhas, kumbhaka, tantra, and other means we use. But we do not use the chakras themselves as the control levers for all this inner development.

In terms of purifying and opening the over all inner neurobiology, the spinal nerve (sushumna) is the king of the hill, with chakras and everything else in the nervous system being connected to the spinal nerve, and subsidiary to it. That is why we do the practices we do in AYP.

To focus on chakras as a primary control lever of the enlightenment process is to risk a tangential path of endless energy manipulations and the experiences (scenery) that come with that. It is beyond human comprehension to cultivate reliable spiritual progress on that level. That is why we regard chakras to be under the hood while we are driving along the road to our destination, using the main controls to do it. And whatever scenery we do encounter along the way, chakra or otherwise, we can enjoy, and then let go again in favor of the procedure of our practice which will carry us further along the highway to ever-greater vistas of inner silence, joy, and outpouring divine love.

All the best!

The guru is in you.

2006/08/03 10:25:42
Support for AYP Deep Meditation and Samyama
http://www.aypsite.org/forum/topic.asp?TOPIC_ID=1296&REPLY_ID=10196&whichpage=-1
Chakra question

Hi All:

Since my background is not in kriya yoga chakra japa, I can't offer much on specifics in this area. I do agree that without meditation in the picture, pranayama is hard pressed to lead us beyond the limits of physical relaxation, and that there are indeed hazards in doing pranayama alone over the long term without effective meditation added, as discussed in the lessons. As you know, in AYP we take the step beyond pranayama with deep meditation right after spinal breathing pranayama, and do not mix the two practices. AYP is different from kriya yoga in that respect.

I also agree that there is a significant difference in the effects of practices before and after the beginning of ecstatic conductivity. This is the advent of vivid inner seeing, and all that "scenery" we talk about. In kriya yoga, this apparently opens the door for chakra japa, if I understand what has been said above. In AYP we just keep going with the same integration of methods, and the experience does continue to advance.

Are there additional opportunities for practice, a la kriya yoga style chakra japa, once ecstatic conductivity is present? We will leave it to the yoga scientists to answer that one. The open source integrators, you know. :-)

Great discussion!

The guru is in you.

Note: First paragraph edited a few hours after original post.

2006/09/20 11:28:28
Support for AYP Deep Meditation and Samyama
http://www.aypsite.org/forum/topic.asp?TOPIC_ID=1523&REPLY_ID=11413&whichpage=-1
Only 20 minutes?

Hi All:

For those interested in "retreat mode," see these schedules and guidelines developed by Trip with my assistance:

Weekend (up to 4 days): http://www.aypsite.org/forum/topic.asp?TOPIC_ID=1416

Extended (5 days or more): http://www.aypsite.org/forum/topic.asp?TOPIC_ID=1428

Trip has experience with the schedule and I'm sure he would be happy to answer any questions.

Note: For a successful retreat involving the AYP practices, it is essential to follow a predetermined schedule, with the associated guidelines. This is because high levels of internal purification will be occurring, and everything must be preplanned and paced accordingly.

There is also the possibility of coordinating "group retreats," physically in one place, or not. As many are finding, group practice (even done long distance) can be very powerful. See here and here. Eventually we will get around to it in retreat mode. All things in their own good time. :-)

The guru is in you.

2006/10/13 11:32:33
Support for AYP Deep Meditation and Samyama
http://www.aypsite.org/forum/topic.asp?TOPIC_ID=1605&REPLY_ID=12262&whichpage=-1
ADD, ADHD, problems during meditation

Hi Hunter:

I'm not an expert on ADD, but can say that deep meditation is not about having an ability to concentrate, or even sit still (movements can be normal). It is about following a simple mental procedure that allows and includes the wandering mind. After a few weeks or months the procedure itself becomes habit, so even it is not a doing.

Interestingly, while deep meditation does not involve the use of concentration, it gradually strengthens our ability to concentrate in daily activity. So this can be a good thing for those with ADD, or anyone who is looking for a way to increase their ability to concentrate.

Of course, it goes far beyond that. The cultivation of inner silence over time opens the doorway to the infinite in us, and ultimately produces "super-normal attention."

No matter what our desire -- for health or for enlightenment -- if we can sustain it enough to keep up a daily practice, deep meditation will carry us forward. The desire for progress is an essential part of the process. That is what enables us to sit daily...

Does ADD limit one's long term desire and commitment to progress in life, or only our ability to focus on the object we are viewing in the moment? If we have the former (ongoing desire), we can easily navigate the latter (attention development) with deep meditation. Once we get to our seat, the procedure of deep meditation takes over. All we have to do is follow it. It becomes easier to get to the seat over time, because inner silence fills us with increasing purpose and laser-like attention. The effect of deep meditation then becomes a cause. But no matter how advanced we become, the procedure of deep meditation is always the same -- not reliant on concentration at all.

The guru is in you.

10/13/06, 2pm eastern -- See update in first paragraph.

2006/11/01 11:48:31
Support for AYP Deep Meditation and Samyama
http://www.aypsite.org/forum/topic.asp?TOPIC_ID=1655&REPLY_ID=12787&whichpage=-1
Breath and Mantra

quote:
_____
Originally posted by Doc

All too often, for example, attempts to consciously force a specific breath pattern to synchronize with a mantra through the course of an entire round or more of practice with a japa mala, succeeds only in reducing the japa yoga to an uncomfortable and counterproductive breath exercise. I have found this to also be true in most instances when practicing hatha asanas, or when meditating, and likewise, particularly during extended practice sessions in which straining is likely at some point.
_____

Hi All:

This is why in AYP we do spinal breathing pranayama and deep meditation in sequence instead of in parallel. The two practices are doing two different things, and are not compatible when done at the same time.

It is the distinction between cultivating inner silence (shiva) and cultivating ecstatic conductivity (shakti). These are separate neurobiological phenomena which mingle and merge after they have arisen.

As for mantras in spinal breathing, likewise, they are left out to maintain the simplicity and efficiency of the practice. In the AYP approach we are dealing with chakra (energy center) and nadi (subtle nerve) purification and opening in a variety of ways, with still more ways to come. So the resonance of chakras and nadis will be there in spinal breathing, in other practices, and in our normal daily activity, with the last being the proof of the pudding -- all occurring "under the hood," of course. :-)

The guru is in you.

2006/11/01 15:55:05
Support for AYP Deep Meditation and Samyama
http://www.aypsite.org/forum/topic.asp?TOPIC_ID=1655&REPLY_ID=12797&whichpage=-1
Breath and Mantra

quote:
_____
Originally posted by Doc

quote:

"....we do spinal breathing pranayama and deep meditation in sequence instead of in parallel. The two practices are doing two different things, and are not compatible when done at the same time.

These are separate neurobiological phenomena which mingle and merge <u>after</u> they have arisen."

_____
It is interesting, however, to observe energetic overlays in the manifested expressions of the two methods while practiced separately....confirming their mutual contributions to a self-disciplined Sadhana. As the yogi/yogini explores profound modifications of Consciousness through Focused Concentration(Dharana), Deep Meditation (Dhyana), and eventual Union with God (Samadhi), breath patterns definitely change along the way to match the neurological, physiological, and psychological fluctuations in the altered states of consciousness (Jivatman). Conversely, the rhythmical breath pattern cycles of various pranayama techniques usually generate a more focused concentration of the mind, and a decidedly meditative mental state as practice skills improve. :-) What's not to like? :-) It's all good! :-)
_____

Hi Doc:

Sounds good to me. :-)

The last three of the eight limbs of yoga you mentioned above (dharana, dhyana & samadhi) also come together in the practice of Samyama. Don't know if you have seen those AYP lessons yet. If not, you might want to take a look at #149, #150, and the lessons that follow. The next AYP book coming out is on Samyama also, looking at it from more angles than we have so far, for additional practical applications. The options really open up as we experience more abiding inner silence (the witness), which increases our ability to relax or surrender into the infinite within us, and act from that level. There are profound implications in this for everyday living.

The fruit of Samyama is "stillness in action," or "outpouring divine love." It is expressed natually through our actions. It is the merging of inner silence with the divine ecstatic flow in all that we do.

What happens with the breath in Samyama, and in this kind of daily activity? Sometimes we breathe, and sometimes breath stops. Breath effortlessly follows the flow of divine consciousness as reflected in the metabolism.

How sweet it is. :-)

The guru is in you.

2006/11/11 09:27:10
Support for AYP Deep Meditation and Samyama
http://www.aypsite.org/forum/topic.asp?TOPIC_ID=1698&REPLY_ID=13143&whichpage=-1
Questions

Hi Comdyne:

There are no restrictions on practice in AYP -- only pointing out the potential issues related to "doubling up" on the same or similar elements of practice found in different systems, and running the risk of excess purification in the nervous sytem, which can be uncomfortable and counterproductive to our progress.

It is up to each practitioner to find their own balance in practices.

The suggestions on this in AYP are based on known probable pitfalls. But it is always up to you. So, what we have in AYP is an open source template that has been shown to be progressive and reasonably stable with prudent self-pacing applied. How you fill it in is up to you. :-)

All the best!

The guru is in you.

2006/12/02 09:00:52
Support for AYP Deep Meditation and Samyama
http://www.aypsite.org/forum/topic.asp?TOPIC_ID=1778&REPLY_ID=13960&whichpage=-1
What is the yantra of the IAM mantra?

Hi Chiron:

I don't know of a yantra (diagram) for the I AM mantra, but have an affinity for the Sri Yantra. See lesson T25. There are links to Sri Yantra diagrams in the lesson. If you have the AYP Easy Lessons book, it will be better to refer to the lesson there, as it was significantly enhanced for the book. Sri Yantra is also discussed in the AYP Tantra book.

As for coming up with a yantra for the I AM mantra, feel free to research it (and let us know). But do keep in mind that we have several enhancements to the I AM mantra along the way, which is AYP's way of sneaking up on the Sri Yantra. :-)

We are That!

The guru is in you.

2006/12/24 14:10:13
Support for AYP Deep Meditation and Samyama
http://www.aypsite.org/forum/topic.asp?TOPIC_ID=1847&REPLY_ID=14817&whichpage=-1

What to watch?

Hi Aditya:

Meditation is not a seeking. It is a doing -- following a simple procedure. All seeking is outside meditation, and it has its place in our life. But not in meditation itself. The same is true for many of the sitting practices we do. We are not there to be analyzing what is happening in the practice -- anything can happen. Whatever happens, we are there to do the practice according to procedure. We can analyse and seek later, when practices are done, and be so much better at it by virtue of the inner silence and ecstatic conductivity we have been cultivating.

When thoughts or other experiences come up in deep meditation, we just easily favor the procedure of meditation, which is easily favoring the mantra with comfort at whatever level our mind is at -- clear, or faint and fuzzy.

We don't deny our thoughts or experiences. We don't try and push them out, and we don't try to hang on to them either. They can be there, and we can still just easily favor the mantra over whatever is happening while we are meditating. Forcing is never part of the process. That is what deep meditation is. Then, after meditation, everything will be more clear.

All the best!

The guru is in you.

2006/12/26 10:43:23
Support for AYP Deep Meditation and Samyama
http://www.aypsite.org/forum/topic.asp?TOPIC_ID=1851&REPLY_ID=14871&whichpage=-1
A.....(yam)?
Note: Topic moved for better placement.
2007/01/04 10:49:27
Support for AYP Deep Meditation and Samyama
http://www.aypsite.org/forum/topic.asp?TOPIC_ID=1853&REPLY_ID=15377&whichpage=-1
what kind of meditation?

quote:

Originally posted by insideout

Shanti,
Where are you? If your group is in Orange County I would be interested in attending.

Hi Insideout:

A deep meditation group in Orange County would be great. Would you like to start one? Shanti and others who have done it can give you the inside scoop. Then we can bring more of the outside in, and more of the inside out. :-)

The guru is in you.

2007/01/17 10:16:57
Support for AYP Deep Meditation and Samyama
http://www.aypsite.org/forum/topic.asp?TOPIC_ID=1960&REPLY_ID=16223&whichpage=-1
Maximizing Samyama practice

Hi Swami Vajra:

Excellent reply from Shanti. I would only add that "default sutra" means the lightness sutra (if no other has been selected) for single sutra usage after the entire list of sutras has been gone through in samyama. This does not mean that the sutra we do at the end replaces the rest of the list. There is no one sutra (or yogic technique) that replaces everything else. It takes an effective integration of methods and tools to achieve the full benefits of yoga.

There is more on this in the new Samyama book, plus expanded applications of samyama available to do in other parts of our practice routine, and in daily life.

All the best!

The guru is in you.

2007/02/13 17:31:10
Support for AYP Deep Meditation and Samyama
http://www.aypsite.org/forum/topic.asp?TOPIC_ID=2049&REPLY_ID=17411&whichpage=-1
Mantra to be given only by a Guru?

Hi EMC:

Of course, all energy experiences and sensations that occur in deep meditation are purification -- part of the "scenery." And we know to easily favor the mantra at whatever level of clarity or fuzziness is comfortable whenever we find ourselves off into whatever may be happening in thoughts, feelings or sensations.

Yes, different inner pronunciations and intonations of mantra can create different energy experiences, but to attempt to supervise or optimize this by tweaking the mantra during meditation is going to be counterproductive. It will also be counterproductive to be adjusting the mantra on a regular basis from session to session, because inner silence is cultivated most effectively as our nervous system develops a deepening familiarity with the mantra as a vehicle of awareness. This takes time -- many months. Keep in mind that because energy experiences and sensations are purification (energy passing through obstructions, causing "friction"), the related experiences will be shifting all the time as the purification advances. So changing the mantra to capture a particular sense of progress in the form of an experience is literally "chasing the ghost" of our karma, which is being dissolved and transformed all the while.

A good way to look at mantra is as an approximate device that can be used as a vehicle for riding or sweeping automatically through the nervous system with increasingly subtle levels of silent awareness. There is no such thing as an "exact mantra" (a point well-taken by David). A mantra's pronunciation may be a little this way or that way. Using the syllables of "I AM" puts us in a ball park of inner sweeping that is known to be more or less effective and safe in the human nervous system. It will never be an exact thing -- only a ball park thing in terms of the quality and effect of the syllables. The same is true of the mantra enhancements, which broaden the sweep of awareness within us, while broadening the breadth of purification. Check lesson 188 for the over all strategy on mantra design in AYP: http://www.aypsite.org/188.html

Because we are using an inexact tool (mantra) doesn't mean that we are not accomplishing profound results. How many straws does it take to make a broom that will sweep our doorstep? The answer is "enough," with a few more or less straws still being "enough." Mantra and mantra pronunciation are like that. The main difference will be when we add an enhancement, which is like doubling or tripling the straws in our broom. That kind of expansion is something different that can be successfully undertaken once we have become well-skilled at using our old broom.

So, it is good to not belabor our current mantra too much, and just carry on with the simple procedure in twice-daily practice. If you are looking for more out of the mantra, then look to an enhancement, after deep meditation with the present mantra has been smooth and stable for at least several months, preferably longer. Of course, enhancements should be taken in order, and not rushed into. It takes time for the nervous system to adapt to fully utilize a mantra or an enhancement, and that is the same reason why we do not keep fiddling with the thing, which I know you aren't -- well, not too much anyway. We have all done our fair share of fiddling, and we are wiser for it. :-)

All the best!

The guru is in you.

2007/02/14 13:37:11
Support for AYP Deep Meditation and Samyama
http://www.aypsite.org/forum/topic.asp?TOPIC_ID=2049&REPLY_ID=17462&whichpage=-1
Mantra to be given only by a Guru?

Hi All:

Kindly shift the guru conversation over to here in the "Gurus..." forum:
http://www.aypsite.org/forum/topic.asp?TOPIC_ID=2054

The related posts (and parts of posts) have been split off or copied and moved there. Let's continue on mantra and deep meditation here.

Good idea, Trip! Oops, that's been moved over there too. :-)

The guru is in you.

2007/04/10 13:18:34
Support for AYP Deep Meditation and Samyama
http://www.aypsite.org/forum/topic.asp?TOPIC_ID=2049&REPLY_ID=20126&whichpage=-1
Mantra to be given only by a Guru?

quote:
_____
Originally posted by riptiz

Namaskars Shailesh,
I completey agree with your post and this is my experience also.
L&L
Dave
_____

I agree too, but how do we cover the world population of 6.5 billion people (and growing) with the venerable old guru system? It is, frankly, a bit petrified, and not yet living in the information age.

All that is good in the guru system, we need much more of that for everyone.

Clearly, something has to change.

The guru is in you.
 <-- more direct access to that One will help. :-)

2007/04/10 14:02:44
Support for AYP Deep Meditation and Samyama
http://www.aypsite.org/forum/topic.asp?TOPIC_ID=2049&REPLY_ID=20130&whichpage=-1
Mantra to be given only by a Guru?

quote:
_____
Originally posted by riptiz

The point is there is room for the old and new and something to be learnt from both.
_____

Hi Dave:

Agreed absolutely. And each ought to keep prodding the other. :-)

I am not anti-guru. I am pro-progress.

As the old saying goes: "Lead, follow, or get out of the way!"

For a bit of perspective, here is some history in an AYP lesson that discusses the progression of the eastern traditions coming west over more than a century, leading directly to the wonderful knowledge we are blessed to be sharing and utilizing today. So, there is no question that we are standing on the shoulders of giants -- and thousands of years of glorious spiritual discovery. That should never be forgotten.

On the other hand, we have to be honest and say to the traditions: "What have you been doing lately?"
Just as the traditions might say to upstarts like AYP: "Better not ignore all this experience."

We are doing the best we can, yes?

The guru is in you.

2007/04/11 12:53:11
Support for AYP Deep Meditation and Samyama
http://www.aypsite.org/forum/topic.asp?TOPIC_ID=2049&REPLY_ID=20188&whichpage=-1
Mantra to be given only by a Guru?

Hi All:

Since I put my toe in here yesterday, maybe it would be good to go back and answer the original question. :-)

"Must a mantra be given only by a guru?"

Well, based on the experiences of many, obviously not, but there may be an initial energy advantage in receiving guru initiation -- at least in the old days there was, when little else was available. It is changing, and the playing field is gradually becoming more level between "transmitted" mantras versus "shared" mantras (see below).

Once a guru initiation is done, it is up to the practitioner. The initial boost and lingering energy connection are a plus. But in the long run it is the aspirant's dedication to daily practice and the effectiveness of the method that will make the difference. It is always about the aspirant. It isn't about the guru. A true guru will be the first to say that, constantly reminding the aspirant to stay on task with the methods that lead to "self-realization." The goal is not "guru-realization."

There is a potential disadvantage to guru initiation that should not be ignored. That is the association with a fixed tradition, with fixed (locked in) methods, and little room for experimentation and discovery of improvements in practice. It has been the job of the traditions to preserve knowledge down through the centuries. And so they have, much to their credit. The problem is that no single tradition has been preserving the total knowledge of human spiritual transformation. There is a noticeable fragmentation of yogic knowledge spread around among the many traditions from which most of our gurus have come.

Tradition "A" is mainly meditation and samyama. Tradition "B" is mainly pranayama and hatha. Tradition "C" is mainly asanas. Tradition "D" is mainly non-dual inquiry. Tradition "E" is mainly bhakti. And it goes on and on. The walls between these highly-focused conservative approaches are quite high. So, when we receive the advantage of guru initiation, we also may find ourselves with the disadvantage of limited opportunity for exposure to all of the methods of yoga in a balanced way. This is especially true when vows of secrecy and loyalty are taken. It can be very limiting.

In the old days, this sort of guru/disciple exclusivity may have made perfect sense, but in the information age it is out of date, at least in the applied science oriented mass markets of the west. We all know of the abuses that have occurred with the guru system being applied in modern times. It is systemic, meaning there is a fundamental incompatibility between the method and the time in which it is being used.

So, change is in the air. It is happening (slooowly) within the traditions. And we also have upstarts moving in quickly to fill the void. AYP is one of many attempts to make spiritual knowledge transmission more open and effective in modern times, while reducing the risk of abuse that has been found lurking in the guru system. It is a shift to the methods of applied science and communications/distribution that take advantage of modern technology. It makes sense -- each generation is entitled to view applied knowledge through its own spyglass, and then to do its best to pass on all that is known to the next generation to look at through their spyglass, and so on...

As shailesh kumar said, we have to learn from someone. While the human nervous system in each of us is the source of all yogic knowledge, we still can benefit greatly from the accumulated knowledge that humanity has assembled on utilizing the mechanisms of spiritual transformation residing in each of us. We should continue to build on what is known, and pass it on as efficiently as possible.

But back to the original question ... if we are learning our mantra through a modern non-guru information system, is something lost? There is that magical energy connection that a guru can give us. What is it? And can we receive it by other means? This is the crux of the question.

There will always be bonafide living gurus, and we are blessed to have them. The energy and knowledge they share help us greatly to uplift ourselves, according to our own spiritual desire (bhakti). It can occur through a variety of means -- mantras, shaktipat, healings, behind the scenes sharing, etc. It is spiritual energy, and it flows in many ways to those who actively surrender to their highest ideal. There is a lot of energy flowing these days, and gurus are no longer the only source of it. They may not even be the primary source of it anymore. Though, still, a real guru who does not tie up his or her followers is a real treasure.

World consciousness is rising rapidly, and more and more spiritual energy is being transmitted through our collective opening. This is a major acceleration in human evolution that is occurring before our eyes. Knowledge that is transmitted through collective means may well someday meet or exceed what the single great guru can provide. Time will tell. The important thing to know is that it is happening, and it will continue to grow. So all is not lost anymore if the guru is not found in an individual person. It can also be found in forward-looking communities, and, most importantly, in ourselves.

See lesson 146 for a discussion on the expansion of energy transmission capability from the individual guru to occurring throughout the society as a whole: http://www.aypsite.org/146.html

Regarding mantra, there is the inherent vibration that is contained within the sound itself, which will provide for effective and balanced purification and opening in the nervous system, if used correctly in deep meditation. This has little to do with how the mantra is transmitted. There are thousands of mantras, and the discussion can be endless on this. In AYP, the selection of mantra and enhancements is based on a particular rationale, and the known causes and effects involved in using the syllables that make up the mantra.

Here are a few lessons that discuss the AYP mantra strategy:
Mantra Particulars: http://www.aypsite.org/59.html
Mantra Design 101: http://www.aypsite.org/188.html
Also see other lessons under "mantra" in the topic index: http://www.aypsite.org/TopicIndex.html

In the end, the proof of the pudding will be in the eating. So eat! :-)

All the best!

The guru is in you.

2007/04/11 14:10:51
Support for AYP Deep Meditation and Samyama
http://www.aypsite.org/forum/topic.asp?TOPIC_ID=2049&REPLY_ID=20195&whichpage=-1
Mantra to be given only by a Guru?

quote:
_____
Originally posted by Mike

The questioning/logical part of my mind tho' was curious as to why you feel/believe that 'spritual energy is increasing' [to be clear I personally have no idea of whether its up down or sideways].
_____

Hi Mike:

To me it is about cause and effect.

It is an observable evolution (or revolution) of access to knowledge on the means of human spiritual transformation (practices). It began filtering over to the west over a century ago, and has been accelerating ever since. In the process, the knowledge is being revitalized in ways that have not happened in India and other parts of Asia, due to the conservative nature of the traditions there.

Millions more people are meditating around the world every year, so there are more results, more inner purification, and more energy flowing. Each individual can gauge it by their own inner openings. Take that and keep reproducing it across the world's population, and we have something remarkable going on.

It is about the numbers of people gaining access, which is why AYP is what it is -- an attempt to expand access to effective practices as much as possible. The more who are opening, the easier it is for others to open, and so on. That is the energy dynamic we can see occurring everywhere.

From an applied knowledge point of view, it is not unprecedented. It has happened in many fields. Faraday was playing around with the invisible forces of static electricity and magnets (spooky stuff in those days), and 150 years later we have electricity available for practical use everywhere, and nearly everyone has a cell phone in their pocket. The application of spiritual knowledge is traveling a similar route.

For those who have been engaged in spiritual practices for the past 30-40 years, the change in the life experience has been pretty dramatic, not only individually, but in the rising receptivity in people everywhere. There has been a lot of change. As Dave pointed out earlier, we are sharing and applying knowledge now that we could barely imagine only a few decades ago. What will it be like 20 years from now? 50 years from now? We'll see...

Looking at it as a practical refinement and worldwide distribution of knowledge puts it within a framework we can easily understand. This is what we have seen already in many other fields of knowledge. In yoga, we should keep going and see where it leads. The least we can do is make sure that everyone everywhere has access to useful knowledge on practices. Then it is up to them. Based on what we have seen going on so far, the prospects are pretty exciting. That is how I see it. :-)

The guru is in you.

2007/02/22 17:20:50
Support for AYP Deep Meditation and Samyama
http://www.aypsite.org/forum/topic.asp?TOPIC_ID=2097&REPLY_ID=17911&whichpage=-1
Practical prayer with Samyama

Hi EMC:

Glad you like the Samyama book. :-)

In using samyama with prayer outside our regular sitting practices, all we want to do is settle into our inner silence for a few minutes. This might take 5-10 minutes of deep meditation (yes, with our mantra), or less if we have been meditating for years. In the latter case, we will have inner silence resident in us all the time, and go to deep stillness as soon as we close our eyes. This is all we need for prayer utilizing the principles of samyama.

So, in meditating for a few minutes before prayer, we don't do it to cultivate inner silence the way we do when we are meditating for 20 minutes twice a day. We only do it enough to settle down. How many times per day can we meditate for a few minutes like this? Well, not too many. It isn't a blank check to meditate 19 times a day to say a prayer. :-) If we do, we will pay the price with extra purification. Self-pacing is necessary in all things yogic, and we each will find our balance.

If we are inclined to pray a lot (a wonderful thing), we will gradually develop the habit of relaxing into our stillness on a moment's notice, without actual deep meditation being necessary to do it. We become stillness. Samyama itself (the act of releasing faint thought impulses into stillness) will promote this also, and move stillness outward as the result (siddhi).

There is a section in the Samyama book that discusses the role of samyama in daily living, which is living our life within moving stillness, acting constantly as That. It is a natural development that occurs gradually over time as we continue with daily practices. By then, samyama becomes part of our way of thinking and acting, and stillness flows as a continuous joyful divine outpouring, naturally dissolving all obstructions within and around us.

Even so, we continue with our regular sitting practices, always favoring our practice over the many wonderful experiences that come up. And always self-pacing as necessary.

All the best!

The guru is in you.

2007/04/09 16:27:16
Support for AYP Deep Meditation and Samyama
http://www.aypsite.org/forum/topic.asp?TOPIC_ID=2400&REPLY_ID=20080&whichpage=-1
so'ham hamsa

quote:
_____
Originally posted by blackmuladar

i have been practicing the SRF hong-sa technique for some years. when i tried the "I AM AYAM" mantra it didn't seem to "reach" or "cover as much ground" as hong-sa did. then i added the Shree Shree at the front of AYAM and it felt as if work was being done. the question is,is it neccessary to start w/the AYAM mantra alone or if it feels right start w/the add ons?
_____

Hi Blackmuladar:

Not sure how you are approaching the use of mantra meditation. It sounds like you might be replacing hong-sau (hamsa/so-ham) with I AM (AYAM) in your present technique. Just in case you are, the I AM (AYAM) mantra is not a breathing mantra, and it is not recommended to use it that way.

As you know, hong-sau (hamsa/so-ham) is a breathing mantra, which involves a different technique from AYP deep meditation. In AYP, we do not mix pranayama with mantra use. Instead, we do spinal breathing pranayama (in kriya yoga, spinal breathing usually replaces the hong-sau method), followed by a separate session of deep meditation with mantra (which kriya yoga does not use). So we are talking about two classes of practice (pranayama and meditation), and the results, while intermingled, are not directly comparable. Each has its own role to play in our purification and opening.

In addition, in AYP spinal breathing pranayama, we do not use mantra (as is done sometimes in kriya yoga), which is a significant difference in approach.

Deep meditation is for cultivating inner silence, and spinal breathing pranayama is for cultivating ecstatic conductivity. Both of these are enhanced with additional techniques as we go through the AYP lessons in order, which is where the mantra enhancements come in on the inner silence side of the equation.

For further explanation on the relationship of mantra and breathing in AYP, see this lesson: http://www.aypsite.org/106.html

So, with all of that, I'm not sure that you would be taking a good step going to the first mantra enhancement, since it is not yet clear what you are practicing. Even using the AYP deep meditation technique, I would not recommend starting with an enhanced mantra.

For those who are using the AYP deep meditation technique, going to the first mantra enhancement is a pretty big step. It may not happen for many months, or even years. It certainly should not be done until our current deep meditation practice with I AM (AYAM) is clear and stable. Of course, it is always up to the practitioner.

Wishing you the best on your path. Practice wisely, and enjoy!

The guru is in you.

2007/04/15 10:57:45
Support for AYP Deep Meditation and Samyama
http://www.aypsite.org/forum/topic.asp?TOPIC_ID=2403&REPLY_ID=20426&whichpage=-1
Will you help me with my Samyama practice please?

Hi Bliss Hunter:

Check this topic for an interesting discussion on samyama results:

http://www.aypsite.org/forum/topic.asp?TOPIC_ID=1034&SearchTerms=sidhi

Also, if you like, contact this forum member -- a TM teacher (one of several who have visited here), who now teaches independently and has recommended AYP samyama to his students.

You can find lots more info by doing targeted searches both in the forums and in the lessons. It takes some work to find out what is going on. It takes some serious study, and dedicated daily practice over time. Rome was not built in a day.

Nearly everything we learn for the first time has a "clunky stage" in the beginning. Just keep going with daily practice and things will refine gradually. That is how it is with all spiritual practices. Samyama is no exception.

As has been suggested already, it is best to start at the beginning of the AYP lessons, and go one step at a time. Then you will have the best chance for results.

If we rely on others too much, expecting instant answers, we will likely come up short, and be disappointed. Disappointed about what? Disappointed because others are not doing for us what we ought to be doing ourselves?

If you don't have the patience for it, then go do the TM/Sid
Hi program -- much more hand-holding there. Ultimately, you will find the same is true there as here. Success in anything takes dedication over the long term.

Don't get me wrong, the TM/Sid
Hi program is very worthwhile, especially for getting a good foundation in Samyama practice. At the same time, we will only get out what we put into it. The same is true of AYP Samyama, and everything else we do in life.

The main difference between TM/Sid
Hi and AYP Samyama isn't in the technique itself. It is in the degree of hand-holding from the TM folks on the front end (for a price), versus the degree of flexibility offered in AYP self-directed practice combined with a wide range of additional practices that complement each other, leading to broad results in full scope human spiritual transformation.

All the best!

The guru is in you.

2010/12/14 17:25:42
Support for AYP Deep Meditation and Samyama
http://www.aypsite.org/forum/topic.asp?TOPIC_ID=2429&REPLY_ID=76752&whichpage=-1
Subtle mantra difference, better results.

Hi All:

A review of this lesson might be helpful:
http://www.aypsite.org/366.html

All the best!

The guru is in you.

2007/04/27 09:18:51
Support for AYP Deep Meditation and Samyama
http://www.aypsite.org/forum/topic.asp?TOPIC_ID=2471&REPLY_ID=21068&whichpage=-1
Merging?

Hi Christi:

If the intention is to serve, there will be no discomfort when we notice that the boundaries we have been living within are a construct. If the intention is to protect, there can be some concern when the clouds part for a moment.

It is an evolution, with adjustments necessary along the way as we unfold from within. The turning point is when we are still/open enough inside to allow it, and that is coincident with the turn to serving more than protecting.

Even so, we will instinctively sustain a boundary to function in the world, and this is where the will comes in. But it is not all or nothing on either side. Stillness knows. The trust we are seeking is trusting our own inner process, and that takes some time. This too is service.

Service/silence also knows when to step back -- self-pacing.

The guru is in you.

2007/04/28 16:04:42
Support for AYP Deep Meditation and Samyama
http://www.aypsite.org/forum/topic.asp?TOPIC_ID=2471&REPLY_ID=21150&whichpage=-1
Merging?

quote:
_____
Originally posted by Christi

Are you saying that if my attitude is to serve (others/ humanity/ The Divine) then everything will be fine, and something in the silence will know when it is apropriate to let the boundaries fall?
Then all I have to do is to change my attitude from one of protecting to one of serving? I guess we all exist somewhere on a spectrum between these two. I take it protecting means fear/ contraction and service means selfless love?

Christi

Hi Christi:

Actually, rising inner silence is what changes our attitude. We can choose to serve, but it will only go as far as our inner opening.

Of course, service is practice also, but will be less a primary cause than deep meditation, for most people anyway.

When inner silence comes, fear goes, That is another way of looking at it. Sometimes acting "as if" there is no fear can help the opening, but this too depends on inner silence.

These are not disconnected events -- your experience of merging, the degree of inner silence, the degree of opening to service, less fear, less need to protect. They are all different aspects of the same multi-dimensional opening that is occurring. Pick parts to do that suit you best. Every aspect of yoga is connected through your nervous system.

Good things are happening! :-)

The guru is in you.

2007/05/31 13:02:43
Support for AYP Deep Meditation and Samyama
http://www.aypsite.org/forum/topic.asp?TOPIC_ID=2624&REPLY_ID=22597&whichpage=-1
I AM or AUM

quote:
Originally posted by salvation

Hi to all

My question is that is "I AM" different from "AUM". I have read about "AUM" everywhere but here I found something different.Does "I AM" produce different vibrations and is it better than "AUM" ?

I apologise if I hurt someone's feelings but I think these type of questions can be helpful for the sadhaks especially like me..

Hi Salvation:

See this lesson: http://www.aypsite.org/59.html

All the best!

The guru is in you.

2007/06/27 17:26:59
Support for AYP Deep Meditation and Samyama
http://www.aypsite.org/forum/topic.asp?TOPIC_ID=2712&REPLY_ID=23612&whichpage=-1
Mantra Repeating

quote:
Originally posted by Anthem11

The only exception to this is sometimes my repetition of the mantra is delayed if I am off in the blissful reverberations of the mantra. Should I come back earlier here if I realize I am off or can I let the reverberations take their coarse?

Yogani, this has been on my mind a lot recently, if this is incorrect can you please correct us?

Hi Andrew:

We can pick up the mantra within the blissful reverberations, or as a blissful reverberation. Then we go from there. We pick up the mantra wherever we happen to be when we realize we are off it. This does not necessarily mean leaving or ending what is happening. It isn't even a shift, only a subtle favoring. We just go in from there.

The guru is in you.

2007/07/03 11:16:19
Support for AYP Deep Meditation and Samyama
http://www.aypsite.org/forum/topic.asp?TOPIC_ID=2727
Samyama Sutras and Language

Hi All:

From a recent email exchange:

Q: My questions about samyama.

1. I can't translate all the concepts (from Cosmic Samyama in the Samyama book) like "cosmos – galaxy – solar system" into my native tongue even though I have mastery over them in a foreign language. What can I do? Begin in one language and finish in the other one? Or simply adopt the foreign language for everything?

2. I do not get the importance of a sutra like akasha – lightness of air (and it is the one we have to repeat for the longest period of time) in the series of the nine that you propose, whereas other sutras like unseen obstructions or renouncement would be much more appropriate to reach the goal of yoga in a more efficient way.
Please comment.

I would like to add identity as a sutra, what do you think ?

Thank you for revealing Samyama in such a clear manner.

A: In samyama, we can go with the words/language that have the clearest meaning within us. Regarding some of the sutras from cosmic samyama from the Samyama book, "cosmos" is the universe containing billions of galaxies. "Galaxy" is our milky way galaxy containing billions of stars, our sun being one of those. "Solar system" is our sun and orbiting planets.

Whatever words or short phrases represent these meanings to you are okay, in the language you choose.

"Akasha - Lightness of Air" is a very powerful sutra, but you don't have to use it if you don't want to. However, I do suggest becoming stable in a basic twice-daily routine of sutras as instructed in the AYP Lessons and Samyama book before changing things around too much. And when making changes, do it in small steps, being prepared to self-pace as necessary. This is discussed in the appendix on Patanjali's Samyama Sutras in the Samyama book, and elsewhere.

"Akasha" means "inner space," so the sutra can also be used as "inner space - lightness of air," translated into one's first language, if desired. The effect of the sutra is to gradually cognize the reality of the body as empty space (it is that), which leads to interesting possibilities. The "inner space" version is how it is used in the Secrets of Wilder novel, which contains no Sanskrit. Whichever version we choose, we should stay with that, as it takes time for the sutra syllables to settle in and increase in their effects over months and years of practice.

I can't predict the effect of sutras you may choose to use outside those in the Samyama book, like "identity." It will be your own research. Do let us know what you discover! :-)

Obviously, it is best to be well-established in a good basic routine of samyama practice before engaging in research, so there will be a solid foundation of practice and experience in place. A long term process of purification and opening finds its best results in stable daily practice, without changing things often.

All the best!

The guru is in you.

Yogani

Note: Basic instructions for samyama practice can be found in the online lessons, and in the AYP Easy Lessons book. Additional instructions and more applications for samyama practice (including cosmic samyama) can be found in the Samyama book.

2007/07/05 16:24:03
Support for AYP Deep Meditation and Samyama
http://www.aypsite.org/forum/topic.asp?TOPIC_ID=2741&REPLY_ID=23861&whichpage=-1
samyama question

Hi Clk1710:

It is an interesting approach to building up your sutras. Nothing wrong with it, if it works for you.

Normally we'd take them all on at once, and self pace the whole set, like Anthem said. But your approach is okay too. Once you have them all, then I suggest keeping them together and self-pacing the whole set as needed, as discussed in the Samyama book.

The guru is in you.

2007/07/08 14:31:37
Support for AYP Deep Meditation and Samyama
http://www.aypsite.org/forum/topic.asp?TOPIC_ID=2758&REPLY_ID=24014&whichpage=-1
Only one samyama

Hi Gentlep:

If you'd like to take the samyama sutras on one (or a few) at a time, like Clk1710 was doing here, I suggest starting at the beginning of the list, so you will be building the sequence habit in the same order. Much easier that way. It takes time for the sutras to settle in, which includes the order of repetition. This is assuming your objective is to build a daily routine of sutra practice for the long term, which is recommended for best results.

See my comments in the other topic linked above.

All the best!

The guru is in you.

2007/07/17 09:32:15
Support for AYP Deep Meditation and Samyama
http://www.aypsite.org/forum/topic.asp?TOPIC_ID=2775&REPLY_ID=24253&whichpage=-1
Deep med versus watching breath

Hi Snake:

...Because it is not possible to do fully effective meditation and pranayama at the same time -- an underlying principle upon which much of the AYP approach is based. It seems to work. :-)

See here: http://www.aypsite.org/43.html

The guru is in you.

PS: A rudimentary proof of this is found in the fact that when breathing naturally suspends, deep meditation will continue. But how can breath awareness continue when that happens? It cannot. Real meditation is beyond breath awareness. That is why pranayama and meditation are two separate limbs in the eight limbs of yoga, with meditation being the limb right before samad
Hi (absorption in inner silence). Pranayama is right before pratyahara (introversion of senses), which is appropriate, since pranayama (spinal breathing especially) opens up inner space to us, and the introversion of sensory perception that comes with it. But this is not meditation -- a good preparation for meditation, but not meditation itself. This is why our routine goes asanas, spinal breathing pranayama and deep meditation, in that order. Each goes progressively deeper. Then, with samyama, we come pouring back out as stillness in action. :-)

2007/07/31 10:58:46
Support for AYP Deep Meditation and Samyama
http://www.aypsite.org/forum/topic.asp?TOPIC_ID=2806&REPLY_ID=24491&whichpage=-1
Mantra question

Hi Jill:

The "inner dialog" as you call it is a normal part of mantra meditation. All thoughts that arise during deep meditation correspond to the release of energy as purification occurs deep in our nervous system when we go to stillness with the mantra. The procedure is to easily come back to the mantra when we realize we are off it. It is a cycle that is repeated over and over for our time of meditation twice daily. We easily favor the mantra over any thought processes that may come up during deep meditation. Thoughts will happen. When we notice, we favor the mantra, which takes us to stillness over and over again. The procedure is very simple. In time, the procedure becomes an automatic habit, which takes us deeper and deeper in our meditation. The whole process and its results become very refined over the long term. It is a journey to abiding inner silence and personal freedom.

If thoughts or sensations in meditation become overwhelming, we have procedures for dealing with that as outlined in the AYP lessons and books. Also, it is very important to take adequate rest at the end of each meditation session to allow the inner releases that are occurring to stabilize before we get up. If we don't rest enough at the end of deep meditation, there can be some irritability in our activity outside meditation.

The experience in meditation can be anything according to the releases occurring. The experience in meditation is not a measure of the effectiveness of the practice. Our experience in daily living outside meditation is the true measure. If there is more peace, joy and creative energy in life, then we will know something good is happening due to our deep meditation practice.

If we find ourselves analyzing during deep meditation, we always just easily come back to the mantra at whatever level of clarity or fuzziness of mental activity we happen to be in. The vibration of the mantra can be entertained at all levels in the mind, from clear pronunciation to very faint and fuzzy. We simply favor the most comfortable level of the mantra. Less is more in this process.

Unlike much of our everyday thinking, the mantra and its associated procedure are designed to travel vertically in the mind rather than horizontally. So when we are meditating, the character of all our thinking will be part of this vertical procedure and process of refinement -- the cultivation of abiding inner silence in our nervous system. With this, the quality of life is uplifted and many positive things become possible. We find ourselves to be increasingly present as the "inner silent witness," and engaging in life more as "stillness in action," or what can also be called "outpouring divine love."

There are many systems that use mantra and many that don't. And no two systems of mantra meditation are the same. The goal in AYP has been to come up with a simple effective approach with mantra that anyone can use. There are three levels of mantra enhancement beyond the basic "I AM" mantra, also covered in the lessons. The over all AYP mantra strategy is summarized in this lesson: http://www.aypsite.org/188.html

As for systems of meditation that do not use mantra, I am not really qualified to speak much about them. They seem to require longer sittings, and the results reported seem to be slower in coming. Which is not to say meditation without mantra does not work. Obviously it does work for those who are consistent in their practice over the years. It is just a different dynamic and kind of journey than deep meditation with mantra, which also depends on steady practice over the long term. Consistency over time is the key to success with any spiritual practice.

If we want to strike water, much better to keep digging in the same place. :-)

All roads lead home, but not necessarily by exactly the same route. It is best to go to a qualified source when seeking information about any given system of practice.

Wishing you all the best on your chosen path. Enjoy!

The guru is in you.

2007/08/14 09:44:08

quote:
_____
Originally posted by Sparkle

Hi Tam Phap

You could have a look at the following lesson and see if it rings a bell for you.
http://www.aypsite.com/92.html

I would personally experience various colours and shapes and lights in the brow area during meditation. Not sure if this is what you are talking about? If it is then Lesson 92 seems to explain it pretty well.

Louis
_____

Yes, the same phenomena can be perceived and described in different ways. But there is only one nervous system and process of purification and opening going on. :-)

The guru is in you.

2007/08/16 10:50:16
Support for AYP Deep Meditation and Samyama
http://www.aypsite.org/forum/topic.asp?TOPIC_ID=2833&REPLY_ID=24838&whichpage=-1
Important Sutras

Hi All:

There is no magic number of sutras, nor is there a perfect blend. The idea is to cover the full scope of the nervous system so outward flowing purification and opening via samyama can be accomplished in a broad-based way.

So, it isn't about any one sutra. It is about the blend. In AYP, we use 9 sutras for regular sitting samyama practice, 16 for cosmic samyama, and have other options for use in asanas, prayer, Patanjali sutra experiments, and in daily living. All of these applications are covered in the AYP Samyama book.

As for redesign, it is really up to the practitioner, but it is not recommended for beginners. It is preferable to have a solid foundation in practice (as in years) before attempting to redesign the practice. Nevertheless, we will all approach it in our own way. That is the nature of self-directed practice. Just don't ask me to do the redesign. You would be surprised how often I am asked to do this (a lot) -- redesign the AYP practices, or redesign someone else's teachings. Yikes! :-)

The guru is in you.

2007/08/23 07:13:22
Support for AYP Deep Meditation and Samyama
http://www.aypsite.org/forum/topic.asp?TOPIC_ID=2859&REPLY_ID=24999&whichpage=-1
I AM GOD

Hi Eddy:

It may be helpful to think in terms of the relationship between deep meditation and samyama. Meditation is about cultivating stillness beyond meaning. This is why we do not use meaning associated with the mantra in deep meditation -- much more refined than meanings that are conjured up in the mind. Samyama is about initiating meaning in stillness and allowing that to express outwardly via the natural flow of stillness into action, which we come to recognize in time as ongoing ecstatic bliss and outpouring divine love. Cultivating stillness consistently over time is the prerequisite for this process, and for all progress in yoga.

Stillness first, and meaning initiated and overflowing from within after that. Not the other way around.

"Seek first the kingdom of heaven, and all will be added to you."

There is nothing wrong with your divine desire. It is only a matter of manifesting it effectively over the long term. It will not happen by following the wanderings of the mind, which change from week to week and month to month. Something systematic needs to be in place to illuminate the mind from within. That is daily deep meditation, consistently taking us beyond the vagaries of the mind each day. In time, it adds up to abiding inner silence. And then we have it -- the whole ball of wax. :-)

All the best!

The guru is in you.

2007/09/12 12:57:27
Support for AYP Deep Meditation and Samyama
http://www.aypsite.org/forum/topic.asp?TOPIC_ID=2915&REPLY_ID=25461&whichpage=-1
Deep Meditation Practice for 1 or more Hours

Hi Sean, and welcome!

In modern terminology, your plan to ramp up deep meditation time to that extent can be said to be, "cruising for a bruising."

It would be like having a very fast car and increasing from a reasonable highway speed of 60 mph at the rate of 10 mph per day to reach a goal of 200 mph in two week's time. There is only one problem with this approach. As logical as it may seem, it is a formula for disaster.

You are the driver and are in charge, and will learn as you go. Just be mindful to avoid flying off a cliff before you have had the opportunity to gain the benefits of safe driving.

Deep meditation of the kind we are using in AYP is very powerful. It is for shorter sittings and then going out and being active in daily life to stabilize the results on an ongoing basis. This is the formula.

If you want to add practice time on (or, more importantly, increase results with safety), consider getting involved in yoga postures and spinal breathing pranayama, also in modest doses as suggested in the lessons. These can add a powerful dimension to your practice. There is a lot more that can be done to enhance practices and their results with relative safety, one step at a time. See the AYP lessons for an integrated plan.

If you are determined to do long sittings of meditation, then you might consider looking at Buddhist and other methods that are more suited for that. However, I would caution about mixing other methods with the AYP practices. Sometimes there can be compounding effects leading to similar issues of excess purification that can occur when overdoing with the AYP practices alone.

As has been said before, the path of human spiritual transformation is a marathon, not a sprint. Rome was not built in a day. :-)

So, consider building a balanced daily approach for the long term that will enable you to carry on in normal life, with steadily increasing inner silence, ecstatic bliss and outpouring divine love. It takes patience and persistence, and is well worth doing.

Other options to consider include joining or forming an AYP meditation group, and eventually AYP retreats which provide the means for an increased number of daily meditation sessions in a carefully regulated routine over days or weeks. AYP meditation groups and retreats will happen as and when practitioners get together and organize them. When practitioners are willing and able to administer such evolutionary group activities, the knowledge and tools to support them will be available within the AYP system of practices.

There is great power in group practice, as many are finding in local meditation groups, and the decentralized web-coordinated group meditation and samyama sessions that have been going on here for some time.

You can see some of the development work that is being done for AYP meditation groups and retreats here:
http://www.aypsite.org/forum/forum.asp?FORUM_ID=41

AYP meditation groups and retreats are still in the embryonic stage. There is a lot of potential there for the future as more and more practitioners are coming along around the world.

As you can see, there are many ways to enhance our spiritual progress, but I don't think driving 200 mph along the curves of purification and opening in our nervous system is one of them. :-)

Wishing you all the best on your chosen path. Practice wisely, and enjoy!

The guru is in you.

2007/09/17 15:09:10
Support for AYP Deep Meditation and Samyama
http://www.aypsite.org/forum/topic.asp?TOPIC_ID=2930&REPLY_ID=25553&whichpage=-1
deep meditation and dreams/vision

Hi Gentlep:

Yes, that is correct, but keep in mind that in deep meditation we are using a specific procedure. We favor the mantra whenever we notice we are off it -- no forcing, no strain. If there is some strain when going back to the mantra, we may be forcing to a less refined (more concrete) level of mental pronunciation. Or there could be a lot of purification going on -- see lesson 15 for what to do if excess purification and discomfort are occurring during deep meditation.

Either way, we take it easy. We just favor the mantra whenever we realize we are off somewhere in the labyrinth of the mind, and the move will naturally be to less activity in the mind. At times, the mantra can be very faint and fuzzy, barely recognizable, a mere nothing. There can be other things going on at the same time -- thoughts, feelings, sensations. It is fine to let the other things be there at the same time, but not deliberately favoring them. When we notice we have wandered off into thoughts or sensations, no matter how refined or entertaining, we just favor the faint vibration of the mantra without undue strain.

Deep meditation is not about deliberately getting rid of thoughts, feelings or sensations, or about forcing our attention to be on one thing or the other. Many experiences will be coming and going during deep meditation, and changing all the time. This is fine. It is part of the process of purification and opening. Everything else will be changing during meditation, but the procedure does not change. It is the procedure that brings us home to inner silence over and over again. Through daily practice we gradually come to know that we are pure bliss consciousness 24 hours a day. This has many practical benefits, going far beyond any experience we may have in any given meditation session. That is why we stay with the procedure.

This is also why we often say, "Favor the practice over the experience."

Forgetting to favor the mantra, getting lost in whatever may be happening, is not being off the procedure. We are only off the procedure when we consciously choose to favor our experiences over the mantra -- you may be flirting with this one a little bit. When we are in our deep meditation session, when we have a choice, the choice is always the same -- favor the mantra on whatever level of the mind we are -- clear or faint. And when we don't have a choice (lost in thoughts, feelings or sensations), no one will come and hit us with a stick, and we don't have to hit ourselves with a stick either. :-)

It is an easy and fun practice, and very powerful too, if done daily.

All the best!

The guru is in you.

2007/09/19 08:32:52
Support for AYP Deep Meditation and Samyama
http://www.aypsite.org/forum/topic.asp?TOPIC_ID=2930&REPLY_ID=25578&whichpage=-1
deep meditation and dreams/vision

quote:
_____
Originally posted by emc

The line between what is "experiences" happening to the person (not to be attached to, just enjoy and then let go of), and what is merely being with what IS (neither thought or feeling nor sensation, no person there, just being the now and therefore impossible to DO anything, no one there to pick up the mantra) is very, very blurry...
_____

Hi EMC:

Being absorbed in "what is," without thoughts, feelings or sensations, is being absorbed in inner silence, which is samadhi, the destination of meditation. Whether we are absorbed in that, or in thoughts, feelings or sensations, there is not a requirement to force our way back to the mantra. But when we realize we have been off into any experience or state of awareness, including samadhi, and have a choice about what to put our attention on next, then that is when we favor the mantra on the level we are at in the mind. Depending on where we are, that can be a clear mental pronunciation of the mantra or a very faint and fuzzy favoring. We will know where we are in that by sensing the lack of strain in picking the mantra up. This a finer point in favoring the mantra, and it takes some practice. Once we are favoring the mantra, it serves as a vehicle to go deep into absorption in inner silence (samadhi) again. We may not even notice until we are aware that we are out on a thought, and then we have the option to favor the mantra again. Very simple.

When we have a choice and instead decide, "I will just be here in the now with no mantra," then this is a choice to do another kind of practice, and this is no longer AYP deep meditation. That may or may not be an effective practice, and I could not predict the long term result. If there is no precedence or other external guidance for the procedure, then it is the practitioner's experiment and it will be what it will be.

It is important to know beforehand what our choice for practice is going to be, and favor that consistently over time. Otherwise, we will be relying on the vagaries of the mind during meditation, or on "automatic yoga." Neither of these is going to be consistent, and will not always be in our best interest.

Again, none of this is to say we are obliged to be yanking ourselves out of samad
Hi or any other condition of awareness with a "mindy" approach to meditation. The mantra can be extremely "unmindy" -- practically no mind at all. From there it is a short hop to absorption in inner silence. If we just "let it be" without mantra, we may or may not make that hop. It is impossible to measure the results of meditation during meditation. The mind will play a thousand tricks on us. We can only know later by how we feel in daily activity. If we have increasing resident inner silence, creativity and energy, then we will know our meditation is working. The results of effective meditation are very practical in daily living.

It has been said elsewhere in the AYP writings that deep meditation with mantra is "proactive" in relation to mindfulness style techniques (letting it be). Mindfulness methods assume that that doing nothing will lead to samad
Hi (it is a big assumption), whereas mantra style deep meditation virtually guarantees samad
Hi by its dynamic nature. This is why deep meditation with mantra may be regarded to be more powerful than mindfulness techniques, requiring shorter sittings and more management of results (cause and effect) through the use of self-pacing. This is as true for practitioners who are undertaking the cultivation of inner silence in a systematic way for the first time as it is for practitioners who are already falling into inner silence at the drop of a hat. Both would like to have the whole enchilada, and the procedure of deep meditation is equally effective for both, assuming familiarity is developed in applying the procedure at all levels of awareness. Like anything else, this takes practice over time.

Do keep in mind that whether we are choosing to do something or not do something in our meditation sittings, we are <u>always</u> making a choice. What we consistently choose to do or not do in our sittings (whenever we have the option) will determine the outcome over the long term. As we develop the habit for the procedure we have chosen, that blurry area between experiences and samad
Hi will become more clear, because the habit of our practice will automatically be taking us to inner silence again and again. That is the case with deep meditation anyway. :-)

All the best!

The guru is in you.

2007/09/19 22:31:58
Support for AYP Deep Meditation and Samyama
http://www.aypsite.org/forum/topic.asp?TOPIC_ID=2930&REPLY_ID=25593&whichpage=-1
deep meditation and dreams/vision

Hi EMC:

Not to worry. I am only describing how AYP deep meditation works, and offering thoughts in general on using a procedure, as I am obliged to do. Systematic and safe so more can fly and arrive. You know, like an airline. :-)

You will choose your own way, and I encourage that. Your bhakti will lead you on. Being an inquiring person, you will continue to explore and gravitate toward the things that work best for you long term, which is how it should be. They are all your choices.

What you may not have thought of before is that using no procedure is a procedure -- maybe a sobering thought. But it could also be called a vacation. :-)

Have fun!

The guru is in you.

2007/09/27 18:36:32
Support for AYP Deep Meditation and Samyama
http://www.aypsite.org/forum/topic.asp?TOPIC_ID=2944&REPLY_ID=25721&whichpage=-1
Bliss: Just More Crap to Get Through

Hi Jim:

A nice piece of self-inquiry.

And from that comes ... outpouring divine love!

The eternal divine paradox. :-)

The guru is in you.

2007/09/27 23:57:01
Support for AYP Deep Meditation and Samyama
http://www.aypsite.org/forum/topic.asp?TOPIC_ID=2944&REPLY_ID=25731&whichpage=-1
Bliss: Just More Crap to Get Through

quote:
_____

Originally posted by Jim and His Karma

quote:
_____

Originally posted by yogani

And from that comes ... outpouring divine love!

_____

I think even that self-identification is an illusion...just another layer of onion.

_____

Hi Jim:

Outpouring divine love and self-identification cannot occur precisely in the same place. One excludes the other. This is the nature of non-duality. It is how we can have all of this going on, and at the same time nothing going on.

The paradox of stillness in action. :-)

You are right. Outpouring divine love cannot be wielded. It can only be allowed. It is the destination of our practices. A natural becoming, not an attainment. Flowers do not attain. They just bloom, filling the air with sweet fragrance and love.

The guru is in you.

2007/09/28 12:52:55
Support for AYP Deep Meditation and Samyama
http://www.aypsite.org/forum/topic.asp?TOPIC_ID=2944&REPLY_ID=25739&whichpage=-1
Bliss: Just More Crap to Get Through

quote:
_____

Originally posted by Balance

Hi Yogani

Would you elaborate on the statement:

"Outpouring divine love and self-identification cannot ~~not~~ occur precisely in the same place. One excludes the other."

Does this say that outpouring divine love and self-identification are mutually exclusive as well as mutually inclusive?

Maybe I'm asking for the unexplainable to be explained, but perhaps you could put a little more light on this one.

Thanks:-)

_____

Hi Balance:

It is a matter of how consciousness is flowing at any point in time. Self-identification is mind identifying itself as consciousness and many other things, as Jim points out in the first post above. Outpouring divine love is consciousness illuminating mind and action, which is a different kind of flow of consciousness, finding its root in expanding inner silence, which gradually becomes dynamic. Each kind of flow of consciousness produces a different point of view as perceived by the individual.

Can both of these be happening in the same instant? I don't think so. It can be flowing back and forth over time (sometimes in a flash) as we are going through the long process of purification and opening, as many of us have noticed.

To bring it closer to everyday living, the same principle can be found in the questions, "Can we be taking while we are giving?" or "Can we be giving while we are taking?" No, we can't. But we can certainly receive while we are giving. This is the principle of giving and receiving (multiplied), also found in "Seek first the kingdom of heaven and all will be added..."

It may seem to be a mixed bag at times, but there is a line in there somewhere, and both of these modes of functioning cannot be found on the same side of that line at the same time. That is the point I was trying to make.

Fortunately, our practices bring us along in the direction of opening without too much fanfare, unless of course, we insist on fanfare. Then it is a matter of easily favoring the practice over the experience. The rest of the time (outside practices) we are naturally integrating as we go about the normal business of life, and this is where we notice a gradual shift in our point of view occurring, on balance (there are many ups and downs along the way).

As for where self-inquiry fits in, this is something we may be drawn to as we have more inner silence available in daily activity. It can't be forced or constructed, though many do try. If we are regular in our practices, in time we can't help but begin to notice "what is," and are drawn to inquire quite naturally.

Self-inquiry is closely related to meditation, in that we will find ourselves consistently making choices that are inclined toward expanding our inner silence. With the awakening of ecstatic conductivity, outpouring divine love will be coming along, which is also the process of samyama (the cultivation of stillness in action). This last stage is seldom recognized by students who adhere (cling?) to a non-dual philosophy, which is kind of impractical. There definitely is life after (and during!) the obliteration of the identification of the mind. And what a life it is.

Enjoy! :-)

The guru is in you.

2007/09/28 14:54:12
Support for AYP Deep Meditation and Samyama
http://www.aypsite.org/forum/topic.asp?TOPIC_ID=2944&REPLY_ID=25744&whichpage=-1
Bliss: Just More Crap to Get Through

quote:
_____
Originally posted by Balance

I think I was confused by your use of a double negative which may have been a writing mistake: "cannot ~~not~~ occur".
_____

Sorry about that. It has been corrected.

TGIIY
2007/11/06 18:50:20
Support for AYP Deep Meditation and Samyama
http://www.aypsite.org/forum/topic.asp?TOPIC_ID=2944&REPLY_ID=26789&whichpage=-1
Bliss: Just More Crap to Get Through

Hi Jim:

To paraphrase Bob Adamson (Sailor Bob):

"What's wrong with bliss, unless you think about it?"

The word "bliss" can be replaced with just about anything we experience in life. The point being, it is not necessary to put a value judgment on anything. And if we do, our value judgment isn't more or less valid than anyone else's. It is what we choose it to be.

Is it so terrible to feel good? Spiritual bliss born in stillness is not a tangent, because it leads directly to union. Spiritual ecstasy born of the body can become a tangent, but it too leads to union when coupled with silent bliss. You can trust the process, and yourself. Just get out of the way and let it happen.

It really boils down to that -- favoring practices and the fullness of daily living over an endless stream of evaluated experiences. We can never get rid of experiences. But we can allow them with infinite grace, because we are That.

We can get used to anything, even ecstatic bliss. Enlightenment is beyond that anyway, in chopping the wood and carrying the water, mostly for others. We can tell others (and ourselves) a thousand times what to let or not let, but in the end it can only be found in our stillness, the witness. That's why I keep telling people to meditate and go out and live. It is profoundly simple.

Practice and do as you are moved, like you are doing now. That is the journey. Sooner or later the intensity of it will pass as inner silence continues to integrate, and you will find yourself relaxing into the whole thing. It could take a while. Paradoxically, once relaxed, you may keep going with intensity in divine flow, and barely notice. Less becomes more.

EMC: Bliss, inner silence and joy are synonymous, while ecstasy is of the body. See here for how the distinction is drawn in AYP:
http://www.aypsite.org/113.html
The emergence of divine love and unity (non-duality, non-identification with objects of experience) may come and go along the way, and then it finally comes and stays for good. Before then, it is mostly an infatuation game we play with the glimpses -- but fun anyway, and part of the journey. Just keep meditating and all infatuations will be fulfilled. The difference between infatuation and fulfillment is found in favoring sound practices over experiences for the long term. Then there can be no doubt because our condition will be alive and unending on the cellular level,

beyond the fickle mind. This is the aim of self-inquiry also.

The guru is in you.

2007/11/07 14:23:02
Support for AYP Deep Meditation and Samyama
http://www.aypsite.org/forum/topic.asp?TOPIC_ID=2944&REPLY_ID=26808&whichpage=-1
Bliss: Just More Crap to Get Through

Hi Jim:

It may be that we have gotten tripped up on terminology here.

"Bliss" is an aspect of inner silence, pure consciousness, and is not intense or overwhelming. Intensity is of the body-mind -- energy moving through the nervous system, which is purification and opening. It may be experienced as intensely ecstatic, overwhelming, or symptomatic in other ways -- pressure, heat, physical movement, emotions, etc.

And, yes, deep meditation cultivating more inner silence can lead to more ecstatic energy flow, seemingly without limit -- those Chinese handcuffs you mentioned. So we self-pace and ground...

Your years in hatha may well have set the stage for what you are experiencing now. Others have come from hatha with similar experiences, sometimes way out of balance. Hatha methods are mainly about the body and energy. That is why the Asanas, Mudras & Bandhas book has the subtitle, "Awakening Ecstatic Kundalini." You are clearly into that. The potential for that kind of experience coming from a strong hatha background is examined in the book.

Pure unadulterated bliss becoming intense to the point of, "Eek! I can't stand it anymore," is not in the cards. Bliss is part and parcel of the "peace that surpasses all understanding." It is inner silence, the witness, sat-chit-ananda, where ananda is bliss. It is pure happiness, an endless "inner smile" -- nothing more, nothing less (check the lesson). Intensity is not part of the bliss of pure consciousness. Intensity is of the body, and the body is the purveyor of ecstasy, not bliss.

The energy side of it is kundalini, which I think is what you are describing. But I could be wrong. It is semantics. It does help to know what is coming from where, making a distinction between bliss and ecstasy, so practices and progress will not be compromised by doubt or fear.

It might be time to take a look at your hatha in relation to the rest of your practices. Less could be more -- more of what you want (inner silence), rather than more of what has been too much (energy). Just a suggestion.

Maybe this topic should be called, "Ecstasy: Just more crap to get through." Whadayathink? Then the kundalini yogis and tantrics will be up in arms. :-)

Happily, there is a marriage of blissful silence and ecstatic energy in the offing, and the child of unifying outpouring divine love to be born from that. Give it some time.

The guru is in you.

2007/11/08 12:28:37
Support for AYP Deep Meditation and Samyama
http://www.aypsite.org/forum/topic.asp?TOPIC_ID=2944&REPLY_ID=26828&whichpage=-1
Bliss: Just More Crap to Get Through

Hi Jim and All:

What we are talking about here is a function of self-inquiry, which is of the mind. Bliss is bliss. Ecstasy is ecstasy. How we engage with these is a mental activity. Obviously, what we'd like is to go beyond identification with these experiences. But this cannot happen until the experience is there and we have enough witness (inner silence) present to "be" beyond the experience.

In AYP, we always say, "Favor the practice over the experience," which is a precurser to self-inquiry.

I would still take issue with bliss being a "layer," since it is an aspect of the witness itself. Any objectiveness or intensity associated with bliss is outside in energy, and in the mind (the "layer" outside the thing itself, only a reflection of it). This is also the age-old argument on whether the ultimate truth is bliss consciousness or the empty void (a soulful versus soulless existence). The Buddhists concede that nirvana is "blissful" (ergo, "conscious"). The hardcore advaitists take a more rigid view, but their arguments sometimes seem a bit strained. I think even Nisargadatta (the hardest of the hardcore) admits to the transcendental nature of bliss, while denying it at the same time. What's the difference? It is what it is. We can experience it for ourselves, and describe it as we wish. :-)

Anyway, what we don't want is to predispose people about experiences they may not be having yet (or just beginning to taste), which is what can turn the path into a mind game of little value, with a lot of confusion and possible loss of motivation to continue along the path, or with anything in life for that matter. That is called "non-relational self inquiry" in the new AYP Self-Inquiry book (no, the book is not ready yet -- give it a month, at least ... it is a tricky one).

Rather, we would like to inquire about things that are actually happening, which is called "relational self-inquiry" in the book. There can be much benefit in this, as it aids us in relating to what is happening in our life right now in an evolutionary way.

Even if we are not experiencing large doses of transcendental bliss (the witness) or inner ecstasy (kundalini), we always have a lot going on in our life in our relationships, with all our desires, actions, etc., for which self-inquiry can have value. This is self-inquiry directed specifically at everyday living situations, like what Byron Katie is doing in her work. Very practical and helpful on that level, and that is "relational self-inquiry," as long as there is a sense of resonance coming when engaging in it.

The path to relational self-inquiry is through cultivation of the witness. Then resonance with self-inquiry methods increases as our perception of truth within and around us is naturally deepening.

I don't think it is particularly helpful for people to be laboring over letting go of things that are not going on, which is building castles of mind stuff in the air. Much better to inquire about what is happening right now. If it feels resonant and good, it is likely relational self-inquiry. If it feels strained and awkward, it is probably non-relational self-inquiry. And we do you-know-what when there is strain in practices -- self-pace accordingly!

What I am saying here is for the benefit of everyone, regardless of location in practices and experiences along the path.

In your case, Jim, self-inquiry about the experiences of ecstasy and bliss may be appropriate, if it is resonant and yielding fruit in terms of finding some release (reduced identification). "Who are you in relation to those experiences?" If you feel like you are banging your head against the wall with that, if there is a lot of struggle about it, then it is likely non-relational self-inquiry, and perhaps consider backing off to something that resonates. It could be as simple as favoring sitting practices over experiences (and balancing hatha) and leaving it at that for a while. There are various grades of self-inquiry, and like with most spiritual practices, one size does not fit all at every point in time along the path.

For this reason, we have to be careful about telling people what they ought and ought not be identified with. Each identification with experience is a rung on the ladder of yoga, and each rung will dissolve as we move on to the next rungs. We are pulling ourselves up by our bootstraps, hopefully with minimum strain and fuss. That is why we always favor the practice over the experience, with or without deliberate self-inquiry in the picture between our daily sittings.

In the case of self-inquiry, there is a sliding scale of intention and practice that can be tricky to match up with the experience where we are. It is very easy to project self-inquiry beyond where we are into bogus analysis and infatuation with imagined certainties, which can be counterproductive. It happens all the time, even with advanced practitioners -- and we may not know it when it is happening. No one is immune from projections of the mind. So we favor the practices that further cultivate the witness. Then we can't miss, and the mind will help rather than hinder.

It is best to keep the witness coming via deep meditation, and take it easy with self-inquiry, favoring relational, which we will know by its natural resonance. It will be there when we need it.

The variety of self-inquiry practice styles happening in the AYP community demonstrates the wide range and relationship of our evolving inner silence/witness to experiences, whether it be in everyday living in dealings with others and our external environment, or in how we relate to our internal mental, emotional and spiritual experiences. Well, it is all "internal," isn't it? In all cases, it takes the witness and an experience playing upon it for relational self-inquiry to occur.

And if we see experiences as "more crap to get through," well, there may be some relational self-inquiry in that. Dissatisfaction is one of the first steps to progress. :-)

The guru is in you.

Edited with additions a few hours after first posting.

2007/11/11 09:02:48
Support for AYP Deep Meditation and Samyama
http://www.aypsite.org/forum/topic.asp?TOPIC_ID=2944&REPLY_ID=26895&whichpage=-1
Bliss: Just More Crap to Get Through

quote:
_____
Originally posted by Jim and His Karma

...I'm letting the bliss be, but deeming it scenery. It happens around me ... but it isn't the defining extent of me. I'm not diving into the scenery just because it's gotten particularly nice.
_____

Hi Jim:

Sounds like some pretty good self-inquiry. AYP-style, of course. :-)

We will know the truth, and the truth will set us free.

The guru is in you.

2007/11/02 10:52:02
Support for AYP Deep Meditation and Samyama
http://www.aypsite.org/forum/topic.asp?TOPIC_ID=3070&REPLY_ID=26627&whichpage=-1
Then What

Hi Eddie:

Much better to keep digging in one place. You pick the place.

Some of us here have been practicing deep meditation with mantra every day for decades. It really does work when the instructions are followed.

I am not aware of a "more advanced" practice, particularly when the mantra enhancements are added on prudently over time, along with the integration of spinal breathing, samyama, tantric methods and other elements of practice. Keep in mind that "advanced" in this case means *very easy to do and very powerful*. Don't take the "very easy" part too lightly, or you might miss out on the "very powerful" part.

As for self-inquiry, it really has no place to go except to building "castles in the air" without the concurrent cultivation of inner silence/witness as the foundation by one means or another (an effective form of meditation). Stand alone self-inquiry by itself is a poor way to cultivate inner silence. Without the expansion of inner silence, moving to "more advanced" forms of self-inquiry will be premature and can lead to much confusion in life and a loss of motivation and effectiveness in conducting our daily activities. If we are experiencing these difficulties, we can be sure we are too far ahead of ourselves with self-inquiry, and it is time to back off.

Once a significant degree of inner silence has been established, then self-inquiry can be very useful. Before then, it is hit or miss, with lots of hazards.

Unlike when assembling a bookcase, with spiritual practices it is a good idea to read the directions that come in the box, and follow them. Come to think of it, following the directions when assembling a bookcase can save time too. :-)

It is your path, and you are free to travel it how you choose. There are plenty of jungles out there to hack through, and lots of quicksand too.

There are roads that have been built that can help us avoid most of the pitfalls and carry us surely to our destination. That is what AYP is about.

All the best!

The guru is in you.

Edited 2 hours later. See paragraph inserted on self-inquiry.

2007/11/02 17:32:52
Support for AYP Deep Meditation and Samyama
http://www.aypsite.org/forum/topic.asp?TOPIC_ID=3070&REPLY_ID=26644&whichpage=-1
Then What

Hi BluesFan:

The main difference between meditation styles with or without mantra is that meditation with mantra enables *proactive* cultivation of inner silence, whereas mindfulness and related meditation techniques are *passive* forms of cultivation. Here is a post that gets into it in more detail: http://www.aypsite.org/forum/topic.asp?TOPIC_ID=598#1578

There is also a marked difference between using mantra and using breath as the object of meditation, particularly as samad
Hi advances and breath may become very slight, or none. This is where breath-based meditation ceases to function, while mantra-based meditation will continue to function far beyond that point into pure bliss consciousness itself.

It is the ability of mantra meditation (with correct technique) to continue bringing the attention systematically and proactively to ever more refined levels of stillness that makes the difference between mantra style meditation and all others.

Of course, meditation can occur using any object. "Meditation" is the natural process of mind dissolving from an object to absorption in inner silence, which is samadhi. It is a matter of optimizing the application of this inherent human ability for efficiency and effectiveness. That is what deep meditation with mantra is about. That is what makes it "advanced" -- meaning, more results can be achieved with less time and effort. Which is not to say everyone ought to be meditating with mantra. But that is the kind of meditation the AYP lessons cover, in relation to a range of other practices that are also optimized within themselves and in relation to the full routine.

The guru is in you.

2007/11/02 18:53:09
Support for AYP Deep Meditation and Samyama
http://www.aypsite.org/forum/topic.asp?TOPIC_ID=3070&REPLY_ID=26647&whichpage=-1
Then What

quote:
_____
Originally posted by BluesFan

So it sounds like when "I AM" does take you to the place of no-mind and complete stillness, you don't force the mantra at that point. Is that correct?
_____

Hi BluesFan:

The mantra can be easily picked up very faint fuzzy in the deepest levels of awareness, taking us still deeper. We do that whenever we realize we have gone off the mantra. In time, it becomes quite automatic to pick up the mantra at all levels in the mind, whether a clear mental pronunciation or very faint and fuzzy feeling. And, yes, the mantra is never forced on any level.

As our nervous system becomes more permanently infused with inner silence over time from daily deep meditation, we will be at that deep level as soon as we sit and close our eyes. And also more and more in daily activity ... which is the beginning of stillness in action.

This makes self-inquiry very easy, because we are becoming the answer to all the inquiries, and our conduct will often automatically precede the answers (rise of yama and niyama). Then it is only a matter of occasionally clarifying "what is," rather then beating ourselves up trying to penetrate the infinite with our little brain, which is not possible. We have to go beyond our little brain to do that. :-)

In AYP, the key word in considering self-inquiry is "relational," which means naturally integrative, or yogic. If the self-inquiry we are doing is "non-relational," meaning of the temporal mind only, or non-yogic, we do not need it, for it will only add baggage. Inner silence (the witness) is the prerequisite for relational self-inquiry. It is both its fuel and its destination.

So, however terrific we might feel about our self-inquiry, being in "the now," or whatever, it is entirely dependent on the resident inner silence we have available. This is why daily deep meditation is so important.

The guru is in you.

2007/11/03 00:30:33
Support for AYP Deep Meditation and Samyama
http://www.aypsite.org/forum/topic.asp?TOPIC_ID=3070&REPLY_ID=26665&whichpage=-1
Then What

quote:
_____
Originally posted by Eddie33

Yeah thinking is a horrible thing. It just get's way out of control.
_____

Hi Eddie:

Thinking is okay. It is what we make of it. The mind makes a good servant, but not a good master. We need to bring the master in to take charge of things -- inner silence. Then the mind will shine. :-)

The guru is in you.

2007/11/07 11:59:24
Support for AYP Deep Meditation and Samyama
http://www.aypsite.org/forum/topic.asp?TOPIC_ID=3107&REPLY_ID=26805&whichpage=-1
Some Questions

Hi Eddie:

See this lesson for an explanation of the I AM mantra (in relation to OM): http://www.aypsite.org/59.html
And, yes, we don't follow the breath with mantra in AYP deep meditation.

There are also enhancements to the mantra, but that is for later. If you can't resist peeking ahead, check lessons under "Mantra" in the Topic Index.

All the best!

The guru is in you.

2007/11/15 12:36:25
Support for AYP Deep Meditation and Samyama
http://www.aypsite.org/forum/topic.asp?TOPIC_ID=3141&REPLY_ID=27049&whichpage=-1
Goal Samyama

Hi Eddie:

Good question -- one we have all pondered at some point on our path.

Actually, the process of "goal samyama" you describe becomes automatic in everyday living with daily structured samyama practice over time, as discussed in the online lessons and Samyama book. The book covers much more than the online lessons, adding cosmic samyama (similar to yoga nidra -- self-directed), as well as the use of samyama with asanas, prayer and in daily activity. Our primary samyama session during sitting practices increases our ability to manifest intentions over all as we go about our life, reducing our expectations while expanding the divine flow coming through us.

The truth about samyama (and divine life) is that, while we may wish for a specific thing, doing samyama on that thing will give us what we need in relation to that desire, which may or may not be the thing itself. Surrender to divine inner silence within, the essential characteristic of samyama in relation to our intentions/desires, has its own dynamic. The end result is a life filled with joy and miracles small and large.

Remember, daily samyama practice is for opening up our natural ability to live our life as "stillness in action," which ultimately is known to be a constant outpouring of divine love.

It is not advised to do samyama on a particular desire while excluding the much broader scope of samyama practice discussed in the AYP writings mentioned above. We are not primarily interested in catching one fish for today. We'd like to develop the ability to catch all fish for all time. Then we will never be hungry. :-)

The guru is in you.

2007/11/16 17:56:16
Support for AYP Deep Meditation and Samyama
http://www.aypsite.org/forum/topic.asp?TOPIC_ID=3141&REPLY_ID=27077&whichpage=-1
Goal Samyama

quote:
_____
Originally posted by Eddie33

...do you think it's a good idea to have goals in general? i mean i see your point on not doing samyama on goals directly but what about just having goals just to work towards something?
_____

Hi Eddie:

Absolutely. Pursue your dreams with all your heart for all your life, and keep up daily practices for years, and years, and years. Then you will not miss on either front. They are one and the same.

All the best!

The guru is in you.

2007/11/26 11:25:32
Support for AYP Deep Meditation and Samyama
http://www.aypsite.org/forum/topic.asp?TOPIC_ID=3186&REPLY_ID=27297&whichpage=-1
Switching mantras

Hi Eddie:

Don't forget the analogy about digging the well. If you want to strike water, keep digging in one place. If practice is related to headaches, then self-pace and ground as needed. And take plenty of rest before getting up after practice. Balance is the key, not more mantras or more practice done randomly.

The guru is in you.

2007/12/01 10:42:21
Support for AYP Deep Meditation and Samyama
http://www.aypsite.org/forum/topic.asp?TOPIC_ID=3204&REPLY_ID=27535&whichpage=-1
Amrita question

Hi Christi:

Radiance of spiritual vitality through the outer skin, which may or may not have a detectable physical component, is described by the term "ojas," mentioned at the end of the quote Shanti gave above.

"Nectar" (amrita) coming down through the sinuses may or may not have a noticeable aroma or taste. The sweetness of it tends to be more noticed by contrast in the early stages, and then fades into the landscape, like so many of our symptoms do as we continue to favor the practice over the experience.

All the best! :-)

The guru is in you.

2007/12/02 09:46:46
Support for AYP Deep Meditation and Samyama
http://www.aypsite.org/forum/topic.asp?TOPIC_ID=3204&REPLY_ID=27584&whichpage=-1
Amrita question

Hi All:

Soma, Amrita and Ojas are aspects of the process described in the DSA book quote Shanti gave above. Each is both effect and subsequent cause, like so many things in yoga are. Everything in yoga is connected within us.

Once inner silence is present from daily deep meditation, then pranayama (kumbhaka particularly), mudras and bandhas are the main stimulants for the energy circulation and radiance described, as are tantric sexual methods in support.

Jala neti (nasal wash) is a helper once ecstatic conductivity begins, as are all the shatkarmas (see the DSA book on that). But shatkarmas are not primary stimulators of ecstatic conductivity and radiance, or of the components of it we are discussing here.

Regarding preserving or rubbing in secretions of the skin, that is a matter of personal choice. For similar reasons, some people prefer to shower before sitting practices rather than after. It is a minor aspect of practice which will not make a big difference one way or the other. Once ecstatic radiance is occurring and ongoing, it will happen regardless of any external treatment. It is not primarily physical anyway.

It is best to regard all of these things as aspects of experience (which they are) and continue to favor the core practices that have brought them about. That is the best way to expand on the process of human spiritual transformation. Zeroing in on particular experiences excessively, to the exclusion of the primary causes of them, is a sure way to stall progress. It is a theme we return to many times along the way -- favoring the practice over the experience.

All the best!

The guru is in you.

2007/12/03 11:22:49
Support for AYP Deep Meditation and Samyama
http://www.aypsite.org/forum/topic.asp?TOPIC_ID=3204&REPLY_ID=27623&whichpage=-1
Amrita question

quote:

Originally posted by Christi

Hi Yogani,

I think I just found out what happens next. I read a quote from Shivananda (of Shivananda Yoga) and he says that as the process of the production of ojas advances, the yogi no longer produces semen. Is this true? Does it mean that I will not be able to have any more children?

_____

Hi Christi:

While Sivananda made many contributions in the field of yoga, his views on sexuality tended toward extremist.

It may be that sexuality can eventually be totally sublimated to spiritual processes for those who seek that, but this is certainly not a primary prerequisite for spiritual progress, or for reaching an enlightened condition. Whatever happens is in the hands of the aspirant, not a foregone conclusion that can be projected on us by others, no matter what their status is perceived to be.

Spiritual development removing the ability to have children is not a risk for yogis and yoginis, since the desire for having children is the underlying cause of having them! :-)

The guru is in you.

2007/12/22 10:34:08
Support for AYP Deep Meditation and Samyama
http://www.aypsite.org/forum/topic.asp?TOPIC_ID=3204&REPLY_ID=28147&whichpage=-1
Amrita question

Hi Christi:

Yes, it is quite possible to notice the inner processes going on, especially by contrast when they are moving to new and unfamiliar levels. Each new development in the neurobiology soon becomes part of the landscape and we notice it no more than we would our heart beating or any other automatic process in the body.

I don't make distinctions between spirit bodies or sheaths much these days (they are classifications of the mind), so can't offer much on this or that body. What I can say is that human spiritual transformation occurs in parallel on every level from gross to subtle, and this is what leads to the natural integration of abiding inner silence, ecstatic bliss and outpouring divine love in daily life. The mechanics are not there to distract from the result. You know, not getting too caught up in the scenery, or what's going on under the hood, and all that.

Of course, scientific research will delve into all of this someday, but that's a different thing.

For most of us, it is enough to know that good things are happening as a result of our daily practices, and we will notice plenty going on to verify that this is so. As we move on down the road, we will come to notice that nothing is happening while everything is happening. That's when self-inquiry comes in handy. :-)

All the best!

The guru is in you.

2008/03/30 12:22:30
Support for AYP Deep Meditation and Samyama
http://www.aypsite.org/forum/topic.asp?TOPIC_ID=3204&REPLY_ID=31947&whichpage=-1
Amrita question
And the reply:

Hi Echo:

Yes, that is a "taste" of the nectar cycle. If you search for nectar, amrita, soma and related terms in the AYP lessons and forums you will find discussions on it. Here is one I recall doing not long ago: http://www.aypsite.org/forum/topic.asp?TOPIC_ID=3204#27584 (check entire topic)

You are wise to let it go and carry on with practices and normal life.

Good things are happening. All the best!

The guru is in you.

2008/11/01 12:57:18
Support for AYP Deep Meditation and Samyama
http://www.aypsite.org/forum/topic.asp?TOPIC_ID=3204&REPLY_ID=39743&whichpage=-1
Amrita question

quote:
_____
Originally posted by Christi

----

quote:
_____

Hi Christi:

Radiance of spiritual vitality through the outer skin, which may or may not have a detectable physical component, is described by the term "ojas," mentioned at the end of the quote Shanti gave above.

_____

Hi Yogani,

I was just wondering.... do you think this is what the term "anointed" refers to in the spiritual world. I ask mainly because you mention the word at the end of lesson 51:

http://www.aypsite.org/51.html

"The truth is that we all have equal access to the divine life through our human nervous system. You can choose to be anointed if you are willing to do the work that goes with it -- the work of applying the knowledge of human transformation, which is doing spiritual practices every day. "

Christi

_____

Hi Christi:

That is one interpretation, though I think being anointed also means to travel a higher path in active surrender to our chosen ideal, not necessarily tied to being physically anointed from the inside or the outside. When we choose, then we are chosen, or anointed. In time, the ojas comes along with that, being a component of the rise of ecstatic conductivity and radiance. The oil anointing ceremonies found in the religions can be viewed as metaphorical representations of that process.

The guru is in you.

2007/12/07 16:08:42
Support for AYP Deep Meditation and Samyama
http://www.aypsite.org/forum/topic.asp?TOPIC_ID=3229&REPLY_ID=27747&whichpage=-1
Mantra Changes (2)

Hi Tallis and All:

Keep in mind that where we start with the mantra is not nearly as significant as where we end up. And on the way there (usually more than once in each sesson), there may be barely any pronunciation at all. Only a faint feeling, and then nothing but inner silence. And then we come back to a faint recollection of the mantra again when we realize we have been off it.

So the pronunciation you are talking about here is what we want to be letting go of nearly from the start. As our mind and nervous system gain experience in this over time (becoming cultivated in the habit of stillness), we will be losing the mantra and everything else as soon as we close our eyes. Pronunciation? What pronunciation? :-)

So the mantra is just an easy direction we take in thought. And then it is refining to stillness. Let it go ... one pronunciation is about as good as the next, because all pronunciations are transcended. Anywhere in the ball park will do fine. If it is easy to let it go to less, then we know it is right.

All the best!

The guru is in you.

2008/01/03 10:52:26
Support for AYP Deep Meditation and Samyama
http://www.aypsite.org/forum/topic.asp?TOPIC_ID=3237&REPLY_ID=28493&whichpage=-1
Meditation Time Length

quote:
_____
Originally posted by yogikanna

Dear Eddie,

I am not very familiar with this particular type of meditation. But In general silent meditation can be done as long as possible. I practise regular silent meditation (not mantra)for 2-3 hrs a day and have been doing so, on and off, for the past couple of year.

It really depends on what you are looking for. If you are looking for complete liberation from the ego, meditation must be done as much as possible, until it becomes 24/7 activity, until it becomes effortless and natural. Michael Langford in his book "The most rapid and direct means to Eternal Bliss" recommends atleast 2 hrs a day and upto 12 hrs a day if it is possible. His realization was complete in 2 years of practising 12 hrs a day. Sri Ramana Mahars
Hi advised that practise of Meditaion, which is focusing on the Self should be unbroken and continuous until realization becomes complete.

You can find more information in the following link.

http://www.albigen.com/uarelove/awa_instructions.aspx

In peace,
Kannan
————

Hi Kannan, and welcome!

While I cannot speak for other systems, what you are suggesting above does not apply to deep meditation as practiced here, or to any of the AYP practices. While very easy to do, these practices are so powerful that a little bit goes a long way in cultivating rapid purification and opening in the nervous system. This is why "self-pacing" of practices receives a lot of attention here.

In AYP, the limiting factor in unfolding enlightenment is not in how much practice time we can put in. It is in how much transformation our nervous system can handle over the days, weeks and months, and regulating that for maximum progress with safety. Everyone is a little different in this, due to unique patterns of karmic obstruction to be dissolved. For all of us, there are definitely times when less practice will yield more results. The rest of the time, we will be wise to stick with recommended times of practice to keep on a steady and stable path of purification and opening.

It is much like driving a fast car. We maintain a good safe speed on the straight-aways, and slow down for the pot holes and sharp curves. If we don't drive prudently we can end up in the ditch for a while, and that will be a slower path, even with the fast car.

There have been discussions elsewhere here in the forums on the relative power and speed of various kinds of meditation. While we have nothing scientific to offer on this, it seems clear that AYP deep meditation is a very powerful and fast one, especially when integrated with the many other methods offered here. So we do not recommend driving with the gas pedal pressed to the floor. Those who do that (we all have!) will often share their crash stories here, and there are a lot of valuable lessons in those for all of us.

We have strategies here to aid folks in recovering from crashes. We also see a lot of crash victims coming here from other systems seeking assistance. Hey, whatever works to get everyone back on the highway and driving safely for a timely arrival. :-)

All the best!

The guru is in you.

2008/01/13 10:32:34
Support for AYP Deep Meditation and Samyama
http://www.aypsite.org/forum/topic.asp?TOPIC_ID=3361&REPLY_ID=28831&whichpage=-1
Mantra and Breath

Hi Bill:

Keep in mind that the mantra is not the mantra when deliberately coupled with breath or set rhythm of repetition. Meaning, we favor the mantra, and not any external criterion or pattern of repeating it. Whenever we notice such a coupling, we can just easily come back to the faint feeling of the mantra. Then it will move and refine as it is inclined to according to the purification and opening that is occurring in our nervous system.

This is not to say we won't experience mantra following breathing, a particular rhythm, or thoughts at times. It will happen. It is normal. But we do not make that our deliberate or fixed procedure of meditation. While thinking the mantra may seem to be connected to thought patterns or external phenomena at times, this is not what we favor. We favor the non-specific in picking up the mantra by itself. Then it will go to transcendence/inner silence quite naturally, again and again.

For those who have a habit of coupling the mantra with breath, set rhythm of repetition, specific pronunciation, or other phenomena, it may take some time to reprogram. That is only a matter of favoring the procedure of meditation consistently in our sittings over time. That is easily favoring the mantra (without the baggage) whenever we realize we are not.

In time, our habit will be moving more and more toward knowing inner silence to be ourselves, and easily resided in that, whether eyes are closed in deep meditation, or open in going about our daily activities. Then all sorts of doors will be opening. :-)

All the best!

The guru is in you.

2008/01/14 19:03:09
Support for AYP Deep Meditation and Samyama
http://www.aypsite.org/forum/topic.asp?TOPIC_ID=3375&REPLY_ID=28894&whichpage=-1
Mantra Clarification

Hi YogaPat, and welcome!

You took the words right out of my mouth. :-)

Yes, the mantra is a thought, the thought of a sound, refining naturally again and again to faint fuzziness and inner silence.

Along the way, the mantra can be experienced in many ways -- visual, auditory, physical feeling, even smell or taste, according to purification and opening that is occurring. But we always easily come back to it as the thought of a sound at a level of clarity or faintness that is comfortable at whatever level we happen to be at the moment in the mind.

All the best!

The guru is in you.

2008/01/15 10:51:13
Support for AYP Deep Meditation and Samyama
http://www.aypsite.org/forum/topic.asp?TOPIC_ID=3375&REPLY_ID=28936&whichpage=-1
Mantra Clarification

Hi YogaPat:

Yes! Now you are taking the spontaneous leap from deep meditation to self-inquiry -- very beautiful. It is your inner silence speaking.

It is a good thing, as long as our self-inquiry (mental analysis) doesn't get too far ahead of our inner silence (the witness). If the inquiry is able to be released in stillness, it will be progressive and evolutionary ("relational"). If the inquiry is moving into thoughts about more thoughts, it will be building castles in the air and be non-progressive and binding ("non-relational"). We each can self-pace our self-inquiry according to the degree of inner silence we have coming up through our daily practice of deep meditation.

We finally have clear documentation on how self-inquiry fits into the AYP approach, in the form of the new Self-Inquiry book. Some suggested guidelines have been much needed, because with deep meditation, self-inquiry comes up as *effect*, which must in turn be self-paced to temper the mental excesses and tangents that can occur on the path. The new book provides metrics (measuring rods) for that.

The best thing about the AYP Self-Inquiry book is that it does not limit the method(s) of self-inquiry which might be studied and utilized. It provides measuring rods that can be used with any method of self-inquiry. Progress is more about navigation in relation to our inner silence than the particular method of self-inquiry being utilized. If the underlying principles are understood and applied, any method of self-inquiry, even one we intuit ourselves (like you are doing), can be used with benefit.

Also, with an in-common understanding of the underlying principles of self-inquiry, we can communicate with each other about it without getting lost in abstraction, which has often been the case in discussions on this subject. Apples for one person will often be oranges for someone else. The trick is to get beyond the apples and oranges to the underlying relationship between the subject/witness and the objects of perception. Then the discussion becomes an in-common one about the rise of our inner silence/witness and how that affects our view of ourselves and the world. Understanding that, it becomes clear what we must do. Keep meditating, and enjoy the divine life that is unfolding before us. :-)

All the best!

The guru is in you.

2008/01/16 12:01:24
Support for AYP Deep Meditation and Samyama
http://www.aypsite.org/forum/topic.asp?TOPIC_ID=3375&REPLY_ID=28999&whichpage=-1
Mantra Clarification

Hi Gumpi:

How about God living in a house with dirty windows? Wouldn't S/He be inclined to clean the windows for a better view of *Self*? God's inclination is our inclination.

Grace is the flow of divine desire for union. And that desire is synonymous with our own. So Grace begins and finds its fruition in us. Bhakti and Grace are two sides of the same coin.

The guru is in you.

2008/01/17 09:46:07
Support for AYP Deep Meditation and Samyama
http://www.aypsite.org/forum/topic.asp?TOPIC_ID=3375&REPLY_ID=29013&whichpage=-1
Mantra Clarification

Hi Gumpi:

Yes, kundalini is necessary for realization, though it may not be called by that name. Mental dodgeball, you know. The rise of whole body ecstatic conductivity and radiance (shakti) in the neurobiology is part of the process of human spiritual transformation. Not the only part, but an essential component along with the rise of inner silence (shiva). It is what it is, no matter how it might be relabeled or avoided.

The new Self-Inquiry book also covers kundalini in relation to the mind, which makes it a bit unusual. Avowed non-dualists (and many others) tend to shun the reality of ecstatic energy awakening. We don't. Much better to deal intelligently with what is actually happening than be hanging people out to dry, which happens a lot when the truth is swept under the rug.

The guru is in you.

2008/01/29 11:49:09
Support for AYP Deep Meditation and Samyama
http://www.aypsite.org/forum/topic.asp?TOPIC_ID=3402&REPLY_ID=29419&whichpage=-1
Metabolism slowing down

Hi EMC:

As the old saying goes, "This too shall pass."

Of course, we all like to watch the scenery as it goes by. Some pleasant, some not so pleasant. We take whatever measures are necessary to keep the ride comfortable, and to assure our arrival at the place we already are. They call it "realization." :-)

The guru is in you.

2008/01/29 13:46:59
Support for AYP Deep Meditation and Samyama
http://www.aypsite.org/forum/topic.asp?TOPIC_ID=3402&REPLY_ID=29430&whichpage=-1
Metabolism slowing down

quote:

_____

Originally posted by emc

But hey, any suggestions on how to do spinal breathing when breath is short, shallow, hasty and full of stops? Just jump up and down with the visualization to root and ajna, or try to do longer, slower breaths?

_____

Hi EMC:

That too shall pass. :-)

Just take it easy, favor the procedure of practice and stay with the daily routine. It will smooth out in time. That is how it goes with purification and opening. It starts out with "friction," and there is less and less friction over time.

If you are getting stuck in the middle, it is fine to go straight to the brow on completion of inhale and straight to the root on the completion of exhale. As long as you are touching both ends in each cycle, the clearing of the middle will come.

Also check "full yogic breathing" in the Spinal Breathing Pranayama book.

The guru is in you.

2008/02/02 12:09:57
Support for AYP Deep Meditation and Samyama
http://www.aypsite.org/forum/topic.asp?TOPIC_ID=3402&REPLY_ID=29590&whichpage=-1
Metabolism slowing down

Hi EMC:

Sorry for the delay getting back.

If full yogic breathing is a stretch for you, that is okay. Just breath normally during spinal breathing, whatever that is for you, and take it easy. If you can slow down and deepen breathing a bit, that is good. If not, don't worry about it. Self-pace as needed. Things will loosen up over time. Friction and obstructions will become less.

Favoring breath suspension is not part of the procedure of AYP spinal breathing, just the way it is not in deep meditation. Breath suspension can happen naturally in either practice. That is fine. When we realize we are off into breath suspension, or anything else, we just ease back to our spinal breathing. There is no right or wrong about it. It is just an easy procedure of favoring one thing over other things when we can choose.

If we are favoring breath suspension beyond its natural occurrence, we can end up with more energy flowing, more friction and more clunkiness. Premature intentional breath suspension can lead to kundalini excesses.

So easy breathing between root and brow is all spinal breathing pranayama is. If anything else comes up, we just ease back to that. It will become smoother and smoother over time of daily practice. And so will our deep meditation sessions, and life in general. It is all connected.

As John Lennon sang, "Your inside is out and your outside is in, so come on and take it easy."

Stillness in action... :-)

The guru is in you.

PS: Regarding the *Secrets of Wilder* novel, keep in mind that John Wilder's journey was one of discovery, with some excesses in practice and resulting difficulties along the way. That is putting it mildly, yes? Those excesses and difficulties are included in the story to offer a heads up on some of the common pitfalls in practice, not so the reader will repeat them! This is especially true of excessive intentional breath suspension, which is a huge energy stimulator. And premature crown practices, which can lead to some difficult traveling. So the Wilder story, among other things, is about what can bring smooth progress and what may not. And the AYP writings are about that too. Carry on! :-)

2008/02/02 13:52:03
Support for AYP Deep Meditation and Samyama
http://www.aypsite.org/forum/topic.asp?TOPIC_ID=3402&REPLY_ID=29598&whichpage=-1
Metabolism slowing down

Hi EMC:

You are really talking about "automatic yoga," which tends to happen more for some folks than for others. It is a karmic thing and it can make the journey seem a bit more complicated while figuring out what to do (if anything) about all the experiences that are going on. But the underlying mechanics of purification and opening are the same for everyone, so it boils down to navigation. Not always easy with so much going on. At the same time, it is very easy as long as we are favoring our center in stillness, including the means that reliably establish us there. All the rest is, yes, scenery! :-)

Fighting automatic yoga is not the answer. It isn't Darth Vader grabbing you by the neck. It is only your nervous system in a rush to open to the infinite divine potential within you. Nothing wrong with that, as long as you can avoid getting frozen or fried in the process. :-)

That is why I say "navigation." We all are obliged to do it by one means or another, no matter how much or how little we have going on symptom-wise.

Here is a lesson on automatic yoga that might help:
Handling Automatic Yoga and Siddhis: http://www.aypsite.org/210.html

While the experience brought up in the lesson is different, the underlying dynamics and measures taken are the same. The lesson takes a fairly broad look at automatic yoga, and can be extrapolated to cover just about any kind of symptom or situation, including breath suspension, etc.

Related lessons can be found in the topic index under "automatic yoga."

All the best!

The guru is in you.

2008/02/05 11:38:17
Support for AYP Deep Meditation and Samyama
http://www.aypsite.org/forum/topic.asp?TOPIC_ID=3414&REPLY_ID=29697&whichpage=-1
Pressure / lump in throat?

quote:
_____
Originally posted by Echo

I tried adding Dynamic Jalandhara to my practice this evening. I had to stop after a couple of rounds. It felt like my tongue was burning!...............interesting.
_____

Hi Echo:

You might try doing a couple of rotations of chin pump (dynamic jalandhara) each day without breath retention ("chin pump lite"). The idea is to continue with the purification process without overdoing -- finding your balance in practice. It does not have to be all or nothing.

Obviously it works for you. It is only a matter of scaling the practice for comfort. That is self-pacing. :-)

All the best!

The guru is in you.

2008/02/05 12:54:51
Support for AYP Deep Meditation and Samyama
http://www.aypsite.org/forum/topic.asp?TOPIC_ID=3414&REPLY_ID=29700&whichpage=-1
Pressure / lump in throat?

quote:
_____
Originally posted by Echo

The pressure, though I can still feel it a little, has almost gone now. I'm pretty sure it was some sort of block as the pranayama seems to going a lot easier now. :-)

I'm just starting to get over the clunky phase of Yoni Mudra Kumbhaka, so am a little reluctant to add anything new just yet!
_____

Hi Echo:

Glad to hear things are smoothing out in the throat area.

Yoni mudra kumbhaka is a big step, and you are wise to give it plenty of time to stabilize. Even after it is stable, ongoing self-pacing will be necessary, because it is a strong energy stimulator, especially when integrated with other practices in the routine.

Industrial strength yoga that won't fly out of control. What we have always wanted, yes? :-)

The guru is in you.

2008/02/05 11:24:24
Support for AYP Deep Meditation and Samyama
http://www.aypsite.org/forum/topic.asp?TOPIC_ID=3420&REPLY_ID=29696&whichpage=-1
eye contact samyama

quote:
_____
Originally posted by cosmic_troll

I tried the **cosmic samyama** 2 or 3 times, but backed off because I wasn't able to sleep afterwards. I'm probably not ready for it yet.
_____

Hi Cosmic:

Keep in mind that cosmic samyama can be done at the end of our twice daily sitting practices, while lying down at the end. This is the best time to incorporate it in our routine. It can also be done at bed time. If it interferes with sleep, then we can skip it at bed time. Doing it with daily sitting practices should not affect our sleep pattern.

As with all practices, if we run into uncomfortable symptoms, we self-pace as needed. This usually means scaling back rather than stopping entirely. It is rarely an all or nothing decision. Always somewhere in-between too much and not enough. :-)

The effect of cosmic samyama is the gradual expansion of our abiding everyday awareness to cosmic dimensions. The entire ocean known intimately in a single drop.

All the best!

The guru is in you.

2008/02/14 10:52:05
Support for AYP Deep Meditation and Samyama
http://www.aypsite.org/forum/topic.asp?TOPIC_ID=3458&REPLY_ID=30051&whichpage=-1
Energy from just DM?

Hi Jack:

One of the first things to check if there is some irritability in daily activity is if you are taking enough rest right after meditation -- at least a few minutes with eyes closed and not engaged in the procedure of deep meditation, just taking it easy. It can also help to lie down for 5-10 minutes immediately at the end of our session, if time and space allow.

Rest at the end of our meditation session allows the internal (and often invisible) purification going on to complete itself before we get up and go out into activity. If we rush the transition going from sitting to activity, the purification can overflow into activity, and that can show up as some dullness, uneasiness or irritability.

So, self-pacing isn't only about regulating the length of our practice. It is also about making the transition from practice to activity as smooth as possible.

Yes, deep meditation can stimulate energy movment. It is in the nature of inner silence to move. All of life and materiality are stillness in motion. The energy-related methods of yoga are for cultivating conscious engagement in the flow of life. But it begins in stillness, in deep meditation. All the more reason to make a smooth transition from sitting to activity. :-)

All the best!

The guru is in you.

2008/02/14 15:39:54
Support for AYP Deep Meditation and Samyama
http://www.aypsite.org/forum/topic.asp?TOPIC_ID=3458&REPLY_ID=30065&whichpage=-1
Energy from just DM?

Hi Jack:

No need to cultivate any special attitude or way of thinking when getting up or in activity. If it is forced it can cause more difficulties. It will come naturally over time from within. The new Self-Inquiry book covers this.

Regarding sensitivity to meditation, check the lessons listed for "Sensitivity to Meditation" in the topic index:
http://www.aypsite.org/TopicIndex.html

And for grounding, which can help when there is unruly energy: http://www.aypsite.org/forum/topic.asp?TOPIC_ID=2165

The good news is that purification is occurring, and it will smooth out in time with regular self-paced practice.

All the best!

The guru is in you.

2008/02/20 09:48:54
Support for AYP Deep Meditation and Samyama
http://www.aypsite.org/forum/topic.asp?TOPIC_ID=3462&REPLY_ID=30295&whichpage=-1
Two options in Samyama

quote:
_____
Originally posted by Emil

Option 1: One repetition of sutras + 5 minutes of lightness sutra
Option 2: Two repetition of sutras + 2 minutes of lightness sutra
_____

Hi Emil:

Option 2 is a more balanced approach. If one repetition is best for you now (option 1), then cut the lightness sutra to a couple of minutes. If you are paring one part of the sequence, you should pare the rest of the sequence.

It's your call, of course. Daily practice (honoring the habit) is more important than how much or how little we are doing. Maintaining your comfort in that is the key. :-)

All the best!

The guru is in you.

2008/03/03 10:23:44
Support for AYP Deep Meditation and Samyama
http://www.aypsite.org/forum/topic.asp?TOPIC_ID=3462&REPLY_ID=30776&whichpage=-1
Two options in Samyama

quote:
_____
Originally posted by Emil

Thanks Yogani,
What I understand from your answer is that the time spent on the lightness sutra needs to be less than or equal to the time spent on rest of the sutras. Is that correct?
I'm looking for a rule of thumb to use for future time adjustments when needed.

_____

Hi Emil:

Not exactly, though the way you are looking at it will yield essentially the same result. I am saying that if you are reducing sutra repetitions to one each, then consider reducing the lightness sutra at the end by one half also, which is a couple of minutes instead of five minutes. That is proportional.

On the other hand, you are free to do less or more of lightness as you see fit. Keeping some proportionality in the sequence is only a suggestion, not an absolute.

Nothing is absolute in AYP except inner silence. :-)

The guru is in you.

2008/02/28 00:11:49
Support for AYP Deep Meditation and Samyama
http://www.aypsite.org/forum/topic.asp?TOPIC_ID=3515&REPLY_ID=30605&whichpage=-1
Samyama produces bad karma

Hi LAMNN:

Doing samyama on "negative words" is discussed in the Samyama book within the context of dissolving the obstacles to enlightenment that such words may imply. This "expanded application" of samyama was covered for those who may be inclined toward illuminating the world's most serious problems with divine light from within. If we have abiding inner silence, there can be a substantial influence.

This aspect of samyama practice, the dissolving of obstructions to enlightenment on any scale, is covered in the Yoga Sutras of Patanjali. Reference is provided in the Appendix of the Samyama book on the "Samyama Sutras of Patanjali," from Chapter 3 of the Yoga Sutras. More importantly, it works! :-)

If someone chooses to increase the negative power of a negative word by doing samyama with it, or even use a positive word for a selfish reason (as we all have), it will not work as intended because of the inherent nature of inner silence (pure bliss consciousness), which is the fuel of samyama.

So, yes, there is a general positive influence that is produced in all samyama practice. What comes through a specific sutra is a flavor of the divine quality flowing from within. No matter where the sutra is pointing, the energy flow coming from within will be radiantly purifying in that direction.

However, this is not so general that it will not matter what sutras we use. In fact, the sutras we use in daily practice matter a lot, and so is maintaining a consistent sutra list for core practice over the long term, because we are engaged in deep and balanced purification throughout our nervous system. This takes consistent practice going deeper and deeper over time.

On the other hand, after our sitting practices, there may be times (maybe often for some of us) when we wish or pray for an end to the maladies of the world, or perhaps maladies closer to home. Our wishes and prayers will be much more effective if we employ the time-tested principles of samyama. We need not be afraid to face the negative energies that may be swirling in the air, or afraid to release their name in our stillness. When our attention is flowing from within stillness, negative energies will hold no sway. They are simply obstructions to be dissolved. When we turn on the light, the darkness will disappear.

Practice is practice and we sit for that in a structured way like clockwork. Then our ability to express ourselves during daily activities will be rooted in the inner silence we have cultivated in practice, and in the ability we have developed to act from within that silence.

Putting it in another terminology, if we surrender the word "disease" to God, will God give us more disease? If we surrender the word "war" to God, will God give us more war? Of course not.

This is why it is said to "Let go and let God." It is not a passive surrender to things as they are. It is an active surrender which has the healing power of all creation behind it. This is what samyama is. Or, rather, this is what samyama becomes for those who systematically cultivate it to its natural flowering, which is unending outpouring divine love. This is the natural obliteration of all negativity, which does not exist in the depths of our being. The ability resides within all of us.

The guru is in you.

2008/02/29 12:15:34
Support for AYP Deep Meditation and Samyama
http://www.aypsite.org/forum/topic.asp?TOPIC_ID=3515&REPLY_ID=30647&whichpage=-1
Samyama produces bad karma

Hi LAMNN:

The word "God" is not used in a relative or philosophical way above, or as a belief. It is used as synonymous with abiding inner silence, as in "Be still and know I am God."

We are talking about the procedure of samyama here, which (with daily practice) leads to natural samyama in all thinking and doing -- stillness in action. In this there can be no negativity, even in the midst of so-called negative events, including some of our own thought streams. It is something everyone will arrive at in time. Before then, our world is seen as relative, as you point out. To bloom spiritually, we must get beyond identification with relative distinctions, so we cultivate the mind to naturally transcend its objects (including thoughts and feelings) with these specialized techniques. Then the objects themselves will be gradually illuminated as they come up, including the so-called negative ones. This is how we come to not worry so much about avoiding "negative thoughts," in samyama or any other aspect of life. Likewise, as we progress in practices, acting on negative thoughts becomes progressively more difficult.

Any thought can be colored negatively in the mind. It is inherent in relative existence. Do the dangers found in relativity pose a danger to our samyama practice, or its results? No, because samyama operates beyond the mind. There are other reasons for choosing our sutras for samyama, having to do with enhancing and balancing the results, but not related to fearing a content-related negative outcome. The latter is not part of the equation for anyone who is familiar with the AYP approach to samyama.

If you are making a case for not doing samyama on certain words because it can lead to negative effects, I must take issue. If such a practice leads to negative effects, it is not samyama. It is something else. It is not possible to amplify negative intentions in inner silence. This is why the practice of samyama is called "morally self-regulating" in the lessons.

Of course, the prerequisite for samyama and its radiating positive effects is abiding inner silence (samadhi). Before that prerequisite condition is available, it is merely concepts we are dealing with, where nothing can be concluded with certainty in spiritual matters, and energy is limited as well. This is why we do deep meditation.

Samyama is amoral, as is deep meditation. Yet, both produce the highest morality (yama/niyama) in the world, because these practices are rooted in *That* in us which is the source of all morality and all life.

It is not a debate that can be settled in external concepts. It can only be settled by direct experience, and that is where we should go to do it. Rather than try to reason it out, let's find out directly, and draw our conclusions from the thing itself, rather than from external concepts. We don't want to miss anything essential because of a particular mindset. :-)

If you think there is something wrong with doing samyama on obstacles to enlightenment as an enhanced application (not core practice), show some evidence that this is so. If you make your case well, we may end up running away from all that is wrong in the world, beginning with our own thoughts. I for one am not for that, and presume that others feel the same way, especially after some time in practices (inner silence/witness coming up). That is why the enhanced applications are offered in the Samyama book.

All the best!

The guru is in you.

PS: Pardon me for hammering away on this, but it is really at the heart of the spiritual path, and is especially relevant when considering samyama, self-inquiry and karma yoga. If there is no chance to cultivate a natural positive outflow from stillness into all aspects of our life, then yoga is not going to be worth the time we are devoting to it. Obviously, many here consider it to be worth the effort, so there must be something good happening.

2008/02/29 17:47:08
Support for AYP Deep Meditation and Samyama
http://www.aypsite.org/forum/topic.asp?TOPIC_ID=3515&REPLY_ID=30659&whichpage=-1
Samyama produces bad karma

quote:
————
Originally posted by Lookatmynavelnow

I am not happy with the practise of samyama on negative words, I think it might be harmful. Until you have other proof, then caution is recommended. Samyama using only neutral or positive words will give the wanted effect without the potential risk.
————

Hi LAMNN:

This has not been suggested as a core practice, and no one is obligated (that goes for anything in AYP). And, yes, kick the tires all you like. But don't expect me to roll over too easily on principles that I can see are operating within us. :-)

The suggestion is that if we happen to be thinking about the maladies of the world, the best place to do it is released in stillness. The emotional charge can be used to advantage, and this crosses over into bhakti -- a subject we can pick up later. All thinking for practitioners of yoga is heading in this direction over the long term. We are deliberately cultivating the ability. So doing samyama on negative thoughts is an inevitability, even if we don't plan on it. Living in stillness is that. Of course, those "negative thoughts" are dissolving already in stillness as our ability increases, so the negativity is a paper tiger, like a shadow on the wall.

So maybe the guideline should be, if it feels negative and scary, avoid it. And it is doesn't, dissolve away! It is really a matter of where our sense of self is. It is like that for self-inquiry too. When we are the witness and operate from there, we call it "relational." The same applies in samyama.

I have pointed this "negative thought" thing out in the Samyama book and in the forums for good reason. We are heading in that direction. It is early to bring it up, but not premature, I think. The controversy was expected. And here we are. Give it some time. :-)

On the evidence side, Check Shanti's excellent topic on dissolving positively and negatively charged thoughts in stillness with equal effectiveness, before they manifest, no less. That is an application of samyama. It is a clear demonstration of how obstructions can be dissolved in stillness, showing that negativity is not amplified in samyama.

Finally, doing samyama on "love" versus "hate" will not be the same, because the object of these will not necessarily be the same, and neither will the energy associated with the thought. Love is opening and hate is obstruction. So there is a difference. Love and other "positive" sutras are best for core practice, for broad purification and opening in our nervous system and surroundings. This does not mean we will never have a negative thought in our mind. When we do, it is far better to let it go in stillness than to act on it. I think most would agree on that.

All the best!

The guru is in you.

2008/03/22 10:56:26
Support for AYP Deep Meditation and Samyama
http://www.aypsite.org/forum/topic.asp?TOPIC_ID=3643&REPLY_ID=31596&whichpage=-1
How did AYAM go I AM?

Hi All:

We use the sound-thought of the mantra in deep meditation. Meaning has no role in it. If meanings come up during practice, we treat them like any other thought and easily come back to the sound-thought of the mantra at whatever level of clarity or faintness we happen to be in the moment.

It is suggested not to analyze the mantra too much. As they say, "Just do it." (meditation, that is) :-)

All the best!

The guru is in you.

2008/03/25 14:04:12
Support for AYP Deep Meditation and Samyama
http://www.aypsite.org/forum/topic.asp?TOPIC_ID=3664&REPLY_ID=31725&whichpage=-1
Small Bright Light

Hi UniversalMind:

Regarding the point of light, you might find these two lessons helpful:
The Star: http://www.aypsite.org/92.html
The Star Revisited: http://www.aypsite.org/179.html

The disorientation (up, down, etc.) will even out in time. Good things are happening -- purification and opening. :-)

All the best!

The guru is in you.

2008/03/31 16:29:44
Support for AYP Deep Meditation and Samyama
http://www.aypsite.org/forum/topic.asp?TOPIC_ID=3696&REPLY_ID=31999&whichpage=-1
Cosmic Samyama

Hi YB:

Any reclined or semi-reclined position will be good for practicing Cosmic Samyama. Hand position is not crucial. Savasana (corpse pose) is okay too. The key is comfort, which helps facilitate the practice.

In contrast, in deep meditation and regular "core" samyama, sitting comfortably upright helps facilitate these practices. Cosmic samyama has the element of yoga nidra (yogic sleep) in it, while deep meditation and core samyama do not, though there certainly can be some overlaps in experience.

Cosmic samyama can be performed right after our sitting practices routine, while we are reclined in rest mode. It can also be done at bedtime by itself, if it does not disrupt sleep. Whether it disrupts sleep or not will depend on the purification and opening that may be occurring in the nervous system. Self-pace as needed.

Cosmic samyama dynamically expands self-awareness to our cosmic dimensions as an ongoing experience in daily life. I happened to listen to the Jill Taylor talk today (excellent!) and she gives a pretty good description of it as experienced during her stroke: http://www.microclesia.com/?p=320 Yes, we can be expanded cosmically like that all the time, even while fulfilling our responsibilities -- a marriage of right and left brain, as she might call it. It has many practical advantages.

As is the case with core samyama, inner silence is the prerequisite for effective cosmic samyama. Even just a little abiding stillness from deep meditation will go a long way with samyama, and everything else too. :-)

As with all yoga practices, daily practice over the long term yields the best results.

All the best!

The guru is in you.

2008/04/02 11:35:48
Support for AYP Deep Meditation and Samyama
http://www.aypsite.org/forum/topic.asp?TOPIC_ID=3704&REPLY_ID=32097&whichpage=-1
Samyama and ecstatic conductivity

Hi All:

What samyama and ecstatic conductivity have in common is that both move from within stillness. So each will naturally facilitate the other. That is true of all aspects of yoga. Everything is connected within us. This is why an integration of practices will be much more powerful than any single practice. "The whole is greater than the sum of the parts."

Inner silence is the prerequisite for samyama. Energy techniques (pranayama, asanas, mudras, bandhas, tantra) are the primary means for cultivating ecstatic conductivity. As we know, it is also possible for deep meditation alone (with or without samyama) to cultivate ecstatic conductivity, depending on the process of purification occurring in the individual nervous system. Inner silence is the common denominator underlying all spiritual progress, including the rise of ecstatic conductivity.

The multiple limbs of yoga provide a full range of connection channels in stillness, leading to *Oneness*.

The guru is in you.

2008/05/10 08:55:51
Support for AYP Deep Meditation and Samyama
http://www.aypsite.org/forum/topic.asp?TOPIC_ID=3875&REPLY_ID=33586&whichpage=-1
Changing my mantra from TM one to I Am

Hi UniversalMind and Kathy:

For going to AYP mantra enhancements, being well-established with the I AM mantra is obviously the logical place to be coming from for known results, since the enhancements are designed for that. So when people come asking about mantra enhancements, I point to that.

On the other hand, I would not recommend outright that anyone change their practice or mantra if following another teaching, since that would be interference with another path, which we avoid doing.

For those who are committed to another path and wanting to add something from AYP, it is possible to use a mantra like a TM one and build the AYP mantra enhancements around that. But the results will be unknown and it would be the practitioner's experiment. So there are several ways to approach it -- some that are straight up and known AYP, and many more that are hybrids with other systems and should be regarded as experimental.

While on the subject of TM and other forms of meditation, AYP spinal breathing pranayama before meditation is a much more clearly defined and easy add-on that can make a substantial difference in results. A lot of bang for the buck available there, with less chance for an unknown outcome. Spinal breathing makes most forms of meditation more powerful. Then self-pacing will likely become the next step on the learning curve.

In applying the AYP methods, it is always the practitioner's choice. What is known (straight up AYP), we can verify and support. What may not be known (innumerable hybrid approaches), we will learn about in time, and share. And the knowledge-base keeps growing. So it goes. :-)

All the best!

The guru is in you.

2008/05/26 10:11:58
Support for AYP Deep Meditation and Samyama
http://www.aypsite.org/forum/topic.asp?TOPIC_ID=3932&REPLY_ID=34060&whichpage=-1
concentration on mantra

quote:
_____
Originally posted by skorpion63

The thing is my mind never goes away from the mantra so there is no question of bringing it back. Does this mean i am doing something wrong or is it not working for me?
_____

Hi Scorpion, and welcome!

It is fine. The fact that you notice the "mind never going away from the mantra" is a thought other than the mantra, right? This is normal. When noticed, just easily favor the mantra over that or any thought. There can be mantra and thoughts mixed together, with the mantra in the background or foreground. It doesn't matter. The procedure stays the same. We never force, just gently favor according to the procedure.

The mantra does not have to be a clear mental pronunciation. In a given session, or over a series of sessions, it will naturally change as purification and opening occur in the nervous system. There is nothing to monitor or judge about it. Monitoring the progress of meditation while doing it is not meditation. We easily favor the mantra over the monitoring. In time, it becomes an easy habit -- it is the habit of stillness we are cultivating. Whenever other thoughts occur, like "I am thinking the mantra all the time," just ease back to the mantra. This can be in a very faint and fuzzy place, and then gone to pure bliss consciousness...

You are doing very well. In some time, the process of daily deep meditation will settle in, and you will notice its affects more and more in your normal daily activity. Carry on, and enjoy!

The guru is in you.

2008/05/26 11:28:07
Support for AYP Deep Meditation and Samyama
http://www.aypsite.org/forum/topic.asp?TOPIC_ID=3951&REPLY_ID=34066&whichpage=-1
meditation vs everyday life

quote:
_____
Originally posted by eputkonen

quote:
_____
Originally posted by Divineis

where lies the difference between when you're sitting in meditation and when you're out and about doing everyday business.
_____

No difference.

"Meditation vs. everday life" is not how it is supposed to be. There is not meditation and then stop and go on with your day. The idea is to resume activity in the day but still in meditation (go from sitting to walking meditation...without a break...to the breakfast table and do eating meditation...etc).

Eventually meditation never stops...and meditation becomes everyday life; even while out and about doing your everyday business.

Namaste,

~ Eric Putkonen
_____

Hi Eric:

Your instruction does not apply to AYP deep meditation. We automatically take inner silence gained in twice daily deep meditation with us into our daily activity, but not the procedure of deep meditation itself (or the mantra). In the AYP approach, there are other means that arise for integrating inner silence in normal daily activity. Additional means include a natural abiding in stillness, the rising habit of samyama (cultivated in core sitting practice), relational self-inquiry, tantric methods, ecstatic conductivity and radiance, and other evolving expressions of "stillness in action."

Just a reminder: The Deep Meditation/Samyama and Pranayama/Mudras/Bandhas forums are primarily for support for the corresponding AYP practices. To be mixing and matching systems of practice (or non-practice) can be confusing for beginners especially.

You are welcome to share your philosophies and methods in other forums here where it is appropriate, including in the "Bhakti/Jnana/Karma Yoga" and "Other Systems of Spiritual Practice" forums. All input is welcome in the appropriate forums where there can be clarity of method while minimizing confusion between different approaches to practice.

And while we are on approaches, you promote Kriya Yoga on your website, but only discuss an advaita/non-duality approach here in the AYP Forums. Perhaps when you have time, it would be nice to clarify your thoughts on kriya yoga practice in relation to your current advaita/non-duality approach, keeping in mind that many readers here are beginners looking for practical methods. Also, many here have broad experience and can spot inconsistencies in a teaching approach in a heartbeat. The fellow who takes a plane to Los Angeles and then preaches that no plane is necessary to get to Los Angeles has some explaining to do. :-)

It is not about where we teachers might happen to be. That is not important. It is about how others can evolve most efficiently in unfolding their own full potential.

A good place to provide the necessary clarifications on the role of Kriya Yoga on your path, if any, is in the "Other Systems" forum. I'm sure it would stimulate a lively discussion on "path versus no path" approaches.

All the best!

The guru is in you.

Hi All:

This recent email exchange might be helpful:

Q: Could you please clarify for me one subtle moment in the practice of samyama ... my "inner light" suggested me in order to refine the sutras, to initially do samyama on each of them for a bit longer, instead of just picking it for a fraction of the second. My experience shows /since my mind is not so fast yet/, that if a hold the sutra for a few seconds /2 to 5/ it refines to a much subtler level, which is on the border of my inner silence and afterwards I transcend to a deeper samadhi. Doing so, seems to leave me with a feeling of great elevation after the practice and during the day. Is it right to do so or shall I strictly abide to the fast form of sutra picking up? I cannot yet pick it up on the finest possible level immediately, it takes a bit longer for it to get there.

A: Like with the mantra in meditation, setting a fixed mode for picking up a sutra in samyama is not the preferred way to go. Due to purification and opening occurring in the nervous system over time, the sutra may sometimes tend to stretch out, and other times be barely noticed (short, faint and fuzzy). Both are correct. We just pick up the sutra at whatever level is comfortable, and let it go. It will not always be the same, and it will interfere with the natural flow of practice to try and make it a particular way. Then we may find ourselves trying to make a longer pronunciation when the nervous system is ready to lightly touch and go into stillness. And the reverse is true also. Sometimes the mind will naturally elongate a sutra a bit (you are experiencing that, right?), and we should not try and force it to be short. It is the ever-changing landscape of purification and opening within us. We just take it all in stride and easily favor our practice without trying to over-control what is happening according to some desired outcome we might glimpse. That can only work against our progress. So we just take it easy and favor the procedure of the practice.

One thing I have said about all the AYP practices is that redesigning them while practicing based on subjective experiences occurring during practice is not a good idea. The experience will always be changing, and the practice should not be changing to follow the experience. Otherwise, we will become like a leaf in the wind, changing our practice every time the winds of inner experience shift. The experience results from the practice, not the other way around. The practice is sufficiently flexible to allow a wide range of experiences. When we realize we are off into an experience (making our strategies, etc.), we just easily come back and favor the practice as we were instructed. That is nearly always the case.

The exception in AYP is "self-pacing," where we may scale back on our practice time for a while if there is excess purification and discomfort occurring in our nervous system. We self-pace with practices for maximum progress with comfort and safety. Self-pacing is an important aspect of AYP, because we are using many powerful practices in an integrated self-directed way. Self-pacing enables us to navigate with much more horse-power in practices than is possible with more rigid approaches. The result of this flexible high-powered approach is much faster progress, and with more comfort as we develop skill in self-pacing our practices effectively.

Another thing to keep in mind in sutra repetition in samyama, particularly if the pronunciation is elongating, is a tendency we all have to "contemplate" the meaning of the sutra on the conscious level of the mind. As you know, samyama is not contemplation. We just pick up the sutra and release it in stillness. Based on our long familiarity with language (in AYP, sutras are suggested to be in our first language) we know subconsciously what it is deep in our inner silence. This is where the sutra finds its manifestation -- in stillness, gradually cultivating "stillness in action."

The fruit of samyama practice is not to be found in the meaning or expression (siddhi) of any particular sutra, but in our gradually rising ability to engage as stillness in action in our daily life with all intentions we have. So, structured samyama practice is not about enunciating any particular sutra or intention, but to gradually develop the ability to naturally manifest all our intentions from within stillness in everyday life. It is about becoming stillness in action. Structured samyama practice plays a key role in bringing about the condition of abiding inner silence, ecstatic bliss, outpouring divine love, and unity ... a life filled with many small miracles, and some big ones too. :-)

There are additional applications of samyama practice provided in the AYP Samyama book. You may find it an interesting read.

Wishing you all the best on your path. Enjoy!

The guru in is you.

quote:

Originally posted by jillatay

...Like when you previously said it is not always in our best interest to automatically do automatic yoga movements. Am I right in seeing this as a similar situation?

Hi Jill:

Yes. Though there is a lot spiritual potential in all of us (sometimes quite visible), we will be able to move the fastest by using an efficient routine of practices. Sort of like burning gasoline in a car rather than throwing it on the ground and setting it on fire. It is all about maximizing fuel efficiency, in this case for our ongoing purification and opening. :-)

The guru is in you.

2008/05/29 10:45:41

Hi YB, emc and All:

The drifting and changes occurring in samyama practice that you describe are normal parts of the purification process. It is natural for the mind to want to add strategies to try and counteract the changes, but the strategies must be let go of too, sooner or later. In time, it all settles in and we find that staying with the original procedure has been the best way all along. Just keep that in mind, and all will work out in time. Samyama tends to have a bigger clunky stage than other practices. This too shall pass, and stillness will rise in all our actions! :-)

On changing sutras based on what feels right, this is altering the practice to suit the subjective experience, which has already been discussed above. Of course, we are all free to tinker as we please, but that will be our research. I do not know the effects of all possible causes in practice.

Maybe go back to Patanjali's Yoga Sutras (Chap 3) and check his original samyama sutras. There is an interpretation of Patanjali's 30 samyama sutras in the appendix of the AYP Samyama book, designed to be an aid for research by well-established practitioners.

Maybe better to wait on altering sutras, at least until past the clunky stage with AYP core samyama practice. It is not necessary to change the core practice sutras at all, but everyone has their own inclinations.

Rather than reinventing core samyama practice, the suggestion is to move to additional applications of samyama once core practice is smooth and stable, i.e., cosmic samyama, asana samyama, prayer samyama, action samyama, and so on, moving steadily toward the actualization of "stillness in action" in daily living.

It's your call, of course. Practice wisely, and enjoy!

The guru is in you.

2008/05/29 12:46:05

quote:
_____
Originally posted by jillatay

Sometimes when it comes time for a new sutra a strange random word pops into my head. What's this?

Jill
_____

Hi Jill:

Purification! :-)

Just ease back to the procedure of the practice, including the sutras.

The guru is in you.

2008/05/29 15:52:32

quote:
_____
Originally posted by emc

Yogani, this is really interesting. Are you saying that it's better to say only one, two or a few sutras and then pass out and wake up 15-20 min later and take a few minutes resting time and consider that to be the samyama session for today, rather than trying to keep aware and say all nine sutras? That would really be a relief if that is considered to be a proper samyama session. Then I can stop counting and just wait for this phase to pass! Have I gotten you right on that?:-)
_____

Hi emc:

Yes, you have it right.

There is no time limit for doing core samyama practice, unless in group practice and/or adhering to a schedule is necessary, of course.

Practically speaking, if you have 10 minutes for samyama and only get through a few sutras in that time, it is fine to lie down and rest whenever you realize your self-appointed time is up. You should not force yourself to do all the sutras in a fixed time frame, devising mental strategies to by-pass the natural purification and opening that is occurring. Just take it easy and enjoy. Samyama practice will smooth out in time, and there will be more awareness of the time and the sutras in turn. :-)

The guru is in you.

2008/05/30 09:10:57
Support for AYP Deep Meditation and Samyama
http://www.aypsite.org/forum/topic.asp?TOPIC_ID=3964&REPLY_ID=34210&whichpage=-1
samyama confusion

quote:
_____
Originally posted by nical ecs

Hello everybody, my problems with samyama have been these:

- Bringing contemplation into practice
- Not letting go easily/clinging on to the words, instead trying to "fill" them with meaning/feeling/intuition
- !...zzz...?...!...zzz...?...!...?...zzz

The first two were mostly dealt with by reading Yogani´s book *"Samyama - Cultivating Stillness in Action, Siddhis and Miracles"*. This book is so good, and very informative regarding context (yogic philosophy) and non-dual dynamics. It made me understand how samyama practice is about establishing pathways for spontaneous expression from within *in general*, not about amplifying this or that concept - unlike many other, non-yogic affirmative/projective techniques. Most of my bad habits in samyama practice stemmed from slipping into the intentions of the latter kind, consciously or not.

For dealing with falling asleep I found another method, of an outlaw variety.

Initially samyama was a powerful practice for me. Especially since it turned out to be "the last bit of the puzzle" in terms of dealing with an over-abundance of pranic energy starting about a year ago. After adding samyama to the routine my "headspace" increased almost explosively (not in the "Scanners" way, though), tensions smoothed out and bliss moved in in a way that has made me faithful to the practice since then, through ups and downs. Yes, I love my samyama!

So, after this "beginner´s luck" abandoned me and I had a phase of falling asleep instead. Similarly to what emc and yogibear relates above, I found it nearly impossible to keep track of time while constantly going into sleep/trance/hypnagogic imagery. I´d be struggling like a fish on land just to remember which word to pick up next. I tried to remedy this situation by cutting down the ordained 15 seconds to about 5 for a couple of sessions. I reasoned it would be better to be able to stay awake all the way through a shortened and incorrectly exercised practice than keeping it up with such an absurd amount of effort and confusion. This strategy turned out to be successful. When I later increased to 15 again, I seemed to have tricked myself, seeing that the aquired habit of staying awake persisted.

By the way, I´ve followed AYP in the recommended order for a little less than a year now, starting it off very slowly shortly after a dramatic K opening. I´ve consulted the forum now and then, but this is my first post here.

I want to express my gratitude to Yogani and those who have helped him provide all the information and guidance on this site, forumites included. The experimental and pragmatic approach around here is deeply appreciated! See you around.
_____

Hi nical ecs, and welcome!

At the risk of contradicting myself (and confusing emc! :-)), let me say there is some merit in the interim strategy you mentioned of temporarily shortening the time between sutras until the question marks are gone, going from this:
!...zzz...?...!...zzz...?...!...?...zzz

to this:
!...zzz...!...zzz...!...zzz

and eventually to this:
!......!......!......

I think one of the reasons samyama remains "clunky" longer than other practices is the time it takes to have the sequence of sutras memorized to the point where they come up automatically, particularly in stillness when the practitioner is "zoning out" or "falling asleep" between repetitions due to purification and/or samadhi. Not a bad thing, but still the next sutra will be needed, and if we are into an internal dialog (the question mark) every time about remembering and recovering the sutra at whatever level in consciousness we happen to be, rather than picking it up automatically, then there is part of the clunkiness. Once sutra recall becomes automatic at all levels, then that part of the clunkiness is gone.

Doing a more rapid repetition of sutras for a while can help ingrain the entire sutra sequence deep in the mind. As long as we are able to return to normal times of stillness in-between, then all will be fine. Of course, the sequence of sutras can also be repeated rapidly outside samyama practice for memorization purposes. In time, such memorization exercises become moot, because the sutras come up automatically. This is also a reason why we do not keep switching the sutras around, so the whole thing will become automatic is stillness. Over the long term, an established series of sutras will become very subtle and deep in samyama practice, facilitating the ongoing process of "stillness in action" in our daily life, much the way long term deep meditation leads to abiding inner silence 24 hours per day.

The main thing is to not get hung up on interim strategies, because samyama is about subtle catch and then release in stillness, with the release being the essence of samyama practice, not the sutra itself. Samyama is not about counting, contemplation, or roaring through the sutras in a minute. Of these, the temporary more rapid repetition of sutras, either inside or outside practice, can support memorization and automatic picking up of the sutras, thus providing a means for building smoothness into the process of samyama.

No matter how we approach it, there will be some time of settling in involved as we move forward with core samyama practice. I don't think we have to be extremely rigid about how the practitioner moves through it, as long as no permanent diversions develop, and effective samyama practice is the result.

And, yes, emc, we can still stop in the middle of sutras when our self-determined time is up. It is good practice. Hopefully this added discussion will help clarity rather than confuse. :-)

Thanks much for chiming in and sharing, nical ecs. We are always looking for better understandings of what we are doing in practices -- optimizing cause and effect.

All the best!

The guru is in you.

2008/06/12 10:28:49
Support for AYP Deep Meditation and Samyama
http://www.aypsite.org/forum/topic.asp?TOPIC_ID=4019&REPLY_ID=34554&whichpage=-1
AYP and breath awareness

quote:
_____
Originally posted by anthony574

I have the book.

Interestingly, I was a bit timid to try self-inquiry. I find that the states it produces tend to happen spontaneously for me - I suspect because of premature openings that occured because of the use of hallucinogens in the past.

When I do self-inquiry I feel it is like doing a stretch. I can go only to a certain point and then it feels "painful", then I back off. I do not know exactly how to intereperet the feeling of "pain" other than perhaps it is the ego "suffering" a blow to its indentity, or perhaps a stretch for its muscles. I feel that each time I reach the threshold of the "stretch" and then back off that something is gained in the same way as one becomes more flexible through stretching - but not through forcing oneself past the point of pain. Does this sound right to anyone?
_____

Hi Anthony:

That sounds just right. This is how self-pacing works in relation to all practices.

Well done! :-)

The guru is in you.

PS: And thanks YB for bringing up the Self-Inquiry book. It can be a useful companion to any kind of inquiry, discrimination or mindfulness practice.

2008/06/12 10:06:16
Support for AYP Deep Meditation and Samyama
http://www.aypsite.org/forum/topic.asp?TOPIC_ID=4029&REPLY_ID=34553&whichpage=-1
Yogani, What is Samadhi?

Hi Neptune:

Samad
Hi is the eighth limb of yoga and means "absorption in pure bliss consciousness," or "abiding in inner silence," "the witness," "stillness in action," etc., all which we talk about so much around here from an experiential perspective. Everyone who loses the mantra during deep meditation enters samadhi.

There are as many types and grades of samad
Hi as one might care to define, and it can get very technical in splitting hairs. It really depends on experience. Before then, it is mostly academic.

See these links:
http://www.aypsite.org/forum/topic.asp?TOPIC_ID=2314
http://www.aypsite.org/forum/topic.asp?TOPIC_ID=667
http://www.aypsite.org/248.html

Carry on! :-)

The guru is in you.

2008/07/11 12:20:53
Support for AYP Deep Meditation and Samyama
http://www.aypsite.org/forum/topic.asp?TOPIC_ID=4119&REPLY_ID=35366&whichpage=-1
Question about kechari activity

Hi Jan:

Sorry for the delay getting back on this.

As ecstatic conductivity begins to stir in the body, one of the possible symptoms can be energy sensations in the area of tongue, mouth and palate. This is discussed in AYP Lesson 108, and has been reported by practitioners from many traditions, both ancient and modern.

Does having such symptoms mean we are supposed to do something with kechari? Maybe. Maybe not. That is a function of our own bhakti. You will know by your inner call.

All the best!

The guru is in you.

2008/07/19 14:27:36
Support for AYP Deep Meditation and Samyama
http://www.aypsite.org/forum/topic.asp?TOPIC_ID=4169&REPLY_ID=35639&whichpage=-1
Meditation over answer of specific question.

Hi equinox, and welcome!

Deep meditation itself is for cultivating inner silence, which then gradually enlivens all aspects of our life, even while increasing our inner stability amidst the constant changes of our external world.

Along with this, there comes a natural inner connection with events that tends to work in our favor over time. Call it being in synch, or being in grace, or whatever. It simply doesn't rain on us as often or as much as it used to. Small miracles, and sometimes some big ones.

Another way we describe it here is that our life gradually becomes an expression of "stillness in action." Deep meditation provides the raw material (inner silence), and what we do with it in life comprises the rest, which is a continuation of our purification and opening on an ever-broadening scale, reaching to the cosmic level. To enhance this aspect of our development, we have the practice of "samyama," which is a structured method we can do as part of our daily sitting practices. Later on, samyama becomes a habit in expressing all of our intentions in life (within inner silence), and that enhances the external manifestation of our inner silence in many ways, as mentioned above.

In other words, in time, we find ourselves able to intuitively know things and do things that we could not before.

If you check out the lessons and forum discussions on samyama (see FAQ links here), you will get a good overview of what it is. Also, there is an AYP book called "Samyama," which goes into more detail on the specifics of practice, as well as expanded applications of samyama. In the appendix of the book, you will see a number of additional "sutras" (formulas) that can be used for "research" in samyama by well-established practitioners, including one for seeing things hidden from view -- those lost car keys... :-)

But, just to be clear, samyama is not primarily about performing miraculous acts at will. It is about purifying and opening our nervous system in a balanced way, and radiating far beyond our body, leading to all aspects of life being lived as stillness in action in a unified way, which is life free from suffering. We also call it living in a state of abiding inner silence, ecstatic bliss and outpouring divine love -- unending happiness.

Wishing you all the best on your path. Enjoy!

The guru is in you.

2008/07/20 10:24:00
Support for AYP Deep Meditation and Samyama
http://www.aypsite.org/forum/topic.asp?TOPIC_ID=4169&REPLY_ID=35654&whichpage=-1
Meditation over answer of specific question.

quote:
_____
Originally posted by equinox

Thank you Yogani!

I have read two of your books-Deep Meditation and Samyama. As far as I understood we start with deep meditation first and then slowly we begin to include the rest of the limbs of yoga. My question is how do we determine when to include a new element to our meditation practice? How long do we practice deep meditation on its own before including the Spinal breathing and Samyama?
In the Q&A section I read that it is up to the individual-but how do you know that it is time to progress further?
_____

Hi equinox:

Yes, it is up to the practitioner. How long is typical between practice additions? A few months is typical, though some may be inclined toward shorter or longer (much longer is fine - it is not a race), according to the experience of the process of purification and opening, which is unique for each nervous system. It is developing the art of "self-pacing," which is the key in conducting effective integrated spiritual practice.

The idea is to reach a stable routine with the practices we are doing and give it some time before moving on, including backing off from time to time as necessary to accommodate short term overdoing. It will happen as our desire for divine union (bhakti) gets ahead of our capacity now and then. The more you read the AYP writings and are engaged in your practices, the more you will get a feel for the unique attributes of your own journey, and develop the ability to accommodate them.

It is like driving a car under varying conditions. The better we get at it and the further we have gone along the road, the more we can relax and enjoy the ride. :-)

The guru is in you.

PS: It is strongly recommended not to add more than one practice at a time. This can muddy the waters quite a bit, and complicate our journey of purification and opening.

2008/08/20 17:52:44
Support for AYP Deep Meditation and Samyama
http://www.aypsite.org/forum/topic.asp?TOPIC_ID=4326&REPLY_ID=36592&whichpage=-1

Trachea sutra

Hi Arim, and welcome!

The sutra "Trachea," alleged to be for subduing hunger and thrist, is in the appendix of the Samyama book, which is an interpretation of the 30 or so sutras in the 3rd chapter of Patanjali's Yoga Sutras on "Supernormal Powers." These are offered in the appendix for "research" by established practitioners.

The word "Trachea" comes directly from English translations of the Yoga Sutras, so I did not change it. Some of the other sutras in the list of 30 in the Samyama book involved more interpretation on my part, but not that one. Refining the sutras for better effectiveness will be part of the long term research that will occur as more and more modern yogis and yoginis come into their own and begin to key off the ancient work of Patanjali to find the real truth by direct experience, which is the only place we will find it. Recorded knowledge can only help point the way. All is subject to verification by the application of cause and effect. Samyama is a wide open area for scientific research looking far out into the future. It will become increasingly relevant as more people cultivate the presence of abiding inner silence.

I have to agree with you that "Esophagus" makes a lot more sense in this case, and this is an area where I'd encourage some research. But only by those who are well established and stable in their core samyama practice. It is very easy to go flying off in too many directions at once with this and that would not serve our purposes in practice very well.

As for when and how to use a sutra for research, it will have the best effect if included (only one change at a time) in our regular series of sutras for core practice and used that way twice each day over a period of time. Keep in mind that it takes time for the inner pathways associated with a sutra to become purified and opened, so it is not a matter of using a sutra and finding its full result immediately. There will be many stages of purification and opening.

By using a balanced range of sutras in the daily practice routine, many pathways are being opened at the same time, leading to a broad-based expansion in consciousness, which is the ultimate purpose of samyama. The list of sutras provided for AYP core samyama practice are arranged with this in mind. Cosmic Samyama is also structured for broad-based purification and opening. Samyama is primarily about increasing our overall spiritual development, not for producing a specific outcome. If we go for the broad-based development, we will gain the specific along with that.

"Seek first the kingdom of heaven, and all will be added..." Like that.

For the very advanced, in whom all thoughts may tend to manifest quickly as evolutionary stillness in action (an outpouring), then once or twice with a sutra might be enough to produce an effect. But for most of us, it is a longer process of purification and opening. That is the reason for daily practice over time, and why research on sutras is probably best done as part of that. In this way we will be building a strong foundation in stillness from which all of our actions can move. And then we will notice that our intentions have an uncanny way of finding fulfillment, though not always in exactly the way we might have imagined.

Stillness in action and outpouring divine love have their own way of doing things, and we may feel like we are just along for the ride. Which goes to show that developing the art of letting go in our inner silence is by far the most important part of samyama. :-)

All the best!

The guru is in you.

2008/08/26 10:48:10
Support for AYP Deep Meditation and Samyama
http://www.aypsite.org/forum/topic.asp?TOPIC_ID=4342&REPLY_ID=36791&whichpage=-1
Mantra Enhancement Issue

Hi Emil:

Any new mantra, or mantra enhancement, will tend to be clunky in the beginning, and refine over time of practice. The advantage of an enhancement is that it covers a wider sweep in the mind and produces broader purification as it becomes more refined, much the way shifting to a higher gear in a car enables us to go faster with no additional effort.

It is suggested to review the lessons on mantra design and enhancements for more on this:
http://www.aypsite.org/forum/topic.asp?TOPIC_ID=2159

All the best!

The guru is in you.

2008/09/07 17:52:17
Support for AYP Deep Meditation and Samyama
http://www.aypsite.org/forum/topic.asp?TOPIC_ID=4407&REPLY_ID=37364&whichpage=-1
Question about using Abundance in Samyama

Hi CarsonZi:

It is the nature of life to evolve, grow and become abundant. It is happening all around us in nature, yes? It is the nature of inner silence to expand in this way, human foibles notwithstanding.

So when we use the sutra "abundance," it is to promote the natural process of life emanating from within stillness. This does not necessarily mean more egoic expansion of human endeavors, or whatever we might imagine. There is a much larger divine agenda bubbling within stillness that is morally self-regulating and in tune with nature.

The worth of a sutra will not be settled in mind by intellectualizing the pros or cons of abundance, or anything else. In stillness it will always manifest for the best, on the side of evolution. That is why the abundance sutra is there, balanced and rounded out by the rest of the sutras on the list. It is not about making value judgments. It is about moving inner silence through a range of channels, purifying them over time. Then all of our desires and actions will be in harmony with divine purpose, even as we go about our normal daily business.

In the Samyama book the optional practice of doing samyama on obstructions to enlightenment is introduced (p68), utilizing sutras that are generally regarded to be very negative in meaning. Yet, by releasing these sutras in stillness, we are purifying the channels that are producing the negative outcomes associated with them -- dissolving those obstructions.

Abundance does not usually fit into that category (as an obstruction), but if it did (as you are suggesting in this case), it would not make any difference. The outcome would be the same, the removal of obstructions and the promotion of evolutionary abundance in all of nature, including in humankind.

Interestingly, one of the best ways to mitigate the non-evolutionary pursuit of abundance by human beings is to do samyama on abundance! :-)

That is how inner silence works when expressing through purifying nervous systems -- it takes all intentions and illuminates them from within, so the outcome will always be divine. Samyama is a powerful means for accelerating the process (after deep meditation), not so much for the specifics of the sutras themselves, but in general so all of our intentions will be naturally illuminated, and we won't have to fear so much about negative outcomes anymore. And as we purify ourselves, we are purifying everyone. It is outpouring divine love...

The guru is in you.

2008/09/08 00:14:05
Support for AYP Deep Meditation and Samyama
http://www.aypsite.org/forum/topic.asp?TOPIC_ID=4407&REPLY_ID=37376&whichpage=-1
Question about using Abundance in Samyama

quote:
_____
Originally posted by CarsonZi

Maybe it is just me and where I am at in my life, but I find the word Abundance to be the characteristic of all that is wrong with us as human beings.
_____

Hi CarsonZi:

Well, anyone might be offended by any word, depending on what it means to them at a point in time, but I can assure you that the words as we use them in samyama have nothing to do with negative outcomes. They are universal in stillness and do not involve value judgments or the furtherance of discordant conditions. It is just the opposite. And, as I said, if a word is emotionally charged as obstruction or disharmony, doing samyama with it will be equally for the good, if not more so due to the emotional content.

But if you just can't stand "abundance" and it grates on your nerves, then leave it out (until later :-)). There is no point fighting with it. Of course, I can't predict the effect of leaving it out, or sutra substitutions, so it will be some research, and that may not be an ideal place to start with samyama. Sutra research is only recommended for well-established practitioners. Before going much further with redesigning samyama, I suggest you read the Samyama book for more detailed coverage of all this. Then you will have the best information we can offer at present, and it will be up to you.

Just to put some perspective on your concern, a number of sutras, both in the AYP system and in Patanjali's yoga sutras, could theoretically be judged to be equally destructive as "abundance," and used to further humankind's mischief. So, this kind of argument could be extended to other sutras that can expand human influence in the world, and therefore an argument against the advisability of samyama in general.

But is this really true? Not according to the experiences of many. The outcome of samyama using a balanced list of sutras is not related to personal interpretations and emotional coloring of specific sutras. Nor is it about extending human power in the world. It is about purifying the human nervous system broadly to be a much better vehicle for stillness in action in all areas, expressing itself as outpouring divine love and unity. Samyama is not about expanding human power. It is about expanding divine power, and that is in accordance with the creative principles originating within stillness and operating in nature everywhere.

All the best!

The guru is in you.

2008/10/15 12:07:11
Support for AYP Deep Meditation and Samyama
http://www.aypsite.org/forum/topic.asp?TOPIC_ID=4572&REPLY_ID=38935&whichpage=-1
external noise while meditating

quote:
_____
Originally posted by YogaIsLife

My friends,

Thank you so much for your advices, they are very good. Scott, how did I not think about that? When we are somehow stressed or anxious we don't even think about the simplest solutions...

Manipura, yes that is very good advice and I thought about it. It is hard though. You know what I mean, when the feelings are very strong, like a wave, it can be hard to remain present. What you suggest would be ideal to do but maybe I won't be able to do it at this stage. I can though do what you suggest plus what jo-self suggests (very good advice as well, thank you), to cutback on meditation time and don't dwell on the irritation feelings for too long, going little steps at the time.

To summarize: I will try a bit of everything until I find my confort! :)

You know what, just the fact that I wrote the post yesterday helped me to feel a bit more secure in a way. It is great to be able to find support, and this forum is great for that. Thank you all for the help and opportunity. I feel blessed.

————

Hi YogaIsLife:

Also, remember that the instruction is to regard external noises just like internal thoughts and sensations occurring naturally in deep meditation. When we realize we are off into them, we just easily favor the mantra again at whatever level is comfortable. Thoughts, sensations, noises, mantra and stillness can be occurring all at the same time. We just gently favor the ever-refining mantra, and we will find more abiding stillness emerging in our life over time. And the many happenings occurring in our environment will have less sway over us.

If there is rising tension during deep meditation that makes it difficult to ease back to the mantra, then we can just be with that tension for a while, and our attention will naturally be drawn to a physical sensation somewhere in the body, and it will unwind by our attention easily observing it. Once it does, we can ease back to the mantra again. We keep our meditation time the same, including any use of the procedure just mentioned.

All the best!

The guru is in you.

2008/11/02 12:00:20
Support for AYP Deep Meditation and Samyama
http://www.aypsite.org/forum/topic.asp?TOPIC_ID=4647&REPLY_ID=39798&whichpage=-1
Second enhancement mantra?!!

Hi Ananda:

The second "NAMAH" is included in the AYP Easy Lessons book as a third mantra enhancement. It is included as an addition to Lesson 188. You can read about it there.

All the best! :-)

The guru is in you.

2008/11/12 15:02:59
Support for AYP Deep Meditation and Samyama
http://www.aypsite.org/forum/topic.asp?TOPIC_ID=4712&REPLY_ID=40381&whichpage=-1
question about rest period

Hi Jill:

If you feel good after getting up and going about your business, who can argue with your long rest in stillness? Self-pace as needed. :-)

The guru is in you.

2008/11/13 14:38:54
Support for AYP Deep Meditation and Samyama
http://www.aypsite.org/forum/topic.asp?TOPIC_ID=4717&REPLY_ID=40448&whichpage=-1
Samyama and 'some inner silence'

quote:
————
Originally posted by Ananda

i'm sorry Shanti to point this out, but in the samyama book yogani doesn't recommend adding cosmic samyama until after years of practice it would be nice if more light could be shed on this point.

————

Hi Ananda and All:

The main thing is to be stable in regular core samyama practice before undertaking cosmic samyama. That is the suggestion, and it could take quite a while because it takes time in daily practice for the nine core samyama sutras to "bake in" and be moving plenty of stillness out through our nervous system. That is when we are ready to take stillness much further with cosmic samyama. On the other hand, cosmic samyama could be tried at anytime. The practitioner is free to choose. No harm done if cosmic samyama is taken on early, but the results would not be guaranteed. :-)

It's best to take things one step at a time.

The guru is in you.

2008/11/21 14:56:30
Support for AYP Deep Meditation and Samyama
http://www.aypsite.org/forum/topic.asp?TOPIC_ID=4778&REPLY_ID=40992&whichpage=-1

getting too much sensitive to light, noise

Hi Peacefollower:

Backing off from practices and becoming more physically active (as much as you comfortably can) would be an appropriate thing to do at this time. That includes reduced spiritual study. Social contact of a non-spiritual nature will be helpful too. You have too much purification going on in your nervous system right now, and self-pacing and grounding are in order.

If you have raging bhakti (spiritual desire), it can aggravate the situation, and it would be wise to temper that also by doing things for a while that will engage the emotions on non-spiritual matters.

Keep as active as you can, be measured, and give the situation some time to recover and stabilize. This will pass, and you will be able to inch back into a comfortable routine of spiritual practice after a while. In the meantime, be sure to take measures to assure your comfort and safety. Perhaps others here will have helpful suggestions also.

The guru is in you.

PS: Regarding your seekingshiva ID, it seems to be in order and I wrote you separately about that.

2008/11/21 18:09:41
Support for AYP Deep Meditation and Samyama
http://www.aypsite.org/forum/topic.asp?TOPIC_ID=4778&REPLY_ID=40996&whichpage=-1
getting too much sensitive to light, noise

Hi Seekingshiva:

Of course, if the symptoms persist and measures you are taking don't offer relief, it will be a good idea to see a doctor.

For some other measures to consider, see this AYP lesson on kundalini remedies: http://www.aypsite.org/69.html

All the best!

The guru is in you.

2008/12/01 12:51:15
Support for AYP Deep Meditation and Samyama
http://www.aypsite.org/forum/topic.asp?TOPIC_ID=4843&REPLY_ID=41640&whichpage=-1
dreams, visions + core and cosmic samyama...

Hi Ananda:

Visions will come and go and we will know their meaning as we continue through life without clinging too much to the ideas we may have about them. I think you know well the relationship between experiences & visions and practices, and how we favor the practices, and self-pace practices if experiences become too uncomfortable or intense.

There will be things that happen in our life that stay with us. Some events we will never really "get over," like the loss of a loved one. But in time they can become a quiet loving part of us in everything we do. The bodies go, but love radiates forever.

If the dreaming is too much, it can help smooth things out if you switch your cosmic samyama to be at the end of sitting practices (before rest) instead of at bedtime. That way you will have more opportunity to ground the expansive effects of the practice in activity instead of taking them into sleep mode. Cosmic samyama is inclined to be a more stable and progressive practice that way.

Keep in mind that in AYP it is suggested we do not do any ongoing practice at the expense of keeping a normal sleep pattern, which is essential for maintaining our physical and psychological well-being.

All the best!

The guru is in you.

2009/02/03 09:05:38
Support for AYP Deep Meditation and Samyama
http://www.aypsite.org/forum/topic.asp?TOPIC_ID=5107&REPLY_ID=44603&whichpage=-1
Yoga Nidra questions

quote:
_____
Originally posted by Shanti

quote:
_____
Originally posted by solo

Thanks again Shanti...you always seem to know just the right lesson to refer me to. You know, I keep getting referred to lessons that I have not yet made it to, maybe a sign that I need to advance my practice a tad?

Nonetheless, things are going well and I appreciate your insights. Thank you.
_____

You are welcome Solo. Glad I can help.:-)

Not sure if this is talked about anywhere in Yogani's lessons.. but it is OK to read ahead. Adding new practices (which would be the ones mentioned in the left hand side panel) will not be done till you feel you are ready for them.. however many of the lessons are just question/answers and do answer many of the questions people ask here. So it will help to keep on reading, just don't add any new practices till you are ready for them.

Yogani, please do correct me if I am wrong.

––––––––––

Hi Shanti:

Good advice. And you just reminded me to add yoga nidra (cosmic samyama) to the key lessons in the left border. Thanks! :-)

The guru is in you.

2009/02/04 15:39:07
Support for AYP Deep Meditation and Samyama
http://www.aypsite.org/forum/topic.asp?TOPIC_ID=5107&REPLY_ID=44660&whichpage=-1
Yoga Nidra questions

quote:
––––––––
Originally posted by Shanti

Yogani, would you say, the order in which the practices show up on the left border is the order in which they should be added to our sitting practice?
(Except, as you mention in Lesson 269 we can leapfrog to samyama.:-))

––––––––––

Hi Shanti:

Not necessarily. The key lessons in the left border are more or less in order, but there are some variations there for presentation purposes. Better to follow the lessons, with suggestions on the sequence of taking on practices as discussed there. Later on, in upcoming lessons, we will get more into sequencing, variations, and other nuances.

Of course, it is always the practitioner's call. :-)

The guru is in you.

2009/02/07 12:19:29
Support for AYP Deep Meditation and Samyama
http://www.aypsite.org/forum/topic.asp?TOPIC_ID=5128&REPLY_ID=44790&whichpage=-1
Rhythmical Pulses count as Mantra?

Hi Mimiron and All:

It sounds like good practice.

In time (months and years), the mantra "bakes in" and it will be common to experience it as a faint vibration beyond pronunciation. We start our session with a clear recognition of the mantra (clear pronunciation if needed), and after that it can be picked up as a faint vibration in the depths of stillness, if that is where we are. If we are in doubt about a faint vibration being the mantra, we can come up just far enough to confirm. In time that will not be necessary, as we become more familiar with our inner silence. This is how deep meditation goes deeper and deeper, beyond any other object of mind or senses, including breath, which will tend to suspend automatically along the way with the slow-down in metabolism. Deep meditation using the ever-refining vehicle of the mantra goes far beyond that, and this is what makes it so powerful.

All the best!

The guru is in you.

2009/02/10 18:52:44
Support for AYP Deep Meditation and Samyama
http://www.aypsite.org/forum/topic.asp?TOPIC_ID=5151&REPLY_ID=45027&whichpage=-1
namah....namaha

quote:
––––––––
Originally posted by riptiz

Hi Ananda,
Why would I talk to Yogani about this? I have just returned from the ashram in Ahmedabad. Both my teacher and guru speak perfect Sanskrit and Namaha is used in several mantras as well as the Divine Sound.I agree with Shanti about the pronunciation.
L&L
Dave

––––––––––

Hi Dave:

This may be so, but the sound is NAMAH in the AYP deep meditation mantra enhancements (#2 and #3), and it always has been in practice here as well. Seems to work fine. :-)

So, to use NAMAHA in AYP deep meditation (assuming a significant variation in pronunciation) is a variation on the system, and results may vary also. It will be for practitioners/researchers to determine over the long term in relation to the AYP system. I really can't say.

This is not to say NAMAHA is not a good mantra component. I just cannot verify it from long term direct experience, which is the only verification that counts, far more important than Sanskrit scholarship. If NAMAHA has been verified experientially over long periods of time in other systems, (presumably so), then this is good. But it is still starting at square one as far as the AYP system is concerned, because the practices and their integration in AYP are different from other systems.

So, what you are talking about is a mantra component used in other systems, not in the AYP system. Let's be clear about that.

There is really no point in debating one mantra component against the other, which would only be academic, and not verifying anything experientially, which takes many years to do. It has been done for NAMAH here, and I presume for NAMAHA elsewhere. And never the twain shall meet, except in stillness, of course. :-)

No one should take this to mean that a modification in AYP mantra components, or any other part of the AYP system is a mortal sin. I just can't verify what every outcome will be. So it will be research.

Sometimes it may be worth trying modifications in the AYP practices, particularly if there are difficulties that are not resolving themselves. Other times it may not be worth it -- if it ain't broke, don't fix it. See here for further discussion on this:
http://www.aypsite.org/forum/topic.asp?TOPIC_ID=5103

All the best!

The guru is in you.

2009/02/10 23:58:21
Support for AYP Deep Meditation and Samyama
http://www.aypsite.org/forum/topic.asp?TOPIC_ID=5151&REPLY_ID=45037&whichpage=-1
namah....namaha

Hi Holy:

The derivation of mantras, at least in the AYP approach, involves three things: Traditional guidelines, inner "seeing" (a function of ecstatic conductivity and refined sensory perception), and the experience of the community of practitioners.

The last is important because there will be many experiences in the same practitioner over time, and many experiences in the community of practitioners at any one point in time.

This is why we start with a core mantra and introduce enhancements in a flexible manner over time. One size does not fit all. The experience of many practitioners is more nuanced than scholarship and fixed teachings can account for, and I think many traditions fall short on this. That is why the AYP system is built primarily around experience, rather than scholarship or fixed by-rote teachings. Surely scholarship has a role to play, but once we have left the dock and sailed off on the boat of practices, it is a different game involving ongoing management of an integration of practices, self-pacing, etc.

So, I think it would be unlikely that one person, no matter how advanced, could intuit every aspect of meditation practice for everyone. Many have said they could, and the roads of history are paved with the limitations of such individuals. No, having a reasonable baseline is the best we can hope for, and it must be adapted for best results by the community it is serving in the present, and also by the community it will serve in the future. That is the logical approach. If we wait for a great savior to give us the magic answer, we will always be waiting. Much better to be doing. :-)

Regarding ALLAH, I do not have a Muslim background, so cannot say much about the long term effects of using ALLAH in meditation. However, it would not surprise me if the Sufis use ALLAH (and other sacred syllables) in a way similar to how we use mantra in deep meditation. Their ecstatic bliss is a clear indication of inner purification, opening, and the outpouring divine.

Btw, the Sufis played a significant role in the development of spiritual wisdom in ancient India, so some conspicuous overlaps should not be surprising.

In any case, from the AYP point of view, meanings are not assigned to mantra and have nothing to do with the process of meditation. If ALLAH is looked at purely from a vibrational standpoint, it has elements not so different from some of the syllables we use. But, again, I have not done the long term research on that. Probably better to consult a Sufi. :-)

All the best!

The guru is in you.

2009/02/11 12:09:34
Support for AYP Deep Meditation and Samyama
http://www.aypsite.org/forum/topic.asp?TOPIC_ID=5151&REPLY_ID=45073&whichpage=-1
namah....namaha

Hi All:

There is a tendency to regard Sanskrit as the last word on mantra definitions and pronunciations. But Sanskrit is a less certain language than many might wish. The very ancient oral traditions of India pre-date Sanskrit, and may or may not be accurately reflected in the Sanskrit writings that later recorded them. There were several versions of Sanskrit that evolved in ancient India, including a version that read from left to right, and another one that read from right to left. Some historians even place the origins of Sanskrit outside India, in central Asia, which is a real heresy. :-)

The truth is that history is always going to be a combination of fact and wishful thinking, with the loudest voice (or military conqueror) usually having had its way. And that is what we will see as we look at history today, not an idealized perfection being magically transmitted to us from the distant past. That only exists in our imagination.

Where does that leave us with mantras, and all other spiritual knowledge? For sure, still with a wealth of resources coming to us from many spiritually advanced people who recorded their experiences in the past. But we must live in the present with the causes and effects that are operating in us now. Each time has its own spiritual dynamic. Therefore, the past is not more significant than the present. It is "now" that matters most. Indeed, "now" is all there is.

So, the suggestion is to use whatever works from wherever we may find it, with reasonable consistency over time. At the same time, if there are useful customizations or improvements that can be made, then make them. Do it as systematically as possible, and share what is learned so everyone can benefit.

All the best! :-)

The guru is in you.

2009/02/21 14:43:14
Support for AYP Deep Meditation and Samyama
http://www.aypsite.org/forum/topic.asp?TOPIC_ID=5215&REPLY_ID=45689&whichpage=-1
Deep Meditation works! - and passing it on

Hi YogaIsLife:

Stories like this make it all worth while. Thank you for sharing, with your mother and with us.

As John Wilder would say, "Pass it on." :-)

The guru is in you.

2009/05/31 16:39:03
Support for AYP Deep Meditation and Samyama
http://www.aypsite.org/forum/topic.asp?TOPIC_ID=5711&REPLY_ID=51697&whichpage=-1
Meditation Problem

quote:
_____
Originally posted by Konchok Ösel Dorje

Vayu is the Hindu god of wind. You a have past-life karmic connection to Vayu and Hindu practice. These memories are stored in your channels and chakras. Thoughts are essentially wind. So Vayu is a fitting ishtadevata. It's nothing to be afraid of. It's just like meditating and hearing a song from a few months ago. Try to sit up in siddha asana or padma asana so that you don't fall asleep. Continue with your mantra.
_____

Hi Osel:

To clarify a key point, siddhasana or padmasana (full lotus) seat are not recommended for those just starting out in AYP deep meditation. A comfortable seat with back support is recommended. If desired, more advanced ways of sitting can can be explored once the basic meditation practice routine has been stabilized. Support for that is provided later in the AYP lessons.

Just a reminder that the AYP Deep Meditation and Samyama support forum category is for AYP deep meditation support only. The same requirement goes for the Pranayama, Mudras and Bandhas support forum category -- AYP technique support only.

It has become necessary for us to insist these two forum categories be reserved for support on the core AYP practices. Many have been coming in from other systems of practice and sending new practitioners off in multiple directions, into other systems/traditions, etc. That only leads to confusion and doesn't help people who are trying to get started. So kindly stick with the AYP lessons and direct experiences with the AYP practices in the two support forum categories mentioned.

There are plenty of other forum categories to discuss comparisons and alternatives to the AYP practices, entire other systems of practice, etc. So please have those discussions there. All input is encouraged, but not in these two forum categories where it can be confusing for those undertaking the AYP practices for the first time.

Many other styles of practice can be found in the "Other Systems" forum category.

Thanks!

The guru is in you.

2009/05/31 16:51:30
Support for AYP Deep Meditation and Samyama
http://www.aypsite.org/forum/topic.asp?TOPIC_ID=5711&REPLY_ID=51698&whichpage=-1
Meditation Problem

Hi kmf333, and welcome!

The key points were well covered in previous posts. When in doubt, check the lessons. It is suggested to follow them in order, where everything related to the AYP system of practices is laid out step by step.

The fuzziness and sleepiness you experienced in your first session will pass (maybe it already has). As mentioned, it is inner purification occurring. You are off to a good start. :-)

If you feel a bit overwhelmed for several deep meditation sessions in a row, or if there is discomfort or irritability during daily activity, feel free to shorten your meditation time temporarily until things smooth out. This is called "self-pacing," and you will see a lot more about this important method for managing practices as you move though the lessons.

By the way, while yoga is used in Hinduism, it is not Hinduism. Yoga is non-sectarian and its elements (sometimes with different names) can be found in all of the world's religions and mystical traditions.

A good way to think of yoga is as a "tool box" of methods that can be used to help awaken our innate spiritual potential, regardless of our religious orientation, or lack of one. It is all within us ... yoga is the technology of inner awakening.

Wishing you all the best on your path. Enjoy!

The guru is in you.

2009/05/31 22:26:01
Support for AYP Deep Meditation and Samyama
http://www.aypsite.org/forum/topic.asp?TOPIC_ID=5711&REPLY_ID=51704&whichpage=-1
Meditation Problem

quote:
_____
Originally posted by Konchok Ösel Dorje

Sorry Yogani, I sometimes forget about your system.
_____

No problem Osel.

It goes with the territory with so much growth in traffic. Not complaining at all. It's great to have so much expertise coming in from so many sources.

At the same time, we'd like to reserve these 2 out of the 22 forum categories for focused support on these core AYP practices covered in the online lessons and books. It seems reasonable. :-)

The guru is in you.

2009/06/04 14:10:05
Support for AYP Deep Meditation and Samyama
http://www.aypsite.org/forum/topic.asp?TOPIC_ID=5740&REPLY_ID=51931&whichpage=-1
Little bit confused with Samyama Sutra's

Hi SeekingShiva:

The idea is to use the sutras in a language that is most comfortable. If that is English in your case, then carry on in English. :-)

All the best!

The guru is in you.

2009/07/16 14:00:01
Support for AYP Deep Meditation and Samyama
http://www.aypsite.org/forum/topic.asp?TOPIC_ID=5954&REPLY_ID=53602&whichpage=-1
I AM Meditation

Hi ZionMe:

No, AYP deep meditation with the I AM mantra is not like So Ham meditation. It is internal (not oral), and is not with the breath. It is recommended to sit comfortably for minimum distraction. For most people that is with back support, and legs either not crossed or crossed, whichever is comfortable.

It is suggested to review the lessons on deep meditation from the beginning in the main lessons linked in the top menu.

The guru is in you.

Note: This discussion is being moved to the Deep Meditation support forum.
2009/07/30 22:28:35
Support for AYP Deep Meditation and Samyama
http://www.aypsite.org/forum/topic.asp?TOPIC_ID=6051&REPLY_ID=54391&whichpage=-1
Mantra Substitution in DM
Welcome Newtoayp!

Thank you for writing and sharing. Happy to hear you are finding the AYP writings informative.

1. AYP deep meditation involves flexible repetition of mantra that will change in both rhythm and clarity. This permits the mantra to serve as a vehicle for attention to move repeatedly beyond thinking to stillness. Therefore, counting mantra repetitions with rosary/mala or any other means is not part of this style of meditation. It can restrict the natural flow of the mantra. And, at times, there will be nothing to count during periods of absorption in silence, and that is good practice. This is why we go by the clock rather than the count for a consistent period of purification and opening. Here is a lesson that discusses mala further: http://www.aypsite.org/86.html

2. Mantra is your choice, and it is not for me to say whether you should stick with a mantra from another system or switch to I AM (AYAM). Whichever works best for you. As you might imagine, it is difficult to predict the results of using a mantra from one system in another system's meditation procedure. It would be your research.
Also, looking downstream, there are some enhancements to mantra in AYP that can have a bearing on what you are starting out with. So maybe take a look at "enhancements" under "mantra" in the topic index: http://www.aypsite.org/TopicIndex.html
There is also an additional small enhancement in the AYP Easy Lessons book.

Wishing you all the best on your path. Enjoy!

The guru is in you.

2009/08/06 19:02:22
Support for AYP Deep Meditation and Samyama
http://www.aypsite.org/forum/topic.asp?TOPIC_ID=6084&REPLY_ID=54774&whichpage=-1
First Mantra Enhancement- When.....how long?

Hi Akasha and Cosmic:

It is good to be stable in our current practice routine before taking on a mantra enhancement. If we feel borderline, and are strongly motivated, it is fine to try and see what happens. In some cases a mantra enhancement can be stabilizing (allowing for an initial "clunky period"), but not always. If it brings overload symptoms, we can back off. No harm done. But we ought not be doing that every other week. A stable routine is much more important than pressing the envelope with new techniques too often.

One thing I would not recommend if a mantra enhancement brings instability in the short term, and that is trying to handle it by reducing meditation time and other forms of self-pacing. Better to back off on the enhancement, re-establish stability with the previous routine, and take it from there.

Onward, and all the best! :-)

The guru is in you.

2009/08/13 12:28:28
Support for AYP Deep Meditation and Samyama
http://www.aypsite.org/forum/topic.asp?TOPIC_ID=6129&REPLY_ID=55048&whichpage=-1
Question on Adding Self-Inquiry to Core Samyama

quote:
_____
Originally posted by Anthem11

Also just wanted to clarify that in the "Adding Self-Inquiry to Core Samyama" lesson you mentioned using "I-thought, who am I". Would "I-thought, what am I" work just the same? I don't resonate with "who" as much as I do with "what".

One other question about Samyama in general. At the end of samyama a daily practice of mine is to contemplate or sit with in silence and go deep into source of "I" or beingness for a couple of minutes. Why does AYP choose touch and release (samyama) over going deep into something particularly in relation to inquiry? Is it a question of style or long term effectiveness?
_____

Hi Anthem:

"I-thought - Who am I?" and "I-thought - What am I" are equivalent. The one to use in relation to Lesson 351 is the one that most resonates with you.

"Who am I?" has been specified because it is the more common way of expressing the inquiry. Indeed, we have been using this phrase since early in the AYP lessons in relation to bhakti, which is a key part of self-inquiry also (Lesson 349). An equivalent phrase for the practitioner is also acceptable. We want to accomplish two things with this sutra in structured core samyama -- tag the I-thought, and inquire its source.

Who can say whether the Self is a who or a what? It is unknowable in the mind. We can only know by Self-realization, which is beyond the mind. And then it cannot be clearly described. All self-inquiry methods are for bootstrapping from the witness stage to Self-realization through intentions released in stillness.

Whichever sutra you choose in relation to the instructions on core samyama in Lesson 351 and Lesson 150, it is suggested to stay with it, as it takes time for any sutra to "bake in" with daily samyama practice. This is how our habit of samyama goes deeper, and then naturally expresses as we release our intentions and inquiries increasingly in stillness in daily life. This is why we do structured samyama.

On your second question about contemplation of the source of "I," this is a different practice. It is a good one ("jnana-transcending" per Lesson 350), and is best pursued outside structured samyama. Soon after is fine if this is your habit. The objective of adding the new sutra to core samyama is to provide an easily incorporated additional tool for strengthening any self-inquiry we may be doing in daily life. It requires a minimal modification in procedure to current core samyama practice, and can bring a large additional benefit in results.

We are aiming to strengthen the connection between structured yoga practice and our normal daily activity. The field of yoga has been somewhat remiss in doing this with self-inquiry, leaving jnana yoga off as a sort of step-child, even though the path of yoga cannot be be complete until it leads us through jnana to direct knowledge/experience of who/what we are. This is the stage of the journey that goes beyond the witness to unity/liberation and beyond, as was discussed in Lesson 350.

There is a lot to be said for having a structured portion of our practice that brings this kind of benefit into daily life, where things tend to be less structured. We already know that core samyama cultivates stillness in action. Now we are strengthening it for jnana.

By building an advanced element of self-inquiry into core samyama, we will be cultivating the capability in daily living, and be less inclined to be walking around all day tending to distract ourselves. We won't have to worry about it, because self-inquiry in stillness will become more a natural part of our life by virtue of sitting practices alone. This is not to replace self-inquiry as we may be approaching it in daily activity. It is only that we are bringing in reinforcements. Kind of like the cavalry, you know. Stillness galloping over the hill to the rescue! :-)

The guru is in you.

PS: It should be added that "touch and release" is "deep" in well-established structured samyama practice, where the sutras are well baked in. It is through daily structured samyama practice that we increase our ability to be "deep" with all our intentions and inquiries during the day. It is the same principle in structured daily deep meditation, which increases the presence of abiding inner silence (the witness) in daily activity. We don't engage in structured practice for its own sake. We do it for the condition it cultivates outside practice.

2009/08/14 11:04:48
Support for AYP Deep Meditation and Samyama
http://www.aypsite.org/forum/topic.asp?TOPIC_ID=6136&REPLY_ID=55102&whichpage=-1
My experience with the I AM mantra

Hi Brian, and welcome! :-)

Thanks for sharing your experience. Just a reminder that picking up the mantra is an easy favoring, and not an "at all costs" kind of thing. When we realize we are off into thoughts, including thoughts about what is happening or supposed to be happening in meditation, we just ease back to the inner mental sound of the mantra at whatever level of clarity or fuzziness we happen to be at in the mind. From there, we will lose the mantra again, and once we notice, we can ease back to it again at that level of vibration, and so on. By this procedure we go steadily deeper during our session. So the mantra is a very flexible vehicle for our attention to go from clear mental pronunciation to very faint and fuzzy barely noticed vibration. In this way, the mantra and the specific procedure for using it take us deep into our inner silence, which is pure bliss consciousness beyond all thinking.

Also, we do not meditate on the meaning of the English words, I AM. We use the sound only. It can be as though we are using a different spelling, AYAM, where there is no meaning.

It is fine to analyze after meditation, but analysis during meditation is to be regarded as just another stream of thoughts, and then ease back to the mantra again. It is a very simple procedure. If we stick with it twice daily, within a few weeks or months, we may notice some changes in our daily life -- more inner stillness, peace, creativity, and energy. This "abiding inner silence" we are cultivating is the foundation of enlightenment, and everything else we discuss in the AYP lessons flows from that.

In the beginning, it is common to think of the mantra as being a kind of battering ram for knocking down the wall between us and our enlightenment. This is what we sometimes call "the clunky stage." Like many things in life we are doing for the first time, meditation can take some getting used to, and then the practice will refine naturally as we settle in. The truth is, we do not knock down the wall. With deep meditation, we become like a very fine vapor and go right through it. In time, the wall (our inner obstructions) is dissolved from the inside, and pure bliss consciousness blooms forth naturally, 24 hours per day, 7 days per week. We are *That*.

Wishing you all the best on your path. Enjoy!

The guru is in you.

2009/08/14 13:24:28
Support for AYP Deep Meditation and Samyama
http://www.aypsite.org/forum/topic.asp?TOPIC_ID=6136&REPLY_ID=55110&whichpage=-1
My experience with the I AM mantra

Hi Grihastha:

Sounds like you are getting some delayed reaction from using a "full boat" of practices earlier. It can seem fine, but underneath a lot is being loosened -- and then one day the dam breaks. This is why we add practices carefully one at a time, and give them plenty of time to stabilize before adding more (months at least, not days or weeks), so we will know what the effects of each practice will be over a longer period of time, and can navigate accordingly.

It will take a little while to settle down, but it will. Be sure to continue self-pacing and grounding as needed. Also keep in mind that bhakti and any other spiritual activities we are engaged in can aggravate an overload. So self-pacing reaches beyond the AYP practices alone.

As for the mantra being a "psychic magnet," I don't think that analogy holds, since we are repeatedly going beyond the mantra and all thinking during deep meditation. So there is no mantra or external (psychic) function we are cultivating. The mantra is only a vehicle into stillness -- a very effective one. Rather, it is the resulting rise of inner silence that loosens everything up.

Obviously, we'd like to be releasing our inner obstructions, but the pace we do it at is important, as too much at once can cause delays while we stabilize excessive energy flows. Keeping a balance between our practices and normal daily life is the key. When the two are kept in balance, spiritual progress can be very fast. That is the advantage of "grihastha" (householder stage of life). :-)

If it is still too much release at the present duration of deep meditation, it is okay to back off more on practice time until things settle down.

Spinal Breathing can provide stabilization in some cases. You will not know for sure until you try a bit of it before deep meditation. See Main Lesson 69 for more discussion on this.

Again, it looks like a delayed reaction from piling on too much before. Live and learn. Have faith ... this too shall pass. :-)

The guru is in you.

2009/11/12 15:00:41
Support for AYP Deep Meditation and Samyama
http://www.aypsite.org/forum/topic.asp?TOPIC_ID=6677&REPLY_ID=59659&whichpage=-1
Ready 4 Samyama?/Adding sutras?/Patanjali's list

Hi Rael, and welcome!

If you are interested in doing research on Patanjali's samyama sutras, the Appendix of the AYP Samyama book is recommended. The Appendix is specifically for doing research with Patanjali's sutras, within the context of a stable overall practice routine. There are 30 sutras there altogether. This is a research list and not the same as the AYP core samyama practice, or cosmic samyama, both which are covered in the book also, as well as in the main online lessons (#150 and #299).

A stable sitting practice with deep meditation is recommended before beginning any samyama practice. This may or may not include spinal breathing pranayama. It is possible to "leap frog" to core samyama practice with a stable routine of deep meditation in place, and abiding inner silence coming up. Stable core samyama practice (Lesson 150) is recommended before attempting research on alternate sutras.

A consistent twice-daily practice over the long term (using essentially the same sutra line-up) is the key to success in samyama. This is true of all practices -- consistency over time.

All the best!

The guru is in you.

2009/11/27 10:15:07
Support for AYP Deep Meditation and Samyama
http://www.aypsite.org/forum/topic.asp?TOPIC_ID=6677&REPLY_ID=60274&whichpage=-1
Ready 4 Samyama?/Adding sutras?/Patanjali's list

quote:
_____
Originally posted by Rael

Thank you both for the guidance on approaching the sutras. i had originally had the book on Samyama, but sent it back in favor of getting the large yellow book, which i thought encompassed the material of all the smaller books. Is there nowhere else to find the listing of thirty sutras by Patanjali?
_____

Hi Rael:

Currently, the only place the samyama research discussion with the 30 AYP-condensed Patanjali sutras can be found is in the appendix of the Samyama book. It will also be included in AYP Easy Lessons Volume 2, due out in about a year.

The guru is in you.

PS: For a recent summary of AYP Vol 2, in development, see here: http://www.aypsite.org/forum/topic.asp?TOPIC_ID=6655#59519

And here is a Dec 2006 discussion on the relationship of the small Enlightenment Series books to the online lessons, AYP Vol 1, and the upcoming AYP Vol 2: http://www.aypsite.org/forum/topic.asp?TOPIC_ID=1830#14599
Note the points of view on the AYP books from others in that topic also.

2009/12/08 23:38:29
Support for AYP Deep Meditation and Samyama
http://www.aypsite.org/forum/topic.asp?TOPIC_ID=6677&REPLY_ID=60969&whichpage=-1
Ready 4 Samyama?/Adding sutras?/Patanjali's list

Hi Tmer, and welcome!

On the 30 Patanjali samyama sutras in the appendix of the AYP Samyama book, these are for optional research for well-established practitioners. It is suggested to read the instructions in the appendix to see how they are recommended to be used. This is not where AYP samyama practice begins. If it were, it would not be the appendix.

As for the order of the core samyama sutras, the order is not as significant as the range of spiritual neurobiology they cover all together.

Real samyama is not about developing individual siddhis (powers) to satisfy our personal will. It is about purification and opening of the entire nervous system to experience all of our life as abiding inner silence, ecstatic bliss and outpouring divine love. This is also called the cultivation of "stillness in action," and unity.

It is suggested to read the book, and you can develop a good foundation for samyama practice and a clear understanding of "stillness in action," "siddhis," and "miracles."

Remember, one step at a time. You should not be considering samyama until you have a stable twice-daily routine of deep meditation in place for at least a few months. As you advance in practices over time, you will be in a much better position to be testing and rearranging things, and by then you may conclude that it is not necessary to do that. :-)

All the best!

The guru is in you.

PS: It is suggested to review the <u>Online Lessons</u> in the order given to get a general idea of the sequence of learning practices in AYP.

2009/12/09 09:04:20
Support for AYP Deep Meditation and Samyama
http://www.aypsite.org/forum/topic.asp?TOPIC_ID=6677&REPLY_ID=60992&whichpage=-1
Ready 4 Samyama?/Adding sutras?/Patanjali's list

quote:
_____
Originally posted by tmer

"As for the order of the core samyama sutras, the order is not as significant as the range of spiritual neurobiology they cover all together."

ok then the order is not the most important?
_____

Hi Tmer:

That's right, but the <u>consistency</u> of our daily practice over time is very important. This is how the list of sutras we are using is "baked in" to our nervous system, yielding the greatest long term results. That's why switching things around often is not recommended. Small steps and steady daily practice is the way to go. That is the AYP approach for all practices, and it is reflected throughout the online lessons and books.

If you have questions on your TM practice, it is suggested to go to your TM teacher for those. Better to go to the source than to rely on speculation from others.

The guru is in you.

2009/11/12 18:54:32
Support for AYP Deep Meditation and Samyama
http://www.aypsite.org/forum/topic.asp?TOPIC_ID=6681&REPLY_ID=59667&whichpage=-1
thank you yogani for solar enhancement

Hi Victor and All:

Glad to hear it. More feedback is welcome as we move along.

"Progress with <u>stability</u>" is our motto for the month, or perhaps for the century. :-)

<u>The lesson (#369)</u> that went up today is for that also.

All the best!

The guru is in you.

2009/11/13 10:14:30
Support for AYP Deep Meditation and Samyama
http://www.aypsite.org/forum/topic.asp?TOPIC_ID=6681&REPLY_ID=59691&whichpage=-1
thank you yogani for solar enhancement

Hi All:

Thanks for the continuing feedback. Sounds like we are off to a good start with the solar centering enhancement. Make sure that you have your mantra well "baked in" (automatic) before attempting this enhancement.

Parallax: Yes, one enhancement at a time. It seems you have three choices at this juncture, since you have barely begun the original first mantra enhancement. You can continue what you have just started, and down the road decide on a next enhancement -- solar centering or mantra.

If there have been stability issues, you can let go of the enhancement you just started and go to the alternate first mantra enhancement for a smoother ride (<u>Lesson 369</u>), or begin the solar centering enhancement instead (<u>Lesson 368</u>). Your choice, according to your experience and preference.

But one thing at a time, and let it bake in for a good long while between enhancements -- months or years, not days or weeks. Very important.

All the best!

The guru is in you.

2009/11/13 14:44:21

Hi SeekingShiva:

The location does not have to be that precise, and neither does the mantra. We don't want to be solidifying them in the mind so much. Both will float and fade, and that is normal. We just easily favor both at whatever level of clarity or fuzziness we happen to be in the moment. That is good practice.

When ecstatic conductivity comes up, we will know the location by feel, and that is not a pinpoint location either. The suggestion is to just be easy with it. If you are favoring the general area mentioned, you will be doing fine.

All the best!

The guru is in you.

quote:
_____
Originally posted by cosmic

Yogani, can the solar enhancement be carried over into our samyama practice? The thought occurred to me, but I decided against trying it until hearing from you about it.
_____

Hi Cosmic:

Yes, as we develop the habit of our meditation procedure, solar centering may naturally find its way into core samyama practice, and it can have stabilizing effects there too. At this time, this is not a formal AYP instruction, but not discouraged either, if it comes naturally.

Obviously, this does not apply to cosmic samyama, which has its own set of locations.

The guru is in you.

quote:
_____
Originally posted by Ananda

Hi Yogani, the mantra is automatic and the concentration on the solar plexus is getting better as it seems for now and as is with every new practice i know that there is going to be a clunky stage but i don't know if this okay but i am tending to visualize a ball of white light at that place and this seems to bring more ecstasy and purification; so is it smthg okay to do or not?
_____

Hi Ananda:

It will be good to let go of the idea of "concentration" on the solar center. It is just an easy favoring, like we do with the mantra. In time, the location will become part of the mantra, and it will be one thing we are favoring.

If visions come, like a "ball of white light," etc., we regard that like any other thought, and ease back to the mantra at the solar location. The experience will be what it will be, changing from session to session. We do not recreate imagery for our own reasons. That is a distortion of the procedure, and will weigh it down. Visions are fine. Hanging on to them and deliberately incorporating them into our meditation procedure is not. Simplicity is the key.

We pick up the mantra so we will lose it again and again. Likewise, we pick up the mantra at a location so we will lose that again and again. Then we will be cultivating abiding inner silence most effectively. The less mental baggage we carry with us, the better it will work. :-)

The guru is in you.

Hi All:

Bravo!

Onward with self-directed practice. :-)

The guru is in you.

2010/03/15 14:58:48
Support for AYP Deep Meditation and Samyama
http://www.aypsite.org/forum/topic.asp?TOPIC_ID=6681&REPLY_ID=66114&whichpage=-1
thank you yogani for solar enhancement

quote:

_____
Originally posted by Ananda

...is the solar enhancement supposed to enhance the nectar cycle?
_____

Hi Ananda

Surely. You have the proof. :-)

The guru is in you.

2009/11/23 11:09:48
Support for AYP Deep Meditation and Samyama
http://www.aypsite.org/forum/topic.asp?TOPIC_ID=6739&REPLY_ID=60105&whichpage=-1
Long break from my practices still having problems

Hi Crazymandrew:

If you have not already, it is suggested to review Lesson 367 on over-sensitivity to deep meditation with mantra: http://www.aypsite.org/367.html

If the "standard methods" for dealing with sensitivity discussed in the lesson are not working, then you may find using breath as object in meditation instead of mantra to be more soothing and effective (covered in the lesson).

Also, if you have been inclined to do pranayama before meditation, and spinal breathing is not helping, it will be best to discontinue that until your meditation practice and its effects are stable.

When considering pranayama, a gentle alternative to spinal breathing can be a few minutes of alternate nostril breathing before meditation.

Most important, be sure to self-pace your practice if having symptoms of excess, as you are doing now.

Stopping and starting meditation every few weeks will make it difficult to find a stable practice routine. I realize you may not have a choice in this right now, if anything you try with meditation is destabilizing. You are right to discontinue that.

Hopefully, breath meditation will help ease the situation (it is suggested to skip the long mantra solution covered in Lesson 367 in this case). If short daily meditation sessions with breath can be maintained with stability, that will be better than doing longer sessions and having to stop completely for a few weeks at a time. Much better to have a daily practice that we can be stable with. With the more gentle methods being suggested, you will hopefully be able to find that. Make sure to take plenty of rest when coming out of your meditation sessions.

On the mental health side, it is suggested to keep in touch with your doctor as needed, and work toward a balance between medical assistance and yoga practices. In relation to any medical measures being considered, it will be good to let him/her know what you are doing in yoga.

All the best!

The guru is in you.

2009/12/03 10:41:29
Support for AYP Deep Meditation and Samyama
http://www.aypsite.org/forum/topic.asp?TOPIC_ID=6739&REPLY_ID=60601&whichpage=-1
Long break from my practices still having problems

quote:

_____
Originally posted by crazymandrew

One quick question, I had also been increasing my pranayama time back in September and in October. Do you think this could have contributed the crash of my practices? I've experienced symptoms of excess from pranayama in the past and it didn't feel like I was over-doing pranayama.
_____

Yes. And delayed reactions are common with pranayama, so it is good to increase in a small increment and wait at least a few weeks to see how it settles in. More than 5-10 minutes of spinal breathing before deep meditation will be too much for most practitioners. If other forms of pranayama are being used in the same sitting or day, the effects will be compounded -- we call that "doubling up" on similar practices.

It should be mentioned that those who are accustomed to doing a lot of pranayama without effects of overdoing will find a different dynamic occurring when spinal breathing pranayama is done before deep meditation. These two practices have a dramatic effect on each other, making them both much more powerful, so less practice will often be more. Without a keen awareness of self-pacing, proceeding with these together in sequence can be like driving a powerful race car for the first time with no brakes.

So you are wise to be self-pacing, using the brakes to slow down when necessary. :-)

The guru is in you.

2009/12/13 11:58:29
Support for AYP Deep Meditation and Samyama
http://www.aypsite.org/forum/topic.asp?TOPIC_ID=6847&REPLY_ID=61254&whichpage=-1
over-sensitivity question

Hi Rkishan:

Sounds like you got off to a bit of a rough start with too much pranayama and some delayed reactions, but now you are getting your arms around it. Good job of self-pacing and balancing your practices.

If you go to breath meditation (does not seem inevitable at this point), you can always come back to mantra meditation later, though it can be a bit of an adjustment favoring mantra over breath again. Whenever we change our practice, there will be an adjustment (clunky) period.

Let us know here how you are doing in weeks to come. It can be helpful to many.

All the best!

The guru is in you.

2010/06/11 10:51:42
Support for AYP Deep Meditation and Samyama
http://www.aypsite.org/forum/topic.asp?TOPIC_ID=6847&REPLY_ID=69757&whichpage=-1
over-sensitivity question

Hi Ram:

Thank you for your feedback. Happy to hear you found an approach that is working for you. Later on, when you consider meditation again, it is suggested to review this lesson for sensitive meditators: http://www.aypsite.org/367.html

Wishing you all the best on your continuing path!

The guru is in you.

2010/01/09 20:26:39
Support for AYP Deep Meditation and Samyama
http://www.aypsite.org/forum/topic.asp?TOPIC_ID=6993&REPLY_ID=62480&whichpage=-1
Meditation Sensitivity?

Hi WSH:

TI's suggestion to learn sambhavi during deep meditation is not an AYP instruction. It will lead to a reduction in the effectiveness of your deep meditation sessions, due to dividing of the mind. This is clearly covered in the lessons.

TI should not be posting these instructions in this AYP only support forum category, as they only serve to dilute the practice and confuse those seeking assistance with AYP deep meditation. So the instructions are being removed, and TI is requested to post practices from other systems in the "other systems" forum category.

For AYP instructions on sambhavi, see Lesson 56. You will see that we learn sambhavi during spinal breathing pranayama, not during deep meditation. This avoids dividing the mind during meditation. Later on, as sambhavi becomes an easy habit in spinal breathing, then it may occur naturally in deep meditation, without dividing the mind.

In the AYP system, sambhavi should not be undertaken until we are stable in both deep meditation and spinal breathing pranayama.

All the best!

The guru is in you.

2010/01/17 12:27:14
Support for AYP Deep Meditation and Samyama
http://www.aypsite.org/forum/topic.asp?TOPIC_ID=7028&REPLY_ID=63049&whichpage=-1
Going into Meditation/Sleep the moment I start SB

Hi SeekingShiva:

The procedure is to favor the practice we are doing when we realize we have gone off it. That can be done on a very subtle level, whether we are in spinal breathing or deep meditation practice.

It is common to "get lost" in spinal breathing or deep meditation practice, where we feel we have gone off somewhere into a deep sleep-like state. Sooner or later, we will realize we have gone off. Then we just ease back to the practice we are doing, without forcing or strain, for the time of our practice. If we force it, some of the difficulty you mentioned may happen in the aftermath. Just be very easy and gentle about it. Good things are happening.

All the best!

166 –   Advanced Yoga Practices

The guru is in you.

2010/01/15 08:00:36
Support for AYP Deep Meditation and Samyama
http://www.aypsite.org/forum/topic.asp?TOPIC_ID=7046&REPLY_ID=62879&whichpage=-1
Ramana's ongoing Self inquiry and Yogani's samyama

Hi Ananda:

On self-inquiry, it is natural that it becomes more powerful when strengthened with abiding inner silence and the habit of samyama. It might seem a bit presumptuous, but Ramana Mahars
Hi probably never counted on these elements coming into play so fast, so the recommendation for self-inquiry all day long in his day was not likely to be an overload. More likely to be non-relational (not in stillness). Not the case with AYP in the picture, where the inquiry becomes relational (in stillness) much sooner, and therefore more powerful.

So self-pace your practice time accordingly. Your choice on whether to do that in sitting practice or in daily activity. Probably some of both. With deep meditation and samyama components involved, you are dealing with a much more powerful self-inquiry practice than Ramana taught. It is a good thing, but don't wear yourself out with it. More time to relax and enjoy (be) the timelessness of non-duality. :-)

The guru is in you.

2010/01/21 10:26:39
Support for AYP Deep Meditation and Samyama
http://www.aypsite.org/forum/topic.asp?TOPIC_ID=7098&REPLY_ID=63394&whichpage=-1
Ayeeeeam

Hi SeySorciere:

When you have a chance, will you email me on an administrative matter?

Thanks!

The guru is in you.

2010/02/27 00:21:27
Support for AYP Deep Meditation and Samyama
http://www.aypsite.org/forum/topic.asp?TOPIC_ID=7246&REPLY_ID=65427&whichpage=-1
pressure in left temple.

Hi Christine:

With the rise of ecstatic conductivity, there is a natural connection between the neurobiology in the pelvic region and in the head, including the palate. Your symptoms are consistent with that. This is discussed in a number of places in the AYP lessons.

This ongoing energetic awakening can also be described as active kundalini, so, yes, you do have one. :-)

Since these developments are universal in all human beings, there is not anything untoward about them in relation to Christianity, or any other religion. My background is Christian also, and over the years I have found many more confirmations than contradictions between my religious upbringing and symptoms of purification and opening.

When it gets right down to it, our experiences as a result of practices (including bhakti and prayer) are the best compass of truth we will find anywhere. With the advancement of our inner unfoldment, to the extent religious teachings are true (or not), we will know by first hand experience, because the divine is awakening in us. This experience of human spiritual transformation is the source of all the scriptures throughout history.

So not to worry. Everything will work out fine. Carry on, and self-pace your practices and activities as necessary to keep on an even keel, as you are doing already.

The guru is in you.

2010/02/24 10:55:12
Support for AYP Deep Meditation and Samyama
http://www.aypsite.org/forum/topic.asp?TOPIC_ID=7330&REPLY_ID=65307&whichpage=-1
Mantra & Sutras

quote:

Originally posted by SeySorciere

Yes guys, but to "favor the mantra", you say /think the mantra inside, it refines itself, surrounded by the silence it has generated and practically disappearing into it.
To release sutras into the silence, it is also saying it/thinking it/ intending it... their effects are different, but the actual thinking it is the same to me.

Moving from DM to samyama, I simply replace the mantra from wherever it was last located with the first sutra (Love)- that's my question.

_____

Hi SeySorciere:

The difference is, in meditation we keep favoring the mantra, even as it is refining. When we realize we are no longer favoring the mantra, we come back to it at whatever level of clarity or fuzziness we left off. In samyama we pick up the sutra and let it go in stillness for about 15 seconds, and then pick it up again. The sutra is picked up at whatever level of clarity or fuzziness we are at, and released. The main difference between mantra and sutra utilization is that mantra is taken within as a vehicle, while sutra is released within like releasing a bird to fly.

These two practices have different functions. Deep meditation takes us inward to stillness using an object (mantra). Samyama brings us out from stillness using an object (sutra). Deep meditation cultivates abiding inner silence (stillness), and samyama cultivates stillness in action, the ongoing expression of our intentions in divine outpouring, which is the rise of the non-dual unity experience in daily life.

The guru is in you.

2010/03/03 01:14:05
Support for AYP Deep Meditation and Samyama
http://www.aypsite.org/forum/topic.asp?TOPIC_ID=7367&REPLY_ID=65572&whichpage=-1
apply samyama on somethin I would like to attract

Hi AYAMER:

Well, it seems you are speaking of two different things. One is for something you want specifically, and the other is for divine grace for whatever or whomever. The grace is easy because it is divine flow. It comes naturally with development of the habit of samyama through structured practice. The specific thing is not so easy because it is a personal desire. Nothing wrong with personal desires, but in real samyama they will turn into divine flow, which may bring a different result than the personal desire. That is fine if we can surrender to whatever comes out of samyama. Surrender is the samyama itself. There is no getting around it.

So it is a mistake to be jockeying sutras around according to what we want this week or next week, thinking that there is a magic formula that will get us what we want. This constant finagling with the mind will dilute the long term effects of structured samyama practice, no matter how good our intentions. Effective healing samyama, prayer, and stillness in action in all aspects of life are in addition to regular structured practice, not replacements for it. These abilities are effects more than causes. It always gets back to daily structured practice over time to build greater divine flow in all aspects of living. Then it just happens. And whatever happens is what we want, not the other way around. :-)

The guru is in you.

2010/03/27 10:24:29
Support for AYP Deep Meditation and Samyama
http://www.aypsite.org/forum/topic.asp?TOPIC_ID=7502&REPLY_ID=66594&whichpage=-1
Samyama: I need help

Hi Sunrise:

Samyama is the art of releasing thoughts/intentions in stillness. The art of it is in cultivating the habit, which structured practice does. In time, with structured practice, our thinking and intentions are originating deep in silence, and outcomes just happen. Life becomes an endless stream of small miracles. And sometimes big ones.

It is in the habit of letting go. We do not control the fuzziness of sutras. They will be where they will be for us, and we can accept that. We just pick one up and then relax. If it isn't refined, that's okay. There is no way we can "make" a sutra be refined, except by leaving it wherever it is. In other words, samyama is not primarily a doing. It is primarily a non-doing. Can you relax with that principle? When you can, you will have it. "Having it" is relaxing and letting it go, wherever it is. :-)

If we have been meditating, and abiding inner silence is there, then samyama is only releasing the heart and mind in that natural condition.

The point of the whole thing is to cultivate spontaneous living from within stillness. This leads to an unending divine flow in all we do. It cannot be done with manipulation, or by fretting over the process. It is about surrender -- letting go. Structured samyama facilitates this through systematic incremental steps. And we don't have to worry about managing the process. It is a simple technique we do, and then we leave it and go out and live.

Samyama is a process of purification. As the nervous system purifies and opens, sutras naturally occur at more refined levels in awareness, as does all thinking and doing. It is a gradual process of transformation. It takes however long it takes. We are each unique in our process of purification and opening, though we share the inner principles of transformation and the basic methods to stimulate them.

If we keep meditating twice-daily, sooner or later all of life will come to be lived in stillness. Samyama aids us in the merging of desiring, thinking and doing in *That*.

It is the cultivation of stillness in action.

The guru is in you.

2010/04/02 14:59:21
Support for AYP Deep Meditation and Samyama
http://www.aypsite.org/forum/topic.asp?TOPIC_ID=7520&REPLY_ID=66808&whichpage=-1
Samyama -Blockages in Neurobiology

quote:
————

Originally posted by Krish and Christi

quote:
_____
Is it useful to do the 2nd mantra enhancement now?
_____

I would say yes. It adds a new dynamic to the mantra. The OM aspect resonates with the brain stem, and also with the root chakra. It is always up to you of course, as you are in the driving seat.
_____

Hi Krish:

You might wish to consider the alternate path for mantra enhancements, as discussed in this lesson: http://www.aypsite.org/369.html

The original sequence is more aggressive, which may be what you prefer, but it is good to be aware of the alternate mantra enhancement sequence also, which is more balanced. Both mantra enhancement sequences are shown in the lesson. Your choice.

Whether we are talking about deep meditation mantra enhancements, samyama, or energetic practices (pranayama, mudras, bandhas, etc.), it is always about stimulating the operative principles in our nervous system for purification and opening. We can try many angles to find our way through. But no matter what techniques we are using, the matrix of obstructions in our nervous system will have to unwind, and that will be the limiting factor in the speed of our unfoldment.

Which is not to say we cannot optimize our practices for maximum progress with stability. We certainly can. That is what self-directed practice with the AYP "toolbox" is all about. However, if we press too hard, we may find ourselves in an unstable opening, and the accompanying discomfort can lead to a loss of motivation to practice, and to our progress. This is why we say less can be more, especially when we find ourselves skirting along the "bleeding edge" of purification and opening. Indeed, we are all pioneers here, on the frontier of human spiritual transformation within us.

Getting back to your original question, it would be very nice if we had a samyama sutra that could "fast-forward" us to enlightenment, regardless of our unique purification and opening requirements. When you discover it, please report back and let us all know. :-)

There are sutra research options in the appendix of the Samyama book, but any additions we may experiment with short term are not likely to exceed the power of a balanced list of sutras used daily in core practice, year in and year out.

All the best!

The guru is in you.

2010/04/03 11:21:03
Support for AYP Deep Meditation and Samyama
http://www.aypsite.org/forum/topic.asp?TOPIC_ID=7520&REPLY_ID=66834&whichpage=-1
Samyama -Blockages in Neurobiology

quote:
_____
Originally posted by krcqimpro1

Hi Yogani, Christi,

I realised, after posting my query re: using Samyama to expedite awakening of ecstatic conductivity, that, all said and done, it is really only pranayama,supplemented with appropriate mudras and bandhas, that is the core practice for raising EC. Samyama is a longer term "technique", for achieving any "effect".
However, if we can identify any "granthi/s" that are causing the obstruction, even after a good degree of purification in the neuro-biology,and that need to be un-knotted,before K can flow freely,then that needs to be addressed,perhaps with some special techniques. Am I right in this assumption?

Krish
_____

Hi Krish:

Generally, it can be a diversion to go looking for specific energy blockages to deal with them individually. It can be like leaving the main controls of the car to individually supervise the engine, transmission and wheels, where we are no longer dealing with the overall operation of the vehicle. The nervous system is like that. Many things are going on, but there are only a few main controlling mechanisms that enable us to facilitate the process of human spiritual transformation in a holistic way.

If we are doing our core practices, the details will be attended to naturally in time. That said, there are a few more intense practices we can use to open the sushumna energetically, but we should be careful not to force things too much. Kumbhaka with mudras and bandhas can be used in this way, and/or with intense asanas like mahamudra. Bastrika and targeted bastrika can also be used for this purpose.

Actually, deep meditation and samyama are the best ways to approach the awakening of ecstatic conductivity, because these put a foundation of abiding inner silence underneath, which is coming into ecstatic energetic awakening from within. We can supplement this with the energy practices for an accelerated balanced opening. The trick is not to get too far ahead of the rise of abiding inner silence with energy practices. If we do, there will be a price to pay in discomfort and slower progress during extended periods of self-pacing.

If we are coming from the outside inward with a primary focus on energy practices, including focusing on what we believe are the knots in our neurobiology, it can end up in quite a mess, as we have seen from time to time with visitors coming here from those kinds of approaches.

So, from the inside out is suggested as the surest course. This does not mean intense energy practices should be avoided. Only brought in when we feel we have the inner silence to support and sustain a balanced opening. Inner silence calls us to these things when we are ready. We will know it when we see it.

The guru is in you.

2010/04/05 10:44:30
Support for AYP Deep Meditation and Samyama
http://www.aypsite.org/forum/topic.asp?TOPIC_ID=7520&REPLY_ID=66924&whichpage=-1
Samyama -Blockages in Neurobiology

quote:
_____
Originally posted by krcqimpro1

Hi Yogani,

I understand what you mean-that developing a solid base of inner silence through DM and Samyama and then, if necessary, aggressively pursuing energy raising practices, is the best way to ensure smooth progress. But again, you say in your lessons, that one should not "overdo" DM, and limit it to 20 mins. twice daily. Is there harm in aggressively doing DM, say, 45 min. twice daily, to accelerate building up of inner silence? I know you have said that "more is usually less", but other systems, like Buddhism, and even Kriya Yoga, seem to advocate more meditation. My purpose in this line of reasoning and querying, is, as must be obvious to you, to try and make up for "lost time".

Krish

_____

Hi Krish:

Deep meditation with mantra is more powerful than styles of meditation that allow sitting for hours. Longer sittings with mantra bring increased risk of overload and instability. If you are increasing meditation time, do it in 5 minute increments, with at least a few weeks in-between to make sure things are stable. Meditation time of more than 30 minutes is not advised, but you are in charge, and are armed with self-pacing. :-)

If substantially more deep meditation with mantra is desired, it is better to do it in "retreat mode," removed from daily responsibilities, with one or two extra cycles of our entire routine done each day in a structured schedule. Guidelines for this are in the Eight Limbs of Yoga book (and Lesson 387), with extra retreat practice routine details here:
http://www.aypsite.org/forum/topic.asp?TOPIC_ID=1416
http://www.aypsite.org/forum/topic.asp?TOPIC_ID=1428

Solo retreats are possible, but it is better to do it with a group. We are not there yet with regularly scheduled retreat events everywhere. In time, we will be...

The guru is in you.

2010/04/24 22:44:21
Support for AYP Deep Meditation and Samyama
http://www.aypsite.org/forum/topic.asp?TOPIC_ID=7672&REPLY_ID=67764&whichpage=-1
How often does one repeat the mantra?

Hi wakeupneo:

The goal during deep meditation is not to "abide in pure consciousness." It is to stay with the procedure of deep meditation, which means easing back to the mantra whenever we realize we are off it into something else, which includes the thought, "Oh, I am abiding in pure consciousness now, and don't need to return to the mantra."

Returning to the mantra is never about forcing. It is about favoring the mantra at whatever level we find ourselves in the mind -- clear or faint and fuzzy. In this way the mantra serves as a vehicle going inward, no matter where we come back into the thought process, and no matter what sort of concept or analysis is vying for our attention. As soon as we give in to the temptation to evaluate what is happening during deep meditation and altering the procedure to suit that, then the effectiveness of our meditation will be less. That is why it is always about the procedure, and never about evaluating experiences occurring during meditation.

We are not after a particular experience in meditation. We are after the results in daily activity. The only way we will have them is by staying with the procedure when we are sitting.

The frequency of mantra repetition will vary widely according to the process of purification occurring within. Some sessions we will pick up the mantra once and be gone for the whole 20 minutes. Other times, we may be coming back to the mantra many times during the session. It will be whatever it needs to be for the purification we are undergoing at the time. It is not something we can regulate. It is regulated by the natural process of purification and opening occurring within us, which the procedure of deep meditation facilitates.

The guru is in you.

2010/05/25 12:39:02
Support for AYP Deep Meditation and Samyama
http://www.aypsite.org/forum/topic.asp?TOPIC_ID=7833&REPLY_ID=69188&whichpage=-1
AYP breath meditation for oversensitive

quote:

Originally posted by innercall

Nonetheless, I have found helpful for the past couple of days to add an extra control over the process of meditation to stay out of the fuzzy state.

Hi Innercall:

Adding "extra control" over the procedure of meditation during sittings can reduce overload because it reduces the effectiveness of the meditation by increasing the role of mind rather than allowing transcendence of mind to stillness. It will be good to be clear about that.

Making distinctions between clear, faint or fuzzy object (breath or mantra) and aiming for one over the other during sittings of meditation is not AYP procedure.

I understand you are seeking to smooth the effects due to sensitivity, and you will do whatever is necessary for that, as you should. However, labeling fuzzy object of meditation as less correct meditation than other manifestations (clear, faint, etc.) of breath or mantra is not AYP procedure. Making these distinctions during practice is reducing the power/effectiveness of the meditation, and that is what you are noticing. It is obviously not what everyone should be doing, as it could lead many away from effective practice.

What others may be teaching about the regulation of states of the object of meditation during practice is for them to teach, and the results will be there accordingly.

By "fuzzy," I mean natural loss of clarity of breath awareness or pronunciation of mantra. Allowing this and coming back to the object of meditation wherever it may be is part of the procedure of meditation. Fuzziness is an indication of attention naturally going deeper and residing in inner silence. For sensitive meditators, this may equate to "fast transcending," with possible excessive purification and opening happening. We looked at several ways to mitigate sensitivity in Lesson 367. Regulating the experience of the object of meditation during sittings was not one of the ways discussed there. Which is not to say it has no merit. From the AYP perspective, exploration of this approach by sensitive meditators would be additional research, and reports on results are welcome.

However, such regulation of states of the object of meditation during sittings is not recommended for those practicing AYP deep meditation who do not have sensitivity issues.

Just wanted to clarify that AYP does not add "extra control" in deep meditation practice. The lack of extra control is a primary reason why AYP deep meditation is as powerful and effective as it is. Sensitive meditators can find less power and more stability in the way you describe, but it is not a habit of meditation procedure I would encourage for most.

All the best!

The guru is in you.

2010/05/25 17:11:38
Support for AYP Deep Meditation and Samyama
http://www.aypsite.org/forum/topic.asp?TOPIC_ID=7833&REPLY_ID=69196&whichpage=-1
AYP breath meditation for oversensitive

Hi emc:

Yes on all counts, with two caveats:

1. Breath meditation does not usually go as deep as mantra meditation, because once breath suspends there is no object. Mantra can go much deeper. This difference is why breath meditation is one of the options suggested in Lesson 367 for those who are very sensitive with mantra.

2. The AYP approach to breath and mantra meditation does not define how other systems of meditation ought to be done. Nor does it invalidate them. One style is not another style, and it is generally best not to mix styles together. That is why I chimed in here. Some procedures have been discussed here that are not AYP. That is okay as long as we are not overrunning one style of practice with another style. That is when effectiveness on both sides can be lost.

Of course, there is always research, and the opportunity for improvement in self-directed practice. In that, it is important to preserve a baseline system of practices, and explore alternatives without distorting the baseline. Otherwise, we could get lost in a sea of alternative approaches, with no "safe harbor" to return to.

The guru is in you.

2010/08/16 11:21:49
Support for AYP Deep Meditation and Samyama
http://www.aypsite.org/forum/topic.asp?TOPIC_ID=8262&REPLY_ID=71965&whichpage=-1
30 sutras

Hi Ayamer:

The most important thing in samyama practice is to have a balanced list of sutras that we can "bake in" over years of daily practice. This is how the effects of samyama are found emerging in all aspects of life, where all of our thoughts and feelings are naturally occurring in stillness. This is the transition of our life to spontaneous divine outpouring and stillness in action.

The number of potential sutras is endless, limited only by imagination. The 30 Patanjali sutras are a general representation of possibilities. They are included in simplified form in the appendix of the AYP Samyama book with some guidelines for those who are inclined to do research on them. Those guidelines honor the importance of maintaining a stable daily practice as the first priority. So if you are inclined to do some research on sutras, it is suggested to follow the procedure there, preferably after you are well-established with your daily core samyama practice.

As you know, AYP is an open resource on practices, so no one will tell you exactly how you should practice. That is for you to decide. For your own benefit, it will be wise to keep a solid baseline practice routine in place for good progress with comfort, and limit research to what can be absorbed in the daily routine without upsetting the apple cart. :-)

Practice wisely, and enjoy!

The guru is in you.

2010/10/25 10:43:34
Support for AYP Deep Meditation and Samyama
http://www.aypsite.org/forum/topic.asp?TOPIC_ID=8623&REPLY_ID=74193&whichpage=-1
Solar centering

Hi Roshan:

The solar centering enhancement is picking up the mantra at the solar center and continuing with it there, as described in Lesson 368. So it is not picking up and dropping the location as in cosmic samyama. It is the procedure of meditation we are doing, with the easy picking up of mantra at that location. Whenever we realize we are off the mantra, we easily come back to it at whatever level of clarity or fuzziness we are at in the mind. If we are doing the solar centering enhancement, that will be automatically included, once we have the habit in place.

If there is discomfort associated with solar centering, this is a sign of purification and opening occurring. If symptoms becomes excessive, to the point where you can't continue with meditation, you can try the procedure in Lesson 15. If excessive sensations continue, then better self-pace solar centering, which you have done already. You can always come back and try again later.

Keep in mind that the fruit of our practice is not in the practice itself, but in daily activity. So if you are having some symptoms during practice that are manageable, and daily activity is good, then it is okay to continue that way. In time, all symptoms settle down as purification and opening advance, and the energy is producing less friction in the neurobiology. That does not mean we should "tough it out" with excessive symptoms in practice. We always self-pace for progress with comfort. Otherwise, we may get discouraged and stop practices altogether, which obviously is not preferred.

As for the eyes, we do not put them in any particular direction (other than closed) in deep meditation, including with solar centering. As we develop sambhavi mudra during spinal breathing, the eyes may tend to naturally drift up during deep meditation, but we do not do that with intention. All of our intention during deep meditation is for the procedure of meditation. This is important, so as not to divide the mind during our meditation with other intentions or procedures. Simplicity yields the most effective results. The solar centering enhancement is the only intention we have added to the basic procedure of deep meditation, other than the optional mantra enhancements.

All the best!

The guru is in you.

2010/10/27 06:29:13
Support for AYP Deep Meditation and Samyama
http://www.aypsite.org/forum/topic.asp?TOPIC_ID=8637&REPLY_ID=74270&whichpage=-1
Can I decrease those 20 minutes in DM?

Hi Natan:

You can tailor your practice time to whatever is comfortable for you.
See Lesson 209 at http://www.aypsite.org/209.html
It can help with prioritizing your practices into whatever time frame you are using.

It is suggested to keep a stable routine as much as you are able, whether is it is 30 minutes, 40 minutes, or whatever.

Also, going to an AYP retreat can help break through any doldrums in a hurry. If there isn't one available near you, then consider setting one up in your area. If you can arrange for a facility, we can probably provide a leader and help find participants.

All the best!

The guru is in you.

2010/12/02 23:55:27
Support for AYP Deep Meditation and Samyama
http://www.aypsite.org/forum/topic.asp?TOPIC_ID=8831&REPLY_ID=76085&whichpage=-1
zoned out?

Hi Nirmal and All:

See this lesson: http://www.aypsite.org/17.html

Does that sound familiar? :-)

It can also go to something we could call "blackout" (seeming loss of consciousness), which is a version of what is described in the lesson. It is normal, a phase, and will pass as those deep obstructions are dissolved. The result will be more clarity and joy in daily living.

The guru is in you.

Forum 4 – Support for AYP Pranayama, Mudras and Bandhas

Spinal breathing pranayama, inward bodily maneuvers, and more.
http://www.aypsite.org/forum/forum.asp?FORUM_ID=15

2005/07/10 13:07:28
Support for AYP Pranayama, Mudras and Bandhas
http://www.aypsite.org/forum/topic.asp?TOPIC_ID=276
Pranayama, Mudras and Bandhas

There are two parts comprising the operative side of the enlightenment equation:

1. The cultivation of inner silence

2. The cultivation of neurological ecstatic conductivity

The first, we have been talking about in the "Deep Meditation and Samyama" forum.

The second is the province of this forum. The cultivation of ecstatic conductivity in the nervous system is accomplished primarily through breathing techniques, called "pranayama," in combination with certain bodily maneuvers, called "mudras and bandhas." Most of these practices have been shrouded in secrecy for centuries, and have been little understood. Furthermore, these practices work best if combined in a routine that also includes deep meditation.

In AYP, we start off with deep meditation. Next we add spinal breathing pranayama, which is the most important of all the breathing techniques covered in the lessons. It is first covered in Lessons #39-41, and developed further in many other lessons. See http://www.aypsite.org/41.html

Spinal breathing pranayama cultivates the entire nervous system so it becomes a much better medium for inner silence, which, in turn, makes samyama practice much more effective. Spinal breathing and meditation are done in separate sessions one after the other -- spinal breathing first and meditation second. In the lessons, you will find out about the timing of learning spinal breathing and adding it in front of your daily meditation session. The practices are learned step-by-step over time like that -- not all at once.

Once spinal breathing has been taken on and stabilized, a series of additional practices can be added over time, including:

Mulabandha (http://www.aypsite.org/55.html)
Sambhavi Mudra (http://www.aypsite.org/56.html)
Siddhasana (http://www.aypsite.org/75.html - technically an asana, but we can discuss it here also)
Yoni Mudra Kumbhaka (http://www.aypsite.org/91.html)
Uddiyana Bandha & Nauli (http://www.aypsite.org/129.html)
Kechari Mudra (multiple stages - http://www.aypsite.org/108.html)
Jalandhara Bandha (see yoni mudra kumbhaka)
Dynamic Jalandhara (Chin Pump - http://www.aypsite.org/139.html)
Spinal Bastrika Pranayama (http://www.aypsitc.org/171.html)
Targeted Bastrika Pranayama (http://www.aypsite.org/198.html)

Spinal breathing itself contains a few nuances: 1) Ujjayi pranayama, and 2) Brahmari Pranayama (not in the online lessons - it's in the AYP book)

So there is quite a lot, and all of it is fair game for discussion here in this forum. The overall effect of these practices can be best described as the rise of "ecstatic conductivity" in the nervous system. This phenomenon will no doubt be discussed in many places in these forums, as will the importance of cultivating inner silence.

As mentioned before, the addition of practices comes logically in a certain order, as discussed in the lessons. We would never try to tackle all of this at once!

Once we have inner silence and ecstatic conductivity coming up together in our nervous system, we find ourselves in a natural joining of these two aspects (or poles) within us. This joining is what produces enlightenment in the human being. These two aspects joining (balancing) within have been called by many names: shakti & shiva, yin & yang, holy spirit & father god, euphoria & emptiness, and so on. Many names -- same inner dynamic in the human nervous system.

And how do we characterize the end result of all this, the enlightenment? It is simple, really. When it is coming to fruition we have unshakable inner silence, ecstatic bliss and outpouring divine love. Then, we do for others as we would do for ourselves, because others become as dear to us as our own self. At the same time, it is complete freedom from the ups and downs of life in this world. We have all known or heard about people with these qualities. We each have that within us, and the methods of yoga are for uncovering it.

The guru is in you.

2005/07/20 14:24:34
Support for AYP Pranayama, Mudras and Bandhas
http://www.aypsite.org/forum/topic.asp?TOPIC_ID=335&REPLY_ID=104&whichpage=-1
Spinal Breathing Suggestion
Interesting suggestion on moving the perineum point forward in spinal breathing to bring sexual energy more into it. Feel free to experiment according to results. You will know it when you feel it. Until then, maybe better to stick to the basics. Once ecstatic conductivity begins to come up, then we are in a much better position to optimize our practice □ having real sensations to follow.

Keep in mind that we eventually are cultivating sexual energy in many ways during spinal breathing. This also creeps out as habit (not necessarily conscious practice) into the rest of our sitting practices, including in deep meditation and samyama.

Other means (habits to develop) we use during spinal breathing that are involved with cultivating sexual energy include mulabandha/asvini, sambhavi, siddhasana, uddiyana (very light) and kechari. After spinal breathing, we go for even more with yoni mudra kumbhaka, chin pump and spinal bastrika. Oddly enough, some of the most powerful practices for cultivating sexual energy in the nervous system are located in the head.

Links to AYP lessons on these practices can be found in the introduction to this forum at http://www.aypsite.org/forum/topic.asp?TOPIC_ID=276

All of these practices are acting to cultivate sexual energy throughout our nervous system, using the spinal nerve as the central transmission conduit ☐ not only up and down, as in spinal breathing-style practices, but also outward via naturally arising ecstatic conductivity. Then we have deep meditation and samyama working within all that inner arousal.

We did not mention tantric sexual practices, did we? That is yet another dimension in all of this. See the forum here devoted to that.

There is a lot we do to promote both the expansion of ecstatic conductivity (the sexual element) and inner silence (pure bliss consciousness). These two aspects of our inner nature join to become unshakable inner silence, ecstatic bliss and outpouring divine love. That is enlightenment. Well, that☐s the big picture on practices. Enjoy!

The guru is in you.

2005/08/03 20:06:30
Support for AYP Pranayama, Mudras and Bandhas
http://www.aypsite.org/forum/topic.asp?TOPIC_ID=335&REPLY_ID=268&whichpage=-1
Spinal Breathing Suggestion

Hello all:

As time goes on, the focal point of rising ecstatic conductivity in the area of the perineum shifts from sexual (the front) toward the anus and rectum (the back). In a very general (and unofficial) way, the perineum represents the distance between root (anus) and second chakra (sexual organs). The perineum is a logical end point in spinal breathing, covering the full scope from genitals to anus.

Kundalini means "coiled serpent," and the scriptural description is specific -- three-and-a-half coils around the root lingam. This corresponds with the neuro-biology in and around the rectum.

As ecstatic conductivity comes to bloom in the nervous system, this spiritual anatomy reveals itself by degrees. Until then, we are taking things a bit on faith when we do our spinal breathing to the perineum. We know something is going on there, but we don't know exactly what until the inner energies are awakened. In the meantime, we want to be careful not to wander too far off in our practice with this or that sensation, or we may end up missing the main event.

Of course, once we have ecstatic conductivity going (an awakened kundalini), we will not be leading her so much anymore. She will be leading us. We just don't want to be jumping the gun on her, running off into myriad sensations, emotions and thoughts with our practices. What I am saying here applies in all the AYP practices. So much can be coming up that can attract our attention. This is why the lessons say so often: When experiences happen in our practice, whatever they may be, we easily come back to the procedure of the practice we are doing.

So, Jim is wise to advise you not to be running too far up the perineum there in your spinal breathing. The real action will be happening in the other direction... But don☐t go charging off there in spinal breathing either. Just stick with the practice as given is my suggestion -- to the perineum. Don☐t forget you will have mulabandha/asvini and siddhasana in there too, along with all the other practices influencing the spinal nerve as well. So it will all work out in the end. Was that a pun?

Ah, adventures in yoga!

The guru is in you.

2006/08/07 11:03:59
Support for AYP Pranayama, Mudras and Bandhas
http://www.aypsite.org/forum/topic.asp?TOPIC_ID=345&REPLY_ID=10303&whichpage=-1
hand positions

quote:

Originally posted by Anthem11

Maybe this was Yogani's intention, not to micro-manage the things that the nervous system will naturally do at the right time to purify itself?

Yep. :-)

We take care of the essentials and the nervous system (inner guru) takes care of the rest.

Wonderful account of the process in action.

The guru is in you.

2005/08/10 14:52:01
Support for AYP Pranayama, Mudras and Bandhas
http://www.aypsite.org/forum/topic.asp?TOPIC_ID=359&REPLY_ID=328&whichpage=-1
Kechari Mudra

Hello Rabar:

Thank you for that.

However, it is not swallowing the tongue. It is going up to stage 2 (and possibly 3). You can tell because the soft palate on top is being pushed forward from behind. If the tongue were going down the gullet, the soft palate would not be pushed forward because there would be nothing behind it. Of course, one can call kechari stages 2-4 "swallowing the tongue" and most would not know the difference. "Swallowing," most people can understand. But up into the center of the head via the nasal pharynx? Few can imagine that, even though it is much easier to do than swallowing of the tongue.

Perhaps this young man has a future in yoga. He has a gift. The question is, will he have the bhakti to go with it?

It is an excellent video of entering stage 2. Thank you!

The guru is in you.

PS -- See these cross sectional sketches for perspective http://www.aypsite.org/kechari_image1.html

2006/01/16 09:32:42
Support for AYP Pranayama, Mudras and Bandhas
http://www.aypsite.org/forum/topic.asp?TOPIC_ID=359&REPLY_ID=2561&whichpage=-1
Kechari Mudra

quote:
_____
Originally posted by Lavazza

Some fellow practitioners are convinced that I must have been practicing in an earlier life, but then I must been quite sloppy concerning many of the other asanas, pranayamas and bandhas, which I do not get at all.

_____

Hi Lavazza, and welcome!

Yes, I would agree. Our tendencies in this life are coming from somewhere, and reincarnation is as good an explanation as any. But that is neither here nor there. The real question is, where do we go from here?

Success with mudras like kechari is a chicken and egg thing. They foster what we call in AYP, "ecstatic conductivity" in the nervous system. That is, a mudra like kechari is both cause and effect. When we are moving into effect mode (and further cause) we will know beyond any doubt that the "secret spot" in about half way up the edge of the back edge of the septum inside our nasal pharynx -- that is the divider between left and right nasal passages. We need go no further than that (stage 2 kechari) to achieve a good connection, and it is very easy to be there once we have gone above the soft palate. The rest after that (stages 3 & 4...) is icing on the cake. Check AYP Lesson #108 for details (diagrams included there).

But how to get that chicken and egg ecstatic conductivity going? It begins with deep meditation, and that is where I recommend you start, just as the AYP lessons suggest if you take them in order. Then there can be a logical buildup from there into spinal breathing pranayama, mudras, bandhas, samyama, tantra, etc. In this approach, it goes from inner silence to ecstatic conductivity and onward to the unity of outpouring divine love, which is working from the inside out instead of the other way around (beginning with physical techniques), which can be problematic.

As it says in the New Testament, "Seek first the kingdom of God and all will be added..." That is the underlying approach in AYP -- inner silence first by very easy means (deep meditation), and all the rest follows naturally.

As for doing kechari now, if you are a natural, it will not hurt. It will have more effect when you have some inner silence coming up and are cultivating ecstatic conductivity with spinal breathing and the additional means suggested in the lessons. It all works together like that.

The most important thing by far is to establish and stick with a stable daily practice. It does not take a lot of time -- just regularity of 20-30 minutes twice each day like clockwork, with a commitment to do it for as long as it takes. With that, we find steady progress over time, and will be in a position to take on more according to our inclinations. Along the way, we also find ourselves developing essential skills in "self-pacing" of practices as the energies begin to move within us, which is navigating the process of purification underway in our nervous system. And so it goes, ever-onward in expressing the infinite divine within us. You can read a lot about it in the AYP lessons, books and here in the forums.

Wishing you the best on your chosen path. Practice wisely, and enjoy!

The guru is in you.

2006/01/16 11:17:23
Support for AYP Pranayama, Mudras and Bandhas
http://www.aypsite.org/forum/topic.asp?TOPIC_ID=359&REPLY_ID=2566&whichpage=-1
Kechari Mudra

quote:
_____
Originally posted by Lavazza

I still do not understand what the secret spot is. I guess I have to get a good dictionary to check up the anatomy. Should it be touched with the top or the bottom of the tip of the tongue? Is it on the the floor, roof, entry or exit of the nasal cavity?

_____

Hi again Lavazza:

See kechari stage 2 in this diagram: http://www.aypsite.org/kechari_image1.html
The secret spot is right where the tip of tongue is there, on the edge of the nasal septum. Or maybe just a tad higher. There can be slight anatomical differences between people.

The secret spot can also be reached indirectly by placing the tip of the tongue up on the roof of the mouth where the hard and soft palates meet.

That's right under the edge of the nasal septum, and is kechari stage 1 (also shown on the diagram).

As for what the secret spot is, it is an ecstatic connection point that promotes the rise of ecstatic conductivity in the entire nervous system. At a certain point on our spiritual journey, the spot becomes as ecstatically sensitive as the genitals, but with a different purpose -- the cultivation of divine ecstasy throughout the nervous system. (Indeed, our sexual function can be directly coaxed in this direction also, but that is a different subject - tantra!) The same is true of all the mudras and bandhas. They become ecstatically sensitive. Sambhavi is a very famous one. We often see the saints depicted with eyes raised. Why? Because it feels extremely good all over!

It's the same with kechari and the secret spot, and all the mudras and bandhas. When they become ecstatic, they combine and work together as one in many subtle ways. In AYP, that automatic coordination of ecstasy body-wide is called the "whole body mudra."

But again, it all rides on deep meditation and the cultivation inner silence, so we are wise to be starting at the beginning.

The guru is in you.

2006/02/10 10:15:21
Support for AYP Pranayama, Mudras and Bandhas
http://www.aypsite.org/forum/topic.asp?TOPIC_ID=359&REPLY_ID=3217&whichpage=-1
Kechari Mudra

Hi SparkyfoxMD:

Thanks for posting that. Below is my reply that was sent when we discussed this in email some weeks ago.

There can be some short term benefit in the spoon technique you mention for stretching the soft palate to achieve initial entry into stage 2 kechari. But I don't see much value in it beyond that, as it is the degree of freedom of the tongue from the frenum tying it down underneath that determines both short term and long term progress in the practice. The soft palate has a certain "home position" that it always returns to (thankfully), so there is no progression of more release or stretching of the soft palate over time. Once the hymen-like band across the back edge of the soft palate has been stretched (by tongue entry which can be with finger help and/or the spoon method you mention), then the deed is done, and it will be the degree of tongue freedom that will determine progress from then on. This can be seen in the kechari diagrams here:
http://www.aypsite.org/kechari_image1.html

Posting the spoon technique would be of interest to kechari connoisseurs in the AYP forum, so please consider doing so. Aside from sharing, I expect you would get some useful feedback, as there are others who are in kechari stage 2 and beyond there. You can pull up numerous topics on kechari by doing a forum search. Some of the methods discussed are quite creative. Where there is a will, there is a way when the bhakti and inner energies are right for it.

The soft palate is much less of an obstacle than it appears. It is a trap door that folds down once the tongue gets behind (left or right side will be the shortest path). I suggest you follow your heart on kechari, taking your time, going step by step. I do not subscribe much to radical means like surgery (see lesson #108 for the "tiny snips" approach), though some are driven to that by their own bhakti. It is a personal choice. You may wish to interact with some in the forum to gain more perspectives.

Keep in mind that AYP is a comprehensive integrated open source on practices, of which kechari is only one aspect. In AYP there are suggested prerequisites to kechari including deep meditation, spinal breathing, other mudras and bandhas and more, all of which work together to cultivate unshakable inner silence, ecstatic bliss and outpouring divine love.

The guru is in you.

2006/02/28 10:14:17
Support for AYP Pranayama, Mudras and Bandhas
http://www.aypsite.org/forum/topic.asp?TOPIC_ID=359&REPLY_ID=3942&whichpage=-1
Kechari Mudra

Hi Alvin:

Those purple lines are blood vessels and you should never snip near those.

The side snipping you are doing is not recommended -- it is not the right place, and is very risky...

If you stay on the protruding edge of the center tendon, at the point of greatest tension, and follow a slow course as per Lesson 108, the blood vessels on either side will not be an issue. If there is no protruding frenum edge in the center, then wait for one -- it will come up eventually as the tongue goes back and upward. If your bhakti and the corresponding energy flow are not yet taking the tongue naturally in that direction, then you are most likely premature with the snipping. My advice is, slow down.

The guru is in you.

2006/03/28 21:19:09
Support for AYP Pranayama, Mudras and Bandhas
http://www.aypsite.org/forum/topic.asp?TOPIC_ID=359&REPLY_ID=5304&whichpage=-1
Kechari Mudra

Hi Alan:

Not to disappoint, but the nasal openings from inside are limited by bone all the way around, including the septum in the center. If you look at a skull you will see the thin bone in the center of the nasal opening. The opening will not change much. The way further in is by whatever can be done with the tongue -- twisting, pushing, stretching, etc.

But it is not that big a deal really. After 20 years of playing with kechari, I stay mostly around the septum -- the "secret spot," and use stage 4 (into the nostrils) sometimes for alternate nostril breathing from the inside when doing chin pump. It can be used that way with any form of pranayama, including spinal breathing. But be careful not to overdo it. Once ecstatic conductivity is coming up, less can be more.

You have the angles and everything right for stage 4. It will go as far as it can go. Up is where there is the most running room in my case. Some don't do stage 4 at all due to anatomy. I don't think it makes a big difference. Many reach higher levels of ecstatic conductivity with stage 1 alone. There are few absolutes in this world, and the level of kechari we achieve is not one of them. (Though getting above the soft palate is obviously a pretty big step.)

The guru is in you.

2006/06/14 10:00:48
Support for AYP Pranayama, Mudras and Bandhas
http://www.aypsite.org/forum/topic.asp?TOPIC_ID=359&REPLY_ID=8056&whichpage=-1
Kechari Mudra

Hi SparkyfoxMD:

A hint that can be helpful: The journey from stage 1 to stage 2 kechari (going behind the soft palate) is actually a thrust forward with the tongue as soon as it clears the back edge. Not up, but forward. The easiest place to do that from (shortest distance to get behind) is on the left or right side of the edge of the soft palate. The tongue can roll right in from either side, while going up the middle takes more length.

Also, keep in mind that the soft palate is not a rigid boundary. As soon as we are behind it, it folds down and forward like a natural trap door. It returns to normal position just as naturally when the tongue is removed from the pharynx. So the idea of the entrance being an opening "way back there" is somewhat of an illusion. As soon as the pharynx is penetrated, the opening expands all the way forward to the edge of the hard palate. See cross-sectional images of kechari here: http://www.aypsite.org/kechari_image1.html

Carry on!

The guru is in you.

2006/06/14 12:49:39
Support for AYP Pranayama, Mudras and Bandhas
http://www.aypsite.org/forum/topic.asp?TOPIC_ID=359&REPLY_ID=8060&whichpage=-1
Kechari Mudra
Just to clarify: The tongue doesn't actually "roll" into stage 2 from the side. It goes in on the side and slides to the center behind the soft palate. A push forward can help once the tip of the tongue has made it behind the edge of the soft palate -- that opens the soft palate trap door (it is usually automatic, but pushing forward with the tongue helps it along). No unusual contortions involved beyond just getting there, which you almost have! :-)

Don't forget, finger help is perfectly legal, especially in the beginning.

The guru is in you.

2006/06/29 11:00:50
Support for AYP Pranayama, Mudras and Bandhas
http://www.aypsite.org/forum/topic.asp?TOPIC_ID=359&REPLY_ID=8560&whichpage=-1
Kechari Mudra

Hi All:

Congratulations ycloutier, and to all who have entered kechari stage 2 lately!

The "tongue swallowing" video was actually first posted by Rabar in this very topic way back on August 10, 2005. Here are a few comments on it that I offered then:

Hello Rabar:

Thank you for that.

However, it is not swallowing the tongue. It is going up to kechari stage 2 (and possibly 3). You can tell because the soft palate on top is being pushed forward from behind. If the tongue were going down the gullet, the soft palate would not be pushed forward because there would be nothing behind it. Of course, one can call kechari stages 2-4 "swallowing the tongue" and most would not know the difference. "Swallowing," most people can understand. But up into the center of the head via the nasal pharynx? Few can imagine that, even though it is much easier to do than swallowing of the tongue.

Perhaps this young man has a future in yoga. He has a gift. The question is, will he have the bhakti to go with it? (and take on the additional practices that are necessary -- deep meditation, spinal breathing, etc.)

It is an excellent video of entering stage 2. Thank you!

The guru is in you.

PS -- See these cross-sectional sketches for perspective http://www.aypsite.org/kechari_image1.html

2006/06/29 16:09:59
Support for AYP Pranayama, Mudras and Bandhas
http://www.aypsite.org/forum/topic.asp?TOPIC_ID=359&REPLY_ID=8578&whichpage=-1

Kechari Mudra

quote:
_____
Originally posted by ycloutier2000

...but one single orifice? So presumably if I were to try to swing my tongue over to the other side, it should just slide over?
_____

Hi Y:

Yes, that's right. However, once behind the soft palate on the side, or anywhere, pushing <u>forward</u> with the tongue will open the soft palate and automatically bring the tongue to the center. So it is not mainly a sideways movement of the tongue, but a forward one that does the deed. Then keep going forward and you will reach the septum (secret spot) and nasal passages which sit right on top of the back edge of the hard palate.

The guru is in you.

2007/04/23 10:40:18
Support for AYP Pranayama, Mudras and Bandhas
http://www.aypsite.org/forum/topic.asp?TOPIC_ID=359&REPLY_ID=20879&whichpage=-1
Kechari Mudra

Hi Le Biotechnomoine, and welcome!

Stage 5 kechari is discussed in the AYP Easy Lessons book as an addition to <u>lesson 108</u>. That is "down the gullet," as per the Hatha Yoga Pradipika. It is one of the more challenging techniques. Its effects can also be achieved by other means -- earlier stages of kechari (with base of tongue pressing down), chin pump, sat karmani (swallowing and withdrawing a long thin cloth), and the use of other prosthetics. In the end, kechari stages 2 & 3 and chin pump will be likely enough to cover all sins in the deep throat. Of course, we will be inclined to go where our bhakti calls us, tempering with common sense for safety.

Thanks much for sharing, and all the best on your path. Enjoy!

The guru is in you.

2007/04/25 14:20:52
Support for AYP Pranayama, Mudras and Bandhas
http://www.aypsite.org/forum/topic.asp?TOPIC_ID=359&REPLY_ID=20970&whichpage=-1
Kechari Mudra

Hi Biotechnomonk:

Yes, stage 5 kechari is tongue folded back and down. Stages 2-4 are up behind the soft palate. Stage 1 is tongue on roof of mouth with tip at the point where hard and soft palates meet. To do stage 5, the frenum must be all but gone -- either born without it, or removed. It is discussed and illustrated in the AYP Easy Lessons book -- the ebook version is pretty inexpensive.

But not to worry about it too much. Kechari stage 5 is not a primary prerequisite for spiritual progress. In fact, neither are kechari stages 2-4. Far more important are daily deep meditation, spinal breathing pranayama and a balance of other practices that anyone can take on step-by-step, with prudent self-pacing.

The journey cannot be made with kechari alone, or, for that matter, with any one practice, except deep meditation. Cultivating inner silence daily over the long term is the key to all spiritual progress -- that is done primarily through deep meditation.

The guru is in you.

2007/10/26 12:24:51
Support for AYP Pranayama, Mudras and Bandhas
http://www.aypsite.org/forum/topic.asp?TOPIC_ID=359&REPLY_ID=26378&whichpage=-1
Kechari Mudra

Hi Le Bio:

Stage 5 kechari (tongue down the gullet) is achieved by eliminating nearly all of the frenum, and with a lot of finger help folding the tongue back and down. This is going far beyond what is necessary even for kechari stage 4 (up the inner nostrils to the brow area).

Stage 5 was included in the <u>AYP Easy Lessons book</u> to provide parity more or less with the Hatha Yoga Pradipika. But, as with some other extreme practices described in the HYP (such as mechanical vajroli), its practicality is questionable. This is why stage 5 is absent from the <u>Asanas, Mudras and Bandhas book</u>, which presents a more targeted and efficient approach to the practices.

We should ask ourselves what kechari stage 5 is doing, and see what easier alternatives may exist for producing the same effects. Perhaps we are doing them already. :-)

Kechari stage 5 is for stimulating the neurobiology in the throat, particularly the higher functioning of the gag reflex, which happily does not involve gagging all the time. This higher function opens the throat, heart and navel areas, and has a significant impact on higher "radiant" digestion occurring in the GI tract, but only if ecstatic conductivity has arisen.

So, there are a few clues. The essential one being that ecstatic conductivity is fundamental to the process, which is cultivated through deep meditation and spinal breathing pranayama. To charge ahead with physical practices (especially extreme ones) before there is a neurobiological basis could be called "premature."

Meanwhile, there are other ways to stimulate the same effects as kechari stage 5. One of the easiest is chin pump (dynamic jalandhara) done concurrently with whatever kechari stage we may be doing. This has a significant impact in the throat area and below, as anyone experienced with chin pump knows.

On the shatkarma side, the more severe forms of dhauti (GI tract cleansing) also have an impact in the throat area. These include ingesting water and deliberately vomiting it out, and swallowing a long narrow cloth and pulling it out. Both of these go after the gag reflex directly. And neither of these are recommended as AYP practices. The form of dhauti in the Diet, Shatkarmas and Amaroli book is less extreme, and more global in its effects.

There is also an interesting recent post by Avatar that has some bearing on this subject (thanks Avatar!):
http://www.aypsite.org/forum/topic.asp?TOPIC_ID=2960

So, there are several ways to skin the cat. The question is, what will be the easiest and yield the best results over time? ... in other words, optimizing cause and effect in our daily practices as much as possible, which is the primary aim around here.

There will be very few who will go for kechari stage 5, and that is okay. Those who do pursue kechari stage 5, or any other extreme practice, should make sure it is not at the expense of maintaining a balanced integrated approach to yoga practices over the long term, which is where the best results will be found.

It is always good to balance our bhakti (spiritual desire) with good common sense. :-)

All the best!

The guru is in you.

2007/11/24 16:29:50
Support for AYP Pranayama, Mudras and Bandhas
http://www.aypsite.org/forum/topic.asp?TOPIC_ID=359&REPLY_ID=27251&whichpage=-1
Kechari Mudra

Hi Joshua:

In the AYP lessons, the presumption is not that neural energy passes between the tongue and tissues of the palate and/or nasal pharynx and septum, though that is put forth by other teachings elsewhere, and some here may believe that, and are free to.

What the AYP writings do describe in both the main and tantra lessons is an ero-ecstatic sensitivity in the septum at a certain point on the vertical back edge especially, which we call the "secret spot," and throughout the tissues of the soft palate, pharynx and the inner nasal passages to varying degrees. The secret spot is accessible for stimulation by the tongue indirectly in kechari mudra stage 1 through the roof of the mouth where the hard and soft palates meet (right under the septum edge), and directly in stages 2, 3 or 4 inside the nasal pharynx. The secret spot in particular has a direct tie-in with sambhavi mudra (third eye stimulation) and the spinal nerve, connecting directly and immediately with the root in the area of the perineum via ecstatic sensations.

Yes, part of this originates near the base of the tongue also (an aspect of kechari), but not all of it. And, yes, a faint impulse of any mudra or bandha can stimulate energy also, particularly in later stages of development. In AYP, we call this the refinement of mudras and bandhas to the "micro-movement" stage. When they all work together in self-coordinated micro mode, we call it the "whole body mudra."

With the root-to-head connection, every nerve in the body becomes activated ecstatically. So while this phenomenon is centered in the spinal nerve and brain, it illuminates every cell in the body, and beyond. This process is progressive and becomes more expansive over time of daily practices. In time, the ecstatic illumination, which is the unfoldment of "inner space," blends with inner silence cultivated in deep meditation, and the whole process moves on to become an endless outpouring of divine love, which will be quite visible in one's daily relations and actions.

The degree to which one experiences these sensitivities, including the direct ecstatic connection and energetic expansion through the spinal nerve, is a function of the degree to which ecstatic conductivity (also called kundalini) has been awakened. It takes some time to reach the stage of directly perceiving it body-wide, and this is dependent on one's daily practices, especially deep meditation and spinal breathing pranayama, which form the foundation for effective practice of mudras, bandhas and additional methods. Once ecstatic conductivity has begun, there is no mistaking it, and it progresses according to the regularity of our practices and ongoing inner purification.

Our perception of sensations and energies at any point in time is going to be a limited snapshot compared to what it will be in the future as we continue with our practices. Therefore, we can't really form any binding conclusions based on our experiences today -- only tentative conclusions are possible, for tomorrow is another day bringing new openings. If we are doing higher stages of kechari and not experiencing an ecstatic connection, that doesn't mean kechari does not work in those higher stages. It just means we may be a bit premature in our level of practice. It is okay. Not a big deal. The nervous system will catch up in time. We just have to keep going with a balanced routine of effective practices and find out for ourselves.

Everyone is looking at something different on their journey, depending on where they are in their process of purification and opening. There are signature experiences that are repeatable and have been discussed in the lessons, and extensively here in the forums, but not everyone will be having these at the same time, or in exactly the same way. No one is asked to believe anything except through their own experience. By the same token, no one's view of what is happening or not happening necessarily decides what will happen or not happen for others.

The yoga scriptures provide some guidelines on what to expect, and this is helpful for motivation and possible confirmation. However, we are engaged real-time in powerful practices here, and experience is the final arbiter of the effectiveness of the practices and their predicted results. We make adjustments accordingly. In AYP this is called "self-pacing" in practices, which is how we build and sustain a stable and effective daily practice routine for the long term. So far in using this approach, we have made quite a few remarkable discoveries about ourselves, and have much more to learn as we continue forward.

The feeling is that daily practice and open sharing on the results over time is a good way to find out what human spiritual transformation is really all about. For that, the lessons and these open discussions can be pretty useful, particularly for independent practitioners. Many thanks for sharing your perspectives. Please continue to do so as you move along.

All the best on your path. Enjoy!

The guru is in you.

2008/02/19 09:36:19
Support for AYP Pranayama, Mudras and Bandhas
http://www.aypsite.org/forum/topic.asp?TOPIC_ID=359&REPLY_ID=30254&whichpage=-1
Kechari Mudra

quote:
_____

Originally posted by Chiron

quote:
_____

Once our bhakti is hurling our tongue back into kechari, breaking the
hymen of the frenum does not have to be stressful and painful. It can
be very easy and gentle. **Above all, it can and should be gradual.**
_____

http://www.aypsite.org/108.html

Does that apply to having the frenum removed surgically? If so, why?

_____

Hi Chiron:

Yes, for those who may be inclined that way.

Why? Because how the frenum is attended to is a personal matter driven by bhakti (spiritual desire), and no reasonable safe option should be excluded.

The emphasis on the word "gradual" applies to self-snipping the frenum, taking small safe steps toward release. A surgical approach would obviously be a large step via appropriate medical procedure.

The "hymen" analogy also may point to the rare cases where opening a woman's hymen might need surgical assistance. In either the case of frenum or hymen, the need for surgical assistance may be rare, but the possibility of it exists nevertheless. It is a matter of the individual's anatomy, need (bhakti), and choice.

All the best!

The guru is in you.

2008/03/14 14:13:04
Support for AYP Pranayama, Mudras and Bandhas
http://www.aypsite.org/forum/topic.asp?TOPIC_ID=359&REPLY_ID=31302&whichpage=-1
Kechari Mudra

quote:
_____

Originally posted by Szu
Where this point accurately is and on which step of ketchari this sprout can be feeled ?

Others sources ?

_____

Hi Szu:

The "point" you are referring to is called the "secret spot" in AYP. It is located on the back edge of the nasal septum just above where the hard and soft palates meet. It is accessed by the tongue by going behind the soft palate and pushing forward. The soft palate then opens downward like a trap door. The secret spot is first accessed in stage 2 kechari (tongue reaching the back edge of the septum). The secret spot may or may not be active (spiritually erogenous), depending on previous progress with a range of yoga practices leading to the rise of "ecstatic conductivity" in the neurobiology.

You did not mention the AYP lessons on kechari which are derived from several of the scriptures you metioned, and a lot of practical experience. The lessons can be found listed in the main website topic index. Lesson 108 is the main one, and there are quite a few others.

It has gone much further in these support forums, with many angles on practice and experience having been explored. Try searching the forums for words like "kechari," khechari," "snip," etc. You will find a lot.

Together, the AYP lessons and forums may comprise the most comprehensive open resource on kechari mudra in the world. If your research has turned up new angles, we'd love to have them posted here in the forums. The learning never ends. :-)

The focus in AYP overall is less on theory and more on methods that produce the best results with steady application over time. So we discuss chakras and other internal machinery less than other approaches. We don't deny the inner mechanics. We just focus more on the main controls of the "car" and leave the inner machinery to do its thing "under the hood." In other words, we don't theorize much about kechari. We just do it as bhakti calls us in relation to the rest of our practices and the rise of ecstatic conductivity.

All the best!

The guru is in you.

2008/03/14 14:17:19
Support for AYP Pranayama, Mudras and Bandhas
http://www.aypsite.org/forum/topic.asp?TOPIC_ID=359&REPLY_ID=31303&whichpage=-1
Kechari Mudra

quote:

_____

Originally posted by Sagittarius

I havn't reached stage 2 of kechari, but with a help of fingers my tongue goes some distance behind soft palate. However if I close my mouth, the tongue immediately drops out of soft palate. How do I avoid this?

_____

Hi Sagittarius:

Try pushing the tongue forward on top of the soft palate. This will open the soft palate downward. Then you will be in stage 2, and closing the mouth while staying in that mode will be easier. It becomes very easy with some practice.

If it doesn't work, some additional stretching and/or trimming of the frenum under the tongue may be be necessary.

All the best!

The guru is in you.

2008/12/21 14:54:09
Support for AYP Pranayama, Mudras and Bandhas
http://www.aypsite.org/forum/topic.asp?TOPIC_ID=359&REPLY_ID=42693&whichpage=-1
Kechari Mudra

quote:

_____

Originally posted by Nitika

Hi all,

This is Nitika here. I have followed the posts on Khechari Mudra on AYP forum for quite some time and would like to say well done to all of you! on the path of your sadhna :)

There is a question inside me which prompted to send this post and that is regd. the laser surgery for frenulum removal.

I wanted to understand that, does the frenulum removal result in losing some control over the movement of the tongue while performing Khechari?

Would the fingers start playing a major part in pushing the toungue behind the uvula, or does a person have full control over the tongue movement without fingers?

Would really appreciate if you could advice me regarding the same.

Thanking you...

Nitika

_____

Hi Nitika, and welcome to the forums! :-)

By whatever means the frenum may be reduced or removed, I am not aware of any cases where this has caused loss of control of the tongue for kechari, or anything else like speech, swallowing, etc. Experience with kechari here goes back back several decades, so this is a long time observation. There are also many in the AYP community who are using kechari mudra who may wish to comment on this.

Finger help may be used to assist with initial entry of the tongue into the nasal pharynx. With practice, finger help may not be necessary later on. See AYP main lesson 108 on this: http://www.aypsite.org/108.html
...and follow-up lessons linked in the website topic index.

There is also a lot of discussion on kechari in these forums, as you know -- many first-hand reports and case histories.

Wishing you all the best on your path. Enjoy!

The guru is in you.

2009/11/09 18:54:18
Support for AYP Pranayama, Mudras and Bandhas
http://www.aypsite.org/forum/topic.asp?TOPIC_ID=359&REPLY_ID=59530&whichpage=-1

Kechari Mudra

quote:
_____
Originally posted by mimirom

Hi,

I'd be grateful for any comments. It's still the same here: energy gets stuck in my jaw during dm and samyama. As soon as I enter kechari it immediately gets nice and smooth and meditation deepens.
I'm not sure how to navigate this situation safely.

Thanks

_____

Hi Mimirom:

Not sure when the energy blockage started in your jaw -- before or after starting kechari. It will be good to be careful about not over-stimulating it with a practice that may be related to its cause.

Have you been self-pacing in practices and grounding in activity in attempts to reduce the discomfort? Blockages in the throat and jaw can be helped with chin pump or chin pump light. Jim & K has a whole topic on front channel blockages, but I'm not sure you are in that category severity-wise at this point.

Remember that trying to "break through" uncomfortable blockages with more practice almost never works. Better to lighten up...

All the best!

The guru is in you.

2009/11/10 15:37:35
Support for AYP Pranayama, Mudras and Bandhas
http://www.aypsite.org/forum/topic.asp?TOPIC_ID=359&REPLY_ID=59582&whichpage=-1
Kechari Mudra

Hi Mimirom:

It is suggested to feel your way along, keeping in mind that while kechari may be giving relief in one area, it is also causing purification and opening in other areas, perhaps not visible at the moment. There can be delayed effects, so it's suggested to proceed with caution (small steps) when increasing practice times. Your call, of course.

Carry on! :-)

The guru is in you.

2005/07/27 20:05:28
Support for AYP Pranayama, Mudras and Bandhas
http://www.aypsite.org/forum/topic.asp?TOPIC_ID=366&REPLY_ID=203&whichpage=-1
kechari -- can't stop pushing the uvula in

Hi David:

Try the "side entrance," meaning near either the left or right connection point of the edge of the soft palate with the extreme back of the roof of the mouth. Depending on personal anatomy, one will be easier to reach than the other, and whichever one it is will always be the shortest route into kechari for you. If you go in with the tip of the tongue there, the tongue will then slide to the center behind the soft palate and uvula. That way you are going around the uvula, so to speak, and it will be less likely to fold up under the tongue, not that there is anything wrong with that. Once stage 2 is in full swing, the uvula will slide back down under the tongue even when it is folded up on initial entry.

Also, once stage 2 and beyond are well established, the practitioner can go in anywhere across the back edge of the soft palate, including "up the middle" through the uvula. The point of entry matters most in the beginning, when minimizing the distance and getting around the uvula can make the difference between getting in and not getting in. This is when finger help (pushing the tongue back from underneath) comes in handy too. Later on, these fine points don't matter much anymore. It is just in we go, wherever and whenever we like. No finger help is needed then either.

Victor's suggestion of "going forward" over the top of the back side of the soft palate is a good one. When we are in stage 2 especially, the feeling is much like the tongue is laying flat on the bottom of the mouth, except it is laying flat on the "second floor" instead, which is the top (back side) of the soft palate. Stages 3 and 4 extend forward and up from there. It is a lot like sticking your tongue out, except the tongue is going forward and up instead of out the front of the mouth.

That way you can stick your tongue out at someone without them seeing it, and be stroking the "secret spot" for ecstatic conductivity and enlightenment at the same time! :-)

The guru is in you.

2006/09/20 19:15:45
Support for AYP Pranayama, Mudras and Bandhas

Hi Yogini:

Welcome aboard!

Thank you for your input on restless leg syndrome. It would be interesting to explore its relationship to the rise of ecstatic conductivity in the nervous system from yoga practices, which can produce similar symptoms for short periods, though often quite pleasurable. That may or may not be a difference ... these two phenomena may or may not be related...

Yes, reading the forums can be a bit confusing in the beginning if the AYP lessons have not been gone through first, at least perused in order for the logical progression in the development of a self-directed practice routine. You may wish to check the lesson menus at the top of this page, beginning with "main lessons."

Becoming familiar with the lessons can help provide a foundation of knowledge, and then there may be more of a "method to the madness" here in the open discussions. :-)

Wishing you all the best on your path. Enjoy!

The guru is in you.

2006/09/21 19:05:41
Support for AYP Pranayama, Mudras and Bandhas
http://www.aypsite.org/forum/topic.asp?TOPIC_ID=431&REPLY_ID=11434&whichpage=-1
Dealing with energy restriction

Hi Yogini:

Glad you have been finding the lessons helpful.

Sounds like you have been through a lot over the years. It is fairly typical around here, so you are among friends who can relate.

It seems like in the past few decades parts of humanity have been leaping ahead of the knowledge traditions that are supposed to be supporting our evolution. It is a good thing, but, to keep up, some fundamantal changes are needed in how spiritual knowledge is transmitted. I hope we will see a continued move toward open source systems of practice with good integration of methodologies across the board. We can't afford to be hanging around anymore begging for what is already ours -- right here within us. It is time to move on.

On your Dutch translation of the lessons, that is great news. Do you have any inclination to post it on a website or moderator-posted only Yahoo group as you go, so others can read it? Of course, in Holland, most everyone reads English already, don't they? So maybe it is not so critical like in other countries. Here is a post on the translations going on that we know of: http://www.aypsite.org/forum/topic.asp?TOPIC_ID=440

In addition, just a few days ago, I received a note from a publisher in Greece interested in doing a Greek edition of the AYP book, and maybe others. We'll see what happens.

Also coming soon are India editions, in English.

Never a dull moment.

The guru is in you.

2005/09/27 13:30:43
Support for AYP Pranayama, Mudras and Bandhas
http://www.aypsite.org/forum/topic.asp?TOPIC_ID=497&REPLY_ID=775&whichpage=-1
"tooled talavya kriya"

Hi David:

Perhaps it should be pointed out that, for vast majority of us, the complete removal of the frenum is not a prerequisite for entering stage 2 kechari and beyond. In fact, some folks (like Victor) do not have to remove any frenum at all to move above the soft palate. In my case, only a little trimming was necessary, and I am still working on it a little bit now and then some 20 years after first entering stage 2 kechari -- driven more by undulating waves of bhakti than any physical requirement.

While trimming the frenum, at least a little, is certainly a factor for many of us in achieving higher kechari, it is not everything. In fact, with some specific knowledge about where, how and in what direction to go, many who may not think they can reach above the soft palate actually can right now -- it is much closer than most people realize. There can be other factors holding us back, and these are more related to our bhakti (spiritual emotions) than to our frenum. There is no doubt that reducing the frenum reduces the challenge of entry. But it is not "all or nothing" with the frenum, and I think you would agree that kechari is not mainly about removing the frenum, but about following the bhakti upward.

I say all this just to reduce the possibility for any confusion to arise about the means and the end. Everyone has their own unique circumstances in this. As you point out -- one approach does not necessarily fit all. You are sharing your experience, which is quite unique. Some might regard it as extreme. But to each their own. A particularly cumbersome frenum might require such measures. Only the practitioner can know for sure.

My suggestion is:

1) Bhakti first - Deep in your heart you are itching to do this kechari thing. Preferably, that will be long after being well-grounded in deep meditation, spinal breathing and other mudras and bandhas.

2) Attempts with finger help going back and up with the tongue to the extreme left or right side of the back edge of the soft plate. You might be surprised what you can do with this.

3) Consider frenum trimming only as necessary to get up there. It may be very little. It was for me all those years ago. Maybe some will need more trimming, but it does not have to be "all" for entry. Once you are in, and on the ecstatic secret spot with your tongue, the frenum will fade in importance, and will only be addressed as and when bhakti to go higher surges. That may be next week, next year or next decade. No need to rush. It is bhakti and our evolving ecstatic experience that will define our progress in kechari, not the imperative of a physical alteration. From the perspective of a seasoned practitioner, kechari is not a physical act at all. It is a spiritual act.

This is not to throw cold water on anything you have shared, David. Your experience is valid for you, and may be for others. It is only to help temper it a bit with a longer view. Practice wisely, and enjoy!

The guru is in you.

2005/10/21 15:00:05
Support for AYP Pranayama, Mudras and Bandhas
http://www.aypsite.org/forum/topic.asp?TOPIC_ID=537&REPLY_ID=1074&whichpage=-1
A lot of questions............

Hi Oli:

There are as many ways to do these practices as there are teachers and practitioners out there. AYP attempts to present the simplest and most effective methods in each category of practice, sticking with the underlying principles, while at the same time allowing some flexibility. For some discussion on principles and practices, see lesson #204 at http://www.aypsite.org/204.html

Some of the things you are suggesting are, in fact, part of other teachings, and diverging pretty far from the simple practices of AYP. I can't cover every variation (I'd be here writing forever! :-)), but can offer a few basic perspectives that I hope will be helpful.

In spinal breathing, the sushumna (spinal nerve) is the "master controller" of energy unfoldment and balance in the entire nervous system. It is not necessary from the AYP perspective to spiral out into the territory of ida and pingala, as these are opened automatically while opening the sushumna. This expansion (the swirling) is not something we have to supervise or worry about. It will happen in due course when ecstatic conductivity comes up. At times, ida and pingala may become very quiet. At other times, very lively. It depends what mode we are in at any given time.

There is much more involved in this process than spinal breathing alone. Particularly important is deep meditation, which is often down-played or even missing completely in the kriya lines of teaching in favor of a singular focus on pranayama.

In AYP, correct use of the mantra in deep meditation is the means by which the sushumna opening is expedited, and everything else along with it. Cultivating inner silence in deep meditation is the first practice we do in AYP, before we even consider working directly with the inner energies. That is why I suggest taking the AYP lessons in order. If we work with the energies first, without deep meditation, there can be that drying up of enthusiastic desire for the divine (bhakti) and clarity (focus). These positive traits are characteristics of rising inner silence, which pranayama alone does not provide for. Man (and woman) does not live by energy alone. It is consciousness that we are, and it is consciousness expanding from within that we need as the foundation of our practice. That is the job of deep meditation.

I do not recommend that we walk around during the day trying to be aware of sushumna, mantra or anything else related to sitting practices. Once we have done our practices, we should go out and engage fully in life's activities. That is the best way to stabilize what we have gained in our sitting practices. As our inner silence, ecstatic energies and increasing flow of love and compassion are coming up, we will find plenty to put our attention on in daily activity along the lines of helping others and doing good in the world. As we engage in the world in accordance with our rising spiritual awareness, that becomes the part of our practice that is action for the benefit of others, or karma yoga.

Well, that is the AYP perspective on what you described. I hope you find it helpful.

The guru is in you.

2005/10/21 23:16:23
Support for AYP Pranayama, Mudras and Bandhas
http://www.aypsite.org/forum/topic.asp?TOPIC_ID=537&REPLY_ID=1084&whichpage=-1
A lot of questions............

Hi again Oli:

As a follow-up, here is an AYP lesson on left side or right side energy imbalances:
http://www.aypsite.org/207.html

If you do some site searches on the lessons or check the topic index, you can find many things that have been covered that may be relevant to your experiences.

The guru is in you.

2005/10/24 23:21:09
Support for AYP Pranayama, Mudras and Bandhas
http://www.aypsite.org/forum/topic.asp?TOPIC_ID=537&REPLY_ID=1147&whichpage=-1
A lot of questions............

Hi Oli:

quote:

Does it indicates something if the swirling happens in counter-clockwise direction (seen from above)? Or is it unimportant which direction?
_____

Actually, when fully active it goes in both directions at the same time: Two distinct energies swirling in opposite directions around the spine, one within the other. This is a symptom of the blending of masculine and feminine energies within us. Among its many functions, the chin pump practice in AYP is related to cultivation of this inner energy activity. But, as mentioned, not to get too involved with the symptoms. Better to be focused on the practices in a logical build-up according to our capacity. Having a few symptoms does not mean we should be jumping ahead too fast. Just take it one step at a time.

quote:
_____
Im more familiar with Vipassana. Is it as effective as the correct use of a mantra in meditation?
_____

I am not an expert on vipassana, but my general understanding of it is that it involves much longer sittings than we do in deep meditation with mantra. I can't tell you if the results are better or not. It can be your experiment. Let us know! :-)

Yes, meditation will make us easier to be around. Others will often notice the difference before we do. It is the power of inner silence coming up in us.

The guru is in you.

2005/10/31 18:05:48
Support for AYP Pranayama, Mudras and Bandhas
http://www.aypsite.org/forum/topic.asp?TOPIC_ID=537&REPLY_ID=1297&whichpage=-1
A lot of questions............

quote:
_____
Originally posted by brauniver
I checked out both methods the last days. For me at the moment it seems that the mantra technique is more energy related and with vipassana I'm more aware, so it seems to me to be more conciousness related. But its just the opinion of a noob.
_____

Hi Oli:

As I understand it, vipassana is following the breath with attention, using breath as the object of meditation.

That is not what we do in AYP mantra meditation. If you are following the breath during mantra meditation (dividing the attention between two practices), that could account for more energy and less inner silence. Check these lessons for more detail on the relationship of spinal breathing pranayama and meditation in AYP:
http://www.aypsite.org/43.html
http://www.aypsite.org/106.html

Your good sense of humor is a help on the path too -- being both cause and effect. When we are laughing, God is laughing. :-)

The guru is in you.

2005/11/09 07:27:24
Support for AYP Pranayama, Mudras and Bandhas
http://www.aypsite.org/forum/topic.asp?TOPIC_ID=582&REPLY_ID=1462&whichpage=-1
to imagine or to feel?-- spinal breathing

Hi Alvin:

Spinal breathing begins as 2 - visualize, moves to 3 - feel and visualize (see lesson #63 for some clues), and ends up almost exclusively as 1 - feel, becoming much more than physical feeling -- more and more to unbounded feeling of ecstatic inner space (inner sensuality). All of this depends on resident inner silence cultivated (separately) in deep meditation.

It is a progression over time. Rome was not built in a day. Lili offered you some good advice in the other topic -- take it one step at a time. You will go far if you go slow and steady. Right now you are measuring in hours and days. That is understandable. This is all new! Later on you will be measuring in months and years. For those who are steady on the path, the experience of yoga keeps expanding endlessly, both inward and outward.

It is a joy to see you here. All the best!

The guru is in you.

2005/11/12 18:05:52
Support for AYP Pranayama, Mudras and Bandhas
http://www.aypsite.org/forum/topic.asp?TOPIC_ID=582&REPLY_ID=1514&whichpage=-1
to imagine or to feel?-- spinal breathing

Hi Anthem:

Yes, ultimately all the senses are involved, gradually refining inward. In AYP terminology that is "inner sensuality." Traditionally it is known as "pratyahara," one of the eight limbs of yoga.

Interestingly, this refinement of the senses inward corresponds with the rise of ecstatic conductivity in the nervous system. In due course, the refinement of sensory perception migrates back outward, and then we experience ecstatic conductivity (and radiance) in all things -- not only within our body.

Along with the outward migration of inner sensuality and ecstatic conductivity, there also comes the expansion of outpouring divine love. So all of these things are tied together, emanating from our expanding pure bliss consciousness -- all coming from our inner silence.

While we are going in, we are also coming out! :-)

The guru is in you.

2005/11/16 10:52:55
Support for AYP Pranayama, Mudras and Bandhas
http://www.aypsite.org/forum/topic.asp?TOPIC_ID=590&REPLY_ID=1540&whichpage=-1
Crown Bastrika

Hi Anthem:

I'll let the lessons speak for themselves on crown openings, including the risks and rewards. We each have to approach it according to our own bhakti, level of purification and known sensitivities.

I do want to add that to the extent one is doing "targeted" crown bastrika, it is okay to put it in front of meditation. In fact, both spinal and targeted bastrika can be done before spinal breathing, if desired. That would be between asanas and spinal breathing, if one is doing postures before sitting practices. There are no hard and fast rules on this. We will have the pranayama benefit whenever we do it. And our meditation will be just as effective over time whether we are doing bastrika before or after. It is a matter of personal choice. That is the advantage of open source knowledge. We can use it however we like. :-)

Of course, there are principles, causes and effects that we are dealing with at every turn, so we can't afford to be careless in our choices on how we do things. With good self-pacing we can regulate our own progress and find our way through. That is the key, and it is especially important in approaching the crown.

Sounds like you are tiptoeing up there with some good results. Keep in mind that there will often be a delayed effect with any crown practice we do. If it feels great today, that does not mean we are in the clear. The suggestion is to continue to step carefully, and enjoy!

The guru is in you.

2005/11/17 11:20:29
Support for AYP Pranayama, Mudras and Bandhas
http://www.aypsite.org/forum/topic.asp?TOPIC_ID=590&REPLY_ID=1544&whichpage=-1
Crown Bastrika

Hi Anthem:

There can be several layers of delayed effect. The most obvious one is doing a crown thing today that feels great, and waking up tomorrow feeling totally reamed. It can take a few days or more to get over that. Needless to say, goodbye crown practice when that happens, and rightfully so.

Then there is the imbalance that sneaks up over days, weeks or months of pushing just a little too much every day. That may not be as acute as the short term overload, but can take longer to smooth out. It is a general feeling of malaise, or worse, that tells us something is not right. There are all sorts of combinations falling between the short term overload and longer term overload.

For those who are crown sensitive and dealing with the ongoing effects of a premature crown (kundalini) opening, all of this gets magnified many times over.

All of which points to the crown being a tricky business. That's why I say, step carefully. The truth of it is, when we become ready via ajna to root practices, we will enter up into the crown smoothly and naturally without much fanfare at all. The fanfare (big energy symptoms, ecstasy, etc.) is the friction of energy passing through unpurified nerves. That is the so-called ecstasy we crave so much. We don't really need those symptoms to progress, but we are all looking for handles on our progress. It is understandable. So we press on... it is the bhakti-ego-practice-purification dynamic that leads us steadily (or not so steadily) toward enlightenment.

Btw, similar imbalance scenarios can be had by overdoing any of our practices. You had that going on a month or so ago, right? The difference between that situation and a crown overload is in the degree of power involved and the recovery time -- much much greater for the crown. The crown is like a spiritual vacuum cleaner that literally sucks all of our pranic energy up and out. This is great when the nervous system is sufficiently purified to handle it. But before that it can be a major reaming -- not very comfortable, and difficult to control if it gets out of hand -- shades of Gopi Krishna there.

On the difference between the brow to root and crown to root, the ajna (brow to medulla) is the area where we have greatest control over our whole body ecstatic energy, including regulating what goes up to the crown. Ajna means "command" for good reason. The crown is just the opposite in that respect. I sometimes call it "the white hole." ... like a black hole, only going up into infinity. Hey, better to get sucked up than to get sucked down!

In terms of characteristics, the ajna has the lore surrounding it about "other realms" and so on. To be honest, all that is pretty miner compared to the ajna's primary earth benefit, which is the rise of spiritual intuition. That has huge implications in our everyday life. Spiritual intuition enables us to know and do things here on earth that we could not even imagine before. To me, that is far more valuable than seeing or traveling in other realms. The here and now is where it is at. The somewhere else is for later when we leave here. There is no escaping the work we have come here to do. We can do it now, or do it later...

In contrast, the crown is a dissolving of everything we are into the great white all-consuming beyond. From there we can come back into the earth plane as that great white beyond. But to function energetically we will have to come back to the ajna, and the heart as well, which is another important aspect. The crown is the doorway to an infinite sea of cosmic energy. We can either draw upon it judiciously or be completely consumed by it. There isn't much in-between. Our surrender to being consumed is best regulated (self-paced) according to the condition of our nervous system, which is indicated by our experiences over time.

The way the AYP practices are set up, we have the opportunity to conduct our unfoldment in a manageable sequence, building all of our energy-related practices and experiences on a firm foundation of inner silence cultivated in deep meditation, and a balanced opening of our sushumna cultivated in spinal breathing.

In the old days, the great bhaktis took a flying leap into spiritual chaos and hoped to come out the other end in one piece. Only a few did. Now we all can.

It is analogous to the lone entrepreneur leaping off the cliff with eagle feathers tied to his arms, hoping to master flight, versus the Wright Brothers spending years systematically developing the easy-to-use controls that would enable all of humankind to take flight. The first approach has led to the second approach. And with the second approach, we don't have to jump off the cliff with reckless abandon anymore, though some may still be inclined to. :-)

So the advice is, don't confuse the flying leap (crown) for the steady joystick (ajna). The crown we can test and enter very slowly as conditions naturally permit us to do so. In that sense, the crown is not really a practice at all. It is a doorway we are opening through a variety of means, so we can pass through easily at some point. The so-called crown practices are the testing of that doorway. At least that is the AYP approach. It is the ajna we can utilize with confidence for a smooth and progressive ride leading to full opening on all fronts.

The guru is in you.

2005/11/18 07:19:59
Support for AYP Pranayama, Mudras and Bandhas
http://www.aypsite.org/forum/topic.asp?TOPIC_ID=590&REPLY_ID=1546&whichpage=-1
Crown Bastrika

Hi again Anthem:

For the sake of clarification, sambhavi eventually goes higher and encompasses both ajna and crown. That resolves the dual focus issue you raised. I don't think folks ought to be encouraged to do that. It comes along naturally as ecstatic conductivity provides a more intimate and stable connection between ajna and crown, and the rest of the nervous system that surges up ecstatically from the root. The safety/stability factor is maintained with both ajna and crown coming together like that -- with the ajna being the point of reference going up into the crown. Interestingly, this provides the same crown vacuum cleaner effect mentioned above, but with much more stability. Such is the stabilizing power of the ajna. So do keep a hand on that joystick.

It is important for everyone to recognize that this sambhavi reference pertains to a natural progression of ecstatic conductivity and not a practice to be pressed beforehand. I don't want to send folks off on a wild goose chase to the crown. Gooses can get cooked prematurely that way!

And to your earlier question, no, I do not recommend more pranayama at the end of practices than has been discussed.

Yes, do take it easy. It is not about having the biggest ecstatic energy explosions. It is about cultivating inner silence and managing a smooth unfoldment from there. Once things get rolling, self-pacing becomes the primary focus. You are doing just right.

All the best!

The guru is in you.

2005/11/22 10:45:18
Support for AYP Pranayama, Mudras and Bandhas
http://www.aypsite.org/forum/topic.asp?TOPIC_ID=590&REPLY_ID=1603&whichpage=-1
Crown Bastrika

Hi Anthem:

The key to the ecstasy thing is in its refinement, which is analogous to purification of our nervous system, the awakening and refinement of ecstatic conductivity (also called kundalini), and introversion of sensory perception which is pratyahara. All of these are aspects of the same dynamic. As the neurological friction becomes less, the expression of ecstatic energy and our experience refines.

On the other hand, bliss is not a dynamic energy-related quality like ecstasy is. Bliss is an aspect of pure "bliss" consciousness, inner silence, which we cultivate (or reveal) in deep meditation. Inner silence does not "refine." Inner silence emerges when we dissolve inner obstructions to it. It is our own inner awareness. It is stillness. Bliss is a resident part of stillness.

So we have these two qualities -- bliss and ecstasy. One is a fixed compass (our awareness) we reveal as inner silence in deep meditation. The other is a dynamic evolution of energy flowing through our nervous system. As ecstasy (energy movement) refines, it comes to reside in silence, or bliss. Then we have "ecstatic bliss," which is a new dynamic in us that brings a "rebirth." It is the joining of "emptiness and euphoria," as Lahiri Mahasaya called it. It is also the joining of "Shiva and Shakti" as Yoga and Tantra call it. And it is the joining of "Father and Holy Spirit," as the Christians call it. The product of this joining is the Jivan Mukti (liberated soul) or Christ, which manifests as the expansion of outpouring divine love. We all know that when we see it, and it is more than enough of a miracle to see in this world. In fact, outpouring divine love brings the miracles with it, and that is the real meaning of miracles.

All of this terminology is to describe a real neuro-biological transformation that we who are doing yoga practices are witnessing at our own particular stage, and describing accordingly. The new AYP book "Deep Meditation" goes into this as well, because I think it is important even for beginning meditators to understand the difference between the qualities of inner silence, the role of energy (ecstatic or not) in navigating the overall purification process, and what the ultimate joining of these two aspects of our nature deep within us is about.

Some may see stillness and energy as mutually exclusive, and paths that attempt to integrate these two aspects of our nature as conflicted. To that, we can only say that the human nervous system operates in a certain way as it evolves spiritually, and all paths are but a reflection of that to greater or lesser degree. The addressing of polarity (silence and energy) found in spiritual paths is there because the polarity is there in nature -- in all of nature, from our human functioning and spiritual mechanics, right down to the inner workings of matter itself. So, to exclude the polarity aspect on our path, whether it be excluding inner silence or ecstatic energy, is to exclude a vital aspect of ourselves.

Having said all that, I recommend that inner silence be given the first priority, as it is the ground state and source of all energy. Yet, once we have inner silence, the witness, we will not find completion until our ecstatic energy function has been refined to marry inner silence, so we can move on to the unity stage, which is outpouring divine love. That's why the sequence of practices in AYP is the way it is -- inner silence first, and all the ecstatic energy development and refinement after that.

And, to bring us back to the topic at hand, the crown and ajna are key players in all of this, as detailed here and throughout the AYP lessons.

The guru is in you.

2005/11/18 11:58:29
Support for AYP Pranayama, Mudras and Bandhas
http://www.aypsite.org/forum/topic.asp?TOPIC_ID=592&REPLY_ID=1549&whichpage=-1
tender pharynx -- surprising cure

Hi David:

Something else that helps is a drop or two of olive oil on the tip of the tongue before going up.

Apologies for not mentioning this much earlier. I have not used it for many years, and forgot about it.

See? I'm not perfect. :-)

The guru is in you.

2005/11/20 23:30:08
Support for AYP Pranayama, Mudras and Bandhas
http://www.aypsite.org/forum/topic.asp?TOPIC_ID=592&REPLY_ID=1588&whichpage=-1
tender pharynx -- surprising cure

Hi David:

It (the olive oil) was helpful to me during a period of sensitivity a long time ago. But it's obviously not for everyone. Better stick with your citrus, and anything else you can come up with that facilitates your practice. Whatever works!

Make sure to report any additional findings here so others will have multiple options to consider.

Over time, a more accommodating biology develops in the pharynx, stimulated by regular kechari practice. It is not only about saliva. It is also lubricaton (often sweet) coming down from the nasal passages. In fact, it is more the latter. So, the need for aids will gradually become less. It did for me anyway. The development corresponds with rising ecstatic conductivity, which is logical from the point of view of the evolving spiritual biology. It becomes a completely natural process, intimately involved with the rise of our inner experience and its steady overflow into our outer life.

In a very real sense, all that I am doing here is an overflow of That. It looks that way from this side of the screen.

The guru is in you.

2006/10/28 15:46:36
Support for AYP Pranayama, Mudras and Bandhas
http://www.aypsite.org/forum/topic.asp?TOPIC_ID=592&REPLY_ID=12652&whichpage=-1
tender pharynx -- surprising cure

Hi Alvin:

You are getting the right advice -- time to slow down and take it easy.

You know, as I look back, significant progress with kechari in my case was measured in decades, not even years, and certainly not in months or weeks. I was on the path 15 years before there was enough ecstatic conductivity occurring to send me in the direction of kechari. And it has been a couple of decades of gradual development since then. The point is, this is a long term gig, not an overnight event.

On the other hand, times are changing, and I think everyone is on a much faster track now. It is obvious around here, isn't it? That is great! But there are limits in everything. We'd like to be on the leading edge, not necessarily the bleeding edge. If kechari snipping is done prudently there will be practically no pain and no blood. If there is much of either, it is a clear signal to self-pace the whole thing. The limiting tendon will present itself when it is time to take the next easy step forward.

I suggest healing up and waiting at least a few months before pressing kechari. Give inner silence and the inner energies a chance to stabilize and mingle, and all will become clear.

Sometimes we need to self-pace our bhakti to balance progress with safety. Kechari stage 1 is a powerful practice also, warranting self-pacing sometimes as well.

Practice wisely, and enjoy!

The guru is in you.

2006/10/30 10:04:00
Support for AYP Pranayama, Mudras and Bandhas
http://www.aypsite.org/forum/topic.asp?TOPIC_ID=592&REPLY_ID=12713&whichpage=-1

tender pharynx -- surprising cure

Hi Alvin:

Check here for my most recent suggestions: http://www.aypsite.org/forum/topic.asp?TOPIC_ID=1649

Don't sweat it too much. You have plenty of time.

The guru is in you.

2005/11/23 10:21:44
Support for AYP Pranayama, Mudras and Bandhas
http://www.aypsite.org/forum/topic.asp?TOPIC_ID=603&REPLY_ID=1622&whichpage=-1
frenum snipping update

Hi Meg:

I agree with Victor. While it is always your choice, common sense indicates that the risk ought not exceed the reward. It is a fact that if we find ourselves forcing our way into a practice, we are probably somewhat premature. It has happened to me along the way too. It happens to everyone. From this we learn to bide our time and take smaller steps. Tempering our bhakti a bit to protect our wellbeing is part of self-pacing. It is balancing the longing of our heart with the evolving abilities of our body, mind and nervous system. Over the long run, the divine will have its way. Gentle persistence over time will yield the best results, more so than short term intensity. The tortoise and the hare, you know. :-)

Having said all that, I'd like to commend you on your wonderful strong bhakti. It will take you far. Practice wisely, and enjoy!

The guru is in you.

2005/11/23 14:28:49
Support for AYP Pranayama, Mudras and Bandhas
http://www.aypsite.org/forum/topic.asp?TOPIC_ID=603&REPLY_ID=1626&whichpage=-1
frenum snipping update

Hi Meg:

If you know you will be hot on the trail of human spiritual transformation for as long as it takes, you can be pretty sure it is bhakti. Either that, or a very special kind of curiosity. :-)

The guru is in you.

2005/11/28 22:48:31
Support for AYP Pranayama, Mudras and Bandhas
http://www.aypsite.org/forum/topic.asp?TOPIC_ID=611
Kechari - Another Creative Approach - Plastic Tube

Hi All:

This email exchange on kechari mudra is offered with permission. I don't know if the author will be available here for questions, but this information is well worth passing on "as is." He has provided details on his method in Email #2 below.

Email #1:

Hi Yogani:

I managed to get the tongue up behind the soft palate aprox. 2 years ago through use of a plastic tube with one end plugged, the other open for insertion of the tongue -- placing tongue in tube and then sucking the air out of the tube, the tongue is drawn deep into the tube and held very firmly and the very bottom of the tube rests upon the frenum ... by slightly sharpening that bottom edge of the tube and gently manipulating the tube up and back, I was gradually able to cut the frenum completely and painlessly. Since then, I have lost my enthusiasm for the kechari somewhat as it did not have the effect upon me that it had on Norm Paulsen (who I went to see and spent some time with last year -- wonderful person!). I was, of course, hoping to have the ecstatic experiences you describe in your lessons (which I just discovered today, incidentally) and Norman describes in his book. I have felt strong movement of prana in the spine at times during kechari practice in the past, but well short of the ecstatic states others describe.

Anyway, my interest/enthusiasm has been renewed by reading your lessons and I've been trying to feel the "secret spot" ("about half way up the edge of the septum is a small protrusion, a small bulge."). I have not yet noticed any bulge along that interior septum ridge. I'm also confused about the "bony protrusion" both you and Norman talk about, above which rests the pituitary ("the throne of the pituitary", to quote Norman). There seem to be 3 different areas or spots being referred to -- the bony protrusion at the very top of the nasopharynx, the "secret spot" in the center of the interior portion of the nasal septum, and, in Kechari stage #4, yet another place to rest the tongue within the nasal passage itself. My nasal passages are still a little too sensitive to handle my inserting the tongue there, but much less so now than the last time I tried some 6 months ago.

I imagine I need to deepen my kriya yoga practice and be a little more regular in it as well to build a foundation upon which the ecstatic connection of Kechari can rise, at least such is my speculation right now. But, be that as it may, where to rest the tip of the tongue??? Very confusing to have the pictures in your lessons where, in stage 3, the tongue clearly rests at the very top of the nasal septum but, in the text on page 456 (of AYP Easy Lessons book), the middle portion of the septum is cited as the location of the secret spot. I wish I could go by feeling and just "know" where that spot is but, for whatever reason, I'm not sure.

Thanks so much for your response and insights.

Yogani Reply:

Hi. Thank you for your kind note and sharing.

That is a very creative approach to achieving higher stages of kechari you came up with. I am sure other readers of AYP would like to hear about it. More on that below...

With regard to the initial rise of ecstatic conductivity in the nervous system, kechari is not necessarily going to be the primary cause of that. I view it more as a "higher gear" practice that takes the process much further once it has been initiated by deep meditation, spinal breathing and other means. Of course, it can happen in a variety of ways, so I am not proposing an exclusive sequence of events or approach to stimulate it. Only an approach that has worked ... and we are always on the lookout for even more effective means.

Kechari is one of several "upper body" techniques we utilize in AYP. Sambhavi and dynamic jalandhara (chin pump) are two others. All of these carry forward whole-body ecstatic conductivity once it gets going. Before we can do much with the upper body techniques ecstatically, we go for "global" purification throughout the nervous system, stimulated by the rise of inner silence in deep meditation and samyama, and clearing and enlivening of the sushumna (spinal nerve) with spinal breathing, yoni mudra kumbhaka, spinal bastrika and other means.

Also, in AYP we directly engage the internal expansion of sexual energy with both yogic and tantric means. Here we are working with lower and middle body methods such as mulabandha/asvini, siddhasana, uddiyana/nauli, navi kriya, and direct cultivation of sexual energy preorgasmically within whatever sexual lifestyle one may be accustomed to.

Well, that is a lot of stuff. Much of it is familiar to you, no doubt, and perhaps some of it is not so familiar. AYP is a refinement and integration of the most effective methods of practice I have come across in my long yoga career. In the lessons, the practices are built up in a logical sequence, utilizing "self-pacing" (an AYP invention) to create a compact and stable routine that leaves us free to continue fully-engaged in our daily activities according to our inclinations, which is how the results of practices (inner silence and ecstatic conductivity) are blended and stabilized in our nervous system.

Given what you have mentioned, you may wish to consider adding deep meditation into your practice routine. In AYP it comes first. It is never too late to cultivate inner silence, also called "pure bliss consciousness," "the witness," "inner stillness," and by many other names. It is the ground state and source of all that goes on in yoga. The time to do deep meditation is right after spinal breathing. You may be doing a form of meditation there already, and it is up to you how to proceed, of course. From your description, it sounds like you could use a boost in the inner silence department. That is usually what is found to be somewhat in short supply in those who have gone far with pranayama and hatha yoga methods alone.

Once we have inner silence/stillness springing into action (a paradox!), then the way will become gradually more clear for the ecstatic elements of our journey. In the end, it is the joining of these two qualities that completes the cycle. The great kriya yogi, Lahiri Mahasaya, called this "The merging of emptiness with euphoria."

On the location of the secret spot in kechari, I find it to be about half way up the edge of the nasal septum -- that's about half way between the floor on top of the hard palate and the top of the nasal pharynx. In my case there is a small protrusion there, but I don't see that as a defining characteristic of the experience. In stage 2 kechari, the tip of the tongue rests right on the secret spot (see diagram). That is the most common advanced kechari position during pranayama and meditation. The secret spot can also be stimulated indirectly in kechari stage 1, through the roof of the mouth where the hard and soft palates meet, right under the edge of the nasal septum.

The secret spot is also stimulated by the back side of the tongue in stage 3 kechari, a position that can occur spontaneously at any time during practices.

Stage 4 (alternating up in each nostril during a practice such as chin pump) covers the secret spot also. In stage 4 we are adding stimulation of the erectile tissues in the nasal passages, which is a new dimension, but not more central (or continuous) than the secret spot on the edge of the septum. I do not find any spot more central than the secret spot in kechari practice, including the top of the nasal pharynx or the top of the nasal passages near the inside of the brow.

There is no special "direct" stimulation of the pituitary gland in kechari that I have found, though it is certainly stimulated indirectly (it is in the bony structure right above the nasal pharynx), and I agree with Norman Paulsen that it is an important seat of divine consciousness. Sambhavi is much involved in this also.

Btw, I have the highest regard for Norman Paulsen and his work -- a true American yoga pioneer!

All of this that I have been mentioning has been determined by direct experience with ecstatic conductivity -- the ecstatic connection between the head, the root, all points in-between, and even the environment outside the body. The secret spot is known by all of those ecstatic connections. A similar kind of ecstatic connection can be found in sambhavi, and these sensations lead us ever higher into divine absorption whenever we are inclined to go there. These ecstatic connections in the head lead simultaneously to the refinement and introversion of sensory perception -- pratyahara.

As a final point on ecstasy, I would add that quite a few involved in AYP have found ecstatic conductivity rising in their nervous system before reaching stage 2 kechari. This is evidence that kechari is not necessarily a primary cause of whole-body ecstatic conductivity. So, perhaps it is better to look back to meditation and other means designed to provide the prerequisite purification and opening of the overall nervous system. Then we can take the upper body mudras and fly!

As you may know, we now have the AYP forums available for anyone who wishes read and interact with many yoga practitioners from beginning to advanced. A search there will yield a wealth of additional knowledge from others on approaches to kechari.

I'd like to ask your permission to post your note (anonymously) and this reply in the AYP forums, so other practitioners can benefit from your unique input on kechari. I am sure they will find it most interesting. Whether or not you choose to participate in the discussion is up to you, of course. As a minimum, I hope we can share this interchange. The goal in AYP is to create an ongoing and evolving "open source" on effective yoga practices that is accessible to everyone. It is my hope that this can be the beginning of real applied yoga science leading to substantial improvements in the application of spiritual practices for present and future generations.

So let me know...

Wishing you success on your chosen spiritual path. With gentle persistence, I know you will find all you are seeking. Practice wisely, and enjoy!

The guru is in you.

Email #2:

Dear Yogani:

I am most grateful for your thoughtful, thorough response to my inquiry and have much more clarity about the placement of the tongue now. As I experimented today at work, I found the best resting place was, indeed, the middle of the septum and was pleased to find your confirmation waiting for me when I got home just now. The reason I had not really experimented with keeping the tongue there in the first place was the notion that it needed to rest at the top of the nasopharynx on the "bony protrusion". Your suggestion to emphasize spinal breathing to prepare for higher states also helped ease my mind and give me some confirmation of direction. And of course you have my permission to share our correspondence on the AYP site.

It was because of a fear I dare say most people will encounter -- that of taking a razor or such directly to the frenum -- that I felt compelled to find some other way (I did try the razor a few times but it was clearly not for me -- i ended up nicking my lips and was very, very squeamish about it). Here's a bit more info on the technique as it may prove useful to some. The tube I used was 1 inch in diameter (you may need a larger or smaller one I imagine, based on the width of your tongue) and can be found in Home Depot or Lowes hardware stores on a spool. I plugged one end of the tube with a bathtub plug which, fortuitously, I noticed in the same aisle as the tubing itself, securing the plug to the tube with super glue. When you get home, use an exacto knife or some such implement to trim to roundness the sharp edges of the tube so as to protect the tongue. Then further trim the bottom portion of the tube so there is a slope to a sharp edge just as wide as the frenum is at it's base. (Side note here: this tube method was engaged secondarily, after talabya-kriya was employed to it's full extent -- pressing the bottom of the tongue against the hard palate with vigor, stretching and gradually tearing the frenum bit by bit -- this process, by the way, produced an amazingly pleasurable feeling in the frenum itself and the craving to tear it further became almost obsessive over time. Dropping the jaw enables maximum extension in talabya and some may not need the tube process after this is accomplished. As for me, my frenum was considerable). Place the tongue into the tube as deeply as you can to begin (mind you, if there are any sharp edges you still need to trim, excepting the small bottom edge over the frenum area although that will perhaps need the most attention to get it just right, you'll feel them and will probably have to make numerous trims to soften the edges of the tube and get a comfortable fit), then simply suck the air out of the tube in successive inhalations. The tongue will produce a secure vacuum and be drawn deeper into the tube with each inhalation. 3 to 5 inhalations, as I recall, is about as much as you can total. Once the tongue is secured in the tube via suction, lift the tube up towards the roof of the mouth and press the sharper lower edge against what is left of the frenum (that is, what is left after maximizing talabya kriya). It basically continues the work of talabya kriya until the frenum is completely severed. There is no pain in the process if performed with care. Take special care to ensure the arteries on either side of the bottom of the tongue are not endangered -- all of the pressure should be and can be isolated against the frenum and, as I already said, keep trimming the edges till it fits properly around the tongue. Considerable force can be used as one gets used to the device. To protect from infection, I applied an equal mixture of turmeric and salt and this also helped keep the "wound" open and ready for the next days efforts, kept it from closing up and slowing the process. The application of the turmeric/salt stings considerably, no doubt about it, but is tolerable and eased my mind somewhat. I used the tube frequently, sometimes 5 times in a single day. I also set the tube and exercise aside for a few days at a time. I let the feeling in the tongue guide my progress. Breaks in the practice will need to take place, in other words. The tongue will actually start hurting from the suction over time, then a break will need to be taken. Or there will be an intuition to simply wait, to let the body "catch up", so to speak. Listen to those intuitions. Oh yes, last thing -- cleaning the tube. I used a baby bottle cleaning brush and anti-bacterial dishwashing soap. You'll have to clean the tube after each use to remove the saliva and I found simply squirting a bit of soap into it, filling it with hot water and inserting the baby bottle brush and scrubbing a very quick and easy way. And one more obvious note -- use the tube over a sink.

Again, thank you so much for your kind response, Yogani. I hope this will prove of some help to someone. Your response has been a great help to me already. Namaste.

2005/11/29 11:49:08
Support for AYP Pranayama, Mudras and Bandhas
http://www.aypsite.org/forum/topic.asp?TOPIC_ID=612&REPLY_ID=1698&whichpage=-1
Kechari Nothin'

Hi Jim:

This is essentially the same question asked in the kechari plastic tube topic, where the practitioner has gone to stage 2 and beyond without much ecstatic conductivity. I did my best to answer it there. http://www.aypsite.org/forum/topic.asp?TOPIC_ID=611

There is a close link between feeling the ecstatic conductivity connection in sambhavi and the connection in kechari. Also, in kechari, ground zero is about half way up the edge of the septum inside, which it seems the practitioner in the other topic is finding now after a couple of years of looking higher up. Once ecstatic conductivity gets going, it becomes much more obvious -- not subtle at all. :-)

The guru is in you.

2005/11/30 15:12:14
Support for AYP Pranayama, Mudras and Bandhas
http://www.aypsite.org/forum/topic.asp?TOPIC_ID=612&REPLY_ID=1722&whichpage=-1
Kechari Nothin'

Hi Jim:

Chin pump will help expand and integrate energies in the head, as well as the connections between head and heart, and lower. Like kechari, it too may need some initial ecstatic conductivity to prime the pump, so to speak. You will know when you try it.

A pitta imbalance can be both effect and cause, so it is important to continue to address it with all available means, including those touched on in lesson #69 -- http://www.aypsite.org/69.html -- and especially judicious self-pacing of practices. Obviously, we do not want that one spinning out of control.

We will know if we are too much or not enough in practices by testing when we feel ready, and backing off if we find we are not.

Like I told "Near" recently on pursuing yama and niyama, we don't want to wait and we don't want to force too much. Somewhere in-between those too is our ideal path. With inner silence coming up and stabilization of that with whatever ecstatic energy we have circulating, the bar keeps getting raised on what we can do. So it is a dynamic process going step-by-step toward the infinite light! :-)

The guru is in you.

2005/12/05 16:08:06
Support for AYP Pranayama, Mudras and Bandhas
http://www.aypsite.org/forum/topic.asp?TOPIC_ID=624
Kechari -- White Spots

Hi All:

Here is another kechari discussion from my email. If the "white spots" mentioned are not callousing related to frenum trimming or tongue stretching, I'm not sure what it would be. Perhaps our resident experts can add some perspective on this.

Q1:
Humbly I am asking you for help, as this is really a very difficult situation for me.

For some time I am practising Khechari, but right now I am at some turning point: I don't know how to proceed as doubts are overpowering me.

First I would like to summarize what I did till today:

Maybe 2 years ago I recognized the necessity of Khechari. So I started bending my tongue back. As time went by, my efforts increased. Sometimes my tongue hearted in the morning, may be because of bending too much. But I never cared too much for that. In this way month by month went by, and there was some progress.

This summer, a dear (who is translating your webpage into German at the moment) has drawn my attention to your webpage. There we studied your recommendations for achieving Khechari. After thinking about it some time, I started snipping a little. Till now I did it 4 times, always carefully and not too much. Sometimes there was very little blood, but not more.

However doubts are overpowering me again and maybe you can help me to overcome them with some additional information.

1. On my tongue's bottom side, there emerged some white dots. I first noticed these dots a long time before I even thought of snipping - to be honest, they appeared slowly after I started bending my tongue back. Did I bend too much? But why are these dots at such a high position? I would have expected that during bending the frenum, most stress is near the tongue's root. However more and more white dots came forward, or existing ones got more detailed, as soon as I started snipping - although I used to cut the frenum at some points closer to the tongue's root. To describe the situation a little clearer, I am attaching some photos.
http://www.imagesharing.com/out.php/i129794_tongueback.jpg
http://www.imagesharing.com/out.php/i129819_tongueup.jpg
http://www.imagesharing.com/out.php/i129832_whitedot.jpg

2. My frenum is not very distinct, more or less it seems to be embedded into the tongue's muscles. How, and where would you recommend may the next cuts? The photos should make a good picture of this, too.

Thank you very very much!

A1:
Thank you for writing and sharing. It sounds like you are determined to move ahead with kechari. That is a good thing if it comes from bhakti (divine desire) flowing out from deep meditation, spinal breathing pranayama and other practices. On the other hand, kechari for its own sake does not do well as a stand-alone practice. Hardly anything in yoga does, except deep meditation. Kechari is very much a later stage development that can take already awakened energies much further. This is discussed in several recent postings I did in the AYP forums,
http://www.aypsite.org/forum/topic.asp?TOPIC_ID=611
http://www.aypsite.org/forum/topic.asp?TOPIC_ID=612

I encourage you to keep up with the kechari (and all) discussions in the AYP forums and raise your questions there too.

On the white spots, I have not experienced that in the same way. Then again, I have not focused on heavy bending of the tongue as you describe, so what you are experiencing may be normal for that. I can tell you that as the tiny tendons of the frenum are snipped and come back up to the surface days or weeks later, they do form a white callous along the ridge of the frenum. So maybe your white spots are related to callous forming like that. If not, then the mystery remains. If you have any suspicion of an infection, I suggest no more heavy stretching or snipping until you address it medically. If there is ongoing inflammation or pain, do see a doctor.

One more thought on this. There are saliva glands in the bottom of the tongue, on either side of the center. It is possible that if you are stretching these that they could show some visual effects like callousing (whiteness). That would be symmetrical on cither side of the frenum. Not sure exactly where your spots are. I experienced that many years ago, and it amounted to nothing.

Regarding what to do next, I suggest taking your time. Rome was not built in a day. That is especially true with kechari. I have been snipping on and off of over 20 years. So be cool, do your meditation, pranayama and other yoga practices, and see what bhakti comes from within. Maybe you are at that stage of bhakti already and that is what is driving you toward kechari. If so, then continue to go for it, but pace yourself. Bhakti is wonderful, but does not always have our health and well-being in mind. All it wants is enlightenment right now and any cost. So there should be a compromise between strong bhakti and common sense to assure that we will be in a long term solution, rather than a shooting star that will light up the night and disappear as quickly as it came.

Your photos look like you are pretty close to going up behind the soft palate. Try that with finger help to the left or right side (shortest distance) as discussed in the lessons. Once you get behind the soft palate, push the tongue forward like you are sticking your tongue out, and it should slide right up into stage 2. That forward pushing is a trick that has helped others who do not get the immediate grabbing of the tongue by the soft palate and are a bit unsure which direction to go once behind there. There comes a time when the focus should shift from stretching and snipping to actually going up there with what we have.

On snipping frenum tendons not clearly exposed, you might want to check David's tooled talavya topic in the forum.
http://www.aypsite.org/forum/topic.asp?TOPIC_ID=497
There are some related and follow-up topics also which you can find with a search. While it is not a technique I can whole-heartedly recommend due to its aggressiveness, tooled talavya is there for anyone's consideration. It will enable you to go deeper and get those tendons. It is your choice.

Would you mind if I post this email exchange (anonymously) in the forum so others might benefit? You may receive some additional feedback that way too. There is at least one doctor reading, and that might bring some answers on the white spots. I can also include the photos as links, or not, let me know. The idea is to share and draw information from as many sources as possible. Then everyone wins.

I wish you all success on your chosen spiritual path. Practice wisely, and enjoy!

Q2:
Thank you very much for your detailed reply, it is really very helpful.

Indeed it is Bhakti that pulled my tongue back during yoga practice. Due to some ecstatic feeling, there is this desire for pulling more and more. And finally it works: I can really feel the increase of progress, when Yoga is practiced with support of forceful Khechari.
But of course you are right: nothing can be enforced over night. I am trying my best not to do too much, but it feels so good.
And I am so thirsty for that freedom; I know it will come as time is getting ripe.

To come back to the white dots, I made some additional photos that show the current situation a little clearer.
http://www.imagesharing.com/out.php/i129952_whitedots2.jpg
http://www.imagesharing.com/out.php/i129960_whitedots3.jpg

Actually the dots are effectively at the frenum's left and right, and therefore it might be logical that they are saliva glands that changed its colour. Only if I touch them, they hurt a little. May be this is a necessary information, too. But there was no infection after snipping, I believe, as I cut at completely different places.

Regarding helping with the finger, I made a photo.
http://www.imagesharing.com/out.php/i129946_fingerback.jpg
There you can see that I am really quite close to move up, but although I tried to push the tongue forward as you described, still my tongue is a little too limited at the bottom and therefore not loose enough for going back behind the soft plate, I think. For sure I will continue practicing.

Interestingly it seems like I am having no problem to go deep and pass through the middle of the soft plate, to move up afterwards. Passing the soft plate at the side seems unnecessary. I really wished the remaining limitations had already disappeared, so that I really could go up...

But as you recommended, I will take the necessary time for the next steps. Carefully I will consider tooled talavya, or may be I will continue by ordinary snipping. If I remove the surrounding tongue's flesh with my fingers, the remaining frenum appears - ready for being cut.

Once again, I would like to thank you whole-heartedly for your great work, and personal support. If you think it will help others, please feel free to publish this mail correspondence (including the photos of your own choice) anonymously on your webpage.

A2:
Those new photos indicate the white spots are along the ridge of the frenum, which may be related to a stretching and callousing effect. So it is not likely the saliva glands, which are further off to the sides on the bottom of the tongue.

If you go to the left or right side and up with the finger help, you will find the distance to be much less for getting behind the soft palate. The time to push forward is after the tip of your tongue goes behind the soft palate.

It looks like you are close. Still, take it at an easy pace, making sure not to overdo.

The guru is in you.

2005/12/07 17:37:21
Support for AYP Pranayama, Mudras and Bandhas
http://www.aypsite.org/forum/topic.asp?TOPIC_ID=627&REPLY_ID=1837&whichpage=-1
Mahamudra

Hi Darvish and Ute:

Sorry I am coming in a little late on this one. Great questions.

It turns out **maha mudra** is covered in the AYP book in the addition to lesson #71 on Asanas. It is in with the "sitting head to knee" postures as a more advanced version. It is mentioned in lesson #183 too, as well as in the glossary of Sanskrit terms both in the AYP book and online.

But you are right, Ute, it is not a regular part of AYP, mainly because all of its elements are covered in other parts of the AYP practices -- forward stretch, siddhasana, kumbhaka (breath retention), mudras and bandhas. etc. Even so, maha mudra can be used in asanas before sitting practices, if desired. Just keep self-pacing in mind for maha mudra in relation to all the other similar practices we are doing, so as not to be "doubling up" on kumbhaka effects.

Maha bandha is doing kumbhaka in siddhasana with mudras and bandhas, which advanced AYP practitioners do all over the place in sitting practices -- spinal breathing (yes, slow breathing has a kumbhaka-like effect), yoni mudra kumbhaka, chin pump, etc. These practices are variations on the same elements, with a different focus in each one.

Maha vedha is essentially maha bandha while dropping the body on the sitting surface from a few inches up with the hands. This is not an AYP practice, however it will happen automatically in samyama at a certain stage when doing the "akasha - lightness of air" sutra. In this particular manifestation it has been called "hopping." It is maha vedha occurring as an automatic yoga in samyama.

When we are doing the core practices of deep meditation and spinal breathing, the nervous system will know what it needs via the connectedness of yoga! :-)

Also, see Victor's topic on doing kechari, kumbhaka and other things during asanas, which has some valuable related insights.

The guru is in you.

2005/12/15 17:27:02
Support for AYP Pranayama, Mudras and Bandhas
http://www.aypsite.org/forum/topic.asp?TOPIC_ID=650&REPLY_ID=1972&whichpage=-1
Siddhasana, Mulabandha and Pulsation

Hi Y:

It is a "kundalini" vibration. I just answered this one recently in email:

Q:
There is something I need to ask you. For the past 2 or 3 days, I have been feeling a constant vibration in my pelvic area, starting from the base of my spine and moving up. It lasts only for a few seconds, but comes back ever min or 2. Not sure if this is a part of meditation ... or should I should go to a doctor. It does not happen during meditation alone, it is happening all the time. It feels like sitting on a machine that is vibrating. Could you help me?

A:
Vibrations in and around the perineum are not unusual when advancing in yoga. It is purification going on and should not last long. I have had it myself many times over the years. If it gets to be too much, then just self-pace your practices, and do some good grounding activity like walking or other exercise. See lesson #69 http://www.aypsite.org/69.html

Sometimes the vibrations will feel physical but will often be more neurological than physical. It can be a mixture of both too. And it can happen during daily activity.

Don't worry, it will pass. If it turns into something that is obviously medical, then be sure and have a doctor's opinion. But just some vibraton coming and going every now and then is normal purification in yoga. As mentioned, if it becomes troublesome, then self-pace practices until it settles down.

The guru is in you.

2005/12/16 13:08:51
Support for AYP Pranayama, Mudras and Bandhas
http://www.aypsite.org/forum/topic.asp?TOPIC_ID=652&REPLY_ID=1989&whichpage=-1
managing the practice of spinal breathing

Hi Alvin:

Ditto on what Anthem said. Also, note that the suggestion on doing spinal breathing "in the car" was for time management in a busy schedule (http://www.aypsite.com/50.html) -- on the way home to sit for meditation. Not ideal, nor recommended for any odd time during the day. Splitting up spinal breathing and deep meditation in time on a regular basis is not recommended.

Spinal breathing during sex is not a strongly recommended practice -- I was commenting on an inquiry received on that subject (http://www.aypsite.com/T33.html). The answer: Try it if inclined, and see if it works, and don't forget to self-pace. If we are being aggressive in practices within or outside our regular sittings, we always keep self-pacing close at hand.

The guru is in you.

2005/12/24 10:09:09
Support for AYP Pranayama, Mudras and Bandhas
http://www.aypsite.org/forum/topic.asp?TOPIC_ID=652&REPLY_ID=2131&whichpage=-1
managing the practice of spinal breathing

Hi Alvin:

I'd leave the spinal breathing out of tantric sex until much later. It is enough to develop the habit of preorgasmic sex. Once you do, then breathing response will become automatic. That is not 100% preorgasmic -- just gradually developing more natural ability than now. It is not an edict, just a favoring with normal sexual activity (whatever ours may be) over months and years.

Spinal breathing is not necessarily for preserving sexual energy -- it is for awakening and balancing ascending and descending pranas in the sushumna between root and brow -- a much broader function than only preserving sexual energy. Once sexual energy is being cultivated via tantric methods, then spinal breathing can do more with it. It comes after certain basics are occurring...

As for losing desire, that may be a shift to inner ecstatic, but it sounds like maybe not. Not sure what is happening there. The spiritual transformation is to more desire, refining to never-ending gentleness of love, becoming divine and going inward and upward feeding into the processes of spiritual biology higher up. All of this requires development of the spiritual biology via the means in sitting practices -- deep meditation, spinal breathing (in sitting practices, not sex), mudras, bandhas, samyama, etc. All this is built up step-by-step over a long time, as we discussed in other topics. Rome was not built in a day.

The AYP lessons provide a recommended sequence and methodology for doing all this.

So, sex is only one aspect, and putting spinal breathing into it in the beginning is premature in my opinion, with so many other important aspects to be addressed first. Just learning gradually to be more preorgasmic via the means in the tantra lessons is plenty for now.

And, no, meditation is not for doing right after sexual activity, tantric or not. Twice per day before morning and evening meal and activities is the formula for meditation.

All the best on your path.

And happy holidays, everyone!

The guru is in you.

2006/03/08 10:38:29
Support for AYP Pranayama, Mudras and Bandhas
http://www.aypsite.org/forum/topic.asp?TOPIC_ID=652&REPLY_ID=4236&whichpage=-1
managing the practice of spinal breathing

Hi Katrine:

It all sounds very good. You might check Victor's topic over here which looks at the relationship of eyes and prana movements, including tie-in of the root. It leads to what I call the "whole body mudra," (see "Micro Movements" in the Topic Index) where all the mudras and bandhas come together automatically in subtle form to advance the ecstatic response in us. Then it all becomes one. It is a stepping stone to merging all that ecstatic activity with inner silence. Then it pours out into our life energetically and in acts of divine love.

The thread to rope to column to whole body consumed spinal nerve/sushumna progression is a parallel process in all of this development. As it advances, the contrasting experiences of energy flow in and around the spinal nerve decrease as there is more purification and less friction. At the same time the energy flow will be 1000 times more, and we will barely notice in our stillness. It is stillness in action! We become a channel of that vast divine flow into the world.

All the best!

The guru is in you.

2005/12/22 17:01:25
Support for AYP Pranayama, Mudras and Bandhas
http://www.aypsite.org/forum/topic.asp?TOPIC_ID=663&REPLY_ID=2098&whichpage=-1
strange "purification?"

Hi All:

I'd be remiss in not confessing to having similar experiences in the past -- mine were mainly brain stem (medulla) related, and have long since cleared up. It is a razor's edge, you know -- when to let symptoms work themselves out and when to go to the doctor. The good news is that, if it is spiritual purification, an episode generally does clear up quickly (assuming good self-pacing in practices), and then we see the world in a new light, literally...

The "gurus" are hands off on discussing things like this (including the gamut of kundalini symptoms) for obvious reasons. I think we have a larger responsibility here in "open source" AYP to develop and deliver a good working knowledge to the public for all that happens on the road to enlightenment. Otherwise, how can yoga ever evolve into a well-documented and successfully applied science?

So, we have to ask the question from time to time -- "Is this particular symptom spiritual purification or is it medical?" and sort through it. I have been in favor of these kinds of public discussions on symptoms since the beginning, as can be seen in the AYP lessons. We can no longer afford to be sweeping the workings of spiritual evolution under the rug, no matter how messy it might be at times. It is certainly not messier than childbirth. It just takes longer... :-)

At the same time, we have to be alert to medical issues that may arise in our life (see this recent post). Interestingly, yoga practices will very often reduce or cure a medical issue, even while occasionally producing spiritual symptoms! So this can be very complicated stuff.

Fortunately, we are getting a good handle on the main controls of yoga in AYP, and so far we have seen fairly few major disruptions from spiritual purification, and lots of visible progress instead. It is my hope that we will continue to refine our ability to manage the process of human spiritual transformation in ways that will enable anyone to approach the task with confidence, safety and good results.

The guru is in you.

2006/01/09 09:09:09
Support for AYP Pranayama, Mudras and Bandhas
http://www.aypsite.org/forum/topic.asp?TOPIC_ID=709&REPLY_ID=2398&whichpage=-1
Questions on Siddhasana

Hi Alvin:

If you sit on a soft surface, like the bed, with back support, the foot will sink reducing excessive pressure and the hips will be level and resting on the bed also. Siddhasana in AYP is intended to be a comfortable seat with some sexual stimulation going upward, overlapping whatever other practice we are doing. The time to build the habit is in spinal breathing. Then eventually it will be comfortable in meditation and other sitting practices too.

Hands can go anywhere that is comfortable. In AYP we regard hand mudras, like chin or jnana, to be effect (automatic yoga) rather than cause.

The guru is in you.

2006/01/09 12:45:55
Support for AYP Pranayama, Mudras and Bandhas
http://www.aypsite.org/forum/topic.asp?TOPIC_ID=709&REPLY_ID=2411&whichpage=-1

Questions on Siddhasana

Hi Alvin and David:

The root of the lingam goes up into the body before the anus and it is in the space between lingam root entry and anus where siddhasana is done, preferably with fairly light and adjustable pressure on the organ itself. With some practice this is quite easy to do on a soft surface with back support. The idea is not to crush the root of the lingam (David's caution on this is well-advised). It is to apply light pressure upward behind it -- the same place where blocking is done in tantra -- the hollow behind the pubic bone and root of the lingam, in front of the anus. This hollow area is analogous with the location of a woman's yoni opening. For further clarification on location, see here for a discussion of female and male aspects of siddhasana: http://www.aypsite.org/T28.html

Mulabandha/asvini joins in the process via the anus.

If you check "siddhasana" in the AYP lessons topic index (near top of list), you will find much more on this: http://www.aypsite.org/TopicIndex.html

The guru is in you.

PS -- Meg, we crossed notes on this one, but I believe the female side of it is covered here, at least as far as AYP goes to date. Lesson T28 above describes the traditional approach to siddhasana for women. Yes, feedback on siddhasana from the ladies would be welcome so we can refine this knowledge. There are yoginis I have been in touch with over the past few years who are using this method (and variations) with good ecstatic stimulation. Everyone has to find their own "sweet spot" in siddhasana.

2006/01/12 07:58:37
Support for AYP Pranayama, Mudras and Bandhas
http://www.aypsite.org/forum/topic.asp?TOPIC_ID=709&REPLY_ID=2499&whichpage=-1
Questions on Siddhasana

Hi Alvin:

The approach to siddhasana in the AYP lessons has been in use here for over 20 years with no deleterious effects. To the contrary, siddhasana has been an essential component in cultivating ecstatic conductivity. But not the sole component -- it is a combination of the means presented that brings about the transformation. In time, these become naturally integrated, forming what the lessons call the "whole body mudra."

The guru is in you.

2006/01/12 10:28:23
Support for AYP Pranayama, Mudras and Bandhas
http://www.aypsite.org/forum/topic.asp?TOPIC_ID=709&REPLY_ID=2505&whichpage=-1
Questions on Siddhasana

Hi again:

There is also the old stand-by, especially favored by the ladies -- the rolled up sock. Where there is the will, there is a way.

The guru is in you.

2006/01/13 23:04:43
Support for AYP Pranayama, Mudras and Bandhas
http://www.aypsite.org/forum/topic.asp?TOPIC_ID=709&REPLY_ID=2532&whichpage=-1
Questions on Siddhasana

Hi Srinivasan:

Sounds like a very good routine. Not sure about the Iyengar anuloma-viloma pranayama. Maybe some of the Iyengar folks here can comment on that. If you find too much energy flowing later on it can be from inadvertently "doubling up" on pranayama. It can happen when using several styles, thinking they are not cumulative. They are, and sometimes it can lead to too much overall "restraint of breath" in a session or day. So be careful with that, and the delayed energy reaction that can happen with pranayama. A reasonable program of spinal breathing (5-10 minutes before meditation) and not overdoing with other styles of pranayama in our early days is the best insurance for avoiding undesirable energy buildups. These buildups are often invisible until a big release happens. Ka-boom! We have seen a few of those around here, and we are all getting smarter about pacing our practices as a result.

Yes, any sensations out of the ordinary are pranic energy flow, unless you are cutting off blood supply to your organ in siddhasana. That has been discussed already -- not the end of the world for short periods, but not something you want to be doing constantly.

You did not mention sambhavi. It is a companion to mulabandha. The two practices cover both ends of the sushumna for aiding spinal breathing in cultivating and balancing the energies in the spinal nerve and throughout the entire nervous system.

You did not mention kechari either -- not necessarily going for a higher stage right away -- just getting started in stage 1 -- tongue up to the roof of the mouth in spinal breathing for starters.

Don't load all of this extra stuff into meditation until it is happening there automatically as established habit. We do not divide our attention with any other practice in deep meditation. That is an important guideline.

I mention developing sambhavi and kechari (in spinal breathing) because, interestingly, it is the upper mudras that ultimately have the greatest influence on lower center (and all) openings -- one of those spiritual paradoxes. That is why we start mulabandha and sambhavi pretty much together once spinal breathing is stable. And siddhasana and kechari add to the simultaneous upper and lower cultivation. It is a sort of layering of increasing stimulation as and when we are ready.

Of course, all of this all depends on maintaining a good and unfettered routine of deep meditation, and the rise of inner silence it brings. It sounds like you have that end of it in good shape.

All the best on you path. Enjoy!

The guru is in you.

2006/01/17 13:40:07
Support for AYP Pranayama, Mudras and Bandhas
http://www.aypsite.org/forum/topic.asp?TOPIC_ID=709&REPLY_ID=2598&whichpage=-1
Questions on Siddhasana

Hi again Srinivasan:

Well, a lack of negative symptoms is certainly not a sign of doing pranayama incorrectly. Progress with pranayama really depends on a well-rounded practice with deep meditation involved. It takes time, according to the process of purification occurring in the individual nervous system. "Progress" does not mean big chaotic energy releases that can disrupt our practice and our life. We are not looking for that. A "break through" strategy with too much breath retention (kumbhaka) will not be a stable path. It is, in fact, slower than a steady less dramatic unfoldment over the long term. So the advice is to aim for the long term rather than the short.

On siddhasana, the same goes -- just easy comfortable sitting. Nothing extreme. This can be aided by using back support on a soft surface for more comfort and better regulation of angle and pressure. Bringing the heel back a bit further toward the anus aids in control too. These means are not mandatory. Nothing is in AYP. Only suggested if better comfort and control are desired. Comfort in siddhasana makes the other sitting practices easier too.

As for what to look for in siddhasana -- some find ecstatic stimulation right away. For others, it takes a while. It is closely related to one's inclination toward tantric methods in general. Siddhasana is a tantric method, though is claimed by several branches of yoga that are non-tantric also. Well, all of yoga and tantra are coming from one place -- the human nervous system. No matter how we slice it, siddhasana is for regulated pre-orgasmic sexual stimulation in sitting practices. We each are free to find it, or not, according to our tendencies. Like pranayama, mudras and bandhas, the effects in siddhasana are dependent on the rise of inner silence in the nervous system. So it always comes back to daily meditation.

The guru is in you.
(you may call me Yogani -- no special titles are necessary. Your appreciation of the knowledge is greatly appreciated here, so the admiration goes both ways. :-))

2006/01/10 11:25:47
Support for AYP Pranayama, Mudras and Bandhas
http://www.aypsite.org/forum/topic.asp?TOPIC_ID=714&REPLY_ID=2440&whichpage=-1
Kechari and spinal breathing

Hi Darvish:

We form the habits of mudra in spinal breathing. When they become automatic, they show up naturally in meditation and other areas of our practice. Yes, that includes kechari.

This is covered in several places in the AYP lessons, including nuances. Perhaps you should review. Check the topic index and site search feature to zero in on particular aspects of practice.

The guru is in you.

2006/01/10 11:03:48
Support for AYP Pranayama, Mudras and Bandhas
http://www.aypsite.org/forum/topic.asp?TOPIC_ID=715&REPLY_ID=2439&whichpage=-1
Mouth of God(medulla oblongata)

Hi Darvish:

The medulla is part of the third eye. See "OM" in the glossary for a quick description and reference to the "mouth of God."
http://www.aypsite.org/glossary.html

Also see "ajna" and "third eye" in the topic index for lots of lessons touching on this from the point of view of practices.
http://www.aypsite.org/TopicIndex.html

Also try a site search on "medulla" http://www.aypsite.org/SiteSearch.html

Anyone who has rising ecstatic conductivity will have experience with the medulla in relation to the opening sushumna and the rest of the neurobiology. This has direct relationship to the AYP practices.

The guru is in you.

2006/01/23 10:55:20
Support for AYP Pranayama, Mudras and Bandhas
http://www.aypsite.org/forum/topic.asp?TOPIC_ID=763
Chin Pump - Where to Put Attention?

Hi All

The below on chin pump is from a recent email. It also ties in with the "under the hood" chakra discussion here:
http://www.aypsite.org/forum/topic.asp?TOPIC_ID=753

Q: Thank you for your lessons. I have begun practicing meditation again after a long period of disinterest and frustration.

One question about the chin pump. The technique is very similar to a traditional kriya method, with one difference. The attention stays at the point between the eyebrows instead of going down to the heart with each swoop. You mention that the chin pump pumps energy between the head and the heart. How does that happen if the attention stays at the point between the eyebrows?

Thank you again for your help.

A: Sambhavi activates the entire sushumna, especially with ecstatic conductivity coming up. This covers the full range from root to brow, including enlivening the energy in the heart area. The chin pump itself is a physical technique, and it is the physicality of it that circulates the enlivened energy between heart and head, and also much broader in the nervous system, as discussed in the AYP lessons. So the physical positioning of eyes (and brow) in sambhavi is opening the full channel, while the physical movement of the head/neck is doing the circulating. The attention traces the spinal nerve up and down on inhale and exhale as in spinal breathing, and stays out the front with sambhavi during breath retention as in yoni mudra kumbhaka. Chin pump lite (an alternate approach also covered in the lessons) does not not involve breath retention, so in that case it is spinal breathing all the way through with attention cycling up and down the sushumna the whole time rather than fixed out through the brow during retention. Sambhavi (eyes up - sushumna enlivened) can be maintained throughout.

The technique works, and is one of the most powerful in the AYP tool kit for building on ecstatic conductivity to more advanced stages. The reality of that dynamic is more important than any explanation of it I can give. AYP chin pump is also much simpler than other forms found in the kriya traditions. Simplicity and effectiveness -- that is what we aim for in AYP.

I should also mention that in AYP we do not do "chakra work," including any particular focusing of attention other than to open the entire sushumna, which covers all of the spiritual neurobiology, including the chakras. In AYP we regard the detailed operations of all that to be "under the hood." We drive the car with the simple master controls (of the sushumna), and do not try and do it with our head in the gearbox (the chakras). This is discussed in several places in the lessons.

In time, chin pump becomes a very organic function, part of our natural spiritual biology. It can be very subtle at times also, not physically noticeable from the outside. The large physical movements we do with mudras, bandhas, etc. in sitting practices lead to ongoing refined activity in the nervous throughout the day which eventually becomes more powerful than the big physical movements have been. That is how it goes with rising ecstatic conductivity. Less becomes more ... it is a natural development inside us that we are cultivating with yoga practices.

Wishing you all the best on your path. Enjoy!

Then guru in is you.

2006/02/05 23:03:59
Support for AYP Pranayama, Mudras and Bandhas
http://www.aypsite.org/forum/topic.asp?TOPIC_ID=792&REPLY_ID=3082&whichpage=-1
How long is one spinal breath?

Hi Bliss:

What Victor has described is also the approach in AYP. The breath will find its own correct length with gentle favoring of slowing down, and it will tend toward a longer exhale than inhale. Ujjayi plays a role in this -- open throat on the way in and restricted epiglottis on the way out. See lesson #41 for the overall spinal breathing procedure. And see lesson #62 for a specific answer to your question on the length of a spinal breathing cycle.

Happy spinal breathing! :-)

The guru is in you.

2006/02/06 12:05:10
Support for AYP Pranayama, Mudras and Bandhas
http://www.aypsite.org/forum/topic.asp?TOPIC_ID=792&REPLY_ID=3105&whichpage=-1
How long is one spinal breath?

Hi Bliss:

That is one covered in the AYP Easy Lessons book. In AYP, ujjayi on the inhale is not suggested because it creates negative pressure in the lungs. So does external kumbhaka (external breath retention), which is not recommended to be done for long periods either. The reason is because the lungs are not designed for long term negative pressure (vacuum), and it can be unhealthy. Safety first, you know.

This does not mean we avoid all negative lung pressure. We use it in uddiyana and nauli. It can happen spontaneously during meditation and spinal breathing (an external suspension of breath -- not much pressure involved with this). That's fine. We can notice it and then easily go back to the practice we are doing. We don't make a deliberate effort to put negative pressure in the lungs over extended periods.

On the other hand, postive pressure (internal retention) in the lungs is natural and we can do that as much as our practices with good self-pacing call for. Hence the use of ujjayi on exhale during spinal breathing. The practice is built on leveraging our natural capabilities for purification and opening to the divine within, just as all yoga should be.

The guru is in you.

2006/02/15 10:48:33
Support for AYP Pranayama, Mudras and Bandhas

Sunburn

Hi Katrine:

I know what you mean about crossing over from chasing after spiritual results (replace with "kundalini" if you like) to having spiritual results chasing after us. It is both a confirmation and a challenge.

On the spinal breathing, make sure you are doing the full cycle, slow and easy, between brow (not crown) and root, and not deliberately stopping in breath suspension on either end. That way you will be bringing energy down from the brow and marrying it with energy being brought up from the root. This is the best inner energy stabilizer I know and can help resolve all sorts of imbalances. But it is not a panacea for everything. Sometimes it just takes time and balanced living to even things out after big new energy openings like you have had.

I had them 20 years ago, initially without the benefit of spinal breathing, and that is reflected in the experiences described in the Secrets of Wilder novel. Talk about sunburn!

While inner silence may be the underlying factor in all of this, it is also what gives us the fortitude (inner center) to weather just about anything that happens. In AYP we work to make the whole process smooth and comfortable. For folks coming in with pre-existing overload (or a strong tendency in that direction), the AYP methods can help, but every case is unique, of course, so we do the best we can. One thing I can promise: Unlike lots of traditions, we will not run away from your (or anyone's) wild kundalini symptoms. We enjoy doing the work and being a mutual support system, you know. What are spiritual friends for anyway? :-) (note the sunglasses)

Maybe you have been through lesson 69 already. If not, check it out -- that is a laundry list of kundalini symptoms and measures that can help. Don't forget physical exercise -- "grounding" is important when the energy is jamming in the upper centers.

Not sure what you mean by "extreme pitta diet," but here is an ayurvedic dosha-based "yes/no" food list that might be helpful: http://www.aypsite.org/ayurveda-diets.html When the energy is running like what you have, the tone of the diet can make a big difference. Also, a heavier diet can help slow down the energies during peak periods.

Well, those are a few suggestions. The most important thing is to be proactive in managing causes and effects as best as possible. In AYP, we call it self-pacing. You are an old hand at this sort of thing, and I know you will be fine. Hopefully we can add a few useful tools here that can help you smooth out the ride.

All the best!

The guru is in you.

2006/03/07 19:04:33
Support for AYP Pranayama, Mudras and Bandhas
http://www.aypsite.org/forum/topic.asp?TOPIC_ID=879&REPLY_ID=4202&whichpage=-1
Eyes as a key to opening prana

Hi Victor:

Are you saying that your eyes stay pretty much in one place relative to a point in front of you as the head goes around? Then the eyes would go up relative to head when the head goes down, and the eyes would go down relative to the head when the head goes back. Left and right too on a chin pump rotation. I have not worked with this, but can see right away that it has a direct effect on the energy flow. Any eye movement will when ecstatic conductivity is present. Then there are all sorts of possibilities.

A more common form of "dynamic" sambhavi is letting the eyes automatically and gently "flex" upward and release in coordination with mulabandha/asvini. With ecstatic conductivity present, this also has a large influence on the pranic energy flow in the body. It is stimulating the spinal nerve on both ends simultaneously. In fact, with ecstatic conductivity, it is difficult not to flex one without flexing the other. The connection is that intimate and instant, not to mention very enjoyable. It is a stepping stone on the way to the merging of our ecstatic energy with inner silence, and then the radiant outpouring that comes from that.

I am sure there will be many further explorations along these lines as more and more yogis and yoginis come into ecstatic conductivity. That is an intimate neurological connection between the third eye (area from center brow to medulla/brain stem) and the root/perineum. Kechari is involved in this also.

Onward and upward! Ecstatically, of course. :-)

The guru is in you.

PS -- Don't forget to self-pace, taking into account time-delayed effects.

2006/03/15 11:20:15
Support for AYP Pranayama, Mudras and Bandhas
http://www.aypsite.org/forum/topic.asp?TOPIC_ID=895&REPLY_ID=4499&whichpage=-1
Perineum Stimulation Tool

Hi Y and all:

The "circuit" of heel on perineum is not a key factor. The gentle pressure is, when one is ready for it, and it sounds like you have a good approach.

There is some benefit in sitting cross-legged. This has to do with opening the hips more than creating a circuit. But, as mentioned in the lessons, crossed legs are not mandatory either.

If a circuit happens later on, fine. If not, that is okay. The rising energy will take care of it as needed, and as one is able. Same thing with thumbs joining index fingers. These are effects (automatic yoga) more than causes. Are these circuit things necessary for enlightenment? Not as far as I can tell. It is much easier to make progress while comfortable. In fact, comfort in sitting practices is more of a prerequisite than any particular body position. Then we can be doing the techniques instead of being excessively distracted by the body.

Enjoy!

The guru is in you.

2006/03/22 10:20:33
Support for AYP Pranayama, Mudras and Bandhas
http://www.aypsite.org/forum/topic.asp?TOPIC_ID=899&REPLY_ID=4877&whichpage=-1
sequencing to extend Kumbhaka effortlessly

Hi Alvin and Vicki:

The interesting thing about bastrika is that the more energy we have flowing, the less intense practice we need to continue with good progress and comfort. The energy takes over the process to a large degree, so we end up tweaking and letting go rather than hammering. This applies with all yoga practices. That is where the "less is more" phrase comes from.

So, as long as you are flexible about it, you will be okay. At the first sign of rapid energy flow, better take your foot off the accelerator a bit, or you could fly off the cliff. Increasing inner flow can manifest as excess emotions, like Shanti suggests, or in many other ways ranging from the sublime to the ridiculous. When it happens, just be a safe driver with prudent self-pacing and you will be fine.

Jim gave you some good perspective on this above. Of course, we all have to go through a certain amount of our own trial and error to find our unique pace and limits. It is usually not good enough to do what someone else says verbatim, based on an experience we have not had yet. So, we push and find out for ourselves. There is nothing wrong with this as long as we know when to lighten up. It is our journey and we have to learn how to travel it within ourselves.

Let me also add that with all practices, especially pranayama and kumbhaka, there can be a delayed effect. So while we may not feel like much is happening right now, if we push too hard, we can find ourselves with too much happening when we least expect it. It is all part of the learning curve. Don't run scared. Just run smart. That's what we are working on constantly here -- practical applications of the means for purification and opening. And then we have it all on our own -- permanent self-contained ecstatic bliss pouring out all over the place! :-)

The guru is in you.

2006/03/22 13:24:06
Support for AYP Pranayama, Mudras and Bandhas
http://www.aypsite.org/forum/topic.asp?TOPIC_ID=899&REPLY_ID=4883&whichpage=-1
sequencing to extend Kumbhaka effortlessly

Hi Alvin:

Yes, we definitely build up according to our inclination (bhakti) and capacity. The latter, "capacity," becomes a much bigger factor once our energy is flowing abundantly. Then we are limited by the energy flow and corresponding rate of purification we can tolerate in daily life, rather than by how much more we can pile on in practices.

Katrine spoke about this shift quite beautifully in one of her early posts. If I can find it, I will add a link here. My own way of explaining it is to say that for years I was chasing the goddess, and then one day I realized she was chasing me! That is what happens when kundalini gets active. We move from being instigator to being partner. Being a partner with kundalini (our active inner energy) is tweaking and letting go, rather than hammering. In that condition, if we are hammering, we will get hammered. That is why the folks around here with active inner energy raise an eyebrow when you talk about doing umpteen rounds of bastrika, kumbhaka, etc. I mean, that is way more than is necessary once the lights go on inside, and probably long before that, as Shanti points out in the previous post.

It is really easy to get the message and ease up on intense practices when the energy takes off (and/or crashes). We learn to let go -- the greatest lesson we can have in life, coming directly from within us. Then we don't need books and all sorts of advice anymore. We become the book and the advice is in our increasingly radiant nervous system. Pretty good deal, actually.

In that sense, yoga is not like physical exercise, though there are still parallels -- conditioning ourselves for a particular function being the most obvious. But once the spiritual conditioning reaches a certain point, a vast energy and intelligence is awakened within us that will carry us forward along with our practices in moderation. That is where yoga departs from the analogy of physical athletics and enters an entirely new realm.

We are obliged to conduct ourselves accordingly. To ignore the reality of where we are arriving and how things work there, hanging on to other models we have been using (like athletic conditioning), can lead to some tough lessons in the school of hard knocks. The lessons don't have to be hard to learn, especially with a few folks around who have already or are currently going through the same thing.

Of course, all of this rides on inner silence, cultivated in daily deep meditation. Have I brought that up lately? :-)

The guru is in you.

2006/03/23 09:14:52
Support for AYP Pranayama, Mudras and Bandhas
http://www.aypsite.org/forum/topic.asp?TOPIC_ID=899&REPLY_ID=4930&whichpage=-1
sequencing to extend Kumbhaka effortlessly

Hi Alvin:

The fastest progress comes with long term stable daily practice, without too much overdoing or underdoing. Either one can bring disruptions in progress. This is why self-pacing is so important.

Jim can tell you about his experience when he stopped for a few weeks. His case is probably more dramatic than most, but illustrates the point.

Sure, there are times when we are all pinched for time, and we do the best we can with our practices. See lesson 209 for a detailed discussion on this -- http://www.aypsite.org/209.html

The guru is in you.

2006/03/31 14:45:51
Support for AYP Pranayama, Mudras and Bandhas
http://www.aypsite.org/forum/topic.asp?TOPIC_ID=1003&REPLY_ID=5447&whichpage=-1
yoni chin pump

Hi Shanti:

No need to rush into yoni chin pump. It is a tool for energy cultivation that is useful when we are pretty far down the road. Regular chin pump is a high octane practice, as many of us know. Adding yoni to it makes it much more powerful, like rocketship powerful. For those who feel stable in all of their practices and wish to try it, just do one or two retentions with yoni as part of the normal chin pump session and see how it feels in daily activity. Then adjust accordingly. Self-pacing.

If I had a dollar for every time I got lost in samyama, we could give AYP books away to everyone. :-) Just easily come back to the practice when you realize you are off it. It is purification you are going through, a natural part of the process. That is good! If time runs short and you have to go, then it is okay not to finish the sutras. There is always next time. Just be sure to take some rest before getting up.

Like everything else, samyama will vary over time according to the cycles of purification that are going on. So, we self-pace that as necessary too.

In the case of getting lost a lot, maybe put a time limit that you are comfortable with, and then stop. It will come back together as the obstructions clear out. If there is no discomfort in activity after a long samyama session from getting lost a lot, then let it take as long as it wants to, or for as long as you have time for. Your choice.

The guru is in you.

2006/04/04 07:18:29
Support for AYP Pranayama, Mudras and Bandhas
http://www.aypsite.org/forum/topic.asp?TOPIC_ID=1014
Emergence of Side Channels in Spinal Breathing

Hi All:

Just a reminder below from my email on favoring the spinal nerve when side channel (ida/pingala) activity begins to emerge. This will expand over time, gradually yielding the rope, column and all-consuming whirling energy vortex experiences. Then it all smooths out as purification advances and friction becomes less. Then we feel minimal friction, even as the whole world becomes contained in our energy field -- stillness moving ever-outward on our ecstatic radiance, the emergence of conscious omnipresence. All the while we continue to favor the spinal nerve in the center during our spinal breathing sessions. There is more on this in the new Spinal Breathing book, which should be on Amazon in a week or two.

Q: For the past 2 days my spinal breathing has been different, moving up and down is like a ribbon, not a column any more, moving up is along the middle and left and is blue, moving down is along the middle and right, and is red. I have been trying to adjust it so it is a column again and is centered, but it keeps going back to a ribbon and off center, should I let it go?

A: The experience sounds nice. However, we always favor the procedure of the practice, no matter what the experience may be. That means favoring the center of the spinal column -- the spinal nerve. No strain. We don't fight the experience, whatever it is. It is just a favoring of the central nerve. There will be many more experiences like this on one, both or all sides. They come from favoring the center channel -- they are effect rather than cause. They are purification and opening

The guru is in you.

2006/04/04 11:32:09
Support for AYP Pranayama, Mudras and Bandhas
http://www.aypsite.org/forum/topic.asp?TOPIC_ID=1014&REPLY_ID=5605&whichpage=-1
Emergence of Side Channels in Spinal Breathing

Hi Katrine:

Isn't it wonderful how so many here are having similar experiences? The telltale signs of the journey are revealed.

It all rides on the cultivation of inner silence and ecstatic conductivity, which we do with the core practices of deep meditation and spinal breathing. All the other methods we use are expansions on or utilizations of these two qualities. In time the two become One, and that is a new dynamic.

This theme of the marriage of polarities is common in the traditions. We are giving it a good dose of practical application and exposure here. One of the best public airings of such phenomena ever. And lo and behold, we find that the metaphorical dance of Shiva and Shakti is none other than the dance of our own emerging enlightenment!

The guru is in you.

2006/04/10 10:18:32

Support for AYP Pranayama, Mudras and Bandhas
http://www.aypsite.org/forum/topic.asp?TOPIC_ID=1029&REPLY_ID=5815&whichpage=-1
Paramhansa Yogananda

Hi All:

Spinal breathing is the mainstay of the kriya tradition, of which Yogananda is an important a part -- the part that came west.

The various lines in kriya teach spinal breathing with different nuances, reflecting style and local culture.

Norman Paulsen, a direct disciple of Yogananda, teaches some deliberate breath suspension in his style of spinal breathing, though I do not believe it is involved in Yogananda's SRF style kriya. See Paulsen's book "Sacred Science" on this. Yoni mudra is a different story, which nearly always involves breath retention, and is part of the kriya lines also.

In AYP we don't use deliberate breath suspension in spinal breathing -- this is reinforced in the new Spinal Breathing book. But we do use it in other practices, as comfortable, like yoni mudra and chin pump, which is standard for these practices in the kriya lines and elsewhere.

So, except for removing the style and cultural add-ons, the AYP treatment of both spinal breathing pranayama and kumbhaka (breath suspension) is pretty standard. What is vastly different in AYP is the flexibility to independently integrate complementary practices (like spinal breathing and deep meditation) and self-pace as necessary. That is a big step forward, enabling highly efficient self-directed practice instead of having to run to "the guru" for every little thing, and then end up in trouble anyway due to the absence of ability to engage in self-pacing on the fly as needed.

With self-pacing, it becomes clear that slow deep breathing and kumbhaka are simply variations on the same principle of restraint of breath, and that we can regulate the application of this principle up or down according to the results we are seeing from our practice -- cause and effect. In this way we can maintain good progress with comfort and safety.

It should also be mentioned that AYP adds back some things that were down-played or removed from many of the teachings that came west from India in the last century. Kechari mudra is one example. A clear presentation of tantric sexual principles is another. Things like these were generally regarded to be "too much" for westerners at the time, and maybe for easterners too. Probably right. But times have changed, yes? :-)

Make no mistake about it, we are standing on the shoulders of giants like Yogananda as we forge ahead into the 21st century. Without them, where would we be? If our successors can benefit half as much from our practical application of the principles of human spiritual transformation, then we will have done our job.

The guru is in you.

2006/04/10 23:40:52
Support for AYP Pranayama, Mudras and Bandhas
http://www.aypsite.org/forum/topic.asp?TOPIC_ID=1029&REPLY_ID=5840&whichpage=-1
Paramhansa Yogananda

Hi Near:

No, deliberate suspension is not part of AYP spinal breathing. It can happen naturally, and then we just favor the procedure of our spinal breathing practice when we notice.

This is not to say deliberate breath suspension is taboo in spinal breathing. It just makes self-pacing more complicated for beginning and intermediate practice, and is not recommended for that reason. In fact, it is not necessary to ever use it to achieve the desired result, because there is plenty of kumbhaka happening in a full scope AYP routine already -- more than most of us need, actually, so it is not a matter of more, but less. Less is more once ecstatic conductivity gets going. And before then we don't want to be forcing it too much.

I agree with what Victor says about it -- keep it as easy and natural as possible. That is the ideal guideline.

The guru is in you.

2006/04/15 11:14:05
Support for AYP Pranayama, Mudras and Bandhas
http://www.aypsite.org/forum/topic.asp?TOPIC_ID=1044&REPLY_ID=6002&whichpage=-1
Spinal Breathing/Kriya Pranayama
Welcome aboard, BluesFan!

You have gotten some good pointers on the hatha extras you can add step-by-step as you go through the AYP lessons that are geared to the cultivation of whole body ecstatic conductivity.

But way more important than that from the AYP point of view is getting established and stabilized in the core practices of spinal breathing and deep meditation, in sequence, not at the same time.

What AYP adds to the scenario is mantra yoga-style deep meditation right after spinal breathing, which is a breakthrough in efficiency and results. While kriya includes meditation after spinal breathing, it is OM nada, which is not nearly as consistent as mantra meditation when done correctly. With deep meditation, the full benefits of spinal breathing will emerge much sooner, because the dynamics of inner silence interacting with ecstatic conductivity are greatly enhanced.

Additionally, in AYP we do not attempt to meditate during spinal breathing (with mantra, chakras or breath), which enhances the cultivation process of spinal breathing itself. Simplicity has its advantages.

Well, these are some differences between AYP and Kriya Yoga, which folks may agree with or not. Just thought I'd point out some of the salient points, which are particularly important to grasp before jumping headlong into the rest of the AYP lessons. Better to have the basics covered first.

AYP is self-directed and open source, so it is always your choice on how to integrate your practices and proceed.

Wishing you all the best on your path. Practice wisely, and enjoy!

The guru is in you.

2006/04/30 12:51:08
Support for AYP Pranayama, Mudras and Bandhas
http://www.aypsite.org/forum/topic.asp?TOPIC_ID=1088&REPLY_ID=6492&whichpage=-1
A couple of questions

Hi Bluesfan, Meg and Shanti:

Some good solid feedback here on spinal breathing and on what to put in the body. It is great to see you all working it out so well, and with good humor too. :-) The same goes for other recent discussions where the questioner needed some clear guidance. You all are making my job easier. Thank you!

On the attention cycling with breath in spinal breathing, if during our journey up and down the spinal nerve during slow deep breathing, we find our attention off into internal or external experiences, sensations or other stimuli, then we just easily go back to our practice of slow deep breathing up and down the spinal nerve. It is normal to lose track of what we are doing and be off into other sensations, thoughts and feelings. When we do, we just simply re-engage the process of spinal breathing again. When we realize we are off it, we just easily come back.

If we have some difficulty visualizing and tracing the spinal nerve as a tiny thread or tube, then it is perfectly all right to follow the spinal column in a less specific way. Over time, we will find more definition in our practice. There is no need to strain or struggle in our visualization. The main thing is that we end up at the brow at the completion of inhalation and at the root at the completion of exhalation. How we get back and forth is less important than traveling from one end to the other without strain during our slow deep breathing. In time, it all comes together.

Sometimes, there can be noticeable resistance in the process of spinal breathing. There can be several causes.

In the beginning, the most common cause of resistance is the newness of it. We all go through a certain amount of awkwardness as we are learning the practice. The first time we got on a bicycle, did we just ride off smoothly? Of course not. It took some practice, some getting used to. Then, after a while, riding the bicycle became easier. Spinal breathing is like that. There will be degrees of awkwardness. Some will take to it easily, while others may need some time to adjust in the beginning. Keep in mind that it is a simple process, and it does not have to be perfect. All of spinal breathing is a favoring – favoring slow deep breathing, and favoring a pathway inside the spine between root and brow. When we wander off, or feel stuck, we just easily come back to it.

There is another reason for resistance in spinal breathing – obstructions in the nervous system. These are neurobiological restrictions within us that we have carried throughout our life. With spinal breathing, we are coaxing them to relax and release. In the beginning, the resistance from these inner knots can be quite palpable. Some people may find it difficult to pass through a particular area of the inner body with attention and breath traveling up and down inside. The resistance can be found anywhere – the pelvis, solar plexus, heart, throat, or in the head. The resistance can be felt as a blockage that we can't get past, or as some pressure.

What do we do? It is simple. If there is a pressure or a resistance, we just go right by it with our attention and breath. Easily right by it. We never try and force through inner resistance. We just stroke it gently with our attention and breath as we go by. This has a good purifying effect, and will not be uncomfortable. Discomfort comes from forcing against an obstruction. We never do this in spinal breathing. We just whisk on through. What we did not dissolve on the first pass, we will get on the next one, or the next, or the 10,000th pass, maybe years later in our practice. That is how we purify the inner neurobiology. And all the while, we will have the experience of less resistance accompanied by more clarity and fluidity. Then traveling the spinal nerve will be easy. Even when there is resistance, we can still cover the full length of the spinal nerve like that.

For more on this, see the Spinal Breathing Pranayama book.

On tracing the spinal nerve physically with the eyes along with attention in spinal breathing, lesson 131 discusses why we'd like to separate the physical position of our eyes from our attention, and provides a practical exercise for easing away from that. It is called, "Coordinating Sambhavi and Spinal Breathing" -- http://www.aypsite.org/131.html

All the best!

The guru is in you.

2006/04/30 13:42:43
Support for AYP Pranayama, Mudras and Bandhas
http://www.aypsite.org/forum/topic.asp?TOPIC_ID=1088&REPLY_ID=6494&whichpage=-1
A couple of questions

quote:
_____
Originally posted by Shanti

I think Bluesfan's question was.. while breathing in.. and following your awareness up the spine.. lets say you are half way up your spine.. and you lung is full.. you cannot breath in any more.. what do you do..
1-hold your breath and finish your awareness travel up the spine..
2-breath out a little so you can continue breathing in and moving up,
3-start breathing out and move your awareness down from where you are.
4-Jump your awareness up and start breathing out and moving your awareness down..
5-None of the above
6-All of the above
Meg's solution is good.. let your awareness lead your breath.. but till he learns how to do it.. what would the right way be?
_____

Hi Shanti:

It is #4 -- jump the attention to the brow before exhalation, and on future inhalations favor bringing the attention to the brow with more continuity by favoring the by-passing of obstructions encountered along the way. It will not necessarily happen overnight, but this is the direction we would like to go in. If we favor it in this way, the habit will develop in time. In the meantime, we can end up at the brow at the end of inhalation and at the root at the end of exhalation. What is in-between we just brush through (or by-pass) along the way. It is inhale root to brow, and exhale brow to root, no matter what else may be going on, or how clucky it may be. With practice, it becomes easier and clarity and fluidity of the spinal nerve gradually emerge. And well-balanced ecstatic conductivity too!

The guru is in you.

2006/05/05 10:13:14
Support for AYP Pranayama, Mudras and Bandhas
http://www.aypsite.org/forum/topic.asp?TOPIC_ID=1099&REPLY_ID=6604&whichpage=-1
Spinal Breathing Pranayama book

Hi Anthem and Shanti.

Thank you for your kind remarks on the Spinal Breathing Pranayama book. Thanks also for the Amazon reviews. Yes, they are really helpful for those who are looking for different perspectives on what a book is about. When I am book shopping on Amazon, I always read the reviews, sometimes even before I read the book description.

Anthem, on the cool and warm currents, it has received clearer emphasis in the book mainly due to better organization of the material. I'm glad it is helping. Maybe if I keep rewriting it in more renditions, it will end up perfect. This was the fourth time through (Yahoo lessons, AYP book, Wilder...), not to mention the endless email exchanges over the past few years. Whew! :-)

Yes, the more refined our combined practices get the more powerful everything becomes. Fortunately, our capacity to conduct all this divine energy becomes much more also. It is a bit of a balancing act. Prudent self-pacing is what keeps the balance as we go ever-onward.

Carry on!

The guru is in you.

2006/05/05 12:18:09
Support for AYP Pranayama, Mudras and Bandhas
http://www.aypsite.org/forum/topic.asp?TOPIC_ID=1099&REPLY_ID=6613&whichpage=-1
Spinal Breathing Pranayama book

Hi Near:

Thanks to you also, and for your great Amazon review too! As far as absorbing knowledge goes, maybe we get it the first time through, or the second, or the third. Going through the lessons more than once, as Shanti suggests, is the traditional way of harvesting knowledge because, as our awareness changes over time, we see more each time through. This is especially true if we are meditating. We will see more when reading any spiritual book the second and third time. As Anthem points out, reading can become spiritual practice, complete with the potential for energy overloads. That goes for writing it too. What's going on here?!

From my side, I felt that something more could be added to help facilitate exposure, plus adding some useful refinements. That is, presenting the AYP knowledge in multiple ways over time so more people would be able to find it -- run across it, if you will. If everyone in the world could run across it somehow, that would be "perfection." Hence, online lessons, a textbook (probably two), a novel, and a growing pile of small practice-specific instruction books (maybe 10 by the time they are done). It is just my way of getting the knowledge "out there" in as many ways as possible.

Next comes the AYP Enlightenment Series books in audio-book form (Deep Meditation, Spinal Breathing Pranayama, Tantra, etc). Beginning next year, I hope.

I even have a crazy idea to write a screenplay for the Secrets of Wilder, and have been studying up a bit for that. Maybe in a year or two, as time permits. Doing a reasonable first pass on a screenplay is the way to help get that ball rolling. A movie could take a very long time to happen -- years and years. The process has to start somewhere, like here on this old computer. Any movie industry people out there? :-)

The guru is in you.

2006/05/12 19:08:42
Support for AYP Pranayama, Mudras and Bandhas
http://www.aypsite.org/forum/topic.asp?TOPIC_ID=1099&REPLY_ID=6866&whichpage=-1
Spinal Breathing Pranayama book

Hi Kathy:

Thank you for that wonderful feedback. I hope we can be helpful to everyone who is looking for paths of least resistance into their pure bliss consciousness and ecstatic conductivity.

Yes, those Amazon reviews do help a lot. We only have 7 on the Spinal Breathing book so far. Spinal Breathing reviews, anyone? :-)

Btw, there seems to be a new beginning of sorts happening in the TM world, or what was the TM world. Friends told us recently that some of the old-line TM teachers are splitting off and regrouping under a new name called "Transcendental Stress Management" and maybe under other names too. Maybe a legal thing has happened that has enabled them to do this? Not sure what it is all about, but, in splitting off, they are apparently opening up to broader teachings of yoga, including joining forces with yoga studios, independent ayurveda clinics, and so on. It sounds pretty good.

Not sure how this relates to what we are doing over here, but perhaps down the road there could be some beneficial synergies. It is too early to tell right now. As far as I'm concerned, the more information on effective practices that is flowing, with the fewest barriers and for the least cost, the better.

The guru is in you.

2006/05/16 13:48:07
Support for AYP Pranayama, Mudras and Bandhas
http://www.aypsite.org/forum/topic.asp?TOPIC_ID=1099&REPLY_ID=7060&whichpage=-1
Spinal Breathing Pranayama book

Hi All:

The Secrets of Wilder movie discussion has been split off and moved to the AYP Helpers forum over here:
http://www.aypsite.org/forum/topic.asp?TOPIC_ID=1154

Feel free to put in your two cents!

The guru is in you.

2006/05/05 10:47:25
Support for AYP Pranayama, Mudras and Bandhas
http://www.aypsite.org/forum/topic.asp?TOPIC_ID=1105&REPLY_ID=6607&whichpage=-1
opposite flow

Hi All:

It obviously works going both ways, and there are venerable traditions going way back on both sides, which raises an interesting question: What is that about?

There is a practical element having to do with advanced practices involving kumbhaka (breath suspension), and which end of the spinal nerve we want to be on with that. That is one reason why AYP goes up on inhalation, though I am sure an argument could be made for the other approach. Here it is from the AYP perspective -- Lesson 46, aptly named, "Which way is up?"

Just to show that AYP is not too terribly biased, we do have it going the other way too in the heartbreathing technique, for sipping some bhakti ishta (chosen ideal) into our heart, as needed -- Lesson 220 (check the next lesson too).

Hey, whatever works! :-)

The guru is in you.

2006/05/05 14:17:25
Support for AYP Pranayama, Mudras and Bandhas
http://www.aypsite.org/forum/topic.asp?TOPIC_ID=1105&REPLY_ID=6627&whichpage=-1
opposite flow

Hi Alan & Near:

I agree that top down inhalation is most common in the traditions and ancient writings. The 4000 year-old Vigyan Bhairava has it that way. The Bhagavad Gita has "surrendering the inflowing-breath into the outflowing-breath" -- don't recall if it specifies direction -- both sides claim the Gita, so maybe it does not. Of course, the nuances and pile-ons begin as soon as people begin playing with these things (ida, pingala, mantras, chakras...), ever-seeking a better way, and complicating things along the way. I have a theory that the traditions became "esoteric" not only to protect the knowledge from the inquisitions and the idle curious, but also because the practices got so darned complicated that only a few could master them anymore! Like trying to squeeze blood out of a turnip, you know. :-)

I am not aware of traditions or writings before the Mahasaya/Babaji line that recommend bottom up inhalation, though there may well be some. Of course, if we believe in the Babaji line, it/he goes waaay back to the Gita and beyond.

Well, who knows? Spinal breathing works, doesn't it? And the more simply it is applied, the better, as far as I'm concerned. We've got other fish to fry practice-wise (like deep meditation) and don't need to be tangling ourselves up in the many nuances (and reductions in efficiency) that can happen in spinal breathing, or any other practice. That is why we stick to the barest essentials of each practice in AYP, so we can do it all across the board and not get ourselves all wound up in one class of practice while making less progress to boot.

Someone said, "It takes a village to raise a child." I think it is fair to say, "It takes an integration of practices to raise the divine child of enlightenment." This is one of the key messages of the Yoga Sutras, and we seem to be verifying it here every day. Bravo for that!

The guru is in you.

2006/05/12 10:00:38
Support for AYP Pranayama, Mudras and Bandhas
http://www.aypsite.org/forum/topic.asp?TOPIC_ID=1134
Ecstatic Energy in Higher Stages of Kechari

Hi All:

Here is an interesting one from my email on the energetic aspects of higher stages of kechari:

Q: I have a question about Kechari Mudra... I have been practicing Kechari for about 4 years and I have a few questions that I am hoping you can answer...

First, I can only get my tongue past the septum and into either of the nasal holes about 1/4 inch; as I keep reaching further, what will I feel inside and where should the tongue finally reach to or rest at?

Second, when I run my tongue up the backside of the septum looking for the "secret spot", I do not find a protrusion half way up; however, I do have a small bump (it actually seems to me like more of a very tiny roll of skin or membrane) about 3/4 or 7/8ths of the way up, almost where the top of the septum reaches the top of the inside of the nasopharynx (where the tongue reaches a dead end when pointed up and forward in the nasopharynx)... Is this the "secret spot" or am I missing something? I don't feel any increase of "spiritual pleasure" at that spot as opposed to elsewhere on the septum so I'm not sure; also, possibly my "secret spot" is higher than average and/or I am not sensitive enough yet?

Could you please clarify and give your experienced opinion?

A: The "secret spot" is more about ecstatic sensation than a physical feature on the septum. It is the same thing with sambhavi. When the sensation is there, it cannot be missed and the physical positioning and movement will follow the sensation rather than the anatomy. Kechari by itself may or may not bring up the sensation. It is part of ecstatic conductivity, which is a whole body phenomenon. Perhaps you have run across the discussions on ecstatic conductivity in the lessons? It also comes under the common term "kundalini."

So, your progress in kechari sensitivity is probably related more toward your meditation, spinal breathing, mudras, bandhas, kumbhaka, tantric methods, etc, than to kechari itself. All of these things work together in the process of over all purification and opening.

Regarding the tongue and nasal passages, if you use the "roll/twist" of the tongue toward the center as described in <u>Lesson 108</u>, that will likely give you the maximum penetration, in and upward. Also check the Secrets of Wilder novel for a personal-style account of entering the nasal passages over time, and many other things discovered along the path. However far you penetrate is far enough. We each have our own natural limit, so there is no standard to be attained in that. The inner nasal openings are not likely to increase in size, as they are surrounded by bone (the septum is bone also). Neither is the tongue going to change much in thickness, except by radical means such as surgery which I strongly advise against. Some advanced yogis can't enter the nasal passages at all due to anatomy, and that does not hold them back.

In your case, it might be that your over all practice, including all of its components, needs some time. That will enhance whole body ecstatic conductivity and then kechari will come into full participation in that. When that happens, the septum is the place to be, so you are ready! :-)

Obviously, you have been doing kechari for some time, since before AYP came along. It is really a question of what else you have been doing in practices over the years, and how you decide to manage it going forward. If you are not doing a twice daily routine of deep meditation preceded by spinal breathing, I suggest you consider going in that direction. Then consider the mudras, bandhas and other methods discussed in the lessons, taking the whole thing in sequence one step at a time. That can do wonders for activating the secret spot and everything else in the nervous system.

All the best on your path!

The guru is in you.

2006/05/24 09:53:28
Support for AYP Pranayama, Mudras and Bandhas
http://www.aypsite.org/forum/topic.asp?TOPIC_ID=1169&REPLY_ID=7288&whichpage=-1
Yoni Mudra and Sinus Infection?

Hi Trip:

I'm no doctor, but don't believe yoni mudra would contribute to a sinus infection any more than going jogging with a fever would contribute to getting sicker. The idea is to give an illness the opportunity to heal without putting excess strain on it. That means rest, so you are wise to hold off (self-pace) yoni mudra until you are feeling better, which I hope you do soon.

Also check this lesson on meditating when sick: http://www.aypsite.org/24.html

All the best!

The guru is in you.

2006/05/25 07:13:01
Support for AYP Pranayama, Mudras and Bandhas
http://www.aypsite.org/forum/topic.asp?TOPIC_ID=1169&REPLY_ID=7306&whichpage=-1
Yoni Mudra and Sinus Infection?

Hi Trip and All:

Another practice that has excellent health benefits, especially on strengthening the immune system, is amaroli (urine therapy).

There are some informative topics on amaroli around here -- just do a forum search. Check "Amaroli Resources" in the <u>AYP links section</u> too. It is also covered in the AYP Easy Lessons book, and slated to be delved into further in an AYP Enlightenment Series book in about six months or so. Our main interest in it in AYP is as a spiritual practice, which it certainly is -- enhancing the nervous system's ability to to radiate the qualities of inner silence and ecstatic conductivity.

The guru is in you.

2006/06/20 14:35:57
Support for AYP Pranayama, Mudras and Bandhas
http://www.aypsite.org/forum/topic.asp?TOPIC_ID=1239&REPLY_ID=8231&whichpage=-1

Kechari problems

Hi Meg:

First, congratulations on your breakthough -- pushing forward to the septum/secret spot. Second, self-pace! You will have this wonderful tool for the rest of your life, and the thing to do now is not run off the road with it. That means easing into it timewise over weeks and months. I know it is a temptation to go all out, but there is only so much energy we can handle at any given time. And don't forget, there can be a delay in the effects, so it is good to step carefully. Even when well-established in advanced stages of kechari, there will be times for backing off. It goes with the territory. The sooner we can nip an overload, the smoother our path will be. As mentioned in the lessons, it is a lot like driving a car.

I suggest you slow down on kechari for as long as necessary and apply the methods of grounding (lesson 69) to spread out the newly circulating energy. As mundane as it sounds, walking, getting out and doing physical things, etc. will help. So can taking a heavier diet for a time until the energy spreads out. The heat is also possibly a call for some attention to diet from an ayurvedic stand point -- pitta pacifying. Here's the food chart: http://www.aypsite.org/ayurveda-diets.html

For the rest, let go of short term expectations and pretend you are in a rocket car that is going a bit too fast at the moment. Time to ease off the accelerator. That could mean slowing down on spinal breathing and meditation for a while as well. All of these practices become more powerful by the addition of a new one like kechari -- the whole is greater than the sum of the parts. So, the more advanced we become with the integration of our practices, the more power each practice will have, and the greater the importance of self-pacing. Less is very often more in a highly integrated practice routine.

It will be okay. You are not off the cliff or anything. Just needing to adjust to the new dynamic of practice and experience you have recently entered. It's good stuff. One small step for a woman -- and another a giant leap for humankind!

Congratulations to Vicki too. :-)

I'm sure others will chime in here...

The guru is in you.

2006/06/21 16:22:15
Support for AYP Pranayama, Mudras and Bandhas
http://www.aypsite.org/forum/topic.asp?TOPIC_ID=1239&REPLY_ID=8259&whichpage=-1
Kechari problems

Hi Tom. Good to hear from you!

Kechari stage 2 is definitely a leaning forward with the tongue, once behind the soft palate. As the tongue goes forward, the soft palate folds down, with a weird stretching sensation the first few times, and then the septum/secret spot is found. In my case this was automatic when I slipped into kechari many years ago. What we are finding more recently is that sometimes it takes a conscious movement of the tongue forward above the soft palate to open it up and find the secret spot. I didn't know it was that secret! :-)

As for snipping, David and others can give you the low-down on the alternatives. You can also find a lot by doing a search on "kechari" or "snip" or "talavya" in these forums. It can be as simple as waiting for the tendon to work its way to the surface again over several weeks or months. For those who are aggressive, there are a variety of other ways, and we have some practitioners here who have been very resourceful with that, while at the same time observing the precautions necessary to keep it as safe as possible.

All the best!

The guru is in you.

2006/06/22 07:13:47
Support for AYP Pranayama, Mudras and Bandhas
http://www.aypsite.org/forum/topic.asp?TOPIC_ID=1239&REPLY_ID=8272&whichpage=-1
Kechari problems

Hi Tom:

The balancing effects of yoga are well known, and can help with allergies, and all sorts of other health issues. The effects can come from one practice, or a combination. In our case we are working with an integration of practices, so it may be hard to tell what is doing what unless we are taking it slow in adding things on -- self-pacing. Not that it matters for positive effects. We'll take them, right? On symptoms of energy overload it is a different matter. We'd like to know what is triggering an imbalance, if possible, and pace accordingly. So we go step-by-step in building up our routine, pacing as necessary -- easy does it...

By the time you add on asanas, refine the mudras and bandhas, and add amaroli and a few other things, you may be rid of your alleriges completely. But you won't squeeze all that in by the weekend. Not without risking life and limb. :-)

The guru is in you.

2006/06/22 07:19:48
Support for AYP Pranayama, Mudras and Bandhas
http://www.aypsite.org/forum/topic.asp?TOPIC_ID=1239&REPLY_ID=8273&whichpage=-1
Kechari problems

Hi Meg:

There is something else you can try for the hot feet. Consider this to be experimental, as I have no scriptural precedent for it, and only limited (but successful) experience with it here for leg and foot pain. Maybe it will work for hot feet too.

Just alter a few spinal breathing sessions (not a permanent change) to be going from feet to brow instead of from root/perineum to brow, and see what happens. Once the problem clears up, or if it has no effect after a few sessions, go back to normal spinal breathing. It is an easy temporary alteration in practice and can have a significant balancing effect on energy in the legs and feet. We just keep going down on the exhale through the legs all the way to the soles of the feet, and back up from there on inhale all the way to the brow. Don't overdo it, just short sessions (5-10 min) until you can see what you are getting out of it, if anything.

Try it and let us know. And keep walking too -- the measure of choice for most foot energy issues...

I have a feeling that once this clears up, your feet are going to feel mighty ecstatic. Meg's lotus feet... :-)

The guru is in you.

2006/06/24 19:00:51
Support for AYP Pranayama, Mudras and Bandhas
http://www.aypsite.org/forum/topic.asp?TOPIC_ID=1239&REPLY_ID=8378&whichpage=-1
Kechari problems

Hi Shanti:

Good advice from Victor. It was about 10 years after stage 2 before I went into the nostrils. There is no rush. Take time to assimilate what you have energetically before moving on. You don't have to wait as long as I did (it was a much lonelier road back then -- all this kechari company we have today is wonderful), but no need to get ahead of yourself either. In time, the mechanics of it will manifest, or maybe not. It is not mandatory to penetrate the nostrils to proceed along the path. In fact, the journey can continue without kechari stage 2. That is the advantage of a diverse integrated system of practices -- one way or another we will continue to move ahead according to our inner light.

Each of us has our own tendencies, and each of us will travel our own path.

The guru is in you.

2006/06/26 11:01:10
Support for AYP Pranayama, Mudras and Bandhas
http://www.aypsite.org/forum/topic.asp?TOPIC_ID=1239&REPLY_ID=8442&whichpage=-1
Kechari problems

Hi Shanti:

Not to be rushing you to stage 4 (see posts above), but a careful reading of AYP lesson 108 can help when the time is right. It is also covered in narrative form in the Secrets of Wilder novel. The stage 4 technique involves twisting the tongue on its side, top toward the center, by following the groove down with the tip of the tongue from the top of the eustachian tube trumpets on either side of the nasal passages.

I am sure there are other ways to do it, just as we have had a breakthrough here recently with pressing forward over the soft palate with the tongue into stage 2. A surge of new stage 2 entries have come from that. Bravo!

Now, it's suggested you give yourself a chance to acclimate before pressing on into stage 4. Stage 2-3 with the secret spot on the edge of the septum is the meat and potatoes of kechari, while into the nostrils to stage 4 is the wild blue yonder of it. Are you the wild blue yonder type? :-)

The guru is in you.

2006/07/02 14:05:10
Support for AYP Pranayama, Mudras and Bandhas
http://www.aypsite.org/forum/topic.asp?TOPIC_ID=1269&REPLY_ID=8777&whichpage=-1
10 month meditation

Hi All:

I read somewhere that this remarkable young man went missing in March, and no one has seen him since. Anyone have more information on this?

The guru is in you.

Sent to me in an email recently -- source of information unknown:

Ram Bahadur Bomjon (born May 9, 1989, sometimes Bomjan or Banjan), also known as Palden Dorje (his official Buddhist name), is a young Buddhist monk from Ratanapuri village, Bara district, Nepal who has drawn thousands of visitors and media attention for spending months in meditation allegedly without food or water. Nicknamed the Buddha Boy, he began his meditation on May 16, 2005, and went missing on March 11, 2006. His present whereabouts, as well as the reasons and circumstances for his disappearance, are unknown...

2006/07/05 10:53:45
Support for AYP Pranayama, Mudras and Bandhas
http://www.aypsite.org/forum/topic.asp?TOPIC_ID=1288&REPLY_ID=8974&whichpage=-1
Kechari Stage 4 + Pranayama

Hi Y:

As mentioned in lesson 108, pranayama can be done with alternate nostrils from the inside using stage 4 kechari. It's not something to jump into on a whim, as it is very powerful, a whole new level of practice involving long term acclimation and self-pacing. Stage 4 kechari can also be used in alternate nostrils during successive kumbhakas in yoni mudra, chin pump and/or yoni chin pump. It is not advised until stability in stage

2-3 kechari is mastered during sitting practices -- which can also take a long time. And, of course, any practice we consider adding kechari to needs to be well established and stable beforehand. There is only so much the nervous system can be absorbing at once. That is why we always go step-by-step in AYP.

In every case, including stage 4 kechari is a major change, like adding a whole new practice. As with any new practice, we begin small and build up very gradually...

It is at the practitioner's discretion, keeping common sense at the fore. Stability and long term daily practice are the keys to progress.

The guru is in you.

2006/07/16 22:19:47
Support for AYP Pranayama, Mudras and Bandhas
http://www.aypsite.org/forum/topic.asp?TOPIC_ID=1288&REPLY_ID=9527&whichpage=-1
Kechari Stage 4 + Pranayama

Hi Loris, and welcome aboard here!

Yes, that's right.

Stage 4 kechari tends to be dynamic (alternating nostrils), and therefore akin to pranayama. As recommended in the AYP lessons, we do not do pranayama at the same time as deep meditation because it divides our attention between the two practices. That is not so bad for pranayama, but can seriously disrupt the simple and delicate procedure of deep meditation. That is why we don't do any of the mudras or bandhas during meditation either, until they become automatic habits that we don't think about when they are occurring. Hence, we use our spinal breathing pranayama session for cultivating the habits of mudras, bandhas and siddhasana.

Now, if kechari stage 4 has reached the level of being an effortless automatic habit for you, then you are welcome to let it be there in deep meditation. But do you really want to be meditating with one nostril blocked for 20 minutes? As soon as you decide to switch, you are not doing deep meditation anymore, but pranayama. nah nah... :-)

So, I'd suggest using kechari stage 4 during pranayama and kumbhaka (breath suspension) related practices where alternate nostril breathing fits in nicely. For most using kechari stage 4, that will be more than enough. Yes, in the practices chart in the Secrets of Wilder, that is how it is shown, without any "secret chamber - upper passages" (stage 4) during i am meditation. On the chart, "secret chamber - altar of bliss" (stage 2-3) is shown during intermediate and advanced stages of i am meditation, meaning, only when it is an effortless habit.

Btw, the same goes for samyama as for meditation. They are in the same class.

I'm really glad you brought up the practices chart from the Secrets of Wilder novel, covering nearly all of the core practices of AYP, applied in routines at the basic, intermediate and advanced levels, all on one page! It is one of the best kept "secrets" of the book, and perhaps in all of AYP. Nothing like it can be found anywhere else in the AYP writings. Maybe I will duplicate it (with the Sanskrit terminology re-inserted) for the ninth Enlightenment Series book next year, which will cover the eight limbs of yoga and the structure and pacing of self-directed practice. That will be the big picture, and the Wilder practices chart is definitely the big picture.

All the best!

The guru is in you.

2006/07/22 09:19:21
Support for AYP Pranayama, Mudras and Bandhas
http://www.aypsite.org/forum/topic.asp?TOPIC_ID=1353&REPLY_ID=9764&whichpage=-1
spinal bastrika pranayama

Hi Meg:

It helps to just let attention go brow, root, brow, root, brow, root, etc. during spinal bastrika. The in-between will fill in later. Same with regular spinal breathing if there is fuzzy or clunky tracing. This is covered in the spinal breathing pranayama book. Fuzzy or clunky tracing is perfectly okay. We just easily favor the procedure when we realize we are off it, with no forcing.

Brow, root, brow, root, brow, root ... and happy ecstatic conductivity cultivating... :-)

Don't forget to self-pace ... spinal bastrika is a very powerful practice for loosening obstructions. Easy to overdo for that reason. Keep in mind delayed effects. A minute or two starting out is plenty -- much less if there is sensitivity.

All the best!

The guru is in you.

2006/08/03 11:14:03
Support for AYP Pranayama, Mudras and Bandhas
http://www.aypsite.org/forum/topic.asp?TOPIC_ID=1381&REPLY_ID=10198&whichpage=-1
Yoni Mudra questions and discussions

Hi All:

The AYP lessons attempt go straight down the middle with practices, with the simplest most effective applications possible. I am forever getting tons of questions on the endless variations. It is impossible to answer them all. :-)

Keep in mind that we are applying techniques to take advantage of the basic principles of human spiritual transformation that exist within us. It is always about that, and managing it in ways to promote good progress with reasonable comfort (self-pacing).

In the case of yoni mudra kumbhaka, it is breath retention and mudras/bandhas combined, which are primarily for raising ecstatic conductivity (kundalini). As that progresses, deep meditation and all other practices are affected as the ongoing blending of ecstatic conductivity and inner silence occurs.

So, whatever your approach to yoni mudra is, take it easy, and work toward a practice you can sustain on a daily basis. Consider the AYP lessons to be a guideline. Less is often more, especially with this practice, and there are no aggressive targets to be met. Gentle persuasion over time will yield the best results. It is like that in all of yoga...

The guru is in you.

2006/08/04 10:01:37
Support for AYP Pranayama, Mudras and Bandhas
http://www.aypsite.org/forum/topic.asp?TOPIC_ID=1383&REPLY_ID=10219&whichpage=-1
Sudden Inhalation

Hi All:

An automatic sudden breath or full blown rapid breathing in yoga can be the phenomenon of automatic bastrika. It is especially common during samyama, where silence is stimulated to move (covered in the lessons). It can also happen in meditation, usually to a lesser degree.

The guru is in you.

2006/08/04 10:59:26
Support for AYP Pranayama, Mudras and Bandhas
http://www.aypsite.org/forum/topic.asp?TOPIC_ID=1383&REPLY_ID=10221&whichpage=-1
Sudden Inhalation

Hi David:

Could be both. Practice yields purification, and purification yields practice.

However, there can more going on here than metabolism alone, or the lack of it. The breath reflex can also happen when there is no lack of oxygen -- a quick and shallow in-breath or out-breath, or a series of both, which is automatic bastrika. In that case, it is an impulse arising from inner silence (samadhi) stimulating it, not necessarily a metabolic adjustment. Bastrika can happen like that, riding on a series of impulses coming from inner silence, and interlacing with whole body ecstatic conductivity.

Whatever the cause, as with any experience, automatic reaction or yogic reflex during practices, we don't charge off into them. When we realize we are off, we just easily come back to the procedure of the practice we are doing.

So, Mufad, you are doing just right. Yes, it's a good thing... :-)

The guru is in you.

2006/08/12 16:11:38
Support for AYP Pranayama, Mudras and Bandhas
http://www.aypsite.org/forum/topic.asp?TOPIC_ID=1415&REPLY_ID=10439&whichpage=-1
a neat pic for kechari
Good one, Kyman!

"A picture is worth 1000 words" -- as in lesson 108, and quite a few words since.

The guru is in you.

2006/08/30 13:37:38
Support for AYP Pranayama, Mudras and Bandhas
http://www.aypsite.org/forum/topic.asp?TOPIC_ID=1474&REPLY_ID=11000&whichpage=-1
spinal breathing versus microcosmic orbit

Hi Snake:

In yoga, the energy coming down the front is regarded primarily as biological, and for that reason is handled mainly with physical methods such as jalandhara bandha, dynamic jalandhara/chin pump, kechari and sambhavi. The lower mudras and bandhas are involved on the other end of the cycle -- mulabandha/asvini (root) and uddiyana/nauli/navi (mid-body).

Obviously, it is the same neuro-biology occurring in the nervous system whether we are in Taoism, Indian Yoga, or any other system of practices. In yoga, the spinal nerve is given preference on the neurological side going in both directions, particularly with spinal breathing pranayama where there is an awakening and balanced blending of ascending and descending pranic energies in the spinal nerve -- an energy dynamic that is apparently not recognized in the same way in Taoism.

The related, but separately regarded "nectar cycle" in yoga is more in line with the Taoist view of the micro-cosmic orbit, with sweet secretions coming down from the brain with the rise of ecstatic conductivity, down through the nasal pharynx, into the digestive system and chest, reprocessed, and cycled back up to the brain again via the spine as a luminous mint-like substance (soma) resulting from "refined digestion" of food & nectar, sexual essenses and air in the GI tract.

I believe the Taoists call the digestive aspect of the cycle, "alchemy occurring in the cauldron," so we are most likely talking about the same process. Only one nervous system, with one process of enlightenment going on...

So, yoga recognizes the cycle. It just divides it into two overlapping components (biological and neurological) and promotes them with an array of practices known to provide the appropriate stimulation.

As they say, "Whatever works!" :-)

The guru is in you.

2006/09/13 17:35:43
Support for AYP Pranayama, Mudras and Bandhas
http://www.aypsite.org/forum/topic.asp?TOPIC_ID=1507&REPLY_ID=11312&whichpage=-1
Breathless state

quote:
––––––––
Originally posted by Yogi

I have a question about the breathless state. I have read somewhere AYP dont give much importance to this state. If someone want´s to master this state, what he would need to change in the basic AYP routine? To increase the time of the spinal breath? I have read people in the Kriya Yoga tradition practice 6 or more hours of pranayama with no ill effects. What do you think?

––––––––

Hi Yogi:

Welcome aboard!

Reduction of metabolism comes primarily from inner silence cultivated in deep meditation, and breath will slow down accordingly. In this case, breath suspension is effect rather than cause. Of course, cause leads to effect, and effect leads to cause.

In AYP spinal breathing pranayama, we easily favor slow breathing, which leads to gradual inner energy awakening. And in several of the mudras and bandhas, we suspend the breath after inhalation, not to the extreme. In both cases the principle of *restraint of breath* (the meaning of "pranayama") is applied for this purpose.

As for doing hours of pranayama, it is not recommended when followed by deep meditation, as the effects will far exceed those of doing the pranayama alone, and likely lead to excessive purification and discomfort. It is a matter of efficiency. The more efficient the practice, the less time it takes to achieve results. Less can be more in that case.

As inner silence rises over time, the breath will naturally become less, even in daily activity, and the mind will become as steady as a crystal clear reflection pond.

The guru is in you.

2006/09/15 10:20:30
Support for AYP Pranayama, Mudras and Bandhas
http://www.aypsite.org/forum/topic.asp?TOPIC_ID=1507&REPLY_ID=11332&whichpage=-1
Breathless state

quote:
––––––––
Originally posted by Yogi

I agree pranayama alone is not the best pratice. I understand in kriya there is deep meditation after pranayama. Lahiri Mahashay stressed this point as essential. I will experiment increasing the time of pranayama very slowly, not to the point of discomfort, and try to find a balance. I understand the more purification your body can handle, faster is your progress, right?

––––––––

Hi Yogi:

Yes, traditional kriya yoga includes meditation after pranayama, but I do not believe it is mantra-based deep meditation of the kind we use in AYP. Rather, it is a nada practice using OM, which I believe is less consistent in its results. In the modern lineages of kriya, pranayama is usually the main focus, as per your post above, and meditation is less emphasized. Please correct me if I am wrong on this.

A balance is essential. This is conveyed in a quote from Lahiri Mahasaya himself (the 19th century father of modern kriya yoga) that is used in a few places in the AYP lessons to illustrate the importance of this balance. He wrote that enlightenment is "a merging of emptiness with euphoria."

From the AYP point of view, this is the merging of inner silence cultivated in deep meditation and samyama with ecstasy cultivated in pranayama, asanas, mudras and bandhas.

In recognizing this dual-pole strategy and exercising prudent self-pacing while using an effective range of practices, we can't miss.

As for how much purification can be achieved by any particular individual, it will be a function of the unique matrix of obstructions (karma/samskara) embedded within the nervous system and the means used to loosen and release them. There is a limit to how much can be done in the present, but there is no limit to what can be accomplished over time. With self-pacing, progress can be maximized. Aggressive practice without self-pacing will lead to excesses that can knock us off the path altogether. It is like driving a car. A safe speed will deliver us to our destination in a timely fashion, while driving at top speed all the time will send us into a ditch or off a cliff sooner or later, probably sooner. So it is suggested to drive safely ... it is the quickest and surest way home. :-)

All the best!

The guru is in you.

2006/09/15 15:27:41
Support for AYP Pranayama, Mudras and Bandhas
http://www.aypsite.org/forum/topic.asp?TOPIC_ID=1507&REPLY_ID=11341&whichpage=-1
Breathless state

quote:
_____

Originally posted by Yogi

The air is sucked out of the lungs and the heart sometimes stops, all body sense is lost, complete sense introvertion. The goal of the Kriya tradition is to achieve this at will.
_____

Hi All:

This sort of experience (sudden exhalation accompanied by inner expansion) is fairly common in the Secrets of Wilder novel -- a story about young Americans charging ahead with powerful spiritual practices. I'm sure we will be seeing much more of it in our non-fictional world too. :-)

Sudden inhalation or exhalation (or both in sequence, which is automatic bastrika) is a normal reflex in the nervous system as it goes through cycles of purification. See here for some more discussion on this: http://www.aypsite.org/forum/topic.asp?TOPIC_ID=1383

There may be a tendency to mythologize these things, where, in fact, they are normal functions of the nervous system when stimulated by yoga practices, past or present, including bhakti. I'm not sure it is a good idea to make goals of particular experiences, as some traditions have a tendency to do. Much better to be focused on the performance of our practices than on creating particular experiences. Everyone's journey will be somewhat different, according to the course of purification going on inside. With sound practices and self-pacing, our inner opening will unfold as it should.

Experiences make much better sign-posts along the way, for inspiration and self-pacing, than they do end goals.

The guru is in you.

2006/09/26 10:07:10
Support for AYP Pranayama, Mudras and Bandhas
http://www.aypsite.org/forum/topic.asp?TOPIC_ID=1544&REPLY_ID=11564&whichpage=-1
kechari and "prana belly"

Hi Victor:

Yes, it is a kind of internal kumbhaka which can happen naturally in the GI tract as part of the "alchemy" going on there -- food, air and sexual essences blending to produce "soma," a biological component of rising ecstatic conductivity. From there, soma can expand air-like throughout the body and out through the pores of the skin, contributing to ecstatic radiance extending beyond the body. The sweet aromas sometimes noticed around yogis and yoginis have been attributed to this.

Muktananda's guru, Nityananda, was known for swallowing large amounts air to accentuate this phenomenon, leading to a large air-filled belly. Not recommended in AYP. It can compromise health.

With kechari and other mudras and bandhas, combined with moderate breath retention during chin pump and yoni mudra, and the slowdown of breathing during spinal breathing pranayama, the retention of air and combined essences in the body will occur naturally. Of course, deep meditation has an underlying role to play in all of this, as in all yogic phenomena we encounter. Inner silence is the foundation of all spiritual progress.

Over time, the internal processing of air becomes more or less a "pass-through," meaning it is not necessary to have a Nityananda (or Buddha) belly to progress with ecstatic conductivity. In fact, an excessively swelling belly or undue pressure anywhere inside is usually a signal to, you guessed it, self-pace our practices. :-)

The guru is in you.

2006/09/26 12:16:30
Support for AYP Pranayama, Mudras and Bandhas
http://www.aypsite.org/forum/topic.asp?TOPIC_ID=1544&REPLY_ID=11578&whichpage=-1
kechari and "prana belly"

Hi Victor:

Yes, kumbhaka can certainly be natural in kechari -- but it is part of a broad process of neurobiological transformation occurring in the nervous system, so it is hard to segregate it. That is why I answered the way I did. Sometimes we may get the same (or similar) kumbhaka effect from deep meditation alone, or any other practice, or group of practices. The cause and effect of it will change as things evolve.

Wish I could be more specific. The vagueness comes along with spiritual progress coloring practices as much as the other way around. Also, the practices color each other, so what might seem to be a kechari effect may actually be other practices coloring kechari, vise versa, and so on. It will shift around according to the unique course of purification in each of us. So, the further along we are, the harder it becomes to nail down one particular cause (practice) relating to one particular effect (experience). A broader view involving multiple practices and experiences then may offer a clearer picture of what is happening.

The guru is in you.

2006/10/14 16:53:13
Support for AYP Pranayama, Mudras and Bandhas
http://www.aypsite.org/forum/topic.asp?TOPIC_ID=1607&REPLY_ID=12295&whichpage=-1
Root to Crown Spinal breathing?

Hi Christi, and welcome!

What a great discussion here. You have been raising some excellent questions and I think you have gotten a lot of good feedback.

The goal in the AYP lessons is to give folks a good appreciation of premature crown opening and its consequences. Most of the kundalini horror stories written over the past 40 years (at least) are related to this. On the other hand, in the lessons, no one is prohibited from exploring their own nature, and the lessons attempt to keep that door open while observing reasonable safety. So those are the two principles that crown discussions are wrapped around in the lessons. I think with a measured approach, we are finally moving beyond the kinds of unwieldy kundalini scenarios that were so prevalent in the past, to something that is much more manageable. It is, after all, our own nature that is manifesting. So we ought to be able to come to terms with it and move forward with reasonable speed and safety. And we can -- fairly gracefully too! :-)

There is really no "formula" practice for the crown that can be recommended whole-heartedly, because each person has a unique matrix of obstructions to be dissolved, and focused crown practices of any kind will not be stable until the matrix is largely dissolved, which can be done with the brow to root oriented practices already given. Going to the crown is then left up to the aspirant, and the suggestion is to wait to do it until ecstatic conductivity is sufficiently advanced so there can be a good awareness of what is happening. That is why prudent "testing" is recommended. And always keep in mind the time delays that are involved in the cycles of ecstasy and letdown.

It is important to note that energy experiences in the crown area (usually mirrored body-wide) are caused by "friction" from remaining impurities in the nervous system. So the energy symptoms themselves can be taken as a caution that there is more work to be done. With crown focus, energy symptoms can quickly turn into roller coaster emotions and all sorts of physical weirdness. Yes, all of this does stabilize later on, but the difficulty of the ride we take is directly related to how aggressive we have been at the crown early on. And it is not necessarily a shorter ride -- it can be much longer due to having to come off a stable routine of practices to deal with the energy dislocations. So, slow and steady (brow to root) will win this race 9 times out of 10.

The best crown experiences are the ones that have gone to dissolution into pure bliss consciousness, without negative after-effects. This indicates body-wide purity. As with all practice, we know it is good if we feel good in regular daily activity.

Once we get to that stage, then what? Well, nothing much really. We just keep going with our stable practice routine (using prudent self-pacing), and our regular life. Contrary to popular belief, there is no place other than here that we have to go to (as Katrine says, just "stay home") -- no exit via the crown to some other exotic dimension. Actually, the opposite happens -- the ecstatic bliss (the exotic) comes in here from out there. That is the thing, you know -- the divine process is not us going somewhere else. It is the divine coming in through us into this life -- this ordinary life. It ends up melting our heart in an extraordinary way and flowing out through our actions. I call it outpouring divine love. That's it...

The crown is a sort of crossroad in all of this, one that takes a long time to purify completely, because to do so, everything else has to be purified, and that cannot be done overnight, no matter what has been promised. The good news is that all the purification we achieve in the sushumna (spinal nerve) and throughout the nervous system with our daily deep meditation, spinal breathing pranayama and other practices is crown opening by proxy. When everything is purified and opened, the crown is open too. In that sense all the practices we do are crown practices. We are just being cagey about it to avoid unnecessary mishaps. :-)

Well, just some food for thought.

All the best!

The guru is in you.

2006/10/15 10:44:13
Support for AYP Pranayama, Mudras and Bandhas
http://www.aypsite.org/forum/topic.asp?TOPIC_ID=1607&REPLY_ID=12317&whichpage=-1
Root to Crown Spinal breathing?

Hi Christi:

Over time of stable practice, the ajna (third eye) will naturally expand to incorporate the crown, and this is the way the whole process can proceed while remaining stable. In other words, as long as the two (third eye and crown) are perceived as distinctly different, favoring the brow will be the more prudent path. When the whole nervous system is becoming gradually more advanced in purification, the third eye and crown will merge energetically. There is little we have to do to promote this, other than maintaining our regular daily practices.

As for what to do between samyama and rest, it is best if we leave that one to you. I am sure your bhakti will help you find your way. Keep in mind that sometimes bhakti itself can use some self-pacing.

In the upcoming Samyama book, something helpful will be added near the end of the practice session, but not as crown concentrated as is being discussed here. We will continue to be very cagey about the crown, which is essentially the same as the whole body and beyond.

Also, more about crown experiences on the edge (and overboard) can be found in the Secrets of Wilder novel, which is a story about the experience of forming this style of application of practices, including mishaps that happened along the way, and what it took to get back on track. It is a story of pioneering work with lots of ups and downs, in contrast to the rather "routine" approach to cultivating enlightenment we take around here. :-)

We'd like for it to become routine. Then the door will be wide open for everyone to do it. Practice wisely, and enjoy!

The guru is in you.

2006/10/15 14:19:28

Hi Christi:

Your experience with naturally suspended exhalation sounds fine.

Natural breath suspension (inhaled or exhaled) is generally not harmful. But if we are engaging in deliberate breath suspension, like in yoni mudra or chin pump, inhaled is better. Deliberate exhaled suspension in practices over months and years can put a strain on the lungs, whereas inhaled suspension (within reason -- not to the extreme) will not. That is the caution that is given in the AYP writings. The lungs are designed to handle positive pressure, and not so much to handle negative pressure (vacuum).

It is a matter of maintaining physical health long term.

If natural breath suspension occurs in deep meditation (very common), or at other times, we just let it be without forcing it or fighting it. It is like any other experience that may occur during practices. Just scenery we will encounter along the way, you know. As we get further along, we may have such experiences in daily activity too, and we treat them just the same and carry on with life.

A good rule of thumb: If it is natural and easy, it is probably okay. If it is a strain, something we are forcing, better be careful. We will not help ourselves by forcing. The path is one of gentle persuasion.

The guru is in you.

PS -- Thanks posting first on this, Shanti. :-)

2006/10/17 14:52:56

quote:
_____
Originally posted by Christi

Hi again, Yogani... before our discussion on crown practices ends (for now), I wanted to say something. It seems to me that your two replies in this thread to my questions on crown practices, add something valuable to what is given in the main AYP lessons on crown practices. They certainly clear up some ambiguities that could arise from lesson 199 ,and they seem to give advice that could be useful to everyone, which is not included in the main lessons. As not everyone who practices AYP yoga is involved in the forum discussions, I was wondering if it would be worth putting some of the advice you gave in this thread in the main lessons?
_____

Hi Christi:

Yes, good point, though I am a little reluctant to (indirectly) send thousands of people toward the crown, for obvious reasons. The original lessons on the crown were a bit muted for that reason. We all will certainly get around to it in our own cagey ways. :-)

The business of preserving the forum writings and making them available to more people is actually a much larger issue, because there is a huge amount of ground-breaking information hidden in these thousands of posts that ought not stay buried. Anything I have written that might be useful has been directly stimulated by the numerous interactions here, so it is a process involving all of us. Likewise, many others have posted excellent insights on practices and experiences too.

These forums are a gold mine for anyone looking to go beyond the foundation AYP lessons. Going the other way, reading the forums first and then the lessons, is not so easy, as many have found out.

It is a process of discovery we are engaged in that can go on indefinitely, leading to steadily improving knowledge of the processes of human spiritual transformation. Applied spiritual science! Very exciting.

In order to capture it all, at least my part of it, an AYP Easy Lessons Vol 2 (another big one) will be published after the Enlightenment Series books are done. It will probably come out sometime in 2008. Vol 2 would pick up all the additional lessons posted online up to that point, my relevant forum writings, and additional material from my unpublished emails that have been piling up here for a long time.

The goal of the AYP books is to capture everything that is useful in a permanent record that is easily accessible by everyone.

Meanwhile, many others are recording amazing insights and experiences here in the forums. Those cannot be easily blended with my writings (copyright issues), beyond the Q&A format that will continue in AYP EL Vol 2.

It is my hope that the useful writings by others here can also be published and preserved in book form someday, some by individuals in their own books, and perhaps many others in an anthology volume with writings from numerous practitioners in it. The copyright issues for an anthology would have to be addressed, of course -- not something I can think about right now with everything else on the plate. Maybe someone else will do it. By then (years from now), participation in these forums and the number of experiences recorded will likely be much larger. It is a long term view for spreading the writings beyond the web to a wider audience, adding visibility and credibility to what we are doing here.

Well, that is a long answer to a short question. Will I put more on the crown in an online AYP lesson? Let me mull it over. Either way, it will be published in AYP EL Vol 2 later on. Perhaps by then many more will find it useful. Let's hope so. The more the merrier, each in their own time... :-)

All the best!

The guru is in you.

2006/10/25 11:47:09
Support for AYP Pranayama, Mudras and Bandhas
http://www.aypsite.org/forum/topic.asp?TOPIC_ID=1607&REPLY_ID=12570&whichpage=-1
Root to Crown Spinal breathing?

quote:
_____

Originally posted by Christi: It seems to me that your two replies in this thread to my questions on crown practices, add something valuable to what is given in the main AYP lessons on crown practices. They certainly clear up some ambiguities that could arise from lesson 199 ,and they seem to give advice that could be useful to everyone, which is not included in the main lessons. As not everyone who practices AYP yoga is involved in the forum discussions, I was wondering if it would be worth putting some of the advice you gave in this thread in the main lessons?
_____

Hi Christi:

As you may have seen, I went ahead and did it here: http://www.aypsite.org/287.html
...with some fine tuning.

Many thanks for the inspiration.

The guru is in you.

2008/11/16 09:50:31
Support for AYP Pranayama, Mudras and Bandhas
http://www.aypsite.org/forum/topic.asp?TOPIC_ID=1607&REPLY_ID=40680&whichpage=-1
Root to Crown Spinal breathing?

quote:
_____

Originally posted by Christi

I have just one question:
If ecstatsy is produced by the resistance caused by prana moving through unpurified nadis, and enlightenment is produced by the merging of ecstasy and bliss, then how can someone become enlightened once the nadis are purified?
_____

Hi Christi:

Ecstasy become refined, less symptomatic, blending with the bliss of inner silence. That is the merging.

Also, the process of purification and opening continues through karma yoga, i.e., service. There are still plenty of obstructions out there, and that is where the energy will flow naturally ecstatically. It occurs through the outpouring of divine love. It flows through each of us into our surroundings in its own way. Samyama (core and cosmic) plays a key role in this also. So does self-inquiry.

Good things are happening. Bravo! :-)

The guru is in you.

2008/11/20 09:00:35
Support for AYP Pranayama, Mudras and Bandhas
http://www.aypsite.org/forum/topic.asp?TOPIC_ID=1607&REPLY_ID=40898&whichpage=-1
Root to Crown Spinal breathing?

quote:
_____

Originally posted by Christi

Hi Yogani,

quote:
_____

Hi Christi:

Ecstasy become refined, less symptomatic, blending with the bliss of inner silence. That is the merging.
_____

Just one more thing. I used to have a strong current of energy which flowed up the centre of my body from the root chakra up to the top of my head. It caused mulabhanda and udyanabhanda to be automatic most of the time (and often sambhavi). Now it is hardly noticeable. Is this flow of energy also part of the purification process which goes (like ecstasy) when the purification process in the body is largely done?

And what about the Om sound? Does that vanish as well?

216 – Advanced Yoga Practices

Christi
_____

Hi Christi:

None of it is ever gone, only refined into stillness. This is what the concept of "whole body mudra" is meant to convey -- a refinement of the energy via purification, and the connected mudras/bandhas along with it. OM is at the heart of that. None of it is gone, only very refined in stillness.

From there it goes outward into action for others, as mentioned. In that sense, the purification process is never done, not until we have become purified everywhere, to the furtherest reaches of the cosmos. It is not so difficult, since mind via samyama travels infinitely faster than the speed of light. Move over Einstein... :-)

The guru is in you.

2008/11/21 09:33:08
Support for AYP Pranayama, Mudras and Bandhas
http://www.aypsite.org/forum/topic.asp?TOPIC_ID=1607&REPLY_ID=40963&whichpage=-1
Root to Crown Spinal breathing?

quote:
_____
Originally posted by Christi

Thanks Yogani. I had thought for a long time that mind was faster than light. I had never heard anyone mention it though.
_____

Hi Christi:

The infinite speed (or omnipresence) of mind becomes much more significant and useful as samyama advances. It is what core and cosmic samyama practices are about. Stillness in action and outpouring divine love everywhere ... and that means everywhere. We are *That*.

The guru is in you.

2008/11/21 10:09:09
Support for AYP Pranayama, Mudras and Bandhas
http://www.aypsite.org/forum/topic.asp?TOPIC_ID=1607&REPLY_ID=40967&whichpage=-1
Root to Crown Spinal breathing?

quote:
_____
Originally posted by Ananda

was that a glimpse of what enlightenment is and can that state stay with the person 24\7, and can we share others a glimpse once we achieve such state of being?
_____

Hi Ananda:

Yes, and of course. :-)

But the latter has more to do with the other person's bhakti than with our own condition. Enlightenment is not something that is sent. It is received through every open heart, regardless of what may be going on in others. There is much misunderstanding about this, in some cases leading to unhealthy co-dependencies. See this AYP lesson on shaktipat: http://www.aypsite.org/146.html

The guru is in you.

2008/11/22 11:25:00
Support for AYP Pranayama, Mudras and Bandhas
http://www.aypsite.org/forum/topic.asp?TOPIC_ID=1607&REPLY_ID=41017&whichpage=-1
Root to Crown Spinal breathing?

quote:
_____
Originally posted by Christi

Hi Yogani,

quote:
_____
From there it goes outward into action for others, as mentioned. In that sense, the purification process is never done, not until we have become purified everywhere, to the furtherest reaches of the cosmos. It is not so difficult, since mind via samyama travels infinitely faster than the speed of light. Move over Einstein...

I think it will be a while before I am zooming around the galaxy purifying every nook and crany as I go. So there is obviously still a lot of work to do here first. :-)

Thanks again for the advice.

Christi

———————

Hi Christi:

The nice thing about it is that we don't have to zoom anywhere. We are already there.

Where do we go when we do group samyama healing? Does it matter where in the world the person is? Nope. We just dial up the name, and we are immediately there, collectively in that case.

So, when we are dialing up "galaxy," "cosmos" and "unbounded awareness" in cosmic samyama, there is no place to go. We are there already. Samyama is about awakening what already is, and it is all here where we are right now. Stillness in action.

The guru is in you.

2006/10/30 09:53:24
Support for AYP Pranayama, Mudras and Bandhas
http://www.aypsite.org/forum/topic.asp?TOPIC_ID=1649&REPLY_ID=12711&whichpage=-1
We Have *SNIPPAGE* (And Related Kechari Questions)

Hi Kirtanman:

See lesson 108 for the original snipping procedure. What you are doing now is consistent with that, more or less. Check "kechari" in the topic index for clarifying lessons, and here in the forums for many additional perspectives -- search on "kechari," "khechari," "snip," "talavya," "talabya," etc.

Hint: It takes less stretch to *be* in kechari stage 2 than to *get* into it. Meaning, once you can get the tip of the tongue past the edge of the soft palate, it is a forward movment of the tongue (to less stretch) to bring the soft palate down like a trap door.

See sketches here for the trap door mechanics. See how the soft palate swings down and forward? That is toward less stretch for the tongue.

Perhaps we focus too much on the snipping, and not enough on the actual getting into stage 2, which is not nearly the stretch that most believe, once the edge of the soft palate has been passed. From there it is a move forward to less stretch. I dare say that most could be in kechari stage 2 now with the stretch they have. Getting behind the edge of the soft palate is greatly aided with finger help. From there it is a cake walk forward (with less stretch) to the septum. The soft palate is a paper tiger, folks. Look at the picture.

Beam us up to inner space, Scottyananda! :-)

The guru is in you.

2006/10/30 11:56:47
Support for AYP Pranayama, Mudras and Bandhas
http://www.aypsite.org/forum/topic.asp?TOPIC_ID=1649&REPLY_ID=12718&whichpage=-1
We Have *SNIPPAGE* (And Related Kechari Questions)

Hi Kirtanman:

By "finger help," I mean pushing the tongue back in the mouth from underneath (your ladder analogy), from whatever point under the tongue that is most effective to reach past the edge of the soft palate with the tip of the tongue. Once that happens, it is a forward movement into stage 2.

The edge of the soft palate may feel stretchy (like a rubber band) as it comes down the first time. That also takes some getting used to -- it stretches out and becomes natural in good time.

Yes, it will sometimes boil down to the limiting tether underneath the tongue, and that is why we focus on the frenum with multiple strategies. But, as Scott and others have pointed out, it is not only about that.

Of course, some are born with less frenum/tether than others. Whatever the anatomy is, there will be several factors involved. It is not only about snipping. It is about all of the factors combined. So we don't want to get too carried away with any one aspect. The two most important factors are bhakti and patience over time (not forcing anything to the point of injury).

With bhakti and patience we will surely move from stage 1 to stage 2 sooner or later. Of course, these two qualities are naturally cultivated in daily deep meditation and spinal breathing pranayama, so there is a logical order in all of this. Kechari is an inner development much more than an outer one.

The guru is in you.

2006/11/04 15:51:08
Support for AYP Pranayama, Mudras and Bandhas
http://www.aypsite.org/forum/topic.asp?TOPIC_ID=1658&REPLY_ID=12924&whichpage=-1

Technological helps for kundalini!?

quote:
_____
Originally posted by yoginstar

Thank you guys!
yoginstar it is!
Now how do I delete the Yogini membership I wonder... I read the FAQ but I guess no one ever undoes their memberhsip here... , I did read how to get smiley's though [:-)}
_____

Hi Yoginstar:

Your old ID can be changed by an admin to the new one if you like (it would change on all the old posts too). The new Yoginstar name would have to be changed or deleted first. Let me know. We'd not like to lose your great posts from before, by whatever name.

The guru is in you.

2006/11/01 12:04:53
Support for AYP Pranayama, Mudras and Bandhas
http://www.aypsite.org/forum/topic.asp?TOPIC_ID=1660&REPLY_ID=12788&whichpage=-1
Secret Spot Troubleshooting

Hi All:

Yes, in kechari, the "secret spot" is the spiritually erogenous area along the back edge of the nasal septum, about halfway up, give or take. Everyone's anatomy is a little different. It is found once ecstatic conductivity becomes active, which is a function of all our daily practices over time. It may not be noticed much before then. We will know it when we feel it. :-)

This is why entry into kechari is closely related to the rise of ecstatic conductivity. Before that, the benefit derived in kechari may be limited. It is sort of like having sex before or after puberty. Obviously, <u>after</u> is how nature intended it. It's the same with kechari and "spiritual puberty," which is the rise of ecstatic conductivity.

The guru is in you.

2006/11/08 10:44:45
Support for AYP Pranayama, Mudras and Bandhas
http://www.aypsite.org/forum/topic.asp?TOPIC_ID=1670&REPLY_ID=13053&whichpage=-1
The amazing kechari method

Hi All:

Lovely and inspiring discussion on kechari here.

Just a reminder that in the overall scheme of things, kechari mudra is a practice we are integrating with spinal breathing pranayama. From there, kechari can overflow gradually and naturally into other practices as it becomes an effortless habit that we do not even think about. This is how we will benefit the most from kechari. It is in the nuts and bolts of daily practice where we find the full results.

Romanticizing or mythologizing kechari mudra to the point that it becomes a fascinating end in itself will not serve the overall integration of multiple practices. This is a common situation in the many traditions, where the teachings tend to get fixated on a few practices and their related experiences, mythologizing them to the hilt, at the expense of the rest of yoga. Here we call it the mythical "magic bullet" syndrome. So be mindful of the potential pitfall.

This is not to say that everyone is running off into distraction. But you know what they say: "A stitch in time saves nine." So, just a little reminder stitch here. :-)

We'd like to be inspired. We'd like to be enthusiastic. We'd like to enjoy! It is fun to romanticize for sure. But we'd not like to get lost, at least not for too long.

Somewhere in all of this is a fine line between useful inspiration (bhakti) and getting lost in the mythologies we all have a tendency to create. In AYP we find the line and use it by easily favoring the practice over the experiences (scenery) we encounter along the way. As we say in the lessons, "experiences do not cultivate enlightenment -- practices do."

All the best, and carry on!

The guru is in you.

2006/11/16 17:23:14
Support for AYP Pranayama, Mudras and Bandhas
http://www.aypsite.org/forum/topic.asp?TOPIC_ID=1710&REPLY_ID=13363&whichpage=-1
Kirtanman 2.0

quote:
_____
Originally posted by Kirtanman

2. I spoke with a medical doctor I know, concerning any health risks, or lack thereof, which might stem from sticking one's tongue up one's own

nose, from the inside (aka Kechari Mudra). He was mildly befuzzled as to the reasons / benefits, but took a moment to consider the attendant physiology (including things like infection risk, etc.), and his conclusion was, "Go it it".

_____

Hi Kirtanman:

We should put him in touch with the doctor who ranted and raved against kechari at one of John Wilder's lectures. :-)

Carry on!

The guru is in you.

2006/11/19 11:49:47
Support for AYP Pranayama, Mudras and Bandhas
http://www.aypsite.org/forum/topic.asp?TOPIC_ID=1738
Another Kechari Story - Stretch, Tear, and Bliss

Hi All:

A recent correspondence from my email, shared with permission:

Q1: I have gotten for the first time (yesterday) into stage 2 past the
tendon that you describe with the help of a finger. I was not liking
the idea of snipping, however I found that after I had gotten into
stage 2 my frenum tissue under the tougue was bleeding (just a drop)
and tore at the stress point. It is sore today. Is it okay that it
tore like this? Is this my own internal unfolding inner snipping, so
to speak, and would it be okay to precede like this? I am missing venturing there, as the soreness and healing are not allowing it.
Would it be okay to go forward in this manner, stretching and
healing and so on and so forth, or did I over do it?
Thank you so much.
Blessings Dear Brother.

A1: Congratulations on your entry into kechari stage 2.

I am sure the frenum tearing approach will work out fine over the long run. Ironically though, tiny snipping can lead to quicker progress with less pain and faster healing, due to its more targeted (localized) approach to trimming the frenum. But your approach will obviously work too.

There are a variety of ways to approach kechari. Where there is a will (bhakti) there is a way. Many of these ways have been reported in the AYP forums. Your approach would be welcome there also. I am sure many would be interested and helped in their perspective.

Q2: Deep thanks for your great service. You have acted as a catalyst for the amazing and wondrous reality of Kechari to unfold in me, just 3 days ago I entered stage 2 for the first time and now it appears (as far as I can deduce) that I am in stage 3 reaching for stage 4. You do know dear brother that words fall short and are inadequate in describing or talking about such events as monumental as this, and please excuse me for all these words, though I can't help express how great and important this feels.

In the spirit of true humility I feel that it is only through Grace that this blessing of far reaching Yoga in the form of Kechari has occurred.

Formal regular practice of yoga for me as been lacking in rigorous
discipline with almost no sitting practices or hatha yoga, yet, for
many many years I have taken a non-physical approach encompassing
the yoga of sound, mantra repetition, different forms of spontaneous
pranayam as well as other forms of spontaneous yoga, sacred study and
devotion. I have been in kechari stage 1 for many many years. What is
so monumental here is how close I have been to stage 2 and how major
the difference and how many other long time seekers also are at the
brink of a divine oppurtunity as this transition.

The effects of the last few days have lit up the inner connection of
the crown to the whole body in a wonderful and dramatic way, a tremendous activation seems immanent it is hard to imagine any practice being
so important.

On another note I really do understand the secrecy factor. As much as
I have been exposed to and its been a lot, the fact of this reality
has been hidden, and literally underneath my nose ... what a wonder
... I am not going to run out and tell everyone I know about it. It is so very special and intimate, spiritually personal, yet in your
case in the right setting their are those that sincerely long for this
in depth connectivity kechari affords.

Brother ... a few questions please. This is so new, a world of
transcendent possibility I want to navigate on an optimum level of speed, efficiency and balance:

1. In addition to sitting practices which I am embracing more than
ever on account of the conductivity of Kechari, I have actually been
there in kechari while driving or doing mundane daily tasks, is this
not recommend? Can it dilute the energetic or the more the better
and as much as possible wherever and whenever.

2. Is the actual mudra arrived at only when fully positioned in

stage 4. And can you share more about the entry into K-4

As of yet I have gone from moving around from one point to another
to remaining stationary on one point or another and of course
endeavoring to enter stage 4 i have read lesson 108 many times (108 is a most sacred number).

For the benefit of others I am all for you posting any part of this
email if you think it would help others but I do not wish to share with my name attached to it. It seems so private and sacred, and I feel so
humbled by the grace of it all.

A2: Sounds very good. Keep in mind that kechari is only part of the program, and it is important to weave it into our overall stable routine of
sitting practices. Once you get used to it, it will become a very normal part of the whole. It takes some time.

You can practice kechari whenever you like. You won't wear it out. :-) On the other hand, be sure to self-pace when signs of overdoing occur.
That goes for all practices, and life in general.

Stage 4 is not the epitome. It is something that can be done during spinal breathing and/or chin pump, or not, depending on bhakti. The way into
stage 4 is by following the groove over the eustachian horn, as described in lesson 108 and in the Secrets of Wilder novel.

The real benefits of kechari come from developing stage 2-3 as a regular comfortable thing in spinal breathing, however long that is for you, and
then letting it overflow naturally (as automatic habit) into deep meditation, samyama and the other sitting practices. Then it all is working
together for the 30-60 minute twice-daily routine. Then go out and live your life normally. The blend of good daily practices with normal living is
how enlightenment is cultivated. Life becomes so sweet in every way...

The guru is in you.

Last note from practitioner: A little bit of an update -- I spent some time reading a lot of references to kechari on the forum and I appreciate the
value of it and benefited by it. It is a good important little or maybe not so little community, eventually I will plug in.

One last thing that I experienced is that while pressing in the middle of the septum in stage 2-3 the septum it seemed to move a bit, having some
give and pushing into the septum in turn pushed into the surrounding area initiating an outpouring of blissful energies saturating my being. I think
I was on that right spot (secret spot) you speak of as well.

Even now just pressing my tongue in stage 1 kechari I can clearly feel the septum above and corresponding feelings.

I will be moderating (self-pacing).

2006/11/29 10:53:01
Support for AYP Pranayama, Mudras and Bandhas
http://www.aypsite.org/forum/topic.asp?TOPIC_ID=1766&REPLY_ID=13877&whichpage=-1
What is beyond the septum?

Hi Kyman:

You might find the following unedited Q&A from my email to be helpful. The septum is the solid center divider wall (made of both bone and
cartilage) between the left and right nostrils, and it goes from the nasal pharynx (back edge -- "secret spot") forward to the center of the visible
nose.

Q: I have a few questions regarding stage 4 and 3 Kechari
I can trace with my toung the length up the septum and above to the roof area
As well as insert my toung (about half of it) into the nostril area,
though (they, the
Nostrils seem to end ? is this right it seems like the toung reaches a
dead end and
It also seems like the top of stage 3 is higher than this dead end spot

Please , if you can shed some light on this,
there is increasing ecstatic response on all levels, I have been
regular in practice also

A: The nasal passages go up above the top of the pharynx to the area behind the center brow and then out through the nostrils, but this is not
necessarily something you need to be concerned with at such an early stage. There is erectile tissue that has to be by-passed along the way (see
lesson 108 on how to do this), which may be what you have run into. Your tongue may or may not ever reach that high point, depending on
anatomy, and it is not crucial anyway. There are other ways to affect that area -- yoni mudra (and variations) in particular. As mentioned, using
kechari stages 2-3 comfortably during sitting practices will produce far more effect over time than occasional use of stage 4. Let your bhakti be
your guide, but also pace it according to common sense. Rome was not built in a day! :-)

The guru is in you.

2007/01/26 12:12:33
Support for AYP Pranayama, Mudras and Bandhas
http://www.aypsite.org/forum/topic.asp?TOPIC_ID=1787&REPLY_ID=16600&whichpage=-1
For the ladies!

Hi All:

I have been following this discussion with interest. Not being a woman, I have been a little reluctant to jump in.

But now I'd like to offer some comments that might add some perspective.

Picking up on blujett8's post over here, where she points to ecstatic connections in and around the perineum:
http://www.aypsite.org/forum/topic.asp?TOPIC_ID=1979#16564 ...

In AYP spinal breathing, the primary lower end point is indeed in the area of the perineum. As we know, the perineum is the crossroad between the anus/rectum and genitals. There have been previous discussions seeking exactly where the bottom end of the spinal nerve is. There has been a tendency by some to take it forward to the genitals, and, in fact, the AYP tantra lessons lean this way with siddhasana for women (Satyananda does too). Yet, as the rise of ecstatic conductivity progresses, the sensitivity tends to move, or spread out, to the anus/rectum area as well.

It is well known that the classical literature places kundalini in the anus/rectal area, wrapped around it 3 1/2 times and all that. We need not get wrapped up in the details :-), but it is good to know that we are talking about ecstatic openings in both the area of the genitals (including the natural vajroli flow of fluid/essence up the urethra to the bladder in both sexes), and the awakening of ecstatic conductivity in the anus/rectal area (that is why we do mulabandha/asvini with our pranayama and kumbhaka). In later stages of root opening, siddhasana may automatically shift from front to back also.

From all of that, we might assume that the perineum, while not necessarily the primary point of awakening (or is it?), is a strategic location that covers, by proximity, the entire territory of root awaking, front and back. So, to borrow from the immortal words of Scott Fitzgerald in the Spinal Breathing Pranayama radio interview: "The perineum tain't in the front and it tain't in the back." (In fact, the perineum is also called the "tain't.")

Regardless of where the perineum is not, it is in the middle, and awakening goes in all directions from there.

And what about the area behind the cervix, or that ecstatic sensitivity somewhere in the middle of the pelvic region? Well, it is the sex center, isn't it? It is similar for men, with radiant ecstatic sensitivity arising in and around the seminal vesicles. It would appear that the similarities between the sexes in these matters are many more than the differences. What might be different is what is awakening when and where in the individual, which is a matter of personal purification and opening, and not necessarily gender related. Such variations are not based on anatomical differences as much as on individual patterns of obstruction we are each dissolving gradually through our daily practices.

In spinal breathing we are enlivening all of these areas as we touch with awareness the root location(s) and the area in the center of the pelvic region, not to mention everything else connected with the spinal nerve between the root and center brow. There is no need to alter our practice to accommodate whatever seems to be ecstatically sensitive in the moment. In fact, this might be favoring the scenery over the practice, something we all need to cognizant of.

So, should the sex center be the terminus of the spinal nerve in spinal breathing? Probably not, but no one is prohibited from experimenting with variations in practice. Satyananda's approach may be a valid variation. The proof of the pudding will be in the long term eating.

My only suggestion would be to not leave the root area/perineum out of the practice. Just because an area does not seem ecstatically active in the moment does not mean there is no gold in them thar hills!

Just some food for thought.

Great discussion and exploration!

The guru is in you.

2007/01/05 14:27:53
Support for AYP Pranayama, Mudras and Bandhas
http://www.aypsite.org/forum/topic.asp?TOPIC_ID=1887&REPLY_ID=15424&whichpage=-1
Spinal Breathing in Siddhasana
Note: Topic moved for better placement.
2007/01/05 14:55:04
Support for AYP Pranayama, Mudras and Bandhas
http://www.aypsite.org/forum/topic.asp?TOPIC_ID=1887&REPLY_ID=15425&whichpage=-1
Spinal Breathing in Siddhasana

Hi Anub3 and welcome!

Somehow your post ended up in the administrator announcements forum, which is supposed to be locked -- not sure what happened there -- tech glitch. That is why your post was moved.

Make sure to take plenty of time between add-ons in practice -- not days, but weeks or months. In some cases it can take years to fully stabilze a new practice element. And do take practices in a logical order. In the AYP lessons we attempt to lay out a logical order. Not sure how you got advanced siddhasana in front of (or coincident with) beginning spinal breathing, if that is what is happening. Maybe you are utilizing other teachings too?

Kumbhaka is especially powerful for stimulating kundalini awaking (yes, that is what it was/is), and it should be undertaken only when our practices and experiences are well-established and stable. If you are prone to having big energy surges, be careful about adding too many additional aggressive practices. All things in good time.

You look to be very much on the right track with bhakti, and with a willingness to act, which is essential. What you need now is a solid grounding in the principles and practices of self-pacing so you can stay on the fast track. Ironically, the more we rush into practices, the slower we can end up going if the energies get out of hand, which they are bound to when pursuing the path of "reckless abandon." :-)

As I often say: "Blasting through does not work."

There are more than a few folks around here who can share very relevant first hand experiences with you. We have a pretty good knowledge-base here for what you are doing and going through.

Wishing you all the best on your path. Enjoy!

The guru is in you.

2007/01/27 15:50:11
Support for AYP Pranayama, Mudras and Bandhas
http://www.aypsite.org/forum/topic.asp?TOPIC_ID=2000&REPLY_ID=16668&whichpage=-1
kechari question...

quote:
_____
Originally posted by Balance

I agree with Victor, the septum continues further up so the tongue is straight up on the bottom of the cranium.
_____

Hi All:

Yes, I believe this is what Mr. Paulsen was writing about -- what we call stage 3 in AYP, which is the tongue rising to the top of the nasal pharynx without entering the nostrils. The roof of the pharynx is bone, and it is right under the pituitary gland.

However, I do not agree that the "bone" is the ultimate connection point in kechari. There are many ecstatic neurological connections that occur in the nasal pharynx and nasal passages. The easiest to reach and most effective one I have found is the "secret spot" on the edge of the septum about half way up. Stage 3 provides more stimulation for that with the underside of the tongue blanketing the back edge of the septum, rather than anything particularly profound happening at the bony top of the pharynx.

As for stage 4, in the nostrils, that is something else -- powerful, but not necessarily conducive for long term stimulation like the secret spot is in stages 2 & 3. So I consider stages 2 & 3 to of greater importance than stage 4 for daily practice, which is essentially what Mr. Paulsen is saying, though from a different angle.

I'm sure a whole book could be written on the nuances of whole body ecstatic energy cultivation in the various stages of kechari. Maybe one of you will write it someday. But don't do it at the expense of maintaining a well balanced integrated practice routine. :-)

The guru is in you.

2007/02/06 14:42:22
Support for AYP Pranayama, Mudras and Bandhas
http://www.aypsite.org/forum/topic.asp?TOPIC_ID=2032&REPLY_ID=17080&whichpage=-1
Spinal Breathing question

Hi Louis:

It is good to end up at the brow and the root at the completion of inhalation and exhalation.

The bogging down that can happen in spinal breathing is due to obstructions encountered, and subsequent purification occurring in the nervous system during practice. Good things are happening, and it will clear up in time.

In the meantime, if we get bogged down going up or down (it can happen either way), we can jump to the brow or root as the breathing cycle is ending in that direction, no matter where we happen to be. So we can always end up at the brow or root, regardless of any bogging down that may be happening in-between. With this approach the clearing of the area in-between brow and root will be facilitated from both ends in every cycle. As anyone with ecstatic conductivity coming up can verify by direct experience, the brow and root are primary instigators of purification in the spinal nerve, so it is very good to touch them both in every cycle of spinal breathing.

What you suggested may also work, though there is the possiblility that the brow will not be reached on the next try either. It will be easier to make the full leap in the current cycle than to save a partial leap for the next cycle. That way we will cover the full distance in every cycle, and can be purifying the full spinal nerve in-between root and brow as we continue.

It is always a matter of personal choice, of course, but the procedure of spinal breathing is to easily favor the journey up and down the full length of spinal nerve whenever we realize we have been wandering or bogging down. Purification occurs as we pass through obstructed areas. In fact, allowing ourselves to pass through, no matter how quickly, is an essential dynamic of the release. It is a letting go! This is the essence of spinal bastrika also, which is very fast and brings an additional dynamic into the practice routine.

So, it is perfectly okay (right procedure) to jump to the brow or root as our breath is reaching the end of its cycle. Spinal breathing can be relatively dynamic like that. We are playing both ends through the middle. To do that, it is important to be establishing our position at both ends in every breathing cycle. :-)

The AYP Spinal Breathing Pranayama book offers more pointers on this and related experiences.

All the best!

The guru is in you.

PS: Thanks much for pulling those posts up, Richard. The more ways we can cover it, the better. :-)

2008/02/20 09:59:35
Support for AYP Pranayama, Mudras and Bandhas
http://www.aypsite.org/forum/topic.asp?TOPIC_ID=2048&REPLY_ID=30296&whichpage=-1
pause before inhalation

quote:
_____
Originally posted by Christi

It (breath suspension) makes SBP into a much more powerful practice energy wise, so proceed with caution.
_____

Hi Christi:

That's why it isn't in the lessons. Though I am not sure it isn't mentioned somewhere in a cautionary way. It is easy for people to get hung up in deliberate suspensions during spinal breathing and overdo (many do).

So "official" AYP breath suspension (kumbhaka) is saved for more discrete practices like yoni mudra, chin pump and nauli, where practice times can be more tightly regulated without having to limit spinal breathing and the many benefits it brings. It is intended to be a smoother approach, with plenty of kumbhaka oomph available outside spinal breathing as desired.

It is always the practitioner's call, of course. :-)

The guru is in you.

2007/09/03 11:19:51
Support for AYP Pranayama, Mudras and Bandhas
http://www.aypsite.org/forum/topic.asp?TOPIC_ID=2076&REPLY_ID=25250&whichpage=-1
fine tuning help please...

Hi Monster:

Yogic breathing is essentially "belly breathing." No attention on the diaphragm is necessary. And yogic breathing is not a prerequisite for spinal breathing, which can be done with our normal breathing slowed down a bit. It is suggested to keep it simple, and not try and take on too much at once. All things in their own time. :-)

All the best!

The guru is in you.

2007/09/04 07:52:21
Support for AYP Pranayama, Mudras and Bandhas
http://www.aypsite.org/forum/topic.asp?TOPIC_ID=2076&REPLY_ID=25280&whichpage=-1
fine tuning help please...

Hi Edmund:

It is suggested to do everything comfortably. Then the next steps will present themselves at the best time. If we are struggling with our body all the time, it will not be ideal. Just relax.

Developing our practice routine is a balance between bhakti (spiritual desire) and self-pacing for progress and comfort. Only you can know when the right time is for you to take a next step. If there is discomfort beyond minor adjustments, then you are probably rushing things.

Three weeks in spinal breathing might be okay for some to add an enhancement, but too short for others. If you are not comfortable in your practice, it is probably too short. Sitting without back support is not a prerequisite for the AYP practices. If it works for you and is comfortable, fine, but if it is challenging, it is okay to use pillows on the bed, or a chair. It is presumed everyone knows how to sit down comfortably somewhere. Do that. :-)

Remember, Rome was not built in a day. It takes years (maybe decades) to build a full yoga routine, while mastering self-pacing along the way. Learning to make choices on practices and managing them effectively is what the game is all about. Once we have become adept at that, there is no limit to how far we can travel. Our possibilities are infinite, but it takes some time, you know.

There used to be a time when just finding effective practices was a major challenge. Now we are moving beyond that into the integration and management of many powerful practices. These days, it is about developing driving skills.

Drive well, and enjoy the ride!

The guru is in you.

2007/03/29 11:35:03
Support for AYP Pranayama, Mudras and Bandhas
http://www.aypsite.org/forum/topic.asp?TOPIC_ID=2355
Kechari Mudra Videos

Hi All:

The following links were received recently from a reader:

Zaadz blog on Khechari Mudra, with a Video: http://t4om.zaadz.com/blog/2007/2/khechari_mudra

Direct link to the video on YouTube:
http://www.youtube.com/watch?v=EJc_LEvTRx4&eurl=http%3A%2F%2Ft4om%2Ezaadz%2Ecom%2Fblog%2F2007%2F2%2Fkhechari%5Fmudra

FYI, the Zaadz AYP page linked to in the blog is compliments of Trip/Brett: http://ayp.zaadz.com

Those who are unfamiliar with kechari mudra, see this FAQ topic: http://www.aypsite.org/forum/topic.asp?TOPIC_ID=2170

All the best!

The guru is in you.

2007/03/30 13:01:04
Support for AYP Pranayama, Mudras and Bandhas
http://www.aypsite.org/forum/topic.asp?TOPIC_ID=2362&REPLY_ID=19685&whichpage=-1
Personal rythm

Hi Leo:

Yes, finding a comfortable rate of breath in spinal breathng pranayama is good, while gently favoring slow deep breathing as we proceed. This is the procedure. Keep in mind that comfortable frequency will change as purification advances. So what is comfortable now will change. And a frequency that is uncomfortable now may be comfortable later. And so on...

The bottom line is that we don't alter our practice or try and "fix it" (as in a fixed breath rate) due to experiences that come up during the practice. That can lead to chasing energy experiences and a loss of effectiveness in our practice. Breath rate will change naturally according to inner purification going on -- sometimes breath will be naturally slower, sometimes faster. We just easily favor the procedure of our practice as given, allowing the flexibilities that are built in. In the case of spinal breathing, it is comfortably favoring slow deep breathing up and down spinal nerve in the center of the spinal column. If we wander off into energy sensations this way or that way, we just ease back to the center of the spinal column, always favoring comfortable slow deep breathing.

If we are feeling some inner pleasure in our practice that is fine. But we don't chase after it, modifying our practice in the process. You can be sure inner sensations will change as purification advances over time, and our practice is designed to accommodate that without being morphed into a different practice that can be less effective over the long term.

We just easily favor the procedure, no matter what is happening. We can enjoy our experiences in-between our practice sessions. How we feel between sittings is the real measure of how effective our practices are. During practices, just about anything is possible, depending on the course of purification occurring in the moment. That is why we favor the practice itself, as this is what is bringing up the experiences in the first place. As we say: "Experiences do not cause spiritual progress. Practices do."

It is important to be clear on what is cause and what is effect.

Many nuances are covered throughout the AYP lessons. It always boils down to favoring the practice while we are doing it, and self-pacing our over all daily routine of practices as needed. And be sure to go out and live life fully between practice sessions, of course. :-)

The new Yoga FAQ offers additional doorways into the AYP writings. Check these FAQ topics:
Spinal Breathing Pranayama: http://www.aypsite.org/forum/topic.asp?TOPIC_ID=2131
Self-pacing: http://www.aypsite.org/forum/topic.asp?TOPIC_ID=2139

Wishing you the best on your path. Practice wisely, and enjoy!

The guru is in you.

2007/04/05 14:22:33
Support for AYP Pranayama, Mudras and Bandhas
http://www.aypsite.org/forum/topic.asp?TOPIC_ID=2387&REPLY_ID=19864&whichpage=-1
Going to a "Professional" for Frenum Removal

Hi Jim:

Here is a topic that goes into removal of the the frenum with a laser: http://www.aypsite.org/forum/topic.asp?TOPIC_ID=460

There have been a few who have gone this route. I don't believe the act of removing the frenum (quickly by surgery, or gradually by tiny snips), or even physically getting into stage 2 kechari, necessarily guarantees immediate progress in ecstatic conductivity. Without some initial ecstatic conductivity, kechari may be little more than a parlor trick, like the kids in the videos are doing. It is the difference between being a contortionist and being a yogi/yogini -- big difference. The same can be said about all physical yoga. Obviously, we are looking for much more.

On the other hand, overcoming the frenum limitation is certainly necessary to physically achieve kechari stages 2 and higher. Yet, the more important factor in this is the rise of inner silence and ecstatic conductivity from within via our other practices, which can then lead to kechari and additional yoga practices. In that sense, true kechari is effect before it is cause, much the way everything is in yoga. It all grows from bhakti, and it all feeds bhakti. Round and round and ever higher the neurobiological transformation goes.

This is not to discourage kechari -- only to suggest that it is not going to be a panacea if regarded mainly as a physical achievment. It depends very much on other non-physical factors. In your case, kechari is likely to be a boost, since you have the energy flowing already. You will know when it is time, and then overcoming the frenum by whatever means you choose will be an incidental detail in the larger scheme of what is happening.

It is also important to note that many have achieved human spiritual transformation without structured practice of kechari, or other specific techniques, though influences are no doubt felt through the urges of automatic yoga rising from within the nervous system as purification and opening advance by whatever means that are applied -- in many historical cases, by blistering bhakti only.

All yoga practices have been derived over the centuries from these natural influences coming from within the spiritually evolving human nervous system. As a result, we have many tools available now to hasten things along, managed for good progress with safety. As far as structured practices go, it is a matter of what tools in the box work best for each individual to maximize progress without blowing the doors off the barn. :-)

All the best!

The guru is in you.

2007/05/31 09:58:27
Support for AYP Pranayama, Mudras and Bandhas
http://www.aypsite.org/forum/topic.asp?TOPIC_ID=2623&REPLY_ID=22593&whichpage=-1
Need suggestions...

Hi Salvation:

Sounds like you are doing something different from AYP, though some of the elements are the same. That's good if it works for you, but there isn't much I can do to advise on the particulars. Better to go back to the source where you learned this approach.

Just to point out a few differences, in AYP we do not "meditate" on the ajna (third eye) -- it is covered in various ways as part of other practices. The only meditation we do is with mantra (I AM), and we take it as separate from pranayama and other energy related practices. This is important for unfettered cultivation of inner silence.

Spinal breathing pranayama is done before deep meditation by the clock (5-10 min) rather than by breath counts, and mudras and bandhas are added on systematically step-by-step over time during spinal breathing, and left to be "automatic" at other times during our routine. The only time we use chin lock (jalandhara) in AYP is in yoni mudra kumbhaka done as a separate practice, and we do chin pump (dynamic jalandhara) as separate from spinal breathing and meditation also. Pranayama, mudras and bandhas are mainly for cultivation of ecstatic conductivity.

That's not all of it, and there are some refinements that are not mentioned, but it gives an idea of the AYP routine, which is built up very gradually over time, beginning first with deep meditation. The routine is more compact than it sounds -- 30-60 minutes twice each day, depending on how many elements of practice are included. It can be streamlined to be much shorter too, as a busy schedule might demand.

The two key elements cultivated in practices, inner silence and ecstatic conductivity, join naturally in us over time to give rise to enlightenment, which is life in unity and endless outpouring divine love. We are designed for that! :-)

If interested, see the main lessons for more detail on all of this. It is suggested to take them in order.

All the best on your path. Enjoy!

The guru is in you.

2007/05/31 11:07:19
Support for AYP Pranayama, Mudras and Bandhas
http://www.aypsite.org/forum/topic.asp?TOPIC_ID=2623&REPLY_ID=22595&whichpage=-1
Need suggestions...
PS: The raising of the tongue (kechari) can happen automatically with the advent of ecstatic conductivity, or with strong bhakti (spiritual desire). It is a natural connection that involves the entire spinal nerve, of which the ajna (third eye) is the top portion. There can be various "automatic yogas" coming up. In AYP we favor the practice we are doing over the experiences, which can include automatic yogas and movements. If the tongue wants to stay up, that is okay. But we should also "self-pace" using good common sense if excess energy symptoms begin to occur either during practices or in daily activity.
2007/05/31 13:14:24
Support for AYP Pranayama, Mudras and Bandhas
http://www.aypsite.org/forum/topic.asp?TOPIC_ID=2623&REPLY_ID=22598&whichpage=-1
Need suggestions...

Hi Salvation:

Here is how we handle chakras in AYP: http://www.aypsite.org/47.html

We use chakras without getting tangled up in them. That is the advantage of using the master controls and leaving the rest of the machinery to do its thing "under the hood." :-)

All the best!

The guru is in you.

2007/06/07 00:08:50
Support for AYP Pranayama, Mudras and Bandhas
http://www.aypsite.org/forum/topic.asp?TOPIC_ID=2648&REPLY_ID=22861&whichpage=-1
is jalandhara required for kumbhaka with kechari?

Hi Victor:

Yes, spinal breathing is normally done with the head vertical, as is deep meditation. And, no, kechari does not replace jalandhara bandha (chin lock). Once we have learned kechari during spinal breathing, we can use it throughout practices if desired as an automatic habit, without any extra attention being devoted to it.

Normal AYP spinal breathing does not include kumbhaka (breath retention). If we are doing yoni mudra kumbhaka (separate practice), that is the time we do breath retention and jalandhara along with the other two locks (uddiyana and mulabandha), plus sambhavi, and kechari to whatever extent we are doing it (stage 1, 2, etc). Dynamic jalandhara (chin pump) is normally an independent practice with kumbhaka (presumably like you are doing now), but can alternatively be done in "lite" mode during part of our spinal breathing session without kumbhaka.

The arrangement of the practice components is like this to make it easy for practitioners to take on new elements of practice step-by-step without overdoing. Once we are familiar with all the components, there can be some flexibiliy in the arrangement according to preference, but never at the expense of deep meditation, which we do not encumber with anything intentional outside the procedure of deep meditation itself.

If you are mixing kumbhaka with spinal breathing, plus jalandhara, and it works for you, then who can argue? But those learning these components for the first time will be wise to take them on in order one at a time, without burdening either spinal breathing or deep meditation beyond what is discussed in the lessons.

It is a matter of building a balanced, effective and efficient integration of practices step-by-step while utilizing self-pacing. This is the mission of the lessons, and why things are done the way they are. As we become more skilled in the use of all the elements of practice, there are more options for using them. Some of these options are discussed in the later online lessons.

But such expertise does not develop in a few months, so newcomers to all of this will be very wise to follow a planned build-up like is given in the AYP lessons. We don't want anyone to be getting indigestion at the spiritual practices smorgasbord table. :-)

All the best!

The guru is in you.

2007/06/07 00:21:56
Support for AYP Pranayama, Mudras and Bandhas
http://www.aypsite.org/forum/topic.asp?TOPIC_ID=2648&REPLY_ID=22863&whichpage=-1
is jalandhara required for kumbhaka with kechari?

quote:
_____
Originally posted by Victor

maybe i should clarify my question. Is spinal breathing always done without kumbhaka and if kumbhaka is used do you require jalandhara even with kechari? I guess that is simpler
_____

Yes, jalandhara should always be used with kumbhaka -- either static jalandhara (during yoni mudra), or dynamaic jalandhara.

The spinal breathing question is covered above. If you are going to be using kumbhaka mixed with spinal breathing, then use jalandhara when in deliberate breath suspension. That is a variation on regular spinal breathing practice -- a major departure actually, which increases the risk of energy excesses for inexperienced practitioners. Ask John Wilder :-).

Jalandhara is not necessary during natural breath suspension, like happens in deep meditation. Sometimes jalandhara (static or dynamic) might happen as an automatic yoga during meditation or at other times during our practices. That is okay, but we don't favor it if it's not specified for use at that time. We treat it like any other automatic yoga, and gently favor the practice we are doing over any experience or automatic yoga that may come up. We don't try and force it out, and we don't indulge it either.

The guru is in you.

2007/06/14 12:45:20
Support for AYP Pranayama, Mudras and Bandhas
http://www.aypsite.org/forum/topic.asp?TOPIC_ID=2670&REPLY_ID=23148&whichpage=-1
Not clear on Mulabandha

Hi Gray:

It is done by pulling the lower abdomen in a bit. It is the beginnings of uddiyana and nauli, which are covered later in the lessons. Mulabandha and uddiyana are connected. All of the mudras and bandhas are connected, and become gradually more subtle (less physical) over time -- even as they are becoming much more powerful in terms of stimulating the ecstatic flow, once ecstatic conductivity is on the rise.

All the best!

The guru is in you.

2007/07/08 00:30:46
Support for AYP Pranayama, Mudras and Bandhas
http://www.aypsite.org/forum/topic.asp?TOPIC_ID=2757&REPLY_ID=24004&whichpage=-1
jerking and twitching
Welcome Doug!

Also see the lessons on "Automatic Yoga and Movements" listed in the Topic Index.

It is the "friction" of inner energy moving through the purifying neurobiology, and it will all smooth out in time. Prudent self-pacing in practices is the key to navigating through over the long term, maintaining good progress with comfort.

All the best!

The guru is in you.

2007/07/12 11:26:58
Support for AYP Pranayama, Mudras and Bandhas
http://www.aypsite.org/forum/topic.asp?TOPIC_ID=2765&REPLY_ID=24139&whichpage=-1

kechari, kumbhaka and thoughts

quote:
_____
Originally posted by gentlep

Hi meg and victor, it's not only during the sitting practices but other times I have observed this as well. I do kechari during the idle moments in the day as well (e.g. while taking a stroll outside or sitting and waiting for someone or something.) It seems a natural position for the tongue and gives a nice buzzing feeling in the head. I don't think I am overdoing as I never had the problem of energy excesses. So it's just the question of excessive thoughts. It seems like rather than being out there, me and my thoughts are trapped inside my head. They say the thoughts come from the heart but I feel everything inside the head.
_____

Hi Gentlep:

Kechari is primarily an energy technique, as are all the mudras and bandhas. The degree to which they enhance (move) inner silence and quiet the mind will depend on the degree to which inner silence is present already, which is a function of daily deep meditation practice, and samyama also.

In AYP we use our spinal breathing pranayama time for the cultivation of mudra and bandha habits, developing them one at a time. Once mudras and bandhas become easy habit, they may happen naturally as a result of our inner energy flows (when they all happen together *subtly* it is called "whole body mudra"). Then mudras and bandhas may appear in deep meditation and in other parts of our sitting practices besides spinal breathing, and in daily activity also. This is fine.

However, we do not "intentionally" practice mudras and bandhas in deep meditation or samyama, because this will divert attention from these specific mental procedures.

The effective development of mudras and bandhas is covered in the lessons, and especially in the Asanas, Mudras and Bandhas book (pages 71-78 - "Filling in the Practice Routine").

As for doing kechari during the day, this is okay if it is not disruptive. "Self-pacing" is the watchword for all of our practices. :-)

The guru is in you.

2007/07/17 00:01:38
Support for AYP Pranayama, Mudras and Bandhas
http://www.aypsite.org/forum/topic.asp?TOPIC_ID=2774&REPLY_ID=24250&whichpage=-1
Spinal Breathing Enhancement

Hi iqtrader, and welcome!

What you are into there is the Taoist microcosmic orbit, which has both similarities and differences with AYP spinal breathing. There has been discussion about it in these topics:
http://www.aypsite.org/forum/topic.asp?TOPIC_ID=1474
http://www.aypsite.org/forum/topic.asp?TOPIC_ID=500
(for related topics, search on "microcosmic")

The additional Taoist physical maneuvers you mention are somewhat analogous to mudras and bandhas in yoga. Nevertheless, these are two different systems, and mixing and matching practice elements can be a bit problematic. That is covered in the topic links above.

It will be your experiment, since no one is able to predict the outcome of every combination of practices from different systems, except in a general way -- be careful not to "double up" in time on similar practices from different systems, and always "self-pace" if energy flows become excessive. Keep in mind that overly aggressive practice can have delayed adverse effects, so be sure to take things one step at a time, stabilizing each new element of practice for weeks or months before adding another. That goes for building up the AYP practices too, which are plenty.

While there can be some benefit in drawing on a few methods from other systems that fill in gaps in our primary approach, trying to do a 50/50 blend of systems is a pretty big challenge, even for an expert. Better to keep both feet in one boat, especially beginners. Less likely to end up in the water that way. :-)

Wishing you all the best on you path. Practice wisely, and enjoy!

The guru is in you.

2007/07/31 13:05:32
Support for AYP Pranayama, Mudras and Bandhas
http://www.aypsite.org/forum/topic.asp?TOPIC_ID=2795&REPLY_ID=24494&whichpage=-1
kechari stage 4 and sushumna

Hi Gentlep:

The purpose of alternate nostril breathing is to stimulate and balance the energies (left and right), which leads to calmness in the center (spinal nerve/sushumna).

Alternate nostril breathing (nadi shodana or anulom vilom) is not critical in terms of counting, timing, etc. It is not that exact, though some into Swara Yoga might take issue. In AYP we don't use alternate nostril breathing, but do respect its prominence, as discussed in an addition to Lesson 41 in the AYP Easy Lessons book. Spinal breathing pranayama without nostril alternation is more than adequate to get the job done. Alternate nostril breathing does happen to be compatible with kechari stage 4, so we can use it there to the degree desired, but this is not regarded as core practice in AYP.

Long before we are playing around with kechari stage 4, we should consider if we have stabilized our practice in deep meditation, spinal breathing pranayama, asanas, mudras (with kechari stage 1 or 2 being plenty), bandhas, samyama, and the application of tantric sexual principles. There is plenty that will be good to put in place before it will be necessary to go deep into kechari stage 4. In fact, kechari stage 4 will not be necessary at all for many people. It is not a prerequisite for enlightenment. :-)

But to answer your basic question, some techniques attempt to quiet the center by directly stimulating and balancing the surrounding energy channels. Alternate nostril breathing is one of those. There are many ways to skin the cat, some more reliable and deeper reaching than others. We will know what works for us as we continue with our daily practices long term.

Wishing you all the best on your path. Practice wisely, and enjoy!

The guru is in you.

2007/08/02 13:31:44
Support for AYP Pranayama, Mudras and Bandhas
http://www.aypsite.org/forum/topic.asp?TOPIC_ID=2795&REPLY_ID=24514&whichpage=-1
kechari stage 4 and sushumna

quote:
_____
Originally posted by gentlep

Thanks yogani for the clarification. As you mentioned alternate nostril breathing with kechari 4 is not part of ayp and can be used outside of practice, can it be used during the day? e.g. while driving the car, waiting or in a meeting etc.
_____

Hi Gentlep:

It is part of AYP, but not a "core practice" like deep meditation, basic spinal breathing, asanas, etc.

It is up to the practitioner if and when to use kechari stage 4 alternate nostril breathing. From the AYP point of view, it is not recommended until core practices are well-established for months or years. The idea is to have a stable daily routine of practices that we can stay with for the long term. That is what will bring real progress. Up and down adventures with any particular practice are not going to make much difference in our long term progress.

It is okay to experiment. But let's not make the mistake of calling that practice. Practice is what we have been doing steadily daily for months and years, with self-pacing as needed, of course. :-)

The guru is in you.

2007/08/30 12:16:56
Support for AYP Pranayama, Mudras and Bandhas
http://www.aypsite.org/forum/topic.asp?TOPIC_ID=2864&REPLY_ID=25151&whichpage=-1
Spinal breathing without bandhas and mudras??

Hi Anthony:

Keep in mind that nearly all practices have a "clunky stage" at the beginning. Everything smooths out in time.

Also check these two lessons, and others listed in the topic index under "mulabandha/asvini."

Hitting a wall at mulabandha -- http://www.aypsite.org/105.html

Some other approaches to mulabandha -- http://www.aypsite.org/119.html

And, yes, spinal breathing pranayama is fine without mudras and bandhas, until you are ready for something more. Ecstatic conductivity may come before, during or after. There is no telling. Ecstasy is a symptom of purification (the friction of energy moving through purifying neurobiology) that may fluctuate up and down over many years before it becomes very refined, steady and radiant. Inner silence is the prerequisite -- so deep meditation is primary. Take it one step at a time, balancing your bhakti (spiritual desire) with your good common sense. Self-pacing! :-)

All the best!

The guru is in you.

2007/09/17 14:04:27
Support for AYP Pranayama, Mudras and Bandhas
http://www.aypsite.org/forum/topic.asp?TOPIC_ID=2928&REPLY_ID=25551&whichpage=-1
Sambhavi and self pacing

Hi Jill:

Sounds like a good beginning with sambhavi mudra. As for how much is enough or too much, it depends on your own experience, with self-pacing utilized as needed.

Beginning sambhavi in our spinal breathing pranayama session is a good place to develop the habit. Going forward (especially in the formative stage), it is a good idea to regulate the daily time for sambhavi, so we can keep track and not to overdo too much. Later on, sambhavi may occur spontaneously as an "automatic yoga." Even then, we should use our common sense in self-pacing to avoid overdoing. Automatic yoga is not necessarily in our best interest at all times, sometimes leading to overdoing. It is a question of how well adapted we have become to the increased ecstatic energy flows within. When we are ready for more, we will know. And when we are not ready for more, we will know also. :-)

As we become more advanced, sambhavi can be used at any time to stimulate and regulate our ecstatic conductivity. This leads naturally to the "whole body mudra." But not to rush things too much. See this related post: http://www.aypsite.org/forum/topic.asp?TOPIC_ID=2921#25495

All the best!

The guru is in you.

2007/11/08 10:32:09
Support for AYP Pranayama, Mudras and Bandhas
http://www.aypsite.org/forum/topic.asp?TOPIC_ID=3109&REPLY_ID=26824&whichpage=-1
Breath Yoga mediation questions

Hi Hahasiah, and welcome!

In the AYP approach, breathing techniques are integrated with many other practices in a step-by-step way. These methods come from bhakti yoga, mantra yoga, kriya yoga, hatha yoga, kundalini yoga, tantra, and other systems of practice. For the sequence of development, see the "Main Lessons" linked at the top of this page.

In the approach here, breathing techniques and meditation are separate, not the same, and not done at the same time. There are specific reasons for this, having to do with achieving maximum effectiveness in both classes of practice.

If by "breath yoga" you mean "swara yoga," that has been discussed here in the forums also (try a search), and it overlaps into several of the disciplines just mentioned. In any case, we do not focus on one particular class of practice to the exclusion of all others here. That has been found to be a less than optimal approach. The human nervous system has a range of capabilities for spiritual transformation, and we attempt to stimulate them all by the most effective means known, in a compact routine of daily practices that can fit into a busy lifestyle.

All of the practices are naturally connected within us, so if we are doing an effective method in one area (like spinal breathing pranayama or deep meditation), then a natural urge will arise to take on other classes of practice. The elements of practice and the natural "connectedness of yoga" are discussed in this lesson on Patanjali's Eight Limbs of Yoga and Samyama here: http://www.aypsite.org/149.html

Regarding astral projection and other "siddhis" (powers), we do not focus on those things here, though experiences do happen from time to time, usually in relation to practical need rather than by curiosity or obsession. What we are interested in here is cultivating enlightenment, which is freedom from suffering through the direct experience of our true nature. While siddhis are part of that, they are incidental rather than a primary objective. The profile of experience in daily living that gradually arises from these practices is abiding inner silence, ecstatic bliss, and outpouring divine love.

You can find more lessons on the integration of practices and siddhis in the Topic Index under "Connectedness of Yoga," "Samyama (near top of page)," and "siddhis/powers."

Wishing you all the best on your chosen path. Enjoy!

The guru is in you.

PS: By the way, "nirvana" is not a place. It is a condition synonymous with enlightenment as described above.

2007/11/19 17:35:48
Support for AYP Pranayama, Mudras and Bandhas
http://www.aypsite.org/forum/topic.asp?TOPIC_ID=3160&REPLY_ID=27132&whichpage=-1
Spinal Breathing and ujjayi

Hi Tosh, and welcome!

Ujjayi is an enhancement to spinal breathing, not a requirement. The style of ujjayi we do in AYP is a gentle restriction of the epiglottis on exhalation only, producing a slight hiss. During inhalation we go for a more open and relaxed throat than usual. Each has its own reason and effect.

Other enhancements from the Spinal Breathing Pranayama book include full yogic breathing, a gentle lifting of the eyes, and noticing cool and warm currents in the ascending and descending breath in the spinal nerve.

All of these are helpful but not essential enhancements. They will happen if and when our purifying nervous system calls for them. Spinal breathing works just fine on whatever level we happen to be practicing it. Not to worry. :-)

Remember, all of our practices will have a "clunky stage" in the beginning, and become increasingly refined over time of daily practice.

The guru is in you.

2007/11/21 11:52:56
Support for AYP Pranayama, Mudras and Bandhas
http://www.aypsite.org/forum/topic.asp?TOPIC_ID=3165&REPLY_ID=27171&whichpage=-1
ways to numb the frenum

Hi Alvin:

Good to see you again. It has been a while.

If you have been trimming the frenum all this time for kechari mudra, with little release of the tongue for going back and up, then this may point to an anatomical difference you have. I don't think it would be wise to force the issue with bigger snips, exposing yourself to greater risks than necessary. And do take Shanti's words to heart and forget about the dry ice!

If your bhakti is burning for kechari and you have to do something, then a better course may be to go see a dentist or oral surgeon with laser capability. Then you can be sure you will not be running an excessive health risk. A few around here have gone that route with satisfactory results. The approach to trimming the frenum in <u>Lesson 108</u> is designed to cover a broad spectrum of people, but obviously not everyone.

Kechari mudra is not an absolute prerequisite for advancement on our spiritual path, and pressing it on principle or intellectual obsession rather than on natural energetic bhakti is not the best approach. Much better to stay focused on our core practices of deep meditation and spinal breathing pranayama for the long term (adding in asanas, samyama and other less extreme measures along the way) -- this combination will take us very far.

It is perfectly okay to be doing kechari stage 1, 1/2, or even 0, as we continue forward. You will know by your own feelings about it. Just self-pace your bhakti to avoid becoming reckless. As we know, bhakti can be reckless sometimes, not minding for our health. It wants it all right now, but that is not how it works on this earth plane, where everything takes time. We are going as fast as we can while preserving life and limb, so we can be here doing practices over the long term. :-)

All the best!

The guru is in you.

PS: Check the <u>Yoga FAQ on Kechari</u> for some more links. Searching the forums for "kechari" and separately for "snip" will turn up many more topics.

2007/12/03 14:27:49
Support for AYP Pranayama, Mudras and Bandhas
http://www.aypsite.org/forum/topic.asp?TOPIC_ID=3215&REPLY_ID=27631&whichpage=-1
Spinal Breathing and Babaji's Kriya Yoga

Hi Sean:

This lesson on varieties of spinal breathing might be helpful: http://www.aypsite.org/206.html

All the best!

The guru is in you.

2007/12/03 14:33:46
Support for AYP Pranayama, Mudras and Bandhas
http://www.aypsite.org/forum/topic.asp?TOPIC_ID=3215&REPLY_ID=27632&whichpage=-1
Spinal Breathing and Babaji's Kriya Yoga
PS: If you are looking at a version of spinal breathing that goes down on inhalation and up on exhalation, check this lesson called, "Which way is up?" http://www.aypsite.org/46.html

2010/08/23 12:35:26
Support for AYP Pranayama, Mudras and Bandhas
http://www.aypsite.org/forum/topic.asp?TOPIC_ID=3215&REPLY_ID=72281&whichpage=-1
Spinal Breathing and Babaji's Kriya Yoga

Hi Viviane:

The primary purpose of spinal breathing (the style used in AYP) is awakening, cultivation and integration of ecstatic energy between root and brow. In order for it to work, both ends of the spinal nerve need be addressed in practice. If it works best for you at present to only use the brow, then maybe that is the way for a while, but that is not spinal breathing. It is a different practice, and the long term effects may be uncertain, so it will be "research" on your part, at least from the AYP point of view.

Ultimately, both ends of the sushumna (spinal nerve) will have to be integrated by some means. Full length spinal breathing is one of the primary ways ecstatic conductivity and radiance are cultivated in a balanced way.

It is suggested to avoid getting overly focused on individual chakras, as this can lead to imbalances. All of the techniques in AYP have been conceived while keeping balanced cultivation in mind, looking far beyond the chakras. This brings natural openings throughout the spiritual neurobiology, and a large payoff in the long run.

If there is too much going on at the root, causing excessive distraction, then it is suggested to employ self-pacing in practice and grounding measures as necessary. Everything will balance out in time.

Wishing you all the best on your path. Practice wisely, and enjoy!

The guru is in you.

PS: For those with awakened ecstatic conductivity (kundalini), one of the most powerful stimulants of the root is sustained attention at the brow (and the crown much more so). Things are not always as they seem. That's why in AYP we suggest balance in all things. Just some food for thought. :-)

2007/12/18 13:11:46
Support for AYP Pranayama, Mudras and Bandhas

When to do Traya (threefold) Bandha

Hi All:

From a recent email interchange, posted with permission:

Q: What do you think about practice of Traya (three fold) Bandha after asana practice instead of performing bandhas with the spinal breathing? The reason this is mentioned is because during the practice of spinal breathing the practice is smooth and it provides good flow of prana as a stand alone pratice. The Bhandas provide good flow of prana by themselves as well, especially when performing Traya Bhanda. So the sequence that feels fit for myself is asanas, traya bhanda and then on to the spinal breathing and meditation. When this order was performed last night there was an inner stillness that came over my mind that was never experienced before. Please let me know is this okay from a practical perspective, and is it correct in terms of systematic practice with wisdom.

A: It sounds okay (it is one way to do it), though you will find over the long term that mudras and bandhas merge into one "whole body mudra" and creep into all aspects of practice and life in automatic "micro movement" form. Therefore, the real purpose for doing mudras and bandhas is not for immediate effects, but to develop the over all ecstatic side of human spiritual transformation. That is why we do them in spinal breathing - - it provides for more practice time of mudras and bandhas without sacrificing the core practice of spinal breathing, which is closely related. We also use them (traya bandha) in yoni mudra, and in a variation during chin pump. We do not focus on mudras and bandhas in deep meditation. If they are occurring there (and they will eventually), it will be as automatic habit and not with a deliberate diversion of attention from the procedure of meditation.

Generally, it is not a good idea to alter the practice routine seeking short term experiences or effects, as these are related to purification and opening, and vary widely over time. We do the practices for the long term effects, not the short term ones. In fact, the suggestion is to always favor the practice we are doing over our experiences. Otherwise, we can end up like a cat chasing its tail, and that will reduce our progress.

It would be great to bring this to the AYP Support Forums, as many others can benefit from the discussion. You will receive more points of view too. The "alterations in practice" discussion is endless. You can find it occurring in many forms in the forums. 95% of the time it is considering altering the practice to chase an experience. The advice from here is always the same -- favor your structured practice (whatever it is) over the experience, and self-pace accordingly.

All the best!

The guru is in you.

Note: Traya bandha is the simultaneous use of mulabandha (root lock), uddiyana bandha (abdominal lift/lock), and jalandhara bandha (chin lock), usually with kumbhaka (breath retention). It is a powerful kundalini stimulator, and should be used in moderation. In AYP, we use several variations of it in combination with certain practices. See the main lessons for details.

2008/02/06 14:21:18
Support for AYP Pranayama, Mudras and Bandhas
http://www.aypsite.org/forum/topic.asp?TOPIC_ID=3436&REPLY_ID=29744&whichpage=-1
Spontaneous pranayama during pranayama

Hi LAMNN:

It is bastrika pranayama (bellows breathing, also spelled bhastrika), and it is covered here with a particular AYP twist, i.e., "spinal" bastrika pranayama:

http://www.aypsite.org/171.html
(and in the next two lessons)

And also here for use in a more "targeted" way:

http://www.aypsite.org/198.html
(and in the next lesson)

Bastrika can occur during practices as an "automatic yoga," as you have described. It is the nervous system cleansing itself, which it is sometimes inclined to do more dramatically as inner silence and inner energy movements are coming up. Be mindful not to overdo. Check lessons with suggestions on how to handle "automatic yoga" in the topic index: http://www.aypsite.org/TopicIndex.html

All the best!

The guru is in you

2008/02/06 20:59:08
Support for AYP Pranayama, Mudras and Bandhas
http://www.aypsite.org/forum/topic.asp?TOPIC_ID=3436&REPLY_ID=29757&whichpage=-1
Spontaneous pranayama during pranayama

Hi LAMNN:

No, automatic yoga is not necessarily a good indicator of where we should be focusing our practices. It is better to regard automatic yoga like any other experience that comes up, and easily favor our normal practices. This is the advice given in the lessons on automatic yoga.

Otherwise, we can find ourselves being dragged from pillar to post by such symptoms of purification and opening. The nervous system is very good at purifying itself when stimulated appropriately, but it is not very good at telling us what is best for us to being doing in practices to stimulate that over all process. If we follow automatic yoga intentionally, it will have us overdoing almost every time. We don't favor automatic yoga, and we don't fight it either when it occurs during the normal course of practices. If it becomes extreme, we self-pace accordingly during our session.

Appropriate stimulation for ongoing long term purification and opening is what the wonderful invention of yoga is for, which took a lot of trial and error to derive over the centuries.

That is why we always favor the practice over the experience, with self-pacing at the fore, of course. :-)

When it comes time to do some intentional tarketed bastrika, you will know it according to your need, and not the need of automatic yoga. It is a subtle point, but an important one.

All the best!

The guru is in you.

2008/02/08 13:54:21
Support for AYP Pranayama, Mudras and Bandhas
http://www.aypsite.org/forum/topic.asp?TOPIC_ID=3439&REPLY_ID=29827&whichpage=-1
siddhasana

Hi Growant:

Yes, the two practices continue normally. Neither is a substitute for the other. In time they both become natural aspects of one thing.

All the best!

The guru is in you.

2008/02/11 10:45:52
Support for AYP Pranayama, Mudras and Bandhas
http://www.aypsite.org/forum/topic.asp?TOPIC_ID=3439&REPLY_ID=29949&whichpage=-1
siddhasana

Hi Avatar:

No, siddhasana as suggested in AYP is behind the urethra (urine tube), not mainly for compressing it, and the energy goes in and up, not out. In AYP we learn siddhasana first during spinal breathing pranayama, and yes, there is a relationship between siddhasana and spinal breathing in guiding the energy in and up, and back down, and back up again, purifying and opening the sushumna (spinal nerve) in the process. All of the mudras and bandhas are for that also.

See the lessons on "siddhasana" (near top of list) in the topic index: http://www.aypsite.org/TopicIndex.html

All the best!

The guru is in you.

2008/02/17 07:01:40
Support for AYP Pranayama, Mudras and Bandhas
http://www.aypsite.org/forum/topic.asp?TOPIC_ID=3464&REPLY_ID=30150&whichpage=-1
Kechari - snips get healed

quote:
_____
Originally posted by Sagittarius

Thokar, I will continue putting the tongue back and forward - maybe one day I will succeed and push the soft palate. Since the end of the tongue tends to roll back it is not that easy to do.
However nobody answered the question I am asking - is it normal that each time I snip the tongue, it gets healed and looks almost like as if it was never snipped, that almost no notch/cut remains present on it? I am doubting whether I am moving anywhere because it looks like I am cutting the same place and it gets healed each time.
_____

Hi Sagittarius:

Thokar offers you good advice on the forward thrust once the tongue is able to get behind the uvula with or without finger help. Once we can reach the back edge of the soft palate, initial entry into stage 2 is not as much about going up as it is about pressing the soft palate forward and down. Going up is more for continuing further into stage 2 and to higher stages of kechari. That is when the frenum will be limiting.

Regarding snipping the frenum, the key in that is to be reducing the tendon which is inside the outer skin. In most people the tendon will present itself on the surface along the narrow edge at the center of the frenum when it is stretched, and it is easy to take small snips from it there, as discussed in Lesson 108 and elsewhere in the online lessons and support forums (try some searches for additional perspectives).

The key to reducing the frenum is in reducing the tendon, which is made of thousands of tiny strands. Those will not grow back once snipped. If only skin is being snipped, then there will not be much release.

In some cases, due to personal anatomy, the tendon will not present itself at the surface at the center edge of the frenum when stretched, and the tendon itself may not be easy to reach in that case. There are ways to do it that have been discussed here, but it may be a more involved procedure (see tooled talavya). Going to these measures may or may not be effective in reducing the tendon, depending on personal anatomy. Tooled talavya is not an endorsed AYP approach, though it has been discussed extensively in the support forums.

Other alternatives consist of relying on stretching alone with traditional talavya (or variations), milking the tongue in concert with other methods, or considering laser surgery by a dentist or oral surgeon.

Each of us will find the best way according to our bhakti (spiritual desire) and personal anatomy. You will know what is right for you as you continue to move along your path. It is suggested to keep a balance in your approach, be patient, and avoid extremes that can bring undue health risk.

All the best!

The guru is in you.

2008/02/17 12:50:06
Support for AYP Pranayama, Mudras and Bandhas
http://www.aypsite.org/forum/topic.asp?TOPIC_ID=3464&REPLY_ID=30175&whichpage=-1
Kechari - snips get healed
PS: A finer point -- for most people the shortest distance to get behind the back edge of the soft palate with the tip of the tongue will be either on the left or right side, not usually the middle. Try and see. This is in the lessons. It is also the natural way to go once we are beyond finger help.

The guru is in you.

2008/02/17 13:31:33
Support for AYP Pranayama, Mudras and Bandhas
http://www.aypsite.org/forum/topic.asp?TOPIC_ID=3464&REPLY_ID=30184&whichpage=-1
Kechari - snips get healed

quote:
───────
Originally posted by emc

I can also easily go behind the uvula. My problem is that if I put a finger in or when I try to push the soft palate back edge I activate the "throw up reflex" or whatever you might call it. Is that reflex naturally going to disappear when it's natural timing for kechari step 2? Or can that be something to practice away? That's what's preventing me from discovering kechari any further...
───────

Hi EMC:

Yes, it will go away. As soon as you are "in" the tongue goes forward and the tickle at the base of the tongue and deep in the back of the throat is significantly reduced, which is where the gag reflex is centered. That, and we acclimate in general to the new positioning of everything in there.

Your bhakti will tell you what to do. :-)

The guru is in you.

2008/02/22 16:55:39
Support for AYP Pranayama, Mudras and Bandhas
http://www.aypsite.org/forum/topic.asp?TOPIC_ID=3480&REPLY_ID=30429&whichpage=-1
practical advice on frenulum snipping

quote:
───────
Originally posted by Lookatmynavelnow

quote:
───────
Originally posted by John C

The frenulum consists of a cord like tether that is pure connective tissue and contains no vital structures like nerve, blood vessels nor muscle.
───────

It is my understanding that the cord like tether is present at the front part of the frenulum. Further back (and to the sides of the cord), there is just soft tissue with blood and stuff.

Once the tongue after snipping have come in to kechari 2 position, from then on what anatomically parts are responsible for the further advancement to position 3 and 4? Is it the soft part of the frenum that will stretch, or is it the soft palate that will flex?

The question is, will there be a need for more snipping, and snipping of the bloody soft part of the frenum, or will all progress be by soft tissue stretching?
───────

Hi LAMNN:

The frenum tether is made of thousands of tiny tendon strands attached between the bottom of the tongue and the floor of the mouth. These are piled up all the way back to where the tongue and floor of the mouth meet, way in the back of the throat. It is a large mass of tendon strands. In that sense, it is not even possible, nor desirable, to remove the entire frenum. Higher stages of kechari will be reached long before.

When a tendon strand is severed, that is it for that strand. It won't grow back. But there are many more strands waiting behind it, going all the way back. They come to the surface in succession at the center edge of the frenum, the place of most tension.

If the frenum is the limiting factor for going to higher stages of kechari (usually the case), then trimming may proceed off and on for many years according to bhakti. Trimming the fleshy part of the frenum for its own sake will not be necessary or helpful, because it is flexible and will stretch as needed. In any case, that kind of trimming is not advised, especially on the sides of the frenum near the tongue, where there are some sizable blood vessels.

The center edge of the frenum at the point of greatest tension is the place, and it can remain the place for quite a long time, as new tendon strands are coming to the surface as we are going to higher stages of kechari. If it is taken in small steps like that, there will be practically no blood and very little risk, because all we are doing is snipping tiny tendon strands nearly exposed at the taunt edge of the frenum under the tongue. Very little flesh is being violated.

Not everyone's anatomy will play out in the above scenario. Some people have very little restriction in their frenum and don't need any trimming, while others may have a larger buried mass of tendon strands that does not come to the surface of the stretched frenum easily and is therefore harder to reach for trimming. In the latter case, a surgical approach may be best considered. The more cutting of flesh that may be involved, the more advisable it will be to leave it to a medical professional.

The guru is in you.

2008/03/27 16:37:42
Support for AYP Pranayama, Mudras and Bandhas
http://www.aypsite.org/forum/topic.asp?TOPIC_ID=3480&REPLY_ID=31836&whichpage=-1
practical advice on frenulum snipping

Hi Scott:

My experience over 20-some years of snipping off and on has been no effect on voice, except sometimes a little out of sorts for a day or two when bigger more aggressive snips were taken (ouch), and then fine with healing. Small snips should not affect your voice at all, and neither should a permanently reduced frenum. The radio interviews are offered as proof. :-)

The guru is in you.

2008/04/02 10:27:46
Support for AYP Pranayama, Mudras and Bandhas
http://www.aypsite.org/forum/topic.asp?TOPIC_ID=3480&REPLY_ID=32092&whichpage=-1
practical advice on frenulum snipping

quote:
_____
Originally posted by John C

You can numb the frenulum/frenum web with Kava Root Extract prior to snipping, each time you wish to re-do it. To lessen the pain. Saturate a cotton tip applicator and apply for several minutes.
This is available at health food stores. What do you think Yogani?
_____

Hi John:

Sorry so late coming back on this. Things have been piling up here lately.

I think anything that numbs the pain of a kechari snip can be helpful, even just a small piece of ice.

The downside is that if there is full numbing, one might be tempted to cut more than is prudent for self-snipping. That could lead to some discomfort during healing for a few days. It is not a very big health risk, but the morning after could be an "ouch." Then some more numbing might be in order without any further snipping for a while.

I prefer the tiny snip approach myself, per lesson 108, which involves minimal pain and practically no blood. It requires very little except persistence and patience over time. That could be said of all yoga.

This is the essence of self-pacing. :-)

See my post to LAMNN above for more thoughts on frenum reduction, and check the main website topic index for all the lessons on kechari mudra.

The guru is in you.

2008/03/13 15:02:15
Support for AYP Pranayama, Mudras and Bandhas
http://www.aypsite.org/forum/topic.asp?TOPIC_ID=3578&REPLY_ID=31254&whichpage=-1
Maha Bandah

Hi Avatar:

It is easy to over do it with this sort of practice and end up in an energy overload, particularly if we are already doing a full daily routine of practices like AYP. So, if you must do it, then small doses are suggested, and always keep self-pacing in mind. Remember that a practice like this can have delayed effects if pursued aggressively.

The key to achieving good results with our yoga routine is building a balanced and sustainable practice over the long term. It isn't about the latest energy surge we may be stimulating. More of that is not necessarily going to be better.

Practice wisely, and enjoy! :-)

The guru is in you.

2008/03/13 14:48:19
Support for AYP Pranayama, Mudras and Bandhas
http://www.aypsite.org/forum/topic.asp?TOPIC_ID=3588&REPLY_ID=31253&whichpage=-1
using breath to cultivate energy

Hi Divineis, and a belated welcome!

Of course, it is up to you what you may try in the way of energy exercises in relation to the AYP practices. You are wise to keep self-pacing in mind.

On the rotating head, it looks like some automatic yoga occurring in the form of chin pump (dynamic jalandhara). Check the main website topic index for lessons on this practice. Also check "automatic yoga" there. Just because we are having some automatic yoga does not mean to charge ahead into that. We can regard automatic yoga to be part of the scenery resulting from purification and opening. We just continue to favor our regular routine of practice over the experiences that come up, and take it one step at time with additions. More self-pacing. :-)

All the best!

The guru is in you.

2008/03/14 14:48:52
Support for AYP Pranayama, Mudras and Bandhas
http://www.aypsite.org/forum/topic.asp?TOPIC_ID=3615&REPLY_ID=31306&whichpage=-1
how do you know there is a "block"

Hi Anthony:

We are not looking for particular blocks, sensations or experiences along the spinal nerve during spinal breathing pranayama. We travel up and down with the breath between root and brow, and that is it. If we have places where we tend to get stuck or distracted, it is best to pass through those areas and continue our journey up and down between root and brow. It is much more important to end up at the brow on completion of inhalation and at the root at the completion of exhalation than to be focusing on particular characteristics of the spinal nerve along the way. These will purify and open naturally with steady practice over time, not necessarily by focusing on them for our own reasons.

In time, the pathway becomes clear and enlivened. It does not happen by "drilling down" in specific locations. It happens by "passing through" without analysis of what is happening along the way. The procedure is simple and we favor it over the experiences that may come up -- very similar to the procedure of favoring the mantra in deep meditation. This is covered in detail in the Spinal Breathing Pranayama book.

The most complicated thing about spinal breathing (and deep meditation too) is our tendency to make it complicated. In time we learn to stay with the simple procedure day after day and let it go. That is when the most progress will be occurring. :-)

The guru is in you.

2008/03/17 15:33:58
Support for AYP Pranayama, Mudras and Bandhas
http://www.aypsite.org/forum/topic.asp?TOPIC_ID=3625&REPLY_ID=31422&whichpage=-1
Sutra Neti suggestion

Hi GreenYogi, and welcome!

You might consider doing jala neti instead. Less physically invasive, and more thorough cleansing and stimulation of the nasal passages and sinuses.

For an intro, see: http://www.aypsite.org/forum/topic.asp?TOPIC_ID=3521

All the best!

The guru is in you.

2008/03/20 12:31:05
Support for AYP Pranayama, Mudras and Bandhas
http://www.aypsite.org/forum/topic.asp?TOPIC_ID=3640&REPLY_ID=31539&whichpage=-1
spinal breathing vs cosmic orbit

Hi Divineis:

You might find this topic interesting:
http://www.aypsite.org/forum/topic.asp?TOPIC_ID=500

(pardon the diversion into kriya yoga there -- it comes back to the topic eventually)

There are many other topics buried here that discuss this from one angle or other. Try subject line searches on taoism, front channel, nectar, amrita and other words that tie in.

Yes, AYP spinal breathing pranayama is up and down the spinal nerve. In the AYP approach, front channel opening is addressed primarily through mudras and bandhas. Seems to work. :-)

All the best!

The guru is in you.

2008/03/26 14:23:24
Support for AYP Pranayama, Mudras and Bandhas
http://www.aypsite.org/forum/topic.asp?TOPIC_ID=3673&REPLY_ID=31792&whichpage=-1
Kechari - where should the tongue rest?

quote:
_____
Originally posted by Sagittarius

What exactly is considered stage 3 of kechari? On which spot should the tip of the tongue rest?

Are little holes on the sides of hard palate - Eustachian tubes?
_____

Hi Sagittarius:

Stage 3 kechari is when the tip of the tongue reaches the top of the nasal pharynx and the bottom side of the tongue is able to touch the full length of the back edge of the nasal septum (center divider). Stage 2 kechari is the tip of the tongue touching part way up the back edge of the septum -- the point we call the "secret spot" in the lessons.

This will happen naturally as ecstatic radiance rises in the body -- our other practices are key in this. Then the nasal septum becomes "spiritually erogenous" and is instantly connected ecstatically with the root at the perineum. That ecstatic pleasure draws us naturally.

Yes, the horn-like structures on either side of the nasal openings in the nasal pharynx are the Eustachian tubes.

For more on all of this, see the lessons on "kechari mudra" listed and linked in the main website topic index:
http://www.aypsite.org/TopicIndex.html (particularly lesson 108)

All the best!

The guru is in you.

2008/03/26 15:39:17
Support for AYP Pranayama, Mudras and Bandhas
http://www.aypsite.org/forum/topic.asp?TOPIC_ID=3673&REPLY_ID=31794&whichpage=-1
Kechari - where should the tongue rest?

Hi Sagittarius:

Best to check the diagrams with lesson 108 for particulars about tongue positions in the several stages of kechari:
http://www.aypsite.org/kechari_image1.html

The little indentations on the top back side of the nasal pharynx are not significant in kechari. Neither are the Eustachian tubes. The ero-ecstatic connection is mainly through the septum, and to varying degrees in the surrounding tissues.

Breathing is not a problem in stage 3 kechari, as there is plenty of room for air to go around the tongue. Anatomical variations could make a difference in some practitioners, but I would be surprised if someone could not breathe easily in stage 3.

The guru is in you.

2008/03/27 13:35:18
Support for AYP Pranayama, Mudras and Bandhas
http://www.aypsite.org/forum/topic.asp?TOPIC_ID=3673&REPLY_ID=31827&whichpage=-1
Kechari - where should the tongue rest?

quote:
_____
Originally posted by Thokar

In my experience the indentation at the top of the nasal pharynx is the most ecstatically charged spot back there... I can still get huge ammounts of ecstatic conductivity just resting the tongue along the length of the septum, but when I push the tip of the tongue up into that little hole at the top (which I believe is anatomically right under the pituitary gland) I receive by far the greatest ammount of energy and bliss and also an extremely strong pulling sensation on the crown..
_____

Hi Thokar:

Following our own ecstasy is always better than following someone else's words and descriptions. With self-pacing as needed, of course. :-)

Thanks for chiming in!

The guru is in you.

2008/03/28 11:11:51
Support for AYP Pranayama, Mudras and Bandhas
http://www.aypsite.org/forum/topic.asp?TOPIC_ID=3678&REPLY_ID=31866&whichpage=-1
Breath Cessation in Pranayama??

Hi Jim and All:

If breath ceases temporarily during spinal breathing pranayama, we are not off the practice. When we realize breathing has ceased, then that is about the time we will begin breathing again, and at that time we just easily favor the resumption of breathing going up and down the spinal nerve. It doesn't matter where we restart our journey between root and brow in the spinal nerve. The same is true if we wander off with attention during spinal breathing. We just easily come back to tracing the spinal nerve. This is part of the procedure of spinal breathing.

Spinal breathing pranayama is very much like deep meditation in this respect. In deep meditation, when we realize we are off the mantra, we easily come back to it at whatever level of clarity or fuzziness is comfortable. Likewise, in spinal breathing, when we realize we are off the spinal nerve (which can be a small or large path in the center of the body, depending on energy flow), we just easily come back. This also applies when we realize breathing has been suspended.

As Jim said, in the AYP approach, we don't make suspension of breath a goal in spinal breathing pranayama. If it happens naturally, that is fine. We don't favor it, or try to prevent it. When we realize it has happened, that will usually coincide with a rise in metabolism, and breathing will be not far behind. So we favor the path of breath again in whatever way it is occurring naturally -- full breathing, or very refined. Whatever the body is needing at the moment.

In the AYP approach, intentional breath suspension is something we use in specialized shorter duration practices like uddiyana bandha (abdominal lift), yoni mudra kumbhaka, and dynamic jalandhara (chin pump). Intentional breath suspension in concert with other yoga practices is a very powerful internal energy (kundalini) stimulator and should be approached with care, and only when core sitting practices like deep meditation and spinal breathing are well-established and stable.

All the best!

The guru is in you.

PS: Just a reminder that we do our spinal breathing pranayama session first for the alloted time and then deep meditation for its alloted time. Pranayama is preparation for meditation. With cultivation of the nervous system during spinal breathing pranayama, deep meditation will be going more smoothly and quickly to inner silence (samadhi), and stillness will be abiding more and more during our daily activity.

2008/03/29 14:02:26
Support for AYP Pranayama, Mudras and Bandhas
http://www.aypsite.org/forum/topic.asp?TOPIC_ID=3678&REPLY_ID=31898&whichpage=-1
Breath Cessation in Pranayama??

quote:
_____
Originally posted by Jim and His Karma

quote:
_____
Originally posted by yogani

If breath ceases temporarily during spinal breathing pranayama, we are not off the practice
_____

Thanks, Yogani

I can easily move prana around without assistance from breath (a product of years of hatha). But I've always been disciplined in respect to AYP's direction to always favor the practice COME WHAT MAY.....and since inhalation/exhalation is a bedrock instruction in AYP pranayama, I'd been very much favoring its continuation.

I guess it will now be interesting to ease that discipline, without mentally injecting encouragement or restraint!

Anyway, now I'm wondering what else I've been taking overly literally in the lessons...!
_____

Hi Jim:

It is true that "inhalation/exhalation is a bedrock instruction in AYP pranayama" ... from the perspective of easily favoring that and the path of the spinal nerve, just the way we favor the mantra in deep meditation.

This does not mean we won't have periods of no breath or no mantra in the respective practices.

The tipping point between doing the practice and not doing the practice comes in what we do with our attention when we notice that we are in a non-breath or non-mantra mode. If we intentionally choose to circulate prana without breath, or continue breath suspension, or in the case of non-mantra in deep meditation go to an "awareness watching awareness" mode instead of easing back to the mantra, then any of these deliberate diversions will be off the practice.

Is this a bad thing? Who can say? What we can say is that if we are not favoring the procedure of practice when we have the opportunity, then we are off the practice.

When I said that natural breath suspension in spinal breathing is part of the practice, I did not mean that not favoring coming back to inhalation/exhalation is also part of the practice. It clearly isn't. That is the tipping point.

There are a thousand ways to divert from practice, all of them legitimate parts of practice until we choose not to ease back with the procedure of our practice from whatever has caught our attention.

Given that spiritual progress is based primarily on maintaining long term consistency of procedure in practices (leading to a stable condition of spiritual awareness in daily living), we have to ask ourselves what we are gaining by doing other things during the short time we have committed to structured practice. It is easy to draw long term conclusions about in-the-moment experiences, but this is no guarantee of anything. It has been said many times here that the worst time to redesign our practice is while we are doing it.

We will only know the effect of what we are doing months and years down the road. It is a very tricky thing. Definitely an area requiring long-term research. We are all guinea pigs in this. AYP is intended to serve as a progressive "safe harbor" from which to engage in purification, opening, and exploration. How far we choose to go from safe harbor will depend on our individual inclinations. As long as communications remain open long term, we will eventually know what works for most people. In the meantime, we are doing the best we can.

So, is favoring energy movement up and down the spinal nerve without breath the same as spinal breathing with breath? Is favoring "awareness of awareness" the same as deep meditation? Is mental kechari the same as physical kechari? These are a few interesting questions that have come up recently, along with the ongoing fare of visions and energy experiences. The answer is always pretty much the same. Cool stuff, but favoring them is not the procedure of the AYP practices we are talking about. It is obvious, isn't it? :-)

There is always room for research. It will be for the benefit and the expense of the researcher. We can all benefit from both outcomes.

The guru is in you.

PS: By the way, the Kriya Yoga portion of this topic was split off by moderators and moved to "Other Systems." This was not done in disrespect to anyone -- only to avoid confusion between AYP and a different system of practice. The best place to discuss other systems is in "Other Systems." It is okay to do comparisons with AYP (or with any other system) there also. It is not ideal to do it in forum categories like this one, which are primarily for support in the AYP practices.

2008/03/30 10:38:34
Support for AYP Pranayama, Mudras and Bandhas
http://www.aypsite.org/forum/topic.asp?TOPIC_ID=3678&REPLY_ID=31933&whichpage=-1
Breath Cessation in Pranayama??

quote:
_____
Originally posted by emc

When I read your post above, Yogani, I felt "oh, what a rigid system". And then it hit me... if we are engulfed in scenery, cool automatic yoga during practices, it's the spiritual ego getting satisfied and seduced by the glitter and glamour comme d'habitude - it's just on the inside now... If we stick to practices no matter what, it's bhakti ruling... Is that somewhat how it is???
_____

Hi EMC and All:

Could be. :-)

Don't get me wrong, the natural breath suspensions are not a bad thing. Quite good actually -- a sign of important purification and opening in the nervous system occurring along the way on our journey. But we don't have to be doing anything with breath suspensions either. What for? Just relax. It is only 5-10 minutes of spinal breathing practice and I don't expect you are suspended the entire time. If you are, great, just take it easy, following the simple procedure of spinal breathing, which involves no strain. Meditation time will arrive soon enough, and then the breath can continue to be suspended if it is natural, and deep meditation can go on normally within that.

Please know that the procedure is the procedure for spinal breathing and I can only describe it for what it is. What you do in practices is your affair. With thousands of people reading, we certainly don't want to be jockeying the procedure around for every individual experience that comes along. If we find in time that everyone is having constant natural breath suspensions, then we may take a closer look at the procedure, or maybe not. Time will tell. Whatever adjustments we might make to the procedure in the future, if any, will be based on the experiences and needs of the many.

Pioneers in consciousness we are. Wonderful new openings happening here every day. Relax and enjoy the ride! :-)

The guru is in you.

2008/09/27 11:54:14
Support for AYP Pranayama, Mudras and Bandhas
http://www.aypsite.org/forum/topic.asp?TOPIC_ID=3721&REPLY_ID=38175&whichpage=-1
yoni mudra kumbhaka before rest

Hi Christi and All:

Cosmic samyama is a practice that is less likely to produce an overload by itself than to contribute to one if purification associated with ecstatic conductivity (kundalini) is accelerating, with self-pacing being ignored. Of course, the crown is central in this, as you point out, and your suggestions are well-informed by experience.

This varied effect, depending on the degree of energy awakening, is why the guidelines on when to undertake cosmic samyama are flexible, depending more on the individual than on a fixed order of learning. Cosmic samyama can, in fact, be taken on fairly early with little risk of mishap, after deep meditation and core samyama are in place and stable. It is an alternate learning track in the AYP system that is alluded to in the Eight Limbs of Yoga book.

Keep in mind that the marketplace is flooded with "guided yoga nidra" CDs and approaches, using attention points, that nearly anyone can indulge in with little risk of overdoing. That's because, for the most part, they do not optimize the samyama effect the way we do with cosmic samyama, and most people are not in a situation of rapid energetic awakening, yet.

AYP cosmic samyama is a different situation, especially when prudently integrated into a daily routine covering cultivation of <u>both</u> inner silence and ecstatic conductivity, and self-paced accordingly. This is how it is presented in the Samyama book. Then this form of samyama becomes truly cosmic. :-)

The guru is in you.

2008/09/27 14:04:42
Support for AYP Pranayama, Mudras and Bandhas
http://www.aypsite.org/forum/topic.asp?TOPIC_ID=3721&REPLY_ID=38179&whichpage=-1
yoni mudra kumbhaka before rest
PS: Tadeas, with chin cump in the picture between spinal breathing and deep meditation, Yoni mudra kumbhaka can be undertaken between core samyama and cosmic samyama. You have that right. :-)

The exact placements of spinal bastrika, chin pump and yoni mudra kumbhaka in the routine are not critical. They are spread out for comfort. In fact, in the Eight Limbs of Yoga book the placement of spinal bastrika <u>before</u> spinal breathing is offered as an option.

It a balancing of methods and personal inclinations. That's why the Eight Limbs of Yoga book has the subtitle, "The Structure and Pacing of Self-Directed Spiritual Practice."

All of these elements are integrated together, with *self-pacing* being the vital link between structure and practice.

The guru is in you.

2008/04/14 16:23:56
Support for AYP Pranayama, Mudras and Bandhas
http://www.aypsite.org/forum/topic.asp?TOPIC_ID=3756&REPLY_ID=32667&whichpage=-1
concerning kechari mudra and the heart!!!

quote:
_____
Originally posted by beirut

i've heard from a friend that the heart and the tongue are physicaly attached and that such a procedure as kechari mudra might have some effects on the heart either good or bad he doesn't know.
_____

Hi Beirut:

Yes, there is a connection, and the effect is good, assuming prudent self-pacing. It is the awakening of ecstatic conductivity between third eye, throat and heart space, stimulated in kechari -- not to mention the simultaneous ecstatic link with the root and other lower centers as well.

The head/throat to heart connection is also directly stimulated in dynamic jalandhara (chin pump), and there is tie-in with bhakti, deep meditation, spinal breathing, sambhavi and the rest of our practices. The amrita/nectar cycle is intimately involved in head to heart awakening as well, on the biochemical level, and is stimulated by the same practices.

When it is all said and done, the whole is much greater than the sum of the parts ... infinite heart opening ... Enjoy! :-)

The guru is in you.

2008/05/14 14:41:19
Support for AYP Pranayama, Mudras and Bandhas
http://www.aypsite.org/forum/topic.asp?TOPIC_ID=3904&REPLY_ID=33763&whichpage=-1
yoni chin pump question

Hi YB:

Adding the eye action makes for a more powerful practice. Nothing wrong with that if you can handle the extra stimulation, and can do it without poking your eyes out. :-)

<u>Don't forget to self-pace as needed.</u>

For those who are interested, the two hybrid practices in the lessons combining elements of yoni mudra with chin pump and spinal breathing are covered here (not for beginners):

Yoni Chin Pump -- http://www.aypsite.org/281.html
Yoni Spinal Breathing -- http://www.aypsite.org/288.html

All the best!

The guru is in you.

2008/05/31 10:02:36
Support for AYP Pranayama, Mudras and Bandhas
http://www.aypsite.org/forum/topic.asp?TOPIC_ID=3980&REPLY_ID=34236&whichpage=-1
Adding chin pump before sidhasana

Hi emc:

The order in which we add practices in AYP is not ironclad, though there is a certain logic to it, and the lessons are laid out accordingly.

We don't want "automatic yoga" to be directing our practice routine, for that will certainly be running us willy nilly. Automatic yoga is great, a clear sign of purification and opening going on, but it wants it all right now. Few practitioners can accommodate that without going though extreme discomfort, and ending up traveling slower while recovering from episodes of excess.

On the other hand, if you want to try a minute or two of chin pump between spinal breathing and deep meditation, it will not hurt, and might help quell the random occurrences of it. That way you will be adding some structure, which you can then self-pace for progress with comfort. The rest of the time automatic yoga may be occurring, we can just regard it as "scenery" and easily favor whatever practice or activity we are doing.

Chin pump is good for helping to clear blockages in the throat, heart and front channel, including bringing energy down from the head, which can help relieve pressure in the third eye area. At the same time, chin pump brings energy up through the spine from root to brow, and when ecstatic conductivity (kundalini) is awake the pumping action can be felt through the entire length of the sushumna (spinal nerve), particularly on both ends.

All the best!

The guru is in you.

PS: A light set of asanas before sitting practices can help calm down/smooth out random occurrences of automatic yoga. And, of course, plenty of grounding activity during the day.

2008/06/01 11:17:13
Support for AYP Pranayama, Mudras and Bandhas
http://www.aypsite.org/forum/topic.asp?TOPIC_ID=3980&REPLY_ID=34251&whichpage=-1
Adding chin pump before sidhasana
PPS: Regarding the above, consider beginning with "chin pump lite" (without breath retention), as this will be less kundalini stimulation. :-)
2008/06/01 15:27:47
Support for AYP Pranayama, Mudras and Bandhas
http://www.aypsite.org/forum/topic.asp?TOPIC_ID=3980&REPLY_ID=34258&whichpage=-1
Adding chin pump before sidhasana

quote:
_____
Originally posted by emc

Good to know that the order of adding practices is not superfixed. I think sidhasana would make my kundalini go crazy since I already have a burning root chakra...
_____

Hi emc:

Yes, siddhasana can do that, though interestingly, in the long run it actually smooths the ecstatic energies, even while cultivating them. In that sense, siddhasana is a really terrific tantra technique.

Perhaps when you consider trying siddhasana, start slow with a soft rolled up sock, or similar. Like everything else in yoga, siddhasana can be self-paced to suit just about any situation.

One thing at a time though... :-)

The guru is in you.

2008/07/12 14:52:54
Support for AYP Pranayama, Mudras and Bandhas
http://www.aypsite.org/forum/topic.asp?TOPIC_ID=4139&REPLY_ID=35423&whichpage=-1
Conversation with an Indian teacher about pranayam

Hi emc:

It is alternate nostril breathing, called "nadi shodana," a very common technique. It is also called "anuloma viloma."

Below is an excerpt from the AYP Easy Lessons book, an addition to lesson 41, which covers it.

As with any pranayama, be careful not to overdo. The combined effects from all pranayamas we do in a given day, regardless of type, will be cumulative. A teacher who offers a limited range of practices may not be aware of the increased potency of any individual practice when combined with a larger range of powerful practices in the daily routine. The same goes for adding intentional breath suspension (kumbhaka) in any part of our routine, which we just covered here: http://www.aypsite.org/forum/topic.asp?TOPIC_ID=4130#35367 (see follow-up posts there as well)

In other words, simple alternate nostril breathing is one thing by itself, and may be something else when added to a full boat of practices like we do in AYP. Always self-pace as necessary.

The guru is in you.

Addition to Lesson 41 – Over the months, several have written and asked about a form of pranayama called "nadi shodana." This is alternate nostril breathing. It is one of the most basic breathing techniques, and is usually the first breathing method taught to beginning students in hatha yoga classes. These days it is also taught by mental health professionals due to its calming influence on the nervous system. Nadi shodana is done by breathing slowly out and then in with one nostril blocked by the thumb of one hand, and then slowly out and in with the other nostril blocked by the middle finger of the same hand. That is all there is to it. It is a well-known practice that brings almost immediate relaxation. Why is it not taught in the Advanced Yoga Practices lessons?

The reason nadi shodana is not used here is because spinal breathing includes the benefits of nadi shodana, plus it is a tremendously more powerful practice with effects extending far beyond those of nadi shodana. The calming effects of nadi shodana come primarily from a reduction of the breath rate by using one nostril at a time – restraint of breath. In spinal breathing, the breath is restrained on inhalation voluntarily with the lungs and on exhalation with ujjayi (partially closed epiglottis), while the attention is used in the particular way of tracing the spinal nerve discussed in this lesson. While spinal breathing does not include alternating nostril breathing, this is not a shortcoming. Otherwise nadi shodana would be included along with spinal breathing. It is possible to do both practices at the same time, but it would be complicating our practice for very little gain. That is one of the guiding principles in all of these lessons – Is there a substantial benefit derived through the addition of an element of practice? If there is not a significant benefit from an additional element of practice, we leave it out. That is how we keep the routine of practices as simple and efficient as possible. Otherwise we would be loading ourselves up with all sorts of supplementary things and risk losing focus on our main practices. There will be plenty of practices added as we go through the lessons that will have huge impacts on results. We want to save our attention, time and energy for those, so we can achieve the most with our yoga.

Still, if you are an avid nadi shodana practitioner, or are strongly attracted to it, it will do no harm to incorporate it into your routine. If you have time, you can do some alternate nostril breathing before spinal breathing. Or you can incorporate it into your spinal breathing session. Keep in mind that nadi shodana is not recommended if you are a beginner in spinal breathing. There is plenty to learn in taking up spinal breathing – new habits to develop – and nadi shodana is not in the mix for the reasons mentioned. But, since it has been asked about by several people, and perhaps wondered about by others, it is covered here.

It should also be mentioned that nadi shodana is sometimes taught in combination with voluntary breath suspension. Breath suspension is an advanced practice and is discussed in detail later in the lessons. Nadi shodana with breath suspension is a different practice altogether, and can be hazardous if done without a good understanding of correct methodology and the effects. If you are a beginner and contemplating using breath suspension (holding the breath in or out) with nadi shodana or spinal breathing, it is suggested you wait until we get into it in these lessons, which is at lesson #91 (on yoni mudra kumbhaka) and beyond. The Sanskrit word for breath suspension is "kumbhaka."

So, for now, it is recommended you develop a good understanding of spinal breathing and get the habit solidly in place, with as few distractions as possible. The following Q&As will help with that. Later on, there will be plenty more to add. One step at a time...

2008/07/12 17:14:35
Support for AYP Pranayama, Mudras and Bandhas
http://www.aypsite.org/forum/topic.asp?TOPIC_ID=4139&REPLY_ID=35429&whichpage=-1
Conversation with an Indian teacher about pranayam

Hi emc:

quote:
Without breath suspension, then...

A modest amount will not hurt, but we all sometimes get carried away. :-)

The guru is in you.

2008/07/12 20:24:19
Support for AYP Pranayama, Mudras and Bandhas
http://www.aypsite.org/forum/topic.asp?TOPIC_ID=4139&REPLY_ID=35435&whichpage=-1
Conversation with an Indian teacher about pranayam

Hi Kadak:

I can't really speak to what others are doing, though I am often asked to. If the results are different, it can only be assumed that they are not doing the same integration of practices we are. We do not focus much on drying clothes here. Cultivating inner silence is the thing here, and maybe that is a significant difference. :-)

In AYP, pranayama plays a supporting role to deep meditation and samyama, whereas in other systems pranayama is primary for energy cultivation.

The actual major overloads that occur here are relatively few, mainly because we discuss a lot about self-pacing. As they say, "A stitch in time saves nine."

More often, we have people coming in from elsewhere with overloads, and deal pretty well with those. Not perfect, but many have found some clarity and balance, and can move ahead. So send your overloaded friends here. We will be happy to help. :-)

All the best!

The guru is in you.

2008/07/13 00:14:45
Support for AYP Pranayama, Mudras and Bandhas
http://www.aypsite.org/forum/topic.asp?TOPIC_ID=4139&REPLY_ID=35438&whichpage=-1
Conversation with an Indian teacher about pranayam

quote:
_____
Originally posted by brushjw

[quote]"By equalising the flow of prana in the ida and pingala nadis, nadi shodhana pranayama rectifies imbalances due to the 'habitual' predominance of the sympathetic nervous system, which is the result of chronic, ongoing stress. The balancing of the flow of prana has a positive influence on the body's stress response activity, and helps to keep levels of stress and tension within a normal range."

http://www.yogamag.net/archives/1991/fnov91/pranstr.shtml_____

Hi Joe:

I am aware of this traditional explanation, but it does not explain why slow breathing without alternate nostril regulation also has a relaxing effect. Isn't it true that the first advice people often give to someone who is highly stressed is to breathe slowly and deeply, not necessarily to breathe slowly and deeply through alternate nostrils? Of course, times have changed, and alternate nostril breathing is recommended more often now than in the past. But why does it work? And why does slow breathing without nostril regulation also work?

We should not take mystical explanations on faith, unless they can be verified, no matter how revered a source scripture may be. That is why the AYP lesson goes with the slow breathing explanation, because it is a characteristic found in both alternate nostril breathing and spinal breathing, and both can be relaxing for those who are comfortable in the practice.

Btw, I did nadi shodana pranayama for over 15 years twice daily before switching to spinal breathing pranayama many years ago, and have found the same benefits from spinal breathing, plus much more. Therefore, I was not comfortable parroting the scriptures on nadi shodana, because I knew something else was going on. So I described my experience as I saw it. If it turns out to be inaccurate, I will be more than happy to correct it.

None of this alters the performance or results of either practice, so it is really a question we can hand off to the scientific researchers. Eventually we will find out what is happening. Meanwhile, and happily, the mechanics of the practices and their benefits will remain the same. :-)

All the best!

The guru is in you.

2008/07/16 14:32:59
Support for AYP Pranayama, Mudras and Bandhas
http://www.aypsite.org/forum/topic.asp?TOPIC_ID=4157&REPLY_ID=35565&whichpage=-1
May Amrit lead to asthma?

Hi panoramix, and welcome to the forums!

While I can't say much about your Kriya Yoga practice, I can say that the sweet secretions (amrita/nectar) coming down through the nasal pharynx will not always be in such contrast. Like many of the experiences we may notice resulting from yoga practices, they are nearly always reflections of purification and opening occurring in the nervous system. As purification advances, they tend to fade into the landscape of our overall experience, which ends up becoming quite vast and diverse, even as *Oneness* arises from within us.

It can be something new every week or month, and it is good to take it all in stride, and keep going. In AYP, we call such experiences the "scenery" of yoga as we travel along our path, as opposed to our continuing "journey," which is associated more with our practices than with the scenery we may happen to pass on the way.

If symptoms become excessive, as might be the case in this instance for you, here in AYP, we advise "self-pacing" in practices (ramping back a bit temporarily). But you'd better ask your teachers about that. I'm the AYP guy, not the Kriya Yoga guy. :-)

Note: Deep meditation with mantra, performed right after pranayama, due to its deeper penetration in the nervous system, will generally help such purification and its associated symptoms become assimilated and balanced more quickly. That is another element to consider, most likely outside the the scope of the practices you are doing now, i.e., not part of Kriya Yoga as far as I know.

All the best!

The guru is in you.

2008/07/18 00:07:54
Support for AYP Pranayama, Mudras and Bandhas

http://www.aypsite.org/forum/topic.asp?TOPIC_ID=4157&REPLY_ID=35596&whichpage=-1
May Amrit lead to asthma?

quote:
_____

Originally posted by panoramix

Thank you Yogani.

What do you think amrit could chemically be, scientifically speaking?

_____

Hi Panoramix:

I haven't the foggiest and could only speculate, but I am sure a team of scientists could have a field day with it. We know there is something happening because the effects of these biochemical changes are quite noticeable and far-reaching. It is not likely that we are imagining these things.

There are many changes that occur in the biochemistry throughout the body as inner silence and ecstatic conductivity/radiance arise. Someday science will get serious about studying this. Our job here as it relates to science is to develop as many credible subjects for study as possible. Sooner or later they will find us, and we will welcome them with open arms. :-)

The guru is in you.

2008/08/04 17:46:51
Support for AYP Pranayama, Mudras and Bandhas
http://www.aypsite.org/forum/topic.asp?TOPIC_ID=4237&REPLY_ID=36034&whichpage=-1
need advice on a huge frenum cut I made

quote:
_____

Originally posted by alwayson

Here is a picture of my frenum, I just took now.

http://img150.imageshack.us/my.php?image=0804081554du5.jpg

What do you all think about the size of my frenum??

Yogani, where are you?

_____

Hi Alwayson:

I'm here! :-)

That's not too bad. Just give it some time. When it's healed and a nice taut edge develops and presents itself again, you can snip a little more if so inclined, probably without pain or blood. The whiteness is normal and will fade along with the frenum over time.

The bigger the snip, the more the initial discomfort, and the bigger the white spot. That's how it goes. So just take it easy. Make sure your daily sitting practices (deep meditation and spinal breathing) are in good shape, and kechari will happen as it should.

All the best!

The guru is in you.

2008/08/04 18:51:34
Support for AYP Pranayama, Mudras and Bandhas
http://www.aypsite.org/forum/topic.asp?TOPIC_ID=4237&REPLY_ID=36038&whichpage=-1
need advice on a huge frenum cut I made

quote:
_____

Originally posted by alwayson

I still have a substantial frenum. Am I right?

_____

Yes. A ways go go yet. But no need to rush, particularly if you are in stage 2 kechari already.

The guru is in you.

2008/08/24 10:30:31
Support for AYP Pranayama, Mudras and Bandhas
http://www.aypsite.org/forum/topic.asp?TOPIC_ID=4237&REPLY_ID=36709&whichpage=-1
need advice on a huge frenum cut I made

quote:
_____
Originally posted by alwayson

Yogani,

I have been snipping like a madman.....My frenum reached a point, where the cuts do not do anything. The frenum tendon just regenerates itself. What should I do?
_____

Hi Alwayson:

The best thing to do is favor your overall routine of practices and daily activities. Then you will have inner silence and ecstatic conductivity naturally rising in everyday life.

Kechari will work itself out in time. It is part of a larger whole. It is suggested not to force it.

The guru is in you.

2008/08/14 08:20:00
Support for AYP Pranayama, Mudras and Bandhas
http://www.aypsite.org/forum/topic.asp?TOPIC_ID=4292&REPLY_ID=36367&whichpage=-1
Spinal Nerve

Hi Neli:

There is no requirement to see or feel anything during spinal breathing. It is just simple tracing of the breath up and down between root and brow. By constantly expecting and looking for a particular experience, we will retard the process of spinal breathing, just as looking for a particular experience in deep meditation will retard the practice. It is about doing the practice, not expecting any particular experience. That is why we say, "Easily favor the procedure of the practice over any experience that may (or may not) come up."

In learning to let go of our expectations we gain everything.

All the best!

The guru is in you.

2008/08/15 09:29:45
Support for AYP Pranayama, Mudras and Bandhas
http://www.aypsite.org/forum/topic.asp?TOPIC_ID=4292&REPLY_ID=36388&whichpage=-1
Spinal Nerve

quote:
_____
Originally posted by neli

Hi Moderator

Sorry for my ignorance, but I don't understand this message, can you explain it ? I have received several of them, but I don't understand what it means.

Thanks in advance.
Sat Nam
Neli

quote:
_____
Originally posted by AYPforum

Moderator note: Topic moved for better placement
_____

_____

Hi Neli:

It just means a topic was moved by a moderator from one forum category to another. In this case I believe from Satsang Cafe to Pranayama..., which is appropriate, yes? Moving topics is how the forums are kept semi-organized by subject matter. Of course, members posting in the most appropriate forum category to begin with is very helpful. :-)

On the sushumna questions, yes, imagining the spinal nerve as a tiny tube during spinal breathing is the original instruction. But if it becomes a bother, then it is okay to simply go up and down the middle of the body between root and brow. That is an instruction also. Ultimately, the sushumna grows to become as big as the cosmos, with many intermediate stages going from tiny tube through gradually expanding energy column and finally to the cosmic. So it is a relative thing. It is an automatic process stimulated by our practices. There is nothing more we have to do about it. So just be easy with it, without expectations. If you are ending up at the brow when filled with air and at the root when empty, that is good spinal breathing practice. Favor that basic procedure over other energy and/or imagery that comes up, and the rest will take care of itself.

As for what other teachings say about the sushumna, I really can't speak for them. Spinal breathing has a very long and varied history, and as far as I know it is the cream of the pranayama methods (when adequately simplified). The results for many practitioners seem to confirm this.

What is new in AYP is the integration of spinal breathing with deep meditation (practiced in sequence, not at the same time), and that is opening a lot of doors for many practitioners, including the infinite inner space of the heart. :-)

All the best!

The guru is in you.

2008/08/16 10:38:15
Support for AYP Pranayama, Mudras and Bandhas
http://www.aypsite.org/forum/topic.asp?TOPIC_ID=4292&REPLY_ID=36421&whichpage=-1
Spinal Nerve

Hi Neli:

The perception of the spinal nerve (sushumna) may remain as a small ecstatic thread or tube, even as the energy is expanding. Or there could be no perception of the tiny thread, with a huge column of ecstatic energy whirling about. All of this is a process of purification and opening, and maintaining steady forward progress with comfort and safety is the priority.

In AYP we always favor the center in spinal breathing, no matter how wide or diverse the energy may become. We also favor the brow as the top point -- over time it may naturally expand upward as inner silence and ecstatic conductivity advance. There can be long term difficulties resulting from favoring the crown as the top point too early -- see lessons under "Crown Opening (avoiding premature)" in the Topic Index of the website or the AYP Easy Lessons book.

It sounds like you are doing a hybrid routine with several systems mixed. That is your choice, and it can work if consistency in daily practice and prudent self-pacing are maintained.

One thing I can tell you is, if you do AYP deep meditation for one or two hours, it will take a spatula to scrape you off the ceiling, sooner or later (probably sooner), so it is not advised. :-)

For the AYP practices, it is best to stick with the AYP instructions. For other systems of practice, I really can't offer much, except the suggestion for maintaining daily consistency, self-pacing, and a caution about doubling up on similar practices, which can lead to overload.

All the best!

The guru is in you.

2008/08/16 14:13:56
Support for AYP Pranayama, Mudras and Bandhas
http://www.aypsite.org/forum/topic.asp?TOPIC_ID=4292&REPLY_ID=36431&whichpage=-1
Spinal Nerve

quote:
_____
Originally posted by tubeseeker

yogani,
when I do spinal breathing if I breath slow enough I feel as if my breath is equal in both nostrils instead of one being dominant. It also actually feels as if the breath is coming in at the thr third eye instead of through the nostrils, I can do this and trace the nerve at the same time.
Thoughts?
thanks
Neil

_____

Hi Neil:

Sounds like good practice. Just remember to keep favoring the practice over the experience, and all will continue to develop naturally.

All the best!

The guru is in you.

2008/09/03 12:05:31
Support for AYP Pranayama, Mudras and Bandhas
http://www.aypsite.org/forum/topic.asp?TOPIC_ID=4389&REPLY_ID=37177&whichpage=-1
A Question about Visualizing the Sushumna

Hi All:

Excellent discussion on a sometimes tricky subject, because the sushumna (spinal nerve) does expand over time, as many have noticed. Nevertheless, the practice remains essentially the same, anchored between root and brow, without excessive imagining in-between being necessary. We just easily favor the center path. As the core grows, we naturally go from being outside everything to being inside everything.

That's why the subtitle of the AYP Spinal Breathing Pranayama book is: "Journey to Inner Space."

This might help:
http://www.aypsite.org/forum/topic.asp?TOPIC_ID=4292#36388

Carry on! :-)

The guru is in you.

2008/09/03 14:01:52
Support for AYP Pranayama, Mudras and Bandhas
http://www.aypsite.org/forum/topic.asp?TOPIC_ID=4389&REPLY_ID=37187&whichpage=-1
A Question about Visualizing the Sushumna

Hi CarsonZi:

Not trivial at all.

Any extra effort of visualizing inside or outside will slow down the process. Just favor the easiest route in the center between root and brow. It is not we who decide what is outside and what is inside. It is the direct perception of the natural expansion of the sushumna that reveals it, as purification and opening advance due to our practices.

It is like AYP-style self-inquiry, where making the thing in our mind is non-relational, and becoming the thing itself is relational. The less forcing there is in any practice, the more relational (in stillness) and effective it will be. Those two words "easily favor" are the key. Add on "twice daily for the long term," and we cannot miss. :-)

The guru is in you.

2008/09/03 16:04:03
Support for AYP Pranayama, Mudras and Bandhas
http://www.aypsite.org/forum/topic.asp?TOPIC_ID=4389&REPLY_ID=37198&whichpage=-1
A Question about Visualizing the Sushumna

quote:
_____
Originally posted by CarsonZi

Thank you Yogani. I figured that would be the answer. Sometimes I feel silly posting here because as I am writing my question I am answering it as well too. But I still end up leaving the question up there for comments and suggestions even though I am pretty sure I already know the answer. I guess I need to TRUST my inner guru a little more, and stop feeling the need for external commendations. Thank you for responding.
Namaste,
CarsonZi
_____

Ah, but think of everyone else who is benefiting from your self-answering questions. :-)

It is simple once we get how utterly straight-forward it is. But not so simple for those who are bogged down in mountains of imagery they feel obliged to maintain. It's not necessary!

This is the primary shortcoming in methods of spinal breathing that have been added on to, and added on to, and added on to some more. So much esoteric mumbo-jumbo. You can see the immovable mental structures cemented in the faces of people who practice this way. Argggh!

Not us. We just dance and sing a lot... :-)

The guru is in you.

2009/07/26 22:09:15
Support for AYP Pranayama, Mudras and Bandhas
http://www.aypsite.org/forum/topic.asp?TOPIC_ID=4779&REPLY_ID=54075&whichpage=-1
How do I get tongue length?

quote:
_____
Originally posted by anandatandava

Can you tell me the title of the Mallinson book you refer to? Looking for help and ideas on how to lengthen.

Thanks
_____

Hi Anandatandava:

Here are a couple of topics on Jim Mallison's book:
http://www.aypsite.org/forum/topic.asp?TOPIC_ID=3891
http://www.aypsite.org/forum/topic.asp?TOPIC_ID=1534
He participated in both of these discussions, as "flying fakir."

Here is an Amazon link for the book, which is called "**Khecarividya**":

It is expensive, priced as a university textbook, not as a handbook for in-the-trenches yogis.

All the best!

The guru is in you.

PS: I don't think tongue elongation is a complete substitute for frenum reduction for reaching kechari stage 2. If the tongue is long and the frenum is limiting, the tongue will be coming up from further forward on the floor the mouth (tied down by the frenum) and will have to compensate for that by bending behind the palate, an awkward maneuver. If the tongue is normal length and the frenum is not limiting, the tongue can go up behind the palate without having to maneuver (bend) around it from a point tied down further forward on the floor of the mouth. An ideal approach is a little bit of of <u>both</u> lengthening and frenum reduction, as needed, with neither measure taken to an extreme. From there, it is largely a matter of technique, i.e., going <u>forward</u> with the tongue as soon as the tip of the tongue gets behind the soft palate on either the left or right side, whichever is the shortest distance and easiest to reach. Then the soft palate comes down like a trap door and the distance to the "secret spot" is very short.

2009/07/27 21:54:48
Support for AYP Pranayama, Mudras and Bandhas
http://www.aypsite.org/forum/topic.asp?TOPIC_ID=4779&REPLY_ID=54118&whichpage=-1
How do I get tongue length?

quote:
_____
Originally posted by anandatandava

My tongue is almost entirely lax with tongue curled back, but I still need a small finger push to get in. Once there I'm above the eustachian tubes and the chamber has narrowed considerably. I can curl my tongue back far enough on the back of my throat so that the soft palate drops back down pushing my tongue out, so I seem real close to success. I need this method very much in high stress situations. Are there any further directions to be given on tongue lengthening such as pulling up when milking? Would a copyright on the Mallinson book allow for copying the portion pertaining to this? Is there anyone who can do this for me?
_____

Hi Anandatandava:

There are very few here who have the book. I don't.

If you are in stage 2 kechari with finger help, it won't be long until you can do it without finger help.

As for lengthening, it is not rocket science, and not nearly as crucial as it is sometimes made out to be. There are plenty of "tongue lengthening" discussions here in the forums. Perhaps some here can pull them out for you. No pun intended. :-)

Honestly, once we are in the nasal pharynx and can spend some time there in relative comfort during spinal breathing, there is not much more needed for good results in kechari. If you are in the area of the eustachian tube openings you are doing fine. The secret spot is right there in-between them on the back edge of the septum.

More importantly, to gain the full benefits of kechari, the beginnings of ecstatic conductivity in the nervous system are necessary, and that is not a function of kechari alone. It is related to all of our practices and our general condition of purification and opening. It is only then that the secret spot becomes an active player in the continuing rise of ecstatic conductivity. Before then, the sensations at the secret spot may be muted, and the whole body connection limited, which begins with root to brow ecstatic conductivity. Mulabandha, sambhavi and siddhasana are at least as important in this as kechari. And, of course, deep meditation and spinal breathing come before that.

So the suggestion is to aim for balance in the overall practice routine and bringing the effects of that into daily activity, where the inner silence and ecstatic conductivity and radiance cultivated in sitting practices will naturally and gradually become stabilized 24/7.

There is no one practice that is going to "save us." If I had to pick one, it would not be kechari. It would be deep meditation. Beyond deep meditation, it is all about developing a balanced integration, not targeting one practice excessively over the others. Of course, at particular times we will be focusing on the practice we are integrating then. Once we have done that we can move on to next things, without becoming too extreme about any particular practice. Step by step. Kechari is one step on the road of purification and opening. The degree to which it is pursued will depend on the individual. Everyone is a little different. It is more about our bhakti than anything.

All the best!

The guru is in you.

PS: If you give it some time, with regular kechari practice you may see a snipable edge of the tendon appearing again at the surface of the center line of the frenum. It can keep coming back like that again and again for years. I snipped off and on for nearly 20 years. So don't write off the frenum too soon. With normal practice of kechari, it will likely be back. :-)

2008/12/19 23:08:08
Support for AYP Pranayama, Mudras and Bandhas
http://www.aypsite.org/forum/topic.asp?TOPIC_ID=4923&REPLY_ID=42628&whichpage=-1
The final Kechari snippings

Hi Carson:

In AYP it is not recommended to snip significantly off the center line of the frenum. You are not in any trouble with what you did, but for anyone who does aggressive deep snipping on either side, there is a risk of hitting the fairly large blood vessels that are located on either side under the tongue.

There are no significant blood vessels in the center, and that is where the edge of the multi-strand frenum tendon is, so that is the safest and most effective place to be with snipping.

Sounds like you are doing great with kechari. Bravo!

Just wanted to give a caution for anyone who might be considering doing deep snipping on either side of the center.

All the best!

The guru is in you.

2008/12/20 10:26:54
Support for AYP Pranayama, Mudras and Bandhas
http://www.aypsite.org/forum/topic.asp?TOPIC_ID=4923&REPLY_ID=42648&whichpage=-1
The final Kechari snippings

quote:
_____
Originally posted by CarsonZi

Hi Yogani,

You know I meant up and down from centre frenulum and not left and right of centre frenulum right? And the reason I did this was not on purpose. I made one snip first and it ended up being a little above centre and not quite as deep as I had desired. So I decided to make a second cut, but didn't want to make it directly in the centre because that would have been too close to the first cut, so I made it the same distance from centre as the first cut, just the opposite side and the right depth. It worked out pretty good. I can appreciate the need to tell other forumites that the way I did it is not the most effective nor the safest way, but it was a little bit of a bumble on my part and not on purpose. Perhaps I should have stated that in my original post. Sorry, I didn't think of it. Thanks for pointing this out though:-)

Love,
Carson
_____

Hi Carson:

Oh, you meant up and down from center, not left and right. There is no undue risk in that. It is fine.

For those considering kechari mudra, it is suggested to review lesson 108, here: http://www.aypsite.org/108.html
...and follow-up lessons linked in the website topic index.

Lesson 108 is also linked in the left side border of this page, along with other key lessons on the AYP practices.

All the best!

The guru is in you.

2009/02/20 10:48:19
Support for AYP Pranayama, Mudras and Bandhas
http://www.aypsite.org/forum/topic.asp?TOPIC_ID=5187&REPLY_ID=45641&whichpage=-1
Kechari Mudra with the index finger!

quote:
_____
Originally posted by Emil

Hi all,
I have been trying to get to the second stage of kechari for the past few months but haven't had any luck yet. I have read some of the forum discussions here as well as the lessons 108 and 205.

A discovery that I made last night was that even though I still cannot perform the second stage of kechari with my tongue, I can actually take the tip of my index finger behind the soft palate and touch the same spot with my finger tip.

My question is: Do you think touching the point behind the soft pallette with finger tip would produce any spiritual benefits?

_____

Hi Emil:

Just a reminder that the ecstatic sensitivity of the "secret spot" on the back edge of the septum in the nasal pharynx does not come primarily from the physical act of kechari. Rather, ecstatic conductivity rises in the whole body through a combination of practices, primarily deep meditation and spinal breathing pranayama, and then the rising sensitivity may draw us toward kechari and other manifestations of yoga. This is why non-yogis who can mimic stage 2 kechari mudra gain little benefit. They should be tipped off about the broader implications of what they are doing. :-)

None of this is to say those who are inclined to pursue kechari should not. Our desire (bhakti) is an essential part of the process. But it is good to know that the physical act of kechari alone will not produce the entire result. Once ecstatic conductivity is present in the neurobiology, then kechari will have increasing effect, as many here have experienced.

Natural kechari also stimulates the deep throat, which is tied in with the rise of the "nectar cycle" beginning in the GI tract, discussed in this recent lesson: http://www.aypsite.org/304.html
This is another way we may be naturally drawn into kechari (the tongue going back), with the throat becoming ecstatically sensitive, along with the septum and many other regions of the neurobiology.

Given these dynamics, I'm not sure that using a synthetic kechari method with finger or mechanical device will contribute much. When kechari is called for, it will come. The results will be there as soon as the tongue naturally goes back to stage 1 (tip of the tongue going toward the point where hard and soft palates meet on the roof of the mouth), so it is not necessary to rush to stage 2 and beyond. We will know when it is time.

Be sure that enlightenment is possible without the full extent of the physical act of kechari mudra. In this sense, kechari is effect as much as cause, largely dependent on on the rise of abiding inner silence and ecstatic conductivity.

Of course, everyone will follow their own bhakti and path, so these are just a few observations for consideration.

When we are inclined to pursue development of the habit of kechari mudra, a good place in our routine to do that is during spinal breathing pranayama, and not during deep meditation. Once the habit is naturally present, then kechari can appear automatically in deep meditation in a way that does not divide the mind. There is only one procedure we can consciously be doing during deep meditation, and that is the procedure of deep meditation (easily favoring the mantra over anything else that may come up). If we are deliberately doing anything else, then we are not doing deep meditation. This is why we consciously cultivate mudras, bandhas and siddhasana outside our deep meditation session. Then when they come up as spontaneous habits during deep meditation, this is fine.

All the best!

The guru is in you.

2009/06/04 13:59:12
Support for AYP Pranayama, Mudras and Bandhas
http://www.aypsite.org/forum/topic.asp?TOPIC_ID=5735&REPLY_ID=51929&whichpage=-1
Support For SBP

Hi Krish:

Some teachings use ujjayi (restricting air flow with the epiglottis) going both ways, but AYP does not. Over the long term, the negative pressure that ujjayi can cause in the lungs during inhalation may not be healthful. Neither are the effects of long term external kumbhaka (breath suspension).

But that is not the only reason why we do not use ujjayi on inhalation with spinal breathing in AYP. Opening the deep throat wider than usual during inhalation has an effect on the medulla oblongata (brain stem) that supports the effects of spinal breathing. Then we use ujjayi on exhalation for its positive effects there.

Using ujjayi just because it helps you track the spinal nerve upward for now may be a false economy, since there are other factors in play that have nothing to do with the energetic scenery we may be experiencing at the moment. This is why we say, "Favor the practice over the experience." The scenery will always be changing, but the underlying principles of practice will remain the same.

It is the same with looking at different modes of spinal breathing, which there are many. An easier tracing of the spinal nerve short term with a more intricate method, may not be easier long term. In fact, over the long term there will be a trend toward less definition of the inner neurobiology, not more. AYP spinal breathing starts with less. Less is more... :-)

If you are getting stuck in-between root and brow, it is fine to skip over the stuck place, being sure to be at the brow at the end of inhalation and at the root at the end of exhalation. This skipping over to the two end points (brow and root) will clear the path in-between, and any stuck place will dissolve in time. If the whole thing becomes too rigid and overwhelming, then stop and let the attention rest easily with whatever sensation is there in the body for a few minutes. This will generally dissolve the obstruction enough to easily continue spinal breathing. Over time, spinal breathing will become much easier, because the inner obstructions become much less with practice. That is the purpose of spinal breathing, and all of yoga.

As for comparing AYP spinal breathing to Kriya Yoga spinal breathing or other methods, it is preferred not to be doing that in this forum category, which is for AYP spinal breathing support, not for analyzing everything else that is out there. Those comparisons are welcome to be done in the "other systems" forum category. There is a recent topic on spinal breathing in there where this was done. It was moved out of here. We'd like to keep support for the core AYP practices as clear as possible in the AYP Deep Meditation and Pranayama forum categories.

In any case, that is the AYP point of view on ujjayi and spinal breathing practice. You are, of course, free to follow whatever path you choose. Better not to try and follow too many methods at once though. Pick your practice and favor it over the long term. That is where the real benefits are. Not in trying to accommodate every energy wrinkle that comes up. Much better to favor the practice than be constantly redesigning it... :-)

The guru is in you.

2009/07/29 11:51:25
Support for AYP Pranayama, Mudras and Bandhas
http://www.aypsite.org/forum/topic.asp?TOPIC_ID=6037&REPLY_ID=54277&whichpage=-1
Mudras and bandhas coming down on exhale?

Hi Tamasaburo:

The mudras and bandhas are intended to be very faint and gentle. They may not start out that way ("clunky stage"), but will naturally evolve to that with the rise of ecstatic conductivity. They are not necessarily tied to the breath, though they may be incidentally at times. We don't make a thing of it.

Mulabandha might be an exception. See this lesson: http://www.aypsite.org/119.html
This instruction on mulabandha/asvini does not apply to all the mudras and bandhas.

The internal integration and refinement of mudras and bandhas evolves to naturally become "whole body mudra."
http://www.aypsite.org/212.html
We avoid building too much structure into the practice of mudras and bandhas so this natural evolution can occur without undue interference. Ultimately, it is driven by bhakti and the resulting flow of ecstatic bliss through the neurobiology. This is the underlying dynamic of outpouring divine love, which is stillness in action, the rise of unity.

All the best!

The guru is in you.

2009/08/28 11:05:37
Support for AYP Pranayama, Mudras and Bandhas
http://www.aypsite.org/forum/topic.asp?TOPIC_ID=6211&REPLY_ID=55848&whichpage=-1
Kechari: Cut, Don't Snip

Hi Yogalearn, and welcome!

I concur with the good advise you have been receiving above.

There have been some who have gone for one-step removal of the frenum that have reported about it here in the forums, and others privately in my email. These have all been professionally done, which is the prudent route to go if you are driven to do this.

There are several topics on professional frenum removal in the forums. They can be found with searches on the appropriate terms (particularly "laser"). Here is one that may be helpful: http://www.aypsite.org/forum/topic.asp?TOPIC_ID=2387

Wishing you all the best on your path. Practice wisely, and enjoy!

The guru is in you.

2009/08/28 11:24:03
Support for AYP Pranayama, Mudras and Bandhas
http://www.aypsite.org/forum/topic.asp?TOPIC_ID=6211&REPLY_ID=55851&whichpage=-1
Kechari: Cut, Don't Snip
Follow-up for Yogalearn:

Here is an aggressive approach to frenum removal that can be self-implemented, and is safer than what you are contemplating:
http://www.aypsite.org/forum/topic.asp?TOPIC_ID=497
I do not necessarily recommend this, but if you must self-implement an aggressive approach to frenum removal, then this approach focusing in the center (where the restraining tendon is) would reduce the risk of cutting the arteries on the sides.

There are a variety of other approaches. If you do forum subject line searches on kechari, khechari, frenum, frenulum, snip, laser and other related terms, you will find dozens of practical discussions on kechari mudra here.

When in doubt, go back to Lesson 108, and check the Topic Index for more AYP lessons on kechari mudra. :-)

It is recommended to keep your yoga practices in balance, and always "self-pace" when things are tending toward any extreme.

The guru is in you.

2009/09/05 15:20:33
Support for AYP Pranayama, Mudras and Bandhas
http://www.aypsite.org/forum/topic.asp?TOPIC_ID=6281&REPLY_ID=56310&whichpage=-1
Has anyone's frenum actually diminished?

Hi Alwayson:

Snipping the flesh over the tendon will not provide any progress, as you are finding. It is the tendon itself that holds the tongue down, and it is snipped a little bit at a time with healing in-between. The AYP procedure in Main Lesson 108 is about that.

In most people, the tendon will come to the surface at the center line/edge of the frenum when stretched, and is easy to snip there. Stretch, snip, heal, stretch, snip, heal. That is the sequence for multiple rounds of gradually reducing the tendon to very little restriction of the tongue's upward and back movement.

For some, the tendon does not come to the surface at the center line/edge of the frenum so easily. Then more stretching will be the way to go. There are some more aggressive means for getting at the tendon, which is made of thousands of tiny strands. It can certainly be snipped a little at at time once it is exposed.

Surgery is another option, and if done, should be by a doctor.

All the best!

The guru is in you.

2009/09/05 15:41:27
Support for AYP Pranayama, Mudras and Bandhas
http://www.aypsite.org/forum/topic.asp?TOPIC_ID=6281&REPLY_ID=56312&whichpage=-1
Has anyone's frenum actually diminished?
PS: See here for a more aggressive method for reaching the tendon, Tooled Talavya: http://www.aypsite.org/forum/topic.asp?TOPIC_ID=497

2009/09/05 16:56:04
Support for AYP Pranayama, Mudras and Bandhas
http://www.aypsite.org/forum/topic.asp?TOPIC_ID=6281&REPLY_ID=56322&whichpage=-1
Has anyone's frenum actually diminished?

quote:
———————
Originally posted by alwayson2

Yogani,

for you personally, did you originally have a frenum, and now it looks as if you naturally didn't have one?

———————

Yes, and much less now. It took several months of snipping to get into kechari stage 2 initially, and more snipping to go to next stages later on. Stretching/milking was used too, but snipping is what made the most difference in my case. That was over 20 years ago. I continued to snip on and off for many years, while integrating a full range of practices. It was never only about kechari, but the integration of all the practices for best overall results in cultivating abiding inner silence and ecstatic conductivity/radiance. That is reflected in the AYP lessons, I hope. :-)

The guru is in you.

2009/09/21 13:06:34
Support for AYP Pranayama, Mudras and Bandhas
http://www.aypsite.org/forum/topic.asp?TOPIC_ID=6375&REPLY_ID=57311&whichpage=-1
Split tongue

Hi Alwayson:

Well, it all depends on where one hails from. Around these parts, this is self-mutilation inspired by an extremist view. Of course, just about anything can be considered extremist, depending on the perspective of the observer.

Suffice to say that tongue splitting is _not_ recommended in AYP. You knew that already, right? I just wanted to make sure that anyone else who looks at this topic will know it. :-)

The guru is in you.

2009/09/21 13:18:49
Support for AYP Pranayama, Mudras and Bandhas
http://www.aypsite.org/forum/topic.asp?TOPIC_ID=6375&REPLY_ID=57313&whichpage=-1
Split tongue

quote:
———————
Originally posted by alwayson2

I am trying to figure out if this is a real historic practice in India. I don't recall it being in James Mallinson's khecharividya book.

I emailed a known academic author.

Hopefully I get a response.
———————

Yes, it is, but that has no bearing on what we are doing here, any more than holding your arm straight up in the air 24 hours per day for 40 years would be. It too is a "real historic practice." That does not make it useful for a community of practitioners.

For most, these are only attention-getters, obtained at a high cost.

The guru is in you.

2009/10/29 18:13:00
Support for AYP Pranayama, Mudras and Bandhas
http://www.aypsite.org/forum/topic.asp?TOPIC_ID=6608&REPLY_ID=59146&whichpage=-1
Breath regulation causes me severe discomfort

Hi IcedEarth:

If you are sensitive to pranayama, it is good to back off it and do what is comfortable, which is what you are doing. It is right practice. Nothing wrong with that. There is plenty else you have to work with.

Deep meditation is a much more fundamental and powerful practice than any form of pranayama. If you are comfortable with twice-daily deep meditation without pranayama, then you can make good progress in cultivating abiding inner silence, clearing out inner obstructions, and in time those emotional (energy) reactions from pranayama will become less. You are wise to be self-pacing now, and it is self-pacing that will carry you forward in managing practices in the future.

Regarding the energization exercises, that is great that they help smooth things out. You may like to try adding a short set of asanas on the front end, before energization exercises and deep meditation. What you cannot do with pranayama right now, you can work on gently with the physical practices coming from the outside, and deep meditation coming from the inside. If that works without discomfort, you have a very good practice, and you can evolve your routine gradually from there.

As for AYP methods being "dark age," that is standard sectarian-speak for, "I don't know anything about that, and don't want to." :-)

All the best!

The guru is in you.

PS: If you find the routine just described to be smooth after a few months, you may like to consider adding samyama. Or perhaps a mantra enhancement. These are ways to gradually broaden the purification coming from inside, from inner silence. One step at a time though...

2009/11/09 12:00:07
Support for AYP Pranayama, Mudras and Bandhas
http://www.aypsite.org/forum/topic.asp?TOPIC_ID=6608&REPLY_ID=59507&whichpage=-1
Breath regulation causes me severe discomfort

quote:
_____
Originally posted by IcedEarth

This is a confusing point for me. Often spiritual teachers will suggest that bringing awareness to places of energy imbalance can result in healing and decrease pain. But then some people from AYP say not to put attention on the areas of imbalance. I think that rather than concentrating solely on the area of discomfort, it might be best to put awareness throughout the whole body. I usually cannot find much discomfort in my body anywhere except my head, and my left hand if I play guitar for several hours.
_____

Hi IcedEarth:

Not sure if the point has been made yet in this topic that there is a difference between focusing attention on a physical sensation (often accompanied by a strong emotion), versus allowing awareness to naturally be with (witness) an emotion/sensation. There is a difference. The first will tend to amplify the sensation, while the second will tend to dissolve the sensation.

This is analogous to clinging to the mantra on the surface in deep meditation versus allowing it to fade, or clinging to a sutra on the surface in samyama versus releasing it in stillness.

It is important to make the distinction between focusing (clinging) versus witnessing (allowing) in these matters. Witnessing may be somewhat problematic before we have some inner silence present, because before then all attention tends to cling (identify with the objects of perception). But as inner silence comes to abide, the process of witnessing gradually takes over and obstructions dissolve much more easily simply by allowing our awareness to be with them. In the meantime, we can intellectually understand the difference between focusing and allowing, and continue meditating within the limits of our necessary self-pacing.

On that, perhaps you have become somewhat sensitive to deep meditation. If that is the case, I suggest looking at Lesson 367.

Other lessons that might be of interest are:

Lesson 15, for using awareness (witness) to dissolve excessive sensations occurring during deep mediation.

Lesson 207, on left or right side imbalances. Not necessarily to encourage spinal breathing if it is not working for you, but to avoid too many attempts to manipulate energy, which does not work in the long run. Much better to be easy and stick with practices that cultivate abiding inner silence (witness), and the natural purification and healing that come with it. This is in line with and supports effective body awareness techniques, no matter who is teaching them.

All the best!

The guru is in you.

2009/11/09 12:04:08
Support for AYP Pranayama, Mudras and Bandhas
http://www.aypsite.org/forum/topic.asp?TOPIC_ID=6608&REPLY_ID=59508&whichpage=-1
Breath regulation causes me severe discomfort
PS: IE, we crossed posts. Sounds like you are on it. You may want to go easy with the energy cultivation (siddhasana) until you know things are stabilizing in the inner silence department. It may be the last thing you need right now is an energy roller coaster ride. :-)

It's up to you.

2009/12/09 10:11:00
Support for AYP Pranayama, Mudras and Bandhas
http://www.aypsite.org/forum/topic.asp?TOPIC_ID=6823&REPLY_ID=61012&whichpage=-1
Bhastrika versus Kapalbhati

quote:

I've also been wondering about bhastrika--when Yogani says that only the diaphragm is moving does he mean that literally only that little band of muscle under the lungs is moving or more that that is the focus but the abdominals will often move somewhat? I feel I have a strong tendency to move the abs in and out somewhat in bhastrika a la kapalbhati, but maybe this is a mistake? Also, is the emphasis more on the inhale in bhastrika as compared to kapalbhati? Or is it just more evenly distributed between inhale and exhale (while kapalbhati focuses very much on exhale)?

Yes, it is really the diaphragm that does it, like a dog panting. People have tried to do bastrika with all the other muscles (abs, chest, etc.), but in the end it is the diaphragm that does it _easily_. It just takes some practice to develop the diaphragm panting habit.

It is different for kapalbhati, which also relies on the abdominals and chest for rapid expulsion of air. The two practices have different purposes -- kapalbhati for brain cleansing, and spinal bastrika (in AYP) for spinal nerve cleansing.

Kapalbhati is covered along with the other shatkarmas in the AYP Diet, Shatkarmas and Amaroli book, and in online Lesson 316.

Spinal and targeted bastrika are covered in multiple online lessons (see topic index), and in the AYP Easy Lessons book.

All the best!

The guru is in you.

2009/12/09 09:57:39
Support for AYP Pranayama, Mudras and Bandhas
http://www.aypsite.org/forum/topic.asp?TOPIC_ID=6825&REPLY_ID=61007&whichpage=-1
Spinal Breathing

Hi SeySorciere:

Here are a few tips from the AYP Spinal Breathing Pranayama book that might be helpful:

From Page 12:

"If we have some difficulty visualizing and tracing the spinal nerve as a tiny thread or tube, then it is perfectly all right to follow the spinal column in a less specific way. Over time, we will find more definition in our practice. There is no need to strain or struggle in our visualization. The main thing is that we end up at the brow at the completion of inhalation and at the root at the completion of exhalation. How we get back and forth is less important than traveling from one end to the other without strain during our slow deep breathing. In time, it all comes together."

From Page 16:

"...There is another reason for resistance in spinal breathing – obstructions in the nervous system. These are neurobiological restrictions within us that we have carried throughout our life. With spinal breathing, we are coaxing them to relax and release. In the beginning, the resistance from these inner knots can be quite palpable. Some people may find it difficult to pass through a particular area of the inner body with attention and breath traveling up and down inside. The resistance can be found anywhere – the pelvis, solar plexus, heart, throat, or in the head. The resistance can be felt as a blockage that we can't get past, or as some pressure.

What do we do? It is simple. If there is a pressure or a resistance, we just go right by it with our attention and breath. Easily right by it. We never try and force through inner resistance. We just stroke it gently with our attention and breath as we go by. This has a good purifying effect, and will not be uncomfortable. Discomfort comes from forcing against an obstruction. We never do this in spinal breathing. We just whisk on through. What we did not dissolve on the first pass, we will get on the next one, or the next, or the 10,000th pass, maybe years later in our practice. That is how we purify the inner neurobiology. And all the while, we will have the experience of less resistance accompanied by more clarity and fluidity.

With each spinal breathing session, we are journeying deeper within ourselves to realms of greater peace and joy."

So it is okay to slip by those stuck places. The procedure is to end up at the brow at the completion of inhalation, and at the root at the completion of exhalation. We can skip over obstructions and go straight to the brow as we complete inhalation, and do the same to arrive at the root at the completion of exhalation. It is not for us to be micro-managing everything in-between. As long as we are comfortably landing at both ends of the spinal nerve, the middle will take care of itself in due course.

And Shanti is right in advising that experiences during practice do not matter. Just easily favor the simple procedure of spinal breathing over whatever may be happening. If we are gradually feeling more centered during our daily activity, that is the proof of the pudding. :-)

All the best!

The guru is in you.

2009/12/13 18:43:49
Support for AYP Pranayama, Mudras and Bandhas
http://www.aypsite.org/forum/topic.asp?TOPIC_ID=6855&REPLY_ID=61277&whichpage=-1
Is it imperative to start with Mulabandha?

Hi The seeker:

It is fine to keep on as you are doing with the eyes during spinal breathing, because it is working for you. At some point you may like to add on some gentle, flexible mulabandha/asvini and see what happens. Lesson 119 offers some options for this. It is in the AYP book, and online here:
http://www.aypsite.org/119.html

Mulabandha comes before sambhavi in the lessons because in many cases sambhavi will not find an ecstatic connection before there has been some direct stimulation at the root. In your case, spinal breathing has been enough to get the ball rolling with ecstatic conductivity. Good things are happening.

Take things at your own pace, and enjoy!

The guru is in you.

PS: For others following along here, the original instructions for mulabandha are in <u>Lesson 55</u>. Additional lessons on mulabandha can be found in the <u>website topic index</u>.

2009/12/15 08:35:34
Support for AYP Pranayama, Mudras and Bandhas
http://www.aypsite.org/forum/topic.asp?TOPIC_ID=6855&REPLY_ID=61353&whichpage=-1
Is it imperative to start with Mulabandha?

quote:
_____
Originally posted by The_seeker

"It is fine to keep on as you are doing with the eyes during spinal breathing, because it is working for you."
Are you reffering to raising the eyes as I do (only at the upper end) or continuously like in full sambhavi as Christi described? (personally I find difficult to keep my eyes up and to focus on breathing in the same time)
_____

Hi The seeker:

What you are doing is fine for now. It is a reasonable start with the spinal breathing enhancement covered in the <u>SBP book</u>, which is an introduction to sambhavi. As you know, there are several enhancements discussed there. It will evolve into what it needs to be as time goes on, with ecstatic feelings and your bhakti, and as you learn more about sambhavi and other mudras and bandhas and their effects. You are doing fine. :-)

The guru is in you.

2009/12/27 18:09:04
Support for AYP Pranayama, Mudras and Bandhas
http://www.aypsite.org/forum/topic.asp?TOPIC_ID=6928&REPLY_ID=61851&whichpage=-1
Soma?

Hi Victor:

The way we discuss the <u>nectar cycle</u> in AYP, your experience would be more on the nectar side, coming down through the sinuses and nasal tissues into the GI tract. With the terminology we use, soma is associated with the higher digestion part of the cycle.

It is true that the energetic side will tend to be more noticeable over time. The biochemistry (nectar cycle) has an underlying role in that which may not be noticed much in advanced stages.

It is all heading in the right direction. :-)

The guru is in you.

2010/01/09 14:40:02
Support for AYP Pranayama, Mudras and Bandhas
http://www.aypsite.org/forum/topic.asp?TOPIC_ID=6988&REPLY_ID=62463&whichpage=-1
Can Pranayama cause mind dullness ??

Hi All:

It should be mentioned that the main difference between hours of pranayama not being enough, versus 20 minutes of pranayama being too much, is deep meditation after pranayama in the second case.

Each of these two practices greatly increase the power of the other, and that largely accounts for the difference in results, and the time it takes to produce them.

Practice wisely, and enjoy! :-)

The guru is in you.

2010/01/16 11:44:13
Support for AYP Pranayama, Mudras and Bandhas
http://www.aypsite.org/forum/topic.asp?TOPIC_ID=7060&REPLY_ID=63001&whichpage=-1
YMK-sequence

quote:
_____

Originally posted by krcqimpro1

Hi Yogani,
Two points I would like your clarification on pl.:
1.Since YMK is a practice more related to Ecstatic Conductivity than to DM, would it not be more logical to do it before DM than after DM as you have recommended in your lessons ?

2. Is YMK considered effective only if, during each breath one sees the annular bright golden ring sorrounding a purple core with a white star in the centre ?
Krish

————

Hi Krish:

1. Yoni mudra can be done anywhere in the routine with equal effect. In the Eight Limbs of Yoga book "practice chart," it is before meditation at the intermediate level and after meditation at the advanced level, mainly to make room for additions of chin pump and bastrika before meditation. How these energy practices are arranged in the routine is more a matter of comfort and convenience than anything. In some systems bastrika is done before spinal breathing, and that is okay too. Whatever works best for the practitioner. However, the sequence of core practices, including spinal breathing, deep meditation and samyama should not be rearranged. The sequencing of these is important.

2. No. Visions or other experiences during practice are not necessarily an indication of the effectiveness of the practice. They are "scenery." With or without the scenery, we are moving ahead. The measure of our practice is in how we feel during normal daily activity outside our practice.

The guru is in you.

2010/01/17 11:43:50
Support for AYP Pranayama, Mudras and Bandhas
http://www.aypsite.org/forum/topic.asp?TOPIC_ID=7060&REPLY_ID=63046&whichpage=-1
YMK-sequence

quote:
————
Originally posted by krcqimpro1

Yogani, thanks for the clarification. I suppose one can consider oneself at the advanced level if one has successfully incorporated all of the concurrent practices in one's routine gradually over 12 months, even if one does not experience any of the "symptoms" of an awakened K, barring, of course, a steady inner silence.
krish.

————

Hi Krish:

And we will be even more advanced when less of everything is needed. We will know it when we see it. Self-pacing is the ultimate spiritual practice. :-)

The guru is in you.

2010/01/22 16:24:35
Support for AYP Pranayama, Mudras and Bandhas
http://www.aypsite.org/forum/topic.asp?TOPIC_ID=7112&REPLY_ID=63556&whichpage=-1
Spinal Breathing

Hi Rael:

Let me point out that there are no "imperatives" in AYP, only suggestions combined with your own common sense.

Whenever someone says something has to be absolutely a certain way, you can be sure you are not receiving AYP advice.

Sure, it is better to do sitting practices on an empty (or nearly empty) stomach. But it is not "imperative." Use your common sense and do what works for you. One size does not fit all.

The guru is in you.

2010/01/24 12:19:20
Support for AYP Pranayama, Mudras and Bandhas
http://www.aypsite.org/forum/topic.asp?TOPIC_ID=7139&REPLY_ID=63712&whichpage=-1
Kriya Yoga and the order they are in. Please Help

Hi Garlic and welcome!

AYP Chin Pump and Kriya Thokar are similar. You can read about chin pump here: http://www.aypsite.org/139.html

It is suggested to read the free AYP online lessons from the beginning, which will give you a good idea how spiritual practices fit together. AYP is not Yogananda's Kriya Yoga, but contains many of the same elements, and much more: http://www.aypsite.org/MainDirectory.html

Also check this lesson on ages to consider the various practices. Your spiritual desire is advanced for your age. That is wonderful. It will be good to be aware of some of the age-related factors. Take your time, and you will save time in the long run, while having a much steadier ride on the way: http://www.aypsite.org/256.html

Practice wisely, and enjoy!

The guru is in you.

2010/01/27 11:36:10
Support for AYP Pranayama, Mudras and Bandhas
http://www.aypsite.org/forum/topic.asp?TOPIC_ID=7155&REPLY_ID=63933&whichpage=-1
kechari stage 4

Hi Victor:

Stage 4 kechari is not critical for effective long term yoga practice. Neither is stage 3. Stage 2, balanced with the rest of our routine will be more than enough, as is stage 1 for those who are drawn to it, and no further.

Ultimately it is our bhakti that determines how far we will go with kechari, and how little of it we may be using in the long run. In the long run, less is more, which doesn't mean we will not be driven to do more in the short run. :-)

The guru is in you.

2010/02/09 14:52:12
Support for AYP Pranayama, Mudras and Bandhas
http://www.aypsite.org/forum/topic.asp?TOPIC_ID=7155&REPLY_ID=64649&whichpage=-1
kechari stage 4

Hi All:

Please, no extreme measures like in the link.

The rolling of the tongue on it's side as discussed in Lesson 108 is the only means recommended for going to Kechari stage 4. As mentioned earlier, stage 4 is not essential. The only time I would suggest doing it, if at all, is during pranayama, not during deep meditation, unless it is happening automatically then.

The guru is in you.

2010/01/27 18:02:03
Support for AYP Pranayama, Mudras and Bandhas
http://www.aypsite.org/forum/topic.asp?TOPIC_ID=7161&REPLY_ID=63958&whichpage=-1
what is Trivangamurari?

Hi Garlic:

It is a term used in Kriya Yoga that refers to "micro movement" beyond physical, ultimately beyond the manifest.

In AYP, the equivalent might be "whole body mudra," which is mudras and bandhas and other aspects of practice integrating (connecting) together naturally and gradually evolving beyond physical. See here: http://www.aypsite.org/212.html

When it has gone all the way, it is existence known as "stillness in action," which is non-duality/unity.

This is a bit advanced. Have you got a daily deep meditation practice started yet? That is the way you will come to to know these things first hand. :-)

The guru is in you.

2010/03/03 12:17:03
Support for AYP Pranayama, Mudras and Bandhas
http://www.aypsite.org/forum/topic.asp?TOPIC_ID=7349&REPLY_ID=65585&whichpage=-1
mulabandha question

Hi All:

The Spinal Breathing Pranayama book has instructions in it on full yogic breathing (belly breathing+), offered as an enhancement for spinal breathing.

It is true that mulabandha involves a slight lift that can bring some compression in the lower abdomen, which can be done near the end of inhalation in a normal full yogic breathing cycle.

As mudras and bandhas refine internally, this compression will be barely noticeable and can be present continuously according to its own need, a mere feeling with little physical manifestation. This is the beginning stage of whole body mudra.

Natural (not exaggerated) full yogic breathing remains primary in spinal breathing and does not conflict with the subtle effects of mulabandha in the pelvic region, or any other subtle mudras and bandhas. In time, all of these elements become quite natural and complementary. It is the inner connectedness of yoga occurring.

The guru is in you.

2010/03/09 10:08:58
Support for AYP Pranayama, Mudras and Bandhas
http://www.aypsite.org/forum/topic.asp?TOPIC_ID=7398&REPLY_ID=65867&whichpage=-1
Taming a wild Horse

Hi SeySorciere:

Ah, the interconnectedness of yoga within us. Can there be any doubt about it?

It is also the beginning (clunky stage) of what we call "whole body mudra" (AYP term):
http://www.aypsite.org/212.html

The good news is that all of this will refine gradually over time and become quite subtle, joyful and natural. It is the evolution of ecstatic radiance and outpouring divine love. In the meantime, self-pace, ground, and know that all is happening for good reason.

Here is a lesson on automatic yogic movements, which may be helpful:
http://www.aypsite.org/183.html
There are more lessons on this under "Automatic Yoga" in the website topic index.

And keep in mind that self-pacing covers bhakti too. :-)

The guru is in you.

2010/03/10 13:32:02
Support for AYP Pranayama, Mudras and Bandhas
http://www.aypsite.org/forum/topic.asp?TOPIC_ID=7398&REPLY_ID=65929&whichpage=-1
Taming a wild Horse

Hi All:

In yoga, mahamudra is an advanced traditional posture (asana), popular in kriya yoga, tantric yoga, and elsewhere. It is discussed in the AYP Easy Lessons book, and in more detail in the Asanas, Mudras and Bandhas book, beginning in the "sitting head to knee" posture description.

In Buddhism, mahamudra is an entire system of practices, not related to yoga mahamudra. Same word -- different meanings.

The guru is in you.

2010/04/20 16:37:43
Support for AYP Pranayama, Mudras and Bandhas
http://www.aypsite.org/forum/topic.asp?TOPIC_ID=7636&REPLY_ID=67506&whichpage=-1
lighter chin pump

Hi kaserdar:

It should also be mentioned that "chin pump lite" does not include breath retention (kumbhaka). This is the primary distinction between regular chin pump and chin pump lite, with the first being more powerful than the second.

All the best!

The guru is in you.

2010/05/04 12:55:33
Support for AYP Pranayama, Mudras and Bandhas
http://www.aypsite.org/forum/topic.asp?TOPIC_ID=7701&REPLY_ID=68189&whichpage=-1
Question about Chin Pumping

quote:
_____
Originally posted by tonightsthenight

One more time, I'm just hoping that somebody has an idea of what the neck crunching is.

Its kept me curious for a long time! Please, anyone, if you know what it might be, or would like to speculate, i would appreciate your input!
_____

Hi tonightsthenight:

Why do bones crunch when we do anything? Probably best to consult a medical source on that. It is not something esoteric. The main thing is not to overdo it with chin pump, or any practice -- self-pace both physically and energetically.

There is also a physical "thump" that may occur in the chest during the downward sweep of chin pump, particularly if kumbhaka is in use. Can't tell you exactly what that is either, but there surely must be an anatomical reason.

It is about cultivating purification and opening in the subtle neurobiology, which is why we use these techniques. In time, with a balanced routine of practices, less movement produces more results, and macro-movements evolve to become micro-movements. More stillness and more flowing ecstatic bliss.

Sorry, not very focused on the bony part of it here.

All the best!

The guru is in you.

2010/05/12 18:17:14
Support for AYP Pranayama, Mudras and Bandhas
http://www.aypsite.org/forum/topic.asp?TOPIC_ID=7756&REPLY_ID=68658&whichpage=-1
kechari mudra stage 4

Hi Alwayson:

Here is a sketch from the Asanas, Mudras and Bandhas book of the nasal pharynx, looking forward:

http://www.aypsite.org/images/kechari-pharynx.jpg

The eustachian tubes are the "trumpets" shown on the outer sides of the nasal passage openings.

I have nothing to add to the instructions on kechari stage 4 in Lesson 108, on rolling the tongue on its side toward the center, except to say it will only make sense once you have identified all the components with your tongue, which is a function of experience in stages 2 and 3.

quote:
_____
...Everyone will be different in approaching it (stage 4). There is a trick to it. The nasal passages are tall and narrow and the tongue is narrow and wide, so the tongue can only go into the nasal passages by turning on its side. But which side? One way works better than the other. The tongue can naturally be turned with the top to the center by following the channel on top of the trumpet of each eustachian tube into its adjacent nasal passage. This naturally turns the top of the tongue to the center and allows it to slide up the side of the septum into the nasal passage. Turning the tongue inward to the center is the way up into the passages...
_____

See the lesson for more details.

You are making a big deal out of kechari, trying to do in a few months what may take a yogi or yogini decades to do as a part of a comprehensive approach to yoga. If you make in into kechari stage 4 soon, you will find it to be only as useful as the rest of your daily practices have facilitated, especially deep meditation and spinal breathing pranayama. The same goes for kechari stages 3, 2 and 1. It is not about what stage of kechari we can reach. It is about how well integrated and effective our overall practice routine is. There are many who can make the entire journey with kechari stage 1, or even no systematic practice of kechari at all, other than the tongue going back from time to time automatically.

Deep meditation and spinal breathing pranayama are essential prerequisites for the systematic practice of kechari stage 4, as is a suitable background in previous stages of kechari.

All the best!

The guru is in you.

2010/05/12 19:24:00
Support for AYP Pranayama, Mudras and Bandhas
http://www.aypsite.org/forum/topic.asp?TOPIC_ID=7756&REPLY_ID=68664&whichpage=-1
kechari mudra stage 4

Hi Alwayson:

It should be added that entering kechari stage 4 is going to be premature if "secret spot" sensitivity (on the back edge of the septum) is not being experienced in stages 2 and 3. This is a function of the rise of ecstatic conductivity, which, again, is a function of our overall routine of practices. It all fits together that way. Honestly, the secret spot is a far easier, more satisfying, and stable place to be for ongoing cultivation of ecstatic conductivity. It is done in kechari stage 2 or 3. The secret spot can also be accessed indirectly in stage 1, through the roof of the mouth.

Jumping to stage 4 before secret spot sensitivity occurs won't harm anything, but it will not be very useful either, until these previous steps of purification and opening have occurred.

The guru is in you.

2010/05/30 10:44:23
Support for AYP Pranayama, Mudras and Bandhas
http://www.aypsite.org/forum/topic.asp?TOPIC_ID=7879&REPLY_ID=69369&whichpage=-1
soft palate was tight. nw it isn't. khechari :(

quote:
_____
Originally posted by fcry64

due to the in n out of teh tonguue into teh nasopharyngx, teh soft palate taht holds teh tongue in place isn't tight anymore. teh tendon lining near teh uvula has lost its tighteness n has elongated.

shouldn't i be bothered about the soft palate this way? wat should i do? should i be lessening khechari practise? should i keep teh tongue stuck to teh uvula for a change? this is happened cause i pushed teh tongue hard up into the sapetum and maybe teh poor palate couldn't take it :(
_____

Hi fcry64:

If you back off kechari mudra for a while, perhaps using only stage 1, you will find the soft palate returning close to its original elasticity. Likewise if you take it easy and enjoy being in stage 2-3, a balance will be found. In any case, whatever we do will not permanently deform the soft palate. At least that has been the experience here over 25 years of kechari practice.

All things in moderation ... and all the best on your path!

The guru is in you.

2010/06/01 10:36:56
Support for AYP Pranayama, Mudras and Bandhas
http://www.aypsite.org/forum/topic.asp?TOPIC_ID=7879&REPLY_ID=69427&whichpage=-1
soft palate was tight. nw it isn't. khechari :(

quote:

_____
Originally posted by fcry64

for stage 4, teh tongue must turn b4 entering the nostril or after entering teh nostril?
_____

During ...

See Lesson 108 on that: http://www.aypsite.org/108.html

The guru is in you.

2010/06/01 12:34:30
Support for AYP Pranayama, Mudras and Bandhas
http://www.aypsite.org/forum/topic.asp?TOPIC_ID=7879&REPLY_ID=69438&whichpage=-1
soft palate was tight. nw it isn't. khechari :(

quote:

_____
Originally posted by fcry64

thank u yoganiji but is there a dead end in stage 4? or the tongue jus keeps going further ?
_____

Hi fcry64:

There are limits to all things in the outer world, but no limit to what we can realize in the inner world. It is suggested to use the tools in whatever way works best to assist your inner awakening, knowing that particular physical attainments are not fixed prerequisites for spiritual progress.

The guru is in you.

2010/07/04 10:33:00
Support for AYP Pranayama, Mudras and Bandhas
http://www.aypsite.org/forum/topic.asp?TOPIC_ID=8069&REPLY_ID=70703&whichpage=-1
Maha Mudra and Maha Bheda Mudra and Om

Hi Chela7, and welcome!

Advanced hatha methods like maha mudra and maha bheda mudra can be incorporated in our asana routine before spinal breathing pranayama and deep meditation. However, keep in in mind that asanas in general become much more powerful when integrated into a full routine with pranayama and meditation, so you may find that "less is more" for the hatha methods in this mode. Not taking this into account could lead to energy excesses. So the advice is to start slow and self-pace as necessary, keeping in mind that excesses often come as delayed reactions to overdoing in practices.

For a strategy on shifting an asana/hatha-based practice to a well-rounded approach to all eight limbs of yoga, see the Asanas, Mudras and Bandhas book. Also see this lesson from not long ago: http://www.aypsite.org/409.html

Regarding using OM versus I AM as mantra in deep meditation, these are not the same, and in undertaking AYP deep meditation it is not recommended beginning with OM. It is incorporated later in a mantra enhancement. For particulars, see this lesson: http://www.aypsite.org/59.html

Of course, it is always your call. Wishing you all the best on your path. Practice wisely, and enjoy!

The guru is in you.

PS: Maha mudra is included as an enhancement in the AYP asana routine in the above mentioned book.

2010/07/04 20:08:26
Support for AYP Pranayama, Mudras and Bandhas

Hi Chela7:

Sorry, I can't offer much more on combining practices from other systems with AYP. The combinations are endless, and it is really up to the interested practitioner to do their own research.

When considering combining practices from two or more systems, I do offer the general caution to be careful about doing two similar practices in the same session or day, as this can lead to overloads due to a "doubling up" effect.

Reporting back in the forums on such research can be helpful to others considering similar combinations. This is best done in the "Other Systems and Alternate Approaches" forum category. The Deep Meditation/Samyama and Pranayama/Mudras/Bandhas forum categories are for support on the AYP system, not combining with other systems. Things can get muddy in a hurry when trying to mix everything together in one forum category. That may go for the practice routine also. :-)

Btw, there have been discussions in the forums in the past on combining Kriya Yoga with AYP. Try a few searches and you can see what has been said about this before. Or maybe a Kriyban or two will chime in. If so, we prefer that discussion take place in the Other Systems forum category.

All the best!

The guru is in you.

2010/07/30 12:31:03
Support for AYP Pranayama, Mudras and Bandhas
http://www.aypsite.org/forum/topic.asp?TOPIC_ID=8069&REPLY_ID=71455&whichpage=-1
Maha Mudra and Maha Bheda Mudra and Om

Hi Chela7:

It looks very good. I see you are making good use of the AYP writings. :-)

Let your experience be your guide for self-pacing and sculpting your daily practice routine for ongoing good progress with comfort.

All the best!

The guru is in you.

2010/07/31 17:35:21
Support for AYP Pranayama, Mudras and Bandhas
http://www.aypsite.org/forum/topic.asp?TOPIC_ID=8069&REPLY_ID=71477&whichpage=-1
Maha Mudra and Maha Bheda Mudra and Om

quote:
_____
Originally posted by Chela7

1.)When doing janusirshasana on each side and then paschimotan asana,as in Maha mudra, should I do it three positions once or three times as in traditional maha mudra?

2.)When doing shambhavi mudra in spinal breathing, I don't knit the brow and my eyes are upturned and half closed, is this practice ok?

3.)When doing deep meditation and the mantra, do I close my eyes and just stare at the darkness in front of me or do I gently lift my half closed eyes as in shambhavi mudra?
_____

Hi Chela7:

1. The baseline instruction in AYP is once for each posture, with a hold of about 10 seconds. If you are expanding into mahamudra with breath suspension (not recommended for beginners), or other expansions of asana practice, self-pace as necessary, keeping in mind the possibility for delayed effects.

2. The knit brow in sambhavi is instructed in AYP to be so slight as to be invisible. However you approach sambhavi in spinal breathing is fine.

3. Eyes closed in AYP deep meditation. Easily favor the mantra over anything visual, or lack of anything visual. :-) If sambhavi or other mudras naturally creep into deep meditation without any intention, that is fine, but we do not intend to do anything in deep meditation except the procedure of deep meditation. Very important.

All the best!

The guru is in you.

Forum 5 – Asanas – Postures and Physical Culture

Many think this is "Yoga." It is, at least in part.
http://www.aypsite.org/forum/forum.asp?FORUM_ID=20

2005/07/11 13:02:41
Asanas - Postures and Physical Culture
http://www.aypsite.org/forum/topic.asp?TOPIC_ID=277
Asanas - Postures and Physical Culture

There is something of a paradox here.

The teaching and practice of yoga postures is a huge worldwide phenomenon. It has even moved over into the mainstream of the physical fitness arena, with numerous kinds of aerobic and extreme yoga regimens now available. This is big business!

Yet, in Patanjali's Yoga Sutras, asanas are one limb out of eight, with meditation, pranayama and the other limbs having equal or greater weight, not to mention samyama. Why the difference between the basic truths of yoga practice and what we see in the world? Some say it is "market driven." We are a culture that craves physical health above all things. It is understandable. We all want our health and well-being, the more the better.

But learning to systematically do less can be much more, you know. That is the secret of yoga. In AYP we use asanas as a limbering, a stretching of the nervous system to warm up for pranayama and deep meditation. Because there is so much about postures on the Internet, asanas are given fairly light coverage in the online AYP lessons. See Lesson #71 for a discussion on asanas at http://www.aypsite.org/71.html

An illustrated "Asana Starter Kit" with fourteen postures is included in the AYP book. And a much abbreviated version is also provided there for those "on the go." Asanas are important in AYP. If possible, we should do a set of asanas before our twice daily meditation sittings. But, when time is short, we do not do asanas instead of meditation. Or instead of pranayama. That is the difference in AYP. For more on fitting practices into a busy schedule, see Lesson #209 at http://www.aypsite.org/209.html

The physical conditioning aspect of life is not ignored in AYP. In the AYP book, a yoga-friendly routine of muscle toning calisthenics and aerobic (cardiovascular) development is included.

In this forum, the doors are flung wide open to discuss asanas and physical culture from every angle. Let off some steam if you like. Build up a sweat, if need be. Then, after you cool down, make sure to check out the Yoga Sutras. See Lesson #149 at http://www.aypsite.org/149.html

May we all find balance in our practices and thereby enter the infinite inner realms of divine joy, and bring that out into our daily living!

The guru is in you.

2005/07/20 12:58:19
Asanas - Postures and Physical Culture
http://www.aypsite.org/forum/topic.asp?TOPIC_ID=336&REPLY_ID=100&whichpage=-1
Please recommend some asanas
I agree with Jim about taking a class on asanas (postures). This is also recommended in the AYP lessons at http://www.aypsite.org/71.html

For those who are chaffing at the bit to get started, an "Asana Starter Kit" is included in the AYP book -- written instructions and illustrations for 14 basic postures that can be done in a short routine before spinal breathing and deep meditation. An "abbreviated" (very short) version is also included for people on the go. The AYP book can be downloaded anywhere in ebook format. See http://www.aypsite.org/books.html

The guru is in you.

2005/08/05 23:21:49
Asanas - Postures and Physical Culture
http://www.aypsite.org/forum/topic.asp?TOPIC_ID=387&REPLY_ID=302&whichpage=-1
Kechari in asana

Hi Victor:

Since I first got into kechari stage 2 some 20 years ago, I have usually let it call me rather than the other way around. The result has been that it is pretty much there throughout sitting practices. Occasionally not. Sometimes it is in part or all of asanas, but usually not. Kechari is a natural for asanas that stretch the sushumna along with kumbhaka and a full array of mudras and bandhas (sambhavi, mulabandha, siddhasana/heel on perineum, uddiyana and jalandhara). Maha mudra is the primary candidate for this. Don't overdo that one...

And who is to say kechari is not okay to do in a shoulder stand, or any other posture? Or, for that matter, while you are driving to work? I'd say it is between your bhakti and your common sense. In other words, self-pacing rules this just like it does everything else we do in yoga, especially when we have such a full tool kit available.

The guru is in you.

2005/10/12 09:48:38
Asanas - Postures and Physical Culture
http://www.aypsite.org/forum/topic.asp?TOPIC_ID=387&REPLY_ID=949&whichpage=-1
Kechari in asana

Hi All:

That's right. We do not want to divide our attention from the simple procedure of meditation by "working" on other practices during meditation. We develop the "habits" of mudras, bandhas, siddhasana, etc. during spinal breathing and at other times, and then they will eventually be

262 – Advanced Yoga Practices

occurring naturally during meditation without any attenion being necessary for them to be there.

So there is no instruction for kechari in meditation. We let it come in naturally as a habit that has been formed elsewhere in our routine. Then it will be easy and not be an attention divider. Recall that anything our attention wanders to in meditation is a cue to easily pick the mantra up again. That goes for wandering off into working on this or that mudra too. So from that you can conclude that I did not recommend holding the tongue anywhere in particular during meditation, except as naturally occurring.

The guru is in you.

2005/10/12 11:48:47
Asanas - Postures and Physical Culture
http://www.aypsite.org/forum/topic.asp?TOPIC_ID=387&REPLY_ID=951&whichpage=-1
Kechari in asana

quote:
_____
I know with breath suspensions that I hardly notice when they occur these days, should it be like that with kechari, because I find this one hard not to notice?
_____

Yes, it will be like that. And we can notice, like anything else that comes up in meditation. Then we ease back to the mantra when we realize it.

We can leave kechari there, or let it subside if need be, like shifting our legs in meditation for comfort. Whatever gives us the clearest attention for the simple process of meditation. Eventually kechari, siddhasana, sambhavi, even mulabandha/asvini will be sneaking into our meditation if we have been developing them elsewhere. We don't let them take over our meditation, any more than we would deliberately sit in an uncomfortable or distracting environment that does not favor easy meditation, though the process of meditation can deal with that, if necessary.

In time, all those yogic elements will naturally be in our meditation to some degree with no effort or distraction. The upshot is that ecstasy via these other methods becomes a regular part of our experience of inner silence in meditation. It is the marriage of shiva (silence) and shakti (ecstasy). It is a fine line getting from here to there.

Btw, sorry to be off topic here, Victor. Your sharing on kechari in asana is both illuminating and appreciated. That is yet another example of practices migrating naturally through the limbs of yoga, demonstrating again the interconnectedness of yoga. It is one tree (one nervous system), after all... :-)

The guru is in you.

2005/10/14 00:08:07
Asanas - Postures and Physical Culture
http://www.aypsite.org/forum/topic.asp?TOPIC_ID=387&REPLY_ID=976&whichpage=-1
Kechari in asana

Hi Andrew:

Kechari in asana. Kechari in meditation. Not such different things. Same tendency -- different practice.

Glad it got around to the clarification you were seeking.

As Victor pointed out, the main obstruction can be our reluctance to do what we are being called to from within due to something someone said, our tradition, or whatever. Clearly our nervous system under the stimulation of yoga has its own evolutionary dynamic -- human spiritual transformation -- and we can seldom go wrong following that, as long as we heed the principles of self-pacing. That is the key, isn't it?

The guru is in you.

2005/08/14 17:52:52
Asanas - Postures and Physical Culture
http://www.aypsite.org/forum/topic.asp?TOPIC_ID=407&REPLY_ID=368&whichpage=-1
painful knees ?

Hello Pala:

See this recent Q&A from my email:

Q: I read your article on siddhasana: http://www.aypsite.org/75.html

I have knee problem due to torn ligament in my right. I cannot bring this leg under. So can I tuck in my left leg instead of my right? Will it effect the efficiency of this posture?

A: Either heel at the perineum will do. If the injured leg won't bend comfortably, it is okay to leave it out straight. With back support it is easy to do this -- one leg under and the other leg straight out. If neither leg will go under, then it is okay to use an object like a rolled up sock at the perineum. In this case you may have both legs out straight. It can be done either on the bed or in a comfortable chair. The key in siddhasana is stimulation at the perineum. The rest can vary according to need.

****

I would add to this a reminder on the basic maxim in all yoga -- Never force beyond your comfortable limit. This applies to postures, and to all other practices as well. This is the essence of self-pacing.

All the best!

The guru is in you.

2005/10/24 12:55:45
Asanas - Postures and Physical Culture
http://www.aypsite.org/forum/topic.asp?TOPIC_ID=543&REPLY_ID=1134&whichpage=-1
kandasana

Hi All:

I can see the picture fine when signed in at the Yahoo AYP forum. Are you sure you are a group member there, Melissa?

I tried to open the photo and files sections for non-member viewing, but Yahoo does not allow it. Sorry for the inconvenience there.

Snitz (this forum's software) does have the ability to include images in posts, but it is turned off because I was warned it could hamper performance and eat up storage capacity and bandwidth. There are potential copyright issues too.

If you all think it is important to have images in here, let me know and I will look into it.

The guru is in you.

2006/01/31 09:27:29
Asanas - Postures and Physical Culture
http://www.aypsite.org/forum/topic.asp?TOPIC_ID=716&REPLY_ID=2914&whichpage=-1
Free cool asana video

Hi Guy:

There is an "asana starter kit" in the AYP Easy Lessons book. There is also quite a lot of other additional material in there beyond the online lessons. Few seem to realize this, as few have been ordering the book. See list of additions here: http://www.aypsite.org/book-additions.html

Later this year a small, low cost AYP Enlightenment Series book on "Asanas, Mudras and Bandhas" will be coming out. Until then, the AYP Easy Lessons book is the only source for AYP instructions on asanas.

The philosophy on asanas from the AYP point of view (putting them in perspective in relation to the rest of yoga) can be found here: http://www.aypsite.org/71.html and http://www.aypsite.org/149.html

The guru is in you.

2006/02/01 10:19:14
Asanas - Postures and Physical Culture
http://www.aypsite.org/forum/topic.asp?TOPIC_ID=716&REPLY_ID=2943&whichpage=-1
Free cool asana video

Hi Kdhanraj:

All of the AYP books are available worldwide in ebook format. That does not seem to stop people from constantly asking me for information that is already in the books.

Since all is done in good faith here, I have stopped everything and assembled the list for the "asana starter kit" from the AYP Easy Lessons book for you:

(about a 10 minute routine)

1. Heart centering warm-up
2. Knees to chest roll
3. Kneeling seat (vajrasana)
4. Sitting head to knee (janushirshasana, paschimottanasana and/or maha mudra)
5. Shoulder stand (viparitakarani or savangasana)
6. Plow (halasana)
7. Seal of yoga (yoga mudra)
8. Cobra (bhujangasana)
9. Locust (shalabhasana)
10. Spinal twist (ardha matsyendrasana)
11. Abdominal lift (uddiyana and nauli)
12. Standing back stretch (urdhvasana)
13. Standing toe touch (padahastasana)
14. Corpse pose (shavasana)

Abbreviated "standing" routine (a couple of minutes for when on-the-go)

1. Standing spinal twist
2. Abdominal lift
3. Standing back stretch
4. Standing toe touch
5. Corpse pose (if a place to lie down is available)

Either of these routines is done before sitting practices. If you would like more details, kindly purchase the ebook, for your own sake and for the sake of others (furthering the AYP work).

264 – Advanced Yoga Practices

All the best!

The guru is in you.

2006/02/02 10:24:17
Asanas - Postures and Physical Culture
http://www.aypsite.org/forum/topic.asp?TOPIC_ID=716&REPLY_ID=2980&whichpage=-1
Free cool asana video

Hi Kdhanraj:

In time, we will succeed in having the AYP books published in India, reflecting local costs, which will solve this. In the meantime, I am looking to see if there is a way to make the ebooks more affordable there.

There is obviously a lot to work with here online at no cost, so please do continue to partake. Your participation in the discussion is much appreciated.

Wishing you the best on your path. Enjoy!

The guru is in you.

2006/02/17 10:25:07
Asanas - Postures and Physical Culture
http://www.aypsite.org/forum/topic.asp?TOPIC_ID=833&REPLY_ID=3459&whichpage=-1
Headstand

Hi Guy:

"Inversion" is one of the basic principles in asanas, and is found in many postures, including the lowly toe-touch (or whatever we can do in that direction).

The headstand is king of the inversion postures, though some would argue that gravity boots (hanging upside down by the boots) is superior. Well, anything can be taken to extremes, and that is what needs to be cautioned here. Seeking a good balance with self-pacing in our routine of practices is the key.

Also, with the headstand in particular, care must be exercised not to place the full weight of the body on the neck. This can lead to a permanent neck injury. So if you are learning headstand, make sure to learn the proper means of supporting your weight with the triangular placement of the arms. This enables the practitioner to regulate the weight placed on the neck. Very important.

As you may know, in the AYP Easy Lessons book, there are some 14 postures which are recommended as an "asana starter kit" -- a well-rounded series that can be done in about 10 minutes before sitting practices. In there is the shoulder stand and several other postures involving inversion. Consider getting comfortable and stable in a routine like that before moving on to more advanced postures like headstand. Just a suggestion.

Do take your time and never force anything in asanas.

I am moving this topic to the asanas forum for better placement.

The guru is in you.

2006/02/17 12:13:23
Asanas - Postures and Physical Culture
http://www.aypsite.org/forum/topic.asp?TOPIC_ID=833&REPLY_ID=3470&whichpage=-1
Headstand

Hi Jim:

If complete weight on the neck can be done safely, I am certainly not opposed. Proper instruction is the key in this, and I bow to Iyengar in all things "asana."

However, do-it-yourselfers beware in taking on the neck-only supported headstand without professional instruction. If training is not available and you must do it, then I still suggest the arm tripod method rather than the neck. It may not be ideal (as per Jim/Iyengar) but much safer for amateurs.

The guru is in you.

2009/07/13 16:04:50
Asanas - Postures and Physical Culture
http://www.aypsite.org/forum/topic.asp?TOPIC_ID=833&REPLY_ID=53507&whichpage=-1
Headstand

Hi All:

What is being suggested recently here is not a recommended AYP practice. Many of the practices offered in the forums are not recommended AYP, and I generally do not comment much one way or the other. It would be a full time job. :-)

But in this case, it is important to mention that permanent neck damage can occur if correct procedure is not followed with headstand, and this should be gotten from a professional yoga teacher who is skilled in this posture. Even a small misalignment in practice without apparent discomfort (especially for long durations) can lead to serious neck problems later on.

For such long durations of practice, an inversion device avoiding neck compression would be a safer approach. Not that this is recommended in AYP either. Three hours per day is enough time to put together a really terrific twice-daily integrated practice routine covering all aspects of yoga, and leading to far greater results than doing any one practice for that duration.

Excess in any individual practice is not the way in yoga. More times than not, it will lead to problems. There are no magic bullets. Only balanced and prudent self-paced practice, integrated with an active life in the world.

Sorry to butt in here, but we don't want anyone going off and hurting themselves unnecessarily.

It should also be mentioned that there are many ways to achieve the beneficial effects of inversion without resorting to extreme measures. Shoulder stand and plow are effective postures for this, as is simply bending over and touching the ankles, toes or floor. These are the kinds of postures that are woven into the AYP approach as part of the broad range of practices designed for good overall results in cultivating abiding inner silence, ecstatic bliss and outpouring divine love. For more on the AYP approach to postures, see the Asanas, Mudras and Bandhas book.

Practice wisely, and enjoy!

The guru is in you.

PS: I also put in my two cents earlier in this topic, back in 2006, here:
http://www.aypsite.org/forum/topic.asp?TOPIC_ID=833#3459

2009/07/13 17:25:09
Asanas - Postures and Physical Culture
http://www.aypsite.org/forum/topic.asp?TOPIC_ID=833&REPLY_ID=53518&whichpage=-1
Headstand

Hi Kadak and ZionMe:

My intention is not to limit personal preferences for practice or discussion here in any way.

However, there will be hundreds of people reading this, and my concern is for beginners jumping into something unaware that they could injure themselves without proper instruction.

So, with that now covered, do carry on.

All inputs are welcome. Many thanks! :-)

The guru is in you.

2009/07/14 11:43:53
Asanas - Postures and Physical Culture
http://www.aypsite.org/forum/topic.asp?TOPIC_ID=833&REPLY_ID=53539&whichpage=-1
Headstand

quote:
_____
Originally posted by kadak

Just to say that my teachers never spoke of overload, they only spoke of practicing more and better.
Maybe western and eastern physiology are very different.
_____

Hi Kadak:

There is no evidence to indicate that geography or ethnicity have anything to do with how aspirants respond to practices -- at least not in the case of the AYP practices, which are being utilized everywhere around the world with the same profile of results. There are differences in response (karmic) in individuals (an area of ongoing research here), but that does not explain why one group will be doing 6 hours of practice, and be needing more, while another group will overload on one hour's worth of practice.

With such a wide variation in duration of sadhana and results between these two classes of practitioners, the arrows point to the practices themselves.

It is already well-known here that kriya yoga style sadhana involving mainly spinal breathing can be practiced for long periods with relatively little impact (no overload), as compared to AYP spinal breathing followed by deep meditation, where much greater results occur with short twice-daily sessions, to the point where prudent self-pacing of practices becomes essential.

Likewise, it is pretty well recognized here that some of the Buddhist styles of meditation can be engaged in for much longer periods without much risk of overload, whereas AYP deep meditation cannot. Again, the implication is that AYP-style deep meditation is more powerful in it's effects.

So, perhaps the difference between your 6 hours and AYP's 1-2 hours is the style of meditation in use. One way to find out is to try AYP deep meditation, as per the lessons, for a few weeks or months and see what happens. You might be surprised. Wouldn't it be nice to be able to go out and live a normal life while having the benefits of powerful sadhana involving much less time? This is a path that fully integrates the fruit of yoga with everyday living. We call it "*stillness in action.*"

Your choice, of course. Just throwing out a few thoughts for consideration.

All the best!

The guru is in you.

Caution: AYP deep meditation will make all other practices we are doing much more powerful. So, if we have been doing long sessions of pranayama, and then add deep meditation to the routine, much less pranayama will be necessary to achieve the same results. The same goes for asanas, and any other practice we have been doing. The efficient cultivation of abiding inner silence changes everything.

2009/07/15 10:32:22
Asanas - Postures and Physical Culture
http://www.aypsite.org/forum/topic.asp?TOPIC_ID=833&REPLY_ID=53555&whichpage=-1
Headstand

Hi Christiane:

I believe the power of the AYP core combination is that it addresses the three key elements of spiritual progress with effective practices in an integrated way, where each element is reinforced by the others. That is the cultivation of inner silence in deep meditation, ecstatic conductivity in spinal breathing, and the permanent stabilization of these qualities in daily activity.

If we focus on one to the exclusion of the others, or water down our routine with less effective elements of practice, something crucial is lost. Evidence of this can be found in other approaches that are skewed in one direction or the other. Keeping a balance in cultivation and stabilization between inner silence, ecstatic conductivity and daily activity is vitally important.

It is also important to maintain that balance when adding enhancements, as with mantra, and additional practices, such as asana, mudra, bandha, tantra, samyama, self-inquiry, service, etc. If we take care of the basics, the additions will take care of themselves according to our particular need and process of unfoldment.

Of course, what I believe is happening is not important. What is important is results, and this is much more in your hands than in mine. :-)

The guru is in you.

2009/07/15 10:48:19
Asanas - Postures and Physical Culture
http://www.aypsite.org/forum/topic.asp?TOPIC_ID=833&REPLY_ID=53556&whichpage=-1
Headstand
Note: The advaita spin-off discussion has been split and moved here: http://www.aypsite.org/forum/topic.asp?TOPIC_ID=5945

2007/04/01 11:52:36
Asanas - Postures and Physical Culture
http://www.aypsite.org/forum/topic.asp?TOPIC_ID=1261&REPLY_ID=19744&whichpage=-1
Longivity?

quote:
_____
Originally posted by Anthem11

Yogani reply from Maximus

quote:
_____
He replied :
The short answer is that there are an unlimited number of forming souls coming up through matter, all which have to go through the same process we are. It is a continuum of pure bliss consciousness evolving toward diverse individuation and then back to unity in self realization.

If the earth blows up, it will continue in the innumerable other places where it is happening. The earth is a special place, but not unique. Evolution proceeds everywhere in the universe. It is inherent in all of creation, not only in the earth. So there is plenty to do for an eternity, and the work of helping each other will not come to an end.

Glad to hear you are thinking ahead. Remember, it all boils down to the practices we are doing today. That is when evolution is at its best -- when we are unfolding pure bliss consciousness and ecstatic conductivity within ourselves today, tomorrow, and every day we we find ourselves in this sacred temple, our nervous system. Let's not waste a minute...
_____

This is a fascinating answer to me and something that feels "right" though I have never read anything about this nor experienced this perception of our reality.

Yogani, are you aware of any books that discuss this perspective of our reality?
_____

Hi Andrew:

It is discussed in great detail in the writings of Theosophy, which also represent (to greater or lesser degree) the esoteric aspects of all eastern (and western?) teachings -- including the practical field of yoga, of course.

AE Powell's book, "The Solar System" is one of the best on this subject. The message is of Oneness continually expressing and evolving in all levels of creation. Stillness in action!

The "cause and effect" in this is that if we each keep moving forward with our evolution, so will everything else. The evolution of consciousness within all forms is connected. So move on! :-)

See Quest Books here: http://www.questbooks.net/title.cfm?bookid=1387

Amazon also has it: http://www.amazon.com/Solar-System-Arthur-E-Powell/dp/0766178633/ref=sr_1_1/002-5079307-9533614?ie=UTF8&s=books&qid=1175442067&sr=1-1

The guru is in you.

2006/07/30 10:22:24
Asanas - Postures and Physical Culture
http://www.aypsite.org/forum/topic.asp?TOPIC_ID=1369&REPLY_ID=10029&whichpage=-1
Mahamudra

Hi Billeejack:

Maha mudra is a great practice, and is included in the AYP Easy Lessons book in the asana instructions, along with other postures covering the same principles of practice in different ways. Also, mudras, bandhas and kumbhaka used in AYP sitting practices stimulate these same principles ... and not to forget siddhasana.

In the beginning, it was decided not to focus the AYP lessons on asanas very much, because it has been done so many times before by others. Instead, the focus in the lessons has been on building an effective integration of powerful sitting practices, which has not been done much before. But none of this is to reduce the importance of asanas in the over all mix -- only to promote a balance.

The Asanas, Mudras and Bandhas book coming out in September will continue with this theme -- balancing a full range of practices for best results.

In AYP we do not think in terms of a "magic bullet." We think in terms of a barrage. :-)

The guru is in you.

2006/09/30 18:36:30
Asanas - Postures and Physical Culture
http://www.aypsite.org/forum/topic.asp?TOPIC_ID=1545&REPLY_ID=11767&whichpage=-1
padmasana or siddhasana

quote:
———————
Originally posted by david_obsidian

Anyone know the sanskrit for sock?:-) Insert here: Padma socki asana is my favorite right now.
———————

Hi David:

How about "sockasana." :-)

Actually, it brings up an important principle that we have been capitalizing on in AYP. That is -- taking elements of traditional practices and applying them in more efficient ways. Padma-sockasana is a good example of dissecting an essential element from siddhasana and combining it with padmasana, or variations. A number of folks have been doing this intuitively. It is easy to do once we know what the elements of practice are actually doing in our nervous system, rather than doing them traditionally by rote.

AYP's deep meditation and spinal breathing pranayama are an example of this kind of application. Rather than combining the two, which some notable traditions do, we keep them separate, with much greater effect in cultivating both inner silence and ecstatic conductivity. Then we layer in the mudras and bandhas like building blocks, to even greater effect. Well, it is an incremental approach, isn't it? And who is to say we can't dissect and rearrange some of the elements for even better effect?

For example, we have begun dissecting yoni mudra by adding the nose-block portion of it to chin pump, yielding "yoni chin pump," a powerful hybrid of chin pump. It can also be done with other elements of traditional practices we have been using, yielding more efficient and effective practice in several areas -- meaning more results with the same (or less) time and effort expended.

There will be more on this in one or more AYP lessons in the months ahead. Some refinements are on the way. Just thought I'd drop a hint.

By the time we are done, anyone can just say "Boo!" and be enlightened. Only kidding. A good concept to aim for though -- more results from less effort, and, of course, easier. :-)

The guru is in you.

2006/12/22 15:47:31
Asanas - Postures and Physical Culture
http://www.aypsite.org/forum/topic.asp?TOPIC_ID=1842&REPLY_ID=14748&whichpage=-1
Numbness after Siddhasana

Hi John, and welcome!

It can happen from time to time, and it can be minimized. Some get pretty wound up over this one. But after 20-some years, I haven't noticed any deleterious effects from doing siddhasana. Just the opposite. It is a very effective tantra practice, and makes a huge contribution to the rise of ecstatic conductivity.

To avoid the genitals falling asleep, the trick is to move the heel back toward the anus a bit, off the back of the pubic bone, which is where the blood supply (and urethra) can be blocked. Also, if you sit on a soft surface, like a bed, with back support, the pressure can be regulated from heavy to almost nothing, depending on how you sit. You will get the hang of it in time.

Here is a lesson with more discussion on this: http://www.aypsite.org/T29.html
Check the website topic index for more lessons on siddhasana.

Btw, if you are doing siddhasana after only a couple months in practices, you are moving very fast. It takes a while to get settled in with each practice. Indeed, you are in the clunky stage of siddhasana now. Make sure your previous practices are stable (beyond clunky) before charging ahead. Otherwise, it could all come piling in on you when you least expect it. We have more than a few with first hand experience with that phenomenon around here. :-)

Carry on, and don't forget to self-pace. All the best!

The guru is in you.

2007/01/17 10:37:31
Asanas - Postures and Physical Culture
http://www.aypsite.org/forum/topic.asp?TOPIC_ID=1955&REPLY_ID=16226&whichpage=-1
Mula Bandha / SB in Vajrasana?

quote:
_____
Originally posted by shivakm

Shanthi,

Your post was very useful. My current pranayama is very helpful to me. I do not want to change it in any way. So, I guess I have to do the spinal breathing pranayama separately.

Thanks,
Shiva.
_____

Hi Shiva:

Of course, you are welcome to experiment with integrations of practice, especially if a time savings can be achieved without significant loss of results, or while improving results! That is one of the primary themes of "R&D" in AYP. However, as Shanti points out, the results of mixing practices from multiple systems can be unpredictable -- "doubling up" effect, especially with pranayama. So any such forays will be your own R&D, whether you are doing the practices in sequence, or combined. Nothing wrong with doing R&D if you have a good foundation in practices (especially deep meditation/inner silence), are motivated, and have a good knowledge of "self-pacing" in your back pocket. There also has to be a willingness to occasionally travel a bumpy road in the interest of science. :-)

Keep in mind that long term effects may not mirror short term effects, so the most meaningful experiments will be the ones that last many months. Please report back here with whatever you find.

All the best!

The guru is in you.

2007/05/04 09:58:13
Asanas - Postures and Physical Culture
http://www.aypsite.org/forum/topic.asp?TOPIC_ID=2520&REPLY_ID=21418&whichpage=-1
Fitness Yoga

quote:
_____
Originally posted by meenarashid

so here in michigan (i dont know if its like this everywhere) there is a large call for *fitness yoga =just the postures

this is not too easy to teach!
always felt and feel it even more now that if people really just wanted a nice tush they would be on a stair stepper reading the gossip column (or whatever) we come to yoga classes for various *reasons* but we all just really want freedom moksha liberation love to feel GOOD to feel aum a while back would not teach these types of classes actually quit at lifetime fitness due to the fact that they say no meditation try not to use sanskrit etc etc
now at a new place same deal going on.. but rather than run am wondering if its not a wonderful challenge to learn to adapt
but it is not easy! but i have to wondr if its not almost snobbishness for me to refuse to share yoga in settings that dont feel like *worship to me... one thing that did come out of lifetime fitness that makes me wonder if i should just go with the flow no matter what ... is that when i taught there i would still get into bandhas & stuff

well when i quit months later a teacher says.. arent you so and so from lifetime? im all yea... he says after you quit we were told to get more into the bandhas cuz everyone really appreciated it

any thoughts on this ?
aum
_____

Hi Meenarashid:

This is true everywhere, and we can be happy that so many are finding a doorway into yoga via the physical route. It is a matter of offering comfortable ways for folks to "spread out" in yoga from there, according to their own inclinations. It can happen quite naturally.

One of the AYP books directly addresses this issue:

Asanas, Mudras and Bandhas - Awakening Ecstatic Kundalini

The title is deliberately provocative, and the contents are fairly logical in terms of presenting the case for looking beyond the mat in yoga, which is looking within, of course.

Don't run. Gently offer integrations of the physical aspects of yoga with deep meditation and pranayama. Everyone has it in them, and it is happening everywhere, even in the most physical studios. People inherently want more. The studios will play to the market as the market evolves. And it is! I am convinced that the yoga studios have a key role to play everywhere, serving as launching platforms to much more. It will take some time. :-)

The guru is in you.

2007/06/29 16:47:04
Asanas - Postures and Physical Culture
http://www.aypsite.org/forum/topic.asp?TOPIC_ID=2714&REPLY_ID=23644&whichpage=-1
heart- warm up
Welcome Flixe!

A way to think of it is gently bringing the blood to the heart from head, arms, legs and lower torso, following the procedure in either the AYP Easy Lessons book or the Asanas/Mudras/Bandhas book. The heart centering warm-up only takes a minute or two, and then it is into the postures. Within 10 minutes, we will be on the way in, and ready for spinal breathing pranayama and deep meditation, which take us much further into inner silence. Then we can be acting from that immovable center of happiness within us in our daily life. Stillness in action! :-)

The guru is in you.

2007/12/30 11:38:51
Asanas - Postures and Physical Culture
http://www.aypsite.org/forum/topic.asp?TOPIC_ID=3311&REPLY_ID=28387&whichpage=-1
I've lost enthusiasm for my asana practice!

Hi All:

This is the kind of balancing and adjusting (self-pacing) that is necessary when spreading out through the limbs of yoga. It is the scenario discussed in the Asanas, Mudras and Bandhas book.

Great job of exploring it here everyone, and thanks much, Echo, for bringing it up.

It is inevitable that the vast asana (yoga posture) movement will gradually transition toward more integrated approaches to practice, as the truth continues to emerge from within us all. Many adjustments will be necessary along the way. It is a good thing.

Per your comments elsewhere, Jim, it is certainly true that Iyengar (and others) in the asana field have been laying the groundwork for much more integrated applications of yoga, and the acceleration of worldwide human spiritual transformation, even if they are not saying that! :-)

The same can be said of every teacher and tradition that has brought useful methods to the table. The unceasing forward march of *open* **Applied Spiritual Science** will continue to bring it all together, and the whole will be much greater than the sum of the parts. Bravo!

The guru is in you.

2008/08/17 10:56:53
Asanas - Postures and Physical Culture
http://www.aypsite.org/forum/topic.asp?TOPIC_ID=4305&REPLY_ID=36458&whichpage=-1
the beauty of asanas in daily practice

Hi Machart:

As with all things in yoga, working toward a balanced integration of practices is the key, no matter where in the eight limbs we have begun our journey. Asanas (postures) are definitely important at any stage along the path, comprising one of the eight limbs of yoga. They evolve as we do, becoming more subtle and refined over time, so there may be less physical emphasis and more refined cultivation of ecstatic conductivity. This is true of mudras and bandhas also.

We live in a culture where the word "yoga" has become synonymous with postures, which has been a limited view, of course. As time goes on there will be a broadening of that view to encompass the whole of yoga. Then when people go to yoga/postures class they will know it is about much more than the body and the mat. This has been happening automatically already as consciousness has been steadily rising around the world. Many are finding by direct experience that all the limbs of yoga are intimately connected within us. Those who begin with asanas are finding more interest in spiritual study, meditation and pranayama, just as those who who begin with meditation find more interest in spiritual study, asanas and pranayama. What goes around comes around. We are all wired for it.

As far as AYP is concerned, I do admit to pushing back a bit on the belief that "yoga is postures only." It has needed to be done. On the other hand, the AYP Easy Lessons textbook and the Enlightenment Series books both provide balanced coverage of asanas in relation to the rest of yoga, including instructions for a basic set of postures for inclusion in our twice-daily practice routine consisting of asanas, pranayama and meditation, in that order (with additional practices added when appropriate). These asana instructions have not been included in the online lessons, so far, which might lead some to believe that AYP does not include asanas. Of course, anyone who digs into AYP will find that this is not true. We love asanas as much as we love the rest of the limbs of yoga. How could we not? All the limbs of yoga are intimately connected within us. They are us. :-)

All the best!

The guru is in you.

PS: See this online lesson on yoga asanas: http://www.aypsite.org/71.html
... and this FAQ: http://www.aypsite.org/forum/topic.asp?TOPIC_ID=2115

2010/01/31 07:58:11
Asanas - Postures and Physical Culture
http://www.aypsite.org/forum/topic.asp?TOPIC_ID=7160&REPLY_ID=64248&whichpage=-1
Asana sequence with picture links

Hi All:

It is suggested to end any asana routine with several minutes of savasana (corpse pose), especially when immediately preceding sitting practices (pranayama, meditation, etc.). This is an important transition posture.

All the best!

The guru is in you.

2010/07/01 11:29:45
Asanas - Postures and Physical Culture
http://www.aypsite.org/forum/topic.asp?TOPIC_ID=7409&REPLY_ID=70618&whichpage=-1
Automatic Yoga / Asanas

Hi uranchan, and welcome!

For the AYP approach to handling instances of automatic yoga, see these lessons:

http://www.aypsite.org/104.html
http://www.aypsite.org/183.html
http://www.aypsite.org/210.html

For more lessons on automatic yoga, see "Automatic Yoga (and movements)" in the Topic Index.

Gently favoring our structured practice routine over automatic yoga, plus self-pacing of practices as needed, are the keys in the AYP approach, not giving over to unrestricted automatic yoga, which can lead to uncomfortable excesses.

The view we take in AYP is that automatic yoga is an effect of practices and/or kundalini awakening, not a primary cause of spiritual advancement. Such symptoms can be wide-ranging, or none at all. It depends on the inner process of purification and opening, which will vary from person to person (and at different times in the same person), according to the inner matrix of obstructions (karma) gradually being dissolved through practices.

Automatic yoga, and other "scenery" (visions, sensations, etc.) we may experience along the way are associated with the "friction" of energy passing through inner obstructions. As we continue with a self-paced, stable and comfortable practice routine over time, the friction/symptoms become less as the obstructions are gradually dissolved. Then our experiences become much more refined, blissful in stillness, and flowing as outpouring divine love. As this progresses we find an increasing sense of Oneness inside and outside. This is the rise of the unending experience of unity and non-duality, which is freedom, even as we remain fully engaged in ordinary daily living. In this situation, we find we have more to give to those around us, and far beyond.

All the best!

The guru is in you.

2010/08/16 11:40:55
Asanas - Postures and Physical Culture
http://www.aypsite.org/forum/topic.asp?TOPIC_ID=8271&REPLY_ID=71966&whichpage=-1
Beginner Asana - er, advise on starting a routine

Hi 11jono11:

The small AYP Asanas, Mudras and Bandhas book offers an approach to asanas that is consistent with keeping a balanced daily routine covering a full range of yoga practices. Included in the book is an "asana starter kit," and an "abbreviated asana starter kit."

Basic illustrations for the asana starter kit can also be found here: http://www.aypsite.org/asana.html

All the best!

The guru is in you.

PS: The book also provides guidelines on how to progressively and safely modify an asanas-only practice to accommodate deep meditation, spinal breathing pranayama and other sitting practices, evolving the practice routine to produce the benefits of full-scope yoga encompassing all eight limbs. As we know, asanas (postures) are but one of the eight limbs of yoga.

2010/08/18 17:06:36
Asanas - Postures and Physical Culture
http://www.aypsite.org/forum/topic.asp?TOPIC_ID=8271&REPLY_ID=72077&whichpage=-1
Beginner Asana - er, advise on starting a routine

Hi 11jono11:

The lessons are the more complete version of AYP, with more techniques and perspectives in most areas of practice than found in the Enlightenment Series books. However, because the lessons have been written "on the fly" over the past 7 years, they are not as well organized as the enlightenment series.

The enlightenment series does a better job of covering the core practices of AYP in an incremental way -- one compact book for each area of practice.

Btw, AYP Easy Lessons Vol 2 is not out yet. Most of it is online here on the website already, and the rest will be included when the complete book comes out in a few months. Once Vol 2 is out, the two Easy Lessons volumes will be the most complete coverage of everything that is in AYP, while the e-series will continue to provide organized incremental coverage of the core practices.

It's up to you whether to go with the lessons or the e-series, or both. If you are into ebooks, we have recently expanded to additional formats covering nearly all e-reading devices, and you get all formats with each ebook when downloading directly through the AYP website. There are also attractive offerings for "bundled" ebook downloads, where some or all of the AYP books can be obtained for substantial savings over buying them one at a time.

If you are into MP3 audiobooks (e-series only), all the "direct download" AYP audiobooks now come with the corresponding ebooks included for free in the zip file.

All of the ebook and audiobook "direct download" offerings can be found here: http://www.aypsite.org/books-xdirdownload.html

Additional retail channels for all the books (paperbacks, ebooks and audiobooks) can be found on the main books page here: http://www.aypsite.org/books.html

If you prefer paperback books, and are looking at getting 5 or more, then take a look at the quantity discount program for possible savings here: http://www.aypsite.org/forum/topic.asp?TOPIC_ID=1248

All the best!

The guru is in you.

Forum 6 – Tantra – Sex and Spiritual Development

What is Tantra anyway? It's about more than sex.
http://www.aypsite.org/forum/forum.asp?FORUM_ID=16

2005/07/11 14:15:51
Tantra - Sex and Spiritual Development
http://www.aypsite.org/forum/topic.asp?TOPIC_ID=278
Tantra - Sex and Spiritual Development

Note: This forum is for mature practitioners, and is moderated to maintain a spiritual orientation and high standard of integrity.

"Tantra" has gotten to be quite a buzz word over the past 30 years. But what does it mean?

Yes, tantra is about sex, but it has a much broader scope, encompassing all of yoga. "Tantra" means "woven together." It is very similar to the word "yoga," which means "to join."

Nevertheless, we still think of the relation of sex to spiritual development when we think of tantra, and that is mostly how we discuss it in AYP. But what kind of sex? It can be summarized in one phrase from a 4,000 year old scripture, the Vigyan Bhairava:

"At the start of sexual union, keep attention on the fire in the beginning, and, so continuing, avoid the embers in the end."

All tantric sexual methods are related to this principle. Put in plain English, it means "preorgasmic sex," or, the simultaneous preservation and cultivation of sexual energy. It is a balancing act that can have a huge impact on our spiritual progress.

But why? When we are sexually stimulated and are able to remain in front of orgasm for an extended period, a spiritual cultivation in the nervous system occurs. This cultivation is closely linked with the natural processes of evolution we are coaxing along in our daily pranayama, meditation, mudras and bandhas, and so on. Not that we do both at the same time. Sex will always be sex, happening as and when it must. We don't regulate that in AYP. But with daily sitting practices happening, combined with an observance of tantric principles and practices in our normal sex life, an important spiritual synergy occurs that accelerates the rise of ecstatic conductivity in our nervous system. This is the spiritual fruit of tantric practices. There are many practical benefits as well -- overcoming sexual dysfunctions, extending lovemaking, greatly deepening the experience for both partners, and profound feelings of love and joy extending throughout the day and night.

Keep in mind that tantric sexual methods alone without meditation and other sitting practices in our daily routine will not be an effective spiritual path. If this were true, we'd have all been enlightened long ago!

Explorations are invited on the full range of tantra, including the principles and practices covered in the AYP tantra lessons, which you can find at: http://www.aypsite.org/TantraDirectory.html

These are:

The holdback method - developing the skill of preorgasmic sex
Blocking of male ejaculation - tantric training for men
The count method - how to stay preorgasmic
Siddhasana - a powerful tantra technique used in sitting practices
Vajroli mudra - the natural upward flow of sexual essences in men and women
Kechari mudra "secret spot" - the "top down" dimension of tantric sex
Amaroli - urine therapy (detailed instructions are in the AYP book) Also see Amaroli resources in the AYP links section at
http://www.aypsite.org/amaroli.html
Brahmacharya - what non-celibate and celibate paths have in common
Sri Vidya - mystical inner lovemaking, the devotional side of tantra

Several of the tantric sexual practices mentioned can be applied in either partner or solo mode.

No doubt the Kama Sutra will come up somewhere along the line. It is good to discuss that too. However, its perceived status as a tantra scripture is in question, because it does not focus on the preservation and cultivation of sexual energy. Without that, there can be no tantric sex.

See also the AYP Tantra Links Section for additional resources -- http://www.aypsite.org/TantraLinks.html

May the discussions here yield new light on this important aspect of our spiritual path.

The guru is in you.

2005/07/17 06:31:31
Tantra - Sex and Spiritual Development
http://www.aypsite.org/forum/topic.asp?TOPIC_ID=304&REPLY_ID=68&whichpage=-1
Swami Atmo Jayakumar

Hello and welcome!

I have great respect for Osho's work (formerly Rajneesh) 20-30 years ago in bringing tantra to public awareness. It was not an easy task! Many have benefited from his open and integrative approach to spiritual development.

You have arrived here just as the new AYP forums are gearing up. I hope we will see many stimulating discussions here in the tantra forum.

Being a sannyasin (renunciate), how would you characterize the differences and similarities in tantric practices between sannyasin and householder ways of life?

Your new topic was moved here from the Yahoo archive forum for a better fit. Once the aypsite.org mail server is tied in with the forum software, an automatic notification will go out to the poster when a topic is moved by a forum moderator.

The guru is in you.

2005/10/13 23:52:34
Tantra - Sex and Spiritual Development
http://www.aypsite.org/forum/topic.asp?TOPIC_ID=344&REPLY_ID=974&whichpage=-1
What happens if you only do sitting practices.

Hello ZN:

Thanks much for chiming in here.

Yes, once the energy is moving it is about flow and balance, which is where sitting practices have a certain advantage -- a daily habit that can work steadily toward promoting the spiritual dimensions of awakened sexual energy (which we also call here, ecstatic conductivity).

Can you share further on the methods you use? As you may have noticed already, we have a lot of tools for this in AYP. But we can always use new perspectives!

The guru is in you.

Yogani

2005/10/17 12:57:39
Tantra - Sex and Spiritual Development
http://www.aypsite.org/forum/topic.asp?TOPIC_ID=344&REPLY_ID=998&whichpage=-1
What happens if you only do sitting practices.

Hi ZN:

Thanks much for the additional detail. Very interesting. It goes to show that there are many ways to skin the "energy cat" while keeping in balance, and living to tell about it.

The fact that you are coming down as much as going up in your practice is most likely the key to your balance. This is similar to the use of spinal breathing in AYP, though we avoid the crown until much later -- using the third eye instead. Your spiraling approach is fascinating, and is consistent with the swirling of energies that occurs as the ida and pingala nerve channels are awakened in conjunction with the spinal nerve (sushumna).

Is there a particular part of your routine that you would say is involved in the cultivation of inner stillness (our unbounded, unshakable inner witness), or do you see this as happening throughout your routine? This gets to a central question that arises when considering all chakra/energy-based paths

In AYP we view the cultivation of ecstatic energy and the cultivation of inner silence to be the two essential poles of enlightenment. This is analogous to setting up for the shakti and shiva union, which leads to the inner rebirthing process and outflow of vast quantities of divine love through our nervous system. Unlimited outflow of divine love into the world is the final stage of all that we are doing in yoga.

So, you can see why I ask about the cultivation of inner silence.

To tie back into the subject of this topic, it is certainly possible to accomplish full ecstatic awakening using sitting practices alone, such as those in AYP, or other methods like those ZN has been so kind to share. The purpose of the tantra lessons in AYP is to provide additional means for those who are sexually active, to whatever degree. In this way, our normal sexual activity can become a periodic aid to spiritual development, rather than be a drag on it. Tantric sexual practices are not a replacement for sitting practices, of course. And neither are sitting practices related to the cultivation of ecstatic energies alone a replacement for methods such as deep meditation and samyama, which are for the cultivation and expansion of inner silence.

I keep bringing up the inner silence component of yoga because it is easy for any of us to forget about it in the face of the huge energy shows we are capable of stimulating within ourselves. So this question about inner silence is not pointed only at you, ZN. It is a reminder to all of us who are inclined to "trip the light fantastic." :-)

It is the blending of these two qualities within us (silence and ecstasy) that will bring us home.

The guru is in you.

2005/10/18 09:26:23
Tantra - Sex and Spiritual Development
http://www.aypsite.org/forum/topic.asp?TOPIC_ID=344&REPLY_ID=1004&whichpage=-1
What happens if you only do sitting practices.

Hi ZN:

Yes, sitting practices are certainly tantra also -- a more refined kind, which is actually the heart of tantra. It is called "Sri Vidya," which means "glorious knowledge" -- knowledge of the inner union of our divine polarities.

If inner silence comes with your practice, who can argue? Presumably it is found in your daily activity as well. That is the test of any yoga practice -- an abiding blissful stillness that elevates the quality of our life. Enlightenment or not, it is quality of life we are all after, yes? And that overflows to others, which is the real fruit -- that infectious bubbling love that can change the world.

So do carry on. There is nothing better to be a lush for than advanced yoga practices. :-)

The guru is in you.

2005/10/18 22:43:38
Tantra - Sex and Spiritual Development
http://www.aypsite.org/forum/topic.asp?TOPIC_ID=344&REPLY_ID=1029&whichpage=-1
What happens if you only do sitting practices.

Hi again ZN:

That is some article on Sri Vidya you found. Quite scholarly... Your own description of what is happening inside is much better.

Here is a much shorter (and hopefully easy to understand) discussion on Sri Vidya from the AYP tantra lessons: http://www.aypsite.org/T25.html

...and also several colored versions of the Sri Yantra diagram, which is discussed in the lesson:
http://www.aypsite.org/sriyantra.html
Here is a blank one for anyone who would like to color their own!
http://www.aypsite.org/sriyantra-blank.html
(click right on it to print it)

Those who have either of the AYP books will notice that the "imprint" (logo) of AYP Publishing is a rainbow colored Sri Yantra. This is a portrait of the human spiritual anatomy from the inside. I think its descriptive relevance will increase in the years to come.

Having a basic familiarity with Sri Vidya and the Sri Yantra can be useful for understanding our inner dimensions and processes in relation to the cosmos, presuming we have the bhakti, practices and inner experiences that directly manifest within us what the wisdom of Sri Vidya and Sri Yantra describe -- human spiritual transformation.

This is why we say that tantra is about much more than sex. It is about getting divinely irradiated and transformed from the inside. :-)

The guru is in you.

2005/10/19 07:55:10
Tantra - Sex and Spiritual Development
http://www.aypsite.org/forum/topic.asp?TOPIC_ID=344&REPLY_ID=1035&whichpage=-1
What happens if you only do sitting practices.

Hi ZN:

You can upload the image to the "files" section of the old Yahoo AYP forum here: http://groups.yahoo.com/group/AYPforum/

Just put the link to it here and anyone can download it.

The guru is in you.

PS -- You can also put it in the "photos" section where it can be viewed online, but there may be less resolution in a download from there.
2005/10/20 07:59:28
Tantra - Sex and Spiritual Development
http://www.aypsite.org/forum/topic.asp?TOPIC_ID=344&REPLY_ID=1053&whichpage=-1
What happens if you only do sitting practices.
It is a nice one ... Thanks much!
2005/07/23 10:10:55
Tantra - Sex and Spiritual Development
http://www.aypsite.org/forum/topic.asp?TOPIC_ID=354&REPLY_ID=166&whichpage=-1
vasectomy and its effect on tantric energy?

Hi Victor:

I am not sure exactly where the plumbing is altered in vasectomy -- before the seminal vesicles or after? Presumably before. In any case, there is some subjective evidence that the upward circulation of sexual energy (semen) comes from the seminal vesicles and up through the urethra into the bladder too. Vajroli mudra (whether manual in the early stages or automatic and ongoing in later stages) is at least in part a drawing up of semen into the bladder.

I emphasis that these are subjective observations, and not scientifically verified. Someday science will have a much better handle on the biology of enlightenment. Until then, we will continue to work with the ancient knowledge and techniques, and the subjective observation of results. It is the best we can do for now, and it can be taken very far forward by those means, obviously. As time goes on, science will fill in the blanks.

Bottom line -- semen in a man (and female essences in a woman) migrate upward via many paths in the biology. It also ends up in the GI track (Chinese ☐cauldron☐) for the biology of soma production, and this continues up into the head and then circulates back down again. I often have had the sensation of the essences of the seminal vesicles being directly involved in this GI track connection. But, again, it is a subjective observation. Needless to say, there is a complex biology that occurs in human spiritual transformation, and while there are many cases of sages who have undergone the full transformation and have tried to describe it (usually metaphorically), we still have much to learn about it.

Not sure where that leaves you with your vasectomy considerations. But it is the best assessment I can give you at this point. We are all spiritual pioneers here.

By the way, the process in women as far as I can tell (even more subjectively) has more similarities than differences to the male spiritual biology, including the absorption of sexual essences up through the urethra into the bladder!

The guru is in you.

2005/07/27 09:18:23
Tantra - Sex and Spiritual Development
http://www.aypsite.org/forum/topic.asp?TOPIC_ID=354&REPLY_ID=193&whichpage=-1
vasectomy and its effect on tantric energy?

Thank you, Lucid, for that informative input.

The question that has emerged here:

Is sperm in the seminal fluid an essential part of the spiritual biology?

Your excellent experiences in yoga indicate not. Of course, one man's experience does not constitute a scientific conclusion, but it is a very useful "data point," as David calls it.

The guru is in you.

2005/08/05 23:45:10
Tantra - Sex and Spiritual Development
http://www.aypsite.org/forum/topic.asp?TOPIC_ID=388&REPLY_ID=303&whichpage=-1
vajroli

Hi Victor:

I used a catheter for a while many years ago, but do not recommend it, or any formal vajroli practice, because I found vajroli to be an automatic yoga coming up once ecstatic conductivity became established. In fact, vajroli is not of much real use until ecstatic conductivity is active in the neuro-biology, with the sexual essences being fully utilized. So, learning vajroli before ecstatic conductivity is getting the cart in front of the horse a bit. See lesson T30 at http://www.aypsite.org/T30.html

Having said that, even if you are effectively using holdback and blocking, you will probably want to learn vajroli anyway. Most men do. But with our daily yoga practices, the reality will come later automatically, and far exceed the mechanical aspects and sexual implications of it now. Real vajroli is a natural, subtle and ongoing mechanism of brahmacharya -- the preservation and unending cultivation of sexual energy in the spiritually awakened nervous system. Anything we are doing mechanically with vajroli before that is a clumsy imitation of the real thing, and possibly even a distraction.

The guru is in you.

2005/08/06 00:15:02
Tantra - Sex and Spiritual Development
http://www.aypsite.org/forum/topic.asp?TOPIC_ID=388&REPLY_ID=305&whichpage=-1
vajroli
I figured you were pretty far along in tantric matters, Victor. It is the connectedness of yoga, you know.

A little air won't hurt, but the other substances definitely can, and are strongly discouraged. Much of the vajroli lore is macho stuff having little to do with real yoga. Similar extremes can be found in the kechari lore too. It is up to modern yoga scientists, like us, to separate the real from the unreal in all of this.

The guru is in you.

2005/08/06 10:52:17
Tantra - Sex and Spiritual Development
http://www.aypsite.org/forum/topic.asp?TOPIC_ID=388&REPLY_ID=310&whichpage=-1
vajroli
Whatever air goes in comes out naturally by the same route it went in. It is like flatulence. Don't be surprised if you see a little blood in the urine when using a catheter. That too is normal, at least in my case it was. I don't encourage this practice, but if you are going to do it, I will be happy to share what I know. I don't consider myself to be an expert on this crude practice, btw. Only someone who took the plunge a long time ago and lived to tell about it. I do not consider it essential for advancement in yoga. Probably the greatest benefit of it was developing an awareness of the inner anatomy of urethra, prostate, entry point of seminal vesicles and the bladder. These are all very sensitive areas, and are crucial in the spiritual transformation process. With awareness of the inner anatomy, the process of transformation seemed to be enhanced, not so much by anything mechanical that was done. As in all things yogic, it is about the blending of inner silence (witness) with rising ecstatic conductivity (kundalini).

I am pretty sure the same end result will occur without deliberate mechanical vajroli practice, because it is a natural evolution that is cultivated by all the rest of our practices, including the tantra techniques in the lessons.

For the ladies, it appears that a similar process of upward absorption of sexual essences from the "G spot" through the urethra to the bladder occurs in the female anatomy, so this discussion may be relevant to both men and women.

Who started this conversation, anyway?

The guru is in you.

2007/10/24 13:23:44
Tantra - Sex and Spiritual Development
http://www.aypsite.org/forum/topic.asp?TOPIC_ID=388&REPLY_ID=26301&whichpage=-1
vajroli

Hi Gentlep:

If you have not already, you might also check these topics on Vajroli for some additional perspective:
http://www.aypsite.org/forum/topic.asp?TOPIC_ID=2951
http://www.aypsite.org/forum/topic.asp?TOPIC_ID=2953

Yes, Avatar, vajroli can be practiced mechanically without ecstatic conductivity, just as kechari can. But neither will do much until ecstatic conductivity arises mainly through deep meditation and spinal breathing pranayama. Before that, these mudras are merely mechanical. There is little harm in this with kechari, but with vajroli with a catheter, there are real health risks. Once ecstatic conductivity arises, natural vajroli will be happening anyway, because it is part of the process of rising ecstatic energy. The same is true of kechari, as anyone knows who has had their tongue automatically "go up" during meditation or pranayama. Vajroli happens naturally that way also, so there is not a need for such extraordinary risky measures.

Inner silence and ecstatic conductivity are the underlying factors in these things, not any particular physical maneuver. When it is time for mudras, bandhas and additional pranayama methods (bastrika, kumbhaka, etc.), we will know and they will come about naturally, with only a pointer or two being necessary. That's what the AYP writings are intended to be -- pointers for those who are ready for next steps on their path. :-)

All the best!

The guru is in you.

2007/10/24 15:53:30
Tantra - Sex and Spiritual Development
http://www.aypsite.org/forum/topic.asp?TOPIC_ID=388&REPLY_ID=26312&whichpage=-1
vajroli

Hi Jim:

The neurobiological changes will happen, and how we engage/cultivate those via this or that practice may happen according to our own unique tendencies, culture and training.

Bhakti (spiritual desire) overrules all of it, turning all mays into wills within the context of our own journey.

This is why bhakti is the cornerstone of all the religions and spiritual traditions, with the rest being about optimizing the details of practice.

Bhakti is the prerequisite, with the many ways to carry out implementation being added after that. With strong bhakti, even one obsessed exclusively with vajroli or kechari (or any singular practice) will get through, because the actions necessary to move ahead will always become obvious to the one who is overflowing with spiritual desire.

Likewise, with strong bhakti, even one completely uninvolved with vajroli or kechari (or any aspect of yoga) will advance for the same reason.

The guru is in you.

2005/08/12 12:01:24
Tantra - Sex and Spiritual Development
http://www.aypsite.org/forum/topic.asp?TOPIC_ID=400&REPLY_ID=346&whichpage=-1
A Woman's Inner Loving

Hello Amaargi:

Thank you for your intimate sharing. It gets to the core of the matter of self-love and self-nurturing, and is at the core of the cultivation of ecstatic conductivity in yoga as well.

Of course, masturbation has been a taboo in many cultures for centuries. It is a two-edged sword. It can be for hedonism (sense gratification) or for divine union (tantra). The first will be leading to the second if we are engaged in daily practices of deep meditation, spinal breathing and other sitting practices. The same can be said for the impact of yoga practices on any sexual activity we may engage in, and on life in the world of the senses in general. What is sensually self-indulgent today can become spiritual practice a short distance down the road if we are seriously engaged in sitting yoga practices. Yoga will transform our experiences in that way.

Obviously, you have found this to be the case in masturbation. It is a profound transformation that is accessible to all of us. The mysteries of sex revealed!

The essence of tantric transformation is a shift from sense gratification to conscious cultivation of ecstatic conductivity, which has a profound effect on our sense of self in the ways you have described. When ecstatic conductivity is blended with rising inner silence gained in deep meditation, then we have the essential elements for the enlightenment process present within us. So the expansion of our sexual function from reproductive urge to spiritual urge has far-reaching consequences.

Whether we are talking about self-pleasuring in masturbation, sexual relations with a partner, or stimulative yoga practices used by both celibates and non-celibates like siddhasana, mulabandha/asvini, sambhavi, kechari, etc., the same principle is involved -- preorgasmic cultivation of sexual energy throughout the nervous system. This applies equally in both women and men. The longer we are cultivating preorgasmically, the greater will be the effect. It leads to a permanent transformation to higher functioning in the neuro-biological functioning throughout our nervous system. This is what the AYP tantra lessons are about. http://www.aypsite.org/TantraDirectory.html

The practice you are describing is in this direction. It is a yoga technique, which, when added to sitting practices, can play an important role in opening our full inner potential. This is not a call to masturbation for everyone. It is a call to take note of what our current sexual habits can become in the future in relation to yoga.

All of this is in addition to the practical benefits you have found in self-nurturing to rise above a tendency toward undesirable relationships. Interestingly, it is the undesirable relationships that have led you to your discovery. So, no matter where we are in our life experience, God is always present showing us our doorways to the divine. All we need to do is notice and walk through them.

As Rumi, the great Sufi mystic, said, Keep walking ... Move within ... But don't move the way fear makes you move.

The guru is in you.

2005/08/17 13:09:38
Tantra - Sex and Spiritual Development
http://www.aypsite.org/forum/topic.asp?TOPIC_ID=412&REPLY_ID=396&whichpage=-1
Sharing Energy

Hello Paul:

As ecstatic conductivity advances, our inward sensitivity in all things increases. Then a glance or gentle touch of our beloved can send us into an ecstatic reverie. Ramakrishna, the great 19th century sage, was famous for literally falling down in bliss at the mere thought of his ishta (chosen ideal), the divine goddess.

This is how progress in tantra expands to greater sensitivity, yielding divine ecstasy. It comes with the opening of inner sensory experience -- ecstatic conductivity throughout the nervous system. And, as you are noticing, all the things we love will touch us more deeply, even in small doses -- our ishta, our lover, our music, our art, our sacred work, etc. In time, all of life can become filled with the many dimensions of ecstatic bliss.

Certainly the flow of energy can be felt coming from us going outward as well. The more pure our nervous system becomes and the more we spontaneously radiate our innate joy, the more will be flowing out in the form of divine love. That will influence everyone around us, and be perceived by others according to their own inner sensitivities.

As for the suction of energy vampires, etc., we become more aware of that too, but our vulnerability to it does not increase. We just have a better barometer on the energy dynamics around and within us, so we are able to manage and navigate through the energies more wisely than we did before. This is covered in a variety of ways in the "Secrets of Wilder" novel.

While we become more sensitive, we also become unshakable like the proverbial "rock" due to our rising inner silence. So, while we are becoming infinitely more sensitive and attuned through ecstatic conductivity, we are also becoming infinitely more stable and peaceful through our inner silence. These two together comprise the two essential poles of enlightenment. That is why we build up the AYP practices the way we do -- so we can cultivate both in a balanced way.

The guru is in you.

2005/08/20 10:34:37
Tantra - Sex and Spiritual Development
http://www.aypsite.org/forum/topic.asp?TOPIC_ID=426&REPLY_ID=420&whichpage=-1
Advanced Siddhasana

Hello Victor.

That is fine, with the following clarifications:

1. Cupping the genitals is an add-on, not to be confused with the main practice of siddhasana. The add-on may be too much distraction for beginners who are not established in siddhasana proper with spinal breathing, meditation, etc. The add-on may also become unnecessary for advanced practitioners later on when the processes of ecstatic conductivity have been almost entirely internalized. Keep in mind that ecstatic conductivity eventually becomes a resident feature of our neuro-biology, requiring little or no external stimulation. At that point, we are in the "doing nothing stage" that David speaks about in another topic, here - http://www.aypsite.org/forum/topic.asp?TOPIC_ID=314

Even so, we will still be wise to be doing something to be doing nothing. At that stage, we will know what to do according to our bhakti and long-established skills in self-pacing.

2. Holding the genitals in public is not recommended. We can leave that to the rock stars. Of course, it is up to you. Discretion is the greater part of valor in many things, including yoga. :-)

3. As for which practices to do this add-on with beyond spinal breathing pranayama, it can be the same as with basic siddhasana, kechari and other mudras and bandhas which we form as habits in spinal breathing pranayama, and may later allow to carry over effortlessly into our other practices. It is matter of effortlessness (no distraction in meditation especially) and personal preference. Our bhakti will let us know.

A man cupping the genitals during siddhasana is an advanced option corresponding with the woman's practice of using the outer heel (or hand) to gently stimulate the clitoris in siddhasana. For details on advanced siddhasana for both women and men, see http://www.aypsite.org/T28.html The beginning instructions on siddhasana are here - http://www.aypsite.org/75.html

The guru is in you.

2005/08/20 15:43:07
Tantra - Sex and Spiritual Development
http://www.aypsite.org/forum/topic.asp?TOPIC_ID=426&REPLY_ID=423&whichpage=-1
Advanced Siddhasana

Hi again Victor:

On the hand positions, balancing the limbs and such, I would put that in the same category as hand mudras -- our inner energy will move us according to our unique patterns of purification. No special instructions needed there, except to be easy with it while at the same time avoiding the extremes of automatic yoga (physical movements).

Yes, I think so much more can be gained by working directly with sexual energy in a systematic fashion. Of course, there is always the risk of running off on tangents. But what in life does not carry such risks?

Perhaps the old-line traditions can't afford the risk, so they avoid sex, kundalini and quite a few other things. A lot gets lost in the watering down of yogic wisdom for the sake of "safety." Here in AYP, we try and face it all head on in a practical integrative way, and so far it has worked out pretty well. May it continue to be so.

By the way, the principles we are discussing here apply in both celibate and non-celibate approaches to tantra. We have not spoken much about the former lately. From the standpoint of yoga, the preservation and cultivation of sexual energy (brahmacharya) is of equal importance to both celibates and non-celibates. The methods vary, but the outcome is the same. Enduring ecstatic bliss!

Siddhasana is a practice that both approaches have in common.

The guru is in you.

2005/08/21 11:46:39
Tantra - Sex and Spiritual Development
http://www.aypsite.org/forum/topic.asp?TOPIC_ID=426&REPLY_ID=425&whichpage=-1
Advanced Siddhasana

Hello Anthem:

If automatic yoga (movements) become a distraction to the practice we are doing, or a physical hazard (in rare cases), we should temper them accordingly. We always have the option to choose what is in the best interest of our practice. While automatic yogas are generally a good sign of the interconnectedness of yoga within us, in the end it is our structured practice that will bring us home.

Of course, those who subscribe to the "no path" approach will not agree. Nevertheless, it is structured practice that fosters automatic yogas, not the other way around. The same goes for all experiences that arise when doing effective yoga practices. The experience is not what will transform us -- the practice is. The same goes for automatic yoga, though the line may be a bit blurred in that case. Still, experiences and automatic yogas are both effects of practice, not causes. It is good to keep that in mind, lest we put the cart in front of the horse.

The best approach to automatic yoga is to utilize it during corresponding structured practices we are doing. For example, if we are experiencing a tendency for head movements, we should not favor this excessively during our meditation -- best to favor the mantra. Better to favor the movements during chin pump practice (if we have added it to our routine), which is a good time for utilizing automatic head movements. As always, we should also apply self-pacing as necessary to regulate the build-up of our practices and correct any excesses. In these ways we can use automatic yoga while keeping structured practices in place.

In the case of siddhasana, we may be squirming around a lot during the formative stages of it, with all sorts of movements. These are normal and may represent identifiable automatic yogas or not. As siddhasana settles in, the movements will subside, transforming to an experience of much more refined internal ecstatic currents -- an inner fountain of ecstasy. This is another aspect of automatic yogas -- they settle down once the inner pathways involved have been opened somewhat. In this settling down, the immensity of joy residing deep within us will emerge.

Whenever we are dealing with automatic yogas or other manifestations of purification in the nervous system, it is a fine balance to allow the expression of our awakening inner energies, and at the same time maintain good forward progress through structured practices. It is like driving a fast car. We'd like to go as fast as possible, while operating within our present abilities so we can stay on the road and reach our destination. Varooom!

The guru is in you.

2005/11/13 10:01:03
Tantra - Sex and Spiritual Development
http://www.aypsite.org/forum/topic.asp?TOPIC_ID=584&REPLY_ID=1515&whichpage=-1
Sex Magnetism

Hello Hendrik:

Hypnosis can go for internal spiritual or external worldly purposes -- usually the latter in our present cultural situation, though it seems to be changing for the better. For more comments on this, see my note of Oct 6th in this topic.

Regarding the cultivation of "sex magnetism" and "personal magnetism" for their own sake, this approach will be a distraction from yoga. Paradoxically, the more we focus on inner development and the less on "powers" such as these, the more we will gain them. This will be in the right direction, because then these natural abilities will come up in support of our increasing inclination for service to others, rather than an egoic manipulation of power, which always leads to more bondage.

More focus on spiritual development = more service to others, more powers in support of that and more freedom.

More focus on development of powers = less spiritual development, less service to others and more bondage.

In a nutshell, that is the case against developing powers (siddhis) for their own sake. So, I do not agree that power should be "directed." Power is a by-product of spiritual development -- not causative at all. If we make the mistake of thinking we are in charge of power as a cause for good, we will end up with less, not more, and so will those we influence in that way. Inner silence (pure bliss consciousness) is the cause of all good and all power.

"Seek first the kingdom of God and all will be added to you."

So the advice is, become firmly established in a routine of daily deep meditation, and then do the other practices (spinal breathing, asanas, mudras, bandhas, samyama, tantric sexual methods, etc.) that cultivate our nervous system as a pure channel for outpouring divine love (divine power). Then things will be in the right order, with the best results for all concerned.

The guru is in you.

2005/11/15 12:09:59

Tantra - Sex and Spiritual Development
http://www.aypsite.org/forum/topic.asp?TOPIC_ID=589&REPLY_ID=1532&whichpage=-1
Ways to relieve sexual urge?
Good question, Alvin. Good answer, David. :-)

I would only add that as you get through the tantra lessons, Alvin, you will gain more perspective on this. Particularly lesson #T46 which ties much of it together in a practical discussion.
http://www.aypsite.org/T46.html

Also, one of these days I will be adding an online lesson on masturbation in relation to the broader topic of spiritual self-stimulation.

The guru is in you

2006/01/07 16:36:17
Tantra - Sex and Spiritual Development
http://www.aypsite.org/forum/topic.asp?TOPIC_ID=704
Lady Questions
From my email:

Q:
I have a few questions that I would like to post on the forum, but I am shy to do it. If you think these are valid and appropriate questions, could you post them for me? Also, I would like your input on these.

1. Has anybody's menstrual cycle changed after starting AYP?

2. Why do they say women should skip yoga practices during menstruation?

3. What is the best birth control method to follow? Pills play with the natural hormones in the system, and cannot be good for you. What other ways are there that a woman can follow for birth control that do not include medication?

A:
Those are good questions for the Tantra forum. I will be happy to post them and hopefully we will receive some suggestions from other yoginis.

As for my thoughts, not being a woman, I can only give you a limited perspective. We need input from the ladies on this one. Here are a few thoughts from this yogi:

1. The menstrual cycle can become less severe with lighter flow as more energy is being drawn upward from the pelvic region due to spiritual practices. Maybe the period will be less often. I have heard of this, but my experience is obviously limited, so your experience (and that of other yoginis) will be a better guide.

2. I don't think normal practices ought to be arbitrarily curtailed during the woman's period, as long as self-pacing is applied if there is any discomfort. Perhaps the advice to curtail yoga during the period is based on a more extreme and less adaptable practice routine -- which is their way of saying, "Pacing of practices may be necessary during menstruation so we are telling you not to practice at all during your period." AYP has a bit more finesse than that sort of rigid dictate, don't you think?

3. On birth control, well, there are many means, some not involving drugs -- but with the obvious sacrifices of naturalness. Tantric lovemaking with good holdback and blocking by the man would be birth control by definition, but we ought not count on that alone, as there can always be a slip-up. The Catholics use "the rhythm method." Maybe the rhythm method combined with holdback would be pretty good birth control, but you need a calendar and good tantric skills in both partners to do that. :-)

This raises the question: Is there such a thing as "natural" birth control? I'm not sure there is, except turning upward to the divine. That is a long term proposition, of course, with birth control being a by-product rather than a primary objective.

For whatever it is worth, my wife and I have three grown children and it all seemed to work itself out naturally over the years. It is between you and your husband, of course. But it can also be helpful to seek advice from friends who can offer additional perspectives. So you are wise to be asking...

The guru is in you.

2006/01/12 08:37:33
Tantra - Sex and Spiritual Development
http://www.aypsite.org/forum/topic.asp?TOPIC_ID=724
If the Goddess cannot withhold orgasm
Some recent emails on tantric practice and female orgasm:

Q: What can I do if the Goddess cannot withhold orgasm during connection?

A: You may find the following interchange helpful. Bottom line: All in her own time...

Q1: First I would like to thank you for your wonderfully organized and informational website. Your thoughts and teachings are easy to understand and very consistent, without using so much traditional language as to be confusing.

Me and my wife have found tantric techniques to bring great pleasure into our lives. For almost two years, we have been using the holdback technique as well as yoni massage and sacred spot massage to create a deeper and stronger bond during our sexual experiences. I truly enjoy staying in front of my orgasm and worshipping her as a divine goddess while she enjoys incredible multiple orgasms. Our union is so strong, it is as if we are one being in total bliss. We do not so much feel a sense of pranic drain from her orgasm, but more of a sense of total and complete mutual satisfaction due to our close coupling. Is there anything wrong with following a path where the man stays in front of his orgasm so that both lovers can enjoy the greatly increased capacity for orgasm in her?

A1: Thank you for your kind note and sharing. I am very happy that you are finding the AYP lessons to be helpful.

On tantric sex, the experience of the man having good ability in holdback and the woman having multiple orgasms is an interim step on the path of tantra. You may both enjoy it as long as you wish. But know that your bhakti will eventually take you beyond that to preorgasmic sex for both partners. Which is not to say orgasms will not happen. It is only that the neurobiology higher up will become much more enjoyable than orgasm for your partner and she will eventually want to go higher with her energy, just as you are.

Of course all of this is predicated on a good routine of sitting practices including deep meditation, spinal breathing and so on. With steady-state inner silence and ecstatic conductivity coming up, the expansion of sexual function to become increasing spiritual will occur naturally.

If you read the **Secrets of Wilder** novel, you will find one scenario of how this can evolve over the years. It is also discussed in the AYP tantra lessons on the website and in the **AYP Easy Lessons** book.

You might like to surface this question in the AYP forums also, where you can receive other opinions. It is a great place to discuss practices.

Q2: Thank you for your answer, it seems our bhakti will eventually lead us to the right path for us.

Reading more and more of your site, I was quite amazed to find I had already instictively discovered Mulabandha, and, partially, Sambhavi without knowing what they were!

I do have one last question - I have realized that for me, orgasm is something from which I must abstain completely - the drain of my prana is far too great, and I don't feel my energy anywhere close to before for even two weeks or more. Will this ever be the case for my wife? I would not want her to have to give this pleasure up forever, and I confess I take great enjoyment in helping her to achieve intense and extended orgasms. Will she still be able to enjoy this pleasure occasionally, or even regularly, without harming our yoga?

Thank you again for your wisdom. There are many "false prophets" out there, and it is clear you are not one of them.

A2: I don't think it is a matter of your wife giving anything up. When the shift happens, she will be going to more via direct perception of that. It can happen gradually over a long period of time, or be a sudden inspiration. It is really up to (and within) her. Of course you can help a lot with that by being open to to what is happening and encouraging her toward more lasting ecstatic bliss. And yes, women generally are less depleted by orgasm, though there are exceptions. In the lessons I say that multiple female orgasms can lead to depletion similar to a single orgasm for a man. A number of woman have told me this. But I am not a woman, so direct experience will be the best guide for women in this matter. For some feminine inspiration on this subject, check out the book The **Art of Sexual Ecstasy** by Margo Anand. You can find it and other books on sexology on the AYP book list http://www.aypsite.org/booklist13.html

One thing is for sure -- there is much more to be found in front of orgasm than behind it for both men and women. To this end, there is a new AYP book coming out in the spring called:
Tantra - Discovering the Power of Pre-Orgasmic Sex

It will be a companion to the new book, **Deep Meditation**, and others that will be coming out this year and next on a wide range of practices, comprising the "AYP Enlightenment Series."

Q3: Thanks again. Clearly the shift will be up to her, and when and if she choses that, I will support her fully. To be honest, this point seems far off for us. We have yet to embrace a truly guided approach; until now, we've picked up some useful information here and there, but some of our practices are confused, some are missing, and some are underdeveloped. She has yet to embrace meditation and breathing practices. To that end, I bought the AYP book today - the online lessons are great and well organized, but it would be much nicer to be able to read and study them together in a book. I see my yoga as starting over from the beginning, and hers truly beginning as we work first on basic practices - any insight we may have gained so far, and my already well conserved prana can only help us.

As far as not knowing if she feels the same energy drain as I do in orgasm, surely this is something I can never know. But I think we both do sense that it is far less (although she does find multiple orgasms to be draining). One thing of which I suppose again, we may never know, but seems to be the case, is that she seems to reach far greater pleasure in orgasm now than I ever was able. If it truly is the case that her pleasure from it is far greater, and her drain far less, this makes me wonder if she might never need or want to stop having orgasms. On the other hand, if her pleasure in pre-orgasm alone can top that, that would be a great delight for both of us to share. Nevertheless, it is clear this must be a decision for her to make when she is ready, and not something I would want to push her towards unless she feels a natural drive for it. Perhaps this is part of the reason why for a couple learning tantra, the man must take the first steps.

In any case, thanks for your time, and I look forward to sharing your book with my wife!

A3: Don't know if you intended to give your wife the new **Deep Meditation** book in addition to having the **AYP Easy Lessons** book on hand (good idea). The former is a short but thorough primer for folks who may have no prior interest in meditation or spiritual practices, and is much easier to digest than the entire body of AYP lessons.

The "more" that pre-orgasmic tantric practice aids in cultivating is found in our 24 hour living. We go from a limited-duration peak experience of orgasm to living in a state of ecstasy throughout our daily life. It is a permanent transformation of the basic functioning of our nervous system. That rise of ecstatic conductivity, combined with the rise of inner silence via meditation is the foundation of enlightenment.

The guru is in you.

2006/01/18 16:47:49
Tantra - Sex and Spiritual Development
http://www.aypsite.org/forum/topic.asp?TOPIC_ID=741&REPLY_ID=2616&whichpage=-1
Hold back method

Hi O4l4:

Take a look at this topic: http://www.aypsite.org/forum/topic.asp?TOPIC_ID=724
While it is not exactly the same situation, the bottom line is the same -- "All in her own time..."

In the meantime, inform her gently and coax her skillfully. Just as you are recognizing her sexual needs, perhaps she can recognize yours. It is a partnership, yes? The truth be told, with skills in holdback you are in a position to give her more pleasure than she can imagine. That is coincident with the spiritual aspect.

And yes, solo practice is a good idea, if you are up for it. :-)

Giving her a copy of the Deep Meditation book would not hurt either. Believe it or not, that has everything to do with what we are discussing here.

Wishing you the best on your path. Enjoy!

The guru is in you.

2006/01/21 09:45:04
Tantra - Sex and Spiritual Development
http://www.aypsite.org/forum/topic.asp?TOPIC_ID=752&REPLY_ID=2698&whichpage=-1
need more advices on tantric practices

Hi Alvin:

A commitment today keeps me from answering in detail right now, but here is a dialog on tantra practice that covers at least part of your inquiry:
http://www.aypsite.org/T46.html

Perhaps others can fill in.

The guru is in you.

2006/01/28 15:49:32
Tantra - Sex and Spiritual Development
http://www.aypsite.org/forum/topic.asp?TOPIC_ID=768&REPLY_ID=2838&whichpage=-1
Why full body orgasm?

Hi Sparkle:

I think you are correct in your conclusion. Energy conductivity is not the primary prerequisite for enlightenment. Inner silence is. Once the foundation has been laid, the house can be built sturdily upon it. A house built without a foundation will not last.

The guru is in you.

2006/02/06 15:20:24
Tantra - Sex and Spiritual Development
http://www.aypsite.org/forum/topic.asp?TOPIC_ID=768&REPLY_ID=3117&whichpage=-1
Why full body orgasm?

Hi Mystiq:

While I am sure some would disagree, I don't think orgasm itself has much to do with yoga. It is related to reproduction -- the ecstatic engine that drives reproduction. And, as we know, it involves body, heart and mind, and all of that is related to the rearing of the family too. That is a crossover of orgasm into the spiritual arena. Whenever we care for others more than ourselves, something spiritual is going on. It can come through the reproductive cycle like that. This is what makes the family sacred.

Beyond that, sex gets truly yogic when we begin to work pre-orgasmincally with it in extended cultivation. This also has a relationship to lengthening and deepening orgasm itself, but if we are aiming for that we are not doing yoga really. So much of modern tantra is like that:

"Come to our tantra class. Learn how to have longer deeper orgasms."

Perhaps those who are born with such tendencies have taken a lot of tantra classes in a past life.

But it (yoga) is not about the orgasm.

If systematic cultivation is done pre-orgasmically, in addition to having an integrated routine of sitting practices (done separately), then something different will be happening. The ecstatic component of that will no longer be for reproduction and will go up toward human spiritual transformation. It is a different thing entirely, though using the same energy that reproduction does. Success depends on the presence of inner silence, and steady commitment and persistence over time.

Siddhasana, mudras, bandhas and pranayama accomplish the same objectives as tantric sex -- cultivation of the ecstatic conductivity (shakti) component of the shakti/shiva duo. Inner silence cultivated in deep meditation and samyama is the shiva component. These means can be used by celibates and by non-celibate tantrics.

If it is an analysis of orgasm we are doing here, that is about as far as we go with it and still be talking about yoga. The rest (the quest for the perfect orgasm) is something else and can be a distraction to yoga, and to everything else we are doing in our life. Maybe that is why many cultures try and put a lid on sex. It doesn't work, of course. It leads to repressed societies and aberrant behavior, or worse.

Sex is what it is. We are all inclined to be obsessed with sex either for or against. It cannot be ignored. I think one of the real strengths of tantra is that is enables serious practitioners to redirect the natural obsession with sex toward spiritual transformation. That is bhakti! Those who really know the methods of tantra, have no fear about sex and less obsession, because the lion's share of it goes toward expansion of ecstatic conductivity within them. It is like a never-ending orgasm, but not really. If it does not end, it is not orgasm anymore. It is a different thing -- a component of enlightenment, life in ecstatic bliss. Then "the act" is about the higher mudras like sambhavi and kechari, and the filling up of the heart to become a channel of endless divine love pouring out into the world. That is the best "orgasm" of all. :-)

282 – Advanced Yoga Practices

The guru is in you.

2006/02/08 14:03:39
Tantra - Sex and Spiritual Development
http://www.aypsite.org/forum/topic.asp?TOPIC_ID=794&REPLY_ID=3170&whichpage=-1
Bhramacharya?

quote:
_____
I am in the initial stage ....I do asanas, pranayama and meditation.... Now i dont release my semen... thats disturbing me after my AYP session
some times.... some times i do blocking method... even that is not helping me ....Urge is devloping daily.... wat should i do now....i think if i can
channelise the sexual energy , problem will be solved.... how to do that.... i thought spinal breathig will help me but i dont think its helping me...Is
it better to release the sperm regularly instead of accumulating it??? if yes what should be the time interval to release the semen????
_____

Hi Thundu:

This one comes up often in my email and it has been discussed here too -- young men doing what young men do, or maybe not so young. It is as
inevitable as the menstrual cycle, part of nature, and certainly not the end of yoga as has been so direly predicted by those celibate yogis who live
in caves off in the mountains somewhere.

I think the dialog in lesson T46 offers some reasonable suggestions on this, as does the discussion here:
http://www.aypsite.org/forum/topic.asp?TOPIC_ID=589
(And Jim is right -- you will do well to read all the AYP tantra lessons for the full picture.)

The key to the whole thing is in what we favor over the long term. If we are favoring expansion of sexual energy upward, we will favor the means
and in time it will happen.

In my case, I had been meditating 15 years, was well into my 30s, and had three children by the time I finally saw a decisive turn in sexual energy
-- and even then, that was only the beginning and it took a long time afterward to develop. I was not really working on it much before then, and
the means were practically unknown. Would expansion of sexual energy (and ecstatic conductivity) have happened sooner if I had known the
means and been working on it in my 20s? Who knows? What was important was that I was meditating all the way through those early years, and
that ultimately led to the process of expansion of sexual function. It always gets back to inner silence, you know.

Things are very different now. If a young man (or woman) is moved to begin working on the expansion of sexual energy upward at an early age,
an arsenal of tools is available, and we have a much clearer understanding of what is involved experientially. This does not mean a nervous
system that needs 10 years to purify and open can now do it in one year. It just means we don't have to spend most of our time trying to figure out
how it is done. That is the benefit of open source information.

Gentle persistence over the long haul and a step-by-step approach are necessary. That is what self-pacing is all about. It will be good to not get
too rushed and stressed about it. Just favor what you know is in the right direction. And when you fall off, just get up and keep going. That is how
it is done.

I don't expect anyone here will have to be meditating for 15 years before ecstatic conductivity begins to stir. On the other hand, it will be what it
will be. It is an interplay of each person's bhakti and the level of purification in the individual nervous system ... combined with application of the
tools available. With these three components well understood and utilized, the task can be accomplished in due course. What that "due course" is
will be different for each of us. Just know that everything we do in that direction will be for the good and we will not lose what we have gained.

The guru is in you.

2006/02/09 13:33:18
Tantra - Sex and Spiritual Development
http://www.aypsite.org/forum/topic.asp?TOPIC_ID=794&REPLY_ID=3200&whichpage=-1
Bhramacharya?

Hi Thundu:

All of the practices have what I call in the lessons a "clunky stage." This is just going through the awkward beginnings and getting familiar and
steady in a new practice. It is wise to move beyond the clunky stage in one practice before considering moving on to the next practice. In fact, it is
even wiser to move well beyond clunky and into good clarity and smoothness in a practice for some months before adding on. That will give the
best chance of not getting too far ahead of ourselves, and bogged down.

As for the masturbation, do your best to have some discipline about it. Holdback and blocking as discused in the tantra lessons can help a lot over
time, and consider the count method in connection with holdback too. All of these methods have a clunky stage as well. Rome was not built in a
day.

It may seem strange, but those who have some excessive feelings in sexuality can have an advantage, IF some disciplne can be brought to bear on
the situation. That is a big IF, of course. What might look like a spiritual liability now, can turn into an advantage later on.

Bottom line: Strong sensuality and sexuality can become strong ecstatic conductivity, if the appropriate means are applied consistently over time.

And all the little bumps in the road you are experiencing? It looks like you are in clunky stages with several practices at once there. Maybe slow
down and take things on one at a time. You can take it all on -- one at a time. :-)

The guru is in you.

2006/02/09 13:43:56

Tantra - Sex and Spiritual Development
http://www.aypsite.org/forum/topic.asp?TOPIC_ID=794&REPLY_ID=3202&whichpage=-1
Bhramacharya?
PS -- Maybe others can chime in on the mantra with thoughts questions, and anything else I left uncovered. Running out the door here...

One more thing: All the AYP books are available worldwide in ebook format, but in western (dollar) pricing, which I know is tough in India. I am working to have the ebooks available in India (rupee) pricing, which will be much more affordable there. Also, there is an ongoing effort to have the physical books published in India. Sooner or later, it will happen, and then we will have overcome the cost and distance barriers.

Anouncements will be put on the AYP web sites and here in the forum when progress is achieved in these things.

Information on the AYP book offerings can be found here: http://www.aypsite.org/books.html

2006/02/14 09:43:01
Tantra - Sex and Spiritual Development
http://www.aypsite.org/forum/topic.asp?TOPIC_ID=813&REPLY_ID=3339&whichpage=-1
Arousal Going Straight to the Heart

Hi Jim:

Nice description of sexual energy expanding upward to become spiritual.

What's next? It is the ecstatic illumination of the heart/body/mind, and a marriage of that with inner silence, leading to an ongoing outpouring of divine love.

For an exploration of the possibilities, check the Secrets of Wilder. The unfoldment can vary from person to person, but the destination is the same.

Hint: As ecstatic conductivity advances, sambhavi becomes an increasing factor in stimulating sexual/spiritual energy.

The guru is in you.

2006/02/12 09:33:04
Tantra - Sex and Spiritual Development
http://www.aypsite.org/forum/topic.asp?TOPIC_ID=821&REPLY_ID=3275&whichpage=-1
some contradictory observations on orgasm!?

Hi Alvin:

The extra energy is an indication that the pre-orgasmic cultivation is outweighing the depletion after orgasm. This is disucussed here: http://www.aypsite.org/T46.html

It is beginning to work for you.

Now, if you add blocking, you will have another leg up in sexual energy management. Yes, I know it is troublesome at first. Clunky stage. You'll get over it. It is much easier than learning vajroli. More effective too, because you don't lose the semen to begin with, so don't have to suck it back up (a really silly macho application of vajroli).

Holdback combined with blocking eventually becomes natural vajroli -- unending automatic upward cultivation, as discussed here and elsewhere in the tantra lessons: http://www.aypsite.org/T30.html
As it advances, this is can be stimulated by sambhavi and/or kechari alone. That is the rise of ecstatic conductivity between head and root.

The secrets of our ecstatic neurobiology revealed and self-evident within us!

The guru is in you.

2006/02/12 14:05:11
Tantra - Sex and Spiritual Development
http://www.aypsite.org/forum/topic.asp?TOPIC_ID=821&REPLY_ID=3282&whichpage=-1
some contradictory observations on orgasm!?

Hi Alvin and Etherfish:

Actually, the bladder plays a key role in the circulation of sexual essences, which corresponds with the pranic flow. Every pranic flow has a neurobiological correspondence. Which is not to say we can always pin-point it, because as it refines it runs deep into the ecstatic realms and marries with pure bliss consciousness which underlies the whole process. Kind of hard to find the bladder, or any other body part, in there.

None of this is to say that we ought to be having lots of orgasms and blocking them up into the bladder. No. What happens is, over the course of our development on all fronts in yoga in relation to our normal life (including normal sexual activity redirected via tantric means), a very refined process develops which involves sexual essences being drawn up through multiple pathways -- the bladder being but one of them, the one most associated with spiritual arousal and flow of the subtle (or not so subtle) sexual essences. This applies to both women and men, though there are differences in method due to anatomy, of course.

After writing this morning, I thought of an analogy that might help with understanding the natural versus not-so-natural approaches that men take to this in relation to vajroli:

If we want to keep the horse in the barn, does it make sense to be letting the horse out of the barn and then devising complicated strategies (macho vajroli) for getting the horse back into the barn? Maybe it would be better to put a good latch on the barn (blocking) and then the problem is solved.

There are those who would say, "Don't go near the barn (abstention), and the horse won't be getting excited and trying to run out."

Maybe so, but that leaves the horse either irritated or asleep, neither of which is tantric or yogic. So we actively engage the horse, teaching it to be active in the barn. Then we find vast new directions the horse can run without ever leaving the barn. Well, am I taking this analogy too far? :-)

Remember, the definition of brahmacharya (from the AYP point of view) is both "preservation and cultivation of sexual energy." That is why we do the practices we do in AYP.

And yes, Alvin, a little inner experience goes a long way toward verifying what is being said here. Otherwise, we'd be wasting our time. Experience is the final arbiter in all of this, and enables us to proceed with confidence in self-directed practices.

For making more progress, you can also add mulabandha and/or asvini into the mix. Take your pick -- both are mainly in the anus/rectum in AYP and from there it naturally goes where it must.

The biggest stimulator of prana in the pelvic region is kumbhaka (breath retention as found in yoni mudra and chin pump), but I suggest you not take that on until you are very stable in everything that comes before. Spinal breathing has a more gentle kumbhaka effect, so that is the place to tackle it with breath first. Pranayama (restraint of breath) is the single greatest stimulant of ecstatic conductivity. When combined with siddhasana and mulabandha and followed by deep meditation, we can't miss over the long term. And that is without even considering tantric sex -- which makes a poor spiritual practice all by itself. There are too many other aspects that have to be addressed to achieve ecstatic conductivity. Tantric sex alone cannot do it. So don't get too carried away with the tantra thing. Keep your practices in balance.

And enjoy!

The guru is in you.

2006/05/25 12:20:57
Tantra - Sex and Spiritual Development
http://www.aypsite.org/forum/topic.asp?TOPIC_ID=1174&REPLY_ID=7314&whichpage=-1
Question about energy loss from orgasm
Yes, Kunsang, blocking reduces the loss, but it is not the whole answer. Neither is mechanical vajroli mudra of which blocking is but a simpler version (and more effective too). The change in the inner neurobiology to upward flowing over time covers the rest of it, and that is mainly a function of deep meditation, spinal breathing, and other sitting practices. That is when internal energy processing gets really efficient -- a natural function that eventually takes over for our crude efforts at priming the pump, so to speak. Then we have the whole body mudra, whole body ecstatic conductivity, and the whole enchilada. :-)

For more on this, see the new tantra book coming out in a few weeks. The ebook version should be up in a few days!

The guru is in you.

2006/06/02 20:46:43
Tantra - Sex and Spiritual Development
http://www.aypsite.org/forum/topic.asp?TOPIC_ID=1195&REPLY_ID=7715&whichpage=-1
PLEASE HELP SEMEN IN URINE

Hi Bindu:

Over the past few years, dozens of young men have emailed me with similar situations, and in the same panicky mode. The first thing to do is calm down and take a logical approach, like others here are wisely suggesting. The chances of you having a serious health problem are slim, but it is good to check things out with a doctor to be sure. Once you have done that, then you can move forward appropriately.

It is a very common thing for young men to think something is terribly wrong when normal sexual functions are exercising themselves to a surprising degree. It certainly does not help to be increasing and distorting the situation with excessive tantric practices. But this is not a fatal condition! You will recover.

Maybe just leave all the energy stimulation stuff alone for a while until things stabilize. Getting into deep meditation would be good, if you haven't already. Doing tantric sexual practices, and even aggressive pranayama, are getting the cart in front of the horse. Cultivating inner silence in deep meditation is the prerequisite for all of the energy-related practices in AYP. That means a stable routine of daily deep meditation well before any energy practices are undertaken. Without that, things can get a bit crazy. You have noticed this, yes?

So take a step back and do what is necessary to take care of business. Then you will be fine.

This is a classic example of why energy practices are not the best place to start on the spiritual path. But it's okay. Just back up, take a break, and when you feel ready to start again, take things in the right order. The AYP lessons can be helpful with that.

This would be a good time to be taking daily physical exercise, a heavier diet and other grounding practices. Engage fully in your regular activities in the world, and also get plenty of rest. See lesson 69 for some more suggestions. http://www.aypsite.org/69.html
You've got everything all jammed up down there, and grounding practices will help spread it out and dissipate it. Don't worry. This too shall pass...

The guru is in you.

2009/12/09 10:06:54
Tantra - Sex and Spiritual Development
http://www.aypsite.org/forum/topic.asp?TOPIC_ID=1195&REPLY_ID=61011&whichpage=-1
PLEASE HELP SEMEN IN URINE

quote:
————

So is this a normal part of the "natural vajroli" Yogani describes (i.e. semen starting to go up there even when you aren't having an orgasm) or is it something I should be concerned about?

_____

Yes, it's a sign of natural vajroli. Good things are happening.

Be sure to keep cultivating inner silence with daily deep meditation. :-)

The guru is in you.

2006/06/12 12:45:13
Tantra - Sex and Spiritual Development
http://www.aypsite.org/forum/topic.asp?TOPIC_ID=1210&REPLY_ID=7969&whichpage=-1
sex and the female

Hi Vicki:

The essence of tantric sex is simply relaxing in pre-orgasmic stimulation. This is the fundamental principle involved. It applies in relations with a partner, masturbation, and in structured sitting yoga practices -- the full range of them, beginning with deep meditation, spinal breathing, asanas, and expanding eventually into mudras, bandhas, kumbhaka, etc. In terms of effectiveness, tantric sexual methods fall into the latter category, after the global techniques of deep meditation and spinal breathing have been well-established. Before that, mudras, bandhas and tantric sex may be premature, which is not to say we should not learn them if so inclined. There are many doors leading in ... we just need to keep in mind that there is a certain natural sequencing in all of this that can yield optimal results.

As Scott mentions, yoga practices play a key role in opening up the nervous system to natural flows of energy in the body, which find their root in the sexual neurobiology. It is a matter of cultivating abiding inner silence, and then the rise of ecstatic conductivity. When these are occurring it then becomes obvious that there is an instantaneous ecstatic connection between head and root. That is when all of the mudras and bandhas, and tantric sex, are acting together in all parts of the body at the same time -- that is ecstatic conductivity riding on an undulating sea of silence. And then it all flows out into the world as divine love.

There is no one thing that will accomplish the "rise" of sexual energy all by itself. It takes a combination of methods. This is the truth of yoga and the enlightenment process. The "magic bullet" is many bullets. :-)

The new AYP Tantra book covers this in more detail for both sexes. Fittingly, it is called: "Tantra - Discovering the Power of Pre-Orgasmic Sex."

The dedication page includes a quote from the 4,000 year old *Vigyan Bhairava* scripture:

"At the start of sexual union, keep attention on the fire *In the beginning*, and, so continuing, avoid the embers in the end."

Though this knowledge has been around for a very long time, it has been difficult for humanity to grasp it. The reasons for this are covered in the book. It has to do with the evolution and maturation of our species, which is directly related to our over all spiritual progress. Maybe now is the time for us to collectively take the leap to the next level ... let's make it so.

Wishing you all the best!

The guru is in you.

2006/06/13 09:17:46
Tantra - Sex and Spiritual Development
http://www.aypsite.org/forum/topic.asp?TOPIC_ID=1210&REPLY_ID=8020&whichpage=-1
sex and the female

Hi Vicki:

Sounds like introducing your husband to sound tantric methods could be win-win all the way around. Your guru may not like it, but is your relationship with your husband really his business?

In fairness to your guru, he is pointing you rightly in the direction of preservation of your lifeforce. He just has not provided you with the alternatives for accomplishing that, some of which are compatible with marriage and an active sex life. Maybe he does not know. It is entirely possible. In not knowing the alternatives, spiritual teachers tend to offer their personal lifestyle as the preferable lifestyle for everyone, which is a mistake. There are many ways to skin the cat of enlightenment. The effective variations of tantric method -- whether conjugal, solo, or celibate -- illustrate the point. As long as the essential elements of preservation and cultivation of the ecstatic lifeforce are present, it is good management of sexual energy. This can be accomplished within any chosen lifestyle by dedicated practitioners.

The guru is in you.

2006/06/14 11:03:16
Tantra - Sex and Spiritual Development
http://www.aypsite.org/forum/topic.asp?TOPIC_ID=1214&REPLY_ID=8057&whichpage=-1
Resistance and hatred of tantra and spirit

Hi emc:

A belated welcome, and thank you for sharing. You have been getting some terrific suggestions here.

Let me add that it is our innate desire for evolution that moves us forward in consciousness. That impulse to grow is found in all of nature, yes? It is part of you, and me, and everyone. Well, maybe you want no part of it, but it is part of you, and here you are. :-)

The difference between not being aware and being aware of our spiritual possibilities is found in our ability in the latter case to apply certain methods that will accelerate the natural processes that are ever-expanding within us. It is evolution moving into high gear via our conscious participation.

If you do not feel the urge to participate consciously in the process, you should not force it. For now, you are compelled to deal with certain energy issues, and so on -- this thing that has stirred and is coming up inside you. But that does not mean you have to continue at such a fast rate. It is always your choice. While others can impact us to a greater or lesser degree, it is ultimately our decision. It is very important to understand this. If we think it is "happening to us" we will continue to be vulnerable and be blown around by the four winds within and around us.

In any case, the sooner you get in the driver's seat the better. Paradoxically, this is a surrender to who and what you are, and to what you can be... You will know what it is as it happens. Daily deep meditation is a good place to start. It opens us to the vast peace, energy and joyous creativity that has been hidden in us all along. From a base of rising inner silence, all that we have been talking about here becomes much easier...

Be careful and measured with the tendencies for purfication and opening you are finding in yourself (breath suspension, etc.) While such tendencies are signs of our spiritual potential, if we over-indulge them, they can eat us alive. "Automatic yoga," as we call it around here, is an indication of our possibilities, but cares not for our physical or mental well-being. That is why you hear so much about structured practice and self-pacing in AYP. If you have over-indulged, check AYP lesson 69 for some additional suggestions on how to stabilize things. The further you get into the lessons, the more on self-directed management of practices and experiences you will find. It goes with the territory.

Finally, you might find some comfort in knowing that there is agreement here with you on the fragility and temporary nature of earthly life, and this is precisely what makes life so special. What came before and comes after is mostly an unknown void. We are here with our awareness, tendencies, possibilities and some accumulated knowledge, and that is all we have to work with. Every moment we have in human form on this world is absolutely precious. The whole idea of yoga is to make the most of it -- experience the truth of it as much as we can ... we are all wired for that.

Wishing you the best on your path. Enjoy!

The guru is in you.

2006/06/16 12:03:19
Tantra - Sex and Spiritual Development
http://www.aypsite.org/forum/topic.asp?TOPIC_ID=1214&REPLY_ID=8118&whichpage=-1
Resistance and hatred of tantra and spirit

quote:
_____
Originally posted by emc

PS:

When I read some messages here in the thread I get energy reactions in my stomach. Is that good or bad? What does that mean?
_____

Hi emc:

It is your inner energy moving - purification. It is good as long as you keep in balance, and comfortable. Keep grounding (exercise, etc.) and limit your exposure to spiritual stimuli (including us!) as necessary to keep things on an even keel. Within that framework, a routine daily deep meditation would be desirable. That way you will be experiencing more abiding inner silence, and more tolerance to the ups and downs of life.

Don't become too much of a stranger here. We are really very nice -- just pretty stimulating sometimes. Welcome to the all-you-can-eat yoga-fest. Dine with care...

All the best!

The guru is in you.

2006/06/25 13:24:44
Tantra - Sex and Spiritual Development
http://www.aypsite.org/forum/topic.asp?TOPIC_ID=1243&REPLY_ID=8392&whichpage=-1
Victim of black magic

Hi All:

"Choice" is the key word in all of this -- what we choose for ourselves.

What do we do when we find ourselves in a situation we'd rather not be in? Do we stay and try to work it out, try and fight off whatever we think is after us, or do we just let it go and move on?

Of course, every situation is different. Often times, working things out or fighting things off can lead to endless complexity and entanglement. Maybe it is worth it if a loved one, dear friend, or our livelihood is at stake. It may be our karma to be in a hazardous environment long term for the sake of the greater good, or at least what we conceive that to be.

On the other hand, there will be times (lots of times) when ignorant forces accost us. Should we bargain with them, marshal an army of ideas and assistants to fend them off, or do we just hang up the phone when that pointless invasion of our life comes?

I mean, the kind of invasion being discussed here is pointless, isn't it? Why give it the time of day? Maybe we should delete this whole topic and be done with it. Poof! Gone.

I once had a powerful guru, or, rather, he thought he had me. It turned out his teachings, on balance, were not consistent with my beliefs or needs, so I decided to disassociate, to step back. But he refused, and cast one of those "You are mine forever!" spells on me. So, over the next year or so, I managed to ignore him, moving on to other things, and in the end he left me alone. He has since passed away. Now I can remember him fondly, and some of his teachings have been a help to AYP, while the rest have been let go.

The point of the story is that if we choose to let something go, and are willing to be consistent in our intention, we can do it. It may take some time for all the psychic hooks to be dissolved, but it can be done, and it is a guarantee of no further hooks, because we have developed the habit of having no attachment.

It is a lot like meditation. In fact, deep meditation builds our ability to let go of negative influences all around, because we learn to let go procedurally in favor of something much more life-supporting and joyful within us -- inner silence/pure bliss consciousness. As mentioned by others in this topic, meditation gradually builds our sense of self beyond all the ups and downs of life. Beyond all the ups and downs.

I know it may be hard to imagine ignoring something like an "evil spell." Yet, it is our attention that makes it stronger. It is like the religious sects that fear the devil so much that the devil becomes their religion. Why is it so hard to see that we can simply walk away and disassociate ourselves from such foolish things?

Well, it will be good to meditate twice daily and work on that over the long haul, along with all the rest we are doing to improve the quality and depth of our life. Fighting devils, demons and evil spells makes for great drama, but doesn't contribute much to our spiritual growth.

Keep in mind that the poisonous snake on the ground there is not a snake at all, only a rope that we have mistakenly identified as a snake, and chosen to make a big drama of.

Suggestion: Favor the practice (the yoga one) over the scenery, no matter how good or bad that scenery is. It is your choice to make...

Just some food for thought.

The guru is in you.

2006/06/25 16:44:19
Tantra - Sex and Spiritual Development
http://www.aypsite.org/forum/topic.asp?TOPIC_ID=1243&REPLY_ID=8405&whichpage=-1
Victim of black magic
Whatever we believe will be true for us in the moment, but whether it is "the truth" or not is another question entirely.

The former is an easy seduction we are all prone to fall into. The latter is a much deeper question that transcends all beliefs, institutions and events, and our physical existence itself...

2006/07/11 11:35:11
Tantra - Sex and Spiritual Development
http://www.aypsite.org/forum/topic.asp?TOPIC_ID=1314&REPLY_ID=9239&whichpage=-1
Amrit / Nectar - Experiences and/or Effects?

Hi All:

These two lessons review the "nectar" cycle within the context of practices and the over all journey:

http://www.aypsite.org/51.html
http://www.aypsite.org/133.html

All the best!

The guru is in you.

2006/09/29 12:23:45
Tantra - Sex and Spiritual Development
http://www.aypsite.org/forum/topic.asp?TOPIC_ID=1553&REPLY_ID=11706&whichpage=-1
porn ?

quote:
_____
Originally posted by paw

I gather from reading "Secrets of Wilder" and "AYP", as well as this forum, that masturbating and tantric partner sex are ok, and sex outside of matrimony is ok too. That is, in AYP there doesn't seem to be any condemnation for those yogis who have sex, or who have sex in "nontraditional" partnerships or methods. I'm trying to understand this, but it's confusing cuz of my lifelong reading of yoga texts that recommend brahmacharya and sannyas (like SRF etc.), or which recommend the householder path of monogamous marriage with sexuality de-emphasized (like Hamsa Yoga Sangh). I gather that Indian society, for example, is sexually conservative, with many no-nos.

Of course, in Xtian USA sex is repressive, with much sexuality equated with "sin".

But then I have read books by Muktananda and Brother Charles that seem to endorse hetero- and homosexual acts outside marriage. Also, Osho is unconcerned with marital status, etc.

Thus my confusion. So I am wondering, is viewing pornographic images also acceptable for yogis? How would viewing porn relate to samyamas and "virtues"?
_____

Hi Paw:

AYP is flexible on lifestyle, sexual or otherwise (nudged persistently higher by yogic and tantric methods), but points to our responsibility regarding conduct that may injure others. That includes lovers, spouses, children (especially), or anyone we happen to be affecting by our actions. Also, the laws of the society we live in should be honored...

Until we have natural **ahimsa** (non-harming) born of inner silence that comes from deep meditation and other spiritual practices, we should at least be aware of the profound value of non-harming. There is great truth in the Biblical injunctions, "Do unto others as you would have them do unto you..." and "Love thy neighbor as thy self."

On "sin," check this AYP lesson for some additional thoughts: http://www.aypsite.org/132.html

Also, here is a lesson on pornography and compulsive behaviors: http://www.aypsite.org/T38.html

The guru is in you.

2006/09/29 15:09:25
Tantra - Sex and Spiritual Development
http://www.aypsite.org/forum/topic.asp?TOPIC_ID=1553&REPLY_ID=11716&whichpage=-1
porn ?

quote:
_____
Originally posted by nearoanoke

Hi Paw, I dont see a link where AYP writings or forums say its OK to have extra-marital sex.
_____

Hi Near and Paw:

I don't know where AYP says that either. :-)
Pre-marital maybe in the Secrets of Wilder novel, but that depends on your definition of marriage. While the novel is very sexy (and eventually quite graphic), it is also very moral. In the process of being morally sexy, it reveals the essential principles of tantric relationship -- the most important being the emergence of bhakti-inspired divine love.

Near, thanks for reminding me about this lesson covering the relationship of sexual fantasies, tantra and extra-marital affairs:
http://www.aypsite.org/T37.html
This link can also be found in the pornography/compulsive behavior lesson referenced above.

The point is, whatever we are doing, whatever our current habit is, it can be turned higher with bhakti and yogic/tantric methods. And no matter what we are doing, we are always responsible for the effects of our actions. What we do to others, we are doing to ourselves. And what we do to ourselves, we are doing to others. We are One.

The guru is in you.

2006/10/09 11:06:24
Tantra - Sex and Spiritual Development
http://www.aypsite.org/forum/topic.asp?TOPIC_ID=1586&REPLY_ID=12121&whichpage=-1
Tantra practice effects?

Hi All:

There is a funny scene (biting satire actually) on the Caduceus in the Secrets of Wilder novel, when John Wilder is being "rescued" from a hospital (how he got in there is another story).

Here is Devi (John's sweetheart) telling it like it is (one of her endearing traits) as she and big Luke are sneaking a very drugged John out of the hospital:

...It was the dead of night, and all was quiet in the hospital. Devi pulled out the I.V. The colorless chemicals dripped slowly out onto the floor. She and Luke got John dressed in his suit pants, white shirt and shiny black shoes left over from the funeral. Soon they were walking out as casually as they could with John in the wheelchair. His head was bobbing on his chest and he was mumbling incoherently. They made it past the nurse's station, down the elevator, and were on the home stretch through the main lobby. On the wall was a big Caduceus, the symbol of the medical profession, a staff with two snakes spiraling up it, biting the wings of an orb on top.

John's head bobbed up. A look of recognition lit him up.
"Thaaaat's meeeeee!" he yelled, pointing at the Caduceus. "Thaaaat's meeeeee!"
"Shhhh," Devi said as they hurried for the front door. Luke led the way, looking a little nervous, as Devi pushed the wheelchair behind him.
"Thaaaat's meeeeee!" John yelled. His arms were reaching back over his shoulder for the Caduceus as they went.
"Yeah, right," Devi said. "These people around here wouldn't know a real Caduceus if it came up and bit them in the ass."

Only a night janitor saw the huge black man and feisty little Indian beauty wheeling the raving lunatic out the front door of the hospital. He watched until they went around the corner of the building, off into the night. He shrugged and went back to his mopping.

I couldn't resist. Oh, and you are definitely not seeing John Wilder at his best here. :-)

There is hope for the medical profession. They are discovering their roots -- slowly -- maybe we are helping.

Also, see these lessons on the Caduceus, sushumna, ida, pingala, and the ecstatic illumination of them:

http://www.aypsite.org/89.html
http://www.aypsite.org/90.html

Good stuff you are sharing, Shanti, on orgasm in relation to the rise of ecstatic conductivity. And great feedback everyone!

The guru is in you.

2006/10/09 11:37:12
Tantra - Sex and Spiritual Development
http://www.aypsite.org/forum/topic.asp?TOPIC_ID=1586&REPLY_ID=12122&whichpage=-1
Tantra practice effects?

Hi again All:

Here are some comments from one of my emails related to Shanti's experience:

There comes a point where whole body orgasm is energizing on the upper end, while at the same time depleting on the lower end. The latter will eventually take over if the strategy goes to more and more orgasms. And, of course, orgasm is a lousy strategy for anyone who has not awakened ecstatic conductivity, which is the key to it.

Is ecstatic-conductivity based orgasm draining or invigorating? Well, both, I think, as is nearly any kundalini surge. So, it is an aspect of tantric practice. But pre-enlightenment. I say this because enlightenment is advancing when the ecstatic merges with inner silence and they move outward together into daily activity, progressing toward the unity state via action. That is ecstatic action moving in stillness, or what I call "stillness in action." The enlightenment paradox!

It is the evolution of the surges into a steady-state flow...

The inner whole-body orgasms are a stepping stone to this. It is all about divine energy purifying and developing the body as a channel into the world. Even reproductive sex is about that, isn't it? The divine projecting itself into the world via reproduction. In yoga it is the same, except it is the divine taking conscious birth in/as the yogi/yogini, and projecting into the world in that way as outpouring divine love.

At first we notice it in bits. Then it is all we notice -- the "gee whiz" stage where we are reminded to favor practices over experiences. In the end, we barely notice it at all -- we just act in that way naturally, and that is life.

Interestingly, some of the upcoming E-Series books will also be stepping through the evolutionary process just described -- samyama, self-inquiry and bhakti/karma yoga. All of these are about taking inner silence and ecstatic bliss (inner orgasmic feelings) out into daily living by various means. Multi-pronged practice, of course, which is the secret of success in yoga.

I would only caution that we not give the impression here that having lots of orgasms is going to be the path. We all know where that leads. It really depends on ecstatic conductivity being present. A good incentive to develop ecstatic conductivity, yes? And, in turn, for developing inner silence, which is the true foundation of ecstatic conductivity and all spiritual progress.

While, at a certain stage, orgasms may add to ecstatic conductivity, brahmacharya remains the underlying tantric principle from start to finish -- that is, preservation and cultivation of sexual energy. There are many aspects to this, and varying approaches to implementation depending on the wide range of sexual preferences among practitioners.

The guru is in you.

2006/11/02 11:35:22
Tantra - Sex and Spiritual Development
http://www.aypsite.org/forum/topic.asp?TOPIC_ID=1659&REPLY_ID=12833&whichpage=-1
tantra book and questions

Hi MathewC:

Thank you for your courageous sharing.

The methods of holdback, blocking and count will aid in reducing the tendency toward premature ejaculation (and wet dreams) over time.

Of course, sexual preferences and limits (or excesses) in opportunity for sexual activity are in the realm of the individual. The principles and practices of tantra will work in just about any sexual lifestyle. This is the approach in AYP tantra -- offering means that can be blended into any sexual situation without pressing for any particular lifestyle change. There is wide latitude for anyone to apply the principles and means with good effect. It is in the hands of the practitioner.

It should also be mentioned that external sexual activity is not a prerequisite for progress in applying tantric principles. There is also the broad field of pranayama, mudras, bandhas and asanas like siddhasana, which can be used for achieving the same end -- ecstatic conductivity. Siddhasana is especially tantric, and I have gone so far as to label it "the best tantric practice" (see lesson T16). Over time, it too will aid in reducing the tendency toward premature ejaculation. So, we don't have to have a particular level of external sexual activity to advance in tantra. It can all be done by internal yogic means as well. There are multiple ways to skin the cat, which can be applied according to individual preferences and situations. Take your pick, or use them all. :-)

The Tantra book is a much tighter presentation of all we have discussed on the subject in the online lessons and AYP Easy Lessons book. It was written primarily to provide a clear doorway into integrated yoga practices via the sexual channel for the many who are interested in "spiritual sex," yet not necessarily drawn to yoga initially. Of course, tantra and yoga cannot be separated -- they are mirror images of each other. And, true to form, the Tantra book is currently the best selling AYP book!

All the best on your path. Gentle persistence will pay off over time. Practice wisely, don't sweat the inconveniences, and enjoy!

The guru is in you.

2006/12/10 14:01:28
Tantra - Sex and Spiritual Development
http://www.aypsite.org/forum/topic.asp?TOPIC_ID=1811
Vajroli
From a recent email exchange:

Q: When an ecstatic conductive state in the nervous system is created either through tantric practice (non-ejaculate) or kechari activity and semen is discharged some time later (could be hours or days later) through the bladder as seen in the urine.

I have heard 2 things, (1) that the subtle energy has already been taken up by the nervous system and transformed into its refined state or (2) that the discharge is of no real consequence or the other point of view is that it is an important loss and to be avoided.

Can you comment from your understanding, both directly as experienced in your own body as well as what do the best (true authentic, based on reality) teachings have to say about it?

I should say thirdly, could it be that it is far far better than an actual ejaculation to discharge in the urine, because in my case there appears to be a great benefit to rouse the pre-orgasmic energies for meditative purposes.

I believe I have been experiencing the upper semen as Shiva refers to it, which is then showering the cells and nervous system with soma.

Especially since being blessed with the unfoldment of Kechari along with regular yogic practice.

Feel free to share the email anonymously as I think it is an important question, although it is not unlikely that you have covered it already, I have not found much anywhere on this important topic.

A: I believe this lesson covers it:

http://www.aypsite.org/T30.html

There is also a clarifying addition to the corresponding lesson in the AYP Easy Lessons book. It is covered in the little Tantra book also.

As the spiritual neurobiology advances and matures, so does the processing occurring within the bladder itself, as well as the process of drawing semen up into it. It becomes an automatic 24 hour process, directly related to the rise of ecstatic conductivity. All of the practices we are using (beginning with deep meditation) contribute to the evolution of this higher biology. Directing semen into the bladder alone will not promote the expansion of sexual function upward -- a common misunderstanding. Neither will celibacy alone. It takes an integration of practices over time to achieve the result.

It is experiential here. In the past I have read many sources on the subject -- yogic, tantric and taoist. While there is the greatest respect here for Svatmarama's Hatha Yoga Pradipika, I believe it is off the beam on vajroli, and this has led to poor understanding and misguided practice in this important area. AYP attempts to clear it up. A sound strategy for keeping the horse in the barn (holdback and blocking combined with a full range of yoga practices) is far superior to a strategy for getting the already escaped horse back into the barn (external vajroli).

You are on the right track. It takes time...

All the best!

The guru is in you.

2006/12/24 14:50:09
Tantra - Sex and Spiritual Development
http://www.aypsite.org/forum/topic.asp?TOPIC_ID=1820&REPLY_ID=14820&whichpage=-1
Immaculate conception and tantra

Hi All:

Please do continue this interesting discussion on Immaculate Conception and Tantra here, and the discussion on Kabbalah, Gnosticism and Christianity (which has just been split off) over here: http://www.aypsite.org/forum/topic.asp?TOPIC_ID=1848

Admittedly, there is some overlap, but I know everyone will do their best to maintain the appropriate distinctions between topics ... and civility, of course. :-)

The guru is in you.

2007/01/02 18:14:25
Tantra - Sex and Spiritual Development
http://www.aypsite.org/forum/topic.asp?TOPIC_ID=1875&REPLY_ID=15304&whichpage=-1
Transgender/Body Questions

Hi Sylvic and All:

In case you have not run across it so far, here is an AYP lesson on homosexuality and other matters: http://www.aypsite.org/T39.html

I think the spirit of the lesson is applicable when considering the transgender question, as well. There is no judgment about such matters in AYP.

We are looking to expand sexual energy to support the permanent rise of ecstatic conductivity in the body. This is beyond gender, and the variations in the gender-specific mechanics and neurobiology of it are very small. From the standpoint of yoga, we all have equal opportunity for spiritual development, including in tantra.

Of course, it all rides on inner silence, so it is good to be engaged in daily deep meditation before tackling tantra. While AYP is not gender or lifestyle specific, it is very inner silence specific. :-)

Along with the rise of inner silence comes ahimsa (non-harming) and other divine qualities radiating from within. Over time, these will temper obsessive conduct issues that might be present in sexual and other kinds of relations. This includes our relationship with ourself, which is the most important one -- everything else we do in life emanates from that.

Wishing you all the best on your chosen path. Enjoy!

The guru is in you.

2007/01/03 16:53:08
Tantra - Sex and Spiritual Development
http://www.aypsite.org/forum/topic.asp?TOPIC_ID=1875&REPLY_ID=15350&whichpage=-1
Transgender/Body Questions

quote:
_____
Originally posted by emc

quote:
_____
Yogani: We are looking to expand sexual energy to support the permanent rise of ecstatic conductivity in the body. This is beyond gender, and the variations in the gender-specific mechanics and neurobiology of it are very small.
_____

This is a bit difficult to understand from reading spiritual literature where the duality of male-female, yin-yang, fire-water is occurring frequently. The taoists describe the two energy qualities quite in detail, the tantrics as well. I am only glad to get to know more about the androgynity of energies. =)
_____

Hi EMC:

That does not mean the inner energy flow involved in ecstatic conductivity itself is genderless -- it is traditionally viewed as feminine -- kundalini shakti. But the cultivation of it by the yogi or yogini is not gender or lifestyle specific. That is what I meant by "beyond gender." The practices don't vary much between genders. Nor does external sexual lifestyle make a difference. The kundalini effect itself is beyond those distinctions.

The corresponding internal masculine pole is shiva, inner silence, cultivated largely in deep meditation. Inner silence merged with ecstatic conductivity/radiance gives birth to the divine child within us -- jivan mukti, christ consciousness, outpouring divine love through us, etc. That is where genders melt to Oneness from a spiritual point of view. Even so, the inner lovemaking of stillness and ecstasy never stops! :-)

On the physical level, pre-orgasmic cultivation of sexual energy is essentially the same act for all of us, leading to the same result -- permanent inner lovemaking.

Internally we are all both divine masculine (stillness) and divine feminine (ecstasy), increasingly engaged in spontaneous inner lovemaking as we move toward advanced stages of yoga/tantra. Whatever our external gender or sexual orientation is, the inner mechanics of spiritual development will be the same. Our nervous systems are wired that way.

Viewed from that grand divine perspective, the external labels really are unimportant. That is what Ram Dass is talking about.

The guru is in you.

2007/02/25 12:21:05
Tantra - Sex and Spiritual Development
http://www.aypsite.org/forum/topic.asp?TOPIC_ID=2119&REPLY_ID=18090&whichpage=-1
Blocking problem

Hi Joti and welcome!

As far as I know, blood in the semen is not usual in using the blocking technique. Others may have thoughts on this. Everyone is different. It is possible for blocking to cause some strain in the beginning, with various symptoms.

Sounds like there could be some strain going on there. Whenever we have strain or discomfort (or symptoms of same) occuring in any practice we are doing in AYP, we self-pace the practice. That means backing off part or all the way until things stabilize, which you have done. It is wise. Then we can inch our way back to a level of practice that is comfortable for us when we feel ready, which you also seem to be doing. That is the way to proceed.

Blocking is actually an interim technique used on the way to automatic internal vajroli (sexual essences rising naturally and continuously with the rise of whole body ecstatic conductivity), which is cultivated by a variety of pre-orgasmic stimulation and other yogic methods covered in both the tantra and main lessons.

In time, the course of that mighty river of reproductive sex can be expanded upward, and there will be much less strain then. But it doesn't happen overnight, and patience and gentle persuasion are necessary over the long term. Self-pacing is part of this.

Perhaps you are having some clunkiness at this stage. It will pass. I suggest you continue to back off in times of strain. And work on increasing the ability to stay in front of orgasm -- holdback technique. With that, you will need blocking less often and the ecstatic results will improve also. As you know, daily sitting practices are an essential part of this process.

An alternative you may wish to investigate is Jack Johnston's multiple orgasm trigger method, which some here have found helpful for reducing ejaculation, and also the need for blocking.

Finally, if you think there might be any health issues involved, it is good to check with a doctor.

Wishing you all the best on your path. Practice wisely and enjoy!

The guru is in you.

2007/03/07 12:20:48
Tantra - Sex and Spiritual Development
http://www.aypsite.org/forum/topic.asp?TOPIC_ID=2119&REPLY_ID=18469&whichpage=-1
Blocking problem

Hi Joti:

Your question is covered in lesson 30 on vajroli mentioned above. There is also an addition to the lesson in the AYP Easy Lessons book.

There is a shift in the neurobiology that leads to natural absorption of sexual essences upward in the body, including through the bladder. It is the semen or white milky substance in both men and women that goes upward. All indications are that sperm itself plays little to no role in this process (see here).

With ecstatic conductivity rising, the milkiness in the urine will disappear (be absorbed in the bladder) within a few hours after blocking. Natural vajroli can be so dynamic during the developmental stage of ecstatic conductivity that some milkiness can appear in the urine without genital orgasm or blocking having been engaged in. This too passes as the neurobiology of ecstatic conductivity becomes more efficient.

Sitting practices (deep meditation, spinal breathing pranayama, etc.) are the primary means by which this transformation is cultivated, with tantric sexual methods being an important support. The process of transformation will happen with sitting practices alone, but is very unlikely to happen with tantric sexual methods alone. This is a main point brought out in the AYP Tantra book, and is why we don't force the issue with tantric sexual practices -- it won't help us much and can lead to strain in the sexual biology. We just gently favor sound tantric methods in our normal sex life as a support to our sitting practices. Gentle persuasion. The synergy between sitting practices and tantric sexual methods can be very good that way.

Our bhakti (spiritual desire) will lead the way in all of this, and prudent self-pacing will keep us from overdoing too much. It looks like you are getting a handle on it.

All the best!

The guru is in you.

2007/03/12 13:58:36
Tantra - Sex and Spiritual Development
http://www.aypsite.org/forum/topic.asp?TOPIC_ID=2229&REPLY_ID=18734&whichpage=-1
lightheadedness and orgasm

Hi Babaly and Chard:

You are both asking essentially the same question (here is the other).

Paraphrasing both questions:
What to do with all this extra sexual energy that can overwhelm me to the point of fainting, or knock me off center for a month if I release it in orgasm?

If the energy build-up is related to spiritual practices (apparently so), then the excess can be regarded as the purification process getting ahead of itself. Too much energy without sufficient opening of neurobiological channels in the body for it to flow freely through the nervous system to express as increasing ecstatic conductivity and radiance. No doubt some of the conductivity and radiance is occurring already, but there is much more, and the energy is welling up and banging into the present limitations.

In the case of a man, venting the energy occasionally in orgasm can help, along with self-pacing in practices, applying grounding methods, and so on. It is the same as kundalini symptom management.

Self-pacing and grounding methods will apply in the woman's case also -- reducing the upward energy flow until a stable balance between energy flow and the ability to conduct the energy is reached. This means backing off on stimulative techniques like mudras, bandhas, siddhasana, kumbhaka, etc. Self-pacing could also involve temporarily backing off on meditation and spinal breathing, if the upsurge is there with only those practices. And applying the grounding methods, of course. You have to find out by experiementing with all of these means.

What seems different here is the lesser role the "pressure relief valve" orgasm approach seems to have. In fact, it may take a woman in the other direction in terms of excess energy. Not being a woman, I do not have an answer for that. Perhaps other women who have been through this can chime in. Does female orgasm relieve excess energy in the nervous system, or increase it? (In some cases it does relieve it -- but apparently not in all cases.) In cases where it increases it, then how does an advancing yogini handle the excesses?

Whatever the answer to that may be, it will be good to emphasize that this is an aspect of purification and opening going on, and, as with all such openings, the adverse symptoms will pass as purification advances and a higher manifestation of the energy emerges. In the meantime, it is a matter of self-pacing and managing the excesses in whatever ways we can, while continuing forward with our process of purification and opening.

If the energies can be brought into balance, one would think normal sexual relations would be possible according to one's desire, and even doing so tantrically. How this situation relates to engaging in tantric sexual methods is another question. Maybe this can be one of those "for the ladies" discussions from which we all can learn. :-)

All the best!

The guru is in you.

2007/03/12 13:53:23
Tantra - Sex and Spiritual Development
http://www.aypsite.org/forum/topic.asp?TOPIC_ID=2230&REPLY_ID=18733&whichpage=-1
what to do with all this energy?

Hi Babaly and Chard:

You are both asking essentially the same question (here is the other).

Paraphrasing both questions:
What to do with all this extra sexual energy that can overwhelm me to the point of fainting, or knock me off center for a month if I release it in orgasm?

If the energy build-up is related to spiritual practices (apparently so), then the excess can be regarded as the purification process getting ahead of itself. Too much energy without sufficient opening of neurobiological channels in the body for it to flow freely through the nervous system to express as increasing ecstatic conductivity and radiance. No doubt some of the conductivity and radiance is occurring already, but there is <u>much more</u>, and the energy is welling up and banging into the present limitations.

In the case of a man, venting the energy occasionally in orgasm can help, along with self-pacing in practices, applying grounding methods, and so on. It is the same as kundalini symptom management.

Self-pacing and grounding methods will apply in the woman's case also -- reducing the upward energy flow until a stable balance between energy flow and the ability to conduct the energy is reached. This means backing off on stimulative techniques like mudras, bandhas, siddhasana, kumbhaka, etc. Self-pacing could also involve temporarily backing off on meditation and spinal breathing, if the upsurge is there with only those practices. And applying the grounding methods, of course. You have to find out by experiementing with all of these means.

What seems different here is the lesser role the "pressure relief valve" orgasm approach seems to have. In fact, it may take a woman in the other direction in terms of excess energy. Not being a woman, I do not have an answer for that. Perhaps other women who have been through this can chime in. Does female orgasm relieve excess energy in the nervous system, or increase it? (In some cases it does relieve it   but apparently not in all cases.) In cases where it increases it, then how does an advancing yogini handle the excesses?

Whatever the answer to that may be, it will be good to emphasize that this is an aspect of purification and opening going on, and, as with all such openings, the adverse symptoms will pass as purification advances and a higher manifestation of the energy emerges. In the meantime, it is a matter of self-pacing and managing the excesses in whatever ways we can, while continuing forward with our process of purification and opening.

If the energies can be brought into balance, one would think normal sexual relations would be possible according to one's desire, and even doing so tantrically. How this situation relates to engaging in tantric sexual methods is another question. Maybe this can be one of those "for the ladies" discussions from which we all can learn. :-)

All the best!

The guru is in you.

2007/03/27 11:51:42
Tantra - Sex and Spiritual Development
http://www.aypsite.org/forum/topic.asp?TOPIC_ID=2345&REPLY_ID=19482&whichpage=-1
What goes up the spine?

quote:
_____
Originally posted by Blue Opal

A Question for Yogani.

I have no semen. What is it that goes into and up my spine? :(
_____

Hi Blue Opal:

I took the liberty of moving your inquiry over here to the tantra forum.

If you are asking how it works for a woman (I'm assuming that, and apologies if this is incorrect), there is a function in the G-Spot (sometimes called the "female prostate") which produces a milky substance which enters the urthrea, and acts in the process of spiritual transformation in the same way semen does in a man. This is the same substance involved in "female ejaculation."

This spiritual process is discussed from the male point of view in the lesson on vajroli: http://www.aypsite.org/T30.html
...also there is some discussion on the process in the woman in this lesson on the evolution of spiritual biology: http://www.aypsite.com/T11.html

...and it is mentioned in this forum posting as well, and perhaps elsewhere in the forums:
http://www.aypsite.org/forum/topic.asp?TOPIC_ID=388#310

Based on private input received from a number of women over the years, the assumption is that the process described in the lessons is what happens in both men and women, including confirmation of a visible milky substance found in the urine at times, due to the ramping up of the ongoing processing of sexual essences. As the process advances with the rise of ecstatic conductivity and radiance, the substance is fully absorbed upward. Higher processing related to this also occurs in the GI tract, which is discussed here: http://www.aypsite.com/51.html

So it isn't only about essences going up the spine, which they do. As a result of our practices, the neurobiology is evolving in many ways within us to support our spiritual transformation.

Further confirmations (or contradictions) on this process are welcome from those who aren't shy about it. All for the cause of advancing applied yoga science. :-)

The guru is in you.

2007/03/27 16:36:00
Tantra - Sex and Spiritual Development
http://www.aypsite.org/forum/topic.asp?TOPIC_ID=2345&REPLY_ID=19500&whichpage=-1
What goes up the spine?

Hi Blue Opal:

Perceptible activity in the pelvic region is not a prerequisite for energy experiences anywhere else in the body. The neurobiology of it can be quite beneath the surface. Such is the case with inner visions and sounds like you describe. And even ecstatic experiences higher up in the body can be quite separate from sexual content. But all of these things find their root (literally) in the pranic storehouse located in the pelvic region. It isn't aways labeled "sexual." It does not have to be. However, the inner mechanics are the same. The spinal nerve (sushumna) goes from perinenum to head and all that happens in there is connected. Plus, every cell and nerve in our body is directly affected by what is happening in the spinal nerve.

As for yoga happening "without practices (meditation)," I'm not sure that yogic progress will. But experiences certainly can, since these are energy movements inside that can happen for a variety of reasons, and are not necessarily indicative of yogic progress occurring. For example, one can be psychic for all their life without progressing one iota in yoga. Yoga is about ongoing transformation (union), and does not happen without some sort of intention by the person involved. Residual symptoms (or gifts) can be the result of our past intentions and actions (maybe forgotten), leading sometimes to the cry, "Why me?!" :-)

Keep in mind that devotion alone (including sincere inquiry) constitutes practice, leading to meditation and other yogic activity. To whatever extent you are emotionally involved with your spiritual development, there is practice occurring. It is called "bhakti." Any sort of longing to know, evolve, or become will result in "yoga."

Also, the focusing of attention within the body is an aspect of practice, and you are seeing cause and effect in that, yes? In AYP we are very specific with the placing of attention in practices, in spinal breathing pranayama in particular. The thing is to do it systematically in conjunction with the cultivation of inner silence via deep meditation. Otherwise things can get out of kilter energy-wise, especially if kundalini is active already, which yours seems to be.

The pain, blue light, inner sounds, ecstatic currents, movements, etc. are likely kundalini symptoms. Kundalini symptoms alone do not necessarily imply ongoing progress in yoga. For progress, we have to steadily move beyond all that through some sort of consistent and effective practice. Here are a few lessons that might help:
Kundalini symptoms & remedies: http://www.aypsite.org/69.html
Blue light (and star): http://www.aypsite.com/92.html
Movements: http://www.aypsite.com/183.html
Deep meditation: http://www.aypsite.com/13.html
Spinal breathing pranayama: http://www.aypsite.com/41.html
Devotion/Bhakti: http://www.aypsite.com/67.html

There are more lessons on these things in the topic index: http://www.aypsite.org/TopicIndex.html

Perhaps if you share some of your history, more light can be shed on what is going on. If you have done so already elsewhere here, just provide a link.

It would be good if you can get into a steady routine of practice of your choosing that will provide some safe regulation of your inner energies and also cultivate inner silence and the refinement of your experiences in a progressive way. Without some sort of systematic daily approach, you might be relating to the present energy patterns as they are for an unnecessarily long time.

By the way, it is not about what is in the books. It is about what is going on in us. You are the book. :-)

Just some food for thought. All the best!

The guru is in you.

2009/09/20 15:09:04
Tantra - Sex and Spiritual Development
http://www.aypsite.org/forum/topic.asp?TOPIC_ID=2345&REPLY_ID=57238&whichpage=-1
What goes up the spine?

Hi Gumpi:

You seem to be misunderstanding the expansion of sexual function in the process of human spiritual transformation, including the reasons for brahmacharya, tantric sexual methods, and the rise of natural vajroli.

Saying it isn't so doesn't make it not so.

Perhaps review this topic for further perspective: http://www.aypsite.org/forum/topic.asp?TOPIC_ID=6326

It is not as cut and dry as you imply. As sexual essences rise, they are sublimated in various ways and function on many levels in the neurobiology. This is not a matter that can be resolved through intellectual debate. It is a matter of direct experience. It is also a matter for scientific research.

As for restraint of breath (pranayama), up to and including suspension of breath (kumbhaka), the knowledge is ancient that it stimulates a body-wide pranic awakening rooted in the pelvic region -- kundalini/ecstatic conductivity. Many of the AYP techniques involve this principle, either deliberately or spontaneously. Someday science will resolve whether or not oxygen intake reduction stimulates the pranic awakening in the pelvic region, and how this relates to the rise of sexual essences via natural vajroli. Until then, anyone can find out for themselves through the use of yoga practices.

The guru is in you.

2009/09/21 07:05:13
Tantra - Sex and Spiritual Development
http://www.aypsite.org/forum/topic.asp?TOPIC_ID=2345&REPLY_ID=57281&whichpage=-1
What goes up the spine?
PS: It should be clarified that the reduction of oxygen intake through pranayama does not directly produce a physical upward "vacuuming" of prana from the pelvic region. Rather, it is a biochemical drawing up, similar to how a food fast stimulates the drawing of nutrients from the fatty tissues of the body. In both cases, there is inner purification and opening, which is why both fasting and pranayama are regarded to be spiritual techniques.

Paramahansa Yogananda asserted that pranayama "purifies the blood" by removing excess carbon. This would be the other side of the same dynamic -- reducing oxygen intake via pranayama would increase carbon dioxide concentration in the blood, and perhaps the subsequent (biochemical) drawing of prana from the pelvic region stabilizes this: Thus, "reducing carbon in the blood." Science will have to answer that one. I can't. Perhaps Yogananda felt it would be less controversial to describe the effects of pranayama as a purification of the blood, rather than a deprivation of oxygen leading to a pranic awakening. The truth is that these explanations are two sides of the same dynamic occurring during pranayama. Either way it is viewed, the beneficial effects of pranayama are well known. We don't have to know all the inner workings of the machine to put it to good use. The actual internal workings will finally be revealed by scientific research, not in intellectual debates that can go on forever. The important thing is that we are practicing daily and gaining the good results.

Natural vajroli is a physical ("vacuuming") process in part, but is a subsequent step after the biochemical drawing up has occurred as it relates to pranayama. Brahmacharya, tantric sex, and hatha yoga methods (mudras, bandhas, etc) also have roles in cultivating natural vajroli, which is more on the physical side of it. It has never been claimed in AYP that pranayama directly produces a physical vacuuming effect. Pranayama produces a biochemical effect as described above. This is true of positive pressure (internal) or neutral pressure (passive) kumbhaka (breath suspension) also.

Negative pressure (external) kumbhaka may be considered to produce a physical vacuuming effect, though such a physical effect may be regarded to be less significant than the biochemical (oxygen reduction) effect. It is another question for science. Extensive use of external (negative lung pressure) kumbhaka is not recommended in AYP, because over time it may have an adverse effect on the health of the lungs. We only use it for brief periods in uddiyana bandha and nauli. It may also occur spontaneously during deep meditation from time to time.

2009/09/21 11:38:46
Tantra - Sex and Spiritual Development
http://www.aypsite.org/forum/topic.asp?TOPIC_ID=2345&REPLY_ID=57299&whichpage=-1
What goes up the spine?

quote:
_____
Originally posted by manig

When I am in Shirsasana... I can feel the prana/energy (or semen?) being sucked from my testicles and going downwards into the head (via bladder?). The testicles feel like a fruit getting its pulp sucked out (it wobbles physically). My breathing also stops before/during this (the belly is already inwards) and the vaccum feeling can also be felt because of this.

However it does not feel like I would die out of oxygen... I am neither out of breath when its over. I rather feel stronger.

Now that I am going through the AYP chapters one by one. I understand that Pranayama, Siddhasana, Kumbhaka, Moolbandha, Vajroli, Shambhavi and many many other asanas, bandhas, mudras happen automatically to me.

I remember the last few times (several months ago) when I had sex, I would go into Shambhavi automatically and it would extend the pleasure and prevent ejacluation.

As you have said in your Eight limbs of yoga book... I realise it was all in the nervous system. Earlier I thought I was possessed by some spirit who was doing all this to me. I still can't fully believe that its all in my nervous system and that I am not possesed. I went to a few Exorcists few years ago but they all said I was not possessed. But I did not believe them and still had a doubt.

_____

Hi Manig:

Yes, inversion postures have this physical effect in the pelvic region also. Asanas, mudras and bandhas help stimulate the awakening of whole body ecstatic conductivity in many interconnected ways.

The reason you do not feel oxygen-deprived during kumbhaka (breath suspension) is because the awakening inner prana is compensating. Be careful about overdoing this. It can lead to excessive purification and imbalance, with recovery time being necessary. In this way, going too fast can slow us down as we overdo, wait to recover, overdo, wait to recover, etc. Much faster (and comfortable) to keep a steady sustainable pace.

Therefore, very important to keep a moderate well-rounded practice routine, balanced with good daily activity for integrating it all into everyday living. Much more fun that way too. :-)

Yes, we are all possessed, by divine evolution longing to express naturally through us. For anyone engaged in effective practices it becomes obvious.

Yoga is derived from the natural evolutionary capabilities observed in the human nervous system. We add structure and self-pacing in an effort to make the journey to enlightenment practical for everyone.

The guru is in you.

2007/05/01 14:14:38
Tantra - Sex and Spiritual Development
http://www.aypsite.org/forum/topic.asp?TOPIC_ID=2412&REPLY_ID=21256&whichpage=-1
tantra- the map

Hi EMC:

It is a natural progression you are going through from erotic to ecstatic, moving ever forward/higher. Your feelings, including doubts, about it are normal too. Nothing is being lost, just continuously spreading out to greater and greater possibilities. The role of sex gradually expands to something beyond sex. You are in good company -- never alone. :-)

The cultivation goes to much finer levels as the progression continues, so you are good on that too. Maybe genital sex continues to play a role -- maybe not. Or maybe not right now, and more later. Everyone is a little different in this.

The good news is that enlightenment is just as accessible to those who are sexually active as it is for celibates, assuming the corresponding means are known. That is the aim of the AYP approach to tantra, to cover the spectrum. We may find ourselves in different places on the spectrum at different times on our path, and each place has a tantric relationship to the over all process of human spiritual transformation.

That is why asanas, mudras, bandhas and pranayama have as significant a role in tantra as sexual activity does, though the line tends to get drawn between sex and everything else. But, in fact, it is a spectrum, a continuum we can address through various means, depending on our current sensitivities and level of purification.

The guru is in you.

2007/05/22 13:11:52
Tantra - Sex and Spiritual Development
http://www.aypsite.org/forum/topic.asp?TOPIC_ID=2543&REPLY_ID=22181&whichpage=-1
A Criticism of Sexual Spirituality

quote:
_____
Originally posted by Hannah

I am so glad someone has the guts to bring this topic up Naz! The "sexual" tantra is the kaula form, which is the lowest form of tantra. Samaya is the highest form of tantra and does not use sexuality at all.
_____

Hi Hannah:

Celibacy is a viable option in AYP, as are tantric sexual relations. There is no one right answer on this. It depends on the individual's bhakti (spiritual desire) and the energy dynamics that are operating within the person due to the level of purification in the nervous system. Of course, deep meditation, spinal breathing pranayama and other practices will shift these dynamics over time. Even then, it is always a matter of personal choice.

For one approach to impose its will on the other will invariably lead to difficulties. Don't we know it?

See this lesson on the relationship of brahmacharya, tantric sex, and celibacy: http://www.aypsite.org/T9.html

All the best!

The guru is in you.

2007/05/23 11:17:05
Tantra - Sex and Spiritual Development
http://www.aypsite.org/forum/topic.asp?TOPIC_ID=2543&REPLY_ID=22223&whichpage=-1
A Criticism of Sexual Spirituality

Hi Hannah:

The thing is, the lower centers cannot be developed spiritually without developing the higher centers. There is a direct connection and interdependence. This is why tantric sexual methods alone do not go far without a daily routine of effective sitting practices, which finally resolves the stigma and failings of "western tantra."

Neither can the higher centers be developed spiritually without developing the lower centers, which is why the "higher tantras" include elements of practice covering the lower centers. To be all one or the other will lead to imbalance.

Regardless of lifestyle preferences (which can surely be accommodated in a flexible self-directed approach), balance in practices is the key, covering the full range of the nervous system.

"Higher tantra" utilizes meditation, pranayama, asanas, mudras, bandhas and other methods to cultivate the whole nervous system, leading to a balanced whole body opening, which includes the rise of both inner silence and ecstatic conductivity. The latter (the expansion of spiritual ecstasy) is an expansion upward of sexual neurobiological functioning, whether it is called that or not. It is clothed in the language of metaphor in the higher tantras (Sri Vidya and Kundalini lore), but it is the same transformation occurring within all devoted aspirants, regardless of preferred method, label, or creed.

The sexual neurobiology cannot be excluded from the spiritual equation any more than can be the body, breath, heart, or mind. All are part of the whole. It is only a matter of natural preference and approach. Still, in that, we cannot exclude an aspect of ourselves as a matter of convenience, or for avoiding karmic obstructions which sooner or later will be dissolved to fully reveal our inner light. Spiritual practices, whether from so-called higher or lower tantra, are for purifying every nook and cranny of our nervous system from top to bottom. With help in purification through effective practices, nature will take her course within us. All spiritual practices are for promoting the natural process of human spiritual transformation.

The path is within us, and not defined by any external source. All external sources, including the much ballyhooed scriptures and external gurus, are but aids to us on our own inner journey of purification and opening.

Certainly we will take advantage of external sources. They are obviously important. Yet, somewhere along the way we will find that the scripture and guru have been stirring within us all along, leading us home. That's why I keep saying...

The guru is in you.
 :-)

2007/05/23 23:44:17
Tantra - Sex and Spiritual Development
http://www.aypsite.org/forum/topic.asp?TOPIC_ID=2543&REPLY_ID=22246&whichpage=-1
A Criticism of Sexual Spirituality

Hi Hannah:

Not a silly example at all, and very worthwhile to bring up. But it is not necessarily related entirely to engaging in simple pre-orgasmic sex.

Just to be clear, the role of tantric sex in AYP is based entirely on one's existing sexual habits and preferences. In other words, if someone is going to be engaging in sex anyway, then why not bring a spiritual benefit along with it? And if sex is not in the picture, that is okay too. We have multiple means for cultivating spiritual progress in either situation.

As you know, AYP is not involved in rituals, and certainly not in working with "lower energies." The act of engaging in pre-orgasmic sex refines and elevates sexual energy to a much more celestial experience, rather than degrading it into lower manifestations. That is why it is done. This is also true of the various yogic techniques coming from high tantra that are stimulating the same energies.

If there is inherent instability in a person, any yoga practice could cause some aggravation of that -- not just tantric sex. Out of all the AYP practices, tantric sex is probably the least risky in that respect. Regardless, in cases where practices contribute to instability, we take immediate action with self-pacing -- scaling back on practices until we find stability in the practice routine and in daily life.

What we are talking about with severe psychological reactions isn't the yoga methods necessarily, but a person's sensitivities and vulnerabilities. We have to be careful when such vulnerabilities are found to be present, self-pace practices immediately, engage in the necessary grounding methods, and seek professional help as needed.

So, this issue you are raising does not have to do primarily with tantric sex, but with all yoga practices in relation to the aspirant's mental health. Extreme instability in relation to yoga practices is an issue pertaining to certain individuals, and we have seen a few cases like that over the past several years. Fortunately only a few. In those cases, yoga techniques were not the initial cause, but may have aggravated a pre-existing condition, particularly if practices were done to excess over a period of time.

Whether or not a person is engaging in tantric sexual methods like the ones presented in AYP is the least of it. The higher techniques can be more risky for those with serious psychologicial issues, because such practices are much more powerful than tantric sex. The truth is, the power of tantric sex by itself is way over-rated.

So engaging in higher tantra (meditation, etc,) is not necessarily going to be the answer in cases where psychological instability is present, though there have been some cases where deep meditation and/or spinal breathing pranayama have helped a lot. Others will say that people with serious psychological issues should avoid meditation altogether, and start with asanas for a good while instead.

Everyone is different, and we are not doctors here. We do our best to provide a self-directed system of yoga practices that will be effective and safe for the vast majority of people. For those who have serious psycholocial issues, specialized attention is required, and we are not necessarily the best qualified for that.

Btw, we have had some pretty good discussions on yoga and mental health in the forums in months past. Pehaps others can point to them.

All the best!

The guru is in you.

2007/05/26 11:24:15
Tantra - Sex and Spiritual Development
http://www.aypsite.org/forum/topic.asp?TOPIC_ID=2543&REPLY_ID=22375&whichpage=-1
A Criticism of Sexual Spirituality

Hi Hannah:

The tantric sexual practices in AYP have been in use here for nearly 25 years (both non-celibate and celibate modes at various times). I've got another 15 years in sitting yoga practices before that. So the sexual aspect came along after quite a long time in sitting practices in my case. I would have done something with it sooner had the info been available. Since there was no obvious organized approach to harnessing sexuality in spiritual practices at the time, it had to be assembled through trial and error with input from many sources over some years. The resulting integration of sitting practices with sexual methods in a logical approach is what I've been doing ever since, with pretty good results.

Btw, celibacy is also a "sexual method." Many around here can confirm that this is so.

So, all that I integrated for myself many years ago is what you see in the online AYP lessons, and expanded on in the AYP Easy Lessons book. It is a sharing.

The small 100 page AYP Enlightenment Series books are being written to offer easier access into the knowledge and practices according to individual interests, so it is not necessary to start out with a 500 page textbook. In the case of the Tantra book, the goal has been not only to discuss tantric sexual methods, whether non-celibate or celibate, but also to point out the necessity of maintaining a daily routine of sitting practices (deep meditation, spinal breathing, etc.) if one hopes to have any real success with tantric sexual methods.

Unfortunately, the book has been categorized by some as the same old "western tantra." Translation: "How to have better sex." I dare say that those who have that opinion haven't read the book, and don't understand what AYP is -- a broad integration of methods on all sides of the human spiritual transformation equation. Ironically, the mischaracterization of AYP-style tantra has led to the Tantra book selling more copies.

But not to worry about money piling up anywhere. More than half of AYP's expenses are still coming out of my own pocket. I hope the book sales will increase enough over the next year to cover current expenses on a month-to-month basis. If sales go beyond that breakeven, then we can do some things to make AYP more visible that are currently beyond our reach financially. I sometimes affectionately call AYP: "A worldwide open-source information strategy being run on a shoestring."

It's been fun so far ... but it can't go on like this forever, or I could end up sitting on the street with a begging bowl. Hey, that might not be so bad. It would be a much simpler life... :-)

The guru is in you.

2007/10/16 14:44:23
Tantra - Sex and Spiritual Development
http://www.aypsite.org/forum/topic.asp?TOPIC_ID=2543&REPLY_ID=26084&whichpage=-1
A Criticism of Sexual Spirituality

quote:
————
Originally posted by mufad

...As I understand, the energy normally (ie for most people in this age) flows downward and outward, we use ayp techniques to reverse this flow inward and upward. This I understand to be transmutation. We try to conserve the vital essence (ojas) so that it may be refined, transmuted and assimilated in our nervous system. Our sitting practice helps in this process.

Kechari Mudhra is sometimes referred to as "Spiritual Sex". I guess we tend to reduce the frequency of 'down and out' sex, when we start experience orgasmic results from 'in and up' spiritual sex. May be yogani can confirm this observation. I doubt if "spiritual sex" is possible with a partner.

In the great vedic epic "The Mahabharata" (of which the the Bhagvad Gita, the bible of Hindu Scriptures forms a part), the war between the pandavas and the kauravas is described in detail. Some teachings (see http://amazon.com/dp/0876120303) interpret this war as an internal war between good and evil that has to be fought by every individual. In this interpretation, each character of the MahaBharata corresponds to an internal quality. "Self Control" and "Desire/Lust" are symbolised by Arjuna and Duryodhana who are the main warriors of each side in the war.

The reason I bring this Epic War here, is that the spiritual path can be seen as war between good and evil and the Mahabharata according to some teachings, is an allegorical detailed description of that war. So physical sex can be seen as one of the great enemies to be defeated before emperor soul can reclaim the lost paradise within. In that view physical sex is bad - something to grow out of as we evolve into more spiritual beings. May be something to be killed? I know it is far easier to make peace with our lower/demonic self but could it be that to eventually overcome maya we will have to destroy that part of our humanity and replace it with another mode of creation at will ? Samayana ?

Acting in Stillness,

————

Hi Mufad:

Kechari mudra is a higher form of ecstatic stimulation, but not the only form. As inner silence rises and ecstatic conductivity awakens, a whole range of techniques and actions become ecstatic and spiritually progressive, including tantric sex. Before the prerequisite inner silence and ecstatic awakening are there, the effects of kechari will be muted, and the benefits of tantric sex will be limited, though there can be some benefit in doing either or both as support to our awakening. However, these methods are not primary awakeners. They find their effectiveness flying on the wings of inner silence cultivated in deep meditation and ecstatic conductivity cultivated in spinal breathing pranayama. When the prerequisites are there, everything becomes ecstatic and spiritually progressive, even taking a walk or eating lunch. :-)

The idea of choosing an "enemy" as spiritual practice, whether it be sex or any other thing we feel may be standing in our way, is contradictory, because it emphasizes divisiveness. There cannot be union (yoga) as long as we hold anyone or anything as separate -- especially as opposed to us.

On the other hand, we cannot deny that we live in duality and must make choices and take sides, even if our inner silence seems not to. In time, the movements of inner silence will make our choices more obvious, which is the natural rise of yama and niyama (spiritual conduct). In AYP, we sometimes call it outpouring divine love.

The scriptures, with their heroes and villains, are acknowledging the fact of our duality. Even so, the call in the scriptures is invariably to go beyond all that. Isn't it so that, in the Bhagavad Gita, Krishna tells Arjuna to forget about making value judgments (pro or con) about the "enemy" and just go do his duty as a soldier? As yogis and yoginis, we can also heed that advice by letting go of making value judgments about sex or anything else, and just do our duty in practices and in life, according to what we know will yield the best results. It is the efficient execution of cause and effect ... with no enemies in sight, even if they may seem to be there from other points of view. We do have some flexibility in choosing our point of view at any point in time. When the clouds have cleared, inner silence is the only point of view. We are That. :-)

The guru is in you.

2007/10/17 14:00:41
Tantra - Sex and Spiritual Development
http://www.aypsite.org/forum/topic.asp?TOPIC_ID=2543&REPLY_ID=26105&whichpage=-1
A Criticism of Sexual Spirituality

quote:
_____
Originally posted by mufad

Do you think the frequency and attraction of 'down and out' sex decreases automatically as we grow in 'in and up' spiritual ecstasy ?
_____

Hi Mufad:

It can be like that. But the timing and sequence of change will depend on the person. Some may be more inclined toward sex for longer, and it will not be a liability if the methods of tantric sex are known -- pre-orgasmic cultivation. In that case, sex can be an advantage.

This is not a call for sex. Just a call for smart sex when engaged as one might normally be in the course of life. This can help cultivate the flowering of ecstatic conductivity and the divine romance within -- the 'in and up' you mention. And if not engaged in sexual relations, that is okay too. There are also tantric methods for sitting practices -- including siddhasana and kechari. The many methods available are more than adequate to get the job done either way. To each their own. One size does not fit all.

Sex is not an enemy any more than gasoline is. If properly utilized, great good can come from both. And if carelessly used, well, you get the idea. Even the celibate will use sexuality in support of enlightenment -- the root source of ecstatic conductivity is sexuality. The dangers in forced celibacy are at least as great as in carelessly expressed sexuality. So it is good for both celibates and non-celibates to know tantric methods.

Each will choose their own path. The methods of tantra and yoga are flexible enough to accommodate any angle of approach to the divine. It can be viewed as war, romance, renunciation, or anything else, as long as practices are going on... :-)

Yama and niyama will manifest differently through each person according to stages of purification and opening. So, while the absolute may be the same everywhere, no two people will express the absolute exactly the same. Neither will two 'enlightened' people express yama and niyama exactly the same. It makes life more interesting, and fun. Stillness in action!

Your equations are very nice. And, yes, AYP is about human spiritual transformation, with each on their own journey of discovery.

The guru is in you.

2007/08/10 10:18:13
Tantra - Sex and Spiritual Development
http://www.aypsite.org/forum/topic.asp?TOPIC_ID=2821&REPLY_ID=24657&whichpage=-1
Tantra: Live Life to the Fullest - Now

Hi Hannah:

I don't believe there is "high" or "low" in tantra, except as may be imagined in an ideology, and that is not very relevant to individual needs, or the wide range of practical methods available for cultivating human spiritual transformation.

If celibacy is undertaken prematurely, without effective means in place for cultivating and expressing the accumulating inner energies, it can end up being a very low path, as the priesthood has clearly demonstrated. So, high can be low and low can be high, depending on the person and the means applied. It does not lend itself to rigid points of view on either side.

Our spiritual progress depends on balanced practice according to our inner condition and bhakti (spiritual desire). Our approach to tantric practice will shift gradually over time as inner purification and opening advance. It is an organic process, not an ideological one.

Avatar makes the point quite well. Two hands are better than one -- less chance of getting stuck using the wrong hand. A key ingredient in self-directed practice is flexibility for the sake of maintaining good progress with safety. We also call it self-pacing. :-)

The guru is in you.

2007/08/10 23:09:39
Tantra - Sex and Spiritual Development
http://www.aypsite.org/forum/topic.asp?TOPIC_ID=2821&REPLY_ID=24681&whichpage=-1
Tantra: Live Life to the Fullest - Now

Hi Hannah:

Actually, all forms of tantra overlap. It is only a matter of emphasis according to the needs of the practitioner. Hopefully, these will be organic needs associated with bhakti (spiritual desire) and the natural processes of human spiritual transformation, rather than ideological.

It should be mentioned that my path for quite a few years has been and is currently along the lines you are seeking, and it is covered in the lessons. So there is a small irony here. It should also be said that it took me many years before that to make the transition, which is why I endorse both left and right handed tantra -- whatever works for the aspirant in the present, and whatever will work for the aspirant in the future. For most people, spiritual transformation is a gradual progression, with much overlap in the many grades of practice and experience along the way. In that sense, each person's path is unique.

There is nothing to defend but what is practical for each person on their path. I am happy to do the same for you, but not at the expense of the spiritual progress of others.

As for Swami Rama, he was a pioneer in his fine writings on the frontier of the increasing transmission of yoga practices in the 20th century. Actually, he is much better in writing than he was in person (just my opinion). As is the case with all pioneers, they provide a foundation and a launching pad for others to carry on to new and broader horizons. If AYP can serve that purpose also, even a little, it will be a success. We are all stepping stones on the way to a more illuminated humanity.

Wishing you all the best on your path. Carry on! :-)

The guru is in you.

2007/08/16 19:05:09
Tantra - Sex and Spiritual Development
http://www.aypsite.org/forum/topic.asp?TOPIC_ID=2846&REPLY_ID=24842&whichpage=-1
Swingers, Crossdressers, bi-sexuals, bdsm etc...

Hi Ventilator:

Who knows why people make the lifestyle choices they do? As it says in the Bhagavad Gita, "Unfathomable are the portents of karma."

No particular sexual lifestyle is more disposed toward kundalini awakening than another. And neither is an awakened kundalini the cause of any particular sexual lifestyle, except perhaps a natural moderation in external expressions of sexuality over the long term, since so much more ecstasy will be occurring inside as inner lovemaking advances with the rise of ecstatic conductivity and radiance. This then expresses more as loving conduct than sexual conduct -- outpouring divine love, which is unity.

From the AYP point of view, ecstatic conductivity can be cultivated equally well within any sexual lifestyle (including celibacy) if the operative principles and practices are applied as a complement to a balanced routine of yoga practices. This is covered in the AYP Tantra lessons and Tantra book.

The preservation and cultivation of sexual energy is the underlying principle found in all tantric sexual practices, regardless of lifestyle.

Energy imbalances can occur in any lifestyle, particularly if practices are not self-paced in relation to experiences.

All the best!

The guru is in you.

2007/10/02 11:23:30
Tantra - Sex and Spiritual Development
http://www.aypsite.org/forum/topic.asp?TOPIC_ID=2951&REPLY_ID=25816&whichpage=-1
Vajroli Again

Hi Tant Rick:

The sensitivity you are experiencing could be caused by the inner stimulation of mechanical vajroli with a catheter. Likely it would pass as you become used to the mechanical stimulation. However, you might reconsider the use of the catheter, in view of the below.

I have experience with use of a catheter also, but do not recommend this as part of the AYP system of practices. It is an invasive approach whose rewards do not warrant the risks of infection and other mishaps.

If you check the AYP Tantra Lessons and Tantra book, you will find that we do not go to the extreme of vajroli mudra given in the Hatha Yoga Pradipika. It is not necessary and can, in fact, be counter-productive in many cases.

What good is a strategy to recover lost semen, when the primary strategy ought to be staying in front of orgasm and preserving semen inside whether there is orgasm or not? This is why in AYP we use blocking in concert with pre-orgasmic cultivation, instead of going to the trouble of trying to recover the horse after it has left the barn. Better to keep the horse in the barn in the first place. :-)

Furthermore, true vajroli is not a practice, per say, but a natural transformation in neurobiological functioning, which arises with deep meditation, spinal breathing pranayama, tantric sexual methods, and other means. So it is not necessary to become a gymnast in physical vajroli to achieve the ultimate result, which is the ongoing automatic rise of sexual essences in the neurobiology. This is part of the rise of whole-body "ecstatic conductivity." Much better to focus on deep meditation, spinal breathing, and the preservation and cultivation of sexual energy in less extreme ways. Then, in time, the best over all result will be there.

Success in yoga comes through a balanced integration of a range of effective practices, not from an obsession with any one practice, or class of practices. The whole is much greater than the sum of the parts. This is very important.

Of course, these are all your decisions, and what you read here is only food for thought.

Wishing you all the best on your chosen path. Enjoy!

The guru is in you.

See also: http://www.aypsite.org/forum/topic.asp?TOPIC_ID=2953#25817

2007/10/02 11:35:52

Hi ParamMudra, and welcome!

You have good feedback from Avatar. For some added perspective, check this post:
http://www.aypsite.org/forum/topic.asp?TOPIC_ID=2951#25816

Also, mudras and bandhas (with some kumbhaka) added over time during our sitting practices (with a foundation of deep meditation) have a large effect on the rise of ecstatic conductivity and natural vajroli -- these include sambhavi, mulabandha, kechari, yoni mudra, dynamic jalandhara (chin pump), nauli (during asanas) and so on...

Sorry, I don't know of any video or graphic illustrations for mechanical vajroli. Maybe someone here does. It is sort of a moot point in AYP, since we don't recommend the athletic version of vajroli -- it can become a tangent in relation to maintaining a balanced routine of integrated practices, which is where the best results will be found.

All the best!

The guru is in you.

quote:
_____
Originally posted by Christi

Hi Guys,

I was just wondering, what exactly is mechanical vajroli? Anyone wish to explain?

_____

Hi Christi:

Mechanical vajroli mudra has been popularized through the ancient Hatha Yoga Pradipika, and is very misunderstood.

It is intentionally creating negative pressure (suction) in the bladder using uddiyana bandha, nauli, mulabandha/asvini, and additional control of the muscles around the bladder and prostate gland. The metric for this is how much fluid can be sucked into the bladder through the lingam. Some may use a catheter to develop this ability.

It is a practice that can bring much distraction in yoga, on the belief that it represents something ultimate in yogic accomplishment. It does not.

Vajroli mudra is only useful when ecstatic conductivity has been awakened, and then it happens automatically, with sexual essences coming into practical utilization in the evolving neurobiology higher up in the body. Until that happens, the forced drawing up of sexual essences is mechanical only, with little spiritual consequence. That is why I call it "mechanical vajroli."

Mechanical vajroli is sometimes viewed by men as a way to exploit women, aiming to literally suck the sexual essences out of women along with their own expelled semen. Some so-called yogis have bragged about this vampire-like practice in their memoirs, much to their discredit. It's got nothing to do with what we are doing in AYP.

As mentioned earlier, natural vajroli occurs (in both men and women!) with the awakening of ecstatic conductivity (kundalini), resulting from a balanced routine of daily practices over time. This is a much more practical and holistic approach supporting the fulfillment of yoga, rather than risking an extended sexual obsession, health problems, etc., for very little return with mechanical vajroli.

Mechanical vajroli (also referred to as athletic or gymnastic here) is not part of the AYP system of practices. Natural vajroli is.

For more on the AYP approach to vajroli, see: http://www.aypsite.org/T30.html
and
http://www.aypsite.org/T46.html

All the best!

The guru is in you.

quote:
_____

Originally posted by yogani

Mechanical vajroli is sometimes viewed by men as a way to exploit women, aiming to literally suck the sexual essences out of women along with their own expelled semen. Some so-called yogis have bragged about this vampire-like practice in their memoirs, much to their discredit. It's got nothing to do with what we are doing in AYP.

_____
quote:
_____

Originally posted by gentlep

Why is that exploitation of women? It's the fluid that would have wasted anyway, correct?

_____

Hi Gentlep:

The exploitation isn't primarily in the act itself, but in the psychology. There is little to no yogic value in this practice. So why do some men go to so much trouble to develop it? ... usually at the expense of developing a more balanced and effective routine of yoga practices. It's a macho thing that's got little to do with real yoga.

There is a logical sequence to the development of yoga practices that is tied to the process and experience of human spiritual transformation, as indicated more or less in the sequence of the AYP lessons, with vajroli being pretty far down the list. So why do some men come in obsessed with such a down the list practice? Sexual issues cannot be effectively resolved in this way. Much better to start at the beginning with deep meditation and spinal breathing pranayama, and then learn the essential principles and practices of (pre-orgasmic) tantric sex as needed. By these means, sexual obsessions will unwind over time, and natural vajroli will be there as part of the evolving ecstatic neurobiology.

Natural spiritual development like this has nothing to do with focusing on mechanical vajroli and developing an ability to suck fluid out of women, which is a gross misallocation of sexual desire. Much better to redirect our desire into the mainstream of spiritual practices, which will facilitate our transformation much more effectively.

To put things in perspective, with the rise of ecstatic conductivity, natural vajroli occurs equally in women as it does in men. If it is not something our women can experience, we probably ought to think twice before running off on an obsessive and exploitive tangent. There are much easier and more pleasurable ways to keep the horse in the barn that will lead to good results for both sexes. :-)

It's always your choice. Practice wisely, and enjoy!

The guru is in you.

2007/10/25 13:17:53
Tantra - Sex and Spiritual Development
http://www.aypsite.org/forum/topic.asp?TOPIC_ID=2953&REPLY_ID=26338&whichpage=-1
Vajroli Mudra Practical

Hi again All:

It can be added that from the point of view of ecstatic conductivity, sambhavi and energy flow in the head have a direct role in stimulating the rise of natural vajroli down below. In fact, with ecstatic conductivity and the accompanying linkage of sambhavi and mulabandha/asvini, natural vajroli is essentially a done deal, because it is the concurrent rise of sexual essences that feeds ongoing ecstatic conductivity. Vajroli is the natural upward flow of sexual essences through the urethra and bladder to support the spiritual biology in the mid and upper body, particularly the radiant form of digestion that occurs in the GI tract.

Of course, all of this is pretty much in the background as inner silence moves outward into daily living on the wings of our expanding ecstatic radiance. Who will pay much attention to the inner biology while dancing joyfully in the light? :-)

The guru is in you.

2007/10/02 13:29:35
Tantra - Sex and Spiritual Development
http://www.aypsite.org/forum/topic.asp?TOPIC_ID=2954&REPLY_ID=25821&whichpage=-1
erection and spinal breathing.

quote:
_____

Originally posted by avatar186

I once heard one should learn to stay "erect" or aroused all the time. I forget what yogi said it, from what ive experiance, the "outer" vibrations are much strong and easyer to produce in this state.
Ive also read that the outer vibrations are created by the out flow i believe it was.

It seems this may be a proficiant way to practise spinal breathing and get the benifits of pranayama.

BUT! i only mean aroused, not the creation of fluids or such.

_____

Hi Avatar:

Forgive me, but that one caused a belly laugh here. Some gurus insist on killing erections permanently with extreme forms of siddhasana, tight strings and other weird devices, while other gurus want us to have an erection during practices.

Well, which is it?
How about letting it be? :-)

The practices we have, including mudras and bandhas in moderation, in addition to our core practices of deep meditation and spinal breathing, are more than enough. Then there is siddhasana (not extreme), tantric cultivation during sexual relations, samyama, and all the rest. A lot of tools...

Erections (or not) are the tail on the dog of yoga, and we can let the tail do what it must. Sometimes the tail will wag the dog, but seasoned practitioners will know better. We just easily favor the practice over the experiences that are continually coming up.

The guru is in you.

PS: If there is a strong desire to experiment with spinal breathing and sexual arousal, consider this lesson, which comes at it from the opposite angle -- spinal breathing during tantric sexual relations: http://www.aypsite.org/T33.html
It also clarifies what has been touched on above about introducing tantric elements (siddhasana, mudras, bandhas, etc.) into sitting practices in a balanced way.

2007/11/12 10:40:52
Tantra - Sex and Spiritual Development
http://www.aypsite.org/forum/topic.asp?TOPIC_ID=3125&REPLY_ID=26942&whichpage=-1
circumcision and tantric sex

Hi Siddha, and welcome!

Results in using tantric sexual methods, or any other aspect of yoga, have little to do with whether a male is circumcised or not.

One's daily practice routine is the primary determinant of progress, i.e., sitting practices, including deep meditation, spinal breathing pranayama, asanas, mudras and bandhas, etc. See the main lessons link at the top of this page.

Tantric sexual methods can be a useful complement to core yoga practices, when applied in concert with one's sexual inclinations. See the tantra lessons link at the top of this page.

The online lessons are expanded on in the AYP books.

Wishing you all the best on your chosen path. Enjoy!

The guru is in you.

2007/11/14 12:29:07
Tantra - Sex and Spiritual Development
http://www.aypsite.org/forum/topic.asp?TOPIC_ID=3138&REPLY_ID=27015&whichpage=-1
mechanics of vajroli

Hi Tadeas:

Good question. It is hoped that as more people are having these experiences, science will investigate and describe what is happening in ways that will strengthen knowledge and conviction on the phenomenon of human spiritual transformation.

Regarding "natural vajroli," I am assuming you read my comments elsewhere here in the forum:
http://www.aypsite.org/forum/topic.asp?TOPIC_ID=2953

Yes, the upward absorption of sexual essences becomes more or less constant as ecstatic conductivity becomes a constant experience. The two go together. It is not only through the bladder that it occurs. Sexual essences also find their way upward through other pathways beginning in the pelvic region. And this applies to both men and women.

It appears that the bladder is not only about eliminating toxins. Otherwise, we would not have the age-old and highly effective practice of amaroli.

When the ecstatic connection is awake, the whole process can be stimulated with sambhavi (easy centering and raising of the eyes). This creates the "whole body mudra" effect, which natural vajroli is part of. Even without sambhavi it will be going on all the time, fed by our bhakti and outpouring divine love. Then it is a closed loop neurobiological operation, where all parts reinforce all other parts for the whole. It is not unlike the rest of our neurobiology, which is all connected and occurring mostly unnoticed within us. Rising spiritual biology is just a refinement and expansion of our neurobiological functioning. When there are more people experiencing this, I am sure science will step in to fully map it, and that will be a wonderful and welcome development.

As for the over all process leading to amrita (nectar) produced in the brain (usually experienced as a sweet aroma in the nasal passages and mouth), and related phenomena., I wrote something on this in the Diet, Shatkarmas and Amaroli book, in this case tying in the relationship of diet, and in the language of kundalini:

"As we engage in our spiritual practices over months and years, we are gradually coaxing our nervous system to move to a higher level of functioning. Many of the characteristics of this are measurable in our neurobiology. And quite a few of the changes that are occurring are directly observable. A complex process of purification and opening is occurring in those who practice yogic methods.

There are two main aspects to our purification and opening, each with its own biological signature.

-- The Rise of Inner Silence – an abiding inner quietness, or stillness, that is beyond our thoughts, feelings and the ups and downs of daily life. We come to know this as our "self."

-- The Rise of Ecstatic Conductivity (Kundalini) in the Body – sensations of pleasurable energy moving within us, penetrating every aspect of our neurobiological functioning. We come to know this as the "radiant aspect of our self."

While diet is not a primary cause of these changes in our inner functioning, it is a participant in them. As we find more abiding stillness within ourselves coming with daily deep meditation, we will naturally be drawn to a lighter more nutritious diet.

Likewise, as the neurobiological changes associated with a stirring kundalini begin to occur within us, our diet preferences may change. In addition, certain diet adjustments may be helpful to aid us in navigating some of the excessive energy symptoms that can occur as our inner experiences advance. The process of kundalini is famous for its many symptoms, which can include sensations of heat or coolness in the body, surging emotions, physical vibrations or bodily movements, visions, occasional dizziness or nausea, etc. Sometimes there can be some pain as inner energy (prana) is moving through areas where there are remaining obstructions in our nervous system. All of these symptoms eventually give way to much higher and enjoyable experiences.

Depending on the pattern of inner obstructions in our nervous system and the degree of prudence we exercise in self-pacing our practices, we may experience little in the way of uncomfortable symptoms – just steadily increasing ecstasy and bliss, which can bring its own challenges (distractions from stable practice). Regardless, when kundalini becomes active, a good knowledge of yoga practices and the methods of regulating them will pay off in a big way. For those who experience an unmanaged kundalini awakening without knowledge of the particulars involved, it can be a challenging experience, lasting sometimes for years.

Once the kundalini process has begun within us, it can be managed by self-pacing our practices in ways that maintain good progress with reasonable comfort. It is a long term transformation we are engaged in, leading to a permanent condition of abiding inner silence, ecstatic bliss, and divine love radiating naturally outward from within us in all that we do in daily life.

Digestion is at the center of the kundalini process and many of its associated symptoms. So it stands to reason that diet has a role to play. And the role of diet will not always be the same, depending where we are on our path. To understand this better, let's look at the process occurring in the gastrointestinal (GI) tract in a person who has an active kundalini, and how this relates to diet.

While there are many aspects to the functioning of kundalini, both physical and non-physical, we will focus on the physical here, as far as we can go with it. For the purpose of this discussion, we will take the view that spiritual experience rises from neurobiological processes occurring in our body. There are more mystical ways of looking at it, and there is nothing wrong with that. It is the same process occurring, no matter how we choose to describe it. When we are reviewing the effects of diet (and shatkarmas and amaroli in the next two chapters) looking at the biology can be helpful, as far as we can trace it with direct perception. There is little doubt that modern science will be taking a much closer look at the neurobiology of kundalini in the years and decades to come. It is the next great frontier of scientific exploration – the causes and effects of human spiritual transformation!

Kundalini is traditionally viewed as the awakening of a vast latent energy located near the base of the spine, which rises up the spine to the head. There, a union occurs between the rising energy and stillness, with the energy being feminine (shakti) and the stillness being masculine (shiva).

When we look at the experiential neurobiology of this, a few more components can be added, which are consistent with the metaphors found in many of the world's scriptures, including the more direct descriptions found in Indian Yoga and Chinese Taoism.

When there is sufficient inner silence present via the daily practice of deep meditation, and then the breath and body are brought into the process via spinal breathing pranayama, asanas, mudras, bandhas, and tantric sexual methods, we will notice three things occurring.

1. An expansion of sexual energy from the pelvic region upward, with part finding its way into the GI tract.

2. The natural retention of air in the GI tract.

3. The interaction of food with the sexual essences and air in the GI tract.

The natural combination of these three elements in the digestive system through an emerging higher form of digestion gives rise to a new substance emanating from the GI tract, which permeates the entire body. Much of this penetration occurs as this substance enters the spinal canal and rises up through the chest cavity to the head. The highly penetrating and sometimes intoxicating substance produced in the GI tract has been given many names. A name prevalent in yoga is soma. The word soma also refers to a hallucinogenic plant, which is not what we are talking about here. In Taoism, the GI tract, when engaged in this higher functioning, is called the caldron, recognizing the alchemy that is occurring there – three ordinary substances (sexual essence, air, and food) being combined to create an extraordinary substance that is a key to the process of human spiritual transformation.

The process continues in the head, with further refinements occurring in the brain, which lead to another substance being secreted through the sinuses, down through the inside nasal passages, into the throat and then down into the GI tract again, where it joins in the process already described. This recycling of subtle essences leads to even more refined processing in the GI tract. The substance coming down from the brain into the GI tract is referred to as amrita (nectar) in the yoga tradition. It can sometimes be experienced as a sweet aroma in the nasal passages and taste in the mouth.

The overall experience of this combining and transformation of substances, and the recycling of the resulting essences in the body leads to large flows of ecstatic pleasure throughout the body, and the radiation of energy beyond the body. This is why those who are advancing in spiritual practices are sometimes said to be radiant. There is a specific neurobiology behind it. In yogic terms, the body-wide radiance of ecstatic energy indicates the rise of the mythical quality of ojas, which is a greatly enhanced manifestation of vitality that is easily noticed by others.

If we begin to understand that such a process really exists and, better yet, begin to experience aspects of it within ourselves as a result of our daily practices, then we are able to look at diet from an entirely new angle. And we can also see the relevance of shatkarmas (cleansing techniques) and amaroli (urine therapy) as well. All of these methods are aimed at enhancing and optimizing the process just described.

As mentioned earlier, diet is not a core practice in yoga, but an important supporting element. If we look at this that way, we can see how our cooperation with inner urges relating to diet can enhance the overall process that is occurring on the road to enlightenment.

The higher form of digestion described above can generate a lot of heat in the GI tract, radiating out to fill the whole body. It is sometimes referred to as the kundalini fire. When the fires are burning, it can be beneficial to eat heavier foods more often. Then the fire (intense digestive activity) can be used to consume the substances in our GI tract in a more regulated way to produce more soma, rather than frying us from the inside, which is the sensation we can get sometimes if eating too lightly when energy is surging within us. It is also possible to quench the inner fires and related inner energy imbalances with application of the diet methods of Ayurveda, which take into account our bodily constitution and inner energy flows, and how certain foods can either aggravate or pacify these. See the appendix for more on ayurvedic diet guidelines.

To keep it as simple as possible, we just listen to what we are being called to do from within with respect to our diet, and in other aspects of our daily activity. When we are engaged in daily deep meditation, we may feel inclined to eat a lighter diet. And when our kundalini becomes active, we may feel inclined to eat a heavier diet at times, and a lighter diet at other times. It will depend on the energy dynamics occurring within us, and the process of purification and opening that is underway.

We learn to become good listeners to the inner voice of our neurobiology as we travel the road to enlightenment."

And, also from the book, covering amaroli in relation to the rise of natural vajroli:

"Vajroli is a practice described in the Hatha Yoga Pradipika, and involves the drawing up of sexual fluids inside the body. In the AYP system of practices we do not go to the extremes that are described in this ancient treatise on yoga. Rather, natural vajroli is achieved through a full range of yoga practices, including deep meditation, spinal breathing pranayama, asanas, mudras, bandhas, tantric sexual techniques, and other methods.

By natural vajroli, we mean a natural drawing up of sexual essences through the urethra into the bladder and through many pathways upward in the neurobiology. This natural upward migration of vital essences gradually evolves to become a full-time occurrence in the life of the spiritual practitioner. This process occurs in both men and women, and is an integral part of the rise of full-time ecstatic conductivity in the body, which evolves further to become ecstatic radiance going out beyond the body.

In conjunction with this evolution in the sexual neurobiology, it may be observed that there is a gradual internalization of amaroli to become an automatic recycling within, which can result in less outflow. While there is no scientific verification of the internal recirculation of urine via natural vajroli, it has been observed in enough cases to be worthy of mention. It is well known that urination can become quite irregular with the awakening and advancement of kundalini (ecstatic conductivity). Whether amaroli itself plays a role in this evolution is not known. It will suffice to say that there is a relationship between amaroli and vajroli. This is pointed to in the Hatha Yoga Pradipika, and has been observed in practitioners in modern times, as well.

The integrated application of a full range of yoga practices gives rise to this phenomenon. It is also related to long term engagement in yoga practices. The changes described do not occur overnight, which is why a steady daily routine of practices that can be sustained long term is advised.

The extreme elements of practice which are sometimes seized upon by enthusiastic aspirants do not make a great difference in the overall scheme of things, because they cannot be sustained over the long term. Nor should they be. It is the practices we can engage in easily in a balanced way as part of our normal daily routine that will carry us steadily forward to the rising condition of abiding inner silence, ecstatic bliss and outpouring divine love.

We will know it is working for us as we find the practical results of the transformation emerging from within us day by day in our daily activities."

All good stuff for the scientific community to be investigating in the years to come. What we need is more people engaging in practices and having the changes occurring so there will be lots to investigate. :-)

All the best on your path. Enjoy!

The guru is in you.

2008/05/18 10:07:52
Tantra - Sex and Spiritual Development
http://www.aypsite.org/forum/topic.asp?TOPIC_ID=3143&REPLY_ID=33873&whichpage=-1
seminal leakage

quote:
_____
Originally posted by mrityunjay_singh_1983

Sir ji

i have some question?????????

Q1.am i eradicate nocturnal emission problem and establish in brahmcharya(no tantrik)?????????????????

Q2.Can i awake my kundalini(ecstatic conductivity) ????????

Q3.Tell some people(in AYP or other) which have problem of nocturnal emission and after some time practicing Yoga establish in complete brahmcharya.

Please ans. these question?????
_____

Hi Mrityunjay:

Occasional nocturnal emissions are common for younger and sometimes older men. It will pass. Not to worry about it. It will not hold back long term spiritual progress.

Yes, you can awaken ecstatic conductivity/kundalini, but not usually by celibacy alone. It also requires a balanced daily routine of practices like deep meditation, spinal breathing pranayama, asanas, mudras, bandhas, etc., plus full engagement in normal activity in the world. Balance in all things is much more important and effective than going to the extreme in any one thing.

What works for you or me may not be ideal for everyone, so it is not a good idea to tell everyone that sex has to be handled a certain way. In AYP, brahmacharya is defined as favoring "preservation and cultivation of sexual energy." There are many ways to accomplish that (see the main and tantra lessons), and celibacy is not an absolute requirement. Many here can verify this.

The suggestion is to build a balanced daily practice that is in tune with your nature, relax, and enjoy life. Everything will be fine. :-)

The guru is in you.

2008/05/21 08:12:09
Tantra - Sex and Spiritual Development
http://www.aypsite.org/forum/topic.asp?TOPIC_ID=3143&REPLY_ID=33956&whichpage=-1
seminal leakage

Hi Mrityunjay

Yes, it is possible with long term practice of effective spiritual methods. But if brahmacharya is the primary goal in practice, the answer will be no.

Can someone obsessed with getting money ever be free from money? Not likely.

The issue isn't money or brahmacharya. The issue is obsession with what we think we do not have. An obsession with lack breeds more lack. All the promises in the world cannot fix that. It will take a shift in attitude, a surrender in stillness...

Read this topic for a balanced discussion on sex and spiritual development -- http://www.aypsite.org/forum/topic.asp?TOPIC_ID=3933
It is a symphony of divine love.

By the way, preservation and cultivation of sexual energy occur simultaneously, not first one and then the other. And this relies on a routine of daily yoga practices.

It is suggested to move beyond the need for hypothetical certainties and into accepting and dealing with today's reality. The answer cannot be found in thinking about the future. Only in picking up where we are today and moving forward with devotion (bhakti) as best we can. Then the future will take care of itself. Today's journey is the destination, not some future imagined perfection.

Have we meditated today and gone out and lived as fully as we can? If we have, that is as good as it gets. As we continue with daily practices and activity in the world, it will get even better. That is the best assurance I can give. The rest is up to you.

The guru is in you.

2008/05/22 11:09:05
Tantra - Sex and Spiritual Development
http://www.aypsite.org/forum/topic.asp?TOPIC_ID=3143&REPLY_ID=33994&whichpage=-1
seminal leakage

Hi Mrityunjay:

With all of these practices, are you finding more happiness in everyday living? This is the true measure of our yoga. The practices can be tallied in a check list (like Patanjali's wonderful eight limbs) and in the formative stage we might even undertake them in a checklist way, but ultimately the application and import of practices can only be measured by how we feel. It is by how we feel that we learn to "self-pace," which is at the heart of effective self-directed spiritual practice.

The technology must be translated into human experience, which means using the technology even while letting it go in stillness. Indeed, the procedures of effective yoga practice always have this at the center -- doing while letting go into non-doing. This is very important if we are to move beyond the mechanical aspects of yoga and into the realm of abiding inner silence, ecstatic bliss, outpouring divine love and unity.

So, yes, the desire for brahmacharya can be an obstruction if it becomes rigid obsession, like anything else. The desire itself is evolutionary, but only if it can be touched and released in stillness again and again. This is samyama, which leads to stillness in action, which is what real brahmacharya is. Then it becomes very natural preservation and cultivation of sexual energy, and the setbacks (energy leakages, etc.) are taken in stride too. Whether we call it "tantra" or something else, that is what happens. By whatever path name, or lifestyle (celibate, hetero, homo, solo, etc.), the expansion of sexual function occurring in the process of human spiritual transformation is the same.

That is why in AYP we do not tell people exactly what to do with sex. We point to the underlying principles and some effective flexible methods for applying them, and the rest is up to each person within the context of their unique preferences and circumstances.

The guru is in you.

2007/11/29 11:55:40
Tantra - Sex and Spiritual Development
http://www.aypsite.org/forum/topic.asp?TOPIC_ID=3191&REPLY_ID=27462&whichpage=-1
ramifications of not coming

quote:
_____
Originally posted by Eddie33

That is it! I'm never jacking off again!!!!

j/k
_____

Hi Eddie:

Keep in mind that Rome was not built in a day. Taking the "I'm never going to..." approach can lead to guilt and other difficulties that can be as disruptive as an excessive energy drain.

There is a middle road.

In the case of Tantra, it is a gentle cultivation of the great force of sexual energy to higher manifestation <u>over time</u>. In addition to tantric sexual methods, an essential part of this is daily sitting practices, including deep meditation, spinal breathing pranayama, etc.

The extreme approach is rarely the right approach. This applies in all of yoga, including self-inquiry, where pounding "Be here now!" or "Who am I?!" can lead to headaches (**!**)

It's the same thing with rigid approaches to sexual abstinence. The priesthood could have used the little red AYP Tantra book. They could have avoided committing a lot of sexual abuse, and stayed out of the headlines, not to mention the enlightenment to be gained.

<u>The middle road</u> ... That is what we are doing around here, though it may not always look like it. It is a road with many aspects, each one with its own middle way. And all these ways are connected within us.

Prudent self-pacing in all aspects of practice enables us to stay on track, steadily opening our inner doorway to divine living.

The guru is in you.

2007/12/03 11:53:51
Tantra - Sex and Spiritual Development
http://www.aypsite.org/forum/topic.asp?TOPIC_ID=3217&REPLY_ID=27627&whichpage=-1
Spiritual sex

quote:
_____
Originally posted by Neesha

I just want ....out
_____

Hi Neesha:

A sure way to get out of such interactions is by not acknowledging them. If someone claims to have done such a thing with you, you do not have to acknowledge it. The claim is part of the interaction, and the claim relies on acknowledgment for its sustaining energy. To not acknowledge the claim is to release the interaction within yourself. It can be as simple as saying, "No thank you."

This is along the lines of discussions on possession that have occurred in the forum in the past.

Whatever we give our attention to in life will grow stronger, and whatever we consistently release will lose its grip sooner or later. We always have a choice.

This is a form of self-inquiry, and true self-inquiry finds its relationship to life in abiding inner silence -- the witness, which is beyond all energy and experience. So deep meditation is an essential ingredient in this as well.

All the best!

The guru is in you.

2007/12/16 09:42:14
Tantra - Sex and Spiritual Development
http://www.aypsite.org/forum/topic.asp?TOPIC_ID=3217&REPLY_ID=27980&whichpage=-1
Spiritual sex

Hi Julied:

Do keep in mind that the "no thank you" is an expression of the person's desire, and not mine. If we don't want to do something, we can always say no, and favor that whenever the undesired circumstance recurs. If we do not give it our energy, its influence will gradually fade. And if we do want to do something, then that is our choice also. The things we favor will grow in their influence in our life. So our choosing each day is what determines our path more so than anything else we encounter in life.

What we'd like to avoid is falling into a victim mentality/habit, where we give our ability to choose over to others, real or imagined. That is a path to nowhere, and something I strongly urge saying "no thank you" to. :-)

The guru is in you.

PS: Surrender to the divine is not the same as victimhood, as long as we are choosing and desiring a high spiritual ideal -- it is the process of bhakti. What often happens in relationships is "the other" is considered to be 100% synonymous with the ideal, which is not true. It is the high spiritual ideal that we seek, not any particular external manifestation of it in another, no matter how perfect they might appear. Others may inspire us with whatever degree of our high ideal they are able to display. That's a good thing. But, in the end, the only true measure of our high spiritual ideal will be in how it is manifesting <u>within us</u>. That is something worth surrendering to.

2007/12/04 11:50:58
Tantra - Sex and Spiritual Development
http://www.aypsite.org/forum/topic.asp?TOPIC_ID=3220&REPLY_ID=27650&whichpage=-1
More Beginner Questions

quote:

I preface my questions with a Namaste and deep bow for Yogani- I have been on the path for 17 years and have never encountered anything like your writings- their simplicity, hopefulness-inspiring, clarity, logic, intuitive correctness, kindness, compassion, non-judgementalness....They deeply resonate with me. I have only been practicing the meditation for a week but already feel the difference. On to my questions-

1 I was under the impression that the holdback method was bad for the prostate (at least until the spinal channel is opened) because, to use the analogy of a rubber band, as the prostate gland is filled with fluid without being allowed to snap back into release/expulsion (i.e., ejaculate) , it is like a rubber band that is stretched repetitively without being allowed to snap back- it ends up stretched out and loses its elasticity.

2 It seems to me that a sensitive lover could 'coax' their partner into tantric states by withdrawing for a time when sensing the others imminent orgasm. Your thoughts on this?

3 You wrote that ultimately vajroli happends automatically/naturally, although you did practice with a catheter. Have you personally known or observed vajroli to happen naturally/automatically in anyone you've known or is this speculation on your part?

4 How would you compare/contrast the efficacy of spinal breathing practices to the running of the microcosmic orbit?

thank you kindly

___

Hi Growant:

Very happy to hear you are finding the AYP writings to be helpful.

Now that is a list of questions. :-)

I'll offer some short answers, and maybe others will chime in with their own perspectives.

1. Holdback will not strain the prostate, as it is only delaying orgasm by discontinuing stimulation. Maybe you meant blocking of male ejaculation? Some feel this can be harmful. Everyone will go through a clunky stage in the beginning, where pressure is more. It becomes much less as progress in yoga continues. There has been no perceptible damage here in over 25 years of use. Quite to the contrary!

2. Yes, this is what is suggested in AYP tantra, both with our own orgasm and with our partner's. This is what holdback is. And it does lead to very high expressions of spiritual ecstasy within us, during and long after the act itself -- eventually permanent ecstatic conductivity and radiance. (This is part of the cultivation of natural vajroli in both sexes.)

3. Natural vajroli was occurring here long before experiments with a catheter were undertaken. It did not add anything, so was discontinued. So much for mechanical vajroli. :-)

4. See here for a discussion on yogic spinal breathing versus taoist microcosmic orbit: http://www.aypsite.org/forum/topic.asp?TOPIC_ID=1474

All the best!

The guru is in you.

2008/01/22 16:09:09
Tantra - Sex and Spiritual Development
http://www.aypsite.org/forum/topic.asp?TOPIC_ID=3398&REPLY_ID=29156&whichpage=-1
Tantric sex and birth control

Hi Echo:

Here are several discussions on vasectomy and yoga:

http://www.aypsite.org/forum/topic.asp?TOPIC_ID=354
http://aypsite.org/forum/topic.asp?TOPIC_ID=785
http://www.aypsite.org/forum/topic.asp?TOPIC_ID=1174
http://www.aypsite.org/forum/topic.asp?TOPIC_ID=1481

Obviously, it can be addressed on the woman's side too, with health and spiritual impacts to be considered. The pill is chemically/hormonally invasive, and even an IUD can affect the spiritual energies in some women, so it is not an easy decision.

Draw your own conclusions. Any additional perspectives are welcome. :-)

All the best!

The guru is in you.

2008/01/29 12:40:28
Tantra - Sex and Spiritual Development
http://www.aypsite.org/forum/topic.asp?TOPIC_ID=3398&REPLY_ID=29426&whichpage=-1
Tantric sex and birth control

quote:
___
Originally posted by afrotantra

The female version of the deer exercise combined with ejaculation control in the male should be sufficient for any couple to prevent conception. Both have to be practiced for at least 2 months. In the meantime, fertility awareness combined with ejaculation control should work. I used nothing external to control birth for five long years, and when I wanted to conceive it took several months to get pregnant, it worked so well. Just a thought. Hope it helped.

Hi Afrotantra, and welcome!

I assume by "fertility awareness" you mean the "rhythm method" -- avoiding sex during ovulation. That is one we have not seen mentioned here. Thanks much for adding it.

Thanks also for bringing up the Taoist deer exercise for women. I was not aware that it could play a significant role in birth control (see article below, dug up from the web).

As with most things yogic, it takes an effective integration of methods to achieve the desired result. Male vasectomy (or female tube tying), while certainly effective for birth control, may not be panaceas. It is a matter of choice, yes? The more information available for consideration the better.

All the best!

The guru is in you.

Note: The below is not an AYP endorsement. Just "Grist for the mill," and plenty of it too. :-)

Deer Exercise for women and men, from: http://iamthegoddess.tribe.net/thread/72c3f610-6651-4d8a-a79b-3f2983911e1e
(see post by Jeremiah on date shown)

Birth Control and The Deer Exercise for WomenTue, February 28, 2006 - 4:22 AM
I noticed that no one has mentioned the Taoist Deer Exercise as a method of birth control. I recommend this exercise to healers as a method of self-healing in the lower chakra and to allow them to hold more c
Hi or kundalini or sehkem. Some have reported that it has regulated their cycles, eliminated PMS and in some cases actually turn back the blood. Please check it out and know that this is a daily discipline, usually done skyclad and occassionally with a partner. There is a similar exercise for men which you should read as well.. I'll paste it after the one for women.
Blessed Be,
Jeremiah

The Deer Exercise for Women

As you do the two steps of this exercise, "feel" the fire or energy generated in your sexual glands and feel it rise upward along the spine into the breasts and the head. (Never try to use visualization to help the energy rise.) Linking mind and body is a prerequisite for the harmonious and powerful functioning of vital energy. Bringing this energy to the pineal gland in the head is the Divine purpose.

First Stage
1. Sit so that you can press the heel of one foot against the opening of the vagina. You will want a steady and fairly firm pressure against the clitoris. If it is not possible to place your foot in this position, then place a fairly hard, round object, such as one of the steel balls commonly sold in boxed sets in Chinese shops, against the vaginal opening. (You may experience a pleasurable sensation due to the stimulation of the genital area and the subsequent release of sexual energy.)
2. Rub your hands together vigorously. This will cause heat in your hands by bringing the energy of your body into your palms and fingers.
3. Place your hands on your breasts to that you feel the heat from your hands enter into the skin.
4. Rub your breasts slowly in outward, circular motions. Your right hand will turn counter-clockwise; your left, clockwise.
5. Rub in this circular manner for a minimum of thirty-six times or a maximum of 360 times up to two times a day. It will not be necessary to do 360 hand rotations once a woman has succeeded in stopping her period. Less than 100 rotations, twice a day, will suffice to maintain a suspension of menstruation once it has stopped. A woman is the best judge of when she should suspend or resume menstruation. Resumption occurs after cessation of the exercise.)

Second Stage This exercise can be done sitting or lying down.
1. First, tighten the muscles of the vagina and anus as if you were trying to close both openings, and then try to draw the rectum upward inside the body, further contracting the anal muscles. When done properly this will feel as though air is being drawn up into the rectum and vagina. Hold these muscles tight for as long as you can comfortably.
2. Relax and repeat the anal and vaginal contractions. Do this as many times as you wish.
NOTE A You may insert a finger into the vagina when you do the contractions, to determine the strength of your contractions.
NOTE B The lips of the vagina are sensitive and must be massaged and stimulated during the Deer Exercise. Sitting on the heel of a foot or a ball serves this purpose. Finger pressure also serves this purpose, but if finger pressure is used on the vaginal lips, it is important to rub the lips and press each of the twelve pressure points surrounding the opening in a clockwise motion. Alternatively, your partner can rub the vagina. This is very beneficial because the energy that flows through the hands of one partner flows into the body of the other. (In the man's Deer Exercise, the woman can do the rubbing and holding of the testicles.)

If a woman finds it tiring to use both hands at once to do the breast rubbing, she can use one hand on the opposite breast while the other hand rests. Or, the free hand can be used to stimulate the vaginal opening in place of the heel. Another method is that the man rubs both breasts while the woman rubs or presses her vagina with her hand. As you can see, this is very flexible exercise which can be adapted to individual preference.

The first few anal and vaginal contractions may be hard to do. Eventually, though, you will be able to increase the number of times you can do it as well as the length of time you are able to hold the contractions. When done properly, a pleasant feeling will travel from the base of anus through the spinal column to the top of the head. This is caused by the build-up of sexual energy and its movement up through the glandular system to the pineal gland at the top of the head.'

The outward rubbing of the breasts is called "dispersion," and it helps prevent lumps and cancer of the breast. It will also decrease the size of breasts that are too large and flabby. Reversing this direction to an inward motion, so that the right hand circles clockwise and the left hand circles counter-clockwise, is called "stimulation" and its effect is to enlarge undersized breasts.

310 – Advanced Yoga Practices

Do this exercise in the morning upon arising and at night before retiring.

When you practice the Deer Exercise, try to avoid touching the nipples. A woman's nipples are very sensitive and easily over-stimulated.

If the exercise is done correctly, a woman will notice an increased sensitivity in her nipples.

Menstruation

A woman's sexual organ system consists of four inter-related parts: the vagina, the uterus, the ovaries, and the breasts. Their inter-relationship can be observed during the course of pregnancy, childbirth, and nursing. Menstruation ceases during these events, and the blood that would be lost during menstruation goes to nourish the baby. After the child is born, the energy is converted to milk for nursing. Menstruation resumes only when nursing stops.

So, stimulating the breasts whether through nursing or massage, as in the Deer Exercise, actually stimulates all the sexual organs. Most women find the exercise very pleasurable, many even reaching orgasm with it.

The Deer Exercise stops menstruation for the same reason that nursing prevents it. When the Deer Exercise is performed, the body reacts just as if a baby were regularly sucking on the breast. The body rushes blood to the breasts rather than the uterus. Taoists refer to this phenomenon as "turning back the blood" because it reenergizes the entire body, expecially the sexual organs.

For thousands of years, the Deer Exercise was used as a technique of family planning. But its main use was for maintaining a youthful countenance. Historical records show that women famous for their beauty consistently use the technique even after giving birth to many children.

The length of times required to stop the menstrual cycles varies by individual. Most women accomplish this within two weeks to six months, but some require as long as a year. All that can be said is that if you practice the exercise diligently, it will happen.

Women should not perform the Deer during pregnancy. The energy generated by the exercise combined with the accompanying increased stimulation of the sexual gland might induce premature labor. Using the Deer Exercise during the menstrual period is permissible., In fact, it usually brings almost immediate relief from menstrual discomfort.

Doing this exercise will correct menstrual irregularities. It will eliminate menstrual cramps and strengthen sexual ability. If you do the exercise with more than the recommended minimum of thirty-six hand rotations twice a day, — as much as 360 times twice a day — you can stop menstruation totally. But on one condition. You must not let your thoughts wander to other matters.

When doing the Deer Exercise, it is important to concentrate on the divine purpose, as it is very easy to become sexually stimulated. If the menstrual period does not stop, practice the Deer more frequently. Work at it a little harder and concentrate on the Divine purpose, even when the body becomes stimulated.

The Deer Exercise will not prolong a woman's fertile period. Menopause will still arrive on schedule at the time specified by the individual's biological clock. However, the problems usually associated with menopause will not appear.

The biological aging process will stop at the point where the Deer Exercise begins to work. If you stop your period at age twenty, you will never look older than twenty years of age. So as you can see, the earlier you begin the Deer Exercise, the younger and healthier you will be. (This also applies to men.)

Furthermore, many students used this method to assist family planning. There were extremely satisfied with it because no chemicals, surgery, or side effects were involved.

www.nine3.com/DeerWoman.html
=======================

The Deer Exercise for Men

The Deer Exercise achieves four important objectives. First, it builds up the tissues of the sexual organs. Second, it draws energy up through six of the Seven Glands of the body into the pineal gland to elevate spirituality. (There is a hormone pathway that leads from the prostate, connects with the adrenal glands, and continues on to the other glands.) Concurrently, blood circulation in the abdominal area is increased. This rush of blood helps transport the nutrients and energy of the semen to the rest of the body.

When energy is brought up into the pineal gland, a chill or tingling sensation is felt to ascend through the spine to reach the head. It feels a little like an orgasm. If you feel a sensation in the area of the pineal gland, but do not feel the tingling sensation in the middle of the back, do not worry. Your sensitivity will increase with experience. If after some time you still cannot sense the progress of energy, certain problems must be taken care of first.

Self-determination is the third benefit derived from the Deer Exercise. If one gland in the Seven Gland system is functioning below par, the energy shooting up the spine will stop there. A weakness is indicated, and special attention should be given to that area. For example, if the thymus gland is functioning poorly, the energy will stop there. The energy will continue to stop there until the thymus gland is healed. When the thymus is again functioning normally, the energy will then move further up along the spine towrad the pineal gland. If the energy moves all the way up to your head during the Deer Exercise, it indicates that all the Seven Glands are functioning well and that there is no energy blockage in the body,. If you do not feel anything during the Deer Exercise, a blockage is indicated. The movement of energy can be felt by everyone if no dysfunctions are encountered.

The fourth benefit of the Deer Exercise is that it builds up sexual ability and enables the man to prolong sexual intercourse. During "ordinary" intercourse the prostate swells with semen to maximum size before ejaculating. During ejaculation, the prostate shoots out its contents in a series of contractions. Then, sexual intercourse ends. With nothing left to ejaculate, induce contractions, or maintain an erection (energy is lost during ejaculation), the man cannot continue to make love. But, if he uses the Deer Exercise to pump semen out of the prostate in small doses, pumping it in the other direction into the other glands and blood vessels, he can prolong intercourse.

Under ordinary circumstances, when the Deer Exercise is not used during intercourse, it will be harmful to interrupt orgasm or prolong intercourse by ordinary means. Under ordinary means, the prostate remains expanded for a long time, unrelieved by the pumping action of the ejaculation, until the semen is carried away by the blood stream. But the prostate is somewhat like a rubber band: it must be allowed to snap back to its original form, otherwise continuous extension will bring about a loss of elasticity. When the prostate loses its elasticity, its function is impaired and it is damaged. The Deer Exercise prolongs orgasm and intercourse, but it protects the prostate by relieving it.

The Deer Exercise is a physical exercise as well as a mental and spiritual exercise. It improves one's sexual abilities as it builds up the energy reserves within the body. Over time, the mental processese are heightened as well, and the outcome is often a glowing feeling of inner tranquility, which is a necessary prerequisite for the unfolding of the golden flower. This exercise may be done standing, sitting, or lying down.

First Stage — The purpose of the first stage is to encourage semen production

Rub the palms of your hands together vigorously. This creates heat in your hands by bringing the energy of your body into your hands and palms.

With your right hand, cup your testicles so that the palm of your hand completely covers them. (The exercise is best done without clothing.) Do not squeeze, but apply a slight pressure, and be aware of the heat from your hand.

Place the palm of your left hand on the area of the pubis, one inch below the navel.

With a slight pressure so that a gentle warmth begins to build in the area of the pubis, move your left hand in clockwise or counterclockwise circles eighty-one times.

Rub your hands together vigorously again.

Reverse the position of your hands so that your hleft hand cups the testicles and your right hand is on the pubis. Repeat the circular rubbing in the opposite direction another eighty-one times. Concentrate on what you are doing, and feel the warmth grow. For all Taoist exercises, it is very important — indeed, it is necessary — that you concentrate on the purpose of the physical motions, for doing so will enhance the results. It will unify the body and mind and bring full power to the purpose. Never tro to use the mind to force the natural processes by imagining fires growing in the public area, or any other area. This is dangerous.

Second Stage — Tighten the muscles around the anus and draw them up and in. When done properly, it will feel as if air is being drawn up to your rectum, or as if the entire anal area is being drawn in and upward. Tighten as hard as you can and hold as long as you are able to do so comfortably.

Stop and relax a moment.

Repeat the anal contractions. Do this as many times as you can without feeling discomfort.

As you do the second stage of the exercise, concentrate on feeling a tingling sensation (similar to an electric shock) ascend along the pathway of the Seven Glands. The sensation lasts for fractions of a second and results naturally. Do not try to force this with mental images.

Some teachings suggest that thoughts should be used to help or guide energy flow. Those who make these suggestions misunderstand the nature of energy. There are six forms of energy: mechanical energy, heat energy, sound energy, radiant energy, atomic energy, and electrical energy. We emit electrical energy. The electrical energy in man differs drastically from that used to run a house, for example. The electrical current in the average house fluctuates at 60 cycles per second; in men, 49,000,000 cycles per second. The latter figure is about half that of light, which travels at 186,000 miles per second. So when a man starts to think or breathe, the electrical energy will have already reached its destination. Our thoughts, breaths, etc. are too slow to guide the flow of electrical energy.

What occurs at the unconscious level was not meant to be subject to the control of the conscious mind. If the conscious mind interfere with something it was not evolved to control — helping or guiding electrical energy through visualization, thoughts, etc., — it can cause a great deal of damage. Its interference with the natural progress of energy can cause schizophrenia, brain damage, and a host of other problems. Taoists call these calamities "Disintegration into Evil."

The Deer Exercise is extremely safe — provided, that is, it is not supplemented with techniques of other teachings. For show, various incompatible techniques are often thrown together to create spectacular techniques, but the results are often disastrous. Lao-Tse said, "My way is simple and easy." And true Taoist methods ARE simple and easy.

NOTE A At first you may find that you are able to hold the anal sphincter muscles tight for only a few seconds. Please persist. After several weeks you will be able to hold the muscles tight for quite awhile without experiencing weariness or strain.

NOTE B To determine whether the Deer Exercise is having an effect on the prostrate gland, try this test: as you urinate, try to stop the stream of urine entirely through anal muscle contractions. If you are able to do so, then the exercise is effective.

NOTE C Pressure is being placed on the prostate gland as it is gently massaged by the tightening action of the anal muscles. (The anus can be thought of as a little motor which pumps the prostate gland.) Thus stimulated, the prostate begins to secrete hormones, such as endorphins, etc., to produce a natural high. When the prostate goes into spasms, a small orgasm is experienced. By alternately squeezing and relaxing the anus during the Deer Exercise, a natural high is produced without having to jog ten miles or endure the side-effects of running.

NOTE D Do this exercise in the morning upon rising and before retiring at night.
www.nine3.com/DeerMan.html

2008/01/29 13:39:02
Tantra - Sex and Spiritual Development
http://www.aypsite.org/forum/topic.asp?TOPIC_ID=3398&REPLY_ID=29428&whichpage=-1
Tantric sex and birth control
Note: It is possible that either of the exercises copied above may cause excessive kundalini energy flows, especially if being added to an existing daily routine of yoga practices -- particularly one involving mudras, bandhas and advanced pranayama methods. There can be a risk of overdoing whenever adding "same in class" practices. In AYP, we call it the "doubling up" effect. So be mindful of the risk and always self-pace practices as necessary to keep things on an even keel.

The guru is in you.

2008/01/30 10:28:30
Tantra - Sex and Spiritual Development
http://www.aypsite.org/forum/topic.asp?TOPIC_ID=3398&REPLY_ID=29457&whichpage=-1

Tantric sex and birth control

quote:
_____
Originally posted by Katrine

So.....is it common, that the "circle" i find myself in (as to Kundalini) eventually ....thins out..... the bleeding?
_____

Hi Katrine:

So it has been said in quite a few writings on advancing spiritual development, including in the above article on the Taoist Deer Exercise, which offers a "cause and effect" (practice) for reducing menstruation. It seems logical that an awakened and advancing kundalini, by whatever means, could have the same effect.

Your experience could be due to a combination of things, as is so often the case. Obviously, the strong emotions associated with the loss of your mother have had an effect, as have likely your dramatic inner energy developments (kundalini) in recent years. Pre-menopause can't be entirely ruled out either.

I can't go too far with this, because I do not have the direct experience to support any conclusions. The main thing is that you are feeling well and moving ahead in life and in spirit. :-)

Perhaps there are other ladies here who can add perspective on this?

All the best!

The guru is in you.

2008/02/21 10:32:15
Tantra - Sex and Spiritual Development
http://www.aypsite.org/forum/topic.asp?TOPIC_ID=3475&REPLY_ID=30362&whichpage=-1
Swollen Lingam

Hi John:

Tantric masturbation is common and well-documented in the Taoist schools, which approach the cultivation of higher sexual functioning with less shyness and secrecy than other traditons. Since human spiritual capabilities are universal everywhere, similar renditions can be found in every tradition, though often less visible.

For example, in yoga, self-cultivation of sexual energy is only thinly veiled in techniquies like mulabandha and siddhasana. Once ecstatic conductivity is awakened, sambhavi and kechari mudras can be regarded as self-stimulation of sexual energy also. And so it goes...

All of this may be regarded as relationship with the divine lover within. This in particularly true as the process advances and becomes more internal. Then it comes to be called "internal lovemaking" and highly charged with bhakti, which accelerates the process of human spiritual transformation. Some of the prominent European nuns of the middle ages were known (through their diaries) to be quite ero-ecstatically involved with Christ within themselves. Was that relationship expressed in some outer ways? Only their habits and confessors knew for sure. :-)

The guru is in you.

2008/02/21 14:22:42
Tantra - Sex and Spiritual Development
http://www.aypsite.org/forum/topic.asp?TOPIC_ID=3475&REPLY_ID=30386&whichpage=-1
Swollen Lingam

quote:
_____
Originally posted by John C

Do you then have a specific reference in the available literature relating to masturbation by Catholic monastics?
_____

Hi John:

"Ecstatic Confessions" by Martin Buber, which covers a range of ascetics over the centuries, west and east. The word "masturbation" is not used as I recall, but the ero-ecstatic element is plainly visible in quite a few of the writings. Highly ecstatic bhakti plays a key role in many cases.

As mentioned, yoga tends to be somewhat indirect on this, though the techniques mentioned already are clear enough in their purpose. If you get into the details of the life of Ramakrisna (see "Gospel of Ramakrishna" by M), the sexual element will be clear enough, though I don't think the word "masturbation" is used there either. However, something that might be called "spiritual orgasm" occurs often without the presence of an outer partner. It is an inside job. :-)

A case for masturbation is not being made here. But the case for expansion of sexual function to higher purpose is -- by whatever effective means that are available within the context of one's sexual preferences. There is no judgment here on methods or lifestyle. We are only interested in results.

The operative principle and the methodologies used are all related to extended periods of pre-orgasmic cultivation. That is the central theme in the AYP Tantra lessons and the AYP Tantra book. It can be found in greater or lesser detail in many traditions.

The guru is in you.

2008/02/21 16:20:47
Tantra - Sex and Spiritual Development
http://www.aypsite.org/forum/topic.asp?TOPIC_ID=3475&REPLY_ID=30395&whichpage=-1
Swollen Lingam

Hi John:

Nothing is new under the sun.

I would not claim that anything has been "invented" within AYP. It is an integration and optimization of methods that have been around for thousands of years, including the spiritual use of masturbation from the ancient Taoist schools, and elsewhere. It is not presented here as a "must do." Rather, it is presented as one of many options for pre-orgasmic cultivation according to one's lifestyle.

If anything is new in AYP it is the flexibility to look objectively across sectarian lines and review causes and effects in relation to known capabilities we all have for human spiritual transformation. That, and open access for everyone to information on the exploration, the means, and the results. Even these elements of AYP are not new. Many have sought to do the same in the past, but were thwarted by the forces of sectarianism and ignorance. Now, in the information age, we can do more, so we will. :-)

The spiritual practices side of what eventually became AYP has been a lone project I was engaged in for many years, based on extensive research, numerous initiations, and personal experiments. All this writing is an attempt to pass it on so others can carry the investigation and applied knowledge much further in the future. It has been happening already through the independent research of many who keep in touch here, which brings me great joy.

The guru is in you.

2008/03/15 13:13:05
Tantra - Sex and Spiritual Development
http://www.aypsite.org/forum/topic.asp?TOPIC_ID=3620&REPLY_ID=31336&whichpage=-1
tantra-sex and spiritual developement

Hi Lambs Bread, and welcome!

With most practices there is a breaking in stage when practice or results can be a bit uneven. We call it the "clunky stage." If there is too much discomfort, then it is wise to reduce practice time until things smooth out. Then practice can be inched up again.

Nothing to fear. Just take some time to adapt and all will be fine.

You will get the most out of tantric practices if you are doing a daily routine of sitting practices -- deep meditation, spinal breathing pranayama, etc. See the "main lessons" link at the top of this page. It is suggested to take the lessons in order for best results.

In the lessons there are many reminders not to overdo, and to "self-pace" practices for good progress with comfort. This goes for all practices, including tantra.

Wishing you all the best on your path. Enjoy!

The guru is in you.

2008/04/01 14:14:43
Tantra - Sex and Spiritual Development
http://www.aypsite.org/forum/topic.asp?TOPIC_ID=3692&REPLY_ID=32041&whichpage=-1
karmamudra in Tantra?

Hi Kris:

Karmamudra is old-fashioned ritualized sex (with young women) for monastic men. Its worth could be debated, not to mention it's obvious chauvinistic characteristics. If a taste of samad
Hi (nirvikalpa or other) were the only prerequisite for karmamudra, many around here would qualify, including many of the women. :-)

In any case, it is not really relevant for yoga practitioners who live in the world, who can integrate effective tantric methods into whatever lifestyle they happen to be living, with good results at any stage of human spiritual transformation. See the AYP tantra lessons and book for more on this.

If "karmamudra" were to be interpreted in a broader more reasonable way to mean "the application of tantric sexual principles and methods for the equal benefit of both genders," then we have it well covered here.

All the best!

The guru is in you.

2008/04/01 17:09:12
Tantra - Sex and Spiritual Development
http://www.aypsite.org/forum/topic.asp?TOPIC_ID=3692&REPLY_ID=32053&whichpage=-1
karmamudra in Tantra?

Hi Kris:

The the role of sexual energy in human spiritual transformation is not that complicated, and it is the same for everyone everywhere. The methods are pretty straight forward also, though culture and religion often cloud the issue with edicts and/or esoteric mumbo jumbo.

The essential principle in practice is "preservation and cultivation of sexual energy," which underlies every true tantric ritual and practice. It can be applied in any sexual lifestyle in modern times (with or without partner), and is also at the heart of the celibate path. Check the AYP writings. :-)

There are many others here who can help with questions on this. All the best on your path!

The guru is in you.

2008/04/02 10:56:41
Tantra - Sex and Spiritual Development
http://www.aypsite.org/forum/topic.asp?TOPIC_ID=3692&REPLY_ID=32094&whichpage=-1
karmamudra in Tantra?

Hi Kris:

It is important to distinguish between the application of tantric principles and lifestyle choices.

Celibacy is a lifestyle choice. So is every other kind of relationship we may be drawn to and choose regarding sexual urges and the energy involved.

All too often, celibacy is taught as technique. It is not technique. It is lifestyle. Likewise, conjugal sex is sometimes taught as tantra technique. It is not technique. It is lifestyle. If lifestyle is taught as technique, sooner or later it will lead to strain and difficulties, because everyone has different lifestyle tendencies and needs.

Whatever sexual lifestyle we may be drawn to can have tantric principles applied within it. Our lifestyle needs and choices may change over time, and the application of tantric principles can be adjusted accordingly as those lifestyle changes occur.

In your case, you are having great inner openings, so you are finding some changes occurring in your inner energy dynamics. Should you change your lifestyle to accommodate that? It is entirely up to you.

On the other hand, you could continue with your present lifestyle with some modifications in conduct to accommodate your inner openings and the need for more vitality to be flowing internally. You don't have to give up sex. You just have to make it more tantric -- leaning more toward preservation and cultivation of sexual energy. Learning the holdback and blocking techniques can help with this. That is where you can start, without upsetting the applecart by making big lifestyle changes, disrupting important relationships, family responsibilities, etc.

Learning and applying sound tantric methods can transform normal sexual relations into spiritual practice.

Your partner should be brought on board. It can bring the relationship to new levels of ecstasy and love. You can also find much better management of sexual energy in solo situations.

If you go through the AYP tantra lessons or the tantra book, then you will be fully equipped information-wise to work the situation from right where you are, without having to make radical lifestyle changes which probably would not stick anyway.

Rome was not built in a day. So take it one day at a time. Nothing to worry about. The tools are available, and things are going to get a whole lot better. Just study up, continue with practices, and give it some time. Good things are happening.

The guru is in you.

2008/04/18 11:40:41
Tantra - Sex and Spiritual Development
http://www.aypsite.org/forum/topic.asp?TOPIC_ID=3786&REPLY_ID=32785&whichpage=-1
Some confusion misconception many-2 things

Hi Mrityunjay:

We take a different slant on brahmacharya in AYP, defining it as "preservation and cultivation of sexual energy," which can be accomplished in either non-celibate or celibate lifestyle. The AYP tantra lessons and book provide means for that.

There are no absolutes in conduct -- only effective application of underlying principles forwarding the ongoing process of human spiritual transformation, which can be accomplished within any culture, religion or lifestyle.

All the best!

The guru is in you.

2010/01/27 11:59:11
Tantra - Sex and Spiritual Development
http://www.aypsite.org/forum/topic.asp?TOPIC_ID=3786&REPLY_ID=63936&whichpage=-1
Some confusion misconception many-2 things

quote:

Originally posted by mrityunjay_singh_1983

Q1.If i do Male NSV(sperm is not add with semen) For birth control.And i still practicing yoga.Am i still progress in yoga(means Mental silence and ecstatic conductivity)?

Q2.Suppose that husband body and wife body both have Ecstatic conductivity.They go to sex for progeny.Is this ecstacy create birth problem?

_____

Hi mrityunjay_singh_1983:

I would say the answer is "yes" to Q1, and "no" to Q2.

Not sure what you mean by "NSV," but sperm in the semen is not a prerequisite for progress with tantric methods and brahmacharya (preservation and cultivation of sexual energy). Several who have had vasectomy here have verified this.

The guru is in you.

2008/05/03 09:52:18
Tantra - Sex and Spiritual Development
http://www.aypsite.org/forum/topic.asp?TOPIC_ID=3843&REPLY_ID=33354&whichpage=-1
An experiment on siddhasana/sex drive

Hi All:

After 25+ years of using siddhasana in sitting practices, there has been no degradation in normal sexual function here. What there has been is a gradual expansion of sexual function upward into the higher neurobiology, tying in with the rest of practices and the rise of inner silence and ecstatic conductivity/radiance. This has naturally led to more focus on radiance (outpouring divine love in activity - stillness in action) and less focus on reproductive sexual function. This in no way limits the ability to engage in sexual activity and have children as desired. It just isn't desired as much, since more engaging and pleasurable things are going on most of the time.

It is the difference between non-stop regenerative orgasm and intermittent degenerative orgasm. With both options available, which would you be doing most of the time? Everyone is free to choose. :-)

The guru is in you.

2008/05/04 11:16:17
Tantra - Sex and Spiritual Development
http://www.aypsite.org/forum/topic.asp?TOPIC_ID=3843&REPLY_ID=33403&whichpage=-1
An experiment on siddhasana/sex drive

quote:
_____
Originally posted by selfonlypath

Do you agree that Siddhasana is more to awaken hence raise up energy to Father Sky but does not resolve the bigger K-symptom which is descend down energy to Mother Earth (grounding then rooting) **once** it has been awakened ?

Maybe AYP through **under the hood** does not have the notion of energy up, energy down then when the system is purified enough, merging safely both flows for self-realisation ?
_____

Hi Albert:

Siddhasana and other tantric sexual methods enliven and make vital essence active and available in the higher-up neurobiology. From there it will go in whatever direction it needs to according to natural development, stimulated by additional practices. The AYP practices are not for taking energy in one direction or the other. They are for enlivening natural balanced flow. More importantly, the whole process resides in inner silence, which is universal without direction, or in all directions -- omnipresent.

Depending on an individual's matrix of inner obstructions, the energy may appear to go one way or the other (sometimes to excess), or get stuck somewhere, and self-pacing and/or grounding may be necessary. As you know, this is discussed in many places in the lessons and forums.

Some may add additional measures, seeking to direct energy in one direction or the other (up, down, or elsewhere). This may be deemed necessary at certain times, but carries with it the risk of creating some distortions even while resolving others. We all do what we must to move ahead.

To the extent directional practices exist in AYP (like spinal breathing pranayama), they are bi-directional or "global," aimed at promoting balance between ascending and descending energies, while enlivening them. Even powerful siddhasana is balanced through integration with the rest of the AYP practices.

Again, the entire process resides in stillness, so the concept of "direction" is a stepping-stone, a construct (literal or imagined) in time and space. That's why we let it go (under the hood) while favoring the practices that stimulate the underlying process of transformation, which is the cultivation and union of stillness with energetic flow, leading to the experience of stillness in action -- non-duality in duality. It is about favoring and releasing -- with releasing being the operative part.

Keep in mind that a sapling will find its natural fruition as a tree when provided with healthy nutrients and environment, and then left to grow, rather than by being managed inch by inch. Unless a Bonsai-style tree is desired, which, while perhaps satisfying in some ways, isn't a very liberated representation of enlightenment. :-)

That's why when we get the thought, "Oh, the energy has to go (or is going) this way or that way," it is wise to just easily favor the practice we are doing. Favor the practice and release...

The guru is in you.

2008/05/05 11:47:45
Tantra - Sex and Spiritual Development
http://www.aypsite.org/forum/topic.asp?TOPIC_ID=3843&REPLY_ID=33438&whichpage=-1
An experiment on siddhasana/sex drive

quote:
_____
Originally posted by selfonlypath

Do you make a difference between grounding and rooting ?

In AYP, what are the specific asanas that helps grounding and / or rooting ?

If there exist such asanas, which one involves sexual energy ?
_____

Hi Albert:

In yoga, "grounding" is a concept implying balance of ascending and descending energies with extra focus on the latter, where-as "rooting" has a marshal arts (or taoist) connotation. In the end, they probably mean the same thing, though the methods of yoga and taoism are markedly different, reflecting their ancient traditional objectives.

To be honest, I can't think of any asanas that are specifically for grounding. Taken together, asanas are for energy awakening and balancing, but not primarily for grounding. Asanas may or may not help an energy imbalance, depending on the type and severity. We find out by trying and self-pacing. Asana experts, please add perspective on this as needed.

In yoga, worldly activity is for grounding, particularly physical activity, though also social and intellectual. Anything that keeps us engaged in time and space will help integrate inner silence and our enlivened spiritual energies into everyday living. It is the evolving dynamic of stillness in action.

Taoist methods are geared more to cultivating rooting prior to engagement in activity, stemming from the marshal arts traditions they come from. Tai C
Hi and related disciplines are both rooting and grounding.

Many asanas (including mudras and bandhas) act directly or indirectly on sexual energy. Siddhasana is an obvious one. As mentioned, asanas are not specifically designed for grounding, but collectively are for enlivening and balancing. So, in yoga, in addition to cultivating inner silence through deep meditation, samyama, etc, and awakening and balancing our energies through pranayama, asanas, mudras and bandhas, etc, we also keep active in daily life for practical integration and grounding.

Bringing in taoist methods, like a daily tai c
Hi routine, can be helpful for grounding/rooting also. Some here have gone much further in combining yoga and taoist methods. And, of course, we self-pace all of our practices as necessary. The measures taken will depend on the individual dynamics of purification and opening.

Where do you see shaman terminology and methods fitting into this, or vise versa?

The guru is in you.

PS:
Hi Alvin: Richard gave you good feedback on siddhasana. It works, doesn't it? :-)

2008/05/05 15:21:11
Tantra - Sex and Spiritual Development
http://www.aypsite.org/forum/topic.asp?TOPIC_ID=3843&REPLY_ID=33443&whichpage=-1
An experiment on siddhasana/sex drive

quote:
_____
Originally posted by Alvin Chan

But I do feel a little uncomfortable in my head which I think is related to it. Something like a pressure, which sometimes annoys me. It's not manifesting any further, just like stucking there. I can bear it and actually, it's not that bad. But sometimes I get a little impatient on whether I'm actually heading anywhere. It feels like it's just a temporary reaction from the practice, rather than a transient state leading to something great.
_____

Hi Alvin:

Don't forget to self-pace. No practice has to be all or nothing. Find your balance -- including with siddhasana. You can use your symptoms (head pressure, etc) as a feedback mechanism for that. It is not a reliable approach to "tough it out" through uncomfortable symptoms. Much better to do what is necessary to stay on an even keel.

As for getting anywhere, it seems you have traveled far in the past few years, in many ways. A few years from now, you will see how much further you have traveled from here. Yogic results do not lend themselves to day-to-day measurement. Though we may see something happening in the short term, it is only in the long term that we come to know what it is. So patience and stable daily practice are the keys. It is a marathon, not a sprint.

Don't build too many expectations for "something great." Just practice and live fully. Then ordinary life will gradually rise to the occasion.

What the ordinary see as great, the great see as ordinary. :-)

The guru is in you.

2008/05/21 11:23:22
Tantra - Sex and Spiritual Development
http://www.aypsite.org/forum/topic.asp?TOPIC_ID=3933&REPLY_ID=33961&whichpage=-1
nonejaculatory orgasm or no orgasm

Hi Anthem:

Favoring pre-orgasmic cultivation is favoring pre-orgasmic cultivation, whether it is genital or higher up. The fact is, we are going to go for what we are inclined toward, and forcing it the other way will not help. But when we have a choice (increasingly with the rise of inner silence), we can gently favor pre-orgasmic cultivation. The tool of holdback works in any situation, always going higher and higher, dissolving in transcendence.

In time, sex expands to become full time ecstatic bliss and almost entirely non-physical, as some of the beautiful posts here have described. Whether we are having orgasms or not in that situation is almost beside the point. We will know what to do based on our own inner process and bhakti.

There is so much psychology in it. It seems in the beginning people on one end either crave or fear going to the other end -- what is not in the present. Having sex versus not having sex, or vise versa. It is really about where we are today, which is always going to be somewhere in-between, and very much a matter of personal choice in relation our lifestyle, present state of consciousness and the methods we have available.

We have been going around on it over here too, from the point of view of having a craving for celibacy:
http://www.aypsite.org/forum/topic.asp?TOPIC_ID=3143#33956

There really are no fixed answers, because everyone is in a different place. Yet, there are underlying principles at work relating to the process of human spiritual transformation. Where there are principles, there can be methods to apply them for benefit, and that is what tantra is about.

I suggest reviewing the tantra lessons (where the key points are covered), and taking it easy. As we practice over time, what is true will certainly emerge.

The guru is in you.

2008/05/21 18:28:08
Tantra - Sex and Spiritual Development
http://www.aypsite.org/forum/topic.asp?TOPIC_ID=3933&REPLY_ID=33971&whichpage=-1
nonejaculatory orgasm or no orgasm

quote:
_____
Originally posted by Anthem11

Hi Yogani,

Thanks for your reply, suggestions always appreciated and I will review the tantra lessons.

Just to clarify, how would you define pre-orgasmic? Does this include orgasmic sensations without ejaculation? Does this also include ecstatic sensations which occur higher in the body during sexual activities?

Starting with where I am now as an example which may be helpful to others? I enjoy favoring not ejaculating, I like the way it feels, but would you also suggest avoiding orgasmic sensations without ejaculation if they come up during sexual activities?

_____

Hi Anthem:

I'd say anything in the nature of a climax is what we can choose to stay in front of. But there are no hard and fast rules.

If there is no depletion, and an increasing energy flow, then what will a climax in that situation matter? If there is depletion, then it will matter more. What we are doing through a range of means is cultivating the neurobiology to continuously expand in ecstasy without depletion. Both the underlying principle and the practical metric are found in that, and the practice can favor it when we are able to choose in stillness. In fact, the entire process depends on stillness, which is the other half of the marriage of stillness and ecstatic conductivity occurring within us.

The guru is in you.

2008/06/03 11:13:27
Tantra - Sex and Spiritual Development
http://www.aypsite.org/forum/topic.asp?TOPIC_ID=3933&REPLY_ID=34343&whichpage=-1
nonejaculatory orgasm or no orgasm

Hi YB, emc and All:

Kumbhaka (breath suspension), or any "restraint of breath" (the definition of pranayama), will draw vitality into the higher neurobiology from the vast pranic storehouse of the sexual function. As many here know, deep meditation helps facilitate this process in a natural way.

Pre-orgasmic sexual stimulation will cultivate vitality into the higher neurobiology.

Orgasm will draw vitality for reproduction, which is its purpose. Hence the often-felt depletion in the higher neurobiology after orgasm occurs. If a sexual "climax" of any kind leads to a sense of depletion, then this we may choose to stay in front of next time, if our objective in sex is enlivening the higher neurobiology.

Kumbhaka and pre-orgasmic stimulation have similar effects, but are coming from two different internal dynamics. We could say that kumbhaka creates a *pull* on the pranic storehouse, while pre-orgasmic stimulation creates a *push*.

Can these two dynamics be combined at the same time for better effect? Perhaps, but it is a tricky business. We will be sure to be getting the best from both dynamics by applying sound pranayama methods during our sitting practices, and sound tantric methods in relation to our sexual lifestyle, whatever it may be (hetero, homo, solo, celibate, etc.)

All the best!

The guru is in you.

2008/06/04 08:45:15
Tantra - Sex and Spiritual Development
http://www.aypsite.org/forum/topic.asp?TOPIC_ID=3933&REPLY_ID=34366&whichpage=-1
nonejaculatory orgasm or no orgasm

Hi YB:

I think you have it. Pranayama (and kumbhaka) restrict our external source of vitality (oxygen) and coax the body to draw on it's internal storehouse of vitality in the pelvic region. That storehouse can also be stimulated directly via tantric sexual means. Orgasm temporarily depletes the internal storehouse. That is the essential relationship between vitality (prana), sexual energy and spiritual development. There are a thousand ways to proceed from there -- many that are practical, and some that are fanatical. We prefer the practical. :-)

The guru is in you.

2008/05/24 16:05:10
Tantra - Sex and Spiritual Development
http://www.aypsite.org/forum/topic.asp?TOPIC_ID=3958&REPLY_ID=34025&whichpage=-1
Loss of libido due to aging

Hi Shakti, and welcome to the forums!

Well, none of us are getting any younger, and I have a few years on you, so don't feel too old. :-)

Active libido is not a prerequisite for progress on the path. Inner silence is much more important, and age is not a restriction on that.

Sex and spirituality are strange bed-fellows. On one extreme we have practitioners trying to kill off libido, and on the other extreme those who want it retained in full force forever. "Energy work" (at all ages) is largely viewed in that sort of love/hate way too. The truth is, if we have neurobiological energy (and we all do) we can use it in natural ways for cultivating ecstatic conductivity and radiance. That is why we have spinal breathing pranayama, asanas, mudras, bandhas, tantric methods, etc. But the core of the journey is really beyond all that, in stillness.

Who is concerned about cultivating inner silence? That is really the key, and it does not depend primarily on energy cultivation. It is great that you are meditating daily. The procedure of deep meditation as covered in the AYP writings will take care of any distractions. Just easily favor the mantra when you realize you are off it. It will become finer with more abiding stillness being present over time. A "clunky stage" with the mantra in the beginning is pretty normal. It will smooth out as your nervous system purifies and opens.

The suggestion is to take it easy, not try and do too many practices (self-pace for progress with comfort), and enjoy!

The guru is in you.

2008/08/01 13:46:44
Tantra - Sex and Spiritual Development
http://www.aypsite.org/forum/topic.asp?TOPIC_ID=4089&REPLY_ID=35938&whichpage=-1
Do Angels have sex?

Hi All:

Great discussion!

This post from this morning in the tantra forum might add some perspective on the celibate non-celibate discussion:

http://www.aypsite.org/forum/topic.asp?TOPIC_ID=4225#35937

The suggestion is for each of us to go with a sexual lifestyle that is natural for us (one size does not fit all), and engage in an effective integration of daily yoga practices. Then we will have the best result, regardless of our chosen lifestyle.

Enlightenment cannot be regimented. It is a process of letting go which, paradoxically, is best accomplished through systematic means that are compatible with the life we are living. :-)

All the best!

The guru is in you.

2008/08/17 14:15:03
Tantra - Sex and Spiritual Development
http://www.aypsite.org/forum/topic.asp?TOPIC_ID=4089&REPLY_ID=36465&whichpage=-1
Do Angels have sex?

Hi All:

So how do we reconcile all these points of view about sex versus no sex, and attachment versus no attachment?

I don't think it can ever be all one way or the other. And neither can we construct it in our mind as such. It is not possible to free ourselves by replacing one mental structure (or obsession) with another one.

From the AYP point of view, we cultivate inner silence in deep meditation, and the whole thing begins to loosen up in stillness. All of our perceptions and notions about things gradually become less rigid and we find that clinging to new mental structures is not needed to dissolve old mental structures -- indeed, that cannot work. Instead, we find ourselves more able to let go into our rising inner silence, and that is the dissolving of attachment to objects -- our thoughts and obsessions about sex (or no sex), and everything else.

It does not happen overnight. It is a gradual development, and it is not reasonable to expect anyone to change instantly from one point of view or lifestyle to another one. That goes for the divine transformation of sexual energy, and for our realization that we are the infinite sea of non-duality (no-thing-ness) that we happen to be swimming in at this very moment.

In AYP we take it gradually, and it all comes in good time with daily practices. When it comes to sex, the methods of yoga and tantra are conducive to this gradual transformation, and able to serve us wherever we may be on the path.

That is why in AYP we do not define brahmacharya as celibacy. The literal translation of "brahmacharya" is "walking in Brahma, the infinite creative stillness of God." There is nothing in this that says sex is bad, though some may insist on making it mean that, at their own peril, and at the peril of those they may be able to indoctrinate likewise.

Rather than go down the sectarian road of insisting on the same lifestyle for everyone, in AYP we identify the working principle of brahmacharya as the preservation and cultivation of sexual energy. This view of brahmacharya opens the door to all lifestyles and to all the tools of yoga and tantra, and there is no conflict. Everyone can walk in Brahma in their own time and in their own way. Favoring the preservation and cultivation of sexual energy with appropriate means can suit the celibate, the heterosexual, and the homosexual.

And guess what? It works, as many here can attest.

I greatly admire the life and teachings of Sivananda, but his views on sex are very narrow, and suitable mainly for those inclined toward an ascetic lifestyle. This is fine, but it is not a valid teaching for the broad population, who, with effective means available, have equal access to enlightenment.

And the angels? Well, I think they have other things on their non-minds. They are surely laughing angel-laughs about our obsession with these things, even as they are wishing to come join us in physical form, so they too can have the opportunity to evolve that we have. Mortality is a great motivator of spiritual progress. Don't we know it? So let's not waste a minute. :-)

All the best!

The guru is in you.

2008/08/01 13:27:31
Tantra - Sex and Spiritual Development
http://www.aypsite.org/forum/topic.asp?TOPIC_ID=4225&REPLY_ID=35937&whichpage=-1
stillness, ecstatic conductivity after ejaculation

Hi Ananda:

It is a revealing experience.

There is obviously more at work here than the relationship of sexual continence with spiritual progress. If that were not true, then those who say "Be celibate!" would be right, and you would not be having this experience. But it is not as simple as adopting a particular mind-set or sexual lifestyle -- celibate, hetero, homo, solo, etc.

The truth is that enlightenment can be cultivated in any sexual lifestyle, as long as there is an effective integration of spiritual practices in use and sexual activity is moderate according to individual need -- not taken to either extreme, which will inevitably lead to difficulties.

Ananda, in your case, I think what you are seeing is the result of your sitting practices (deep meditation, spinal breathing, etc) in relation to your normal sexual activity. As the neurobiology becomes accustomed to sustaining inner silence and ecstatic conductivity, then the sexual function will be expanding naturally as part of this transformation. So then any sexual stimulation will become naturally tantric in nature (even with orgasm/ejaculation), with part of the energy automatically supporting our spiritual experience. That is what happens as our neurobiology awakens. The role of sex naturally expands into the spiritual realm. I think everyone knows this intuitively. Sometimes there is fear about it, but there is nothing to fear. Sexual energy is an expression of our divine Self, like everything else is.

It is not the orgasm/ejaculation that is feeding the process as much as the nervous system's expanded capacity to express stillness and ecstasy. If we overdo with too many orgasms/ejaculations in a given time, we will find out that depletion will still be there. The reproductive biochemistry can only be pushed so far before the limitation on the spiritual side will be felt, and then some recovery time will be needed. So moderation is the key.

As the AYP tantra lessons and book say, preservation and cultivation are something we can favor in our sexual lifestyle, whatever it happens to be. That, combined with an effective integration of yoga practices, will take us where we need to go, as you are seeing first hand. Bravo! :-)

As a side note, the expansion of sexual influence in our spiritual experiences is a sign of natural vajroli occurring in our nervous system. This is the rise of sexual essence into our higher neurobiology, where it plays a role in the broad expression of our spiritual experience. In time, vajroli becomes a full time event, part of the neurobiology associated with the ongoing experience of stillness in action and outpouring divine love. This applies equally in both men and women. The idea that vajroli is a mechanical "guy thing" is a myth that has little relevance in the effective application of spiritual methods, as has been discussed in the AYP writings and elsewhere in this tantra forum category.

What Ananda describes above is the effect of natural vajroli brought on by an effective integration of yoga practices, and not a mechanical fabrication. The inner mechanics have not even been noticed, but they are there as evidenced by the experience. Simply put, vajroli is the expansion of sexual function from reproduction to also encompass the neurobiology of enlightenment.

So keep on with daily yoga practices and continue to be moderate in sexual activity. Of course, learning about the principles and practices of tantric sex and favoring them as comfortable within our lifestyle (even if celibate) will be helpful also. As we advance in our yoga practices it becomes steadily more clear what will support our evolution and what will not. As with so many other things, the cultivation of abiding inner silence through deep meditation is the key to good tantra. Then we can't miss.

All the best!

The guru is in you.

2008/08/04 11:00:57
Tantra - Sex and Spiritual Development
http://www.aypsite.org/forum/topic.asp?TOPIC_ID=4236&REPLY_ID=36025&whichpage=-1
tantra and fertility

Hi Glow:

I don't have any special knowledge on fertility, but do concur with Mikkiji.

Doing tantric sexual methods should not interfere with conception as long as your husband ejaculates at the end. That could be after a long time in lovemaking once he develops some skill with holdback, etc. The suggestion is to enjoy the intimacy you have, and nature will take her course. The deep relaxation gained in tantric sex can be an aid, since everything will flow more naturally. Like samyama, just pick it up and let it go. Nature will take care of the rest.

If fertilization is not happening, there are things that can be done to help it along. Our oldest son and his wife were having a similar issue for over a year, and as soon as they began to think seriously about taking additional measures with a doctor's help, they got pregnant (before any measures were taken). Now we have a cute little grand-daughter. It happens like that sometimes, when you might least expect it. Give it some time... :-)

All the best!

The guru is in you.

2008/09/17 07:50:55
Tantra - Sex and Spiritual Development
http://www.aypsite.org/forum/topic.asp?TOPIC_ID=4420&REPLY_ID=37746&whichpage=-1
Can you hurt yourself with "Blocking" technique?

Hi All:

I concur with Christi's comments, with one addition. As ecstatic conductivity is awakened and advances, sexual essences are absorbed increasingly upward through the bladder as part of the corresponding higher neurobiological functioning (natural vajroli), even when there is no external sexual stimulation. In the case of blocking in this situation, only part of the semen will be expelled during urination, due to the constant upward absorption of sexual essences, and depending on how much time passes until urination after blocking.

I have been using blocking for about 25 years with no adverse health effects. Just the opposite. That is why it is in the lessons, and why it has been called "poor man's vajroli." It gets the job done. :-)

Note: Tantric sexual methods work best in conjunction with a daily routine of sitting practices, including deep meditation, spinal breathing, etc. Without these, all bets are off on the effectiveness of tantric sexual methods.

The guru is in you.

PS: As discussed in the tantra lessons and elsewhere in the forums, I believe simple blocking is superior to the much-ballyhooed method of mechanical vajroli. Why develop an elaborate strategy for getting the horse back in the barn when we have a perfectly good strategy for keeping him in the barn in the first place? In any case, neither of these methods are the primary cause of natural vajroli. Sitting practices are the primary cause of natural vajroli, which is a component of the awakening of ecstatic conductivity and radiance (kundalini).

2008/09/17 09:14:38
Tantra - Sex and Spiritual Development
http://www.aypsite.org/forum/topic.asp?TOPIC_ID=4420&REPLY_ID=37749&whichpage=-1
Can you hurt yourself with "Blocking" technique?

Hi Albert:

Blocking or simple blocking (same thing): http://www.aypsite.org/T5.html (plus related AYP tantra lessons) Note: It is pressing and blocking the urethra against the back side of the pubic bone during ejaculation.

<u>Mechanical vajroli:</u> an ancient method of sucking fluid up the urethra into the bladder. See the Hatha Yoga Pradipika.

<u>Natural vajroli:</u> automatic and ongoing uptake of sexual essences into the bladder and beyond, an aspect of rising ecstatic conductivity. A natural result of sitting practices in both men and women.

The guru is in you.

2008/09/18 07:40:27
Tantra - Sex and Spiritual Development
http://www.aypsite.org/forum/topic.asp?TOPIC_ID=4420&REPLY_ID=37789&whichpage=-1
Can you hurt yourself with "Blocking" technique?

quote:
_____
Originally posted by selfonlypath

quote:
_____
Originally posted by yogani
<u>Natural vajroli:</u> automatic and ongoing uptake of sexual essences into the bladder and beyond, an aspect of rising ecstatic conductivity. A natural result of sitting practices in both men and women.
_____

Thx for your clarification Yogani.

One last question, do you consider my practice of *PC muscle self-locking, using deep breathing, tongue touching the roof of my mouth, eyes looking up to have energy go up & relaxing while maintaining high arousal* to be a Natural vajroli ?

In Shakti, Albert
_____

Hi Albert:

Pranayama, mudras and bandhas (basically what you are describing) are part of what cultivate natural vajroli, along with deep meditation, samyama, etc. You will know it is becoming natural vajroli when "whole body mudra" begins to happen, without external sexual stimulation. That is when the internal movements become automatic and very small (micro), and there are ecstatic waves coursing through the body, and beyond. This is the rise of ecstatic conductivity and radiance. It is a second puberty, an awakening. From here, our life gradually transforms to become *stillness in action*, non-duality in the field of duality -- outpouring divine love...

All of this is in the lessons, from many more angles than I can cover here. :-)

The guru is in you.

2008/09/27 12:32:11
Tantra - Sex and Spiritual Development
http://www.aypsite.org/forum/topic.asp?TOPIC_ID=4501&REPLY_ID=38176&whichpage=-1
Genital Pain

Hi Michael Beloved, and welcome!

Just to clarify, the AYP holdback technique is not for blocking, but rather about cultivating in front of genital orgasm, whereby the sexual function is gently coaxed to natural expansion upward in the direction you describe. This is most effective if other yoga practices are engaged in daily, including deep meditation, spinal breathing pranayama, and other methods you have alluded to, which are covered in the AYP Main Lessons linked at the top of this page.

The approach to sex and human spiritual transformation in AYP relies on the same principles you have mentioned, but works within the framework of normal sexual relations, whatever those may be for the practitioner, while easily favoring a course of methods that will aid in expanding the sexual function upward. In this way, the expansion of normal erotic life to normal spiritually ecstatic life will happen in due course, without imposing fixed rules of sexual conduct, which do not work for the broad population. The goal is to provide a clear and do-able path for people, beginning with wherever they happen to be in their sex life today.

Here, we define "brahmacharya" as the preservation and cultivation of sexual energy, and there are effective ways to accomplish this within any sexual lifestyle. For more on the AYP approach to sex and spiritual development, see the Tantra Lessons linked at the top of this page.

Eddie, the discomfort you are experiencing could be associated with your back injury, or it could be congestion from overdoing with tantric methods. Maybe a combination. In either case, the discomfort should be temporary. If it persists, then see a doctor. If there is energetic congestion, then it is suggested to self-pace practices (as you are doing) and make sure to get plenty of <u>grounding activity</u> (walking especially), minding not to aggravate your back, of course. There are more comfortable days ahead.

All the best!

The guru is in you.

2008/09/27 14:43:35
Tantra - Sex and Spiritual Development

http://www.aypsite.org/forum/topic.asp?TOPIC_ID=4502&REPLY_ID=38181&whichpage=-1
Help: Brownish discharge in urine

Hi Anil, and welcome!

Not time to worry yet. Depending on what your tantric practices have been (you should let us know), there can be some discoloration in the urine from time to time. If practice has been intense, then this could be a signal to scale back a bit -- self-pace.

If the symptom persists after self-pacing, especially if there is ongoing discomfort, then it will be good to check with a doctor.

All the best!

The guru is in you.

2008/09/27 17:19:25
Tantra - Sex and Spiritual Development
http://www.aypsite.org/forum/topic.asp?TOPIC_ID=4502&REPLY_ID=38191&whichpage=-1
Help: Brownish discharge in urine

Hi Anil:

Just to clarify, holdback is not the same as blocking. Holdback is a technique for remaining pre-orgasmic, and Blocking is the perineum press method you described, which can be used to aid in retaining semen during and after orgasm. Both practices have their use. See also today's post here: http://www.aypsite.org/forum/topic.asp?TOPIC_ID=4501#38176

In your case, it is probably only a matter of terminology, since you seem to be familiar with both favoring pre-orgasmic sex and blocking.

In time, your occasional symptom should fade as you gain more experience and there is more natural uptake of sexual essences. The suggestions given above still hold.

Also, you will gain the most from tantric sexual methods if you have a daily routine of sitting practices in place -- deep meditation, spinal breathing, etc.

Carry on! :-)

The guru is in you.

2008/10/02 18:06:43
Tantra - Sex and Spiritual Development
http://www.aypsite.org/forum/topic.asp?TOPIC_ID=4502&REPLY_ID=38430&whichpage=-1
Help: Brownish discharge in urine

quote:
_____
Originally posted by Anil

Hi Yogani,

thank you so much for your help. Recently I had an orgasm and I saw some blood along with semen, No pain and no discomfort.
I remember once that I have used extreme force in blocking (perineum press) method.
probably might have ruptured some nervous at the perineum.

Please let me know what should I do now.

Love
Anil

_____

Hi Anil:

It would be prudent to discontinue blocking and any other practices that place stress in that area, until the symptoms normalize. Give it a chance to heal up. Once things get back to normal, then you can consider bringing practices back bit-by-bit in moderation, if so inclined. This is the essential procedure of *self-pacing*, and it applies in any case where practices may be causing symptoms of excess that may cause us discomfort or concern. If the symptom persists, it will be good to see a doctor to get it checked out.

All the best!

The guru is in you.

2008/10/10 11:26:24
Tantra - Sex and Spiritual Development
http://www.aypsite.org/forum/topic.asp?TOPIC_ID=4553&REPLY_ID=38757&whichpage=-1
urinating after tantric practice

Hi Ananda:

It should also be pointed out that with the rise of inner silence leading to ecstatic conductivity, the body-wide neurobiology moves gradually into a new mode of functioning. This is what is behind the beautiful ecstatic experiences you have been describing in other forum topics lately. Many things occur in the body, including the advent of "natural vajroli," which is the automatic uptake into the bladder of sexual essences in both men and women. Some or most of this will be absorbed further upward (our ecstatic experiences are the tell-tale sign), but there will always be some residual left in the urine in the bladder, which is routinely expelled. This is why, even in advanced practitioners, the urine may appear milky and/or foamy from time to time, depending on variations in the process of purification and opening occurring throughout the body. It is normal, and nothing to worry about.

The same thing can happen when the tantra blocking technique is applied, which is less natural, but heading in the right direction in support of an overall routine of yoga and tantra practices. Those who practice old-fashioned Hathayogapradipika-style "mechanical vajroli" (not recommended here) will have this experience also. Obviously, natural vajroli is the best kind of vajroli, because it is a normal part of the much broader process of human spiritual transformation.

Note: Natural vajroli will occur in both celibate and non-celibate practitioners. It is part of our spiritual biology.

The phenomenon of sexual essences showing up in the urine also has some implications for amaroli, but that is a another subject. :-)

All the best!

The guru is in you.

2008/10/10 12:42:40
Tantra - Sex and Spiritual Development
http://www.aypsite.org/forum/topic.asp?TOPIC_ID=4553&REPLY_ID=38764&whichpage=-1
urinating after tantric practice

quote:
_____
Originally posted by Christi

Hi Yogani,

quote:
_____
The phenomenon of sexual essences showing up in the urine also has some implications for amaroli, but that is a another subject.

_____

What implications does it have for amaroli? Presumably it means that anyone practicing amaroli, once natural vajroli is taking place, will be drinking their own sexual fluids, which would end up in the stomach and then be transformed into soma?

Yes?

_____

Hi Christi:

Yes. However, the role this might play in the overall process of human spiritual transformation is not known, so not to get too carried away with it. The symptoms of internal natural vajroli feeding ever-expanding ecstatic conductivity are far more profound than any noticeable symptoms coming from ingesting sexual essences during amaroli practice. I see no "magic bullet" here. :-)

It should not affect normal amaroli practice one way or the other, for those who are doing it. It was mentioned only in passing, as anyone doing amaroli will be sure to think of it in relation to the vajroli discussion. There are implications in the ancient scriptures that vajroli and amaroli have a connection, and this is probably it. If anyone has further revelations on the amaroli aspect, do let us know.

The guru is in you.

2008/11/07 11:05:40
Tantra - Sex and Spiritual Development
http://www.aypsite.org/forum/topic.asp?TOPIC_ID=4656&REPLY_ID=40109&whichpage=-1
Tantra and Homosexuality

Hi Carson:

Here is an AYP lesson that covers tantra and homosexuality:
http://www.aypsite.org/T39.html

The guru is in you.

2009/04/16 11:38:01
Tantra - Sex and Spiritual Development
http://www.aypsite.org/forum/topic.asp?TOPIC_ID=5461&REPLY_ID=48752&whichpage=-1
major case of prostate congestion ?

Hi Non:

Are you practicing deep meditation and spinal breathing pranayama? These (or practices producing similar global effects) are essential for long term progress with tantric sexual methods.

It is not easy to purify and open the upper neurobiology with tantric sexual methods alone. Hence the resistance.

Once a balance of methods is established, then, in time, the resistance gives way to abiding whole body ecstatic conductivity and radiance. It takes an effective integration of practices <u>over time</u> to get the job done.

When we meet with excessive resistance on one front, it can signal that we are neglecting other important fronts. Then it is time to self pace where our intense focus and resulting discomfort is and consider a broader view.

All the best!

The guru is in you.

2009/04/16 16:26:51
Tantra - Sex and Spiritual Development
http://www.aypsite.org/forum/topic.asp?TOPIC_ID=5461&REPLY_ID=48772&whichpage=-1
major case of prostate congestion ?

quote:
_____
Originally posted by Non

I would just love to see a scientific biological viewpoint of tantric practices...
_____

Hi Non:

I am sure it will happen. Maybe it already has. If anyone runs across useful research, do let us know.

The logical place for science to look for the effects of tantric sexual practices is in the rise of "natural vajroli" in spiritual practitioners, and the broader scope of it manifesting as the "nectar cycle" throughout the body. Sooner or later, measurable parameters for these neurobiological/spiritual phenomena will be discovered.

Both of these have been discussed from time to time in the forums (try a few searches). And here are a couple of lessons:
On natural vajroli: http://www.aypsite.org/T60.html
On the nectar cycle: http://www.aypsite.org/304.html

The rise of natural vajroli corresponds with a reduction of resistance to upward flowing vital essences and the rise of ecstatic conductivity throughout the body, beginning between root and brow. As mentioned earlier, this is tied in with our overall approach to spiritual practices, of which tantric sexual methods are one part.

The guru is in you.

2009/04/25 14:53:18
Tantra - Sex and Spiritual Development
http://www.aypsite.org/forum/topic.asp?TOPIC_ID=5508&REPLY_ID=49350&whichpage=-1
Sexual symptoms?

Hi Solo:

Yes, there is a possibility that it is kundalini related, particularly if you are having other kundalini symptoms occurring at the same time.

On the way to <u>natural vajroli</u>, there can be some stinging sensations in the urethra from time to time, even if one is not involved in tantric sexual practices. Deep meditation, spinal breathing and a few mudras and bandhas can produce the same effects.

This is not a diagnosis, just some feedback on spiritual possibilities. It could also be a UTI (urinary tract infection). If the symptom persists, it will be good to get it checked out by a doctor.

All the best!

The guru is in you.

2009/07/18 15:36:41
Tantra - Sex and Spiritual Development
http://www.aypsite.org/forum/topic.asp?TOPIC_ID=5957&REPLY_ID=53679&whichpage=-1
loss of prana

Hi Phoenix:

There is little to no loss of pranic energy in the pre-ejaculatory fluid. In fact, full ejaculation every so often will not be a hazard on the path. Like with anything else, it is the extremes that carry the most risk. That applies to <u>both</u> extreme sexual drain and extreme abstinence. The suggestion is to find your middle path, your balance in normal life. The AYP Tantra writings are designed to be an aid in that for anyone.

Everyone has a different tendency. Fighting that tendecy with the mind for too long can lead to distortions. Much better to gently coax in the direction of our bhakti and chosen ideal, within the context of the life we are living.

The guru is in you.

2009/07/17 11:06:21
Tantra - Sex and Spiritual Development
http://www.aypsite.org/forum/topic.asp?TOPIC_ID=5960&REPLY_ID=53630&whichpage=-1
even the greatest yogi has his seed jump?! :P

quote:
_____
Originally posted by fcry64

by mastery i mean the mastery over the desire itself, not the methods to control it... in the lessons it was given that kundalini awakening or the upturning of the muladhar due to the passage of kundalini through it is the only way to get past the sexual desire.
_____

Welcome Fcry64!

The methods of yoga are what enable us to reach "mastery over the desire," as you call it. It would be more accurate to call it "transcending the desire." The AYP approach to full-scope yoga covers the preservation and cultivation of sexual energy (regardless of sexual lifestyle) along with the necessary cultivation of inner silence and ecstatic conductivity and radiance. Prior to and during all of that is our bhakti (spiritual desire). The combination of all these means leads to a transcendence of the dominance of reproductive sex.

Sex will always be there in the neurobiology, but our intention with that energy and its manifestation can be transformed in stillness, as Etherfish has discussed. In time, it becomes automatic. Then there need not be any fear or obsession about the biological response. Like everything else in time and space, it becomes a wave on the ocean of our infinite Being, and we cannot be swept away by it any more than the ocean can be swept away by one of its waves.

When Shankara's statement is taken in this context, it makes perfect sense. Remember, he was still a young man at the height of his great mission. From the standpoint of self-identified awareness ("I am the body"), I can see that Shankara's statement could be disturbing. But here we are talking about going far beyond the limits of self-identification with the body, and that is where Shankara was speaking from also. It is much better to be honest about our urges and transcend them by effective means, than to be fighting with them on the surface level of mind where they can never be mastered.

Wishing you all the best on your path. Enjoy!

The guru is in you.

2009/07/23 16:58:52
Tantra - Sex and Spiritual Development
http://www.aypsite.org/forum/topic.asp?TOPIC_ID=5960&REPLY_ID=53981&whichpage=-1
even the greatest yogi has his seed jump?! :P

Hi All:

I have moved this interesting topic from Gurus to Tantra, so it will be easier to find in the future.

Also, I have taken my first response here, added additional details, and included it as a Q&A in the online tantra lessons (#T67):
http://www.aypsite.org/T67.html

All the best!

The guru is in you.

2009/07/27 21:09:34
Tantra - Sex and Spiritual Development
http://www.aypsite.org/forum/topic.asp?TOPIC_ID=6024&REPLY_ID=54112&whichpage=-1
Can a non-ejaculatory orgasm impregnate a woman?

quote:
_____
Originally posted by lover

Hi Folks,
Can a non-ejaculatory orgasm impregnate a woman?

You know,This is assuming after months to years of cultivating pre-orgasmic sex without having waking orgasm between,can a woman be impregnated by this?'

Thanks all...:-)

_____

Hi Lover:

Effective tantric practice (holdback and blocking) may reduce the chance of conception, but it would not be as reliable as other methods of birth control.

The guru is in you.

2009/07/28 10:27:43
Tantra - Sex and Spiritual Development
http://www.aypsite.org/forum/topic.asp?TOPIC_ID=6024&REPLY_ID=54144&whichpage=-1
Can a non-ejaculatory orgasm impregnate a woman?

quote:
_____
Originally posted by lover

hello,

Thnx guys...
Glad to read from you..:-)

To Yogani and others:
This is regarding brahmacharya..
I've read that ejaculating once every 2 weeks is not such a big deal in Yoga..specially if the kundalini is not yet active,right?
So,assuming comparing the two situations of two men practicing AYP in which they are both neophytes and have exactly the same obstructions in their nervous system,almost in everything but only differ in the frequency of ejaculating.That is,the first man ejaculate every two weeks while the other one ejaculate only once a year.
My question is,who among them has a better spiritual perspective?

_____

Hi Lover:

With two men the same in their nature, purification and practices, their need for sexual release will be the same. If one forced celibacy and the other did not, the first would find distortion and delay on their path, while the other would not, assuming the latter favored tantric techniques. Things are rarely what they seem in this business. Much better to go with the flow while favoring practices without forcing. Change occurs by consistent favoring over time, not by forcing.

Celibacy is only the right answer when it is the right answer. The rest of the time, it isn't. So the exhortations for celibacy for everyone are a lot of hot air. This error is common prior to the rise of inner silence, ecstatic conductivity and stillness in action. When the times are right for sexual continence, it will come without any fanfare. It is more about process than choice. If we choose the process, the outcome will be assured according to the characteristics of our unique unfolding.

In AYP, we do not define brahmacharya as celibacy. We define it as favoring preservation and cultivation of sexual energy with effective techniques in whatever sexual lifestyle one is living. That also includes during times of celibacy when it occurs naturally. See here:
http://www.aypsite.org/T9.html

All the best on your path!

The guru is in you.

2009/09/11 15:04:50
Tantra - Sex and Spiritual Development
http://www.aypsite.org/forum/topic.asp?TOPIC_ID=6326&REPLY_ID=56731&whichpage=-1
Sex has nothing to do with Kundalini

Hi Alwayson:

Whether there is a relationship between sex and kundalini or not is not a philosophical point. It is an experiential one.

For those who experience kundalini as an expansion of sexual function, that is what it is. And for those who do not, it isn't.

Either way is fine. Practice, and it will be what it will be. There is no point in debating what someone else's experience ought to be, or how they ought to interpret it. Better to practice, and encourage others to do the same. Then it will all come out in the wash.

The best knowledge is found in direct experience, not from anywhere else. All the great scriptures of the ages are a second-hand shadow of the eternal light shining in every one of us here and now.

The guru is in you.

2009/09/12 14:31:44
Tantra - Sex and Spiritual Development
http://www.aypsite.org/forum/topic.asp?TOPIC_ID=6326&REPLY_ID=56811&whichpage=-1
Sex has nothing to do with Kundalini

Hi Alwayson:

As I said early in this topic, feel free to share your experiences and interpretations of them. It will be honored here. But be careful about dishonoring the experiences of others and arguing against them in an "ad nauseum" fashion. It is not appropriate.

As mentioned elsewhere, these forums are for support of the AYP system of practices, not for promoting endless arguments, Buddhist or otherwise.

If you take a closer look at the AYP lessons, you will see that all of the practices on the ecstatic conductivity (kundalini) side are related to the cultivation of higher pranic/energetic expression, beginning and connecting with the pelvic region, i.e., the storehouse of sexual energy. This is a fundamental principle (and experience) in AYP, and not subject to endless arguments. It is what it is, just as core Buddhist principles are what they are, and not subject to ad nausem arguments in any forum that aspires to be useful to its readership.

Practices such as spinal breathing pranayama, mulabandha/asvini, sambhavi, siddhasana, yoni mudra kumbhaka, kechari, uddiyana/nauli, chin pump, nauli and shatkarmas, tantric sex, and others are all related to cultivating ecstatic conductivity within us. From there we find natural vajroli arising (continuous upward absorption of sexual essences), whole body mudra, and other developments throughout the body, which, taken all together, we call the "nectar cycle." This is the AYP view of the ecstatic neurobiology which underlies the energetic evolution we call kundalini. This leads to ongoing ecstatic radiance, which we also call outpouring divine love, stillness in action, the rise of unity, non-duality, etc.

None of this on the ecstatic side will go very far without concurrently cultivating abiding inner silence, and there is also a list of practices for that (deep meditation, samyama, etc). All of it can be integrated and condensed into a relatively short twice-daily practice routine. From there we can go out and live fully, which is how enlightenment is gradually baked into our life. That is AYP.

While all of this fits together conceptually and, more importantly, experientially, no one is asked to take any of it on faith. Practice and find out for yourself.

If you have a different view and approach to kundalini and the role of sexual energy, that is fine. Share it for practical benefit, not to "be right." Kindly do not engage in endless arguments here aimed at redefining what AYP ought to be, or how anyone ought to experience the cause and effect of their practices. It is not appropriate.

Thanks!

The guru is in you.

PS: Traditional definitions of Tantra (left or right handed) are interesting, but not relevant for labeling or redefining what the AYP system is with endless doctrinal arguments. Better not, Alwayson. Practice and enjoy!

2009/09/12 19:07:29
Tantra - Sex and Spiritual Development
http://www.aypsite.org/forum/topic.asp?TOPIC_ID=6326&REPLY_ID=56835&whichpage=-1
Sex has nothing to do with Kundalini

quote:
_____
Originally posted by alwayson2

Yogani,

I apologize. AYP is very important, because of kechari mudra which you brought out of the shadows into the light of day. Kechari mudra is a big deal, and is directly related to kundalini, according to James Mallinson's kecharividya book.
_____

Hi Alwayson:

Not a problem. We just have to make sure to keep our eye on the ball here, or we could lose it. It happens. :-)

Somewhere you made a comment that you feel kundalini is not about the genitals. That is essentially correct. Kundalini is about the vast pranic storehouse within the pelvic region. The genitals are on one side of that and the rest of the neurobiology is on the other side. So there is that connection, the vast storehouse of prana that both reproductive sex and spiritual evolution draw upon. The energy dynamic may be experienced going all the way from one end to the other, or not. Hence the possibility for occasional sexual arousal during "non-sexual" spiritual practices like deep meditation.

When the energy is felt moving in the genitals, it is erotic. When it is felt moving in the higher neurobiology it is ecstatic. Kechari is related to the latter, though it may also be erotic in the beginning due to the aforementioned connection. Pranayama, kumbhaka, asanas, mudras, bandhas, and tantric sexual methods (when genitals are engaged), are all for cultivating the higher manifestation of the pranic energy (kundalini) originating in the pelvic region. None of these practices stand alone. The key is a practical and effective integration. The whole of the resulting cause and effect is far greater than the sum of the parts.

The guru is in you.

2009/09/12 23:41:34
Tantra - Sex and Spiritual Development
http://www.aypsite.org/forum/topic.asp?TOPIC_ID=6326&REPLY_ID=56842&whichpage=-1
Sex has nothing to do with Kundalini

quote:
_____
Originally posted by Konchok Ösel Dorje

Wow... This is going well.

So when I meditate, I feel the kundalini spontaneously rise through the central channel, and a powerful sense of love. But I don't call it ecstatic,

Yogani. It feels a lot more like deep empathy in a powerful way.

When I release that feeling, my awareness blends into everything and I basically feel my kunda diffuse everywhere, into a sphere all around. And everything seems to be happening within that sphere.

Ecstasy is so strong. What I feel when the diffusion happens is more like "aaahhh..., so wonderful." Whenever I feel ecstatic, I feel like the feeling is too strong, and I want it to burst already or subside a bit.

_____

Hi Osel:

Good stuff. :-)

It can be called many things. The more refined it gets, the more it equates to outpouring divine love, expanding emptiness, stillness in motion, unity. This is the blending of ecstasy and abiding inner silence.

In its more raw forms, what we call ecstasy is a symptom of energy passing through inner obstructions. It can be pleasurable, intense like ero-ecstatic. Or if we have overdone in practices, recently or in the past, it can be uncomfortable -- the classic kundalini symptoms. It is all energy, moving in relation to our process of inner purification and opening.

As the obstructions clear away through practices over time, the energy refines and becomes those qualities of love, expansion, wholeness... The dynamic aspect (energy) serves as the vehicle for the stillness aspect, enabling divine expression in the world, which is the same as the expression of unending compassion in the Buddhist sense.

One nervous system, one evolutionary outcome. Many angles on how it comes about, with first-hand experience being the final arbiter of the process. The greatest scripture is in us. :-)

The guru is in you.

2009/12/29 11:05:44
Tantra - Sex and Spiritual Development
http://www.aypsite.org/forum/topic.asp?TOPIC_ID=6931
Tantra and Post Prostate Surgery

Hi All:

The following was received in email, and is being posted with permission, along with my comments.

Additional input is welcome.

The guru is in you.

Q: U may may post this in forum.
Read you book Tantra best definition of Bhramcharya preservation and cultivation of sexual energy after all Bharma is creator. Ordered almost all your books.

I had radical(total) removal of prostrate last year.It was cancer but it all gone t Now I finally get erections (with Viagra) main question is I have NO ejaculate with orgasms all dry. As no prostrate and sperms can-not come up as seminal vesicles all tied up. They die in testis. So where do I fit with preservation of Shukra and transformation to Ojas -Tejas and in Tantric practices. Now am I naturally conserving sexual energy as nothing comes out even with genital orgasm.

Also have lot of problems with urinary incontinence and impotency, bladder and urethra pain etc etc.. All this was not supposed to happen. I guess this is life..

Now can you please recommend any specific yogic practices to help with the healing above problems , of Urinary system of the second chakra related organs.

A: Sperm does not play a significant role in tantric sex. There have been cases documented in the AYP forums where vasectomy has no effect on the awakening of ecstatic conductivity. Whether prostatic fluid does or not has not been reported on to date. I doubt it will make a difference, as the energy is still in the system and will find its way where it needs to go with yoga practices engaged. There are many with physically compromised body parts who are not impaired spiritually. That is because it has more to do with bhakti and cultivating abiding inner silence than anything. All else follows from that, including the natural emergence of the ecstatic component.

That said, I see no reason why you could not practice pre-orgasmic sex with the holdback technique in whatever sexual lifestyle you are drawn to. The brahmacharya effect would still be present -- the preservation and cultivation of sexual energy.

Regarding healing, time will bring things back into balance, as long as you "self-pace" your practices and life. Be sure to take it easy and not press too hard. It is time to heal. Obviously, you should also seek additional medical advice as needed. You may wish to sign up for the global group meditation and healing samyama program, where healing assistance is available. Many participants have reported postive results.

With your permission, I will post your question and my comments in the Tantra category of the support forums, and perhaps there will be additional views on this.

All the best!

The guru is in you.

2010/01/28 09:16:11
Tantra - Sex and Spiritual Development
http://www.aypsite.org/forum/topic.asp?TOPIC_ID=7173&REPLY_ID=64007&whichpage=-1
Tantra and Single Women

quote:

Originally posted by SeySorciere

And how come nothing is said on the breasts?

_____

Hi SeySorciere:

Funny you should mention this, because an upcoming tantra lesson on breast and nipple stimulation is planned, for both women and men.

Regarding the rest, AYP attempts to present traditional methods for most effective results, including the use of mudras and bandhas, which are not primarily genital-oriented for the man either.

Siddhasana does have an angle specific for women, and you may wish to check it out here: http://www.aypsite.org/T28.html (the main siddhasana lesson is here)

Admittedly, yoga has been largely a man's field over the centuries, and I am all for leveling the playing field. In time, it will happen. Maybe AYP can serve as a catalyst for continuing development along these lines.

There are some excellent books on tantra by women. Margo Anand is one of the prominent authors and teachers in the field. Perhaps others here who are up-to-date on tantra from the womans's point of view can recommend more resources.

Thanks for bringing this up. :-)

The guru is in you.

2010/02/05 10:26:12
Tantra - Sex and Spiritual Development
http://www.aypsite.org/forum/topic.asp?TOPIC_ID=7221&REPLY_ID=64501&whichpage=-1
Caught between the devil and deep sea

Hi vd007, and welcome!

Sounds like you need to find a balance in all of your practices. In AYP, we call this "self-pacing," which you have been obliged to do by necessity.

I can't really comment much on vipassana in relation to tantric sexual practices, but can tell you that well-paced AYP deep meditation, spinal breathing pranayama, and other elements in the AYP system are compatible with both tantric sex or celibate lifestyle choices.

It seems your challenge isn't only about the tantric aspect, but balancing your entire routine in relation to your family life. I am sure you will find a way forward. Most here have been doing the same thing with reasonable success. It takes some time. This awkward stage will pass, and new openings await you and those around you.

On tiredness after tantric sex, this lesson echos some of the same points: http://www.aypsite.org/T72.html

You can find many similar discussions here in the tantra forum. Feel free to chime in anywhere. You are not alone. :-)

All the best!

The guru is in you.

2010/10/01 11:25:14
Tantra - Sex and Spiritual Development
http://www.aypsite.org/forum/topic.asp?TOPIC_ID=8499&REPLY_ID=73411&whichpage=-1
Wow i feel like im going to blow up ,

Hi dnice, and welcome!

Your symptoms are related to inner energy build-up and a need for more purification and opening so the energy can flow into higher expressions without that sense of impending "blowup."

A daily routine of deep meditation and spinal breathing pranayama will help smooth this out, leading to higher expressions of your inner energy and less pressure occurring against inner obstructions. It is suggested to start at the beginning of the AYP lessons here: http://www.aypsite.org/MainDirectory.html

You may also wish to review the tantra lessons, which offer practical methods for cultivating and managing sexual energy for spiritual benefit: http://www.aypsite.org/TantraDirectory.html

Wishing you all the best on your path!

The guru is in you.

PS: You might also find this recent discussion on pressure build-up and sexual energy management to be helpful:
http://www.aypsite.org/forum/topic.asp?TOPIC_ID=8485
Similar discussions have occurred many times here in the forums. The mechanics of this are well-known around these parts, so there is plenty of help available.

2010/10/25 11:22:47
Tantra - Sex and Spiritual Development
http://www.aypsite.org/forum/topic.asp?TOPIC_ID=8621&REPLY_ID=74194&whichpage=-1
Meditation after tantric practice?

Hi All:

All references to following spinal breathing pranayama with deep meditation are in relation to our twice-daily sitting practices. It does not necessarily apply to pranayama we might choose to do in tantric sexual practice, or at other times. In AYP, spinal breathing is not strongly recommended for use during tantric sex. The pros and cons if it are discussed here: http://www.aypsite.org/T33.html
It is a matter of personal preference...

While the relationship between pranayama and meditation described in the lesson quotes in previous posts above is real, keeping a balance between the cultivation of ecstatic energy and inner silence is not mandatory for minute-to-minute practice. This means that having deep meditation in our twice-daily sittings will aid in balancing the effects of pranayama at any other time. Abiding inner silence is what balances and enhances the effects of pranayama. However, this is not a license to be adding pranayama sessions willy-nilly throughout the day. It will be a formula for overload, and doing extra meditations will only amplify the overload.

For those who are looking for enhancements in practice outside normal twice-daily sittings, moderate tantric sex, and the occasional group meditation, it is suggested to look into structured retreats. That is where big leaps in spiritual progress can be accomplished while maintaining relative comfort and safety. See a lesson on "Retreats" here: http://www.aypsite.org/387.html
Anyone can organize a retreat for their local area/region, and if you contact me, we can see about arranging for an experienced leader to come and run it.

All the best!

The guru is in you.

Forum 7 – Yamas & Niyamas – Restraints & Observances

Personal habits, ethical conduct, diet, cleansing methods for the body, and more.
http://www.aypsite.org/forum/forum.asp?FORUM_ID=42

2005/07/13 05:02:54
Yamas & Niyamas - Restraints & Observances
http://www.aypsite.org/forum/topic.asp?TOPIC_ID=283
Yamas & Niyamas - Restraints & Observances

The Yamas and Niyamas are the first two limbs of the eight limbs of yoga from Patanjali's Yoga Sutras. They have to do with codes of conduct and various methods of preparation of the body, mind and heart for yoga practices. In AYP, we devote selective attention to the yamas and niyamas, as necessary, to support a quick start in meditation, spinal breathing pranayama and other practices. Then the yamas and niyamas are greatly boosted by these powerful practices and blossom of their own accord. This is discussed in Lesson #149 on the eight limbs of yoga, at http://www.aypsite.org/149.html

The yamas and niyamas comprise the following:

Yama - It means "restraint," and includes ahimsa (non-violence), satya (truthfulness), asteya (non-stealing), brahmacharya (preservation and cultivation of sexual energy), and aparigraha (non-covetousness).

Niyama - It means "observance," and includes saucha (purity and cleanliness), samtosa (contentment), tapas (heat/focus/austerity), svadhyaya (study of scriptures and self), and isvara pranidhana (surrender to the divine).

Saucha (purity and cleanliness) includes the shatkarmas (bodily cleansing techniques) and diet.

The shatkarmas (most commonly used ones) include: jala neti (nasal wash), dhauti (intestinal wash), nauli (churning of abdominals, see Lesson #129 at http://www.aypsite.org/129.html), basti (colon cleansing/enemas), trataka (steady eye gazing), kapalbhati (sudden exhale/blowing)

Diet is of interest to many. The basic AYP advice on diet is in Lesson #30, here: http://www.aypsite.org/30.html
Ayurvedic diets to aid in quelling excessive kundalini symptoms are discussed in lesson #69, here: http://www.aypsite.org/69.html

Again, in AYP we rely primarily on the rise of inner silence and the natural purifying tendencies contained within it to inspire our conduct and personal habits to higher expression. This is why in AYP you do not find many rules of "do's and don ts." Paths that focus heavily on yamas and niyamas tend to be filled with rules and regulations -- highly regimented. And initiations into additional yoga practices (like those we discuss openly in AYP) are contingent on following the requirements of yamas and niyamas to the satisfaction of the guru. This works for some people, but not for most.

This forum is for discussing the particulars of the yamas and niyamas. Should they be enforced from day one on the spiritual path, or allowed to rise naturally with the expansion of consciousness occurring from deep meditation, spinal breathing pranayama and other yoga practices? When we feel the urge coming from within to undertake shatkarmas, diet changes and other yamas and niyamas, what should we do? Where do the principles of "self-pacing" fit into all of this? There is plenty to discuss here.

The guru is in you.

2005/08/03 11:18:56
Yamas & Niyamas - Restraints & Observances
http://www.aypsite.org/forum/topic.asp?TOPIC_ID=376
12 Step Programs for Compulsive/Addictive Conduct
A few days ago, AYP Lesson #272 was posted on **"Addiction, Abusive Conduct, Tough Love and Yoga."** See:
http://www.aypsite.org/272.html

The lesson is an account of the challenges faced by a woman with a boyfriend with addiction issues relating to drugs and sex. My response recommended firmness and the use of a 12 step program for dealing with the compulsive behavior and addiction. Firmness on the part of loved ones and the 12 step program are the most effective known means for dealing with such issues. The 12 step program has non-sectarian spiritual principles behind it and is compatible with yogic methods. That is why this topic is posted here in Yamas and Niyamas.

A revealing reply to the inquirer in Lesson #272 was received from a reader in long-term recovery from addiction and is posted anonymously below. It sheds light on the difficult journey that addicts must take before life can move forward.

These are stories of great courage and I wanted to offer the thread started in Lesson #272 for continuation here in Yamas and Niyamas. These are important matters of conduct -- daily choices we make that can either hold us back or transform us in positive ways as we move forward in life and in yoga.

I hope this lesson and feedback will be helpful and that this topic and others like it will continue for the benefit of those with compulsive/addictive difficulties and their loved ones who are facing these issues and choices every day. The stakes are high.

For more on 12 step programs, see "Twelve Step Recovery Programs " in the AYP links section at http://www.aypsite.org/Links.html

The guru is in you.

****
Reply to Lesson # 272 on Addiction and Yoga:

Hi Yogani,

I wanted to respond to your correspondent (in lesson 272) regarding addiction in relationship. As someone with long-term recovery from my addiction to sexual stimulation and romantic fantasy, caffeine, and work, I concur with your call for firmness.

For me, and I suspect for other addicts, the substances and hormones that are produced by overstimulation mask emotional pain that we're afraid will destroy our spirits. Asking us to give them up sounds like a request that we succumb. When the traumas that created such pain in us occurred, we might not have had the inner development to cope. However, in time we develop other resources. By the time we bring people into our lives who call us to something higher in no uncertain terms, it is a blessing. It indicates that we are, in fact, ready to face the pain even though we might not be aware of that readiness.

I would never have gotten my life in order had I not been confronted with a make-or-break choice. Unfortunately for me, I was not able to preserve the relationship that revealed the truth of my spiritual condition to me. However, I know of others who have been able to. Though I cannot give her hope that her relationship will survive. But I do not think she needs to despair over it either.

It seems to me that we bring people into our lives who mirror us to some extent. When she stands firm with respect to his inappropriate behavior toward himself and her, I believe as one who's been there that she will be fulfilling the love she feels toward him in the highest degree. My suggestion to her would be to make ongoing participation in an anger management program a bottom-line requirement for continued contact. Her physical safety simply must be guaranteed. Beyond that, a genuine effort to apply the 12 steps to his addictive sexual behavior is the only method I know of to ensure that a person can gain a measure of freedom from that particular form of addiction. Unfortunately, addicts lie to protect what they unconsciously believe is their only reliable source of comfort. After more than a decade I still have trouble with that at times. But sustained progress is an indication of devotion.

I hope that he is strong enough to one day dissolve the hard crust of his conditioning. I hope that she is strong enough to tend to her own growth in the meantime. Why she brought in someone with such difficult issues is a question that only her soul can answer. But I can just about guarantee that it wasn't so that she would succumb to despair--though that risk certainly seems present.

I guess what I most want to say is that her love will leave its mark on him whether he can respond in a time that harmonizes with her spiritual development or not. If she needs to move on for her own sake, she can rest assured that her involvement with him will have been a blessing to him whether he is ever able to recognize it and express his gratitude or not. I know, because I've been in his shoes.

My question for her now is this: is her relationship with him proving to be a blessing to her or not? Sadly, from what I read, my guess is that at the moment it is not. She cannot expect anyone to change that and especially not him. She can certainly ask him to correct what is wrong. But, if he isn't ready to do what it takes to sustain the relationship and she secretly knows that, it might already be over. If so, it might be time for her to acknowledge that, grieve her grief, and move on.

Sometimes, an addict will do what it takes to recover after enduring the loss and realizing exactly what it was that the addiction has cost him. Sometimes the threat of such a loss is enough for an addict to wake up. For his sake I hope the latter. But if he doesn't change his behavior, sooner or later that loss will come. She cannot save him from it. What she can do is protect herself from the abuse that is beginning to degrade her.

All the best,

Anonymous Recovering Male Addict

2005/08/03 16:24:29
Yamas & Niyamas - Restraints & Observances
http://www.aypsite.org/forum/topic.asp?TOPIC_ID=376&REPLY_ID=267&whichpage=-1
12 Step Programs for Compulsive/Addictive Conduct

Hi Lily:

It does not hurt for non-addicts to become familiar with the 12 step program. Very practical stuff for just about any kind of dysfunctional behavior we might find in our life. We all have something amiss, or we would not be here on earth for the big yoga cleanout!

In the cases mentioned, the behavior was/is extreme and destabilizing to relationships and health, not to mention yoga. To those with strong addictive tendencies, normal things can become obsessions -- far beyond the normal cup of coffee, hard day's work, sexual fantasy or experiment with a recreational chemical.

There have been some admitted alcoholics very interested in AYP, but not able to get very far with the practices. Yet, they keep drinking. There are also smokers in AYP who have difficulties in yoga. These conducts retard the effects of yoga, sometimes to the point of making progress impossible.

Meditation, spinal breathing and the other techniques are very refined tools for purifying the nervous system, and cannot do the job if impurities are being thrown on the window faster than they can be cleaned off.

In the later stages of yoga, even caffeine or a heavy diet may be found to be obstructions to growth. These are not necessarily "addictions," but it all gets thrown into one barrel called "yama and niyama," meaning the things we do in life that tend to advance (purify) or retard (clog up) spiritual progress in yoga.

Interestingly, as we move forward in yoga, and give our nervous system half a chance by not polluting it too much, many of these "good habits" come up all by themselves, and the "bad habits" tend to go away. I call it "the connectedness of yoga." See lesson 149 at http://www.aypsite.org/149.html for a discussion on the connectedness of the eight limbs of yoga.

That is why we don't harp on the issues of diet, conduct, personal hygiene and habits, etc. too much in the AYP lessons. Deep meditation and spinal breathing alone go a long way toward bringing the yamas and niyamas naturally into our life.

Hardcore addictions are a much tougher nut to crack, and that is why they are getting some extra attention here. We won't shy away from it. Everyone is entitled the best opportunity possible to pursue their spiritual destiny. There are sound means to deal with addiction, so we mention them.

In time, the full scope of yamas and niyamas will be discussed in AYP too. There is a lot in there, and middle to advanced AYP practitioners will be especially interested because the connectedness of yoga will call us to these things. With most traditional approaches to yoga, the yamas and niyamas come first, and much later we may get to learn the things we do first in AYP. In AYP we are going the other way.

The guru is in you.

Hi Lili:

Not having been through the 12 step program in-depth myself, I am not the best one to describe it. May others come forward like Ranger (thank you!) with their own stories. It is not something you do by yourself without a support group, though I expect once one is solidly grounded in the principles, it becomes a part of the individual daily living experience -- more a way of thinking and feeling than a "practice" as we think of it in AYP. Of course, bhakti is that sort of ongoing thing in AYP, and there is a close relationship between the principles of bhakti and the 12 step program.

Below are the 12 steps as laid out by Alcoholics Anonymous (AA) back in the 1930s. The words "alcohol" and "alcoholic" can be replaced with "addiction" and "addict," and have been by hundreds of groups that use the 12 step program for every kind of compulsive and addictive behavior imaginable. It is a very successful program in many arenas of conduct.

The 12 Suggested Steps of Alcoholics Anonymous

1. We admitted we were powerless over alcohol--that our lives had become unmanageable.

2. Came to believe that a Power greater than ourselves could restore us to sanity.

3. Made a decision to turn our will and our lives over to the care of God as we understood Him (or Her).

4. Made a searching and fearless moral inventory of ourselves.

5. Admitted to God, to ourselves and to another human being the exact nature of our wrongs.

6. Were entirely ready to have God remove all these defects of character.

7. Humbly asked Him to remove our shortcomings.

8. Made a list of all persons we had harmed, and became willing to make amends to them all.

9. Made direct amends to such people wherever possible, except when to do so would injure them or others.

10. Continued to take personal inventory and when we were wrong promptly admitted it.

11. Sought through prayer and meditation to improve our conscious contact with God, as we understood Him, praying only for knowledge of His will for us and the power to carry that out.

12. Having had a spiritual awakening as the result of these steps, we tried to carry this message to alcoholics, and to practice these principles in all our affairs.

****

The guru is in you.

PS -- I'd say a "middle" level AYP practitioner is anyone who is feeling the connectedness of yoga and is able to act on those urges, i.e., meditation leading instinctively to more practices (step-by-step via self-pacing), including yamas and niyamas -- purer habits of living coming up naturally without forcing the issue. It can happen with beginners too, and often does. So, at the beginning you can be in the middle and at the end. The flavors of enlightenment have many overlapping layers. Enjoy!

Here is an account of 12 step recovery by the same person who gave the feedback on lesson #272 in the first posting of this series. Some feedback on the role of AYP is given at the end.

****

The 12 Steps are all about redirecting intention away from gratification and toward the cultivation of serenity. In my experience, the relief that comes from surviving withdrawal, an addict's worst fear, produces a profound and lasting state of gratitude that makes service a priority--as an expression of that gratitude. I think that the 12-Steps might well be a form of Bhakti.

Believe me, I'd never wish withdrawal on anyone--unless that person happens to need it to get free. I like what Yogananda says about freedom: it isn't the ability to do whatever one wants, it is the ability to do what is in one's best interest.

I wonder if obsessions are conditions that we actively choose. For me, and for the other addicts whose stories I've been privileged to hear, obsessions arise as survival mechanisms. An emotional trauma occurs, a child (or childlike sub-personality) goes into shock and gets stuck in the denial or bargaining stage of the grieving process. The pain remains unbearable and the adaptive personality (ego) begins a desperate search for relief.

Conditioning being what it is, the first thing that numbs out the particular form of pain becomes the target of an obsession. When we don't understand or find support for the grieving process, anesthesia looks like the best option available and so we seize upon it. It is a very fortunate person who finds appropriate guidance and a safe haven for grieving life's traumas fully as soon as they occur. Oh for a culture in which this basic need was fully appreciated! Working from a place of serene gratitude is a different experience than working from a place of suppressed despair.

To me, obsession is about seeking relief from a trauma, a terror, that my ego might not be willing to risk acknowledging. Because of the phenomenon of spiritual materialism, I'm not sure that an obsession for yoga is necessarily a good plan for coping with that sort of terror. Yoga is safer than drugs and legal, and it can certainly lead to improved physical health and mental acuity, but that does not mean it brings serenity or peace. I did Hatha and T'ai C

Hi compulsively before I got into recovery, and all it did was increase the intensity of my dysfunction. Well, that's not all it did, but it didn't get to the root of my pain and so I experienced life as a treadmill. The stronger I got in my practices, the stronger my pain grew until one day my ego just came apart at the seams. I experienced a true spiritual emergency. Because I had no faith in a Higher Power and only meager guidance, the best I could do at that time was to piece myself back together as I'd been before. Thus the cycle started over again and it was another 10 years before I was able to find help in the 12 steps. I had no idea at the time that the grieving process includes a stage in which a person experiences utter disorientation. Had I known that that was normal, and that all I needed was a fair witness who could look after my safety and reassure me that I'd get through it, things would have been much better for me.

So, I think there's a bit more to it than redirecting an obsession for something that some consider "negative," like drugs, sex, or gambling, toward something "positive," like "service," or "God," or "Yoga." I think that the bottom line is about being able to recognize when, and with whom, it is safe to grieve whatever damage one has done or experienced. I say "done" first because it is usually the guilt and shame over our misbehavior that comes first. Those losses are typically much easier to acknowledge than the damage that was done to us--the damage that produced the need for an obsession/compulsion in the first place.

When a person decides, once and for all, to get to the bottom of her or his condition, it is then that the Divine energies really get to work. They don't have to keep hammering it with karmic consequences to get our attention, so the whole process shifts toward more positive development. To me, the trick is recognizing when I'm operating out of an obsession vs. when I'm operating from a place of serenity. I like the perspective of AYP because the meditative practices help bring that distinction into focus. The ecstatic practices help to maintain that focus even in the presence of intense stimulation (bliss). The balance is lovely, and builds confidence that I can stay serenely myself in the face of whatever might come.

It is only in that frame of mind that I become truly available.

All the best,

Anonymous Recovering Male Addict

2005/08/05 14:13:42
Yamas & Niyamas - Restraints & Observances
http://www.aypsite.org/forum/topic.asp?TOPIC_ID=376&REPLY_ID=293&whichpage=-1
12 Step Programs for Compulsive/Addictive Conduct
Here is more from our anonymous friend:

****

I'd like to further comment about the 12 steps and 12-step groups. The steps are tools, and they're very effective. However, as with any tool they take a bit of practice and guidance to apply well. That's why the groups recommend getting a sponsor. Choosing a sponsor carefully is important. They say that a good sponsor is someone who demonstrates the qualities that you want. The steps were worded in a way that is a bit arcane. It took me a long time to figure out why they're set in the past tense. The steps work, but they must be applied with some insight and judgment. That's hard to do when a person realizes that her or his judgment has been severely impaired by addiction! Steps 1 through 3 are all about coming to terms with that apparent paradox.

As with yoga, compulsively working the 12 steps to avoid the scary process of grief slows the healing/rebuilding process. It's still better than the previous addictions, which is why the presence of 12-step cultists in meetings is still a positive thing. Better that they remain obsessed with the 12 steps than that they continue to wind up in the gutters or other outposts of hell. Even the cultists contribute useful tips for dealing with addiction.

Also, most 12-steppers use a simple criterion to evaluate habits that they question: Can I count up to 1 when I'm under the influence of the particular substance (or hormone). For instance, if I can feel satisfied with 1 cup of coffee or 1 drink and can easily stop there without engaging in a struggle of will, then I'm probably not addicted to it. That doesn't mean my yoga practices wouldn't improve if I quit, but it does help me set priorities about what aspects of my behavior I want to work on.

What I love most about the 12 Steps are the promises:

If we are painstaking about this phase of our development, we will be amazed before we are half way through. We are going to know a new freedom and a new happiness. We will not regret the past nor wish to shut the door on it. We will comprehend the word serenity and we will know peace. No matter how far down the scale we have gone, we will see how our experience can benefit others. That feeling of uselessness and self-pity will disappear. We will lose interest in selfish things and gain interest in our fellows. Self-seeking will slip away. Our whole attitude and outlook upon life will change. Fear of people and of economic insecurity will leave us. We will intuitively know how to handle situations which used to baffle us. We will suddenly realize that God is doing for us what we could not do for ourselves.

I can honestly say that most of those promises have been fulfilled in my life so far. I am embarking on things that I would never have believed possible while I was actively engaged in my addiction. I still regret my past, but I do not wish to shut the door on it because remembering how I was, and how it was for me, allows me to respond with compassion. What I grieve now is the potential for what could have been had I not been so damaged or so damaging.

I might not become what I could have been had I not gone down the path of addiction, but I'm doing my best to become all that I can be now. We all have a Divine calling in this life, one that fully engages our strengths and talents while providing a safe avenue for addressing our weaknesses; my prayer is that each of us finds that calling. I'm grateful for the help that AYP provides in that regard.

All the best,

Anonymous Recovering Male Addict
2005/08/15 22:35:52
Yamas & Niyamas - Restraints & Observances
http://www.aypsite.org/forum/topic.asp?TOPIC_ID=410&REPLY_ID=384&whichpage=-1
Moral discussions

Thank you, Frank.

You beat me to the punch on that one, and I agree. :-)

Pure bliss consciousness is the source of morality (oneness), just as being obstructed from it is the source of immorality (separateness).

Patanjali provides specific guidelines -- the 1st and 2nd limbs of the 8 limbs of yoga (http://www.aypsite.org/149.html), which are symptomatic of the rise of the inner light. In AYP we regard them as signposts of spiritual transformation more than edicts, though at certain times firmness of will in a particular yama or niyama may be in the best interest of all concerned (like in our recent 12 step discussion http://www.aypsite.org/forum/topic.asp?TOPIC_ID=376) --

Yama ☐ It means "restraint," and includes ahimsa (non-violence), satya (truthfulness), asteya (non-stealing), brahmacharya (preservation and cultivation of sexual energy), and aparigraha (non-covetousness).

Niyama ☐ It means "observance," and includes saucha (purity and cleanliness), samtosa (contentment), tapas (heat/focus/austerity), svadhyaya (study of scriptures and self), and isvara pranidhana (surrender to the divine).

Interestingly, these bear resemblance to the 10 commandments of Moses and the beatitudes of Christ. The truth is the same everywhere...

The guru is in you.

2005/08/16 10:56:19
Yamas & Niyamas - Restraints & Observances
http://www.aypsite.org/forum/topic.asp?TOPIC_ID=410&REPLY_ID=387&whichpage=-1
Moral discussions
"I reach for a piece of wood. It turns into a lute.
I do some meanness. It turns out helpful.
I say one must not travel during the holy month.
Then I start out, and wonderful things happen." ~Rumi

Like that, if we meditate and keep dancing, we will find our way. That is where our responsibility lies. Divine life is filled with paradox, and ever opening. Better not to second-guess it too much ... though that too is part of it.

The guru is in you.

2005/08/17 11:26:39
Yamas & Niyamas - Restraints & Observances
http://www.aypsite.org/forum/topic.asp?TOPIC_ID=410&REPLY_ID=395&whichpage=-1
Moral discussions

Thanks, Anthem, for your kind note. If we keep up practices over the long term, the decision-making gets easier -- obvious even. Not that we know the outcome of all things, or that it will always be what we want. We just come to know that inner silence is the best launching pad for all outcomes. Experience bears this out over time. This is how abiding inner silence gained in deep meditation fulfills yama and niyama. But more than that, we become our own compass at the deepest level of morality, which is beyond yama and niyama. Freedom...

The guru is in you.

2005/11/04 16:58:08
Yamas & Niyamas - Restraints & Observances
http://www.aypsite.org/forum/topic.asp?TOPIC_ID=490&REPLY_ID=1385&whichpage=-1
Protecting the Senses
Oh Lili:

You'll have to read the new book coming out in December called, "Deep Meditation - Pathway to Personal Freedom."

I am doing the part today on how inner silence leads us to "right choices."

Pretty good timing on your part bringing that up. I am feeling lighter now that the book is coming together on time. Can you tell? :-)

The guru is in you.

2005/11/20 10:56:49
Yamas & Niyamas - Restraints & Observances
http://www.aypsite.org/forum/topic.asp?TOPIC_ID=597&REPLY_ID=1577&whichpage=-1
Discipline of the senses

Hi Lili:

It is the path of the renunciate, which does not fit well into everyday living. In fact, in ordinary living, to take this approach is divisive -- just the opposite of yoga, which means union.

Interestingly, if we are established in inner silence through daily deep meditation, we will inwardly be doing all that Sivananda recommends, not engaged on the level of our inner Self, even as we are enjoying life in the world. More than that -- with inner silence coming up, whatever we do in the world will enhance our growth -- stabilize our inner silence and stimulate the rise of ecstatic bliss and the flow of divine love from within. That is union.

I have the highest regard for Sivananda, but to apply this advice in everyday living would be to take it out of context. This lifestyle is consistent with the life of a renunciate -- not for householders.

We have to ask the question: What are renunciates doing anyway? Seeking enlightenment, or hiding from life? While some are sincerely engaged in the former, many are doing the latter. It is a problem for all monastics to deal with.

For householders, the question of personal motivation is also there. But at least we can do our yoga practices and then go about our business the rest of the time without being haunted by rules about what we can and cannot do with our lives, knowing we will grow simply by doing our practices and engaging in life however we see fit -- no self-judgement necessary...

The guru is in you.

2005/12/26 11:51:04
Yamas & Niyamas - Restraints & Observances
http://www.aypsite.org/forum/topic.asp?TOPIC_ID=668&REPLY_ID=2171&whichpage=-1
Shatkarma

Hi Alvin:

I moved this topic from healthcare into yamas and niyamas...

Basti and dhauti are the shatkarmas to consider for cleansing and improving GI tract function. See the summary in the yamas and niyamas introduction.

Shatkarmas are especially helpful if one is well-established in a steady routine of sitting practices, because there is a substantial spiritual dimension to them -- they are an aid for cultivating ecstatic conductivity in the neurobiology. The GI tract plays a central role in this, but not necessarily in the beginning days of our practices. It is much more important to become stable in our core practices.

The shatkarmas are an area slated for detailed coverage in the AYP writings, but are down the list from all the rest that is being covered, so it will be a while longer. I am planning a book on them for 2007.

That does not help your immediate need, I know. Perhaps others can step forward on this until I can get an online lesson together to help folks develop some practical familiarity with the shatkarmas. One reason I have been slow on shatkarmas is I want to be careful not to distract folks from the core practices (meditation, spinal breathing, etc.) with what are ancillary hatha yoga methods. From the AYP point of view, they are middle stage practices, not needed much by most yogis and yoginis at the beginning or at the end of the journey. They are very helpful in the middle when ecstatic conductivity is coming into play.

Of course, for health reasons shatkarmas can be useful anytime, so they straddle the spiritual and medical arenas, as do all yoga practices. In AYP we focus primarily on the spiritual side...

The guru is in you.

2005/12/28 10:11:34
Yamas & Niyamas - Restraints & Observances
http://www.aypsite.org/forum/topic.asp?TOPIC_ID=668&REPLY_ID=2229&whichpage=-1
Shatkarma

Hi Alvin:

Basti is simple warm water enema with a gravity bag, hose with clamp, and an insert fitting at the end. Tap water can be used if it is free of bacteria. If not, use bottled water. Just fill up (a quart or so), either leaning over on the toilet or lying down, and wait for a few minutes before expelling. It is a good colon clean-out.

For spiritual purposes basti is done every morning before bathing and sitting practices, along with jala neti (nasal wash, discussed here). However, as mentioned earlier, this is not a routine for beginning yogis/yoginis, nor needed for advanced practitioners with ecstatic conductivity well established. That is mainly what these practices are for, middle stage cultivation of ecstatic conductivity, done in conjunction with a full yoga routine.

However, basti will clean the colon for sure, which is a useful side effect for health.

Can basti become a habit that we cannot let go of, so we are bound to the bag forever to eliminate? Not in my experience. I used it for a solid 3 years in the 1980s and it was an important part of ecstatic awakenings back then. Then it dropped off and I have used it only occasionally since then. Elimination becomes part of the overall ecstatic neurobiology, but it takes a transition (with a full range of practices) to get there. The cleansing shatkarmas are part of that transitional phase.

So you can see why I am dragging my feet on basti and cleansing shatkarmas in general. If you start with daily basti now, when will you stop? How far off is middle stage? That is the question. But if you need it for health, it can work. Obviously, you don't want to become dependent on it for elimination forever. If it is used mainly for health purposes, then maybe once or twice per week will be plenty. When the inner energies are moving (kundalini), your rising bhakti will let you know to do more basti and other shatkarmas.

Dhauti is the intestinal wash -- drinking salted water for a full GI tract flush. Is that what "Laghoo Shankprakshalana" is? Dhauti should not be done often. It does deplete the system much more than basti. Weekly would be a lot. Monthly is even too often for some. I rarely used it. It is drinking 2-4 quarts of salted water (about the same salt concentration as used in comfortable jala neti) over 10-15 minutes, and then lying down on the left side (best flow through intestines) for 20-30 minutes. Then run for the toilet. It's best to plan on at least a half hour of eliminating off and on, and then lie down and rest afterward. The salt causes the water to pass straight through the entire GI tract for a big flush out. Besides the cleansing, this can be very depleting. This is what hospitals have you do before major surgery -- complete emptying of the GI tract.

Basti is the more practical method, I think -- it can be done daily with relative ease (not a big operation like dhauti) and is not depleting. In fact, basti brings energy once ecstatic conductivity gets going.

Alvin -- As for all those cramps and difficulties in the colon, it sounds like stress. The cure for that is deep meditation and spinal breathing, and some consideration of lifestyle. Besides keeping up your spiritual practices as simple and relaxed as possible, you will be making choices as you move forward in life with education, career, living space, friends, lover, etc. How those choices are made will have a bearing on how you feel inside. Right now you are living a rather cramped and stressful life. Is it surprising that you feel cramped and stressed inside? Maybe you have not had a choice so far, but you will as time goes on. So choose wisely! :-)

The guru is in you.

2005/12/28 14:07:26
Yamas & Niyamas - Restraints & Observances
http://www.aypsite.org/forum/topic.asp?TOPIC_ID=668&REPLY_ID=2242&whichpage=-1
Shatkarma

Hi Alvin:

This is what I used for basti:
http://www.optimalhealthnetwork.com/product.asp?specific=jnkqnoo0

It can be found at drug stores in the West. Not sure about Hong Kong.

I found this page with a Google search on "enema bag." Lots of info came up. The internet is great, isn't it?

As for constricted anus, mulabandha/asvini can help in time.
See http://www.aypsite.org/55.html and follow-up lessons later on.
But again, that is a spiritual practice more than a medical remedy.

All the best on your continuing journey!

The guru is in you.

2006/05/24 10:17:12
Yamas & Niyamas - Restraints & Observances
http://www.aypsite.org/forum/topic.asp?TOPIC_ID=1165&REPLY_ID=7290&whichpage=-1
What is your daily food plan?

Hi Yoda and All:

If there are inner energy issues, make sure to take into consideration the ayurvedic aspects of diet. See this chart for some suggested guidelines on the ayurvedic properties of many different foods: http://www.aypsite.org/ayurveda-diets.html

For example, spinach can be pitta aggravating, causing excess fire in the body. Carrots can be pitta aggravating too. This does not mean do not eat spinach or carrots. It only means "self-pace" them if there are some excess energy effects. Using a little olive oil can reduce the effects of pitta aggravating foods. If that does not work, then try some of the foods that are pitta pacifying. Cabbage juice anyone?

Ayurvedic diets were first covered in the lesson on managing kundalini symptoms, here: http://www.aypsite.org/69.html

A little background on ayurveda, doshas, etc., is given there. Diet is one of the immediate things we can address to quell energy flare-ups, often with immediate results.

For the rest, the sum total of my recommendations on diet are -- Favor "light and nutritious." http://www.aypsite.org/30.html

All the best!

The guru is in you.

2006/06/01 12:47:51
Yamas & Niyamas - Restraints & Observances
http://www.aypsite.org/forum/topic.asp?TOPIC_ID=1193&REPLY_ID=7622&whichpage=-1
Anyone here practicing Amaroli?

quote:
_____
Originally posted by meg

quote:
_____
Originally posted by Shanti

Meg that is going to be a part of his 6th book in his AYP Enlightenment Series ...
Diet, Shatkarmas and Amaroli – Yogic Nutrition & Cleansing for Health and Spirit (#0978649648 -- Due out first half 2007)
_____

Well, there you have it. Amaroli rocks! Or, amaroli on the rocks.

_____

Hi All:

338 –   Advanced Yoga Practices

Amaroli is covered in the AYP Easy Lessons book (addition to tantra lesson T32) -- nearly did not make it in due to the gross-out factor, and that is discussed in there too. And, yes, it will be given treatment in the E-Series book Shanti mentioned, at the risk of staining all of AYP yellow. :-)

But seriously, one way to find out what amaroli is doing for us at a point in time is to stop for a while after doing it for a few months. From that angle, the effects can be quite noticeable. It is an important practice, for both health and spiritual progress, though certainly a controversial one.

As with all of the AYP practices, the results are also related to the integration of practices we are doing. Deep meditation works better with spinal breathing in the picture, and vise versa. Mudras and bandhas work best with deep meditation and spinal breathing going on. Tantric sexual relations are much more effective when daily sitting practices are being done also, and so on...

It is like that with amaroli too, which is not to say that any single practice is not beneficial by itself. But an integration can accomplish so much more. Taking practices on in a particular order helps a lot too -- deep meditation, spinal breathing, mudras/bandhas, etc. This suggests that amaroli may not be the first thing to be doing, and that our rising bhakti will bring us to it naturally, like it brings us to everything else.... Of course, there are many ways to skin this cat, and many places one can start and progress from. That is why we call this "self-directed practice." Pick your doorway and stroll on in. Each doorway inevitably leads to more doorways. It is the nature of purification and opening in the human nervous system on the road of spiritual transformation.

Cheers!

The guru is in you.

2006/06/01 13:34:51
Yamas & Niyamas - Restraints & Observances
http://www.aypsite.org/forum/topic.asp?TOPIC_ID=1193&REPLY_ID=7632&whichpage=-1
Anyone here practicing Amaroli?

Hi Meg:

It is a personal self-paced thing, and you should follow your inner lead on it. If you feel the need to increase, try it ... and if it is too much, then back off accordingly.

In truth, with the rise of inner silence and ecstatic conductivity, less can be more for all the practices, including amaroli. Until that situation and a realization of it dawns, things can be a bit choppy now and then...

So it is all about taking it easy with our long term persistence in practices -- gentle persuasion, you know ... doing whatever is necessary to keep moving steadily and safely along.

Unlike some traditons, we do not have goals here to reach certain durations or quantities of practice, as this could be counter-productive depending on the course of our purification and opening.

Once we have the tools in hand and are familiar with how they work, the game is almost entirely in the self-pacing. This is where the science of yoga gives way to the art of yoga. The practices are the brushes and colors and we are the living canvas that reacts to the various stimulations by the artist.

The guru is in you.

2006/06/01 15:52:21
Yamas & Niyamas - Restraints & Observances
http://www.aypsite.org/forum/topic.asp?TOPIC_ID=1193&REPLY_ID=7643&whichpage=-1
Anyone here practicing Amaroli?

quote:
_____
Originally posted by azaz932001

Changes in your mind and body occur and then become so much the norm so much the essence of you that you forget they ever happened :-)
_____

Hi Richard:

Yes, it is amazing how quickly we can get used to a particular level of progress. It can even become like, well, God, what have you done for me lately?

And God answers back, "Well, what have you done lately to move on?" :-)

The guru is in you.

2006/06/01 17:09:14
Yamas & Niyamas - Restraints & Observances
http://www.aypsite.org/forum/topic.asp?TOPIC_ID=1193&REPLY_ID=7646&whichpage=-1
Anyone here practicing Amaroli?

quote:
_____
Originally posted by Shanti
Yogani is this the reason you chose that color for the cover of your 6th book?:-) http://www.aypsite.org/books.html
_____

Hi Shanti:

This one will be about the "nine gates" and what connects them. What goes in, what comes out, and what sometimes goes back in again. :-) It will explore the odd contraditons we live with -- the common obsession with what we put in and the common revulsion with what comes out.

In truth, the inner neurobiological processes are where the action is, and helping optimize them for spiritual functioning will be the focus of the book, as is always the case in the AYP writings.

Just a word on laying out the E-Series titles in advance -- "Samyama." They are happening already ... well, they are done already. All I have to do is type the 600 pages.

The guru is in you.

2007/06/18 09:53:46
Yamas & Niyamas - Restraints & Observances
http://www.aypsite.org/forum/topic.asp?TOPIC_ID=2677&REPLY_ID=23295&whichpage=-1
do no harm and prayer--

quote:
Originally posted by NagoyaSea

From the Dalai Lama:
"Develop a strong desire to refrain from harming others either physically or verbally, no matter whether you are embarrassed, insulted, reviled, pushed or hit."

Hi Kathy and All:

Regarding conduct, I have often said that practices will elevate our conduct over time due to the rise of inner silence. It is true. But before that can happen, we have to want it.

Bhakti (spiritual desire) is the prerequisite for success in spiritual practices, even deep meditation. It is in the AYP lessons. If we are obsessively focused on contracted attitudes and conduct, expansion will be very difficult, even with spiritual practices in the picture. The habit of contraction cannot be broken until we make a choice for expansion. If we can shift our obsession to that, then expansion will happen much faster from within, and spiritual practices will be much more powerful.

Obsession is not a bad thing, if pointed in the direction of expansion. That is what bhakti is.

It has been said that people can't change, and it is true for those who don't want to change. Nothing much will happen until a conscious choice for something more is made, and acted upon.

On the other hand, people who really want to change can, and are readily expandable to infinite abiding inner silence, ecstatic bliss and outpouring divine love. That is what AYP and these forums are about. If we can bring a sincere desire to the table, and are willing to apply proven methods to assist us in letting go of our contractions, then AYP can help a lot. An outright obsession for inner expansion (flowing out) is even better, with self-pacing applied as needed, of course. :-)

It is our choice. We can raise the bar of our bhakti whenever we decide, which will lead to the full time habit of favoring expansion over contraction. Then it will show up in our conduct in many ways.

All the best!

The guru is in you.

2007/08/20 15:22:41
Yamas & Niyamas - Restraints & Observances
http://www.aypsite.org/forum/topic.asp?TOPIC_ID=2827&REPLY_ID=24937&whichpage=-1
Fine Book: Diet, Shatkarmas and Amaroli

quote:
Originally posted by bewell

I tried it. First, to create a new account, they required another email address, which I had. Then they required that I had bought a book from that account. I had not. Next time I buy a book from Amazon, I'll buy it with that account, then I'll do the anonymous review.:-)

Hi Bewell:

Thank you for your kind comments.

There is a way to set a separate (anonymous) name for doing Amazon reviews, but I can't seem to find it.

Another way is to change your account name in "my account" information. This does not affect sign-on (which is by email address), or anything else in the account.

Amazon reviews are very important for reaching beyond the AYP community, and the AYP books have been receiving fewer and fewer of them for the past several books. Here is how many we currently have on Amazon USA:

AYP Easy Lessons - 21
Secrets of Wilder - 12
Deep Meditation - 18
Spinal Breathing Pranayama - 11
Tantra - 9
Asanas, Mudras and Bandhas - 8
Samyama - 6
Diet, Shatkarmas and Amaroli - 0

The Amazon international sites have far fewer reviews -- none in many cases.

Some balance is much needed. It would be greatly appreciated if everyone who is on Amazon and enjoys the AYP books will chime in with reviews. Only a few words are necessary for a review. In many cases, it can be a matter of copying your comments from the forums or private emails to me to an Amazon review. Limited visibility compliments are very nice, but for best results it is the general public that really needs to see them.

Many thanks for helping out in this important area!

The guru is in you.

2007/08/22 09:39:24
Yamas & Niyamas - Restraints & Observances
http://www.aypsite.org/forum/topic.asp?TOPIC_ID=2827&REPLY_ID=24979&whichpage=-1
Fine Book: Diet, Shatkarmas and Amaroli

Thank you! :-)
2007/08/22 18:06:50
Yamas & Niyamas - Restraints & Observances
http://www.aypsite.org/forum/topic.asp?TOPIC_ID=2827&REPLY_ID=24990&whichpage=-1
Fine Book: Diet, Shatkarmas and Amaroli

quote:
_____
Originally posted by anthony574

I got your back, Yogani :-)
_____

Thank you too, Anthony.

Glad to hear amaroli is helping with a long time health issue. Sometimes an answer is literally right in front of us. :-)

And certainly within us...

The guru is in you.

2007/10/26 12:31:15
Yamas & Niyamas - Restraints & Observances
http://www.aypsite.org/forum/topic.asp?TOPIC_ID=2960&REPLY_ID=26379&whichpage=-1
To clear the stomech and its track.

Hi Avatar:

Thanks much for this sharing.

See here for a related discussion:
http://www.aypsite.org/forum/topic.asp?TOPIC_ID=359&whichpage=7#26378
All the best!

The guru is in you.

2007/10/12 13:42:32
Yamas & Niyamas - Restraints & Observances
http://www.aypsite.org/forum/topic.asp?TOPIC_ID=2981&REPLY_ID=25973&whichpage=-1
Living on light

quote:
_____
Originally posted by Christi

p.s. I must strongly advise anyone reading this not to try this practice, as you could just get thin and die, which really defeats the whole point of the exercise.
_____

Hi Christi:

Wishing you the best in your exploration. Do keep us posted.

It should also be pointed out that there is no procedure in the AYP writings for discontinuing food consumption on a long term basis. It is touched on in several places in the Diet, Shatkarmas and Amaroli book, including in the sections on fasting, avoiding obsessive "flights of fancy" in practice, and the importance of favoring balance via self-pacing in all that we undertake in yoga.

The guru is in you.

2007/10/12 23:39:08
Yamas & Niyamas - Restraints & Observances
http://www.aypsite.org/forum/topic.asp?TOPIC_ID=2981&REPLY_ID=25998&whichpage=-1
Living on light
PS: Also, this lesson might be helpful:
http://www.aypsite.org/167.html

Let the divine inner light shine! :-)

The guru is in you.

2008/03/29 11:36:02
Yamas & Niyamas - Restraints & Observances
http://www.aypsite.org/forum/topic.asp?TOPIC_ID=2981&REPLY_ID=31894&whichpage=-1
Living on light

Hi Nirodha and Christi:

Interesting discussion. However, it is not clear to me if you are talking about meditation OR other methods (like pranayama), or meditation AND other methods.

While this old yogi can't put it in Buddhist terms, there is an opinion here. :-)

If the question is, which is more progressive, meditation OR pranayama? (for example), then I'd have to agree with Nirodha that meditation is the more sure path to samadhi.

If the question is whether meditation AND pranayama is more powerful than meditation alone, then I'd have to agree with Christi, assuming he means that pranayama (and other methods) are practiced in addition to meditation, and not instead of it.

Of course, an integration is what we are doing in AYP, using a full range of methods in a self-paced way, with deep meditation at the center. An integrated approach like this has been demonstrated time and again to be more progressive than using any any single practice by itself, including meditation.

This is why Patanjali documented eight limbs of yoga, instead of only one, and I believe an equivalent multi-tool kit can be found in Buddhism too.

Of course, if I had to pick just one practice, I'd be back with Nirodha with meditation. Happily, we can do much more to accelerate our progress, and do not have to rest on our laurels for long before finding openings to new levels of "stillness in action" with the many tools we have available nowadays. :-)

The guru is in you.

2008/04/01 23:00:52
Yamas & Niyamas - Restraints & Observances
http://www.aypsite.org/forum/topic.asp?TOPIC_ID=2981&REPLY_ID=32069&whichpage=-1
Living on light

quote:
_____
Originally posted by Christi

I remember you once said that at some point Tantric practices are dropped. Is this because the job of purifying the subtle nervous system has been done? And does this correlate to any point of Samad
Hi having been reached?
_____

Hi Christi:

Not dropped, only transformed over time into something much more refined. Erotic becomes ecstatic, and outer lovemaking becomes inner lovemaking. Then a glance or a touch from our Beloved sends the infinite cosmos into ecstatic waves of bliss. It is ecstatic conductivity becoming ecstatic radiance, and then constant outpouring divine love -- stillness in action.

This is what the whole universe is about. Not so far fetched, considering the infinite power of Love. An effective integration of practices opens the door. All practices become refined along the way. Nothing is dropped. Everything is transformed until it is all samad
Hi -- living moving samadhi. There is no end of the journey. The journey is the destination, just as unending becoming is the destination of the universe.

Except, of course, for those who want to check out. That is an illusion. There is no checking out. Only more and more becoming what we are.

One part cannot be separated from the other parts, even if we call that part absolute. What is has no name, and it is everywhere. We are *That*. :-)

The guru is in you.

2008/04/02 11:03:19
Yamas & Niyamas - Restraints & Observances
http://www.aypsite.org/forum/topic.asp?TOPIC_ID=2981&REPLY_ID=32095&whichpage=-1
Living on light

Hi Christi:

Yep to all you said. :-)

The guru is in you.

2008/04/05 11:40:14
Yamas & Niyamas - Restraints & Observances
http://www.aypsite.org/forum/topic.asp?TOPIC_ID=2981&REPLY_ID=32233&whichpage=-1
Living on light

quote:
_____
Originally posted by Nirodha

I'd like to share an insight I gained during meditation one night: When a contemplative is residing in Samadhi, that contemplative is simultaneously exercising, refining his/her acquisition of and fulfilling the Noble Eightfold Path.
_____

Hi Nirodha:

Yes, I agree (from a yogic point of view).

But it is also true that "magic bullet" thinking will more often be wrong than right, which is why the greatest sages documented multi-fold paths rather than singular ones.

Our wisdom is limited in direct proportion to the degree we believe it to be complete. Speaking only for myself on that, of course.

The less we know, the more we know. Another of those divine paradoxes. :-)

The guru is in you.

2008/04/07 10:46:53
Yamas & Niyamas - Restraints & Observances
http://www.aypsite.org/forum/topic.asp?TOPIC_ID=2981&REPLY_ID=32330&whichpage=-1
Living on light

Hi All:

If we are clear about our path and what works for us, that is great. However, when sharing, it is incumbent on us to offer what can work for others, rather than only for ourselves at our present stage. This is especially true for advanced practitioners who feel they have "IT" figured out, who may have more credibility and hence more responsibility.

It is particularly an issue in teaching non-dual self-inquiry (the Krishnamurti conundrum), but also for anyone who feels like they have reached a level of understanding that others should "get" straightaway without having to travel their own path. It doesn't work like that.

The AYP Self-Inquiry book goes into the "wise teacher few can benefit from" scenario in some detail, because this is a common problem in the field of self-inquiry. But it can happen with anyone who has a revelation about "what works."

This is why we have multi-fold paths and, nowadays, open source knowledge, so everyone will have an opportunity to find their own way, rather than spending too much time listening to some fool on a hill. :-)

The guru is in you.

2008/04/07 21:48:59
Yamas & Niyamas - Restraints & Observances
http://www.aypsite.org/forum/topic.asp?TOPIC_ID=2981&REPLY_ID=32369&whichpage=-1
Living on light

Hi All:

No accusations were intended by the phrase "some fool on a hill."

It is anyone we may listen to beyond the bounds of our good common sense. It is we who create the fool on the hill in how we listen. We can turn the fool into a wise person just as easily, simply by accepting what is true in them and letting go of what is not.

There are no absolutes, though we often crave certainties to the point of distraction. There is wisdom and foolishness in everyone. Life is a never-ending process of separating wheat from chaff. The more abiding inner silence we have, the easier it becomes.

It isn't about the teacher, after all. It is about the student, where the process of human spiritual transformation is occurring. It is good to keep that in mind from both the student's and the teacher's point of view. If all parties approach it like that, everyone will win.

We are all students, and the teacher lives in us too. But, in either case, only to the degree we long for our opening and move in surrender to the flow. All yoga practices are expressions of that dynamic.

The guru is in you.

2008/10/10 13:14:31
Yamas & Niyamas - Restraints & Observances
http://www.aypsite.org/forum/topic.asp?TOPIC_ID=2981&REPLY_ID=38767&whichpage=-1
Living on light

quote:
_____
Originally posted by gumpi

How do you know that semen is going up inside your body? Is it nothing but an opinion?
_____

Hi Gumpi:

The tell-tale sign is the body-wide ecstatic connection. It is admittedly subjective, but those who experience it can "see" what is happening. This is one that the scientists will be able to measure, whenever they get around to it.

See here also, and other topics on vajroli in the tantra forum: http://www.aypsite.org/forum/topic.asp?TOPIC_ID=4553

The guru is in you.

2008/10/11 10:17:47
Yamas & Niyamas - Restraints & Observances
http://www.aypsite.org/forum/topic.asp?TOPIC_ID=2981&REPLY_ID=38783&whichpage=-1
Living on light

quote:
_____
Originally posted by Christl

Hi Yogani,

quote:
_____
The tell-tale sign is the body-wide ecstatic connection. It is admittedly subjective, but those who experience it can "see" what is happening. This is one that the scientists will be able to measure, whenever they get around to it.
_____

Why do you say that the whole-body ecstasy is proof of automatic vajroli? I always thought it was caused by the nadis being pure enough and wide enough to channel large amounts of prana after kundalini awakening. Could this not happen even before vajroli sets in?

Wouldn't the release of amrita and ojas in the brain be a more sure sign of vajroli occuring?

Christi
_____

Hi Christi:

The short answer is that the sexual essences <u>are</u> the prana in motion in the nervous system on the physical level. The ecstatic experience is a symptom of this flow. Because of that connection, I think it is safe to say that anyone experiencing whole body ecstasy also has natural vajroli occurring. And, yes, this is a function of the purification of the entire nervous system (nadis).

It is really a question of how far we carry the neurobiology/prana relationship. Neurobiologically speaking, sexual essences are the source of ecstatic conductivity (kundalini), and the purification of the nervous system (corresponding nadis) by a full range of practices provides the opening for the process to move forward, yielding the spiritual experiences.

I am not saying that this physical/spiritual connection is absolutely how it is, going all the way in, but there is strong evidence that the connection between the neurobiology and spiritual experiences goes pretty far. Soma, amrita and ojas can be seen to be subdivisions of this, going to very refined substances finding their origin in the neurobiology also, as we have discussed previously. And you are right -- the presence of these substances is also evidence of natural vajroli, as is whole body mudra and other indicators of ecstatic bliss permeating the body and beyond.

Whether the neurobiology model of enlightenment turns out to be true in the long run is the question, isn't it? By taking this approach, many are given a handle on their experiences in terms of understanding the symptoms and underlying neurobiological changes that are clearly occurring. I have been asked literally hundreds of times in private, "Why is my spiritual ecstasy accompanied by sexual arousal?" The rise of natural vajroli is the reason. It is a component of kundalini awakening.

Putting the neurobiology out in front also hangs a <u>big carrot</u> out there for modern science to grab on to. There are plenty of things here that can be measured, and sooner or later science will get around to it. As many more practitioners come on line having these experiences (inevitable now), and the general lay of the land of the enlightenment process becomes more familiar everywhere, a fertile new field for scientific research will emerge.

Those who are more mystically inclined can ignore all the neurobiology and simply enjoy the ride, laughing all the way. :-)

Either way, our bhakti and the maintenance of an effective daily practice routine will continue to be the engine for human spiritual transformation in individuals and the population at large.

Onward!

The guru is in you.

2008/10/11 11:24:33
Yamas & Niyamas - Restraints & Observances
http://www.aypsite.org/forum/topic.asp?TOPIC_ID=2981&REPLY_ID=38786&whichpage=-1
Living on light

quote:
_____
Originally posted by Anthem11

Hi Yogani,

It has been my observation that when the inner energy changes (openings or directions of flow etc.) that the physical body follows in time to match. It appears from my current perspective to have more power when it comes from this direction.

So the work we do, the sitting practices, the self-inquiry, seems to have greater impact than the physical efforts we make: asanas, the physical practice of vajiroli, diet, etc. These do impact the energy body but more like using a teaspoon to empty a barrel of water whereas inner energy changes internally punch giant holes in the barrel emptying it in a far more straight-forward manner.

Would you say this is an accurate perspective?
_____

Hi Andrew:

Yes, I agree. But an avid hatha yogi may disagree. :-)

All roads lead home. An effective integration of all roads leads home even faster. :-)

The guru is in you.

2007/11/04 10:55:21
Yamas & Niyamas - Restraints & Observances
http://www.aypsite.org/forum/topic.asp?TOPIC_ID=3037&REPLY_ID=26702&whichpage=-1
amaroli and diet

quote:
_____
Originally posted by gentlep

I just got the Diet,shatkarma and amaroli ebook. It mentions that on days of fasting amaroli can be used several times during the day. But why not on regular days. Is taking amaroli during the day while not fasting is not helpful? How about before going to bed at night?
_____

Hi Gentlep:

Just about anything can be tried with prudent self-pacing of practices in relation to our daily activities. Balance...

You decide. :-)

The guru is in you.

2008/04/22 15:35:14
Yamas & Niyamas - Restraints & Observances
http://www.aypsite.org/forum/topic.asp?TOPIC_ID=3209&REPLY_ID=32935&whichpage=-1
The karmic price of meat

quote:
_____
John wrote: And that night I was sitting and meditating, and I had forgotten about what we had for dinner, but I noticed how the kundalini/prana was not flowing at all, not even a little. That's very unusual for me. And then I remembered we had split that chicken breast on our salad, and realized all over again why I was feeling no energy flow. But it was OK, what ever happens or doesn't happen is OK. It becomes a teachable

moment not to have any energy flow, and re-experience what things used to be like, and to realize that it doesn't really matter whether we can perceive the kundalini or not. It's there resting at muladhara then I suppose. I know that tomorrow, I will notice it again.

———————

Hi John:

For those who have kundalini energy overloads, this is why a temporary heavier diet may be utilized, along with other means. It is part of self-pacing and grounding.

Of course, it works the other way too, as you are pointing out. That is why the main AYP diet suggestion is "light and nutritious" ... except when we need to be going the other way. :-)

The guru is in you.

2008/04/22 23:53:48
Yamas & Niyamas - Restraints & Observances
http://www.aypsite.org/forum/topic.asp?TOPIC_ID=3209&REPLY_ID=32947&whichpage=-1
The karmic price of meat

quote:
———————
Originally posted by Steve to John

One person's chicken and broccoli is another's 'nuts and sprouted alfalfa'. As you said, it's best to quiet down and listen to what our body is telling us about our individual needs.

———————

Hi Steve and John:

That sums up the diet section of the "Diet, Shatkarmas and Amaroli" book -- in a nutshell, of course. :-)

Bon appetite!

The guru is in you.

2007/12/18 09:35:38
Yamas & Niyamas - Restraints & Observances
http://www.aypsite.org/forum/topic.asp?TOPIC_ID=3270&REPLY_ID=28028&whichpage=-1
abstentions and purification

quote:
———————
Originally posted by John C

Another idea for you is that the book I mentioned above in the original post, talks about a plain salt water solution recipe.

———————

Hi John:

What you mention above (plain saline solution) is what is suggested for intestinal wash in the Diet, Shakarmas and Amaroli (DSA) book. And more than once or twice per month for intestinal wash would be considered very frequent, with potential diminishing returns due to the temporary depletion of natural biochemicals in the body that occurs each time the procedure is done, with some recovery time being necessary.

A less invasive approach to GI tract cleansing is basti (colon cleansing enema) which can be done as often as daily for months on end without negative effects, as inclined by the call of emerging ecstatic conductivity (kundalini). Basti is not as complete a cleanse as intestinal wash, but is much less taxing on the body.

A balanced "self-paced" approach is what is suggested in the book, using shatkarmas (cleansing techniques) during times when the neurobiology is calling for them, which for most is "middle stage" in the process of human spiritual transformation -- during the rise and stabilization of ecstatic conductivity. Of course, this is a spiritual point of view. These methods can also be undertaken for health reasons, which could include factors other than supporting the biochemistry of ecstatic conductivity/kundalini in the GI tract.

This is also the approach to diet in the DSA book -- learning to listen and respond to what the body is calling for, which can vary over time as our practices and spiritual development advance.

The book also covers fasting, ayurvedic diet considerations for helping stabilize kundalini imbalances, other shatkarmas, and, of course, amaroli, which helps open more refined functioning in the neurobiology for sustaining both abiding inner silence and the flow of ecstatic energy.

All the best!

The guru is in you.

2008/01/27 17:31:32
Yamas & Niyamas - Restraints & Observances
http://www.aypsite.org/forum/topic.asp?TOPIC_ID=3409

Diet and Cost for 9 Families Around the World

Hi All:

Here is an informative and thought-provoking email attachment I received recently on the weekly diet and food cost for nine families from around the world (photos included):

http://www.time.com/time/photogallery/0,29307,1626519,00.html

They are listed from the most to the least spent on food, if not from the healthiest to the least healthy diet.

Let us ponder these things...

The guru is in you.

2008/10/06 12:07:20
Yamas & Niyamas - Restraints & Observances
http://www.aypsite.org/forum/topic.asp?TOPIC_ID=3409&REPLY_ID=38632&whichpage=-1
Diet and Cost for 9 Families Around the World

Hi CarsonZi:

"...if not from the healthiest to the least healthy diet" means the families with more will not necessarily be more healthy than those with less, a fact that is becoming well-known in the modern world. So we are saying the same thing.

It's an amazing montage of humankind, isn't it? We are so different, yet so much the same. I am sure the need for spiritual practices is also present in every one of those cultures. We all share in that, not living by bread alone.

With increasing inner silence around the globe, those with too much will tend toward less, and those with not enough will tend toward more. The rise of stillness in action on all sides brings *balance*, which is the essence of health, happiness and enlightenment.

The guru is in you.

2008/03/17 13:36:16
Yamas & Niyamas - Restraints & Observances
http://www.aypsite.org/forum/topic.asp?TOPIC_ID=3626&REPLY_ID=31412&whichpage=-1
Yama and Niyama

quote:
_____
Originally posted by brushjw

I have been going through a somewhat protracted dark night of the soul. I think this may be because my ability to concentrate on meditative absorption has leapfrogged my ability to dissolve my karmic traces.
_____

Hi Joe:

Remember to self-pace in all things as necessary (including bhakti), to maintain good progress with safety. Sometimes the best thing to do is just go out and dig in the dirt (or equivalent) for a while for some solid grounding. Everyone deserves a break once in a while. :-)

Our rising awareness of yama and niyama (restraints and observances in conduct) is a direct result of bhakti and our daily practices. It is suggested to approach matters of conduct with gentleness as and when it feels natural. Forced conduct is not much help on the spiritual path, and can in fact have the opposite effect if it becomes obsessive. This is the main risk in overdoing yama/niyama.

It does not look like that is where you are coming from. Sitting practices will lead to yama/niyama much more assuredly than the other way around, as your experience indicates. As yama/niyama is coming up, there will be some clunky stages involved. It goes with the territory. So be kind to yourself and take your time.

Btw, karma will not go away. It will be transformed to higher purpose through your inner silence and increasingly inspired actions. All that has been sour and dark will become sweet and luminous.

All the best!

The guru is in you.

2008/03/18 11:08:47
Yamas & Niyamas - Restraints & Observances
http://www.aypsite.org/forum/topic.asp?TOPIC_ID=3626&REPLY_ID=31456&whichpage=-1
Yama and Niyama

quote:
_____
Originally posted by Maximus

quote:
_____

It is suggested to approach matters of conduct with gentleness as and when it feels natural. Forced conduct is not much help on the spiritual path, and can in fact have the opposite effect if it becomes obsessive.

_____

Hi Yogani
But doesn't Patanjali say to practice continous non-attachment without a break? I take conduct to mean how we handle fears, attractions and aversions.

_____

Hi Maximus:

Times have changed considerably since Patanjali's day. The order of the eight limbs of yoga can be approached in different ways to optimize results. The "yama/niyama first" approach is a difficult path, as anyone who has tried it knows. Btw, practicing "non-attachment" is a form of self-inquiry. In the language of the AYP Self-Inquiry book, it will be "non-relational" without the presence of abiding inner silence, the witness. Non-relational is mind playing on mind, which does little to cultivate inner silence and spiritual progress. It can be a strain and create obstructions to progress. That is what I meant.

The suggestion is to do deep meditation daily and take it easy in our thinking and doing, keeping active each day, favoring what we know is right conduct (this awareness will expand with time in practices). Then the integration of stillness will come naturally, and everything we do will become "relational," meaning, performed in stillness. Then the flow into yama/niyama (spiritual conduct) will be easy.

We can't consistently think our way past fears, attractions and aversions, but we can permanently dissolve them in our abiding silent witness. That is the key point. It is a process of purification and opening in our nervous system, best undertaken in a balanced way.

The issue brought up by Joe at the beginning of this topic has more to do with self-pacing in practices and grounding in daily activity than with yama/niyama. Adding regimented conduct (mental or physical) on top of an uncomfortable energy excess is not going to help much -- might even make the energy excess worse, since parts of niyama are focused on more intense bhakti and more spiritual stimulation! Self-pacing and grounding are the ticket when things are getting to be too much. This is not anti-yama/niyama. It is just putting the emphasis where it is needed to deal with circumstances in the moment, which is what we should always be doing on our path.

The guru is in you.

2009/05/17 20:02:23
Yamas & Niyamas - Restraints & Observances
http://www.aypsite.org/forum/topic.asp?TOPIC_ID=4086&REPLY_ID=50948&whichpage=-1
atkin diet yes or no, with kundalini process

Hi All:

Everything you ever wanted to know about diet, but were afraid to ask -- a 4 minute AYP video called "Are we what we eat?" :-)

http://www.youtube.com/watch?v=64rz_nX-kLE

The guru is in you.

2009/05/18 09:49:13
Yamas & Niyamas - Restraints & Observances
http://www.aypsite.org/forum/topic.asp?TOPIC_ID=4086&REPLY_ID=50981&whichpage=-1
atkin diet yes or no, with kundalini process
:-)
2008/11/12 19:18:55
Yamas & Niyamas - Restraints & Observances
http://www.aypsite.org/forum/topic.asp?TOPIC_ID=4714&REPLY_ID=40386&whichpage=-1
Sharing of amaroli experience

Hi Holy:

Sounds like you should have been doing less rather than more, and perhaps even going with micro quantities and diluting with water. This is a case where some self-pacing (scaling back) would have helped a lot.

Regarding meat-eating and amaroli, with a more measured approach it should not be a problem. The urge to eat meat may become less during the natural course of practices.

In any case, sorry you hit a wall with it. A clear sign of overdoing, I'm afraid. Maybe try again later starting with much smaller quantities. But there is no rush. There is plenty else to do in AYP. :-)

All the best!

The guru is in you.

PS:
Hi Machart. Amaroli has been discussed extensively in the forums in the past. Try some searches and you will find some long topics on it. Doing "subject only" searches helps narrow it down.

2009/01/19 12:39:06

Hi All:

Interesting discussion.

Ruiz's "Four Agreements" are useful guidelines for conduct too.

However, having such guidelines for conduct is not the whole answer. If it were, the world would be a much better place, because the spiritual traditions and religions have had plenty of guidelines for conduct in place for centuries.

Since codes of conduct (yama and niyama) are already part of many spiritual traditions, they alone having limited effect on the course of human spiritual evolution, then we have to ask ourselves what might be missing.

I believe the lack of fully-integrated systems of spiritual practice is the greatest shortcoming in the traditions, not necessarily a lack of guidelines for conduct. Ironically, it seems most traditions reach a limit in the scope of spiritual practices they are able to offer because they become preoccupied with matters of conduct. In that sense, too much attention on yama/niyama can be a pitfall, like the many other pitfalls of the mind.

With many of the later practices we have presented in AYP (samyama, self-inquiry, karma yoga, etc.), having them become "relational in stillness" is the key. This is the direction we want to go in approaching yama/niyama -- moving steadily toward "stillness in action" in all aspects of our practice and our life. This places sitting practices, especially meditation and pranayama, at the center. From such a foundation in practice, all the rest can flower naturally, as these discussions indicate. :-)

All the best!

The guru is in you.

2009/01/19 15:33:49

quote:
_____
Originally posted by Anthem11

I am suggesting that the roots of the action that people take (verbal, physical) are a more accurate and more meaningful measures of a person's inner condition and spiritual progress. If there are still actions based in ignorance which are reactions to emotions such as anger, jealousy, hatred, greed, fear, etc., then there is still work to be done despite levels of ecstasy, bliss or understanding of the unity of all things. Action born from love, compassion and understanding being the other end of the spectrum and only the one acting can know if their actions truly stem from these sources even if they appear otherwise from the outside.

Yoga holds inner energy development, ecstasy, bliss and unity consciousness as sign-posts and no doubt there are strong correlations to overall inner condition but these can be very misleading when certain practices accelerate certain experiences. I think we have seen this often and from the experiencer's perspective they can be misleading too, how much, how often etc., I must be enlightened, I had bliss, I saw the unity of it all etc. From my perspective it appears to me the root of action doesn't lie and is a more accurate measure.

Of course all of the measures rely on self-truth but yoga practitioners would be better served in many ways from my perspective focusing on the degree to which they act in the world from a place of love, understanding and true service.
_____

Hi Anthem:

No disagreement there. However, as you point out, this kind of measurement is ultimately internal. While our external behavior may seem to be improving, the real dynamic is occurring inside. Perhaps, in time, science will develop objective ways for measuring this.

Meanwhile, the further we go in cultivating inner silence and ecstatic conductivity/radiance, the more acute our awareness of evolutionary and non-evolutionary action becomes, and our actions are affected accordingly. When our actions are in disharmony, we will feel the pain of it to the end of the earth. And when our actions are in harmony, we will feel the joy far out into the cosmic regions. So our choices become relatively easy, and codes of conduct may become somewhat incidental, but not necessarily to be ignored.

Because of the internal dynamics, it is difficult to measure external acts as being evolutionary or non-evolutionary. Nevertheless, there must be some measurement by someone to limit the ignorant abuses that happen in this world. That is what the law is for.

As for the internal fireworks and other experiences associated with the purification and opening of spiritual development, we have been calling these things "scenery" for a long time around here, haven't we? We acknowledge such experiences, and enjoy them if they come, but...

Spiritual development is about improving the quality of everyday living. Those who think it is a thrill ride will get over it eventually. The more effective the system of practices we are using, the sooner we will get over the thrill ride aspect of it, which is not a prerequisite for enlightenment. Going off on tangents tends to delay the process, as many here know. :-)

We will know we are making progress as we become less concerned about our own spiritual condition, and more concerned about helping others. That's the bottom line.

The guru is in you.

2009/01/20 11:08:47

Hi Anthem and All:

It is important to acknowledge all experiences that may come up along the path, so there can be understanding of them, and so they can be used to fuel bhakti for daily practice. All experiences are valid for the person who is having them. If we are not feeling inclined to go out and serve humanity, it is not a shortcoming. Whatever experiences we are having today will suffice to help us stay motivated on our path. The flashy experiences of purification and opening are as valid as any other. We can acknowledge them, enjoy them, and move on.

Along the way on the path of daily practices, a gradual shift occurs from small self (me) to big Self (we), and our motivations in action naturally shift to a service mode. The indicators for this latter stage are covered in the AYP Bhakti and Karma Yoga book.

The thing is, every stage has its own signature, its own milestones, its own validity, and it is not appropriate to measure one stage with another stage's milestones. This is the same issue we run into when "enlightened" teachers tell us that we should be seeing the world as non-dual now rather than later. If the milestones are not geared to the experience of the practitioner, then the teaching will be lacking in that time and place, creating expectations that are not reasonable or practical. We should be careful about this.

So, I don't think we can come up with a single set of criteria that can be applied to all practitioners. One size does not fit all. Broadly speaking, there is the inner silence stage, the ecstatic conductivity stage, and the unity stage. Each has it own characteristics. Shades of all three stages may be occurring at the same time to one degree or other. So, as we move along on our path, we may be noticing the presence of inner silence (witness), having waves of ecstasy or other energy events, and wanting to serve others, all at the same time. This mixture can be a normal experience for us as we move along on the path of practices. One part of the experience is not superior to another part. Any or all of these characteristics can be acknowledged as progress. The feedback is very useful for sustaining our motivation to go on with practices.

This is a very interesting topic, and an opportunity to clear up misunderstandings about what the enlightenment process is. It is a continuum, with many characteristics that we may experience along the way. Or we may not experience much that is dramatic, and only find life gradually getting better in ordinary ways. This too is rising enlightenment. All experiences we have are milestones, but not conditions to be clung to by us or anyone else. There is always a next stage, and we will be wise to continue beyond the inner adventures of the moment.

Hanging on will hold us back. Moving on is living in the now. That is why we always favor the practice over the experience. :-)

The guru is in you.

Hi Anthem:

There is much to be said for the "life improving in ordinary ways" approach for assessing our spiritual progress. All things being equal, it is a good way to view our path, with the least distraction.

However, when inner experiences (symptoms) occur involving the rise of inner silence (witness), or dramatic energy events (ecstatic or not, sometimes physical), then practitioners will ask about these. I don't think it is an effective approach to push them off, as many traditions do. This does not resolve whatever concerns a practitioner may have. As long as there are unresolved concerns, then there will tend to be a focus on the experience. That is a distraction, and can reduce motivation to practice.

This is also tied in with self-pacing in practices. If we understand the general nature of the excesses in purification that can occur within us, and know how to regulate our practices to mitigate such excesses, then maximum progress on our path can be sustained in a balanced way over the long term. We can acknowledge experiences for what they are, and then favor our practice over them, including self-pacing as needed.

So there are several reasons why we would like to have an understanding about anything that might happen, and that is a difference between AYP and other approaches.

If we can understand the process of human spiritual transformation as a whole, it can help us to be less fixated on the various experiences we may encounter along the way. That goes for service (karma yoga) also, which is largely an effect of abiding inner silence and its movement outward through us into the environment.

The guru is in you.

Hi Solo:

Traditionally, kapalbhati is considered a shatkarma, and it is covered in the AYP Diet, Shatkarmas and Amaroli (DSA) book from that perspective.

Of course, there is overlap in many things in yoga. Nauli is also a traditional shatkarma, but is normally done as part of an asana routine. Siddhasana is technically an asana, but is closely associated with mudras, bandhas and tantric sexual methods. And so it goes...

I agree that kapalbhati belongs back in an AYP practice forum, since we do cover it in the DSA book and in the online lessons (in Lesson 316). I'll put it in "Yamas and Niyamas," which is where the shatkarmas are usually discussed (they are niyamas).

The AYP Pranayama, Mudras and Bandhas forum category is reserved for support on spinal breathing pranayama, spinal bastrika, and related

AYP pranayamas, mudras and bandhas. Likewise, the AYP Deep Meditation and Samyama forum category is reserved for support on those practices. Other things tend to get moved out of these two forum categories for clarity sake, so it was appropriate for kapalbhakti to be moved out. Now we will send it to its right home. :-)

If we don't do this kind of housekeeping, things can get rather confusing for those seeking support on AYP-style deep meditation (DM), spinal breathing pranayama (SBP) and closely related practices. The rest of the forum categories have a lot more diversity in them, discussing many things. But those two, in particular, we try and keep as focused as possible, because DM and SBP are the foundational practices of AYP, and we'd like to have clear support for them.

Hope that clarifies things a bit. Thanks much for your contributions to the forums!

The guru is in you.

2009/10/12 07:48:53
Yamas & Niyamas - Restraints & Observances
http://www.aypsite.org/forum/topic.asp?TOPIC_ID=6512&REPLY_ID=58317&whichpage=-1
white tongue

Hi Sage:

"Tongue scraping" can be added as part of daily oral hygiene, though ultimately the amount of material collecting on our tongue will be related to other things, as Christiane points out.

Here is an excerpt on tongue scraping from the AYP Diet, Shatkarmas and Amaroli book:

"*Mouth and Tongue*
We have all been brought up (hopefully) to practice good oral hygiene by brushing our teeth every day and flossing regularly to remove tartar (plaque) from our teeth. There are varying opinions on using antiseptic mouthwashes, so it is suggested to go with the intuition on that. Our habits of oral hygiene will improve as we advance in yoga.
A yoga method that can be added to daily oral hygiene, which few may be exposed to in modern society, is tongue scraping. Sometimes brushing the tongue with the toothbrush is advised after brushing the teeth. The yogic equivalent of this is tongue scraping, which is far more effective for removing tartar and its resident bacteria from the tongue. This involves using the edge of a straight piece of metal or plastic to scrape the top of the tongue forward from the area right in front of the taste buds. A more effective tool for this is a flat strip of metal that has been bent into a "U" shape. The curved edge can be used to scrape forward on the top of the tongue, covering the full top surface with a single stroke, or several repetitions.
The amount of tartar collected with tongue scraping in this manner will far exceed what can be accomplished with a brush, and will greatly reduce the amount of tartar collecting on the teeth as well.
Of course, excessive tartar on the tongue and teeth can be a sign of an imbalance in the diet and/or general health condition. If that is the case, we can step back further and look at our lifestyle to address the root causes of excess proteins and bacteria (tartar) building up in the mouth. If we do this, we will find ourselves with a much cleaner mouth, and much better all around health as well.
The condition of our mouth at any point in time is a visible indication of the condition of the rest of our body, and the quality of life we have been living."

All the best!

The guru is in you.

2009/10/12 11:43:51
Yamas & Niyamas - Restraints & Observances
http://www.aypsite.org/forum/topic.asp?TOPIC_ID=6512&REPLY_ID=58323&whichpage=-1
white tongue

quote:
―――――――
Originally posted by Yonatan

Way cool, this is exactly what I need, as I have dental implants which the doctor can't open or it takes much pressure to open each time because of a lot of calculus that builds up.

One question.. When you say to scrape the area in front of the taste buds.. Is it the area with not many taste buds on the top of the tongue?

Here, the green area?
http://pactlab-dev.spcomm.uiuc.edu/classes/08SP/280blogs/first_weblog3/tastebud.gif
―――――――

Hi Yonatan:

In front of the big ones in the back. Those can't be scraped. Everything in front can. Not too hard ... self-pace. :-)

The guru is in you.

2010/01/01 08:54:14
Yamas & Niyamas - Restraints & Observances
http://www.aypsite.org/forum/topic.asp?TOPIC_ID=6944&REPLY_ID=61989&whichpage=-1
Revenge and Justice..

Hi FrancoHolland, and welcome!

Self-defense is appropriate in many cases, and in the ideal situation will be a positive karmic outcome, where all involved will move forward spiritually.

Revenge is not self-defense. It is aggression, and will lead to complications down the road.

It all depends on our spiritual condition. We act as we must.

In truth, no one is injured, for ultimately we are beyond events occurring in time and space. We are pure bliss consciousness. As we advance in practices and on our path, we find this as direct experience, and act accordingly.

On the other hand, current perception is 100% of our reality, and we must live from where we are. In that case, some common sense can help keep us out of the ditch -- paying some attention to the basic precepts of yama (restraint) and niyama (observance), and to the laws of the land wherever we are living.

Acting with intent to injure others will injure us. Breaking the law will lead to unwanted complications in life. And so on...

If someone is harming you, it is reasonable to protect yourself, and take steps to prevent repeat injury from the same source in the future. However, it is not in your best interest to attempt to injure the other for revenge. That kind of "justice" is fleeting, and will only lead to further cycles of injury to you and others.

Prudent self-defense and forgiveness make good partners. "I love you, but will not permit you to do that" is the way to handle those who are prone to violence. It may mean exiting a situation altogether, with no hard feelings. Actions performed on that basis are not personal. They are divine flow. But we may find anger mixed in, so it is good to pause to consider the consequences of our actions beforehand.

Moderation is the prudent course, but no one is required to be a doormat. We have a choice, and the high road is always available to us.

The main thing is to keep meditating daily. Then these choices become easy, because we will know through direct perception what is the high road and what is not. No one will have to tell us.

Wishing you all the best on your path. Practice wisely and enjoy!

The guru is in you.

2010/01/06 17:28:38
Yamas & Niyamas - Restraints & Observances
http://www.aypsite.org/forum/topic.asp?TOPIC_ID=6973&REPLY_ID=62264&whichpage=-1
Amaroli and conception

Hi Ram:

On amaroli and reduced ovulation, there is some mention in yoga lore about it (besides Satyananda). Is it true? I'm not aware of any scientific research on it. On the other side, there are opinions out there that amaroli aids fertility and makes birth control pills less effective. What to believe? It needs some science.

For those who are having difficulty conceiving, it may be wise for the woman to discontinue amaroli until there is conception, while recognizing that this is only one of many factors.

There are also mixed opinions on whether a woman should be doing amaroli during pregnancy. It has been pretty common in the East for centuries.

Btw, amniotic fluid is mostly fetal urine. We were all made in our own urine. :-)

Note: Amaroli and ovulation were also discussed here: http://www.aypsite.org/forum/topic.asp?TOPIC_ID=6594

All the best!

The guru is in you.

2010/03/26 12:07:12
Yamas & Niyamas - Restraints & Observances
http://www.aypsite.org/forum/topic.asp?TOPIC_ID=7493&REPLY_ID=66562&whichpage=-1
Miserable

Hi SeySorciere:

Low blood pressure for someone who normally has high blood pressure, doesn't sound like a bad thing. If it persists, then maybe a fundamental change is happening in your nervous system toward more balance. Then it might be time to visit your doctor to discuss your medication.

Change is not always comfortable, but if it is for the good, then there is cause for optimism.

You are wise to self-pace practices. Too much change all at once is not always in our best interest, not the best for our ongoing inspiration and stability.

This too shall pass...

The guru is in you.

2010/05/12 00:32:00
Yamas & Niyamas - Restraints & Observances

http://www.aypsite.org/forum/topic.asp?TOPIC_ID=7759&REPLY_ID=68592&whichpage=-1
wondering if any can advise

quote:
_____
Originally posted by denislav12

Hi,

I have been doing some cleansing techniques and the results are interesting so far.
I am just wondering if any of you have some experience and maybe can give me some guideline...
How frequently should one do the Kunjal? Is it something that can be performed at least 3 times a week , or maybe because the intestinal wash flashes the bacterial flora of the intestine such a procedure has to be limited? I know the idea about self pacing but if maybe there are some tips of general essence, i will appreciate those.
Also, I am interested if it is ok to combine and do Kunjal first and then perform Laghu shanka prakshalana. Would it be ok to do those two one after another?
Also, isit ok to do amorali after those cleansing techniques?
thanks in advance

_____

Hi denislav12:

Kunjal (swallowing and vomiting out a large amount of water) is not included in the AYP system, so I can't comment much about it.

Laghu shanka prakshalana (intestinal wash) is included in the AYP shatkarmas, and it is suggested not to do it more than once or twice per month, as it requires recovery from the depletion of natural essences in the GI tract. Basti (enema) is less invasive and can be done much more often. For details, see the AYP Diet, Shatkarmas and Amaroli book.

All the best!

The guru is in you.

2010/05/12 09:43:44
Yamas & Niyamas - Restraints & Observances
http://www.aypsite.org/forum/topic.asp?TOPIC_ID=7759&REPLY_ID=68611&whichpage=-1
wondering if any can advise

quote:
_____
Originally posted by denislav12

Thank you for the replay.
I only skimmed through your book Diet Shatkarmas and Amorali so initially I did not see the (intestinal wash) explained but it is good to know that it is recommended to do only twice a month.
thanks again

_____

Hi denislav12:

In the book, it says that weekly intestinal wash would be very aggressive. Even twice-monthly or monthly could be questionable unless there are overriding health or spiritual reasons. Basti (enema) is healthier for frequent use. But there should be a need.

It is not like deep meditation, where if you just keep doing it on a schedule, all good things will happen automatically. Intestinal wash can be very depleting if overdone. Kunjal (forced vomiting of water -- not in the AYP system), could also be depleting if overdone.

Speaking of "need," it should be mentioned that shatkarmas have a particular role to play on the spiritual path -- middle stage support of the rise of ecstatic conductivity and the nectar cycle. Before or after may have less relevance from a spiritual point of view. This is discussed in the book, and here: http://www.aypsite.org/312.html

Of course, for health reasons, shatkarmas may be helpful at any time. It is your call.

The guru is in you.

2010/06/29 14:16:47
Yamas & Niyamas - Restraints & Observances
http://www.aypsite.org/forum/topic.asp?TOPIC_ID=8040&REPLY_ID=70503&whichpage=-1
Vegetarian or non-Vegetarian

Hi All:

Here is a lesson summarizing the AYP approach to diet, which avoids the extremes on either side of the debate that can actually retard spiritual progress if over-emphasized and/or forced on others: http://www.aypsite.org/305.html

As with so many things in spiritual practice, one size does not fit all. Tolerance for varying approaches to diet in the community of practitioners is therefore encouraged. This provides everyone the opportunity to evolve according to their own process of purification and opening, which is the fastest path.

The guru is in you.

Forum 8 – Jnana Yoga/Self-Inquiry – Advaita (Non-Duality)

The rise of the witness in self-inquiry brings awareness of our true Self, and the unity of all.
http://www.aypsite.org/forum/forum.asp?FORUM_ID=54

2005/11/27 11:41:39
Jnana Yoga/Self-Inquiry - Advaita (Non-Duality)
http://www.aypsite.org/forum/topic.asp?TOPIC_ID=608&REPLY_ID=1665&whichpage=-1
Neutralizing negativity

Hi Lily:

Between the two approaches you mentioned for dealing with negative thoughts, the thought replacement strategy is not as effective as the witnessing strategy. However, the witnessing strategy depends on the degree to which we have developed our inner silence, and witnessing by itself is not the best way cultivate inner silence. As we have been discussing lately (here and here), while passive witnessing does have some affect on increasing our witnessing quality, deep meditation is a more direct approach to cultivating it as a full time presence. Then we are in a position to observe, enter into and dissolve negative mental and emotional activity without experiencing inner fluctuations in our awareness (sense of self).

The rise of the witness also leads to the ability to engage effectively in "self-inquiry," which is the ability to proactively question and dissolve the non-reality of negative thoughts, feelings and perceptions. This is the shattering of illusion. What remains is our eternal pure bliss consciousness.

Interestingly, the rise of the witness, combined with the intellectual process of self-inquiry, leads to increasing bhakti (desire for truth) and surrender to what is real within us and our surroundings. The most basic form of self-inquiry is the inquiry, "Who am I?" That single question, released deep within our inner silence, can move mountains. In fact, every other form of self-inquiry is a variation on "Who am I?"

There is the samyama connection here -- our ability to effortlessly release thoughts and feelings within our inner silence where they have the greatest evolutionary power. Negative thoughts and feelings have no evolutionary power, and have no influence in inner silence. They are dissolved and transformed to evolutionary energy there. This is why I have said that samyama is a morally self-regulating process.

There is a book called "Loving What is," by Byron Katie, that offers a simple approach to developing a habit of self-inquiry. When combined with daily deep meditation and rising inner silence, self-inquiry can be a viable approach for dealing with the negative thoughts and feelings that come up in daily life. Self-inquiry is a proactive form of witnessing, just as mantra meditation is proactive cultivation of inner silence (the witness itself).

All the best!

The guru is in you.

2005/11/27 14:46:53
Jnana Yoga/Self-Inquiry - Advaita (Non-Duality)
http://www.aypsite.org/forum/topic.asp?TOPIC_ID=608&REPLY_ID=1669&whichpage=-1
Neutralizing negativity

Hi Lily:

Though the approach Feuerstein (who is a respected yoga scholar) promotes is the common traditional one, I don't know anyone who has had success with it going the distance in yoga, which again begs the question: "Where's the enlightened?"

The premise in traditional yoga is that learning to behave enlightened (yama and niyama), doing neuro-energy practices (asanas and pranayama) and draconian sensory deprivation (pratyahara) are the prerequisites for learning the most powerful enlightenment practice -- meditation that directly cultivates inner silence. Perhaps the reference here is to a method of meditation that does not go immediately deep beyond the thinking process, and therefore it requires "preparation" so we will not get hung up in it. Well, who needs forms of meditation that place the burden of their ineffectiveness on the practitioner? This entire process seems backwards to me, and leading nowhere fast.

Oddly enough, the mainstream traditional approach to yoga is highly esoteric because it leaves ardent seekers hankering indefinitely outside the door of deep practice. Add to it that only a "guru" can impart the "advanced" teachings of meditation, and you have a sure-fire formula for not much happening.

The traditional eight limbs "in sequence" approach to yoga that Feuerstein and others promote is the least risk, least results strategy. It reflects the condition of yoga around the world today where nearly everyone is left wallowing in physicality and intellectuality -- barely scratching the surface of the vast potential for human spiritual transformation. Then add to that the kundalini messes associated with premature crown practices, and who would even want to look further?

The shortcoming is not in the practitioners. The shortcoming is in the teachings!

The limbs of yoga need not be taken in sequence. In fact, the best results are found by taking them in a more practical order, with effective deep meditation first. There is more discussion on this in the lesson on the eight limbs of yoga and samyama (#149) at http://www.aypsite.org/149.html

The bottom line is, we ought to be optimizing the application of yoga practices in ways that are results-oriented, rather than blindly following approaches and practices that are slow and produce sub-par results. There is no time to waste.

The guru is in you.

PS -- Btw, the answer to the question, "Where's the enlightened?" is to be found right where each of us is sitting... :-)

2005/11/29 22:45:21
Jnana Yoga/Self-Inquiry - Advaita (Non-Duality)
http://www.aypsite.org/forum/topic.asp?TOPIC_ID=608&REPLY_ID=1710&whichpage=-1

Neutralizing negativity

Hi Near:

The answer is the same for all the yamas and niyamas -- "Don't wait and don't force." Waiting is not so good, and neither is forcing. It is the procedure we use in all of our AYP practices -- gentle persuasion ... or proactive letting go toward more of inner quality of life, which enhances outer quality of life. Simply knowing the guideline is enough. Rising inner silence will do the rest. When we find ourselves on the fence, we can easily choose the guideline. That is how yamas and niyamas can be used in AYP, without waiting or forcing. When the choice is easy, we make it for purity, evolution and for the good. We don't wait...

An exception to this procedure would be in the case of harming others. If we do not firmly guard ourselves from harming others, then others should, and will. This is the value of laws put in place to safeguard the common good.

Happily, yoga will bring up ahimsa (non-harming) pretty fast. In fact, those attracted to yoga usually already have it, and the other yamas and niyamas to a degree as well. Bhakti alone will bring that degree of purification, as well as bringing us to our path, or our path to us!

The guru is in you.

2006/03/24 20:19:08
Jnana Yoga/Self-Inquiry - Advaita (Non-Duality)
http://www.aypsite.org/forum/topic.asp?TOPIC_ID=968
Self-Inquiry -- A Practice Between our Meditations

Hi All:

Every now and then, I get asked what practice we can do all day long between our meditations. As you know, what I always say is , "Go out and be active." That really will do it, because as our inner silence rises and we integrate it into our daily life through normal activity, we will become more aware of the relationship between our self and our inner and outer environments. Add to that the cultivation of ecstatic conductivity via spinal breathing and other means, and our inner silence will be come active, riding on our ecstatic radiance flowing everywhere in and around us.

Well, I think it is time to expand on this discussion a bit, and look into the primary practice of Jnana Yoga -- Self-Inquiry. Jnana yoga is the yoga of the intellect. It involves the ways that we can think throughout the day that can be used to promote our spiritual growth, happiness and enlightenment.

Below is an email Q&A on this that sums up where I hope to go with self-inquiry in relation to AYP. All thoughts and inputs on this are welcome!

Q: I read the book "The Power of Now" by Eckhart Tolle, and I am trying to incorporate that into my life. Have you ever thought about writing something on what we could do during the times in-between the meditations, when we add all the mud that we are trying to clean off during meditation? I mean, this book on "Power of Now" is good, but like so many other books -- very vague -- not how you give instructions on how to do something. It says, "Observe your mind, don't identify with it." How?

A: I have been through Tolle also. He strikes me as being one of those mountain climbers who woke up on top of the mountain not knowing exactly how he got there and is now trying to tell everyone how to get there too. But he doesn't know, really. He is very sincere, and trying very hard. I give him a lot of credit for that. But he knows little about yoga practices, so he is working from a disadvantage. The fact that he has become extremely popular is a testament to how much people would like to have what he has -- inner silence, living in the now. Good stuff.

What to do between the meditations? Live life as fully as you can, and pay attention! If you are looking for a way to keep the mud off during the day, I suggest reading "Loving What Is" by Byron Katie. It is the best book on self-inquiry I have seen -- Tolle even endorses it. It is not easy to read and absorb -- but worth the effort. The bottom line is that we make all our own mud, and all we have to do is develop good habits of noticing how we do that. Then the mud machine grinds to a halt. Of course "noticing" is a function of our awareness, our inner silence. It always gets back to that.

Another one is "The Four Agreements" by Ruiz, which is a Shaman book. Very good and to the point advice on how to live daily life. It is a form of self-inquiry also -- always asking ourselves if we are doing thus-and-so that leads us to greater peace and happiness. His four guidelines are excellent. See here: http://www.aypsite.org/forum/topic.asp?TOPIC_ID=466

Self-inquiry is really the best practice to do during the day. Ramana Maharis
Hi is the most famous promoter of it, and it is what Tolle is trying to get across. I think Katie actually does a better job, with practical instructions, though a bit messy.

Next year I will take a crack at simplifying self-inquiry in an AYP Enlightenment Series book -- one of those little skinny ones, you know. If I can do in 100 pages what Katie did in 250 pages, making it much simpler and easier to apply, then that will be a useful addition to the literature, and will help round out AYP as well. It won't be easy, because self-inquiry does not lend itself to a simple practical application. At least not until now.

In truth, self-inquiry relies on the presence of inner silence (the witness) to work at all. Both Tolle and Katie have it, but many of their students do not, so the results are mixed. That is why I have not tackled self-inquiry so far. Solid grounding in deep meditation and samyama should come first. With inner silence coming up, a lot more is possible. Everything is possible! The AYP approach will be from that angle -- meditate and do samyama, and then do self-inquiry during the day. Then maybe the whole operation can be made more reliable. Before a systematic cultivation of inner silence is brought in, structured self-inquiry is pretty much hit or miss. That's not what we want in AYP. We want to hit the target every time.

Going out and living fully while paying attention is self-inquiry too -- if inner silence is coming up from sitting practices, we naturally see more and inquire more about the relationship of our self with our environment. It is all about becoming *stillness in action*. There is enough in AYP now to get it done. But I will keep adding more. I hope eventually to make AYP absolutely airtight, so no one will be able to ignore the practicality of it. Give me a few more years at this keyboard. :-)

The guru is in you.

2006/03/24 23:55:56
Jnana Yoga/Self-Inquiry - Advaita (Non-Duality)
http://www.aypsite.org/forum/topic.asp?TOPIC_ID=968&REPLY_ID=5058&whichpage=-1
Self-Inquiry -- A Practice Between our Meditations

Hi Shanti and Weaver:

Oh, jnana and self-inquiry are a can of worms until inner silence is brought in. Then, eventually (all by itself), it turns into a cake walk, because the witness puts us beyond our thinking process, and we can really see it for what it is -- a bunch of knee-jerk reactions coming out of the subconscious. From the position of the untouched observer, new and healthier habits of thinking are much easier to cultivate. The mind becomes like dust that vanishes in the breeze of our awareness, instead of like a brick wall that seems impenetrable. Such is the power of deep meditation and growing inner silence.

Self-inquiry is getting inside the thinking process with certain kinds of questions, exposing it piece by piece to unbiased observation, during which the machinery of self-made illusion can be gradually dissolved. It is the kind of thing we can do all day long if we want. :-)

Some of the most basic general questions are "Who am I?" (Ramana Maharishi's favorite), "Why am I here?" "Is there something more?" "What is real?" (neti, neti -- not this, not this), etc. Personally, I never found these very helpful in dealing with the specifics of daily life, but very helpful for inspiration to meditate, which is not a small thing at all.

Katie's work in "Loving What Is" is impressive, because she boils it down to a sequence of a few practical questions that can be applied to any situation in daily life, including very difficult challenging ones. No matter what the problem is, it always comes back to identifying a contracted thought process in the observer that is revealed for what it is, and then it dissolves. So it is intellectual, in that the inquiry is via the mind. But the inner observer of the revealed dysfunction ("story") is ultimately what dissolves the contraction, kind of the way we do when there is a big disruptive knot in deep meditation that we rest on with our awareness and watch dissolve. That sort of benign observation is a big part of self-inquiry. So, yes, jnana is mainly about the processes of the mind rather than intellectual analysis. That is absolutely correct. As soon as we turn it over to western-style intellectual analysis, the whole thing is lost in building huge castles in the air. That is not jnana, though many think it is.

Just to make it interesting, there is desire involved in the self-inquiry process also. This is a bhakti component. It is touched on in the lessons, here: http://www.aypsite.org/185.html If we long deeply for answers to our inquiries, this does facilitate the process -- there is the element of surrender involved in self-inquiry. That is a quality of the witness also.

I avoided diving headlong into self-inquiry when writing the original AYP lessons for the reasons mentioned in the Q&A above. It is a really complex subject, and very dependent on the presence of the witness. But maybe over the next year it can be gradually developed into something simple and practical that can be useful to anyone who is meditating and having some inner silence coming up. I would certainly like to do that. It is much needed. In the meantime, there are the other resources, and whatever else we can cook up here. And, of course, the natural self-inquiry we gain with the rise of inner silence. That is why I say, "Between your meditations go out and live life fully, and pay attention!"

If anyone knows of additional approaches to self-inquiry, please do share them. I view this as a long term boiling-down process on this end -- an ongoing inquiry! :-)

The guru is in you.

2006/03/25 08:02:16
Jnana Yoga/Self-Inquiry - Advaita (Non-Duality)
http://www.aypsite.org/forum/topic.asp?TOPIC_ID=968&REPLY_ID=5065&whichpage=-1
Self-Inquiry -- A Practice Between our Meditations

Hi Sparkle:

We are treading into fuzzy territories of yoga here. Jnana, bhakti and karma yogas have so much overlap, and in some ways could be considered as one. That is why this particular forum was originally set up to cover all three. I knew we'd get to it sooner or later. All three of these can be used "between the meditations."

In practical application, what we are talking about is cultivating methods/attitudes of self-inquiry, devotion, and service to others. All of these are highly dependent on the presence of the witness. Without the witness, it is just more "gee whiz" mind and heart games. AYP is not about that, though it sure does sell well in the mainstream.

My limited understanding of vipassana is that it is a sitting practice. Is there a walking around version? If so, then maybe there is some further overlap there, because the success of all these methods depends on the presence of the witness. In AYP, we do that in deep meditation, and then stabilize it in activity. In Buddhism, they do "mindfulness," a different kind of practice. I don't think that is what I am suggesting for AYP -- we have the witness already from deep meditation. It is mindfulness. I think we are looking for elements of practice that are much easier to latch on to in daily life. Specific techniques, you know, like we have been doing so far. This may or may not work when addressed in daily living. It is one thing to sit and do a specific practice for 20-30 minutes. We know that works. But when we are at work or walking down the street, doing other things, it is a different matter.

One thing I am against is turning us into highly disciplined all day long "practice robots" like we see in some of the European systems of the past century. Not only does that not work, it is not much fun either. I strongly believe that whatever we do ought to be a joy in daily life. Meditating and then going out to live life fully certainly accomplishes that. Maybe in the end the conclusion will be, "If it ain't broke, don't fix it." That is why this is only an inquiry, for now.

Meanwhile, in the AYP lessons there are discussions on all of these branches of yoga and their role as they relate to progress in cultivating inner silence, ecstatic conductivity, the joining of these two, and eventual endless outpouring of divine love. This evolution includes within it the natural development of all the elements of yoga we are looking at here -- self-inquiry, devotion and service.

The guru is in you.

2006/03/26 01:18:33

Jnana Yoga/Self-Inquiry - Advaita (Non-Duality)
http://www.aypsite.org/forum/topic.asp?TOPIC_ID=968&REPLY_ID=5127&whichpage=-1
Self-Inquiry -- A Practice Between our Meditations

Hi Anthem:

If it resonates in stillness, it will not be a castle in the air. That is the appeal that Tolle or any teacher has -- the extent to which their teachings resonate in stillness. In his case, it is a huge audience. So he must be doing something right. But for practice-oriented yogis and yoginis there is sometimes that feeling about unclear guidelines that Shanti described.

I agree with you that multiple approaches will bring the best results, and that we should go with what resonates for us always.

Times have changed a lot in that respect. It used to be that if you signed on with a tradition, you were literally banned from studying anything else. Of course the black market for eclectic spiritual knowledge thrived anyway. What is denied is sought all the more!

The guru is in you.

2006/03/26 01:28:29
Jnana Yoga/Self-Inquiry - Advaita (Non-Duality)
http://www.aypsite.org/forum/topic.asp?TOPIC_ID=968&REPLY_ID=5128&whichpage=-1
Self-Inquiry -- A Practice Between our Meditations

Hi Jim:

I agree that each will find a different manifestion of the characteristics of yoga, particularly bhakti, jnana and karma, as these are intertwined with lifestyle. The question is how to offer simple guidelines that will both recognize this diversity of individual natures and offer clear pathways of practice at the same time.

I guess my job is to identify the clear pathways, and then individuals will pick and choose according to their nature. In fact, that has been going on in AYP from the beginning, hasn't it? It works for me. :-)

The guru is in you

2006/03/26 12:59:07
Jnana Yoga/Self-Inquiry - Advaita (Non-Duality)
http://www.aypsite.org/forum/topic.asp?TOPIC_ID=968&REPLY_ID=5160&whichpage=-1
Self-Inquiry -- A Practice Between our Meditations

Hi Satyan:

Bhakti is always a stimulus to other actions in yoga, because all the limbs of yoga are connected within us. It is the ultimate stimulator of practices -- it is our desire for freedom manifesting. That is why it is covered first in the AYP lessons, and developed further along the way.

Which practices your bhakti will lead you to is a matter of your personal style. If you are inclined to worship, which is regarded by many as a bhakti-only path, then that is a style thing. On the other hand, don't be surprised if you wake up in the middle of the night doing an asana, or advanced pranayama technique. Reading the life of Ramakrishna (the ultimate bhakti yogi) is very instructive on things like this.

In AYP, we try and create a template of reliable practices that will address the primary aspects of the process of human spiritual transformation, with deep meditation being the central practice after spiritual desire (bhakti) arises, because the cultivation of inner silence is the primary mover of enlightenment. At least that is my opinion. Can this be done with bhakti/devotion only? Sure, but the odds of it are less than when using a broad systematic approach utilizing our bhakti plus a full tool kit of time-tested methods.

As for the role of self-inquiry in all of this, I am sure it can be done with bhakti and self-inquiry only. I just don't have any examples to give you to support that opinion. In fact, traditionalists would argue that bhakti and jnana are incompatible. That is sectarian bickering, of course, because bhakti and jnana are two sides of the same coin, and we are that coin!

On silence, a fellow came to my email a month or so ago who felt like he had a lot of resident inner silence, and ecstatic energy moving besides. Indeed, he seemed to. His conclusion was that he did not need to do sitting practices at all. Instead, he was determined to stop eating, because he had read somewhere that enlightened sages can live on sunlight alone. He had lost a lot of weight and was betting on achieved his goal of living on sunlight before he expired. I did my best to talk him out of that and into taking a more centered course of sitting practices and going out and living life to the fullest to stabilize and expand on his inner silence and ecstatic conductivity.

The point is, just because we feel some inner silence, we do not have a blank check to ignore sitting practices and be a success in any other practice we choose, including self-inquiry. Better I think than we keep cultivating our inner silence to such a level that all the rest will happen automatically. I think it is the closest we can come to a guanrantee of success in yoga. Then if we want to play around with self-inquiry (or living on sunlight), any success we have with those things will be the icing on the cake. Of course, the prerequisite for anything we do in yoga is <u>desire</u>, and that is where bhakti comes in.

Note: One key word I have left out of the self-inquiry discussion so far, and I don't think anyone else has mentioned it yet either, is "discrimination." When we talk about jnana and self-inquiry, what we are really talking about is <u>choosing</u> particular inquiries and organic responses deep within us, as opposed to <u>analyzing</u> them in thought. So, as our inner silence provides an infinite screen of stillness, we then are in a position to choose according to resonance in stillness. External analysis is a choosing also, but not necessarily in the direction we want to go for maximum progress in yoga.

So, let's throw discrimination/choosing into the mix here and see what comes out. Gee, sounds like samyama. Well, we'll save the discussion on the relationship between samyama and self-inquiry for another time. :-)

The guru is in you.

2006/03/27 10:28:11

Jnana Yoga/Self-Inquiry - Advaita (Non-Duality)
http://www.aypsite.org/forum/topic.asp?TOPIC_ID=968&REPLY_ID=5214&whichpage=-1
Self-Inquiry -- A Practice Between our Meditations

Hi Sean and Katrine:

All I can say is, Wow! Wonderful perspectives. And you have both confirmed that it was the right thing not to tackle self-inquiry in the original AYP lessons.

The basics of cultivating inner silence and ecstatic conductivity are so much more fundamental. Once that is going on, then we can use them in self-inquiry and other real life oriented (between the meditations) yoga methods.

Yes, Sean, those are all self-inquiry methods, and Katrine has really refined the focus on what is involved. If we have some inner presence of witness, then these methods work. And if we do not, it is problematic.

Maybe self-inquiry is best thought of as being like a higher gear in a car, or an afterburner in a jet. Once we reach a certain velocity (with inner silence) then the higher gear or afterburner will add a lot. But before then, it will not work so well. Of course it never hurts to try, and we should, as long as we do not spend years in a technique that is not working for us because we have not cultivated sufficient inner silence first. Self-inquiry, when working, is a confirmation of our inner condition. If it is not working, that is a strong signal to get on that twice-daily deep meditation seat.

Now, how to simplify all this even more? As mentioned, I'd like to condense it into a 100 page book that anyone can use after getting settled into a stable deep meditation routine. I think we have taken a few steps in that direction already.

Thank you, Shanti, for inspiring this "between the meditations" topic. We've all got an oar in the water, and the boat is moving. :-)

The guru is in you.

2006/03/27 15:28:19
Jnana Yoga/Self-Inquiry - Advaita (Non-Duality)
http://www.aypsite.org/forum/topic.asp?TOPIC_ID=968&REPLY_ID=5232&whichpage=-1
Self-Inquiry -- A Practice Between our Meditations

Hi Lili:

Nice to see you again. Yes, creating some separate topics for the different methods may be a good approach, as each method is a world in itself. I don't know how deep we will end up going into each method. It is up to all of you. I have been looking to light this one off for some time, as I know everyone is interested in "what more" can be done during the day. Hopefully, we can put a good foundation under it -- inner silence. Then it will be okay, and all of these methods will be at their best.

Anyone wishing to start new topics on various approaches involving discrimination and the intellect (jnana), feel free. Bhakti and karma yoga topics are good too -- there is plenty of overlap.

The guru is in you.

2006/03/28 09:51:41
Jnana Yoga/Self-Inquiry - Advaita (Non-Duality)
http://www.aypsite.org/forum/topic.asp?TOPIC_ID=968&REPLY_ID=5273&whichpage=-1
Self-Inquiry -- A Practice Between our Meditations

Hi Near:

The difference between this discussion and others in AYP is that we are investigating various approaches to self-inquiry with the aim of distilling out a simple and practical approach that will be useful for people who are already practicing AYP deep meditation. So, in that sense, your concern is being addressed. The systems we look at here are not being endorsed necessarily, only examined for their value. In the end, I hope something useful will come out of it. In the meantime, everyone will no doubt develop their own opinions about self-inquiry, which is very good too. AYP does not dictate any particular style for our daily living. These approaches are for daily living, so variations in style are to be expected.

Whichever way it goes, as inner silence rises, most of us are inclined to do something useful with it. Samyama is for that. And so is self-inquiry.

I have seen cases like Sean mentioned, in cloistered meditative environments, where meditators with lots of inner silence could not handle the fact that the salt shaker had been moved to the wrong end of the table. That is a very limited and conditioned enlightenment. We want to take our inner silence and develop it into unconditional enlightenment. That means getting involved in life. That is why I say go out and engage after meditation, and pay attention (inquire). Whether we are using other systematic approaches to living or not, this alone will produce an integration of inner silence into our life. And also ecstatic conductivity, when it rises -- there are interesting new perspectives on the relationship of ecstatic conductivity and inner silence in activity in the new AYP Spinal Breathing book coming out in a few weeks -- explaining much better what we mean by "stillness in action."

The guru is in you.

2006/04/18 10:29:00
Jnana Yoga/Self-Inquiry - Advaita (Non-Duality)
http://www.aypsite.org/forum/topic.asp?TOPIC_ID=968&REPLY_ID=6107&whichpage=-1
Self-Inquiry -- A Practice Between our Meditations

Hi Ether:

I believe we all have "errant thought or perception patterns" and one of the primary effects of yoga is the dissolving of these. Inner silence via deep meditation will do much of the job on its own, but we can certainly add to our progress by choosing when we can, which is also a function of inner silence, our ability to witness how we relate to our thoughts and feelings, and the world around us.

The primary feedback we can use in this is how we feel. If we feel bad (i.e., "suffering"), then it is a signal of an errant pattern of thought or perception. If we are making others feel bad, it is the same thing, except we might not notice as easily -- an errant perception for sure. To get around this we can develop the ability to see the world through the eyes of others as well as through our own eyes. This too is a function of inner silence -- the witness. It always comes back to that.

In any case, once we can see our suffering, and the suffering of others (which is also ours), we are in a position to question the thoughts and perceptions that have created that suffering. Life is not inherently suffering. It just is. It is we who do the coloring of it.

Self-inquiry asks us to notice our thoughts and feelings, and question their validity when they create suffering. We can ask ourselves if we need a specific thought that is creating suffering, is it true, and what would we be like without that thought? Then we can turn the thought around and look at it 180 degress the opposite, like a mirror on ourselves instead of focused on the other. This is the Katie approach (in her book -- "Loving What Is"), which works like a razor. It is event-specific and therefore practical in the now. Is this the kind of mechanism you use, Ether?

Once we have isolated a thought or perception that brings suffering and sincerely questioned its validity, we can then rest our attention on it, and it will tend to dissolve much the way knots dissolve in meditation when we allow our attention to rest on them when they dominate our session to the extent we are not able to pick up the mantra easily. Like that, errant thoughts and perceptions can dominate the clarity of our life experience at times. And, like that, they can be dissolved once they have been recognized for what they are -- isolated and errant, outside the sphere of who we really are.

Of course, this is a simplification of a very complex dynamic. The errant thought and perception patterns are seemingly endless streams rooted in deep traumas of the past. We don't have to ferret out what all these roots are, thank goodness. But we should recognize that self-inquiry is a long term cultivation of habit in the way we look at ourselves and the world around us, so as to gradually dissipate the energies that are "errant." The more inner silence we have, the easier this will be, and the more often we will be having those "Ah Ha!" type releases. We do not have to travel down the same errant roads over and over again as we have in the past. We do have the option to choose something more -- a road of happiness for ourselves and those around us.

As soon as our inner silence affords us the growing discrimination that comes with the rise of the witness, we can take advantage of it. That too is a choice we can make -- to use the witness. It is the big one that changes everything. A sea change in our perception of ourselves and everything around us. Once that happens, self-inquiry becomes pretty much a cake walk, like washing the dishes and taking out the trash. We realize we don't have to be hanging on to the trash anymore -- our ego-driven errant thought and perception patterns. We just let them go in each moment, and find that right underneath them we are an endless sea of ecstatic bliss. In time, we are easily dissolving the errant stuff like patches of brown foam floating on our infinite crystal clear sea.

This is self-inquiry, karma yoga, and bhakti all rolled into one. And thank goodness for inner silence! :-)

The guru is in you.

2006/05/05 15:42:51
Jnana Yoga/Self-Inquiry - Advaita (Non-Duality)
http://www.aypsite.org/forum/topic.asp?TOPIC_ID=968&REPLY_ID=6631&whichpage=-1
Self-Inquiry -- A Practice Between our Meditations

quote:
───────
Shanti wrote: These days, as soon as I realize I am thinking, I bring my mind back to where I am.. so if I am driving.. I watch the cars, the tree, listen to the music on the radio ... Just like I do in my meditation.. as soon as I realize I am off the mantra, I go back to the mantra.. so too during the day.. as soon as I realize I am off on one of my thought trips.. I come back to what I am doing.

───────

Hi Shanti:

You are on to something important there. The gentle persuasion of attention over thoughts. It is a choice we can make. No sledge-hammer needed. Only some inner silence and an easy intention. In time it becomes a habit we do not even think about. Keep up the good work! :-)

The guru is in you.

2006/06/06 10:54:01
Jnana Yoga/Self-Inquiry - Advaita (Non-Duality)
http://www.aypsite.org/forum/topic.asp?TOPIC_ID=968&REPLY_ID=7786&whichpage=-1
Self-Inquiry -- A Practice Between our Meditations

Hi Sadhak:

Yes, for many, self-inquiry is a mind swamp full of mosquitoes, quicksand and alligators. No place to stand except on egoic suppositions, which will take us on wild goose chases through the swamp every time.

Real self-inquiry is beyond all that. It rests in our silence, which means the entire process depends on something that came before, another method, deep meditation, which brings about the rise of the witness. That is the thing, you know. Either that, or the witness is present already (via previous efforts), a la Tolle, Katie and others who wake up one day like that, and they tell us all about how to take it from there, from their waking-up point. Well, fine, but from where is that?! So we end up genuflecting at the altar of their mysterious condition -- a condition we could easily cultivate for ourselves, if only we knew how. Meditate!

Just as you say, without inner silence it is pretty fuzzy. But look what happens with some simple inner silence creeping up. Shanti manages a stage production without even trying. Bravo! Stillness in action! Encore!

So what do we need self-inquiry for? Well, for the same reason we need bhakti. These things will move us forward if taken to our deepest levels in stillness. Besides making the day (between the meditations) much more interesting, these processes give us understanding and perspective on the gift within us. More than that -- they give us *energetic stillness*, alive and moving outward from us into the world. There is no doubt we can make better use of our stillness if we learn a few good methods (or non-methods), and self-inquiry is about that.

Stillness blends with mind, emotions and ecstasy, and that is the process of enlightenment going forward. It is an automatic process. There is little we have to do but let go into what we are, once we experience that we are That ... all the strategies are for That. Enter Tolle, Katie, Ramana Maharishi, et al. Until then, it is all a big fuzz, a mind swamp. Inner silence is our boat. Let's arrange for the boat before we go too far into the swamp. It is common sense... :-)

The guru is in you.

2006/06/06 13:08:54
Jnana Yoga/Self-Inquiry - Advaita (Non-Duality)
http://www.aypsite.org/forum/topic.asp?TOPIC_ID=968&REPLY_ID=7789&whichpage=-1
Self-Inquiry -- A Practice Between our Meditations
Etherfish said: "So I decided to put ALL my energy into doing what I'm doing at the moment instead of splitting some of it off on worrying. I decided I don't care if it all goes wrong. It had an interesting outcome. I found I was actually doing better than before because the worrying was taking some of my energy."

Hi Etherfish:

You are absolutely right. Self-inquiry is about choice. And so is bhakti/karma yoga, which you are also touching on there.

Traditionally, jnana yoga/self-inquiry is called the "path of discrimination."

But on what basis are we choosing? Knowing that rational thinking is a minefield, it would seem that choosing the path of least complication, least worry and angst, would the most rational (!) way. At least until our deepest hot buttons get pushed, and then we are back into the mire.

What we need is that which is beyond all thinking, inner silence. That is the table upon which everything else in us rests, hot buttons and all. Once we know we are the table (a permanent state of being), it is much easier to move the stuff around on the table to suit the need of the moment, or clear it all off the table at will. It is our choice.

Become inner silence and the choices become easy -- self-inquiry becomes easy. Everything we do before that is a temporary solution -- a negotiation of thinking with thinking.

There is no negotiation between the witness and thinking. The witness permeates thinking and thinking (and all resulting action) dissolve into pure divine purpose. Then there can be lots of thinking and action coming through us as the divine flow pours out. And all we do is watch, in a continual state of ecstatic bliss. That is what we are...

The guru is in you.

2006/11/19 10:14:42
Jnana Yoga/Self-Inquiry - Advaita (Non-Duality)
http://www.aypsite.org/forum/topic.asp?TOPIC_ID=1136&REPLY_ID=13467&whichpage=-1
Detachment (vairagaya)

Hi Doc:

I believe "witnessing" as stand-alone practice tends to be overrated, especially as a first stage approach where we have little more to work with than the intellect and ego consciousness. It is a tough road to hoe from there with no other methods in hand. But it can be done if enough bhakti is present. Ask any dedicated Buddhist.

If we are using additional practices such as deep meditation and samyama to cultivate inner silence directly, then witnessing arises naturally along the way, and we can do much with it then. That kind of doing will be with less attachment, the essence of "dispassion," which is at the heart of progressive karma and jnana yoga. The interesting thing about these yogas, when undertaken propitiously, is that they are beyond duality, even though they are in the field of doing. This is possible only when the witness is already present, previously cultivated as "effect." Only then can the witness become a "cause" in our further development. Before then it is much like pushing on a string.

Of course, those born with a degree of witness consciousness already present have a "leg up." The rest of us have to develop it. Those who are born with, or have reached a high level of witness consciousness early on in life ("old souls"), tend to teach from that level, and then many begin to regard witnessing practice as the primary path to enlightenment. Well, it is a stepping stone for sure, but not a very good place to start for most of us. Better to reduce duality (bring up the witness) by more direct means before diving into the methods of non-duality. Keeping the horse in front of the cart, so to speak.

Thanks for your great perspectives, Doc and All. Very stimulating! :-)

The guru is in you.

2007/03/25 11:26:59
Jnana Yoga/Self-Inquiry - Advaita (Non-Duality)
http://www.aypsite.org/forum/topic.asp?TOPIC_ID=2315&REPLY_ID=19330&whichpage=-1
Yogani's Dual/Non-Dual Distinction

Hi All:

To help clarify, consider a seed becoming a flower.

Is a seed a flower? Can it become a flower instantly? In potential, the seed is everything the flower is. But it is a process for the seed to become the flower -- sprout, leaves, stalk, bud, blossoming, and finally ... flower! The process can be facilitated with good fertilizer and water -- not too much and not too little. Then the flower will come. Near its end the seed can proclaim, "I am the flower!" And, poof! It can be imagined to be an instant transformation. But was it really? No. It took some time. Nature operates that way on the physical plane. Only in vain can natural process be denied, which is very frustrating. So forget all that "instant" nonsense, and let the process happen naturally. Give the poor seed a break, and have some fun along the way. Each stage is a blooming. It is divine joy in motion. :-)

In AYP we attend to the process by facilitating with practices, and taking it out into our activity every day without thinking about it too much. We just go within and then come out and do. It is daily union by degrees, which is yoga. If our methods are good, the becoming happens. But any appearance of "instant" is illusion. Our neurobiology doesn't operate instantly, and neither will our emerging enlightenment, which is entirely dependent on our nervous sytem.

So, "crossing over" is the process we are all engaged in as we practice. Better to engage in effective methods than labor over the process itself. The process is "under the hood."

Dual and non-dual are seed and flower. It is not black and white. The journey is through much overlap and blending -- a crossing over through many shades of gray. In the end, the seed is burnt and we are the eternal flower.

It is not complicated. Natural process does not need our supervision. Only the right amount fertilizer and water. The rest will take care of itself.

Self-inquiry is part of this. But like all of our practices beyond deep meditation, it only offers significant help when we have reached a certain stage of purification and opening. Before that, self-inquiry is building castles in the air and like pushing on a string, which many who pursue self-inquiry prematurely have found. When it is time for non-dual self-inquiry, it will happen all by itself, and few pointers will be necessary. You can be sure that if it is a big deal, it is too soon, and it will be an unnecessary distraction.

Self-inquiry will happen naturally as inner silence and ecstatic conductivity rise. Then the heart and mind will be infused with the necessary prerequisites, and it will happen. First things first.

The guru is in you.

2007/03/25 16:17:53
Jnana Yoga/Self-Inquiry - Advaita (Non-Duality)
http://www.aypsite.org/forum/topic.asp?TOPIC_ID=2315&REPLY_ID=19344&whichpage=-1
Yogani's Dual/Non-Dual Distinction

quote:
_____
Originally posted by Jim and His Karma

Do you agree with the classic view that enlightenment is an experience of non-dualism (i.e. non-dualism is how it really is)? In other words, when you characterize AYP as a dualistic system, is it correct to say it's dualistic as an APPROACH, rather than as an ultimate understanding of the universe?
_____

Hi Jim:

Yes, I agree that the destination is non-dual. But I do not agree with the over-simplified "quantum leap" way in which it is often presented. Neither do I agree that non-dualism is a static transcendental condition. That view discounts the natural processes of evolution occurring in creation, including those processes that deliver the realization of non-duality.

I see "non-dual" as a relative term. While it represents undifferentiated oneness beyond all action, it also represents stillness (oneness) in action. That's why in AYP we do our practices and then go out and live our life in a normal way. If we do that, then the rest will happen naturally.

And therein lies both the simplicity and the mystery of non-dual duality. :-)

The guru is in you.

2007/04/26 00:41:58
Jnana Yoga/Self-Inquiry - Advaita (Non-Duality)
http://www.aypsite.org/forum/topic.asp?TOPIC_ID=2477&REPLY_ID=21000&whichpage=-1
radical no holds barred self enquiry

Hi Eddy:

There is nothing wrong with wanting to get on with it. No argument there. That is bhakti, which is the underlying cause of self inquiry, and of all spiritual practice. But if we want progress, we have to be smart about it. There is much more going on than meets the eye.

Self-pacing is not something we do because anything is feared or imagined. We don't do it because someone says we are supposed to, or because it is fashionable. We do it when our rate of inner purification is slowing our progress, while making us pretty uncomfortable and/or unhealthy at the same time. It is a very common problem that all serious aspirants run into at one time or other on the path. Self-pacing is a practical measure that speeds our progress -- not slowing it down.

In theory we could drive from New York to Los Angeles in about 30 hours at 100 miles per hour. Maybe someone has done it. The mythological Nisagadatta/Ramana of the highways! But more than likely anyone who tries that will get tickets (delays), end up in jail (longer delay), or have a really bad crash (maybe not get there at all).

The smart driver knows that sometimes 100 mph will work (in the lonely desert), other times 65 mph will work (thank you interstate highway system), and other times only 25 mph will work (oops, rush hour in the city). It all depends on the conditions.

Yoga is like that. It is about reacting to what is going on within us as we apply powerful spiritual practices that purify and open us from within. Cause and effect. That is the real world of our evolving neurobiology. It can be done by most anyone, but not very well by those who choose to ignore the mechanics involved.

Do you think the Wright Brothers would have gotten off the ground if they had ignored the aerodynamic principles they were attempting to harness? Remember the guy with the feathers glued to his arms jumping off the cliff? We learn from our mistakes. Well, maybe he didn't, but the rest of us did.

The best person to compare yourself to on the path is yourself, over weeks, months and years. There isn't anything wrong with being inspired by the great ones. But we have to deal with where we are, not with where we imagine someone else was or is. Enlightenment is a state of being, based on a cultivated inner receptivity. It takes whatever it takes for as long as it takes (Alan's point). That is an attitude that will lead to real and lasting results. It has been the attitude of all saints and sages, including the ones you mentioned.

"Magic bullet" instant enlightenment (as in, "You are there already!") is a flawed approach for the vast majority of people, without other methods being employed. Stand-alone self inquiry often will lead to time-wasting fantasies and/or ogling around those who are on the mountain top (or claim to be). Other times it can lead to excess purification causing long delays, because the process of purification is being ignored. To be sure, the shortest distance between two points is a straight line, but we have to walk that line. The line is our own nervous system, and we should come to understand its transformative powers and limitations well. Then we can travel it.

Spiritual transformation is not an instant event. It only may seem like it is sometimes. If we are seduced by an inner experience, we can fall into an ongoing non-dual rationalization or energy obsession. This can hold us back, as we favor our illusion of attainment over real practice. That is why in AYP we favor our practices over our experiences. Then we will have constantly expanding results. The real signal of enlightenment is the emergence of unending loving service to others. Odd as it may seem, this is the only unmistakable manifestation of enlightenment. Actions over time speak much louder than words.

Self inquiry can be very valuable if it is engaged in with the rise of our inner silence. More than a few around here are doing that. It is beautiful to observe, like watching butterflies emerging. This is stillness in action. It gets back to daily deep meditation and the additional methods for moving stillness out into everyday living. Self inquiry is one of those methods. Only when we allow stillness to move as it must will we be going beyond all movement to non-duality. It is the paradox of enlightenment.

It is great to see more young folks here in the forums these days. The future belongs to the young, just as it once belonged to we who are older now. Keep banging on the door. Do it wisely, and pass on what you learn in this life so the coming generations will benefit. We are benefiting today because those who came before remembered to pass on their well-earned knowledge.

Looking forward to your report three years from now. Wishing you good driving between now and then. Enjoy the ride! :-)

The guru is in you.

PS: Rumi said, "I have lived on the lip of insanity, wanting to know reasons. Knocking on a door. It opens. I have been knocking from the inside!"

2007/04/26 14:47:10
Jnana Yoga/Self-Inquiry - Advaita (Non-Duality)
http://www.aypsite.org/forum/topic.asp?TOPIC_ID=2477&REPLY_ID=21047&whichpage=-1
radical no holds barred self enquiry

quote:
_____
Originally posted by Scott

Self pacing applies to AYP style meditation and practices, not to Ramana style self enquiry practice. The more self enquiry you do, the better. My energy problems have actually totally disappeared due to taking on this type of practice.

These are good instructions:
http://uarelove1.tripod.com/imposter7.htm
_____

Hi Scott:

Interesting perspective and experience.

The question that is at the center of all this is:

Does self inquiry cultivate inner silence, or does inner silence cultivate self inquiry?

As you know, I lean toward the inner silence cultivating self inquiry scenario, and that is why we emphasize simple daily deep meditation around here. Self inquiry emerges pretty naturally that way over time, and we can see evidence of it in many meditators.

On the other hand, the non-dualists emphasize self inquiry as a starting point, an ending point, and the only point. While it can be stimulating and inspiring because it is philosophically sound, I have not seen any evidence that it actually works in practice as a starting point and sole ongoing practice for large numbers of people.

In fact, I don't know of any teacher who practiced strict self inquiry as their primary path from the beginning. There may an exception or two -- the born enlightened, which isn't you or me, or even Buddha or Jesus. Yet, self inquiry is always presented as the logical thing (and only thing) for everyone to be doing from the beginning, usually from the perspective of a teacher who has umpteen years of previous multi-faceted practice and experience under their belt. While infinitely altruistic, it does not make practical sense.

It always seemed odd to me that someone skilled in the high-wire act would ask beginners to start way up near the top of the tent. Is there any solid evidence that this really works? Any such evidence would have to be over years of experience by numbers of people. It isn't going to be sufficient to say, "I have been doing this for a few weeks or months, and it works." It is encouraging, but not conclusive. It is not sufficient to make conclusions that way about any practice, including deep meditation. The proof of the pudding is in the eating by many, and that eating takes time.

I regard this to be a very important discussion, because it involves reconciling self inquiry with all other yoga practices. It is something which must be done. Not to do so leaves yoga in a state of separation. And as we know, separation is not yoga.

Interestingly, hardcore forms of self inquiry involve a complete denial of manifest existence, which is non-duality built on separation. Ironic, isn't it?

Case in point: Nisargatta's talks shortly before his death read like little more than rationalizations -- mental gymnastics:
"I am dying, but nothing is here so I don't care."

Is pure self inquiry pure rationalization without engagement of any kind? It seems cold and loveless, doesn't it? The witness is about more than that. Stillness is always longing to move as outpouring divine love. Otherwise, absolutely nothing would be here. In our essential nature, we are that also. Can true enlightenment be based on denial? When does denial cease to be a mind game?

None of this is to deny the non-dual (unified) nature of existence, or the role of self inquiry on the path. But it has to be real, not only for the sage, but for the aspirant, and consistent with the rest of yoga. Otherwise, it doesn't hold up.

The guru is in you.

2007/04/26 15:20:22
Jnana Yoga/Self-Inquiry - Advaita (Non-Duality)
http://www.aypsite.org/forum/topic.asp?TOPIC_ID=2477&REPLY_ID=21050&whichpage=-1
radical no holds barred self enquiry

quote:
_____
Originally posted by Scott

The question is: does self enquiry awaken too much energy at once? I suppose someone would have to devote their entire day to the practice to find out. I have in the past, but back then the kundalini wasn't awakened for me, so it'd be difficult to say for sure. I don't have time to do it these days.
_____

Hi Scott:

See this topic: http://www.aypsite.org/forum/topic.asp?TOPIC_ID=2202

The person in question in that topic is still having challenges two months later, following an Adyashanti (leading non-dualist) retreat. It may have also been other factors on the retreat, but the experience was handled strictly from a self inquiry perspective while there, which only aggravated what was already a major overload. She has been self-pacing ever since.

There have been other non-dualist types having problems in my email here. The causes of energy difficulties are often rooted in individual tendencies in relation to practices undertaken. The jury is still out on whether self inquiry is a remedy or a cause in these cases -- maybe it can be either, like spinal breathing can be. I'm glad self inquiry has been of some help to you. We'd like to get more data points on that over time.

Human spiritual transformation is ultimately the same neurobiological process no matter who is doing it, how or where. It is the same nervous system we are working with in every case. Regardless of the method, some management is going to be necessary for every aspirant, depending on individual tendencies in practice. No shortcuts ... just optimizing the process for speed and safety through self-directed practice.

The guru is in you.

2007/04/27 10:15:04
Jnana Yoga/Self-Inquiry - Advaita (Non-Duality)
http://www.aypsite.org/forum/topic.asp?TOPIC_ID=2477&REPLY_ID=21070&whichpage=-1
radical no holds barred self enquiry

Hi Mike:

Well, you know, we are all among friends, and working with the same inherent capabilities of the human nervous system.

We have far more in common than culture and creed often dictate. Differences are to be honored, of course. Each of us chooses our own path. Yet, artificial human barriers must be crossed if we are to have a chance of finding the whole truth. It is human nature to make such explorations, and this hunger for truth has been the genesis of all the great traditions. Traveling the dusty corridors of time, the traditions may stray from their own roots, so constant inquiry and rediscovery are necessary to keep knowledge fresh and flourishing in the present.

Einstein, when asked in later life why his greatest discoveries were mainly in his youth, said: "Discovery comes from defying authority. The reward for discovery is to become an authority, and that is the end of discovery."

If AYP is a sect, it is a sect of evolving applied knowledge. A secular sect. This may shake a few boundaries, because the evolution of applied integrated knowledge is ever-expanding. But there is nothing to worry about. It is ourselves we are discovering, and we will always be here, so nothing is lost.

In the case of non-dual inquiry, if it has apparent inconsistencies in its application (such as exclusivity), it should be questioned, not to undermine what is valid, but to get at the truth. No applied knowledge should be immune from such scrutiny. It is about understanding cause and effect, and integrating applied knowledge to optimize both.

No one gets to stand on their laurels with this approach, and that is a good thing. Hopefully any discoveries we make here will not cripple us by making us an "authority." I am not for that. This is why it is important to keep bringing in new blood and fresh points of view. It keeps us all on our toes.

The guru is in you.

PS: Scott, "enquiry" and "inquiry" mean the same thing (the latter is twice as common in Google). I use the "inquiry" spelling because of the "in." :-)

2007/04/27 16:45:57
Jnana Yoga/Self-Inquiry - Advaita (Non-Duality)
http://www.aypsite.org/forum/topic.asp?TOPIC_ID=2477&REPLY_ID=21109&whichpage=-1
radical no holds barred self enquiry

Hi David:

Obviously, those who defy authority for the sake of defying authority aren't going to progess much more than those who uphold authority for the sake of upholding authority. Both are out on the edges and can't see the middle.

In Einstein's case, he was considered a misfit and a never-do-well, flunked math (famously now) and was kicked out of school. When he put together the theories of relativity, he was working as a bureaucrat in the Swiss patent office. No doubt he was a creative genius all along, but his disregard for authority was obviously going on for a long time too. Or maybe he just didn't care what people thought. Is that defying authority? It is said he didn't even speak as a child until much later than usual.

The relevance of his idea on authority usurping creativity, as used here, doesn't have much to do with your well-stated argument about the abuses. Rather, it is about how when new innovations happen and are finally accepted (usually after a struggle), they then become the status quo, and the window for further new innovations looking beyond the original one tends to close. Einstein felt this was true of him personally, and it is obviously true of many institutions as well. As something or someone becomes prominent, a kind of paralysis creeps in. Maybe it is like an actor being type cast.

It is very difficult to change what has been established in the public mind, unless an environment fostering constant innovation can be established and sustained. In that case, the status quo can be constant innovation. That is the hope for this AYP community.

Einstein became the icon of a certain scientific ideology (mythologized!), and he was not able to go much beyond it. When quantum physics came along, introducing probabilities into the exploration of the inner energy realms, Einstein dismissed it out of hand by saying (famously again), "God does not play dice." He was wrong, and that is where the forward march of physics into the subtle realms started to leave him behind.

The point being that if knowledge is being calcified by the status quo (or for any other reason), we'd better be prepared challenge that if we want to advance. That is why I used the quote.

It has certainly been true in spiritual circles, where the problems have been much more severe, because so few have come along in history with innovations. The traditions have been bastions of authority with very few coming along with new approaches to aid spiritual progress. Those who did were treatly very unkindly, like crucified or burned at the stake. Come to think of it, some forward-leaning scientists were burned at the stake too. Fortunately, times have changed, in many places anyhow.

Meanwhile, the wheels of progress just keep turning, because human beings simply must know the truth about themselves and everything else. The good news is that we can not only know the truth, we can live it too.

The guru is in you.

2007/05/01 13:45:54
Jnana Yoga/Self-Inquiry - Advaita (Non-Duality)
http://www.aypsite.org/forum/topic.asp?TOPIC_ID=2498&REPLY_ID=21251&whichpage=-1
self enquiry : positive and negative

Hi Eddy:

Not to sound like a broken record (or coffee perculator :-)), but consider just moving step-by-step toward a good balance between practices, daily acitivity and sleep at night, and all will be well. This is what the AYP lessons are about, assuming they are taken in order.

If there are shortcuts, you can be sure they have been considered long ago, and, if practical, are included already. Anything beyond balanced self-paced practice is likely to be "cruising for a bruising." This is as true for self inquiry as for any other practice.

Another way we describe it in AYP is to say that we move past the beginning "clunky stage" to a stable daily practice we can do (and gradually build on) long term. The results come with long term practice, and, for that, establishing and sustaining stable daily practice is essential.

Practice wisely, and enjoy!

The guru is in you.

2007/11/19 09:59:33
Jnana Yoga/Self-Inquiry - Advaita (Non-Duality)
http://www.aypsite.org/forum/topic.asp?TOPIC_ID=3148&REPLY_ID=27124&whichpage=-1
Non-duality - multiplicity

Hi EMC:

Scenery is scenery, but our relationship to it is different in practices than in regular daily activity.

In sitting practices, it is pretty cut and dry -- we favor the practice over the scenery (experiences). This is what brings us the best results from practice.

In daily activity is is not so cut and dry, because we are engaged in living, active in the scenery even while letting it go. This is what makes self-inquiry so tricky, and sometimes counter-productive. It is a matter of how much we have become inner silence via sitting practices. When we have become "stillness in action," then the process of doing while living in non-duality becomes natural -- "relational." If we are prematurely pressing for that intellectually (building castles in the air), it can become strained and disruptive in our daily activity, which is "non-relational."

The simple solution is to engage in sitting practices and go out and live fully. Then self-inquiry occurs relationally and non-duality (unity) is realized naturally.

See the differences in considering scenery? It is the unfoldment of non-duality in duality. It takes an integration of practices to cultivate it, for most of us it does anyway. It is not for prodigies only, who are often mimicked. With effective means, the real thing is for everyone! :-)

The guru is in you.

2008/01/17 00:27:49
Jnana Yoga/Self-Inquiry - Advaita (Non-Duality)
http://www.aypsite.org/forum/topic.asp?TOPIC_ID=3380&REPLY_ID=29010&whichpage=-1
A Self-Inquiry, relational inquiry (hopefully)

quote:
_____
Originally posted by YogaPat

When you observe thoughts, feelings, and objects as separate from self do you also eventually view your human self this way? Seeing your mind/body as an object separate from your awareness. Is this kind of thinking Intuitive relational inquiry or is it just a distraction from practice?
_____

Hi Patrick:

The answer is "yes" in the beginning, and "no" later on. All objects of perception, including body/mind may be noticed to be separate from awareness in the beginning stages of witnessing. At the same time, and going forward, it is all merging back together again in a unifying non-dual way. This is the journey through the stages of mind discussed in the book.

If self-inquiry is relational (with the witness) it will be natural and not a distraction. If self-inquiry is non-relational (without the witness) and labored on as a mental construct, it will be a distraction, or worse.

As you can tell from reading through the book, relational self-inquiry (with the witness) cannot be conjured up in the mind. This is why we keep meditating. It takes time to cultivate the witness, and this is first and foremost in considering self-inquiry. It is hoped that the benchmarks and pointers will be helpful as you travel along.

An interesting thing to observe in these forums is that many who begin meditating may have little resonance with self-inquiry. It seems like voodoo. Either that, or they are beating themselves to death with it.

Then, as inner silence is noticed to be coming up, they begin to engage in self-inquiry naturally (usually the every day variety -- enter Byron Katie style self-inquiry), because a new perception of self and the world is gradually emerging during daily activities and relationships. In that evolving situation, not much guidance is necessary. We will know it when we see it. The Self-Inquiry book offers snapshots that can help us recognize and take advantage of the stages we are traveling through along the way. It also gives us tools to help evaluate the current applicability of any method of self-inquiry we may wish to consider.

The important thing is to just keep on living a normal life between our sitting practices. We will not gain much by stopping to inquire about everything -- it can be counterproductive. We will know when self-inquiry is right, because it will simplify and resolve whatever situation we happen to be in, rather than complicate it. When things are getting confusing and complicated, that is a sign of non-relational self-inquiry. Then the best thing to do is lighten up and move on through, and be sure not to miss our meditation. :-)

All the best!

The guru is in you.

2008/01/17 10:26:17
Jnana Yoga/Self-Inquiry - Advaita (Non-Duality)
http://www.aypsite.org/forum/topic.asp?TOPIC_ID=3380&REPLY_ID=29018&whichpage=-1
A Self-Inquiry, relational inquiry (hopefully)

quote:
_____
Originally posted by YogaPat

Thanks Scott and Yogani-

I see how it can get a little tricky, as the mind likes to keep running with these new discoveries once they have been revealed. I Guess the idea is to acknowledge natural realisation when it happens and then let it go and continue with the practice that got you there in the first place.

Cheers,P
_____

Yep, you got it. :-)

The guru is in you.

2008/01/17 11:42:56
Jnana Yoga/Self-Inquiry - Advaita (Non-Duality)
http://www.aypsite.org/forum/topic.asp?TOPIC_ID=3380&REPLY_ID=29023&whichpage=-1
A Self-Inquiry, relational inquiry (hopefully)

Hi Mac:

The idea is not to intentionally locate the mantra. Wherever it happens to go on its own is fine. But we do not pursue any particular location or attitude. We treat any tendency to physically locate the mantra the same way we treat anything else that comes up in the mind. Ultimately, the mantra does not have a specific location, and this is one of its strengths. The more we add to it with extra intentions, the less its abliity will be to transcend identification with external perceptions. We just easily favor the mantra and let it go.

If we are drawn into sambhavi (eyes going to center brow), or we find other mudras or bandhas occurring naturally during meditation, this is okay. But we do not entertain them intentionally. In deep meditation, our attention is for the simple procedure of easily favoring the mantra whenever we realize we are not. In time, we find that the mantra is not associated with any physical location or mental activity, because the mantra will take us beyond indentification with all perceptions during practice. This condition will carry over into daily activity, and this is the rise of abiding inner silence -- the witness. :-)

The guru is in you.

2008/03/10 10:46:23
Jnana Yoga/Self-Inquiry - Advaita (Non-Duality)
http://www.aypsite.org/forum/topic.asp?TOPIC_ID=3429&REPLY_ID=31096&whichpage=-1
In the sky of your mind you are the sun.

Hi YB:

"Jnana Yoga" includes these elements:

1. Inquiry -- "Who am I?" etc.
2. Discrimination -- "Not this, not this." (neti neti), etc.
3. Affirmation -- "I am *That*." etc.

They occur more or less in order as we develop along the path, with some obvious overlaps. The trick is to keep it relational (evolving in stillness), or mental tangents will begin to dominate. With daily deep meditation, samyama, etc., the evolution occurs naturally. The more we think about it, the less it will be working for us. That's why the suggestion is to engage in sitting practices and then go out and do. The mental component will become illuminated naturally then, and we will know it when we see it. :-)

The guru is in you.

PS: There is also "dispassion," which is a phenomenon we will be discussing more as we move forward, I'm sure. :-)

2008/03/24 10:56:55
Jnana Yoga/Self-Inquiry - Advaita (Non-Duality)
http://www.aypsite.org/forum/topic.asp?TOPIC_ID=3429&REPLY_ID=31676&whichpage=-1
In the sky of your mind you are the sun.

Hi VIL:

The next stage after dispassion is outpouring divine love and unfolding unity. This is about going out and being active in the world. Then we find the rise of passionate dispassion. :-)

The guru is in you.

2008/07/15 13:32:03
Jnana Yoga/Self-Inquiry - Advaita (Non-Duality)
http://www.aypsite.org/forum/topic.asp?TOPIC_ID=4142&REPLY_ID=35538&whichpage=-1
Non-duality

Hi Joanna, and welcome to the forums! :-)

There is no doubt that non-duality rules in the realm of mind. How can we ignore it, now that science has informed us that all things are the expression of one thing? Of course, the sages have known this for centuries, by direct perception.

I think most of us would prefer to be perceiving non-duality directly, rather than be thinking about it in ways that deny our current life experience, or putting that burden on others. Changing our perception requires some means, and an inner process of transformation, since perception is a function of our neurobiology. It takes some time. That is not a bad thing.

No one can become an olympic athlete overnight. This is a downside found in many non-duality (advaita) paths, where practical methods for unfolding the direct perception of non-duality are often shunned, while the mind is left to run in circles with concepts. Little will change. Ask around, and you will find that this is true. Never mind the glowing proclamations of instant enlightenment written in books, or offered by a self-assured person sitting at the front of the room. Go see what is really happening out there among the people. It is not so clean and neat.

With rare exceptions, the great advaita teachers themselves went through years and years of arduous practices in their lifetime (and those who didn't, likely did it in previous lives), to finally arrive at their often-touted "instant transformation." Come on ... is that true?

Now-a-days, more practical approaches to the matter of realization are coming forward. Like maybe meditation can help in our realization of non-duality? If all this is stillness, wouldn't it make sense to directly experience IT abiding within us first? Then the inquiry, discrimination, or affirmation can proceed much more effectively from there. Abiding inner silence/stillness is, after all, the essential ingredient in letting go of the habit of perceiving and identifying with duality as being outside the play of unity.

The AYP Self-Inquiry book is about this, designed to be a helpful companion to anyone on any non-dual/advaita/jnana path.

And what is non-duality really like? Why, it is *stillness in action*, of course. A never-ending ecstatic dance of the *One*. We are *That*.

It is not a matter of mind, though the mind can provide the logical inspiration for pursuing realization, and the means for transcending itself (which by any other name is still meditation). Realization is a matter of direct perception, and that means purifying and opening the neurobiology. There is no way around it. Realization is a whole body/mind/heart experience. The good news is that we are wired for it. We all sense this inside. It is just a matter of doing what is necessary to unfold our natural condition. Fortunately, we have many effective tools available today to aid in this. Why not use them?

As far as I know, taking an airplane is still the fastest way to get from New York to Los Angeles. If there were a way to get there (or anywhere) instantly, we'd all jump on, right? Likewise, as far as I know, daily spiritual practice over time is still the surest way to realize enlightenment. If there were an instant way to realize it, I'm sure we'd all jump on. Maybe someday for both, but not yet.

The fact is, today, the "instant approaches" take much longer, because they tend to be sectarian and closed to innovation. Much better, I think, to take a more pragmatic and effective approach. When it comes to advaita, it often boils down to a choice between embracing a philosophy (for better or worse), versus approaching the thing itself in a more flexible manner. It does not have to either/or. Integrated solutions are often found to be the best solutions.

We tend to be doers here in the AYP community, driven ever-forward by the intensity of our spiritual desire (bhakti). Of course, we are always looking for faster ways. We'd all like to be there like right now, but not by make-believe. We want the real thing. So we stay on the path, and notice as it is gradually disappearing beneath our feet along the way. That is the fun part...

Wishing you all the best on your path, non-path, or disappearing path, whichever the case may be. Whatever works! :-)

The guru is in you.

PS: This topic is being moved to the "Bhakti, Jnana and Karma Yoga" forum category. Be sure to check related topics there.

PPS: See also: http://www.aypsite.org/forum/topic.asp?TOPIC_ID=3610

2008/07/17 13:28:43
Jnana Yoga/Self-Inquiry - Advaita (Non-Duality)
http://www.aypsite.org/forum/topic.asp?TOPIC_ID=4142&REPLY_ID=35584&whichpage=-1
Non-duality

Hi All:

It might be good to add that the experience of non-duality will always be a paradox in concept, because it cannot be captured by the mind.

Does the phrase "*stillness in action*" make any sense? Maybe not. But that is what the experience of non-duality is. It is not a sterile condition, detached from life. It is just the opposite. It is the fullest possible engagement in an unending flow of Love, because we are *That* in everything we see everywhere we go. It is unity lived in diversity. More paradoxical words...

We often hear that non-duality is non-existence and that nothing else is really happening. This boggles the mind too, no doubt, because it defies our everyday experience. Personally, I think the "nothing is happening" description is a poor way to explain it, because it tends to place people in denial of their direct perception of life. This is not healthy. It is non-duality based on a divisive thought. That makes no sense at all. It is the very thing it is denying -- a dualistic view!

If we are going to speak in paradoxes, let it be in ones that include our everyday experiences, and not denying them. It is only a matter of expanding our perception. Then we gradually come to see the unity in all things -- the appearance of duality residing and playing within non-duality. Then we come to know we are *stillness in action*, and we don't have to be embarrassed about it, deny it, or pretend it isn't there. It is what it is.

The nature and flow of life can't be negated by philosophical proclamations or games of logic. But it can be directly perceived and lived in non-duality without even thinking about it. That is the "immovable and moving" silent witness "seeing and being seen" in all that is, and there is no fear in that. It is freedom.

That's why the AYP Self-Inquiry book has the subtitle, "Dawn of the Witness and the End of Suffering."

Regardless of the descriptions we may come up with for non-duality, the actual experience of it will not be changed. It is an evolution in functioning of the nervous system that is accessible to everyone. We may as well use descriptions that are inclusive and inspire us to take the journey of expanding our perception, rather than attempting to deny everything that is going on around us. The latter, when taken as a singular approach, is a very tough road to hoe.

The interesting thing is that yoga can easily accommodate advaita (non-duality), but advaita sometimes has a hard time accommodating yoga. What's that about? :-)

The guru is in you.

2008/11/17 10:46:40
Jnana Yoga/Self-Inquiry - Advaita (Non-Duality)
http://www.aypsite.org/forum/topic.asp?TOPIC_ID=4743&REPLY_ID=40728&whichpage=-1
Inquiring the personal will

Hi emc:

Human will becomes divine will when we are able to let go of analyzing for its own sake and just do or not do according to whatever circumstance we are in. Then the divine flow is happening, and it is us. :-)

The guru is in you.

2008/11/17 14:12:18
Jnana Yoga/Self-Inquiry - Advaita (Non-Duality)
http://www.aypsite.org/forum/topic.asp?TOPIC_ID=4743&REPLY_ID=40738&whichpage=-1
Inquiring the personal will

Hi emc:

But it is all personal and it is all divine. One cannot be separated from the other. There really isn't any difference. The only difference happens when we finally are able to accept it as it is, and that we can easily do in stillness. All of the discussions about ego and getting rid of ego are fabrications of the mind. The concept of ego itself is a fabrication. If a realized person acts egotistically, then that is what is happening at the moment. We can debate endlessly whether or not that is a realized person acting that way. The question (if there is one) is whether action is undertaken with attachment to the outcome or is occurring in stillness, i.e., radiating divine essence/love, even if it seems not to be. There is no answer to that riddle!

Everyone wants a good parking place, even the realized, but it is not life and death for them. The bad parking place will surely have a silver lining, because everything does. So in stillness we choose, and accept what comes.

It will never be captured in the mind, because it is a complete paradox. Realization is not about "getting it." It is about "becoming it," and that is why we do practices, which unravel and simplify the whole thing.

No matter what path we are on, the mind always has a lesser role to play, not a greater one. We use the mind to take actions that lead to transcendence of the mind. The mind will still be there as stillness in action, and it will then still be us making the choices as *That*.

Things do not change that much. We just see more clearly, that's all. When we can see, the struggle and the suffering end, even as we go on doing what we are called to do.

The guru is in you.

2008/11/17 16:49:47
Jnana Yoga/Self-Inquiry - Advaita (Non-Duality)
http://www.aypsite.org/forum/topic.asp?TOPIC_ID=4743&REPLY_ID=40743&whichpage=-1
Inquiring the personal will

Hi emc:

Yes, we can inquire about our will and our actions that bring discomfort. In stillness, we can inquire into the truth of such impulses and actions. We can release what is untrue in them even as they are occurring, much the way we can release our attachment to the motives and actions of others, or whatever else might be happening.

But that does not mean we will not continue to act as we did before for some time (maybe indefinitely), or that others will not continue to act as they did before. We will only be less attached to the impulses occurring within and around us. Self-inquiry can help with that.

Patterns of identification will tend to weaken over time as we no longer feed them, and then behavior can change (maybe long after the fact). The weakening of identification and eventual behavior change are not primary causes. They are effects. Better to attend to causes. Then the effects will be there sooner or later, and we don't have to dwell on them in the meantime.

It always gets back to cultivating stillness and acting from there, allowing life to happen while participating fully in the mode we are in, whatever that is, warts and all. Then it gradually becomes easier to let go of what is untrue. As we are more in stillness, we reside in untruth less, even as its residual may still be occurring there within us. We can let it go even as it happens. This change cannot be conjured up in the mind. It can't happen much until we have abiding inner silence. So we meditate. Then the inquiry will be increasingly in relationship with stillness rather than identified with the thing we are inquiring about, or tangled up in the process of inquiry itself.

The guru is in you.

2009/01/10 11:39:27
Jnana Yoga/Self-Inquiry - Advaita (Non-Duality)
http://www.aypsite.org/forum/topic.asp?TOPIC_ID=5006&REPLY_ID=43257&whichpage=-1
From attachment and aversion be free..

quote:
_____
Originally posted by Shanti

So how do you break free of attachment to the highs?
_____

Hi Shanti:

Just keep giving it away in service to others. Then it becomes a flow, a divine outpouring, and our attachment gradually goes. This is karma yoga, an important aspect of later stages on our path. Less thinking ... more ecstatic doing ... in stillness.

Here is a lesson on it: http://www.aypsite.org/120.html
Just replace the word "enlightenment" in the lesson with "high." Same thing. :-)

Enjoy!

The guru is in you.

2009/01/11 10:39:21
Jnana Yoga/Self-Inquiry - Advaita (Non-Duality)
http://www.aypsite.org/forum/topic.asp?TOPIC_ID=5006&REPLY_ID=43305&whichpage=-1
From attachment and aversion be free..

Hi Shanti:

Sorry, I was away for a while. Looks like you figured out there is nothing to figure out. :-)
We just do it, first through our practices, and then in becoming stillness moving out into daily living.

Enlightenment isn't enlightenment until we let it go -- give it away. Neither does a "high" have much significance until we let it go -- give it away. Before that, it is just scenery. The giving away is scenery too, but that is not our concern. It is the divine flow emerging through us.

This process is wrapped up with advancing samyama in daily living (cultivated in structured daily practice), which is releasing and moving in stillness. Then it flows out. It is the concurrent rise of relational self-inquiry also. Paradoxically, our ongoing desire (bhakti) to move through the transformation is the essential ingredient in all this.

It all merges together into one thing -- surrender in stillness. The act of giving it away (karma yoga) is part of the process. But it is not something we can conjure up until the flow is happening. We are priming the pump with our daily practices. Once the flow starts, it expands indefinitely. As Katrine says, you have been moving in this direction for a long time already. Thank you. :-)

It is the shift in our internal flow mentioned in lesson 120 -- the natural shift from getting to giving. It is a relaxation of heart and mind in stillness and the ecstatic flow. With that, the attachment is dissolving, even to the most glorious highs. Along the way, the question is naturally shifting from "How do I keep this?" to "How do I give this away?"

In time, there is no question about it. We just flow out with no attachment. Divine outpouring!

Meanwhile, our life continues in its ordinary ways. Chop wood, carry water...

High? What high? The world is becoming illuminated within and all around us. It is normal. Time to brush teeth again (practice). It is all in a day's work.

The guru is in you

2009/07/28 17:12:27
Jnana Yoga/Self-Inquiry - Advaita (Non-Duality)
http://www.aypsite.org/forum/topic.asp?TOPIC_ID=5330&REPLY_ID=54210&whichpage=-1
Awareness!

Hi emc:

You might find Adyashanti's book "The End of Your World" helpful, particularly the chapter called, "I got It, I lost It." :-)

The book is about the ups and downs of "stabilizing enlightenment," and points to the same kinds of messes that you have described.

From my perspective, none if this is necessary, as it is what happens when the cart gets in front of the horse in lopsided advaita (non-duality) approaches, relying largely on "guru-energy." It is certainly not representative of my experience, and I hope not for others who are utilizing the AYP approach without excessive exposure to the powerful energies that are being thrown around these days. It is a sign of the times. When enlightenment is approached backwards (starting at the end instead of the beginning), this is what often happens.

When a teacher effectively (or actually) tells you, "I am here to chop off your (ego) head," it is the practitioner's choice whether to dive into that mess or not. There is very little practical infrastructure provided to support it (a la self-pacing). Let the buyer beware.

Just a point of view from a quiet place that seeks not to run people more ragged than they wish to be.

The guru is in you.

PS: You are not the only one riding the yo-yo. Many are who follow this kind of approach. I don't think it is faster. Maybe slower, with all the backing and filling that goes on.

PPS: As someone else pointed out recently, lamenting the loss of bhakti is bhakti. :-)

2009/07/28 18:39:04
Jnana Yoga/Self-Inquiry - Advaita (Non-Duality)
http://www.aypsite.org/forum/topic.asp?TOPIC_ID=5330&REPLY_ID=54221&whichpage=-1
Awareness!

Hi emc:

Oh, no one likes to get their ego head cut off. But there are plenty of teachers out there now who find pleasure in it, without much concern for the near term consequences: Big highs and big lows for the practitioner. I have seen enough over the years to know it has become pretty common. Your posting here only reminded me of the chaos. Who is looking to smooth that out? Can it be smoothed out?

At least here you are advised to self-pace, and you should whenever necessary. :-)

All the best!

The guru is in you.

2009/05/19 12:16:40
Jnana Yoga/Self-Inquiry - Advaita (Non-Duality)
http://www.aypsite.org/forum/topic.asp?TOPIC_ID=5657&REPLY_ID=51068&whichpage=-1
Choices.....

Hi Carson:

Choice is entirely relative, depending on our state of consciousness and point of view.

If we are living mostly outside stillness (non-relational), we make all our choices and live with the consequences (karma). The choices are ours, because we see ourselves as material beings. Our reality is defined by our state of consciousness, not by an outside force, including God.

If we are living increasingly in stillness (relational), we make our choices just as we did before, except they are gradually merging with the divine flow and becoming stillness in action. There is karma here too, aligning with the divine flow coming through us.

If we are a pure advaitin, having fully realized the non-duality of life, then choices are going on outside the field of our Self. In that situation, action, karma, even God, are perceived to be outside what we are. The advaitin regards all this manifestation as a veneer, an illusion playing on the unmanifest Self behind it all, even while engaged fully and compassionately in it. It is a paradox. By then, choice is not an essential part of life, but the advaitin doesn't care. Choice keeps happening, but is transcended because he/she has transcended.

So it isn't that choice is ever going to be out of our reach. It is we who eventually evolve beyond the field of choice!

We cannot play this game from the point of view of a state of consciousness we are not in yet. In other words, it is not useful to take the point of view of an advaitin if we are operating outside stillness, or even engaged relationally seeing ourselves as increasing stillness in action. We will do best to be honest about where we are and operate from there. As soon as we project in mind outside our present reality we are nowhere (out of our "now"), and this is where the difficulties arise.

Therefore, it is much better to be fully living the life that is before us, while engaging in practices and moving gradually toward higher stages of consciousness. We will be making choices along the way, even when our choice is active surrender to the divine flow coming through us, and finally choosing non-duality, where we see the choices occurring outside our nature.

When we reach the advaita (non-dual) stage, we will see that all is happening automatically, and we are the eternal awareness (void) behind it. But this cannot be imagined. Those who try and live it in the mind will be in a disconnected state, worse off than the "unenlightened" person making an honest effort to move ahead by every means available.

The suggestion is to be where you are, make the best choices you can for betterment, and by all means, enjoy the ride!

The guru is in you.

2009/05/19 12:59:22
Jnana Yoga/Self-Inquiry - Advaita (Non-Duality)
http://www.aypsite.org/forum/topic.asp?TOPIC_ID=5657&REPLY_ID=51072&whichpage=-1
Choices.....

Hi Carson:

Identified awareness (ego) isn't an illusion at the point it is occurring. It is a condition of consciousness. It is as real as what we are perceiving in the moment. If that is what we are at a point in time, I don't think it is wise to label it as "an illusion." We can only play from where we are. If we negate where we are, we've got nothing to work with, and will be prone to get stuck in that mind set.

Ultimately, it is all an illusion, but what good does it do to dwell on that? Without the dawn of the witness, it will lead to mental paralysis, because it cannot be solved in the mind. It can only be solved in stillness. Effective self-inquiry dances along the edge of this.

Can a realized advaitin create negative karma? He/she would not make the distinction between positive or negative, and would not claim to be creating anything. The point of view is that the entire universe is going on by itself within him/her/it. This point of view is totally confounding to anyone but another realized advaitin. It takes One to know One. :-)

Fortunately, yama and niyama are operating in the grand illusion of the universe, according to the degree of presence of the witness, which includes the realized advaitin, of course.

The guru is in you.

2009/05/19 14:28:57
Jnana Yoga/Self-Inquiry - Advaita (Non-Duality)
http://www.aypsite.org/forum/topic.asp?TOPIC_ID=5657&REPLY_ID=51080&whichpage=-1
Choices.....

Hi Carson:

If an inquiry into "illusion" promotes an expansion in consciousness (more peace and happiness in life), then it is in stillness (relational). If it becomes a mental proclamation about life being illusion, and only that (becoming more misery in life), it will not be in stillness (non-relational). That is the edge, and we are all obliged to find it for ourselves.

The realized advaitin does not recognize karma as being positive or negative, or karma at all. All actions and choices are seen as instinctively played out within their field of awareness, like a dream. If you apply all these questions to the dream state, it is a pretty good analogy for the advaitin's point of view about life. That is assuming the advaitin is not one of those people who is obsessed with their dreams, which would be a contradiction. :-)

The guru is in you.

2009/05/19 14:41:02
Jnana Yoga/Self-Inquiry - Advaita (Non-Duality)
http://www.aypsite.org/forum/topic.asp?TOPIC_ID=5657&REPLY_ID=51082&whichpage=-1
Choices.....
PS: Someone may consider what an advaitin does to have a "negative" karmic effect. Like pushing beginners into premature (non-relational) self-inquiry leading to lots of misery. Kicking the dog, whatever... But the advaitin would not consider the consequences of their actions. They just act instinctively. That's why I say thank goodness for the natural presence of yama and niyama in the enlightened, because they are no longer discriminating like the rest of us. So, which advaitin can you trust? This is a can of worms, isn't it? :-)

2009/05/19 14:51:58
Jnana Yoga/Self-Inquiry - Advaita (Non-Duality)
http://www.aypsite.org/forum/topic.asp?TOPIC_ID=5657&REPLY_ID=51084&whichpage=-1
Choices.....
:-)
2009/05/19 15:20:36
Jnana Yoga/Self-Inquiry - Advaita (Non-Duality)
http://www.aypsite.org/forum/topic.asp?TOPIC_ID=5657&REPLY_ID=51088&whichpage=-1
Choices.....
PPS: The good news is that the guru in you knows...

2009/05/25 17:17:29
Jnana Yoga/Self-Inquiry - Advaita (Non-Duality)
http://www.aypsite.org/forum/topic.asp?TOPIC_ID=5657&REPLY_ID=51445&whichpage=-1
Choices.....

Hi Carson and All:

I took our interchange from this topic, added to it, mainly at the end, and posted it as a new lesson called:

"Advaita (non-duality), Free Will and Karma"
http://www.aypsite.org/334.html

More nitty gritty on self-inquiry. :-)

The guru is in you.

2009/05/26 09:11:34
Jnana Yoga/Self-Inquiry - Advaita (Non-Duality)
http://www.aypsite.org/forum/topic.asp?TOPIC_ID=5657&REPLY_ID=51468&whichpage=-1
Choices.....

quote:
_____
Originally posted by emc

Yes, Yogani, thanks a lot for that! I had the same question a while back (http://www.aypsite.org/forum/topic.asp?TOPIC_ID=4743) but were mostly confused by the answers I got then which were sort of just encouraging me to stop writing or minding about it as if it was hardly worth discussing, and I'm glad to finally get a really clearcut and elaborated answer. Thank you Carson for bringing the topic up again!

Yogani, your latest lessons are absolutely fabulous! :-) I enjoy to read immensely!

_____

Thanks All...

Hi emc:

The recent lessons are not saying much different than replies I wrote in the topic link you gave, except perhaps becoming more proactive with the mind.

Honestly, I have some reservations about it, because as soon as we begin describing the "nitty gritty" of self-inquiry, many people may run off into mental circles -- non-relational self-inquiry -- at the expense of prerequisite cultivation and natural outward flow of inner silence (witness), which is what naturally produces relational self-inquiry.

For me, self-inquiry has always been an organic process, emerging naturally with the rise of inner silence and ecstatic conductivity over the years. A gradual development. Not the slam-bam-boom kind of enlightenment that is offered by so many advaita teachers these days, which is often chaotic, requiring a lot of backing and filling, and I think not faster than the smoother path that AYP aspires to be, putting in a firm foundation of the witness first. I'm not sure that proactive self-inquiry is suitable for the masses, even though it has obvious mass appeal -- "mind candy."

So I have these reservations about slam-bam-boom "neo-advaita" -- with houses too often built on sand, rather than on the rock of abiding inner silence.

Nevertheless, with so many here moving ahead quickly with clear experiences of abiding inner silence (stage 1), ecstatic conductivity (stage 2), and even unity experiences (stage 3), I felt it was time to do more nitty gritty on self-inquiry in the lessons. I hope it does not produce too much grinding of the gears -- non-relational grinding that is. :-)

Thanks for the opportunity to express these thoughts. We'll keep on and see how it unfolds -- a work in progress. It's a community thing, you know.

May all the flowers bloom in their own way. Enjoy!

The guru is in you.

2009/05/18 13:22:16
Jnana Yoga/Self-Inquiry - Advaita (Non-Duality)
http://www.aypsite.org/forum/topic.asp?TOPIC_ID=5658
Jnana Yoga - Advaita Vedanta (Non-Duality)
Note: As of May 18, 2009, the "Bhakti, Jnana and Karma Yogas" forum category has been split in two, to better accommodate the expansion of practitioner experiences and the AYP lessons. Happily, both are moving steadily deeper into non-duality/unity topics of discussion. As advanced experiences and our collective understanding of them continue to unfold, the forums are being adapted accordingly. The two forums are:

Jnana Yoga - Advaita Vedanta (Non-Duality):
http://www.aypsite.org/forum/forum.asp?FORUM_ID=54

Bhakti and Karma Yoga:
http://www.aypsite.org/forum/forum.asp?FORUM_ID=23

Here is the introduction from the original "Bhakti, Jnana and Karma Yogas" forum category. It is as relevant a starting point as ever:

Way back in the 1890s, a great sage named Vivekananda came from India to the West. He was the first from India who became widely known, and he paved the way for the many more sages and teachers who would follow throughout the 20th century.

Vivekananda spoke about the eight-limbed path of Patanjali's Yoga Sutras. He called it "Raja Yoga." He also spoke about three additional paths of yoga: Jnana, Bhakti and Karma. These correspond to the yogic roles of mind, heart, and our actions. The first two limbs of Raja Yoga, the yamas and niyamas, actually include these, but Vivekananda separated them out, perhaps because they have to do more with our ongoing thoughts, feelings and conduct throughout the day, rather than with the sessions of yoga postures and sitting practices which make up the rest of the eight limbs.

Jnana has been called the path of the intellect, the path of discrimination. Discrimination of what? Of truth. And what is the truth? According to great sages like Ramana Maharishi, the truth is found in inquiry -- in the simple question, "Who am I?" If we ask this question in earnest, repeatedly, with an intense longing to know (a blending with bhakti), then truth will come up in us and around us. Jnana is not primarily about gathering intellectual information, or building big philosophical structures. True jnana is a process of thinking the mind beyond itself. The best job of the mind in yoga is to think itself out of a job! If we can decide to practice meditation and other yoga practices, and stick with a daily routine of practices over the long haul, the mind will be serving us well in yoga. And in all other areas of life too, because our thinking will come into harmony with our inner silence. A mind moving in silence is divine mind, the field of Oneness, or unity. See Lesson #185 at http://www.aypsite.org/185.html

Bhakti is called "the science of devotion" in AYP. It truly is a science, because it has known causes and effects which can be harnessed by diligent practitioners. If we know how to redirect our emotional energy toward our highest ideal, whether it be "God" or "Truth" or "Love," then huge invisible forces will be turned loose that bring knowledge to us in an avalanche. Such is the power of bhakti. See Lesson #67 at http://www.aypsite.org/67.html

Karma means action and its effects. Karma is what we do and how it affects us and others. The action side of karma yoga is found in gradually gravitating toward an attitude of serving others. No one can force this on us. It comes up naturally in us when we have been doing yoga practices -- meditation, pranayama and asanas. Then the karmas (effects) residing in our nervous system are illuminated from within and we cannot help but care more for those around us, in our own way. Then karma yoga really shines and is not an obligation or drudgery. Just the opposite. Service becomes pure joy! See Lesson #228 at http://www.aypsite.org/228.html

This forum is for discussing our practical experiences in applying our emotions, mind and daily actions to help us along the path of yoga. It can be as simple as saying "Yes!" to the voice inside that is calling us to do what is necessary to grow, and making the choices that will propel us forward.

Each of these three categories of yoga can stimulate many dimensions of discussion and spiritual progress:

Jnana Yoga -- The intellectual examination (and release) of the nature of existence.
Bhakti Yoga -- The role of desire in our daily spiritual practices, and the many devotional paths of worship.
Karma Yoga -- The natural rise of outpouring divine and service to others (who we see increasingly as out own *Self*) as our spiritual progress advances.

Feel free to indulge. Enjoy!

The guru is in you.

2009/05/22 17:35:47
Jnana Yoga/Self-Inquiry - Advaita (Non-Duality)
http://www.aypsite.org/forum/topic.asp?TOPIC_ID=5666&REPLY_ID=51300&whichpage=-1
an inquiry on the witness state and emptiness

Hi Ananda and All:

I took our original interchange from your first post here, expanded my reply, and posted it as a new lesson (#333) called "Dissolving the Witness in Unity" here: http://www.aypsite.org/333.html

Getting into the nitty gritty of self-inquiry a bit. :-)

Enjoy!

The guru is in you.

2009/05/23 10:55:39
Jnana Yoga/Self-Inquiry - Advaita (Non-Duality)
http://www.aypsite.org/forum/topic.asp?TOPIC_ID=5666&REPLY_ID=51328&whichpage=-1
an inquiry on the witness state and emptiness
Whatever comes out on the keyboard here is inspired by all of you. So thank you, and keep going. :-)

The guru is in you.

2009/06/03 14:19:22
Jnana Yoga/Self-Inquiry - Advaita (Non-Duality)
http://www.aypsite.org/forum/topic.asp?TOPIC_ID=5666&REPLY_ID=51840&whichpage=-1
an inquiry on the witness state and emptiness

quote:

Originally posted by Konchok Ösel Dorje

Ananda, there's no need to quip. I can accept your words are from your experience. Can you accept that my words are from mine?

I just meditated. I can't put it into words. It was an experience. Now that I'm writing, I can't say it wasn't a mind, just not my ordinary one I'm writing with now.

I know Yogani has been implying that I'm espousing ideology that I heard from someone else. That's unfair. I am sharing my experience. This may not be the place to share. Considering. Applying wisdom. Perhaps taking a break from this forum. I wish you all safe passage.

Ösel Dorje

Gee Osel:

One of the few times I sense your real 2 cents, and now you are running away? Maybe inquire a bit on it. It is an opening, so why run?

Whatever the case may be, I greatly appreciate all efforts you make toward your awakening, as this is also everyone else's awakening. It takes a village, you know, present and accounted for or not.

Carry on! :-)

The guru is in you.

2009/06/03 17:46:39
Jnana Yoga/Self-Inquiry - Advaita (Non-Duality)
http://www.aypsite.org/forum/topic.asp?TOPIC_ID=5666&REPLY_ID=51865&whichpage=-1
an inquiry on the witness state and emptiness

quote:

Originally posted by Konchok Ösel Dorje

I know Yogani has been implying that I'm espousing ideology that I heard from someone else. That's unfair. I am sharing my experience. This may not be the place to share. Considering. Applying wisdom. Perhaps taking a break from this forum. I wish you all safe passage.

Hi Osel:

I'd like to try and address this.

There is nothing wrong with espousing the teachings of another, as long as we do not present them as a foregone conclusion, or as our own knowledge. Either way, that is espousing ideology, no matter how intimate we may be with the source. It creates a false sense of authority, which isn't good for the writer or the reader.

If the experience is there, it will not be necessary to verify it, because the vibe will be there in every word. The words will be original, not echoing the vocabulary of a third party source. Once the thing is seen, original descriptions will flow like water. That's why realization is nearly always

374 – Advanced Yoga Practices

expressed with a mixture of old and new terminology.

In any case, I did not point this out to belittle or offend you. Nor did I do it to one-up you in any way. I pointed it out because it is not real spirituality, and I think you and everyone here deserve better. You are not the first here to project third party knowledge with an air of certain authority, and you will not be the last. Don't get me wrong, it is fine to read some rhetoric in order to get to some real stuff. We'd like to maximize the real stuff, because that is what we are here for. If it takes a two-by-four to get 2 cents worth of real stuff, maybe it will happen sometimes, though I am not much into Zen. :-)

So the suggestion is to share what is in your deepest heart -- if not here, then somewhere where there is a suitable mirror (everywhere?), because those are the most pregnant opportunities for inquiry. That is what we are looking for, right?

And if you want to share everything you ever heard about spirituality from your teacher or anywhere else, then feel free to do that here also. But share it as what it is (third party knowledge), not as something absolute that we should all accept at face value, because we will not. There is an awareness here that reaches far beyond what I may contribute. Your experience we can easily accept, no matter what it is, but that is only possible when you are coming clean with it.

These forums are experience-based from top to bottom and from beginning to end. That is how the online environment can serve as real satsang, and sometimes much more. This is, after all, a node (connection point) in the vast <u>global web of awakening</u>.

If all you have presented here with authority in the past is based on your direct experience, then I stand corrected and apologize. If not, then let's inquire on it in stillness. It's the least we can do. :-)

The guru is in you.

2009/06/04 00:11:23
Jnana Yoga/Self-Inquiry - Advaita (Non-Duality)
<u>http://www.aypsite.org/forum/topic.asp?TOPIC_ID=5666&REPLY_ID=51879&whichpage=-1</u>
an inquiry on the witness state and emptiness

Hi Osel:

I have failed to reach you on this matter. It is my fault and I take responsibility for it. It should not have been brought up in the forum in the first place, and for that I apologize.

If you would like clarification on what this is about, I will be happy to provide it in email.

Thanks for your contributions, and all the best!

The guru is in you.

2009/07/07 11:03:21
Jnana Yoga/Self-Inquiry - Advaita (Non-Duality)
<u>http://www.aypsite.org/forum/topic.asp?TOPIC_ID=5907&REPLY_ID=53268&whichpage=-1</u>
Kundalini and Vichara

Hi Vicha:

Thanks for writing and sharing.

Actually, your "kundalini" symptoms are a sign that your self-inquiry sadhana is working, producing some inner purification and opening. Where it happens in the body will depend on your unique pattern of inner obstructions. It is a natural process that will evolve according to its own inner dynamic. The symptoms are a sign of energy producing "friction" when passing through and purifying the subtle neurobiology. In time it will smooth out. In the meantime, make sure to self-pace your practice and get plenty of "grounding activity" to stabilize the process for progress with comfort. Additional information on managing kundalini symptoms can be found here: <u>http://www.aypsite.org/69.html</u>

A careful reading of Nisargadatta's "I Am That" reveals that he has all the elements of yoga in there, including bhakti, meditation, and energy (kundalini) experiences. Much of this has been minimized for consistency with a "pure advaita" approach. Yet, the first things he often asked new visitors to his satsangs were, "What is your sadhana?" and "What is your experience?" He himself ran meditation classes and bhajans when not waxing eloquent on advaita. So let's not over-simplify the teachings of Nisargadatta, even though advaita (non-duality) may seem to demand it. In truth, Nisargadatta is quite consistent with AYP. It is only a matter of what is being emphasized when. It is good to put things in a logical order to avoid unnecessary confusion. :-)

No matter what the path or approach, the inner processes will be essentially the same. All effective systems of practice are working with the same human nervous system.

You might find the writings of American teacher Adyashanti helpful. He is zen/inquiry/advaita, has a strong affinity with Nisargadatta, and teaches in a modern down to earth way. His latest book, "The End of Your World" has many helpful chapters in it for those who are experiencing degrees of non-duality, including one on the "energetic component of awakening" (kundalini).

Also see this AYP online lesson on "non-duality and ecstatic kundalini": <u>http://www.aypsite.org/331.html</u>

From the AYP point of view, kundalini, or ecstatic conductivity and radiance, provides the vehicle for stillness to "move" outward into a full expression of unity - outpouring divine love - which is the fulfillment of "I am That" in all aspects of everyday living. The application of self-inquiry in AYP is covered in the <u>Self-Inquiry book</u>, which can be a helpful complement to any approach to self-inquiry.

Carry on, and all the best!

The guru is in you.

2009/07/14 15:14:37
Jnana Yoga/Self-Inquiry - Advaita (Non-Duality)
http://www.aypsite.org/forum/topic.asp?TOPIC_ID=5945&REPLY_ID=53543&whichpage=-1
Practice Shifting Toward Advaita (non-duality)

quote:

_____
Originally posted by Ananda

...after being involved in a large set of ayp practices, i don't know why but automatically or unconsciously when i added samyama i started cutting down practices more and more and tending to go toward mindfulness and self inquiry more and more to the extent where i am only doing spinal breathing and deep meditation and even those i've cut back to 15 to 20 minutes of DM and 7 to 8 minutes of SBP with a last round of kumbhaka and this feels like more than enough for me it just fills me up.

i mean i don't experience any overloading symptoms and i can play around the crown with no uncomfortable symptoms it's ecstasy the other way around but it feels like this is what i need to evolve at the steady rate i am going just that and no need to add any new techniques and my bhakti is leading me toward a burning search for an advaita guru and more inquiry and affirmation and away from new practices even though i was having some extraordinary results with some of them.

i know that there are others here like Katrine who started cutting back on practices as well and i know you're saying about less is more at a certain stage but in the case of others like our good friend Christy it doesn't seem that way.

any feedback about the mechanics of this would be appreciated.

namaste,

Ananda

_____

Hi Ananda:

It is interesting, isn't it? Perhaps verifying the statement: "The efficient cultivation of abiding inner silence changes everything." :-)

A couple of years ago, advaita (non-duality) was a source of non-relational irritation to many around here. Now it is emerging as a full-blown trend. Clearly, chosen ideals are migrating for some here, which is not to say it will be the same for everyone. All things in good time.

I think the increasing tendency toward advaita and non-dual self-inquiry is good, as long is it is not pressed too much outside the presence of abiding stillness (witness). When it is, it becomes a mind game (non-relational), as you know. So it is important to keep a foundation of practices to support the cultivation and movement of stillness. Samyama is a key in this, obviously, and it leads naturally to relational self-inquiry.

Energy-related cultivation (kundalini) is important too. It is on the wings of energy that sensory perception and self-identification are refined, and by which stillness pours into the world in the form of divine love. We each will find what is necessary for us to address the energy aspect. It may be as simple as some light spinal breathing followed by deep meditation, or as involved as extensive additional pranayama, asanas, mudras, bandhas, etc. We will travel as we are inclined, and self-pace accordingly. It is fascinating to see how paths are evolving among the practitioners here.

And if at a stage on our path we find headstands helping to bring us closer to liberation, then so be it. :-)

The guru is in you.

2009/07/15 12:25:49
Jnana Yoga/Self-Inquiry - Advaita (Non-Duality)
http://www.aypsite.org/forum/topic.asp?TOPIC_ID=5945&REPLY_ID=53558&whichpage=-1
Practice Shifting Toward Advaita (non-duality)

Hi Ananda:

If you are letting go of intentions in abiding stillness and experiencing a natural flow into self-inquiry, service, etc., then this is samyama also, expressing in everyday living.

The structured procedure of samyama during daily practices is for promoting this natural ability, and the condition of freedom it leads to. It produces a lot of purification and opening, within and beyond the body. You are wise to self-pace according to your ongoing experience. :-)

The guru is in you.

2009/07/16 11:05:25
Jnana Yoga/Self-Inquiry - Advaita (Non-Duality)
http://www.aypsite.org/forum/topic.asp?TOPIC_ID=5949&REPLY_ID=53596&whichpage=-1
Spontaneous Non-attachment

Hi All:

The view from here is that emotions do not cease, but self-identification with them does. All it takes is abiding inner silence (witness), and progressing gradually from there to the direct experience of radating divine love and all-inclusive unity.

It can happen with leaps (awakenings), followed by retracements -- ups and downs. A smoother unfoldment might be preferred, which is what the AYP approach aims for.

Along the way, the base emotions are transmuted to divine purpose, just as all karma is. So there is a noticable change in conduct. But at other times base emotions may seem to be expressed, like Jesus driving the money-changers from the temple in a rage, or expressing fear about his impending execution. The difference is the lack of self-identification, so such episodes leave little or no samskara trace. This dynamic imbues even the base emotions with divine purpose. In the enlightened one, compassion and outpouring divine love will utilize the full range of human attributes.

This is not something out of reach for anyone in this lifetime. All it takes is a sincere commitment to a chosen ideal, and daily engagement in effective practices. A normal life need not be left behind. Indeed, enlightenment is normal life. What most in the world are living is abnormal. The secret is out... :-)

The guru is in you.

2009/07/30 10:32:33
Jnana Yoga/Self-Inquiry - Advaita (Non-Duality)
http://www.aypsite.org/forum/topic.asp?TOPIC_ID=6046&REPLY_ID=54353&whichpage=-1
Mind is the Enemy

Hi YogaIsLife:

Should the hammer become our enemy just because we keep hitting our thumb with it? It is only a hammer after all. Maybe take a closer look at who is using it?

Likewise, the mind is only a thought machine, a marvelous computer. If we confuse our identity with it and allow it to run our life ragged, is that the mind's fault? Maybe take a closer look at who is using it?

By making enemies of things like that, we are only reinforcing duality and suffering, the very situation we'd like to transcend. I am reminded of a certain famous teacher who has descended into long writings on demonizing the ego in every avenue of life. To what avail?

Yes, we can drop what is not in our best interest, and we should. But it is very difficult to drop (let go of) something we are hanging on to as an enemy. Witness is the key, the cultivation of abiding inner silence.

Then find out "who" is behind all these desires and fears. That One is easily found by releasing the inquiry in stillness. Let go and let God. :-)

The guru is in you.

2009/08/02 23:55:48
Jnana Yoga/Self-Inquiry - Advaita (Non-Duality)
http://www.aypsite.org/forum/topic.asp?TOPIC_ID=6062&REPLY_ID=54509&whichpage=-1
Why Yoga if inquiry/vedanta/ gets you there...
Welcome, Beetsmyth!

Yoga and self-inquiry are not different systems. They are both part of the same system. That is the way it is viewed in the AYP approach. One of the branches of yoga is called "jnana yoga," dealing with self-inquiry. Advaita-vedanta and jnana yoga are the same. Splitting off jnana (self inquiry) from the rest of yoga as stand-alone greatly reduces its effectiveness, not a complete path for the vast majority of people, and there are good reasons for this. When properly integrated, all aspects of yoga (including self-inquiry) are highly complementary, and much faster than any one branch by itself.

If you review 15 or so online lessons, starting here, you will get an idea on the AYP approach to integration of yoga and self-inquiry:
http://www.aypsite.org/321.html
There is also an AYP book on Self-Inquiry, which covers the relationship between self-inquiry and the rest of yoga, particularly the importance of cultivating abiding inner silence (the witness) in daily deep meditation as an essential prerequisite for effective self-inquiry.
Current and upcoming online lessons are going to take the use of self-inquiry in the AYP system significantly further. It is time. So stayed tuned. :-)

Wishing you all the best on your path!

The guru is in you.

2009/08/04 11:46:14
Jnana Yoga/Self-Inquiry - Advaita (Non-Duality)
http://www.aypsite.org/forum/topic.asp?TOPIC_ID=6074&REPLY_ID=54606&whichpage=-1
A Word on Yogic Practices in Advaita

Hi All:

A few more cents on this topic over here:
http://www.aypsite.org/forum/topic.asp?TOPIC_ID=6062#54509

:-)

The guru is in you.

2009/08/06 13:11:02
Jnana Yoga/Self-Inquiry - Advaita (Non-Duality)
http://www.aypsite.org/forum/topic.asp?TOPIC_ID=6092&REPLY_ID=54751&whichpage=-1
Dropping the "me"

Hi Shanti:

You are homing in on it. This is much in line with the lesson posted yesterday, where a progression of self-inquiry methods is explored: http://www.aypsite.org/350.html

We all begin self-inquiry somewhere, and it evolves as we do. I'd like to say that self-inquiry evolves us, but there is limited evidence to support this, at least not for many people. Rather, it is inner silence that evolves us, and self-inquiry is part of the movement of stillness, and the merging our our I-sense with stillness that comes as a result of cultivating the ability of samyama (releasing intentions/inquiries in stillness).

The reason self-inquiry was not working for you with the "flutters" is because you were reaching a limit with the particular style of self-inquiry (neti neti) you have been using. How many identifications of awareness can we drop? How many stories? How many manifestations of fear? How many flutters? They are unlimited, as you point out. This is a weakness of the "negating" (neti neti) style of self-inquiry. Which is not to say it ought to be thrown out. It is a stepping-stone to a more fundamental (transcending) practice, which you are finding now.

There is one thing that is behind all this, and that is the I-sense, or I-thought. Who is experiencing all these stories? Who is having all these fears? These memories? These anticipations? It is "me," as you say. It is "I." We can see that in every experience we have in life. We can develop it as a feeling: It is "I" to which all these things occur. It is "I" who perceives all. Everything can be traced back to the I-sense.

Then ... Who or what is "I?"

Let that one go in stillness, and you have it. The trick is to feel the "I-sense" as that which is experiencing whatever is happening. Therefore, "Who am I?" must be preceded by, "To whom is this experience occurring?"

This is not an intellectual exercise.

Both questions evolve to become feelings, and become essentially one inquiry that is released in stillness (samyama). This can be taken deep, deep, deep. The procedure will transcend itself, because we can keep asking on ever-finer levels, "Who is having this most subtle feeling about 'Who am I?'?" ... It is "I." ... And "Who am I?" -- Release. It can be taken to pure radiant emptiness with absolutely nothing manifesting. Not one story, not one thought. It is the light of the *Self* nipping everything in the bud before any object can be perceived.

In time, this can become our attitude in life, and this is life lived increasingly on the level of the *Self*, which is unending joy and freedom in whatever may be happening in time and space, even as we are fully engaged in life. Who is engaged?...

So, yes, you are on to something big. So big that it will disappear into the infinite *Self*, and take everything with it. Slurp! ... and gone to infinity. You are *That*. Welcome to advaita/non-duality. Now go do the dishes. :-)

The question arises, why can't we all start with this style of self-inquiry (what I call "jnana-transcending" in the lesson), instead of spending years and lifetimes getting around to it? The fact that we all get around to it in our own time and way has made the stream-lining process of self-inquiry in the lessons very tricky. It is not like deep meditation, where most of us can start more or less with the same thing, and then here comes the witness. On the other hand, self-inquiry is all over the lot. In AYP we got underneath it by identifying abiding inner silence (the witness) as the common denominator for success with all forms of self-inquiry. But even with that, everyone seems to have their own progression.

I think now we are finally homing in on it, both in the lessons, and experientially, as you have so eloquently described. Nevertheless, it remains a process we each will approach in our own way. This is why self-inquiry will continue to have various styles and stages that make up a progression that each practitioner is going through in developing understanding and experience.

Hopefully, the AYP writings will offer some practical help in this, with Lesson 350 being the most recent addition. More is to come!

The guru is in you.

2009/08/16 18:20:52
Jnana Yoga/Self-Inquiry - Advaita (Non-Duality)
http://www.aypsite.org/forum/topic.asp?TOPIC_ID=6156&REPLY_ID=55179&whichpage=-1
Latest lesson 354

Hi emc:

It may be that the best way to recognize relational self-inquiry is in noticing what it is not. If there is strain, expectation, judgment, headache, etc., those would be signs of non-relational self-inquiry, and it is best to lighten up (self-pace) in those instances. In time, those things will be absent, and we will simply be noticing thoughts and feelings to be more like objects in our awareness, no longer classifying them or hanging on to them, no longer seeing them as extensions of our self, or even as "baggage" to be carried around. They will be seen to be outside our sense of self.

If inquiry is increasingly joyful and luminous, through both "good times" and "bad times," we can be pretty sure it is becoming relational. That is, released in stillness (the witness).

For those who are interested in a possible progression of stages in self-inquiry, see Lesson 350. It is a long lesson, but perhaps one of the clearer ones so far on the various stages of self-inquiry from the AYP point of view: http://www.aypsite.org/350.html

The guru is in you.

2009/08/16 23:42:32
Jnana Yoga/Self-Inquiry - Advaita (Non-Duality)
http://www.aypsite.org/forum/topic.asp?TOPIC_ID=6156&REPLY_ID=55188&whichpage=-1
Latest lesson 354

Hi Kirtanman and All:

The term "relational" was coined to identify a relationship between abiding inner silence (the witness) and thoughts. That relationship consummates with the release (letting go) of thoughts in stillness, the blending of one into the other, which is samyama. It is the basis of effective self-inquiry, divine outpouring, stillness in action, spontaneous siddhis (small and large), etc.

Prior to the rise of inner silence as an abiding presence, this relationship cannot occur. Then it is thoughts interacting with thoughts with the aforementioned difficult symptoms. The term for that is "non-relational," meaning thoughts not occurring in relationship to stillness.

The reason why I came up with these terms is to clarify the essential point that self-inquiry is not a viable practice without at least the beginnings of the witness stage, which is not difficult to cultivate in deep meditation, but is often ignored in neo-advaita teachings. I say "neo-advaita" because if we dig a bit we will find that the great advaita and jnana yoga teachers clearly recognized the role of the witness, bhakti, and yoga practices. Neo-advaita is prone to strip it all down to the the bare logic and expect that to be a viable "stand-alone" approach for everyone at every point on the path. Clearly it is not.

So "relational" and "non-relational" have been born in an attempt to make the distinction between self-inquiry with witness and self-inquiry without witness as clear as possible. The experiences of many here have verified the development of this dynamic going from non-relational to relational. Whatever we may choose to call it, the shift is quite noticeable. Many here are delving into self-inquiry these days with pretty good results, whereas a few years ago it was, well, non-relational. :-)

What we don't want to be doing is turning these terms into have and have-not labels. That is not their purpose. The purpose is to inspire the continued favoring of daily deep meditation (and samyama) when self-inquiry is not yet working for us as well as we would like. If there were no clear guidance offered on this, there may be a tendency to beat our head against the wall for a long time in thought-based only self-inquiry, or drop spiritual practices altogether. We'd like to avoid that situation, so point to a more viable approach as clearly as we can.

The recent addition of a powerful self-inquiry sutra to core samyama practice in Lesson 351 is also for the purpose of helping smooth the transition from non-relational to relational inquiry. This can be included as soon as we are able to undertake core samyama practice, and it does not carry the risks of outright non-relational self-inquiry, even if the presence of our abiding witness is at an early stage.

The wise farmer drives the plow around the stump, and not through it, right Ether? :-)

The guru is in you.

2009/08/31 10:41:33
Jnana Yoga/Self-Inquiry - Advaita (Non-Duality)
http://www.aypsite.org/forum/topic.asp?TOPIC_ID=6247&REPLY_ID=56051&whichpage=-1
Ramana Mahars
Hi on Meditation Experiences

Hi All:

Very good, but such inquiries should not be favored during AYP deep meditation or other sitting practice procedures. Before or after, but not during. This would be diluting the cultivation of abiding inner silence and ecstatic conductivity, the very foundation of effective (relational) self-inquiry.

The hour or so we spend in structured sitting practices each day sets the stage for clear experience and understanding of our non-dual nature (radiantly free *Self*) in everything else we do.

An effective integration of practices (involving mind) means doing each one in its own time, not at the same time. :-)

The guru is in you.

2009/09/22 17:11:38
Jnana Yoga/Self-Inquiry - Advaita (Non-Duality)
http://www.aypsite.org/forum/topic.asp?TOPIC_ID=6247&REPLY_ID=57395&whichpage=-1
Ramana Mahars
Hi on Meditation Experiences

Hi Beetsmyth:

Do you think refining the I-thought is not an object/subject practice?

Non-duality teachers so often dismiss meditation as an object/subject practice, while tying their students up in endless loops of mental gymnastics and call it "self-inquiry." Often it is an object/object (mind/mind) practice, which is much worse. That's not real self-inquiry.

There is an important point being missed all right. The process of self-inquiry you are describing cannot be undertaken with any degree of success until the witness quality is already present. We cannot transcend the witness in self-inquiry until we have the abiding stillness to do it in.

True meditation is not about object and subject. It is about refining object into subject, until only subject remains (stillness). This is how the witness is cultivated.

The process of refining the I-thought (object) in stillness is actually meditation. It is what Ramana Mahars
Hi taught, and it is an excellent practice for those who are ready for it.

The difference between Ramana's practice and AYP deep meditation is that it has a "meaning component," the concepts of "I" and inquiring as to who or what that is. The Ramana practice is attempting to do several things at the same time:

1. Cultivating stillness through meditation on the I-thought.

2. Inquiring as to who or what that is, to its source.

3. Attempting to do that all day long in the midst of daily activity.

It is a bit much to take on for those who are beginning without significant spiritual background, for those who are not already "ripe." See this lesson.

AYP breaks this up into digestible components which can be incorporated into the daily routine one step at a time:

1. Cultivation of abiding inner silence in deep meditation with a mantra having no meaning, in two short daily sessions. Much more efficient than attempting to use an object with meaning all day long. Reminder: This is no more an object/subject practice than using the I-thought in the Ramana technique. Actually less so, because meaning is not included.

2. Developing skill in samyama, which is the ability to release intentions and inquiries (meaning) in stillness, both in structured practice and ad-hoc during the day. This integrates all thinking and activity in stillness, making life "stillness in action."

3. Incorporate structured self-inquiry into samyama practice with a sutra such as: "I-Thought - Who am I?" Equivalents can be derived, but it is important to settle on one for structured practice, so the inquiry can be "baked in." This has a profound effect on #4.

4. Inquire ad-hoc during the day as so inclined, based on a strong foundation in both abiding inner silence (witness) and deep self-inquiry cultivated in structured practices.

If you are interested in more detail on this, see these two lessons:

Self-inquiry practices for transcending the witness: http://www.aypsite.org/350.html

Structured self-inquiry samyama: http://www.aypsite.org/351.html

Both Ramana Mahars
Hi and Nisargadatta Maharaj were well aware of the importance of "ripeness," and were supportive of practitioners undertaking whatever means necessary to become ripe. Their successors have not been nearly as understanding, and that is why the field of non-dual self-inquiry has remained esoteric and problematic. There is no need for this. Only an understanding of the means for becoming ripe should be added. Then non-dual self-inquiry will become a rich field of realization for everyone.

None of this need alter anything you are doing now, assuming you are ripe and happily dissolving the "I" in the heart of non-duality. This has been posted for everyone else. :-)

The guru is in you.

PS: Carson, you beat me to the punch.
Beetsmyth, you see where we are coming from? Ultimately, it is not about our own experience. It is about everyone else. :-)

2009/09/23 10:44:40
Jnana Yoga/Self-Inquiry - Advaita (Non-Duality)
http://www.aypsite.org/forum/topic.asp?TOPIC_ID=6247&REPLY_ID=57446&whichpage=-1
Ramana Mahars
Hi on Meditation Experiences

Hi Chinna:

I hung a sign in front of the house:

"Inquire within for the path to enlightenment based on cultivating futility."

So far, no one showed up.

Like I said: "esoteric and problematic" ... and also unnecessary. Earnest bhakti can be utilized in much more effective ways, by many many more people.

This isn't for you who may already be ripe. It is for everyone else. :-)

The guru is in you.

PS: Perhaps the sign needs an addition, in fine print: "Only the ripe need apply."

AYP is mainly concerned with helping all people become ripe. Once that is being accomplished, the harvest is inevitable. Jnana/advaita is a good harvesting tool. We are on the same team.

2009/09/23 20:40:35
Jnana Yoga/Self-Inquiry - Advaita (Non-Duality)
http://www.aypsite.org/forum/topic.asp?TOPIC_ID=6247&REPLY_ID=57488&whichpage=-1
Ramana Mahars
Hi on Meditation Experiences

Hi Chinna:

I don't think we have any disagreement on the value of non-dual self-inquiry. Only on how and when it might be applied. With the multiple points of view expressed here, anyone reading can find some assistance for making decisions about it according to their own inclination and need.

Many thanks for sharing!

The guru is in you.

2009/09/24 10:56:10
Jnana Yoga/Self-Inquiry - Advaita (Non-Duality)

Ramana Mahars
Hi on Meditation Experiences

quote:
_____
Originally posted by chinna

quote:
_____
Originally posted by yogani

Hi Chinna:

I don't think we have any disagreement on the value of non-dual self-inquiry. Only on how and when it might be applied. With the multiple points of view expressed here, anyone reading can find some assistance for making decisions about it according to their own inclination and need.

Many thanks for sharing!

The guru is in you.

_____

"He who has ears to hear, let him hear."

_____

Hi Chinna:

AYP is more concerned with helping everyone find their ears. :-)

The guru is in you.

2009/09/25 12:32:35
Jnana Yoga/Self-Inquiry - Advaita (Non-Duality)
Ramana Mahars
Hi on Meditation Experiences

Hi Chinna:

All in due course...

Yes, there is a difference. All approaches rely on prerequisites, whether they choose to admit it or not. AYP is about covering prerequisites for as many people as possible. The goal is to leave no one to rely on "the stars" for finding salvation. Rather, it is a longing heart which can find its legs and its "ears," if provided enough effective means for doing so. It is really only about attending to the nuts and bolts (of which jnana/advaita is a part), and self-realization will fly.

I am not much interested in an "AYP point of view," or any other point of view. I am interested in opening doors. For this, the integration and transcendence of all points of view is essential. If this is in agreement with the sages, that's great. And if not, well, we are still going ahead with it.

Therefore, I do not see jnana/advaita as a specialized stand-alone approach that is only for those of a particular intellectual or philosophical bent. In fact, intellectual indulgence is well-known to be an obstruction to awakening. This is not to deny a stand-alone intellectual approach. As the saying goes, "Knock yourself out." :-)

But know this. With the pre-cultivation of abiding inner silence, much of the futility can be by-passed. This is a fact that has been demonstrated again and again. But no busy intellect wants to hear it. That's fine. Each will choose their own way. Live and let live, which is what you are asking. Fair enough.

Now here's the rub. When jnana/advaita claims exclusivity and superiority over a broad range of methods, then you must expect some push-back, for that is nothing but ideological posturing. I am not directing this observation specifically at you, for you have been very kind and generous, and it is much appreciated. However, for many, jnana/advaita is adopted as a "magic bullet" ideology that breeds a false sense of sectarian superiority, which, ironically, is duality to the extreme.

True non-duality is the way of absolute inclusion, whether the ideology-clinging mind likes it or not.

So, regardless of our persuasion, it is good if we can ask ourselves regularly, "Am I in love with enlightenment, or only with 'an idea' of enlightenment?" If it is the latter, and we are not applying systematic means for transcending it, we are at risk of becoming a hazard to ourselves and others.

While jnana/advaita may seem to you an innocent endeavor, a wonderful playground promising "instant enlightenment" for curious minds, it also, with its ideological matter-of-factness, often finds itself debunking the realms of spiritual practice that benefit the vast majority of the population. This does not help anyone.

I'm not much concerned about it. We are just going to keep working on the prerequisites, and the rest will take care of itself. The truth will prevail. It is not about "this or that." There is only *This*, which we also call *That*.

All in due course ... and all the best! :-)

The guru is in you.

2009/09/25 20:39:06
Jnana Yoga/Self-Inquiry - Advaita (Non-Duality)
http://www.aypsite.org/forum/topic.asp?TOPIC_ID=6247&REPLY_ID=57634&whichpage=-1
Ramana Mahars
Hi on Meditation Experiences

quote:
_____
Originally posted by chinna

Thanks for your reply. But you caricature what I say, every time. You seem to be responding to something very different from what I am actually saying. You compare the best of what you offer (which is extraordinarily sane and good) with the worst of neo-advaita. History suggests that there are just as many misleading advocates of every path as there are skilfull guides.
peace
_____

Apologies, Chinna.

It is not my intention to offend. At this stage of the game, given the nature of the work here, it is very difficult for me to resonate with a spiritual approach that is hard-pressed to produce real change in the population at large, no matter how skillfully it is presented. Therefore, it is impossible for me to endorse jnana/advaita as a stand-alone. This is not to diminish what jnana/advaita is for you or anyone else who benefits from it as a stand-alone approach. The knowledge you share is precious, but only under very special circumstances. That simply will not do for the whole of humanity, which is the focus here.

On the other hand, the natural inclination toward self-inquiry that evolves with the rise of the witness and the underlying principles of jnana/advaita are highly relevant to what we are doing here, and AYP has moved to incorporate those aspects. As has been the case with all of the AYP practices, this often involves a stripping away of traditional elements to facilitate an effective integration into the whole of the open source practice system. Traditionalists often do not like that. Hopefully, the end result in the hands of many will help to compensate. Again, apologies...

While we may have a parting of the ways, we do not have a parting of the principles.

The guru is in you.

2009/09/08 14:08:25
Jnana Yoga/Self-Inquiry - Advaita (Non-Duality)
http://www.aypsite.org/forum/topic.asp?TOPIC_ID=6299&REPLY_ID=56497&whichpage=-1
The Habit of Narrating

Hi Carson:

There is nothing wrong with narrating if that is what happens. I'm a pretty good narrator myself. Let's see, now there is typing, now there is sending, now it is off for a walk -- doop-de-doop. :-)

The fact that you are questioning all this simply means you are moving beyond it already. No need to dive back in to manage it all. That sort of defeats the purpose, doesn't it? It is just the opposite. You can let it go as it likes. What has it got to do with your witness, your Self?

Your activities, outer or inner, don't have to change one iota, though they might. Whether or not they change isn't anything you have to be judging, or supervising, though it might seem like you are.

In the end it will all still be happening, and it will be okay. We gradually learn to be "in it but not of it." The "it" will not necessarily change.

We are finding our existence to be the depth of the ocean. Just because the ocean realizes itself does not mean the waves on the surface will suddenly be doing something different or going away. Of course, as the ocean radiates, there will be that divine outflow for the betterment of all. So the waves will tend to line up for evolutionary purposes. Then the narration becomes interesting, kind of like watching a cool movie. That guy who keeps narrating and questioning what is happening is part of the movie too. Relax and enjoy the show. :-)

The guru is in you.

2010/02/22 12:08:11
Jnana Yoga/Self-Inquiry - Advaita (Non-Duality)
http://www.aypsite.org/forum/topic.asp?TOPIC_ID=7320&REPLY_ID=65220&whichpage=-1
Is Self-Enquiry really necessary?

Hi Krish:

If a serious meditator using an effective daily practice never gives self-inquiry a second thought, it will happen anyway, because it is perceptual -- naturally seeing all objects from the point of view of rising inner silence (the witness) more and more. When that is happening, one "notices," and that is automatic inquiry. Noticing the objects of perception in stillness is enough to advance the process on non-dual enlightenment. It may become structured self-inquiry, or not, depending on the background and inclination of the practitioner.

This is why, in the AYP writings, a particular mode of self-inquiry is not put forth as "the method." Once the witness is coming up, perception will become relational (in stillness), and from there the approach will be quite personal, depending on the practitioner's ishta (chosen ideal) and resonance found with one or more approaches to self-inquiry, or no structured approach at all. This range of possibilities for self-inquiry was covered in Lesson 350, on the various ways one may move beyond the witness/object relationship into direct experience of non-duality.

And, yes, Lesson 351 referred to by Cosmic above is a very easy and effective way to engage in the self-inquiry process as part of our structured samyama practice, with no mess and no fuss -- a good place to start self-inquiry if we are well-established in core samyama practice. It gets right down to it -- releasing the most basic inquiry in stillness. In time, this practice leads to an intuitive sense of relational self-inquiry during daily activity, without accumulating a lot of non-relational mental baggage to be carried around all day long. We become the automatic inquiry in motion, which is stillness in action, the non-dual condition. :-)

All the best!

The guru is in you.

PS: For more lessons on "self-inquiry," check for links in the top "main techniques" section of the Topic Index.

2010/02/22 15:24:24
Jnana Yoga/Self-Inquiry - Advaita (Non-Duality)
http://www.aypsite.org/forum/topic.asp?TOPIC_ID=7320&REPLY_ID=65229&whichpage=-1
Is Self-Enquiry really necessary?

Hi Krish, and thank you.

AYP is a fresh look at venerable spiritual approaches across the board, minus the traditional limitations. Someone had to do it sometime. Why not us? And why not now?

If we dig into jnana and advaita teachings, we find that meditation and yoga have always been regarded as preparations for self-inquiry. It can be found in the teachings of both Ramana Mahars
Hi and Nisargadatta Maharaj, two 20th century giants of jnana/advaita, though hardly at all in the teachings of their many successors.

It has been a bit of a shadow game the great advaita teachers played, speaking of the uncompromising immutability of the non-dual nature of existence, while at the same time looking the other way, or outright encouraging practitioners to engage in the systematic methods of yoga. This contradictory approach has been confusing for many practitioners, often misleading them to believe that they must "walk the talk" of non-duality before they really can. It leads to what we have called "non-relational self-inquiry," lacking abiding inner silence (witness), and a formula for building thought-form castles in the air.

While the truth of the interconnectedness of yoga and advaita has always been there, it has been obscured, perhaps because the methods of practice have not been very effective on either side of that philosophical divide for large numbers of people.

The very few who manage to make it through this contradictory approach are the ones who were ripe and ready to fall off the tree anyway. Then, generally, they teach from that perspective of ripeness, with no systematic yoga practices recommended, which does not reach the vast majority of people who are yet to become ripe. This is essentially a denial of what is, in favor of the teacher's perspective: The proverbial forgetful mountain climber.

The more flexible advaita teachers do get this in time, and end up teaching meditative practices of one kind or other in an attempt to fill in the gap between the majority of their followers and the condition of ripeness (abiding witness) necessary for engaging in effective non-dual self-inquiry. Less flexible advaita teachers just keep hammering away at their followers with non-duality concepts, sometimes accompanied by bursts of shaktipat energy, which can be a rather chaotic approach.

In AYP, we put the entire process in the practitioner's hands, with lots of tools and self-pacing guidelines available. By utilizing effective daily practices and the unique experiential track of the practitioner, where the regulation of practices and measure of progress is according to direct experience rather than arbitrary external guidelines, we are finding many people experiencing the natural emergence of relational self-inquiry, with results that are quite fruitful. With effective tools, each will find it for themselves. Spiritual unfoldment on that basis is real, as many have verified.

And why not? Yoga has always been an integrated experience-based (scientific) approach. It is the unruly mind that has tended to dis-integrate it into conceptualizations of little value. Yoga is very smart about taking us beyond the mental mish-mash to ripeness, and beyond... :-)

The guru is in you.

2010/08/18 14:39:19
Jnana Yoga/Self-Inquiry - Advaita (Non-Duality)
http://www.aypsite.org/forum/topic.asp?TOPIC_ID=8276&REPLY_ID=72066&whichpage=-1
Walking the Line

quote:
_____
Originally posted by CarsonZi

In Yogani's recently posted lesson 426: http://www.aypsite.org/426.html he says; "A few are born to become enlightened in this life, while for the rest of us it may be only a possibility."
_____

Hi Carson and All:

The most important part of that quote is what comes right after. For context, here is the whole thing:

quote:
_____
A few are born to become enlightened in this life, while for the rest of us it may be only a possibility. Yet, for all of us the possibility is clearly there, and that is very significant. Where there is the possibility, there will be ways that can be devised to bring it into manifestation. It is a matter of having good tools available, and having the desire and willingness to put forth the effort toward the goal through daily practice.

So we are all special, and we live in a time when many more of us have the opportunity to live the fullness of enlightenment in this life. It is a matter of having the technology, and the willingness to use it to its full capacity.

In the old days, it was primarily those born ripe who fell off the tree. Now we all can. It is in our hands. :-)

The guru is in you.

2010/08/18 15:08:08
Jnana Yoga/Self-Inquiry - Advaita (Non-Duality)
http://www.aypsite.org/forum/topic.asp?TOPIC_ID=8276&REPLY_ID=72068&whichpage=-1
Walking the Line

quote:
_____
Originally posted by CarsonZi

So...... just ego :-)

Thanks Yogani:-)

Love!
_____

Hi Carson:

The ego can be very useful.

Who else would be sawing that limb, sitting on the part that will fall, if not the ego? :-)

The guru is in you.

PS: For those who might worry about this, the fall is into infinite peace and happiness. :-)

2010/08/18 16:28:30
Jnana Yoga/Self-Inquiry - Advaita (Non-Duality)
http://www.aypsite.org/forum/topic.asp?TOPIC_ID=8276&REPLY_ID=72075&whichpage=-1
Walking the Line

Hi Carson:

The ego acts not for cutting off its own head, but for expanding its view. What is the ego anyway, but identified awareness? It is the same awareness that we find in enlightenment when identification has faded. Same awareness -- much happier situation.

As for cutting the limb, if ego were not the one cutting it while sitting on it, there would be no limb, because limitation is what the limb is. We must operate from limitation to move beyond limitation. That is the rationale for practices also, and it works.

Attacking the ego does not help much. It never has. It is like saying, "Someday I will be able to fly to California without an airplane, so I will dump this crummy airplane today." Where does that leave us? Nowhere.

The ego is our airplane to enlightenment. We have to operate from where we are. It is not possible to operate from where we are not.

Someone wrote me recently asking if it was okay to meditate to be more successful in business. I said, sure, go for it. Meditating for business will be sure to lead to a broader view. If that person were discouraged from meditating for business, how would he ever get beyond that need? Meditating is the fastest way to do it, not by condemning or trying to ignore the attachment to business.

It is the same thing for health. Millions take up yoga for health. Why not? It can lead to much more than health.

If it is the ego who wants to meditate, that is great. It will lead beyond whatever the imagined reason is -- even the concept of enlightenment. Hard as we may try, we cannot imagine our way beyond the fact of what it is. We can only purify the vehicle (this nervous system) and become a fuller expression of our essential nature, which is pure bliss consciousness.

Honestly, I can think of nothing that would want to meditate besides ego (identified awareness). If that were not the case, there would be only pure awareness, and meditation would not be about purification and opening, but about basking in the infinite. Even then, it is the person who sits down to meditate. Or is it stillness in action sitting to meditate? Does it even matter?

We can only operate from where we are, and there is no practical reason to divide ourselves into good and bad, ego and non-ego. It's all one thing (one awareness) in the process of transformation from expressing with identification to expressing without identification.

As you know, I consider it counterproductive (non-relational) to be inquiring about these things too much before abiding inner silence is present. It is ego that brings us to the meditation seat to get us to that stage. Bravo! :-)

The guru is in you.

2010/08/18 17:31:22
Jnana Yoga/Self-Inquiry - Advaita (Non-Duality)

Walking the Line

quote:
_____
Originally posted by CarsonZi

There are differing degrees of abiding inner silence though right? It isn't an "on/off" sort of thing is it? Meaning, am I too early to be properly utilizing self inquiry? (I know you can't really Know this) I'm not doing "active" self inquiry...I'm letting it happen as and when it does....but I guess I can get a little carried away with it once the process begins.
_____

Hi Carson:

Self-inquiry can be very helpful once we are able to release our inquiry in stillness, no matter what procedure of inquiry we may be using. That requires some abiding inner silence, obviously. It is abiding inner silence that draws us to self-inquiry.

We will know it is time for self-inquiry if we feel the identification of our awareness fading when we engage in inquiry. If we are feeling confusion, strain, headache, etc., then we can be pretty sure we are getting ahead of ourselves, and it is time to self-pace.

This lesson offers additional perspective on relational vs. non-relational self-inquiry, and technique suggestions as well:
http://www.aypsite.org/356.html

Enjoy the ride. :-)

The guru is in you.

2010/10/14 11:14:17
Jnana Yoga/Self-Inquiry - Advaita (Non-Duality)
http://www.aypsite.org/forum/topic.asp?TOPIC_ID=8571&REPLY_ID=73794&whichpage=-1
What do you find significant?

quote:
_____
Originally posted by CarsonZi

So, I'm wondering how you would answer the "What do you find significant?" question. Does it turn your mind off? I know there are hundreds of questions that are "designed/capable" of creating this effect ("Who am I" kind of questions), but none of these have ever shut down the mind like this question did. Which begs (IMO) a few other questions..... Does it matter which question is used? Is there even a point to consciously asking these questions, or is this "shutting down of the mind" effect only going to happen when the question comes to you on it's own?
_____

Hi Carson:

Yes, the question(s) may be unique to each individual. This is why AYP takes an open approach to self-inquiry, focusing instead on the enabling principle of systematically cultivating abiding inner silence (the witness), and "activating stillness" through structured samyama practice. From there, the flow into self-inquiry will be natural, according to individual inspiration and preference.

Btw, as a rule, it is best to save self-inquiry for after sitting practices. It is good to keep in place the underlying cause of effective self-inquiry (cultivation of the witness), and then capitalize on the effects afterward. There will be rare exceptions, like your dramatic experience described above, but we don't want readers to think that continually pursuing thought processes during deep meditation will be an aid to practice, because it will not.

The guru is in you.

Forum 9 – Bhakti and Karma Yoga

The evolutionary roles of desire and devotion, and the rise of divine love and service flowing through us.
http://www.aypsite.org/forum/forum.asp?FORUM_ID=23

2005/07/12 11:03:34
Bhakti and Karma Yoga
http://www.aypsite.org/forum/topic.asp?TOPIC_ID=280
Bhakti and Karma Yoga

Note: As of May 18, 2009, the "Bhakti, Jnana and Karma Yogas" forum category has been split in two, to better accommodate the expansion of practitioner experiences and the AYP lessons. Happily, both are moving steadily deeper into non-duality/unity topics of discussion. As advanced experiences and our collective understanding of them continue to unfold, the forums are being adapted accordingly. The two forums are:

Jnana Yoga - Advaita Vedanta (Non-Duality):
http://www.aypsite.org/forum/forum.asp?FORUM_ID=54

Bhakti and Karma Yoga:
http://www.aypsite.org/forum/forum.asp?FORUM_ID=23

Here is the introduction from the original "Bhakti, Jnana and Karma Yogas" forum category. It is as relevant a starting point as ever:

Way back in the 1890s, a great sage named Vivekananda came from India to the West. He was the first from India who became widely known, and he paved the way for the many more sages and teachers who would follow throughout the 20th century.

Vivekananda spoke about the eight-limbed path of Patanjali's Yoga Sutras. He called it "Raja Yoga." He also spoke about three additional paths of yoga: Jnana, Bhakti and Karma. These correspond to the yogic roles of mind, heart, and our actions. The first two limbs of Raja Yoga, the yamas and niyamas, actually include these, but Vivekananda separated them out, perhaps because they have to do more with our ongoing thoughts, feelings and conduct throughout the day, rather than with the sessions of yoga postures and sitting practices which make up the rest of the eight limbs.

Jnana has been called the path of the intellect, the path of discrimination. Discrimination of what? Of truth. And what is the truth? According to great sages like Ramana Maharishi, the truth is found in inquiry -- in the simple question, "Who am I?" If we ask this question in earnest, repeatedly, with an intense longing to know (a blending with bhakti), then truth will come up in us and around us. Jnana is not primarily about gathering intellectual information, or building big philosophical structures. True jnana is a process of thinking the mind beyond itself. The best job of the mind in yoga is to think itself out of a job! If we can decide to practice meditation and other yoga practices, and stick with a daily routine of practices over the long haul, the mind will be serving us well in yoga. And in all other areas of life too, because our thinking will come into harmony with our inner silence. A mind moving in silence is divine mind, the field of Oneness, or unity. See Lesson #185 at http://www.aypsite.org/185.html

Bhakti is called "the science of devotion" in AYP. It truly is a science, because it has known causes and effects which can be harnessed by diligent practitioners. If we know how to redirect our emotional energy toward our highest ideal, whether it be "God" or "Truth" or "Love," then huge invisible forces will be turned loose that bring knowledge to us in an avalanche. Such is the power of bhakti. See Lesson #67 at http://www.aypsite.org/67.html

Karma means action and its effects. Karma is what we do and how it affects us and others. The action side of karma yoga is found in gradually gravitating toward an attitude of serving others. No one can force this on us. It comes up naturally in us when we have been doing yoga practices -- meditation, pranayama and asanas. Then the karmas (effects) residing in our nervous system are illuminated from within and we cannot help but care more for those around us, in our own way. Then karma yoga really shines and is not an obligation or drudgery. Just the opposite. Service becomes pure joy! See Lesson #228 at http://www.aypsite.org/228.html

This forum is for discussing our practical experiences in applying our emotions, mind and daily actions to help us along the path of yoga. It can be as simple as saying "Yes!" to the voice inside that is calling us to do what is necessary to grow, and making the choices that will propel us forward.

Each of these three categories of yoga can stimulate many dimensions of discussion and spiritual progress:

Jnana Yoga -- The intellectual examination (and release) of the nature of existence.
Bhakti Yoga -- The role of desire in our daily spiritual practices, and the many devotional paths of worship.
Karma Yoga -- The natural rise of outpouring divine and service to others (who we see increasingly as out own *Self*) as our spiritual progress advances.

Feel free to indulge. Enjoy!

The guru is in you.

2005/08/12 10:36:49
Bhakti and Karma Yoga
http://www.aypsite.org/forum/topic.asp?TOPIC_ID=390&REPLY_ID=345&whichpage=-1
Opening the heart chakra

Hello Frank:

While jyotish/astrology has some merit in pondering general trends, I don't recommend it for determining such specific things as one's ishta (chosen ideal). That is a contradiction, isn't it? Ishta means one's chosen ideal -- not an ideal chosen by an astrologer or anyone else. It is entirely personal, based on the deepest longings within one's heart. Indeed, one's ishta may begin as one thing (like the burning question, "Who am I?"), and end up as something else later on (a particular deity or an intimate relationship with the truth of one's own inner silence and ecstatic energies.) Who can decide these things but the person involved? Enlightenment is not gained through consultants, but through developing self-reliance in matters of our own spirit.

Add to this the fact that some of the major schools of jyotish cannot agree on what yuga (age) we are in, or even how long a yuga is! Are these the people we should be entrusting our spiritual destiny to? I think not. Much better to listen closely to the voice of divine longing within us. The heart is a better doorway to the cosmos than the mind.

The guru is in you.

PS -- For more on the AYP approach to bhakti and ishta, see main lesson #67. http://www.aypsite.org/67.html

2005/11/18 15:14:17
Bhakti and Karma Yoga
http://www.aypsite.org/forum/topic.asp?TOPIC_ID=594&REPLY_ID=1563&whichpage=-1
Importance of Purpose/goal

Hi Near:

Rather than a specific objective, what is most important in yoga is spiritual desire, or bhakti, which is by nature always looking for more growth. That is the engine that drives all spiritual development.

And yes, the level of our bhakti will color the results in our practices. It is our heart instinctively calling for God or Truth within us that increases the effectiveness of our yoga. It is not that we engage in inner rituals in our practice. It is the innate resident attraction we feel for the divine that has the effect. So be mindful not to burden the specific procedures of yoga practice with mental exercises that are not resident bhakti -- only ritual trying to stimulate bhakti. Better to be doing our bhakti generating activities outside our other yoga practices. Review lesson #67 on that. http://www.aypsite.org/67.html

It is a fact that if we fix our desire on a single outcome, like physical health, we may not be motivated to do the practices that reach beyond physical health all the way in to our inner divinity. Bhakti is the prerequisite for making those choices, and it is also a product of sound spiritual practices...

Bhakti has an object, called "ishta" (chosen ideal), but it is not fixed. Rather, it is constantly expanding and morphing toward the infinite. That is the nature of the object which we imbue with divine qualities within us. Bhakti is a process going on deep inside us that yields divine results, much like samyama. That is the difference between having a material goal and having bhakti. Bhakti has no limits. So much so that we have to self-pace bhakti sometimes to keep from frying in our own spiritual enthusiasm!

What is the source of bhakti? Our own inner desire for freedom, which is an aspect of our inner silence. That is why meditation invariably lights the fire of bhakti. Rising bhakti is a symptom of rising inner silence. It is the guru moving within us. And it is pure love.

I once knew a sage who used to say: "Oh God, Thou art the goal in me!"
That is the kind of goal-setting yogis do. It leaves the field wide open for treading the path by whatever means that will bring the desired result.

The guru is in you.

PS -- Btw, "enlightenment" as an object is a material goal. But it is a good stepping stone goal on the way to something more -- surrender to God or Truth. So, "enlightenment" is not anything really. Just a word. That is why I say we can't have it until we give it away. See this lesson on "getting enlightenment." http://www.aypsite.org/120.html

2006/04/21 10:29:42
Bhakti and Karma Yoga
http://www.aypsite.org/forum/topic.asp?TOPIC_ID=1062&REPLY_ID=6234&whichpage=-1
Role of Bhakti in yogic sadhana

Hi Satinder:

I agree with you very much that bhakti is the fuel of all spiritual progress.

In AYP we take a direct angle on using bhakti (spiritual desire and devotion) to inspire daily spiritual practices, which completes the connection between our spirtual longing and effective implementation of sadhana. The ecstatic bliss and all of that are but the result of that process. See these lessons for more on the use of bhakti in AYP:
http://www.aypsite.org/12.html
http://www.aypsite.org/67.html
Also see "desire/bhakti" in the topic index (top of list) for more lessons on this.

With this integrated approach of using bhakti in direct relation with a full program of spiritual practices, there is great power for transformation -- so much that we will sometimes be called to temporarily self-pace (tone down) our practice, and even tone down our bhakti, which is a great force for transformation within us. In doing so, we assure the maximum spiritual progress we can absorb in a given time within safe limits.

All the best!

The guru is in you.

2006/07/12 09:33:49
Bhakti and Karma Yoga
http://www.aypsite.org/forum/topic.asp?TOPIC_ID=1316&REPLY_ID=9266&whichpage=-1
Kirtanananda - The Joy of Kirtan

Hi Kirtanman:

There are no taboo practices in or in relation to AYP. It is simply a matter of the practical aspects of managing the cause and effect of practices in our lives. Yoga is a process of purification and opening, and that is what we each are obliged to manage prudently to sustain steady, safe progress over the long term. This applies to the level of intensity of our bhakti, as well as all other practices. The more advanced we become, at least through the late intermediate stages of unfoldment, the more critical self-pacing will be.

It is what we do over the long term that will make the difference, not so much the glories of the moment, though we can certainly enjoy them. :-)

Carry on!

The guru is in you.

2007/06/27 15:42:08
Bhakti and Karma Yoga
http://www.aypsite.org/forum/topic.asp?TOPIC_ID=2684&REPLY_ID=23608&whichpage=-1
Resistance, fear and control issues

Hi All:

I don't think karma is actually "eradicated." It is transformed by the divine flow pouring out through it. In this sense, individuality is not lost either, only expressed increasingly divinely -- through expanding love from within, which is the simultaneous fading of contracted perception.

So where does the karma go? No place. We are only passing through it with expansion rather than contraction. So the expression of karma becomes purified. In fact, this is the meaning of "purification and opening" occurring in our practices, and flowing out into our everyday activities.

The same goes for creating new karma. As long as we are here on earth, we will be creating karma. Each breath we take creates karma. For every action there is reaction. The question is: What is flowing through us in our actions and reactions? This will be the product of our spiritual condition (our abiding inner silence and ecstatic radiance), which is cultivated via effective practices.

Note: Here is something I wrote on transforming karma back in 2005: http://www.aypsite.org/forum/topic.asp?TOPIC_ID=301#65

It could also be regarded as a matter of semantics. If our fear subsides and our conduct becomes more positive and radiant, is our karma gone? I suppose we could say so, at least the negative rendition of it. But, at the same time, we will continue to act through the very same inner impulses we have experienced with fear and loathing in the past. Only now with joy and forbearance. Is that no karma, or transformed karma? You decide. :-)

It was never about the karma, or getting rid of it, was it? We can no sooner get rid of the devil by focusing on getting rid of him. It will only make the contraction stronger. But we can transform the devil into an angel by going beyond to the realm of inner silence, pure bliss consciousness -- becoming That.

All karma (and life) is a sweet little puppy dog when we have become That. Then our karma is the impetus and opportunity for service, so there is no need to get rid of it. In fact, our karma becomes a blessing to us and everyone else. The divine flow is always looking to expand -- it is stillness in action.

Karma, past and present, provides the necessary channels for this.

All the best!

The guru is in you.

2007/06/29 17:53:22
Bhakti and Karma Yoga
http://www.aypsite.org/forum/topic.asp?TOPIC_ID=2684&REPLY_ID=23646&whichpage=-1
Resistance, fear and control issues

Hi Christi:

Yes, fully aware of objects and influences, and totally free (and constantly inspired) to act for the common good through those same objects and influences. That is what it is.

There are so many ways to describe the same thing. But there is only one thing going on -- human spiritual tranformation, assuming effective means for purification and opening are being consistently applied.

Whether karma (or its absence) is described as what someone is inclined to be doing or not doing (attached or unattached), or as the objects and influences themselves, doesn't change the reality of what is happening, which is a changing relationship with all that is going on within and around us. As we operate increasingly as stillness, our choices are affected accordingly, and the grip of cause and effect becomes less. The only grip was the one we created ourselves via contracted awareness, anyway. Karma? What karma? Maybe that is what the Buddha was talking about. Karma is only karma when we are reacting to it. But won't a sage also react within his or her surroundings to remove suffering, just as the Buddha did?

Do we become free from the influences of action and reaction? And is karma the influences or the conduct? It does seem to be semantics.

The truth is, as time goes on we can choose more easily to act as part of the natural divine flow expressing through whatever is happening, and that will illuminate all our actions and reactions. We will still chop wood and carry water, just like we did before, but the suffering will be less and less. The things we may wish to avoid now may be very things we will choose to fully engage in a freer state, filled with ecstatic bliss instead of the revulsion of the past. Ironic, isn't it?

It is the paradox of divine flow, which raises the question, "What is freedom anyhow?" Is it freedom to do or not to do? I don't think so. It is the freedom to love and give infinitely, and not suffer in the process. Happiness is becoming a channel of infinite giving. Everything else is a strategy based on limitation.

I agree that static samad

Hi (the witness) is not enough. It is a good first step. The non-dualists make a big hoopla about unconditioned awareness, but it is incomplete without full engagement in the world. Even total absorption (nirvikalpa) is not complete. We will not be penetrating the karma thing (by whichever definition) until we are wide awake in the world and moving in samad

Hi (sahaj) -- stillness in action.

Wisdom is both cause and effect in this. We learn by doing, without doing. :-)

The guru is in you.

2007/12/31 11:31:11
Bhakti and Karma Yoga
http://www.aypsite.org/forum/topic.asp?TOPIC_ID=3318&REPLY_ID=28411&whichpage=-1
Spiritual Envy and Jealousy

Hi Louis:

Thanks very much for your courageous sharing. It is purification and opening on the move for sure. Let's just let it happen, while self-pacing as needed.

The progress that matters most is our own in relation to where we were last month and last year. Everyone is on their own journey. And, ultimately, everyone's progress is our own also.

The phenomenon of widespread human spiritual transformation, which used to creep imperceptibly from century to century, shifted to being observable over a few decades during the past 50 years. Now, amazingly, the same multi-decade process can be observed to be happening over a few years!

We seem to be heading in the right direction. It's a great time to be on the path, yes? :-)

Onward into 2008, and beyond, and all the best to everyone!

The guru is in you.

2008/01/01 12:50:46
Bhakti and Karma Yoga
http://www.aypsite.org/forum/topic.asp?TOPIC_ID=3318&REPLY_ID=28457&whichpage=-1
Spiritual Envy and Jealousy

quote:
_____
Originally posted by Sparkle

quote:
_____
Recently I have heard "The love that you withhold is the pain that you carry". I figure it is the same thing with jealousy and praise. The more praise you offer to the people that exceed you in spiritual merits and soul maturity, the less jealousy you will feel towards them. Something to meditate upon.
_____
I see it from the point of view that it actually has nothing to do with the person or people I would feel envy or jealousy for, and everything - 100% - to do with me. I am just projecting these thoughts and feelings onto them.
If I cop on to myself and realise that it is just a story of the thinking mind, which feeds and fuels the emotions and feelings. When I do this then inner silence is given a chance to purify, open and expand the consciousness.

I think too that "withheld love" is another story we all have. If we see it as a story and just feel the effects of it in the body without attaching anything to it - just be present in the moment, when we eat our dinner, be fully conscious in eating our dinner, when we walk -feel the pavement with our feet, see the trees, be present to people passing by etc etc.
In this way those feeling, which we are also aware of in the present moment, will dissolve away, sometimes quickly, sometimes slowely.

Of course the base practice, of the AYP deep meditation and spinal breathing, maintains and developes the inner silence necessary for all this to happen.
Just my 2 cents
_____

Hi Louis:

You have just summed up the new Self-Inquiry book. Good job! Especially since the book isn't out yet. :-)

The book focuses on underlying principles and common sense applications of self-inquiry, while avoiding giving "cookbook" approaches. Key measuring rods are included covering the relationship between rising inner silence (the witness) and self-inquiry, to aid us in *seeing* where we are in the over all process, so we can self-pace our practice accordingly.

The book will be out in a few weeks.

All the best!

The guru is in you.

2008/02/22 17:35:29
Bhakti and Karma Yoga
http://www.aypsite.org/forum/topic.asp?TOPIC_ID=3494&REPLY_ID=30430&whichpage=-1
question regarding bhakti

Hi SeekerofTruth:

If we have desire, we can use it to advance ourselves on the path by aiming it at a high ideal -- our ishta (chosen ideal). Of course, we must be willing to act also, and practices are a direct manifestation of our desire.

To form the habit of a regular routine of practice is important, because it is regular practice over the long term that will make the difference, whether we have strong spiritual desire or not. In that sense, our daily routine may be like "brushing teeth," performed like clockwork.

If we have strong desire for advancement, it should not affect the procedure of our practice. However, the presence of bhakti (spiritual desire) in general will make all of our practices more powerful.

So ongoing bhakti and a regular habit of practice are both beneficial. At times we may be obliged to use self-pacing with both, but that is another story. :-)

The long run scenario is that practices will continue according to habit, and the results and influences of practice will show up more and more in daily life (see my other post today touching on that). A central part of this evolution will be increasing bhakti on a higher level, which can reach far beyond our person. This will become known as an outpouring of divine love. So personal bhakti gradually becomes universal bhakti -- this is a "letting go," but the bhakti becomes even more. By then, it has become a constant pouring of love for the divine, coming from the divine. It is the melting of the heart to become a pure channel of divine love in the world, which is anything but wishy-washy. Mountains can be moved with such love, and entire civilizations can be illuminated from within.

So it is good to bring our bhakti along with us all the way to the end, while keeping our daily routine of practices intact... :-)

Bhakti comes in many forms. It can be very quiet and determined, or gushing all over the place. Bhakti might even seem selfish. It is a personal thing, as is our choice of ishta. Anyone who is engaged in regular spiritual practices has bhakti. Without spiritual desire there can be no spiritual practice. And spiritual practice brings more bhakti, spiraling higher and higher. Meanwhile we just keep doing our daily practices without fanfare. So it goes...

The guru is in you.

2008/04/05 10:52:03
Bhakti and Karma Yoga
http://www.aypsite.org/forum/topic.asp?TOPIC_ID=3716&REPLY_ID=32229&whichpage=-1
Bhakti - getting a new picture of it

quote:
_____
Originally posted by emc

The disturbed emotions function as fuel to bhakti. Not long ago I found myself quite ishtaless (see http://www.aypsite.org/forum/topic.asp?TOPIC_ID=3389#29079), and was confused over that concept. Now my ishta is clear. Superclear. I just didn't see it before! I don't care if it is an illusion or not. It's working! My journey is going very fast forward, always burning the tires in the curves. I see now why that is! It's the beautiful hatefulness!
_____

Hi emc:

Yes, all emotions will be harnessed for divine purpose, even our most negative ones. It is stillness in action. All of our seeking and running away are for *That*. As soon as we realize it, Whooosh!

That is bhakti. Bravo! :-)

The guru is in you.

2008/04/15 15:57:21
Bhakti and Karma Yoga
http://www.aypsite.org/forum/topic.asp?TOPIC_ID=3782&REPLY_ID=32697&whichpage=-1
Understanding

Hi Katrine:

Very beautiful. Isn't it wonderful how understanding resides beyond ideas in the radiance of love? It is not a process of mind, but an Ahhhh...

It is not something the intellect can grasp, but we know it when we feel it -- presence in silent radiance -- all-knowing, all loving. That's it, and we just continue to go about our business, and there is no separation. As soon as we draw conclusions, normal activity stops, and so does union.

I have been corresponding with someone recently about the Self-Inquiry book, and the same kind of thing came up. We were discussing the "idea handles" that are provided in the book to aid in "understanding" the complex process of inquiry melting in stillness, even as normal functioning in the world continues.

Strangely, people who read the book find openings happening according to their need. Nothing I ever could anticipate. Yet, it happens. We consider a few ideas related to the process of self-inquiry occurring in stillness, and when we "understand," the ideas are gone, replaced with loving radiance. So the Self-Inquiry book isn't about ideas at all.

Go figure. On second thought, don't bother. Just meditate, go out and do, and enjoy! :-)

Your lovely sharing reminded me of this. It is all around us. It is what we are.

The guru is in you.

2008/06/04 08:22:07
Bhakti and Karma Yoga
http://www.aypsite.org/forum/topic.asp?TOPIC_ID=3988&REPLY_ID=34364&whichpage=-1
Karma & Spiritual Progress

Hi All:

Since the role of karma has been brought up here, I can't resist sharing that the **Bhakti and Karma Yoga book** will be out in a few weeks.

In fact, it is already available through some third party ebook vendors -- see the list of sources for ebooks and audiobooks near the bottom of the AYP Books Page. Once the paperback edition shows up on Amazon, we will do an official roll-out.

Below is the table of contents, and an excerpt.

Yes, the more inner silence we have, the quicker we will learn the lessons that karma brings to us. We find new meaning in the phrase "instant karma." :-)

The guru is in you.

Table of Contents

Chapter 1 – Desire and Action

Chapter 2 – Bhakti Yoga
Bhakti – Up Close and Personal
Ishta – The Chosen Ideal
The Systematic Transformation of Emotion
Bhakti and the Limbs of Yoga

Chapter 3 – Karma Yoga
Action and its Consequences
The Spiritual Evolution of Action
The Role of Service

Chapter 4 – Passionate Living
A Journey from Here to Here
The Dance of Unity

Further Reading and Support

From Chapter 3 on Karma Yoga

Transcending Karma and Putting It to Good Use

While, on the one hand, it is not possible to fathom the full consequences of karma, on the other hand it is quite possible to influence all outcomes of karma through our actions. We have a choice about how we view the world and what we do in our life each day. The actions we choose to undertake will have short term and long term consequences.

Our choices will be colored by the many influences in our lives (unfathomable karma!), and the ingrained habits we live by, so we might question whether our supposed free will is an illusion. Do we really have a choice about the things we do? If we have given the time and effort to strengthen a higher ideal in our life, we will have a choice. Our ideal, our ishta, will be our choice. From that, everything else will flow. This is the vital connection between bhakti and the actions we undertake, which determine our relationship to the karmic machinery of cause and effect that is constantly operating in life.

Whether our chosen ideal is for God or for Truth, in whatever form we may be drawn to, the effect will be the same. Ideals like these reach beyond the limiting aspects of karma. Having a high ideal is the sure way to reach beyond whatever limitations we are facing in life. Devotion to a high ideal is the way by which we can transcend karma, even while we are making good use of its underlying principles.

There is free will. However, exercising it effectively requires some finesse. If our chosen ideal inspires us to make choices that take us beyond the influences that distract us, then we will be on our way.

Developing bhakti in relation to our chosen ideal is the first step. Then we will be presented with opportunities and act in ways that promote the process of our spiritual development. In the AYP approach, we use an integrated system of practices, beginning with deep meditation. This first step in practice is a key one, once we have found the will to act on our spiritual desire.

With deep meditation, we are cultivating the natural presence of inner silence within ourselves, an abiding stillness that penetrates all of our thoughts, feelings and actions. This innate stillness, also referred to as pure bliss consciousness, is beyond the ups and downs of life. Life goes on as it did before, but stillness resides in us as a silent witness that we recognize as our own self. As we come to know our Self beyond the many influences in our life, it has a profound effect on the way we view events. We see life occurring as change on the ocean of our stillness. Even catastrophic events will be unable to touch us in our deepest realm of Self-awareness.

This is the transcendence of karma. It is not the elimination of karma. Karma will go on, but our relationship with it will change, and it's role in our life will change also.

Once we have begun daily deep meditation, we will be on the road to becoming the master of karma, rather than its servant. When we act from the perspective of inner silence, our actions will be capable of transforming the influences of karma in ways that are evolutionary and joyfully liberating, rather than in ways that are darkly limiting. For one who is awakening in the fullness of expanding inner silence, the mechanics of karma become a vehicle for spiritual development. Likewise, the expansion of inner silence through daily deep meditation provides for constant expansion of bhakti. It is a cycle of desire, action and consequences leading to a life of ever-expanding peace, creativity, and joyous service.

This shift is a gradual one, occurring over years of daily deep meditation, increasing bhakti and the normal course of our life's activities. Steadily, our actions in daily life rise to the level of divine relationship. While, before, we may have spent significant energy attempting to either reclaim or change the past, we now spend our time in the present, enjoying what is, and engaging in conduct that is both immediately fulfilling and sowing the seeds for a better future. Both our past and future can be made better by living increasingly in the now.

We do not do this by trying to. It cannot be done that way. We can't will an immediate shift in our quality of life, because the life we are living has been structured in us for a long time. But we can gradually unwind the structures within us through the power of bhakti and yoga practices. And, in doing so, we can transform our relationship with karma. Karma will not be eliminated. It will be transformed. There is the idea that karma can be erased, made to go away. This is not so. As long as we have action, we will have consequences, the process of karma. But we can transform karma's influence to be uplifting and divine – this is just as true for so-called negative karma as it is for so-called positive karma. The fact that consequences are coming to us from past actions does not mean any particular coloring comes with it. It is we in the present who do the coloring. All karma can be seen as being for good or ill. As our inner silence grows and matures, all karma will become a positive springboard to new openings in spirit.

This is not a passive experience. It is not the killing off of desires. It is the transformation of desire to divine purpose. Then we find that our ever-seeking desire has been the guru in us all along, carrying us steadily forward into fullness. Then all events become opportunities.

The blend of bhakti, spiritual practices like deep meditation, and our actions in ordinary life, leads to a harmonizing of influences sown in the past, and the fulfillment of openings in the future. It is all happening in the now. While it has been said that we should "Be here now," this can be expanded to say, "Be and do here now."

Our active devotion to our chosen ideal is what makes the difference. Once we have realized our abiding inner silence, we can make good use of karma, no matter what it is bringing us in life.

....

2008/06/06 12:35:02
Bhakti and Karma Yoga
http://www.aypsite.org/forum/topic.asp?TOPIC_ID=3988&REPLY_ID=34399&whichpage=-1
Karma & Spiritual Progress

Hi emc, Kathy and VIL:

Thank you. Glad to hear you find it interesting. :-)

Even though the *Bhakti and Karma Yoga* book is not quite out yet, I am finishing up the draft for the *Eight Limbs of Yoga* book here, which will have us all caught up with the scheduled Enlightenment Series books this summer.

Then it is back to online lesson posting, leading eventually to *AYP Easy Lessons Volume 2*.

Keeping busy here. Not sure where all this is coming from.

Karma transforming?

All the best!

The guru is in you.

2008/07/16 10:34:52
Bhakti and Karma Yoga
http://www.aypsite.org/forum/topic.asp?TOPIC_ID=4155&REPLY_ID=35557&whichpage=-1
Bakt
Hi clarification

Hi Mani:

It is good progress, with more purification going on. The discomfort should pass (if it does not, it will be good to check with a doctor). Be sure to self-pace your practices (and bhakti) for progress with comfort.

You may also be interested in this lesson on "heart breathing," which can be used with ishta (our chosen ideal): http://www.aypsite.org/220.html (see the following two lessons also on "heart space")

But not to overdo. One step at a time. :-)

The guru is in you.

2008/08/11 18:16:11
Bhakti and Karma Yoga

http://www.aypsite.org/forum/topic.asp?TOPIC_ID=4266&REPLY_ID=36226&whichpage=-1
right and wrong/ karma

quote:
_____
Originally posted by tubeseeker

from what I am gathering, reading on here, yoganis book and some other books it seems that some gurus dont believe in sin, and the concept of right and wrong. so if there is no such thing as sin or right and wrong, then what is karma. If someone kills somebody that will be on their karma and they will have to fix their karma and may suffer because of it.
thanks
Neil

_____

Hi Tubeseeker:

The implication is not that the kind of action we undertake doesn't matter. Certainly it does, and the longer we have been meditating, the better we come to know that from within. It is the rise of evolutionary conduct (yama and niyama) directly from inner silence. With inner silence (the source of all morality) the message comes very quickly, and we find ourselves adjusting our conduct accordingly.

Before then, conduct will be regulated by whatever conscience we have, our willpower, and the laws of right and wrong in religion and society. All of these serve a purpose. However, distinctions of that kind are often on the level of mind, and are therefore subject to misallocation and abuse, as is so often the case where people are judging each other from artificial ethical platforms -- "good and bad," "winners and losers," "sinners and the righteous." It is the division of humanity, which is directly opposed to its unification. This is how many well-meaning systems have gone wrong. The way to fix it is by bringing in more inner silence through the people on all sides, i.e., more people engaged in daily spiritual practices, regardless of religion, culture, or position in society. It has been improving that way for some time, and there is much further to go.

Regarding karma resulting from past harmful actions, there are many ways that karma can unwind, depending on how much inner silence is coming up in the person. Karma does not produce fixed outcomes, as is often believed. It is highly variable, depending on our own spiritual condition. The choices we make about our spiritual path and our practices can dramatically alter the effects of our karma. All karma can be transcended and put to good use. The AYP Bhakti and Karma Yoga book goes into this in some detail. There is an excerpt from the book on the transformation of karma in this post.

Other excerpts from the book (text and audio) can be found here.

All the best!

The guru is in you.

2008/09/17 20:16:07
Bhakti and Karma Yoga
http://www.aypsite.org/forum/topic.asp?TOPIC_ID=4454&REPLY_ID=37774&whichpage=-1
What can I DO in daily life to further humanity?

Hi CarsonZi and All:

If you have not seen the movie "Pay It Forward," consider taking a look. It really captures the essence of service in a practical way. There is an AYP lesson on it here: http://www.aypsite.org/166.html

Many small acts of service, paid forward, add up to big change.

All the best!

The guru is in you.

2008/09/22 15:19:38
Bhakti and Karma Yoga
http://www.aypsite.org/forum/topic.asp?TOPIC_ID=4454&REPLY_ID=37966&whichpage=-1
What can I DO in daily life to further humanity?

Hi CarsonZi:

I think it is important to know that we cannot create desire in another person. It is desire coming from within the person that precedes everything else they may do on the path. It comes from surrender to their higher ideal -- their higher ideal, not ours. We can certainly inspire others to consider this, and that you are doing wonderfully by your own example. But beyond that, it is up to each individual. Whenever it happens, it is within the framework of each person's life aspirations and challenges.

To the degree our own expectations get tangled up in whether someone else is desiring spiritual unfoldment as much as we might wish them too, there is our lesson and our self-inquiry for today. When we can live amongst a crowd of people who care nothing about the spiritual path, and keep radiating and smiling in stillness, then we are really getting somewhere. It is a letting go, which is part of our surrender to our ideal. And that energy will continue to radiate out to everyone else, and have its appropriate effect. How others may eventually manifest it, who can say? We are doing our part.

Of course, a little satsang (spiritual company) now and then doesn't hurt. That is what we are here for, and why we start meditation groups, teach, engage in retreats, and inspire research by the professionals who can inform the public. :-)

Carry on!

The guru is in you.

2008/12/06 11:40:17
Bhakti and Karma Yoga
http://www.aypsite.org/forum/topic.asp?TOPIC_ID=4852&REPLY_ID=41954&whichpage=-1
The chest, the iron dust and the magnet

quote:
_____
Originally posted by Katrine

quote:
_____
Anthem wrote: I see that white pinpoint of light randomly throughout the day as well as in lucid dreams and sitting practices. I have gone there or at least tried to and if the path isn't clear enough it can feel awful. I recently had some intense clearing in the Ajna, but have not had the opportunity to try going there again since. I also associate that blue/ violet color with Ajna.

I wish I could read about this somewhere, it would be helpful. I don't want to make any mistakes while exploring, there can be consequences!
_____

Yes....I guess this is why I don't feel drawn to go there. Maybe I am not ready for the impact. But also.....when resting as heart....nothing is lacking. There is absolute contentment.....and I *see*.....I love....even in great pain the resting is fully possible. I *experience* that I am not the feelings. I cry - and I experience that nobody is crying. All is allowed now! I can let my human nature be completely as it is! The feelings are just here...they belong to noone in particular. So why would I need to go out the Ajna door? I trust that the Ajna will fully open by itself.....that the opening will widen along with the resting as heart.

Yogani:

How do you feel about this exploring that Andrew is talking about? Are there written materials on it? Is it safe to explore?

_____

Hi Katrine and Anthem:

As we know, the way is a letting go, not a doing. It is always safe to explore letting go, guided by prudent self-pacing. One of the most reliable and safest ways to do this is to favor our practice over our experience (in this case, spinal breathing).

If all that sounds like paradox, it is. Doing without doing. Stillness in action. "Unpractice" -- the Zen of yoga. :-)

The guru is in you.

2008/12/07 10:06:36
Bhakti and Karma Yoga
http://www.aypsite.org/forum/topic.asp?TOPIC_ID=4852&REPLY_ID=41984&whichpage=-1
The chest, the iron dust and the magnet

quote:
_____
Originally posted by Anthem11

Hi Yogani,

Thanks for your reply to Katrine's post, it makes perfect sense to me.:-)

_____

Hi Anthem:

Cosmic samyama is another practice that expands our perception in stillness beyond this body and this dimension of time and space, though not in a singular direction like spinal breathing does in sushumna/ajna, root to brow and beyond.

All of the AYP practices do it in one way or other. Then we gradually find ourselves living IT naturally, with no striving necessary. It becomes a natural outpouring of divine love, rather than a striving to go in. The essence of freedom in all realms is found in this non-striving outpouring, even as we favor the means of producing that condition. We don't have to go There. IT is coming here. IT is already here. Paradox strikes again. :-)

The guru is in you.

2009/01/16 10:25:59
Bhakti and Karma Yoga
http://www.aypsite.org/forum/topic.asp?TOPIC_ID=5028&REPLY_ID=43580&whichpage=-1

Karma Yoga Self-Pacing

quote:
_____
Originally posted by emc

I clearly remember Yogani having talked about overload from karma yoga! I think I got the suggestion to go do some dirty work for someone else when I had overload once, and then he added a comment of the type: "Just don't overdo that either" since karma yoga also is about being "spiritual".

.

_____

Hi emc, Carson and All:

Yes, I did say it, but I don't remember where at the moment.

It is covered from the standpoint of self-pacing in bhakti (spiritual desire) in the Bhakti and Karma Yoga book, which also covers our inclination to engage in karma yoga (service).

There is a difference between pure grounding activity (physical exercise, digging in the dirt, etc.) and service (doing for others). There is certainly a positive and useful overlap between these two activities as well.

The basic difference is that in grounding activity we are simply bringing our energy down, while in service we are letting our energy flow out into our environment for the benefit of others. Grounding is much more localized in our nervous system, whereas in service our energy is going out and engaging with other energies, specifically the needs of others. The latter can bring a grounding effect in simple serving situations (like doing chores for someone else, etc.), but in more complex serving situations, the demands on our energy can be considerable. This is certainly the case in the service you are doing with addicts, Carson.

This increased demand on the energy flow coming through us brings purification and opening like in any other spiritual practice, and it is possible to overdo.

"Burnout" is a well-known phenomenon in the serving professions. It is a visible indication of overdoing in karma yoga. So, yes, self-pacing is appropriate in karma yoga. It means backing off a bit when needed and doing some simple grounding activity that does not involve the needs of others so much. It is about finding our balance.

As we advance in our spiritual practices and experiences, our ability to serve will increase. The divine outpouring grows year by year, and in time the energy coming through us can help many without undue strain on our nervous system.

We will be called according to our capacity, and more. It is a form of automatic yoga that is tied in with our bhakti. As with any automatic yoga, there will be a limit to how much growth we can accommodate in a given time period. The signals of overdoing will be clear, and we should honor them accordingly with prudent self-pacing. Then we will be able to contribute the maximum over time. The idea is to avoid burning out in the short term, which will enable us to continue to purify and open as a channel of the divine outpouring over the long term. In this way, our capacity will keep increasing gradually, rather than being interrupted for extended periods by overloads. It is the same principle we find in utilizing all of our practices, as discussed throughout the lessons.

Yoga is a marathon, not a sprint, and that applies in karma yoga too.

All the best! :-)

The guru is in you.

2009/01/16 11:03:38
Bhakti and Karma Yoga
http://www.aypsite.org/forum/topic.asp?TOPIC_ID=5028&REPLY_ID=43585&whichpage=-1
Karma Yoga Self-Pacing

quote:
_____
Originally posted by CarsonZi

Hi emc,

quote:
_____
Originally posted by emc

I clearly remember Yogani having talked about overload from karma yoga! I think I got the suggestion to go do some dirty work for someone else when I had overload once, and then he added a comment of the type: "Just don't overdo that either" since karma yoga also is about being "spiritual".
_____

Thanks for this....you have any reference thread I can read? There doesn't seem to be much on pacing karma yoga in the karma yoga lesson. #120 I believe?

Love,
Carson
_____

Hi Carson:

We may have crossed posts. Take a jump back up here: http://www.aypsite.org/forum/topic.asp?TOPIC_ID=5028#43580

Carry on! :-)

The guru is in you.

2009/01/16 11:18:14
Bhakti and Karma Yoga
http://www.aypsite.org/forum/topic.asp?TOPIC_ID=5028&REPLY_ID=43587&whichpage=-1
Karma Yoga Self-Pacing
PS: Yes, Carson, if we are purifying and opening through karma yoga, it may limit what we can do with other practices. There is only so much growth the nervous system can accommodate in a given time period. On the other hand, the growth of inner silence and ecstatic conductivity in sitting practices is what enables the effectiveness of other practices, like karma yoga, so I don't think we should regard the rise in effectiveness of these outward flowing practices as a replacement for sitting practices. It is a matter of keeping a balance between them.

The guru is in you.

2009/01/23 12:01:32
Bhakti and Karma Yoga
http://www.aypsite.org/forum/topic.asp?TOPIC_ID=5065&REPLY_ID=44041&whichpage=-1
Karma yoga and Samyama

Hi Ananda:

The dynamic involved in samyama, prayer, karma yoga and even self-inquiry, is that all of these things find their effectiveness and fruition in the rise of abiding inner silence.

Before then, these kinds of activities will be more involved with mind, emotions and the flow of energies back and forth. Then they are more transactional (this for that, one object for another), rather than "relational in stillness," which is an endless outpouring. The outpouring is the result of the application of the principles of samyama, which underlies all of these practices mentioned. It is the rise of stillness in action on all levels of our daily life.

Do energies still flow when we are moving into stillness, when it is the process of samyama - intentions surrendered in stillness? Yes, and we may see some depletion, or challenging karma flowing. At the same time, the further we progress in our practices and our inner purification and opening, the less we will be touched as these reactions occur, and we will learn to self-pace when the reactions are too much.

As we grow with our practices and their effects in daily living, there will be a mixture in the purity of our actions, gradually evolving toward more outflowing of stillness in action, and less action producing reaction. We will know by the increasing joy we find before, during and after our spontaneous acts of service, and fewer challenging karmic reflections coming back. This is another way of saying that the more advanced we become, the more we can handle.

Another way of looking at this process of transformation is as a rising innate ability to transform all karmas in and around us to a more immediate evolutionary purpose. Then it will not matter what karma is coming back. It will automatically be transformed into a positive influence, and not weigh on us as before. That is the power of mature abiding inner silence that has been activated and is moving in daily living. This is discussed in the AYP Bhakti and Karma Yoga book.

Along the way at every stage on our path, we are called according to our capacity, and usually more. We do all that we can, and self-pace the rest, so we can come back to serve another day. :-)

All the best!

The guru is in you.

2009/02/21 11:50:15
Bhakti and Karma Yoga
http://www.aypsite.org/forum/topic.asp?TOPIC_ID=5210&REPLY_ID=45682&whichpage=-1
bhakti questions

Hi Gayle:

All of our desires (and frustrations) are for wholeness, and the central "technique" of bhakti is favoring a gradual recognition of this, and, most importantly, acting on it. We have to begin somewhere, putting one foot in front of the other, and we keep going. Yoga practices will accelerate the process. Then emotions of all kinds will increasingly coalesce around the formation of our ideal representing our wholeness. It is called our "ishta," our "chosen ideal."

Over time, every feeling we have is increasingly redirected toward our ideal, and our ideal also gradually expands as we expand within. It is not all or nothing at any point in time. It is a gradual shift we find occurring in our life. Like all yoga practices, the growth of bhakti is gradual and cumulative. Which is not to say it cannot be momentous at times. Like all other practices, bhakti requires some self-pacing to even out the ups and downs, so our steady progress can continue over the long term.

Many of the discussions around the forums deal with bhakti, the translation of emotions, how it drives our practices and life choices, self-pacing, etc. You are on your path, and you will witness your process with more clarity with every passing month. As you do, the mystery of redirecting emotional energy will become much more clear. It is more about seeing than applying a mechanical technique. We will know it when we see it, and act accordingly. This is the process we favor.

Take the bhakti you have now and act on it. In time it will expand to encompass everything you do. The rise of inner silence is what facilitates this. Bhakti is the first manifestation of stillness in action. From that, all the rest will flow.

The AYP Bhakti and Karma Yoga book provides a layout of the path of bhakti, and how it relates into our actions, which is the karma yoga aspect -- the movement of our inner silence as a divine outpouring in daily living. Step-by-step, bit-by-bit, this is what happens.

"From a small acorn does the mighty oak tree grow."
Bhakti is like that. More experiential than conceptual. :-)

Enjoy!

The guru is in you.

2009/06/02 10:53:08
Bhakti and Karma Yoga
http://www.aypsite.org/forum/topic.asp?TOPIC_ID=5660&REPLY_ID=51753&whichpage=-1
Karma

Hi Osel:

Karma may be immutable, but its outcome is not. Outcome is dependent on the state of consciousness of the individual, as is how it is seen -- being "positive" or "negative." For the sage-in-the-oven, all karma is positive. The AYP Bhakti and Karma Yoga book goes into this in some detail. It will be showing up in the online lessons soon too.

War? What war? It is all in the mind. Is cleaning the windshield of the soul a war? If so, now there are two things to do -- clean the windshield and get over the war mentality. Maybe better to clean without making war. Just clean and let go...

I don't have much background in Buddhism, but do know that the idea isn't the thing. The more we get stuck in the idea, the further we are from the thing itself. It is like looking in the mirror and not seeing ourselves. How silly is that?

How many layers of ideology does one need to be "spiritual?"
None. Less is more. None is All.

If I had to pick a Buddhist teacher, it would be Adyashanti. He may be off the beaten track of traditional (idea encumbered) Buddhism, but he has got it right. And he happens to be sitting in your backyard. Whoa! :-)

But ya gotta be ripe for it... You will know when it is time.

The guru is in you.

2009/06/02 23:22:58
Bhakti and Karma Yoga
http://www.aypsite.org/forum/topic.asp?TOPIC_ID=5660&REPLY_ID=51778&whichpage=-1
Karma

Hi Osel:

With respect, truth is surrendering our deepest questions and longings in stillness, which then blossom from within. Ideology is being satisfied to provide someone else's answers.

Karma does not rule our heart or our will. In this way karma is transformed. Perhaps this is what you are talking about. But is it your own discovery? Until it is, it will be second hand information, no matter how venerable the source.

The greatest compliment we can pay our teacher is not to create a web with their ideas, but to unfold the truth from within ourselves. Then the divine love will be pouring out.

The guru is in you.

2009/06/03 10:12:08
Bhakti and Karma Yoga
http://www.aypsite.org/forum/topic.asp?TOPIC_ID=5660&REPLY_ID=51801&whichpage=-1
Karma
PS: Not intending to give you a hard time, Osel, but there is hazard in advising others to inquire about karma if it is not based in stillness. In AYP, this is what we call "non-relational self-inquiry," and it can lead to hopelessness and despair. It is easy to fall into victim mode if we get caught in the karma mind trap.

Presumably the prerequisite stillness cultivation aspect is covered on your path, but I see no clear emphasis on that here. For everyone's sake, it is best not to be putting the cart in front of the horse. Karma is transcended and transformed in stillness, not in any other way. The same goes for self-inquiry of any flavor.

And, of course, it is best to speak from our own experience rather than someone else's. That is not only a heads up for you, but for everyone who is utilizing AYP. Two cents worth of our own experience is worth $10 of anyone else's. The two cents of honest sharing on our inner condition is spiritual technique. The $10 on someone else's stuff is ideology. I will take the two cents over the $10 any day. :-)

The guru is in you.

2009/06/03 11:30:35
Bhakti and Karma Yoga

Hi Osel:

Thanks for the clarifications. It is fair to request that if you are advising people to analyze their karma, then it should be made clear how it is done without undue risk to the psychology and motivation to practice over the long term.

What you call "letting go" is analogous to what we do in samyama in the AYP system. We do not attempt that until there is some abiding inner silence cultivated in deep meditation over a period of time. It doesn't take long to put in a basic foundation.

This is at the crux of it in comparing inquiry-style meditation with mantra-style meditation.

In inquiry-style meditation, transcendence is achieved through dissolving many objects, the numerous manifestations of karma as you call them. There is nothing wrong with this, assuming the practitioner has the where-with-all to weather the many vagaries of the mind through a long and arduous process. Few do. I see now where the word "war" comes from. :-)

In mantra-style meditation, one object (the mantra) is dissolved repeatedly for a couple of short sessions per day, whereby abiding inner silence is cultivated. Then that abiding inner silence can be used to transcend everything else with much greater ease (no war). In this case, it may not be called "meditation" anymore, but samyama, or self-inquiry, or devotion to ishta, depending on one's nature and inclination. It doesn't matter what it is called. Stillness, once present, has its own agenda in us, and "letting go" (surrender) in any system will be much easier.

In Buddhist methods, including Adyashanti's style of meditation which is similar to what you describe, and in advaita in general, it is assumed that the average practitioner can navigate the transcendence of many objects through inquiry without inner silence being brought to the abiding state beforehand by other more focused means. This is a huge assumption, and accounts for the small percentage of the population having access to self-realization through Buddhist/advaita methods alone.

One has to somehow become "ripe" beforehand for these methods to work, which is exactly what we talk about in AYP, whereby abiding inner silence is cultivated quickly and easily, and then all the methods of Buddhism, advaita, samyama, self-inquiry, bhakti, service, etc., become much more accessible.

So I don't see an either-or situation here. No competition at all. Only the potential for a better integration and sequencing of existing methods across the board, regardless of tradition, that can enable many more people to have rapid access to the liberation we all seek.

That's all. :-)

The guru is in you.

2009/06/03 11:36:48
Bhakti and Karma Yoga
PS: Parallax and I cross-posted. He eloquently makes the same point. It is not a competition. Not an either-or. It is an efficient integration of methods coming from all sides for the benefit of all. May applied spiritual science continue to march forward. :-)

2009/06/03 13:38:22
Bhakti and Karma Yoga

quote:
_____
Originally posted by Konchok Ösel Dorje

Wouldn't you agree that once the practitioner has "abiding inner silence" they can drop the mantra and just "abide"?
_____

Hi Osel:

No, I would not agree, because this throws out the benefits of the advancing effects of mantra meditation, which have many subtle nuances. The cultivation of abiding inner silence is not a one time event. It is an endless continuum that is dependent on the ongoing use of a procedure. The expansion of abiding inner silence supports powerful additional methods of practice. So why on earth remove that support that clearly works?

We can "abide" for 23.33 hours per day, doing or not doing whatever we choose. Why throw out the 40 minutes (2 x 20) of structured practice that is forever increasing our presence as *That*? It makes no sense, even for someone who has been using mantra meditation for many years.

This does not preclude us from doing anything else in spiritual practice, coming from any source, assuming we use good common sense and are prudent in self-pacing. Besides the many additional methods within yoga, there is much in Buddhism (and other systems) that may be useful to one who has become the witness. The abiding witness is only the first stage after all. :-)

The guru is in you.

2009/06/03 14:38:26
Bhakti and Karma Yoga

Hi Osel:

Whatever cultivates abiding inner silence is good, mantra or no mantra.

But let's face it, multi-object self-inquiry is not the best place for most people to start. If it were, Eckhart Tolle would have millions of enlightened followers. He doesn't, though he is inspiring many on their path. No doubt about that. But how to get from inspiration to realization? That is the question.

Daily scheduled sit-down meditation with a specific procedure is a much better place to begin cultivating inner silence (abiding witness). Then the role of karma can be more easily known. There are a variety of styles of sit-down meditation found in all the traditions. Most people with some motivation can handle sit-down meditation if the instructions are simple, and the results noticeable.

Everything I am saying here is with the average seeking person in mind. Those who are already "ripe" are going to fall off the tree of illusion one way or another. It is everyone else that concerns me. The simpler we can make it, the better.

The guru is in you.

2010/05/14 13:46:07
Bhakti and Karma Yoga
http://www.aypsite.org/forum/topic.asp?TOPIC_ID=7733&REPLY_ID=68783&whichpage=-1
Bhakti for nothingness???

Hi Ananda:

The higher we go, the more in the trenches we are with everyone else. And that is exactly how it is supposed to be. :-)

The guru is in you.

2010/11/09 16:30:20
Bhakti and Karma Yoga
http://www.aypsite.org/forum/topic.asp?TOPIC_ID=8709&REPLY_ID=74993&whichpage=-1
Selfless Service??

Hi Carson:

It is always about the "self." With practices, the small (personal) self keeps getting smaller and the big (universal) Self keeps getting bigger. The only real say we have in it is our choices to practice effectively and go out and do in the world. The rest is in the hands of the emerging divine flow. Best not to judge too much. It only gets in the way.

Every ugly duckling (personal self) is destined to become a swan (universal Self). If we accept the ugly duckling as it is and keep going with methods that we know will work, it will happen. Doubt is an ugly duckling thing, and all we have to do is walk (or stumble) through it to our meditation seat each day, and keep active serving others as so inclined.

We all need a reward. The other person's happiness is a pretty good reward. Not needing a reward is a good reward too. It is okay to need something, and okay to need nothing. It all evens out in the long run. :-)

The guru is in you.

PS: Like self-inquiry, karma yoga is not a very effective stand-alone path. But with abiding inner silence coming in, both of these become spontaneous, and much more powerful. That is how swan-hood happens.

2010/11/17 17:43:47
Bhakti and Karma Yoga
http://www.aypsite.org/forum/topic.asp?TOPIC_ID=8757&REPLY_ID=75413&whichpage=-1
Fuel the Desire

Hi Kite:

What are you most passionate about deep in your heart? That is where your path is. It is up to you how to follow your passion. You can trust yourself in that.

The guru is in you.

2010/11/17 18:40:43
Bhakti and Karma Yoga
http://www.aypsite.org/forum/topic.asp?TOPIC_ID=8757&REPLY_ID=75417&whichpage=-1
Fuel the Desire

Hi Kite:

That need to know the truth is fundamental in all of us, whether it is seen clearly and raised to a passion or not. It is the seed of our awakening.

Meditation brings it out and makes it more passionate. It is an aspect of inner silence. We call it "bhakti."

The best way to view our progress with practices is in terms of our own journey -- where we are now versus last year, etc. Comparing to others (even a biological twin) can be a formula for frustration. We can only be who we are and travel our path, not be someone else and travel their path.

There are many helpers, tools, and fellow travelers, but the journey is our own. Taking responsibility is the key. Once we have done that, there is no stopping, no turning back. :-)

The guru is in you.

Forum 10 – Building a Daily Practice with Self-Pacing

Managing practices for maximum safe progress on the road to enlightenment.
http://www.aypsite.org/forum/forum.asp?FORUM_ID=18

2005/07/12 09:14:12
Building a Daily Practice with Self-Pacing
http://www.aypsite.org/forum/topic.asp?TOPIC_ID=279
Building a Daily Practice with Self-Pacing

In the old days, aspiring seekers were lucky if they could find someone who would teach them one, two or maybe three advanced yoga practices. And that was only if both the teacher and the student lived long enough for the several transfers of knowledge to happen. According to tradition, the transmission of spiritual knowledge could only occur over many years, and only to those who had "qualified" themselves through rigorous devotion and austerities. No wonder the world has seen so few enlightened people!

Now we find ourselves in the twenty-first century, catapulting headlong into this still-young information age. The knowledge of humanity in all fields is expanding at a mind-boggling rate. And, as the knowledge expands, the world is shrinking. Thanks to the Internet, the distance between opposite sides of the globe has been reduced to nothing. We are all close neighbors living on the same street in this medium.

It was inevitable that the free flow of information around the planet would wear away the boundaries that have kept the knowledge of advanced spiritual practices divided and unavailable to most of the people in the world. AYP is one example of how ancient spiritual knowledge can be integrated and opened up to all using modern technology. It's a good thing, and the time is right...

Along with the free flow of powerful knowledge comes responsibility -- an obligation we all have to put safety first, taking things in a logical sequence and not overdoing. We have a long list of practices here in AYP which we are free to undertake at our own discretion. Can we take them all on in a year? Five years? Ten years? It will depend on each person. Everyone has a unique capacity for spiritual practices, and we find out what ours is when we commit ourselves and begin the journey. This is the building of our daily spiritual practice routine.

We all have a present limit on how much we can undertake in practices. It is determined by the remaining obstructions in our nervous system. If we are doing too much, we will know soon enough, and then it is time for us to act according to the principles of "self-pacing."

Most of the questions that come to me are related to balancing practices with each other and daily activity. Overdoing or having an imbalance between practices and activity can yield a wide range of symptoms -- some extremely pleasurable (at least for a while), and some not so pleasurable. Yoga practices affect us in every way -- mentally, emotionally, physically and sensually, and the symptoms of imbalance can show up in any or all of these areas.

When there is an excess in our experience, the advice is to "self-pace," meaning ease back a bit on the practice that is causing the excessive purification. Bring it back to a comfortable level of inner purification. Then we can continue our practice at that level for a while, and consider creeping back up when the symptoms have stabilized. The same applies to taking on new practices. We only do what we can assimilate, taking it step-by-step, always. It is a never-ending balancing act -- a vitally important balancing act on the path of yoga. Without a good awareness and application self-pacing, it will not be possible to progress steadily on this path, or on any path for that matter.

So, in AYP, with so many powerful practices available, everyone is in the position to move forward at their own pace, and that is what this forum is about. Do share your experiences with overdoing, and how you have self-paced your practice to correct any excesses. If you are having symptoms of excess now and do not know what to do, you should be able to find help here.

Practice wisely, and enjoy!

The guru is in you.

2006/01/26 14:49:57
Building a Daily Practice with Self-Pacing
http://www.aypsite.org/forum/topic.asp?TOPIC_ID=321&REPLY_ID=2810&whichpage=-1
Reply Topic - Daily Practice & Self-Pacing Intro

Hello YogaMaya:

If you have extra time on your hands, that is a yogi/yogini's dream. You do not have to use it overdoing in practices, or sitting around twiddling your thumbs either. You can add some light asanas in front of your sitting practices, take a nice long time coming out at the end, and spend some extra time in service to others if so inclined. There are plenty of things to do that will help stabilize the progress gained in spinal breathing and deep meditation.

You don't have to wait forever to add on either. If things are smooth and you are spiritually hungry, it is okay to experiment according to your inclinations. In doing so you will find your limits. Just be prudent as you do so, knowing that in some cases (with pranayama especially) there will be a delayed effect.
Note: It is pretty easy to leapfrog to samyama without upsetting the applecart. See this lesson: http://www.aypsite.org/269.html
and followup in my July 20, 2005 note here: http://www.aypsite.org/forum/topic.asp?TOPIC_ID=306

Practice does not have to be so intense so as to be difficult. Nor does it have to be too slow and boring. It can be whatever you like it to be. That is the beauty of self-directed practice, and having a full tool kit available as needed.

The guru is in you.

2006/01/27 10:51:32
Building a Daily Practice with Self-Pacing
http://www.aypsite.org/forum/topic.asp?TOPIC_ID=321&REPLY_ID=2830&whichpage=-1
Reply Topic - Daily Practice & Self-Pacing Intro

Hi Weaver:

The so-called delayed effects of excessive pranayama come in the form of various kundalini symptoms, like what has been described in the forum by several recently. The same effects as from the other means. They are all tied together.

It is not necessarily purification of the spinal nerve that causes this. It is the energy going elsewhere due to a buildup that is beyond what the spinal nerve can conduct between root and brow. This is right in line with your suggestion to wait for some clearing and clarity in the spinal nerve in spinal breathing before pressing too hard to awaken the energies further.

To clarify, it is not the tracing of the spinal nerve in pranayama that causes the potential difficulty. It is the restraint of breath that does so, especially kumbhaka, which is suspension of breath. But even slow breathing for long periods has a kumbhaka-like effect, because it produces a prana deficit in the nervous system that is ultimately responded to by the huge storehouse of prana in the pelvic region. This is a primary way that kundalini is awakened, in conjunction with the mudras and bandhas. Spinal breathing is both awakening the energy and opening the channel of the spinal nerve for it, so it is by far the safest and most effective means to conduct this operation. It clears the channel (spinal nerve) and awakens the energy at the same time. All other forms of pranayama (and kumbhaka) in AYP also incorporate spinal breathing (tracing the sushumna) for this reason.

The "doubling up" effect that is warned about has to do with adding more restraint of breath on top of the AYP basics, without spinal breathing incorporated. It may well be that opening of the spinal nerve (sushumna) achieved with the AYP methods can absorb additional energy flow from other causes -- but we do not know that for sure. We only find out when there is a buildup and a release (often time delayed), which can be quite uncomfortable. The caution on doubling up on restraint of breath is for that.

In the Secrets of Wilder, the discovery of spinal breathing came after extensive kumbhaka had been practiced which led to a major kundalini event that took a long time to recover from. The sushumna was not ready for this -- no spinal breathing. Once spinal breathing was discovered and added, the imbalance cleared up quickly and the capacity for energy flow was vastly increased, leading to a resolution of the kundalini issues and opening the door to tremendous progress toward enlightenment. This scenario mirrors what my own path was many years ago. In the case of John Wilder (and me) long time practice of deep meditation preceded the kundalini releases, which made the whole thing bearable (presence of the witness).

The Gopi Krishna case was similar except he instigated the release of kundalini using crown practice, ultimately far more problematic than the kumbhaka approach which tends toward more controllable imbalances. Crown practices can lead to far more chaotic situations, especially if there has been no work to open the spinal nerve, which was the case with Gopi Krishna. What made matters worse for him was the fact that he found no help -- he never did have a systematic approach involving spinal breathing, though he did ultimately use his attention to redirect the energies up the middle channel, which was a sort of poor man's spinal breathing approach.

It is very important for us to be having these conversations, so the process of energy awakening in the nervous system can be fully understood and the most effective means for promoting and managing it applied.

Weaver, the formula is as you suggested: Take it one step at a time, beginning with deep meditation, adding spinal breathing when ready, then looking for signs of spinal nerve (sushumna) clearing and conductivity before charging ahead, self-pace, and, of course, have fun! It does not have to be a perilous journey if one is familiar with the parameters and observes good common sense in applying the means for purification and opening.

The guru is in you.

2005/09/08 11:31:59
Building a Daily Practice with Self-Pacing
http://www.aypsite.org/forum/topic.asp?TOPIC_ID=469&REPLY_ID=601&whichpage=-1
Can you overdo without adding anything new?

Hi Lili:

Yes, it can happen that we have new purification symptoms or breakthroughs in experience with no change in practices. This is what yoga will deliver in time at any fixed level of practice.

In your case, it is a sense of separateness, which is a good sign of rising inner silence in your nervous system. It will integrate and feel normal soon enough and you will be able to go about your daily activities effectively with a stronger inner center of stillness, and getting stronger all the time. Bravo for that!

It can also happen that we may have purification symptoms that are more than we'd like. In that case, we will be wise to self-pace our practices, even if we have not added anything on lately.

The car analogy can help with understanding self-pacing. If we are driving along at a fixed speed (our current practices) and the road (our purifying nervous system) becomes bumpy or goes into a sharp curve (uncomfortable purification symptoms), can we continue driving at the same speed? Not in a car without increased risk, and not with practices either. In both cases we let up on the gas a bit until the road smoothes out, and then we can speed up again. This is safe driving, and we are least likely to end up getting banged up too much.

I am happy to see self-pacing coming up here as a dedicated topic. It is so important, and I hope others will share their stories relating to self-pacing too. It does not matter how advanced we are. The regulation of practices is always central to what we are doing in yoga, just like the gas pedal is in the car. In fact, the faster we are going, the more we need to be aware of the fine points of self-pacing.

Self-pacing is not only a factor for beginners. It is the constant reality for everyone at every level, whether adding on new practices or not. It is at the heart of AYP, because here we do not have to spend most of our time looking for practices -- we spend our time applying them. That really brings self-pacing to the fore, and our accelerated progress along with it.

The guru is in you.

Yogani

Edit PS --

Hi David. We posted simultaneously. Right on the beam there. Carry on everyone! :-)
2005/10/07 11:23:43
Building a Daily Practice with Self-Pacing
http://www.aypsite.org/forum/topic.asp?TOPIC_ID=506&REPLY_ID=881&whichpage=-1
Perverse Practice Observation

Hi All:

Very interesting experiences.

It goes to show what expectations can do, and the lack of them. It is normal enough. I'm the one who said, "You will be rushing to your meditation seat." It is one more step to let go of that and move beyond. In time we can develop an equanimity about practices, while at the same time remaining 100% committed. That is the benefit of keeping a steady "habit" that transcends how we are feeling at the moment.

Like so many things spiritual, there is paradox here. By the time we are experiencing stillness and ecstatic bliss around the clock, we will be pretty calm about it. Just another day of the divine, and just another day of cultivating cosmic life on the cushion.

We can get used to anything , yes? :-)

The guru is in you.

2005/10/07 13:16:59
Building a Daily Practice with Self-Pacing
http://www.aypsite.org/forum/topic.asp?TOPIC_ID=506&REPLY_ID=888&whichpage=-1
Perverse Practice Observation

Hi Jim:

Well, as we settle in over the long term, that is how we even out the expectations. Like a 747 jet pilot with lots of experience. For him or her, flying that thing is just another day at the office. For you or me it is like, "Holy mackerel! We'll never get off the ground with this thing!" Training is important. But, ultimately, the difference is experience ... time in the practice. When it becomes part of us, we no longer anticipate anything, not even subconsciously ... that's why I used the word "habit."

On asanas, pranayama and meditation, these each go progressively deeper, in that order. That's why they are separate limbs in the Yoga Sutras. They work together in sequence. Maybe one or two will be enough, but all three is optimal. If I had to pick one, it would be meditation. If I had to pick two, it would be pranayama and meditation. Asanas come into it third, with all due respect to the vast and thriving asana industry. It doesn't take much to stretch the nerves out enough for a smooth transition from on-the-go activity to pranayama and deep meditation: 5-10 minutes, which most hatha yoga teachers would scoff at. But that is all it takes with all the other horsepower we have here.

The guru is in you.

2005/11/14 09:58:08
Building a Daily Practice with Self-Pacing
http://www.aypsite.org/forum/topic.asp?TOPIC_ID=587&REPLY_ID=1521&whichpage=-1
problem on managing practices

Hi Alvin:

Irritability or other excessive emotions in activity can be an overflow of purification from deep meditation or other practices.

The first thing to be sure of is that you are taking at least a few minutes "coming out" of meditation, with no intention to pick up the mantra during that time -- just easily resting. If there has been some roughness in the session (or even if not) it is good to lie down for 5-10 minutes at the end. Not resting enough at the end of meditation is the most common cause of overflow of unwinding purification into activity, which can manifest with some emotions in the way you described.

Less common is a sensitivity to meditation in the individual. If irritability continues in activity even with good rest at the end of meditation, then sensitivity to meditation may be the cause. The way to find out and deal with it is by scaling back the time of meditation a bit (5-10 minutes) and see if that helps. If it does and the emotions smooth out, then we can try inching back up with meditation time when we are feeling better to fine tune our time to the right amount for ongoing smooth purification.

Of course, meditating for more than 20 minutes twice per day is asking for irritability, for just about anyone. That goes without saying, yes?

There can be many ups and downs along the path of inner purification, and we can navigate them by regulating our practice a bit up and down along the way, much like driving a car along a winding road and adjusting our speed to match the varying conditions along the way. This is the art of self-pacing.

Finally, inner energy excesses can also happen by adding other practices, and/or by doubling up on practices, especially when using several pranayama methods in the same session or day. Of course, I cannot speak to all the other practices you may be inclined to try in addition to AYP. These will be your individual research. Let us know of your discoveries! But do keep in mind that beginning stage is not necessarily the best time to be doing research on the effects of diverse practices. Better to get a foundation of inner silence underneath with deep meditation, and then you can tolerate much better the inevitable excesses one is bound to encounter when doing research – trying new things. That goes for taking on new practices within AYP too.

It is good to be aware that there is only so much purification our nervous system can handle comfortably on any given day, and ongoing irritability or other energy upheavals are the common symptoms of continually overdoing in some area of our practice.

Other than that, it sounds like you are having some good benefits already in your life. As you stabilize your routine it will become even better!

The guru is in you.

2005/11/26 10:54:03
Building a Daily Practice with Self-Pacing
http://www.aypsite.org/forum/topic.asp?TOPIC_ID=587&REPLY_ID=1657&whichpage=-1
problem on managing practices

Hi Alvin:

20 minutes twice a day still works fine for me, after 30-some years. Of course, all the other practices are there too, so overall sitting time is more. Good activity is essential to stabilize the results of sitting practices. It is a balance we each have to find for ourselves, applying the principles of self-pacing.

On longer sittings with other styles of meditation, that is certainly true. I touched on "witnessing-sytle" meditation in your topic over here:
http://www.aypsite.org/forum/topic.asp?TOPIC_ID=598

Mantra yoga-style deep meditation is unique when correctly performed -- it is pro-active meditation with great power, so a little bit goes a long way.

The guru is in you.

2005/11/29 10:31:51
Building a Daily Practice with Self-Pacing
http://www.aypsite.org/forum/topic.asp?TOPIC_ID=587&REPLY_ID=1693&whichpage=-1
problem on managing practices

Hi Alvin:

Yes, "regularity" is a matter of keeping up daily practices. If that is at irregular times it can still work, though it does make it a bit harder to keep the habit -- more difficult to infuse it into the biorhythms. That is the main reason for developing a steady routine. Insuring longevity!

The business of keeping the habit of regularity is discussed in lesson 209 - "Fitting daily practices into a busy schedule"
http://www.aypsite.org/209.html

The guru is in you.

2005/12/01 10:29:54
Building a Daily Practice with Self-Pacing
http://www.aypsite.org/forum/topic.asp?TOPIC_ID=614&REPLY_ID=1731&whichpage=-1
Too early to add yoni mudra kumbhaka?

Hi Weaver, and welcome!

On your questions:

1. If you feel stable in your routine and are hungry to move on, then by all means, test the next step. If it is too much, you can back off as needed. No harm done. Keep in mind that a "stable routine" can be a bit illusive, meaning, practices may have a delayed reaction in effects. You will usually know within a few weeks or months what the short to intermediate term effects are from adding new practices, but some cycles of purification are longer. It is like driving a car through a changing landscape. Sometimes the road is straight and smooth. Other times it will be winding and bumpy. We adjust our speed accordingly, yes? Same in yoga. The longer you are doing this, the better you will get at self-pacing.

2. While traditionalist teachings put a lot of weight on keeping straight posture without back support in sitting practices, I think it is highly overrated -- the equivalent of a puritan fixation or something. Certainly not worth sacrificing comfort, which diverts the attention from our practices to the discomfort. Who needs that? The AYP approach is comfort first and posture second. It works quite well that way.

3. We all have what we have time-wise, and we will be gaining every day we are in practices. I think the "here and now" of yoga is most important. It is an improvement in the quality of life we can be cultivating and enjoying today. Looks like you have at least 20 years to work on it. That is a lot of "todays."

The maturing of sexuality (less reproductive urgency) is actually an advantage. It makes the tantric aspects of yoga more manageable. The most effective tantra is pretty laid back. And don't worry, you will not "run out" of the energy.

Finally, whatever we accomplish here spiritually we take with us. Nothing is ever lost. All the more reason to get on with it. See this lesson:
http://www.aypsite.org/74.html
Bottom line, whether we have one year to live or 50 years, yoga is worth it -- for today, and for ever more.

Will you finish in this lifetime? Not sure. It depends on how much housecleaning is necessary. Everyone is different in that. One thing is for sure -- a couple of decades is a lot of housecleaning, especially now that we are getting more efficient practice-wise, and certainly even more efficient in the years to come as applied yoga science takes off.

Wishing you the best on your path.

The guru is in you.

2005/12/30 12:26:42
Building a Daily Practice with Self-Pacing
http://www.aypsite.org/forum/topic.asp?TOPIC_ID=679&REPLY_ID=2271&whichpage=-1
changing routine dynamics

Hi Anthem and David:

Excellent points.

There is also the macro-phenomenon of rising world consciousness, which means more inner silence and spiritual energy coming up with the same practices. World consciousness affects our practice in this way, and we (all spiritual practitioners of all kinds around the world) act on world consciousness. Indeed, the entire globe is in a state of rapid purification these days, as we can see in the news reports.

All the more reason to be skilled in self-pacing.

The guru is in you.

2006/01/01 18:32:24
Building a Daily Practice with Self-Pacing
http://www.aypsite.org/forum/topic.asp?TOPIC_ID=679&REPLY_ID=2310&whichpage=-1
changing routine dynamics

Hi Anthem:

It is logical that as we advance we will become more sensitive to perturbations in world consciousness, like a new year shift. :-)
Our own expanding awareness is the same as the expanding inner being of the world. The more we come into the living reality of that, the more we become the world and the more the world becomes us.

As for what to do about it, nothing different than we are naturally inclined to do. It is only our expanding sense of self occurring. While the world might seem a huge responsibility to take on, from the standpoint of inner silence it is just the same as we have been doing all along. It is business as usual with daily practices and going out and living life according to our natural inclinations.

There are the practices we always favor and there is the ever-changing scenery passing by. We know all about that, yes?

Wishing everyone the best in this exciting new year!

The guru is in you.

2006/01/11 10:59:32
Building a Daily Practice with Self-Pacing
http://www.aypsite.org/forum/topic.asp?TOPIC_ID=679&REPLY_ID=2470&whichpage=-1
changing routine dynamics

quote:
_____
My outside life is going very well and smoothly though and when self-pacing I have been feeling an inner joy throughout my days that I have never known as consistently. So it is just my practices that are out of kilter at the moment should I be concerned?
_____

Hi Anthem:

This is the acid test. No matter what happens in practices, our results in activity are what matter. This is an excellent example of how prudent management (self-pacing) of a rough patch in practices still will yield continuing progress in daily activity.

The bucking bronco in practices will come and go. It is all purification. A cycle of heavy symptoms of purification can go on for some time, though it is rare to last for weeks and months. It will change -- guaranteed.

You are doing a good job navigating it. Do whatever is necessary to keep on the track. I have had some similar periods in the past, and sometimes practices do have to be scaled way back for a while. We just keep testing and doing what the nervous system can tolerate under present circumstances. Have faith. This rough patch will pass and the inner sun will shine ever brighter. :-)

These are wonderful sharings. The mystery of the process of human spiritual transformation is unraveling a little more each day. My goodness, this is real science!

The guru is in you.

2006/01/20 18:17:31
Building a Daily Practice with Self-Pacing
http://www.aypsite.org/forum/topic.asp?TOPIC_ID=750&REPLY_ID=2687&whichpage=-1
Consolation for Backtrackers

Hi All:

Here is what I wrote on this earlier today. Common threads in the postings here. Experiences in common, which is confirmation.

Hi Jim:

Ah, but you are noticing. Do you feel you can watch all of this a little clearer than before? That is the "keeper." Our practices may give us the illusion of instant relief from the woes of mundane life. It's a nice side benefit. But the real benefit is found in what has been permanently stabilized whether we are practicing or not -- inner silence.

Well, it is never enough, so we loath stopping once we have tasted the nectar of our inner possibilities, no matter how much inner silence we have to keep. Ultimately, that is why John Wilder ended up doing what he did -- or allowing it to happen to him is a better way of putting it. Butterflies are free, and he would settle for nothing less...

Just remember that practices are not all or nothing. Honoring the habit is the first step. That takes a few minutes twice per day. We all have to eat. We all have to sleep. We all have to brush our teeth. And we all have to evolve... There is time enough in the day for all of these. Some guerrilla yoga tactics can help when we are living in the corporate jungle. See http://www.aypsite.org/209.html

And, by all means, side-step the energy-wasting skirmishes in life if possible. That means adopting a flexible point of view on everything. That too is a characteristic of rising inner silence. Until it fully blooms, Ruiz's "Four Agreements" can be helpful. As inner silence blooms, the agreements (yama/niyama) become automatic.

The guru is in you.

2006/01/23 19:18:16
Building a Daily Practice with Self-Pacing
http://www.aypsite.org/forum/topic.asp?TOPIC_ID=765&REPLY_ID=2745&whichpage=-1
Energy experience and thoughts on self-pacing

Hi Weaver:

Thanks so much for taking the time to record your experiences over the past year, the snags you have encountered recently, and how you have been addressing them. This will be very useful information to many who are traveling on the AYP fast track. And it is the fast track, for sure.

Your suggestions 1-6 at the end are excellent refinements on the big picture of self-pacing practices over the long term -- building a stable routine that is flexible, progressive and safe.

This is real pioneering work going on here. The "leading edge" in modern yoga. We do not want it to become the "bleeding edge," so this kind of sharing and reflection on what we are doing is very important.

Consider this. It took me over 30 years to take on and assimilate all the practices in AYP. Of course, I spent a lot of time searching and researching, so I am sure I could have done it in much less time had the knowledge been readily available. How short a time? That is what all of you are finding out. This degree of fast track has not been done before. Not that I am aware. So there is a lot of research yet to be done on the cultivation of human spiritual transformation, and you are the ones doing it. I can't experience it the same way you are. It is too late for me. I'm too far down the road at this point. Hopefully not too far gone. :-)

So, AYP can be very speedy, limited only by the steps of purification that each person must go through. Something is happening. We know that for sure. Now we have to systematize it in ways that will keep everyone off the guard rails on the curves.

How long is the journey going to be? Five years? Ten years? Twenty years? More? We'll find out from all of you.

In the Secrets of Wilder, I assumed a 10 year journey for John Wilder, which was a big compression of my 30 years. Well, he is a fictitious prodigy -- a mythic figure on a fantastic inner journey. Now we have to bring it to earth and make it real. It is going to take some doing, and no doubt some more scraping of the guard rails. Are you all up for it? Or are we going too fast here? Some might be feeling a little weak in the knees and thinking we should pull the plug on all this and go back to the slow track. What do you think?

Weaver, I believe the kind of excess you have experienced can be settled down fairly easily. It is a crown opening that brings the greatest risk. Yours does not sound like that. Your suggestion is a good one, to look for more clarity and fluidity (conductivity) in spinal breathing before turning up the heat with mudras, bandhas and kumbhaka. Then you will have a clear route up and down (it goes both ways). You just got a little ahead of yourself, so turning down the heat for a while is the right thing to do. You will be back.

What we do not want is to be like the guy who strapped some feathers on his arms and jumped off the cliff hoping to take flight. It did not work. Can man fly? Absolutely. We know that now. Can he fly like that, with feathers strapped to his arms? No. With a hang glider? Yes! But only if he knows how. The key is in developing the "know how."

It is the same thing in this no-nonsense AYP approach to fast track yoga. Do we know that humanity can cultivate enlightenment? Well, we are not as sure about that as we are about man flying. But there is plenty of evidence that a thing called "enlightenment" is inside us somewhere. Will we find it by jumping off the cliff with a smattering of ill-applied practices? Not likely. We have to fully explore the means available, apply and integrate them judiciously, optimize them over time, and so on. Then we will have it.

These kinds of discussions are just for that. Thanks again for sharing ... great stuff!

The guru is in you.

2006/01/24 10:27:37
Building a Daily Practice with Self-Pacing
http://www.aypsite.org/forum/topic.asp?TOPIC_ID=765&REPLY_ID=2758&whichpage=-1
Energy experience and thoughts on self-pacing

Hi Anthem:

It is good to know some are game for the fast track aspect of AYP, risks included. Of course, it can be used much more gradually too. Weaver's first post here counsels wisely for a measured approach. Each step is a matter of personal choice. When I first started writing a few years ago, I did not really know how all of this would be received. Not too bad so far. The level of responsibility exhibited by everyone has been outstanding. See http://www.aypsite.org/217.html

As for what is to come in AYP, yes, there are more techniques in the works for both sitting practices and in-between. But first, it would be good to see some more formation in the application of the core practices we are working with now. It is a grand experiment whose results are yet to be fully known. Plus, there is a lot of writing and practical dissemination work to do on this end to spread the knowledge out into the mainstream as much as possible -- a lot of "catch-up" in the documentation and publishing end of it. That is what the AYP Enlightenment Series books are for, and there are a bunch of those to do. So time is becoming quite crunched here. Logically, the more help there can be from practitioners on the dissemination end of AYP, the better.

So, more techniques? Yes, in time... The scope of AYP will eventually broaden to integrate and optimize additional elements of practice. The project continues!

The guru is in you.

2006/03/04 10:54:18
Building a Daily Practice with Self-Pacing
http://www.aypsite.org/forum/topic.asp?TOPIC_ID=865&REPLY_ID=4087&whichpage=-1
Super Time Delayed Reactions

Hi Jim:

Rapid increases in practice times or the number of practices is an area where tracking the relationship of practices and experiences is tricky, because the cause/effect dynamic can be spread out in time.

The phenomenon does exist, as anyone who has had a big energy surge coming out of nowhere can attest (sometimes uncomfortable).

Think of the situation as being like a dam where the water is steadily rising behind it. The spillway of the dam has a certain limit for water to pass through the dam safely. Once the water reaches a level well beyond what the spillway can handle, the dam becomes strained and can break apart in large pieces. Until then, there may be no sign of the impending break -- the delayed reaction to the rising water. When the break finally does happen, it is not usually an orderly event, and not even progressive, as the dam can be damaged in the process.

The dam is our nervous system with impurities still in place. The water is our spiritual energy wanting to flow through the dam. The spillway is our present capacity to handle the flow, which we are working to increase with our daily practices. The rising water behind the dam beyond what the spillway can comfortably handle is what happens when our practices produce energy exceeding the openings we can handle in the present -- a pile-up behind the dam. The pile-up can be quiet and unnoticed, like water steadily rising behind a dam. We may only notice the pile-up of inner energy when there is finally a crumbling from the build-up in the pressure and a chaotic breakthrough -- the delayed reaction.

Of course, what we are trying to do is a smooth purification of the dam of our nervous system, without causing undue stress and damage to the dam itself, or our confidence and ability to continue with the dam purification project on a daily basis. We are gradually increasing the spillway to handle the infinite divine flow that is available within us at all times. It does not work so well with cycles of big inner pile-ups and big crumblings. Hence, we go gradually, increasing our practices in small steps to make sure we do not exceed the capacity of our nervous system (our spillway) to purify and open in a smooth and safe manner.

This is what self-pacing is all about. We each have our own inner dynamic, and self-pacing is about matching our practices and experiences to be both progressive and manageable. Taking delayed reactions into account as we ramp up practices is part of this process, one of the more tricky aspects. But we learn quickly after getting ahead of ourselves with practices and having a few unexpected time-delayed sunburns from the inside, yes? :-)

The guru is in you.

2006/07/31 08:21:44
Building a Daily Practice with Self-Pacing
http://www.aypsite.org/forum/topic.asp?TOPIC_ID=1222&REPLY_ID=10075&whichpage=-1
Housecleaning?

Hi Shanti:

Longing is a key part of the path -- without longing there would be no path. And the further we go on the path, the more longing there is. What is it?

Longing and the inner guru are one and the same. Our longing for completeness is the divine longing for expression. It is sacred.

In AYP we say, "Pace bhakti as necessary." How do we do that? The most obvious way is to do "other things." Work in the garden. Take walks. Help another. Watch life ... and see that it is who we are.

There is something going on underneath, something wanting to come out. Meg hit on it -- ultimately, longing is not about adding something, but about giving something away, about expressing from within, whether it be in our art, or our service. It is both. There is a close connection between bhakti and karma yoga. Service as divine outflow is the final destination of surrender. That is why the AYP book slated for next year on Bhakti Yoga has Karma Yoga in the title also. What we long to know and be, longs to know and be from within us. It is a process of unfoldment from within -- it is our purification and opening ... our union.

Here is another Rumi quote (thank you for the beautiful one above, Ranger) that captures it. It was posted here in the forum last year and is copied again:

"I have lived on the lip of insanity,
wanting to know reasons,
knocking on a door.
It opens.
I've been knocking from the inside!" ~Rumi

If you have great longing, you are blessed. Reading some Rumi can help. He is the master of longing and surrender. See here for more. Keep refreshing that page for more quotes.

The guru is in you.

PS -- "You are broken-hearted too, you shall find cure in love;

If you listen to me and pursue this ailment." ~Rumi

2006/09/19 18:08:21
Building a Daily Practice with Self-Pacing
http://www.aypsite.org/forum/topic.asp?TOPIC_ID=1519&REPLY_ID=11394&whichpage=-1
Progression

Hi Kyman:

You are part of a new breed of yogi and yogini, and it will be very interesting to see how things progress in the years and decades to come.

There are plenty of folks around from my generation (baby boomers) who have been doing practices of one kind or other for a long time. Yet, the results have been mixed -- some would say disappointing in relation to the claims that were made early on. I believe this has been due to a lack of full-scope integration of powerful methods that have not been brought together before now. Outside AYP, I don't know of anyone who has been integrating practices across rigid traditional lines the way we have been doing.

It is silly really. In this scientific age, we are only now beginning to effectively combine the essential methods of human spiritual transformation, even though these methods have been around for thousands of years! Well, better late than never.

The experiences being recorded here after a year or two (yours are beautiful) are the kind one might hear from old-style long term practioners, if at all.

Of course, in quite a few cases, long term practitioners involved in one class of practice are coming into AYP and adding on, with big leaps forward in a very short time. That is because they have been selectively purifying for a long time with the one class of practice, and suddenly a new element of yoga is brought in and it can go pretty fast from there. So nothing is ever wasted on the spiritual path. My own practice evolved like that over some three decades, picking up essential pieces along the way as AYP slowly crystalized into an easy-to-use integrated system. And I believe there is much more to do yet. Science is never satisfied and never sleeps. It's a good thing too ... now that we are getting it all out in the open, it means much more progress will be coming.

So, it will be folks like you who are giving the 10, 20 and 30 year perspectives on self-directed integrated practices. It is a real adventure that has the potential to exceed the greatest achievements of humanity so far. We just need to get everyone into the act, and the divine synergy will take over. :-)

Of course, there are always a few enlightened people around. That is not really a big deal in the overall scheme of things. But thousands? That will be something else entirely.

The guru is in you.

2006/11/30 09:44:22
Building a Daily Practice with Self-Pacing
http://www.aypsite.org/forum/topic.asp?TOPIC_ID=1771
Flywheel Effect
An interesting Q&A from the email:

Q: In your lessons you talk about about practicing spinal breathing 10 minutes and deep meditation 20 min. But if you see any famous books of any Yogi, all of them have been meditating you long intense hours for a long time. Because you have a lot of experience in this, have you been increasing the times on spinal breathing and deep meditation during the years or you continue practicing 20 minutes?? I suppose then when your are are more purifized your body is capable to support more long sesssions. Is it like that?? When you are more purified, is possible practice more time on each sitting??

If it is possible to increase the times, is it correct to increase in 5 min spinal breathing and deep meditation each month??

A: Actually, it is just the opposite. Less can become more practice-wise the further we go along the path. A wide range of practices can continue, with small doses of each being all that is necessary to keep moving at a heady pace. It is a "flywheel" effect -- it takes less to keep it going once it is spinning fast. Self-pacing becomes very important as we advance, so as not to overdo with the inner energies, which become quite dynamic as ecstatic conductivity rises in us.

The AYP practices in combination are much more powerful than the normal fare, so a little will go a long way. Anything over 10 min spinal breathing pranayama followed by 20 min deep meditation will be pushing the envelope for most people, especially as additional practices are added. You are welcome to try more time, but be sure to self-pace at the first sign of overload. And keep in mind the delayed effects of practices. Overdoing today might hit us three weeks from now. That is why we make changes in small increments and allow plenty of time for things to settle in.

It is much better to be moderate and consistent in twice-daily practices and lead an active life. This combination will produce more spiritual progress than more time in practices and less activity, because the balanced integration of inner and outer life will be enhanced.

This is really the kind of question that should be brought up in the AYP forums so everyone can benefit. Consider doing that in the future.

All the best!

The guru is in you.

2007/04/19 10:30:02
Building a Daily Practice with Self-Pacing
http://www.aypsite.org/forum/topic.asp?TOPIC_ID=2444&REPLY_ID=20630&whichpage=-1
Request for Guidance in Meditation Practices

Hi gm chaudhari, and welcome!

It sounds like you have been moving with steadiness through some difficult times. May you continue to do so and may your wife have a full recovery.

These lessons may help add some perspective on your experience with the sun/light:

The Star: http://www.aypsite.org/92.html
The Star Revisited: http://www.aypsite.org/179.html

Whatever inner experiences we may encounter, it will be our practices and our continued dedicated activity in the world that will carry us forward. Inner experiences can inspire us in these things, solidifying our faith in the divine, and our surrender to the process of our transformation. As we continue to practice and serve others, we will become the divine light in action in the world, even as we become the One that comprises all and never acts.

All the best!

The guru is in you.

2008/02/24 10:53:26
Building a Daily Practice with Self-Pacing
http://www.aypsite.org/forum/topic.asp?TOPIC_ID=2884&REPLY_ID=30500&whichpage=-1
The "Overdoing Symptoms" Thread

quote:
_____
Originally posted by emc

In short... I never thought I'd suffer from overload symptoms like this. Haven't happened since the start of it all 2 years ago... One month with a cold that never gives up, feeling so tired and mindy... The victim getting recharged here! Mr Smith and the agents multiplying...:-) Gosh, it's really slowing the path down.
_____

Hi EMC:

Keep in mind that while heart and mind may wish to soar, the body needs some time to catch up.

Your bhakti is nothing short of spectacular, and I seem to recall you adding a mantra enhancement not long ago. Combine all that with your weekends with Bernie and whoever else, and it makes for a nervous system facing transformational challenges.

So maybe do take a closer look at the physical exercise/grounding side of it, getting more rest, and digging a few holes in the garden (when the snow melts). If I had to guess, I'd say it is your unbridled bhakti that is getting you ahead of your body more than anything else. That can translate into getting to far ahead in practices too, which can compound the overload.

If you can't turn down the bhakti, then one way to divert it is to take it to others in mundane service mode. That can be very grounding, taking some of the energy load off your nervous system. If we are directing bhakti inward, the load will be more in us. If we direct our bhakti outward, the environment will share more in the transformation. That is where it must go eventually anyway.

Note: I am not talking about "blazing light" service here -- more along the lines of changing dirty sheets and scrubbing toilets -- just being there for the other in need. Forget the blazing light for a while...

Service is spiritual practice also, as you well know. So even that may need to be self-paced if the body is struggling too much in becoming a divine channel. We will know we are making progress when it is becoming pretty ordinary.

It all takes time. It is amazing how far we have traveled in a very short time, yes? Let's do what is necessary to keep it on the rails. :-)

All the best!

The guru is in you.

2007/09/14 10:26:55
Building a Daily Practice with Self-Pacing
http://www.aypsite.org/forum/topic.asp?TOPIC_ID=2921&REPLY_ID=25495&whichpage=-1
Self-pacing lessons with ecstasy and the crown

Hi Andrew:

Glad to hear you are feeling better. Make sure to give yourself some "headroom" going forward, meaning, room to go over a bit without going over so much that it will require a long recovery. Of course, sometimes it is hard to tell. But going to the crown for extended periods poses obvious risks under any circumstances.

A good and generally safe place to go during ecstatic reverie is sambhavi - to the brow. Once ecstatic conductivity is resident, it is also a good place to stimulate it in the whole body. This is the "mainstream" approach on the energetic side of yoga. Isn't it interesting that there is no mainstream mudra identified for the crown? ... though the crown is obviously involved in any ecstatic event. This is also true for what we call the "whole body mudra" in AYP, which is not crown focused, but involves the crown.

With long term practice, sambhavi tends to expand upward toward the crown, where both ajna and crown are involved, a kind of merging. But this is not something we can advise to do arbitrarily. If we do, we face the same risks of going directly to the crown. However, when it evolves naturally, there is generally little or no crown backlash. In short, sambhavi, besides being the master controller of ecstatic reverie in the nervous system, is also a means for naturally approaching the crown.

Of course, we can overdo with sambhavi also (headache is the most common symptom), but generally the recovery is much quicker than overdoing at the crown. In both cases, grounding methods and self-pacing in practices are utilized.

As we know, quite a few people who come to us with energy overloads have been involved in crown practices and/or premature crown openings. So it is a real issue. But not one to demonize and run away from. There is a time and place for everything in yoga, and that is certainly true of crown openings too. That is why the lessons do approach the crown later on, with caution. The crown is also incorporated into cosmic samyama (yoga nidra procedure), stimulating the flow of awareness both within and outside the body. I'm not aware of anyone having overload issues with cosmic samyama. It generally has a balancing effect on the energies, while expanding and stabilizing inner silence.

There are those who claim easy crown opening with certain types of practices, particularly spinal breathing to or from the crown -- not an AYP method. I am not sure if this is true over the long term, since we have seen a significant number of energy overload refugees from such approaches. Any clarifications that can be offered on these approaches will be welcome. If we are missing something, it would be good to pin point the dynamics involved. We are not resting on our laurels here, and are always looking for ways to further optimize cause and effect in our practices. The more everyone knows about the journey and its means, the better. Much better we face the issues as they arise and resolve them.

Our goal is to make the full path easily accessible for everyone, leading to the flowering of acts of kindness and loving service, spreading naturally across humanity like an invisible wave. Stillness in action. This will be the outcome of effective spiritual practices occurring in every household.

The message is simple: Enlightenment is for ordinary people living ordinary lives. We are getting our arms around the technology that can enable it to happen surely and safely on a wide scale. This is what will change the world. Not gurus sitting on pedestals.

The guru is in you.

2007/11/19 08:51:29
Building a Daily Practice with Self-Pacing
http://www.aypsite.org/forum/topic.asp?TOPIC_ID=3155&REPLY_ID=27122&whichpage=-1
Voice

Hi Julie, and welcome!

I don't recall any of the AYP lessons being specifically about relating to inner voices, unless having our divine savior ride up in a golden chariot to offer us a ride during practices counts. In that case, we just easily favor the practice we are doing. Our savior can wait until afterwards. :-)

This is the formula for handling all experiences during practices, assuming our practice is stable and not causing excessive discomfort, particularly in daily activity between sessions, which is where the rubber of practices meets the road.

It is the same advice we give for all experiences occurring during practices, whether they be visual, auditory, physical, mental or emotional. Handling experiences during practices is covered from many angles in the lessons, and all of those situations could be regarded to be more or less analogous to your situation.

Practices are what produce our spiritual progress. Following experiences during practices does not produce significant spiritual progress, so we favor the practice while we are doing it. How we relate to visions, voices, energy experiences, etc. outside practices is another matter. That is our own business, and we will find our way with increasing inner silence and ecstatic radiance over time. If there is instability in daily activity resulting from our practices, then self-pacing should be applied accordingly.

If the AYP practices are helping our life to become better, this is the desired result. Then go out and live fully! But if practices are causing problems in daily activity, then we take responsibility for that and apply the best solutions that are available -- the methods of self-pacing, grounding, etc.

There are some discussions here in the forums on "voices," and you can find them by doing a search. Most of those are related to mental health issues, discussing whether or not practices would be an aid in those situations -- not an easy question to answer. But that seems not to be what you are asking about at this time.

EMC has offered some interesting perspectives on this from her experience. Something to consider outside practices. But while sitting, I suggest favoring the practice over the experiences, no matter what they may be. That applies to all of us.

Wishing you all the best on your path. Enjoy!

The guru is in you.

2009/10/20 12:52:11
Building a Daily Practice with Self-Pacing
http://www.aypsite.org/forum/topic.asp?TOPIC_ID=6555&REPLY_ID=58727&whichpage=-1
This Freaking Rash Will Live On After I'm Dead

Hi Jim:

If rash is the only symptom, it could still be an underlying contraction. Heat is friction, and friction is energy passing through obstructions. Mentally excluding a symptom from the whole can limit its resolution, at least for a while.

Treating the heat with a pitta pacifying diet from ayurveda and natural remedies you have available from Chinese medicine can temper the symptoms for sure. Do it. I stayed on a pitta pacifying diet for years after my peak rash episode in 1990, and continued to self-pace and ground as well. That's also when I was doing Tai C
Hi daily.

As mentioned, I lightened up on the bhakti attitude, which included going back to full time employment in the corporate world after being in a yoga-soaked self-employment lifestyle for 10 years.

Eventually the underlying contraction went, and eventually I was able to eat spicy food again with no problem. Spicy food is the canary in the kundalini coal mine. This is an indication that the delicacy of the overall situation became much less touchy.

So it isn't only about the heat. It is also about the underlying condition that is causing the heat, which I call "contraction." In my case, attitude (and lifestyle) played a significant role in normalizing things, even as big energy flows continued to occur, becoming much less restricted, with far fewer adverse symptoms. That's also when the energy began flowing out to others, steadily increasing over time. It continues today, except I retired from the corporate job along the way, and here I sit typing. :-)

So we grow into it gradually is my point. Some of these issues just take time to resolve themselves, and taking a longer more relaxed view is a help in that. This doesn't mean taking no remedial measures as needed. It just means broadening our life out in time and space, opening to avenues that we might not have considered to be "yogic" before. Ironically, being intensely focused in the now isn't living in the now.

I can't really tell you specifically what is going on there. I can only share what it has been here, and offer some extrapolations. I'd guess your symptom is more deeply rooted than you can readily access right now. I am also confident you will get to the bottom of it sooner or later.

Couldn't it be possible that your intense focus on this issue is adding energy to it, rather than resolving it? Letting go a bit with the problem solving attitude, combined with other measures you are taking, might offer some relief. Only guessing. You never know until you try, or untry. It's a balancing act. Solving without solving. Doing without doing. Seeking without seeking...

It is taking each step, knowing that it will land in the right place, no matter what it looks like. That kind of letting go is not necessarily kundalini aggravating. It is stillness in motion.

The guru is in you.

PS: Throughout all of this, sitting practices continued here, self-paced as necessary.

2009/10/20 15:27:04
Building a Daily Practice with Self-Pacing
http://www.aypsite.org/forum/topic.asp?TOPIC_ID=6555&REPLY_ID=58742&whichpage=-1
This Freaking Rash Will Live On After I'm Dead

quote:
_____
Originally posted by Jim and His Karma

Yogani, two quick follow-ups:

1. were you able to in any way locate the contraction, even vaguely? When it evaporated, was there an opening sensation in a particular place, or a change in the direction of flow (i.e. an easing of one direction), or other sensation of specific opening? Or was it all just...one of those undefinable things?

2. Am I correct in concluding that once this contraction evaporated, you could have - if it was practical at the time - gone back to your yoga-centric, "bhakti-first" lifestyle without suffering problems? E.g. I'm assuming your current lifestyle (even with all the activity of writing and running AYP) is fairly similar to your self-employed period?
_____

Hi Jim:

1. No, not any one or few things that could be said to be specifically definable as "the thing." Except after so many years the acorn has become an oak tree. So that is something noticeable. If you take the sum total of the Wilder story and the the AYP writings, that defines it more or less. And the writings aren't done yet, so neither is the definition. It probably never will be. Better to just live it.

I should add that kundalini is a means to an end, not an end in itself. The further we go, the clearer it becomes that ecstatic conductivity and radiance (kundalini) are the means by which stillness expresses in the world as divine love, and this is what is stimulating world consciousness. All of the kundalini symptoms, etc., are part of that transformation: a purification and opening, a birthing process. Yoga adds a lot on that side of it. But all too often the cultivation of stillness is left behind for the energy work, the experiences, the tantra, the self-inquiry, or the whatever. Without cultivation of abiding inner silence, none of it is going very far. I love to harp on that, as you know. :-)

2. Yes, but it took a change in attitude and years of doing other things lifestyle-wise to get there. Now I can do pretty much anything practice-wise without getting into trouble. But who has time? Happily, my path has a lot of karma yoga in it now, so my sitting practice is pretty typical AYP. Once in a while I red-line it a bit, but can generally recover in a day or two. A good excuse to lighten up on everything for a few days and take some long walks.

The guru is in you.

2009/10/21 17:24:53
Building a Daily Practice with Self-Pacing
http://www.aypsite.org/forum/topic.asp?TOPIC_ID=6555&REPLY_ID=58797&whichpage=-1
This Freaking Rash Will Live On After I'm Dead

Hi Jim:

Meditation surely is a stimulator of kundalini. The speed and degree of symptoms is a primary way we might conclude someone is sensitive to meditation.

There is also the aspect of delayed reactions, which can occur with pranayama or deep meditation, or any spiritual practice. If you were "meditating up a storm" without the rash symptom, you should not rule out a possible delayed reaction. This would not necessarily mean someone is sensitive to meditation. It could simply be a matter of overdoing while not taking into account a possible delayed reaction. It is very common.

I'm not saying that is what happened. But it is a possibility whenever we do any practice "up a storm." There are many here who can attest to it, myself included. And John Wilder too! :-)

The guru is in you.

2009/11/06 09:09:42
Building a Daily Practice with Self-Pacing
http://www.aypsite.org/forum/topic.asp?TOPIC_ID=6637&REPLY_ID=59384&whichpage=-1
Giving it all away, the ultimate self-pacing?

Hi Anthem:

Yes, we humans are designed to be channels for the divine, our true nature. Yet, we are so often inclined to try and put it in a bottle, which creates all sorts of challenges. Once the bottle breaks, we become a river of stability and love. As you know, there are many stages of breaking.

It's summed up nicely in the Rumi quote on the dedication page of the AYP Bhakti and Karma Yoga book:

"I have lived on the lip of insanity, wanting
to know reasons, knocking on a door.
It opens.
I have been knocking from the inside!"

:-)

The guru is in you.

2009/11/06 08:53:51
Building a Daily Practice with Self-Pacing
http://www.aypsite.org/forum/topic.asp?TOPIC_ID=6639&REPLY_ID=59383&whichpage=-1
Latest lessons 366-367

Hi emc:

You have good suggestions from Miguel and Yonatan, both who have traveled a similar road.

In your case, it seems you went from normal sensitivity to over-sensitive. It is hard to know exactly why. Maybe you were wired for it from the start. Or maybe it was all the powerful additional things you did -- the "anything goes" approach. Maybe a combination of both.

In any case, there's no reason to cry over spilled milk. You have gained valuable experience. Now it is time to use what you have learned and move ahead. It will be alright.

While spinal breathing may have been a help earlier with kundalini, it may not be now with the over-sensitivity to deep meditation.

Cultivating inner silence is the priority, and it can't be done very well with such a short meditation practice. So, I suggest following the line in Lesson 367, and see how it goes.

Some feedback here from time to time will be helpful to everyone, and much appreciated.

All the best!

The guru is in you.

2009/11/06 11:18:36
Building a Daily Practice with Self-Pacing
http://www.aypsite.org/forum/topic.asp?TOPIC_ID=6639&REPLY_ID=59388&whichpage=-1
Latest lessons 366-367

Hi Holy:

I agree that 5-10 minutes of easy alternate nostril breathing pranayama can be calming before meditation, and an aid to those with unruly inner energy.

Whether alternate nostril breathing can help reduce over-sensitivity to deep meditation is another question. Or would it aggravate the situation, as spinal breathing can? Feedback on that is welcome.

The guru is in you.

PS: For over-sensitive meditators who find alternate nostril breathing to be a help, I'd suggest it instead of spinal breathing, not in addition to spinal breathing. One or the other. Or neither, if it doesn't help with stability in meditation.

PPS: The majority of practitioners will be able to follow the baseline AYP system. What we are discussing in Lessons 366-367 is extra measures for those who may be under or over-sensitive to deep meditation with mantra. Lesson 365 lays out the reality of a range sensitivities being observed, followed by specific suggestions in the next two lessons. Whether such measures turn out to be short term or long term solutions is not as important as finding the solutions for those who can use them. I am very happy to see such additions to the AYP toolbox.

It is much better than saying, "Gee, tough luck. There must be something wrong with you." Not true! We are all spiritually gifted. It is only a matter of finding what works best for each of us in self-directed practice. That's the mission. :-)

2009/12/10 11:59:02
Building a Daily Practice with Self-Pacing
http://www.aypsite.org/forum/topic.asp?TOPIC_ID=6639&REPLY_ID=61056&whichpage=-1
Latest lessons 366-367

Hi emc:

The answer is at the end of your question. It is stillness that enables the purification process to advance. Without abiding inner silence, it really isn't purification. It is just energy running around, and that can keep on for a long time.

The key is to keep cultivating abiding inner silence. That is what enables all the rest to happen, including becoming an untouched witness to it. Then as the "friction" becomes less, the energy is transformed gradually into ecstatic bliss, and beyond ... stillness in action.

The guru is in you.

2009/12/11 11:12:57
Building a Daily Practice with Self-Pacing
http://www.aypsite.org/forum/topic.asp?TOPIC_ID=6639&REPLY_ID=61134&whichpage=-1
Latest lessons 366-367

Hi emc:

There will be ups and there will be downs. No one is exempt. We can dance through them both, for in truth (stillness) we are neither. Remember that the next time you are up, and it will soften the down. :-)

The guru is in you.

2010/09/15 11:06:14
Building a Daily Practice with Self-Pacing
http://www.aypsite.org/forum/topic.asp?TOPIC_ID=8435&REPLY_ID=72892&whichpage=-1
Finding the time, when, where to practice?

Hi Jono:

Sounds good.

You might find this lesson on time management helpful:
http://www.aypsite.org/209.html

It is your call, of course. It will work out all right as we "honor the habit" with whatever time we have each day, no matter how little.

All the best!

The guru is in you.

2010/11/22 14:14:36
Building a Daily Practice with Self-Pacing
http://www.aypsite.org/forum/topic.asp?TOPIC_ID=8780&REPLY_ID=75598&whichpage=-1
Self-Pacing for the Under-sensitive

Hi Kami:

Under the category of under-sensitivity to deep meditation, Lesson 366 is offered, which is good for anyone looking to fine-tune the effectiveness of their deep meditation practice.

But your inquiry seems broader than that, as in asking, "How do I speed things up overall?"

Well, going through the lessons and adding practices on step-by-step is one way. But as Carson, Ananda and others (including me) will tell you, it can't be done overnight. And there are delayed effects associated with taking on practices too quickly, so a gradual approach is advised. You will have to find your own pace in taking on new practices in a way that will be stable for you. It is generally not advised to take on a new practice or enhancement to practice more often than every few months (one at a time). And even that is quite aggressive by traditional standards in yoga and spiritual practices. (Note: There are additional suggestions in Lesson 366 also.)

On the retreat side, yes, much can be gained by going several times per year to keep that deeper cycle of cultivating and stabilizing inner silence going. It is generally a stable way of moving ahead in larger steps without upsetting the apple cart, assuming additional practices are not being piled on when in retreat mode. Lessons 387 provides an overview on AYP retreats.

It is normal to notice some fade in the results of a retreat after a few months, and that may be a good time to think about doing another one. It should be mentioned that we get used to new openings pretty quickly, and what we might perceive as a fading in results from a retreat may actually be an acclimation to new openings that have not faded as much as it might seem. The people around you will know best. :-)

In any case, it is normal for the results of practice to fade (and stabilize) in activity, whether from daily sittings (short cycle) or a retreat (long cycle). The fading will not take us all the way back to where we were before practice, but to a new level of opening that is stable within our normal daily routine. It is like a staircase, where we go 4 steps up and 2 steps back again and again, gaining a net of 2 steps every time we go through the cycle of practice and stabilizing the results in daily activity. There is a daily cycle in this with daily practices, and there can be a deeper cycle of several months also, corresponding to retreats we may undertake.

All the best!

The guru is in you.

Forum 11 – Kundalini – Inner Energy Ecstasy

Considering "the awakening," while keeping in balance.
http://www.aypsite.org/forum/forum.asp?FORUM_ID=22

2005/07/13 08:50:30
Kundalini - Inner Energy Ecstasy
http://www.aypsite.org/forum/topic.asp?TOPIC_ID=284
Kundalini - Inner Energy Ecstasy

There are two ingredients in the enlightenment equation -- the rise of inner silence and the rise of ecstatic conductivity.

While inner silence cultivated in deep meditation is the foundation of all progress in yoga, the occurrence of ecstatic conductivity gets much of the press. That is because it is immediately noticeable to the inner senses and can be dramatic, especially if it is prematurely awakened or spontaneously occurring in the nervous system due to past practices engaged in, even before this lifetime. When in its dramatic form, the movement of inner energy is often called "kundalini." But kundalini is a term that applies to all phases of energy awakening, and even to unawakened energy residing in our sexual biology in the pelvic region. AYP Lesson #54 discusses the sexual origins of kundalini, here http://www.aypsite.org/54.html

In AYP we engage in practices that gradually awaken our inner energies in a balanced way. The main practices for this are pranayama, mudras, bandhas and certain asanas. Tantric sexual practices play an important role in the awakening of the inner energies as well. Meditation and samyama stimulate the awakening at very refined levels in the nervous system (the level of pure bliss consciousness), which is essential for the enlightenment connection to occur. The natural outcome of all this is a gradual awakening of an abiding inner ecstasy throughout the nervous system -- and we call that "ecstatic conductivity." The blending of this with our rising inner silence gives rise to the alchemy of enlightenment. The end result is a combined state of unshakable inner silence, ecstatic bliss and outpouring divine love.

There are other kinds of inner energy awakenings that fall outside what we would call an orderly progression. The fundamental causes of these have not been in the AYP style of practices, but have originated in past practices and tendencies some people have been born with. Quite a few have come to AYP with kundalini symptoms of the more extreme variety already in full flame, with an array of dramatic symptoms -- some not very pleasant. For that reason Lesson #69 is included in AYP, which deals with kundalini symptoms and remedies. See http://www.aypsite.org/69.html

Along with a good grounding in AYP-style "self-pacing," Lesson #69 also comes in handy if things go a little out of kilter due to overdoing in AYP practices.

This forum is for discussing energy experiences that can be classified as "kundalini." The initial intention here is not to set up a "kundalini clinic," though that will be up to the participants. While many teachings avoid kundalini difficulties like the plague (too much controversy), that is not the approach here. If something in our experience needs addressing, we should address it as best we can. This is not a guarantee that all energy difficulties can be solved here. In some cases, seeking professional medical help will be the best course to take. But, as a minimum, there is the opportunity here to find good listeners and others who are having similar experiences, along with basic measures for dealing with energy imbalances. It is the least we can do.

There are quite a few kundalini Q&As in the AYP lessons. You can find direct links to them by looking up "kundalini" in the topic index at http://www.aypsite.org/TopicIndex.html

The challenge of dealing with severe kundalini excesses due to wrong sequencing of practices is covered in the Secrets of Wilder novel. See http://www.aypsite.org/books.html
In that case it was the late discovery of spinal breathing pranayama, which is one of the best practices for cultivating and balancing the inner energies.

The guru is in you.

2005/08/04 09:59:45
Kundalini - Inner Energy Ecstasy
http://www.aypsite.org/forum/topic.asp?TOPIC_ID=326&REPLY_ID=275&whichpage=-1
Reply Topic - Kundalini Intro

Thank you, Paul.

Very nice progress with kundalini in the gentle, progressive ways AYP is designed to cultivate. John Wilder could have used your help in the chaotic early stages of his transformation!

The guru is in you.

Yogani
2005/08/27 10:31:06
Kundalini - Inner Energy Ecstasy
http://www.aypsite.org/forum/topic.asp?TOPIC_ID=435&REPLY_ID=453&whichpage=-1
Current of Kundalini

Hello Oliver:

Thank you very much for raising these important questions on the inner pathways and risks of kundalini. Keep in mind that we are all dealing with the same nervous system, and all of the descriptions and practices are working with the same principles and neuro-biological dynamics.

The differences come from interpretations based on individual observations and discoveries, geo-cultural factors and traditional approaches that have been passed down for many generations. The efficacy of them is best judged on experience rather than blind faith acceptance. That is what we try and do here in AYP with a full range of integrated advanced yoga practices.

No doubt you have noticed that all of the variations of the path of kundalini you have mentioned have one thing in common -- part or all of the path is in the vicinity of the spinal cord. This is a pretty big clue on where the center of kundalini activity lies, and where the master control switch is. Certainly kundalini can be observed moving in many other nerve channels (nadis) in the body -- some major ones and many minor ones. Of course there is nothing "minor" about kundalini flowing anywhere. But it emanates primarily from the spine. Anyone who has awakened kundalini will tell you that. While some traditions go beyond the spine in their systems of practice, it is safe to say that the spinal cord is the master channel and controlling mechanism on the kundalini journey. In the yoga traditions, it is called □sushumna.□ In AYP we usually call it the □spinal nerve.□

In AYP we work almost exclusively in and around the spinal nerve with all of our practices, with noticeable results. Make no mistake about it. It is results we are after, first and foremost. Progressive and safe results.

There are a couple of other factors that should be mentioned.

There are two primary aspects of the spiritual transformation we are cultivating. First is the awakening of □inner silence,□ which is done primarily through deep meditation and samyama. Second is the awakening of what we call □ecstatic conductivity□ in the nervous system, which is done mainly with pranayama, mudras, bandhas, asanas and tantric sexual methods. The first is the awakening of the □Shiva□ principle within us. The second is the awakening of the □Shakti□ principle, which is kundalini. There is overlap between all these methods on both the Shiva and Shakti sides because we are neuro-biologically "interconnected" inside.

On the kundalini side of this, yes, you are right that there can be difficulties if the path is not correct and the awakening is not measured (□self-paced□) according to one□s capacity. The most common cause of difficulties has been demonstrated to be □premature awakening of the crown.□ For that reason, here in AYP we do not approach the crown directly until very late on our journey, if at all. Instead, all the practices in AYP are geared to the root to brow (third eye) spinal nerve route, which has been found to be a very stable and progressive route for the vast majority of practitioners. Interestingly, by taking the root to brow approach in our practices, we also are opening the crown □by proxy,□ without incurring the dangers to which you refer.

Once we have effectively cultivated both our inner silence and ecstatic conductivity, then we find a merging of these, which produces a condition where we are experiencing unshakable inner silence, ecstatic bliss and outpouring divine love, all resident in us on an ongoing basis. This we call □enlightenment.□ And all of this will be found to be emanating from the spinal nerve, flowing endlessly outward into the physical environment around us, and inward to the unbounded reaches of inner space. In the end, the outward and inward journeys are found to be one and the same. We become one with all, and that is Unity. Kundalini is but one aspect of the journey, dealing with the transformation of the neuro-biology to a permanent ecstatic condition.

That is a quick summary on how we view the path of kundalini in AYP, and how we cultivate it while minimizing the risks that are often associated with this important aspect of our enlightenment.

For further reading, check the AYP topic index at http://www.aypsite.org/TopicIndex.html which provides many lesson links on all that has been touched on here. If you are new to AYP, it is suggested that you also start at the beginning of the lessons and work your way straight through. There is a logical build-up of both knowledge and practices in the lessons.

Wishing you ongoing success on your chosen path. Practice wisely, and enjoy!

The guru is in you.

2005/08/29 10:24:51
Kundalini - Inner Energy Ecstasy
http://www.aypsite.org/forum/topic.asp?TOPIC_ID=435&REPLY_ID=471&whichpage=-1
Current of Kundalini

Thank you, Oliver. I'm very happy we found you too. May you find the AYP lessons, books and forums to be good resources as you move forward on your chosen path.

Yes, this is much more than a forum. At least we aim for it to be. It will depend on what everyone brings to it. The hope is for it to evolve into a large community of practitioners giving and receiving "horizontally" rather than rigid top-down from a "vertical" hierarchy of teachings. The AYP lessons are designed to be a touchstone for these horizontal communications, not an absolute. The only absolute is your experience with the practices. As they say, "The proof of the pudding is in the eating."

By the way, I have the greatest respect for Swami Satyananda. His book, "Kundalini Tantra" (1984) is a milestone in breaking the secrecy barrior on esoteric practices. If he is off on spinal breathing pranayama or other practices, we can look at all the options and make corrections based on logical assessments of causes and effects. But he broke the secrecy barrier on many practices, you know, and that is very important. Because of people like him, we are now able to have these comparative discussions leading to maximum effectiveness of our yoga practices.

There is more on the gradual shift of yogic writings over the past century from philosophy-oriented to practice-oriented in AYP lesson #253 at http://www.aypsite.org/253.html Philosophy is great. Practice is even better!

The guru is in you.

2005/09/19 10:50:16
Kundalini - Inner Energy Ecstasy
http://www.aypsite.org/forum/topic.asp?TOPIC_ID=485&REPLY_ID=697&whichpage=-1
to heal kundalini syndrome
Hello 2002:

Victor has asked you just the right question. If your kundalini imbalance is related to recent practices, we obviously need to know what they have been in order to offer suggestions. If this is a tendency you have been born with, then it will probably also be practice-related from a previous lifetime you may not remember. Either way, there are measures you can apply now to find relief.

On the religious aspect, keep in mind that "kundalini" is the same as the "Holy Spirit" in Christianity. There is no difference. Only a different name. It is the same human nervous system we all have expressing the same energy. Yoga methods are for advancing the process of spiritual transformation in the human being without regard to race or creed, and this can be seen through eyes that are Christian, Jewish, Hindu, Buddhist,

Muslim or any other religion. There is nothing opposed to God in yoga or kundalini. It is only a matter of right management of practices and experiences. Then the truth contained within our religious orientation will become much stronger.

It seems you have moved too fast somewhere in the past (perhaps doing certain practices too much, or in the wrong order) and that is why you are having difficulty now. That is why the first thing to look at is your practices, and consider making necessary corrections. Also, additional help for managing kundalini energy symptoms can be found in AYP lesson #69 at http://www.aypsite.org/69.html

Do continue with your story here, and I know we can offer some helpful suggestions. I wish you all success on your chosen spiritual path. It will get better!

The guru is in you.

2005/09/23 12:11:42
Kundalini - Inner Energy Ecstasy
http://www.aypsite.org/forum/topic.asp?TOPIC_ID=485&REPLY_ID=744&whichpage=-1
to heal kundalini syndrome

quote:
_____
...another question is the hate for "serpent." I think what you see as serpent as a imagery of nerve channels in your body suddenly you have become more aware of what it happening in your body and started hating it.
_____

Thank you, sauravu, for your fine contributions across the board in the AYP forums. In a very short time you have brought a new dimension to the conversations here. It is always good to hear it from those who grew up in Santan Dharma, Hinduism, or whatever you choose to call it. However it may be named, I have the deepest respect and gratitude. Without it, we would be a few thousand years behind where we are now in putting the practical methods of human spiritual transformation to good use.

Your quote above is especially important, as it points to the role of illusion (maya) in life. How easy it is to mistake the image or metaphor for the reality, and personify it as something opposed to us -- or evil. I think all the human suffering in the world can be traced to this kind of misinterpretation.

The fact is, the "serpent" is none other than the enlivening of our own spinal nerve and other nerves spinning off from it. If we interpret that as something other than our own inner process (or positive divine process in bhakti mode), that is the illusion. A few weeks or months of daily deep meditation can go a long way toward clearing up such misinterpretations. A mind illuminated with inner silence sees the truth of things much more clearly. That's why in AYP we get grounded first in deep meditation, before we attempt to awaken the ecstatic (kundalini) side of our nature. Spinal breathing (root to brow) is also an important prerequisite because of its powerful energy balancing properties.

Just as these core practices can clear up the illusions associated with events inside us, so too do they gradually clear up the illusions on the outside. As Jesus said, "The truth shall set you free." Inner silence and a balanced unfoldment of ecstatic bliss is the truth inside all of us.

I am reminded of the old Indian story about the rope lying on the ground. Someone yelled, "It's a snake!" and everyone went running hither and yon yelling, "There's a snake in the village! A snake in the village!" Many plans were made to get rid of that snake. Finally, someone dared to go close to the rope lying on the ground and saw it was just a rope. Do you think it was easy for her to convince everyone else that it was not a snake? Well, you know the story. We live it every day in real life with all sorts of ropes and imaginary snakes. All the more reason to meditate...

I hope 2002 is still reading. The times when we see a "serpent" in yoga, and think it is a real serpent, are the times when we are a bit ahead of ourselves in practices, or perhaps bumping up against an old sensitivity we have in our nervous system. This does not mean that the serpent is out to get us or our religion. It just means we need to tend to our practices and experiences with a level head, using tried and true methods to bring things back into a tolerable range of inner purification so we can proceed ahead on our journey as smoothly and safely as possible.

The guru is in you.

2006/03/01 23:19:08
Kundalini - Inner Energy Ecstasy
http://www.aypsite.org/forum/topic.asp?TOPIC_ID=527&REPLY_ID=3992&whichpage=-1
Currents while asleep

quote:
_____
Katrine wrote: I tried to meditate with a mantra this morning. It was impossible - completely out of place....it felt meaningless and superficial. The sound wants me to hear it. So I relaxed...and let myself be embraced by it. This immediately results in ecstasy. I have a question for Yogani here: There is no limit now to how high I can go with this sound. But I am a little hesitant....if I let go all the way; will I harm myself? Am I ready for this, or should I still only do 10 min meditation and 5 min pranayama (I love pranayama). And should I "hold back" while meditating? Also: Since the sound is there all the time: how to self-pace?
_____

Hi Katrine and all.

See my comments today on nada (inner sound) versus mantra meditation here: http://www.aypsite.org/forum/topic.asp?TOPIC_ID=860

Let me add that if the sound/energy is taking us up and out the crown, we will be wise to do some grounding instead, as discussed in lesson 69. If we go high without a gradual buildup and balancing of the energy over time, there can be the classic kundalini overdose syndrome. It is rare to have all of a sudden up and out one time and "they all lived happily ever afer." It is more like up and out and crash, and up and out and crash. If the crown is seriously involved, the recovery from this rollercoaster cycle can take a long time. That is not what we are looking for in AYP. More of a smooth and steady development is preferred. Then going up and out will come on gradually via root to brow practices and be light and easy, and so will the aftermath. In fact, eventually we will not know the difference between being up and out the crown and being down here. It will all become the same whole body illumination and divine flow. Then the intensity will be far greater than the crashing version, but we will not notice the intensity, because the energy will be streaming through us with very little friction. Others will notice more than we do. Achieving smooth and stable purification of the vehicle, the human nervous system, is the key in all of this. If we can do that, then there is no limit to how far we can go. We just have to build up to it gradually.

Keep in mind that "automatic yoga" does not put our safety first. It is up to us to do that. We always have the option to ground our excessive energy flows, when necessary. There are many ways to do this. It is good to become familiar with the means, just like it is good to know where the brake pedal is in our car. :-)

The guru is in you.

2006/03/04 10:11:38
Kundalini - Inner Energy Ecstasy
http://www.aypsite.org/forum/topic.asp?TOPIC_ID=527&REPLY_ID=4085&whichpage=-1
Currents while asleep

Hi Katrine:

The mantra knows where to be and how to be according to the course of our inner purification, which is automatic, riding on the wings of inner silence.

The mantra may seem to be somewhere, or nowhere. It matters not. It is the process of easily picking it up and letting it refine that takes us forward in silence. If we notice locations it is okay, but we do not determine them for the mantra. In other practices -- spinal breathing in particular -- we locate with attention. But gently, not to overdo in that. Even spinal breathing has its own inner scheme -- our glorious divine flight through inner space -- opening, balancing, transforming!

The guru is in you.

2005/12/05 16:21:55
Kundalini - Inner Energy Ecstasy
http://www.aypsite.org/forum/topic.asp?TOPIC_ID=625
Kundalini Imbalance

Hi All:

Here is an interchange from my email:

Q1:
I have just ordered both your books and look forward to receiving them. A search on Kechari Mudra led me to your site.

I have a question about Kundalini.

I had always been a very relaxed and laid back guy. Slowly I got interested in Yoga, then meditation, pranayam...As my practice deepened, I became more and more calm, more content and peaceful. Then one day, about 2 years after starting my practice, all this changed.

I started feeling a pressure in the throat area, as though someone was gripping my throat. It feels somewhat like having a lump in the throat, when someone is about to cry. I started becoming very anxious and mentally agitated. I also started suffering from insomnia. Since that day (almost 2 years ago) I have been trying to cope with these things. To this day I still feel as though there is a blockage in my throat. I don't remember the last time I felt physically relaxed.

I was wondering if it's possible my symptoms might have been triggered by kundalini coming up to fast. I am a sensitive Vata type person and perhaps my nervous system was not strong enough to handle the kundalini what was being roused from all the pranayam and to a certain extent, meditation.

Would starting my practice up again only agravate the these symptoms if in fact it were related to kundalini?

A:
Thank you for writing and sharing, and welcome to AYP!

Yes, it does sound like a kundalini imbalance and/or energy blockage in the throat area. Since I do not know the particulars of your practices in the past, it is hard to say what has caused the difficulty -- how things got to be imbalanced. However, the important thing is to to move forward correctly from here, and AYP can offer quite a few suggestions on that.

AYP includes a lot of preventive and curative measures for kundalini, including managing the inner energies in a progressive and safe way. Check lesson #69 for a review of some of the factors and possible measures for dealing with an energy imbalance. Near the top of the list for remedies is spinal breathing, which is a core practice in AYP. It has very good balancing properties and can help resolve blockages like you have described, and also help with the emotions and sleep problems that often come with energy imbalances. These are caused by having too much energy running around inside without balancing the ascending and descending energies in the nervous system. Spinal breathing addresses this directly and immediately.

Also, in the particular case of a throat blockage, the "chin pump" practice, done in moderation, can be very effective for clearing up the problem. See lesson #139 and related followup lessons on that.

Normally I would not recommend jumping around in the lessons like that, but these are two that come to mind that might offer you some measures for immediate relief. It would also be wise to take the lessons from the beginning and go straight through. That way you will have the whole picture and see how all the practices are interrelated and logically managed in AYP using "self-pacing." It will also give you some useful perspectives on the practices you have been doing in the past, and help you reach decisions on where your practice should go from here. These are all your choices. AYP is not a rigid tradition. It is an open resource for independent practitioners.

If you don't mind, I'd like to post our interchange anonymously in the AYP forums so others can benefit from this discussion. You can read and interact with many practitioners from beginning to advanced in the AYP forums.

Please let me know if it would be okay to post this there.

I wish you all success on your chosen spiritual path. Practice wisely, and enjoy!

The guru is in you.

Q2:
Thank you for your advice. I have no objections against posting our exchanges on the forum. I felt it was somewhat strange that I had felt so peaceful and calm, and that in one instant, that all changed. hopefully, with your suggestions, I will be able to go back to remove any blockages in the throat and help the energy circulate more freely.

2005/12/06 08:32:13
Kundalini - Inner Energy Ecstasy
http://www.aypsite.org/forum/topic.asp?TOPIC_ID=625&REPLY_ID=1802&whichpage=-1
Kundalini Imbalance
Here is more with the same correspondent:

Q:
Prior to my problems arising, I was well established in abdominal breathing. I was breathing from the belly most of the time. Since that day, it seems my breathing has been confined to the area of the upper chest and just below the adam's apple. Trapped. Even when trying to consciously breathe from the belly, it is difficult and not as natural as it had once been.

A:
That also should become better as the energies are balanced via the means suggested. Everything is connected -- mind, body, emotions, breath, etc. This connectedness throughout the nervous system is a fundamental principle in yoga. See "connectedness of yoga" in the topic index for lessons on that.

All of your symptoms point to energy being "up" without enough downward flow to balance it. This is a common ailment in a yoga culture that is dominated by the idea that enlightenment is a one way journey -- upward, with practices skewed that way also. The worst in all of this is often a premature focus on crown practices which can create a real kundalini mess, epitomized in the problematic journey chronicled by Gopi Krishna about 50 years ago. The problems associated with premature crown practices are discussed in the AYP lessons. Check the topic index again, this time for "crown practices (avoiding premature)."

Lesson #69 on kundalini symptoms and remedies is mostly about "grounding" the energies by various methods, some quite mundane (yet effective) like exercise and diet, and then picking back up with practices that are more balanced for moving forward.

Also, if you are going to use chin pump as mentioned in the first posting above, I suggest you do the "lite" version without breath retention (kumbhaka), at least starting out. This is covered in a follow-up lesson to the main chin pump lesson (#139). Breath retention is a kundalini stimulator. While breath retention is fine when everything is going in the right direction (and chin pump will help with that), it is not necessarily the best thing to be doing during a period of imbalance.

All the best!

The guru is in you.

2005/12/06 12:32:03
Kundalini - Inner Energy Ecstasy
http://www.aypsite.org/forum/topic.asp?TOPIC_ID=625&REPLY_ID=1808&whichpage=-1
Kundalini Imbalance

Hi Y:

Yes, food sensitivities and anal itching can be common kundalini symptoms too. Which is not to say these things can't happen for other reasons.

The good news is that the practices here in AYP, if done with good self-pacing, do lead to many fewer uncomfortable symptoms, while at the same time much more energy flowing and refining to ecstatic bliss. It takes some time though, depending on how far out of kilter things are now and what the underlying state of purification in the nervous system is.

Keep in mind that the cultivation of inner silence in deep meditation is the ground state of all the progress we are discussing here. Kundalini is really the tail on the big dog of pure bliss consciousness. If we put the tail in charge of the dog, what happens?

That's is why I am frequently cautioning folks about doing energy practices without deep meditation in the picture. Most kundalini cases demonstrate this point.

The same can be said of spinal breathing, which is by far the most effective means for awakening the ecstatic energies in a balanced way. But even that should not be the primary focus over deep meditation. That is the AYP point of view.

There is lots of hope around here. Dip in and take a nice long cool drink. :-)

The guru is in you.

2006/01/04 11:07:25
Kundalini - Inner Energy Ecstasy
http://www.aypsite.org/forum/topic.asp?TOPIC_ID=686&REPLY_ID=2339&whichpage=-1

Move over Tesla, here she comes ("K" reminders)

Hi Yves:

That was a beaut. Balance and self-pacing in practices are the first things that come to mind on reading your dramatic kundalini experience.

That, and a reminder that the idea of "breaking through" to higher levels in the body with these kinds of experiences is somewhat of an illusion. I know this is not your intention. It just happened, right? Yet, the idea can creep in that "this is it," and we should now focus on cultivating these kinds of dramatic breakthrough events. To be honest, there is no such thing as a final opening of this kind, and there is barely such a thing as a significant incremental opening. These things rarely happen in quantum leaps, even though they might appear to be doing so. There is the idea out there that all we have to do is bring the energy up to the top and then we are done -- enlightened. Not so.

Rather, there are endless degrees of purification and opening going on to infinity. The *Secrets of Wilder* novel provides a scenario representing this process. No matter how big a jolt we might get, or how high up, we are still only at the beginning of the next stage. So there is no rush to open a particular physical area and break through into higher centers with all this. We can arrive there via natural means (a la AYP style practices), and be much more comfortable going at it that way.

Of course, our bhakti will always be begging for more, and therein lies the balancing act. John Wilder had a tough time with this, balancing his bhakti with his sometimes frenetic pace, learning his lessons as he went along. We all have to do this...

I mention all this because, while the big experiences may seem like a lot progress-wise, they are all baby steps. The real big progress comes from long term stable daily practice. And that can be with no big jolts at all. In fact, the big jolts can lead us into energy overdoses that can delay our practices for days, weeks or months. An intentional big jolt breakthrough approach is a slower path!

Which is not to say we will not ever have them. It can can happen sometimes, as you have experienced, even with a stable practice routine. It is a reminder that we are dealing with powerful forces within, and should keep that in mind as we manage our practices day-to-day. If we are pushing too hard in practices, we can have this kind of delayed reaction. Therefore, it is good to keep a smart foot on that accelerator (our practices).

So now you have some proof that something is really going on in there. You have become a believer in your own inner potential. :-)

May it be an inspiration to settle down into a long term stable routine that will steadily open things up. Then, one morning you will wake up and realize that without even noticing you traveled a thousand miles further than all the jolts in the world could take you.

If we are steadily cultivating inner silence, and gently coaxing up ecstatic conductivity, all will unfold naturally and more quickly than any energy breakthrough experience can deliver.

Thanks for sharing that one, and all the best as you move ahead from here.

The guru is in you.

2006/01/04 23:46:29
Kundalini - Inner Energy Ecstasy
http://www.aypsite.org/forum/topic.asp?TOPIC_ID=686&REPLY_ID=2352&whichpage=-1
Move over Tesla, here she comes ("K" reminders)

Hi Yves:

Is this the Tesla you are talking about? Interesting story.

http://www.thevillager.com/villager_44/pennypost.html

Note also the Gopi Krishna reference in the article.

Yes, kundalini is like that -- it produces huge flows of creative energy, and can burn one out from the inside if the ground of the nervous system is not prepared. Hence, self-pacing in our advanced yoga practices. When the nervous system is prepared it definitely becomes a case of "Move over Tesla." :-)

I must say there would be no AYP bubbling out without this sort of thing going on here. It is much more than the raw creativity and insight that Tesla and Gopi Krishna exhibited and described. It is also a boundless outpouring of divine love. That is a higher manifestation of the energy -- turning it all toward loving service and the inevitable unity experience for everyone -- the conscious joining.

"I am That. You are That. All this is That."

Or -- The One is the many and the many are the One.

The guru is in you.

2006/01/05 00:05:56
Kundalini - Inner Energy Ecstasy
http://www.aypsite.org/forum/topic.asp?TOPIC_ID=686&REPLY_ID=2354&whichpage=-1
Move over Tesla, here she comes ("K" reminders)

Hi Anthem:

We posted at the same time.

Yes, AYP-style practices are for making the journey smoother and safer -- more balanced. We can also say that the practices facilitate the journey itself -- that the journey would be much much slower for most of us without the practices. That is, after all, what yoga is for -- union -- though Krishnamurti types pooh-pooh the idea of yoga practices. What do they know? We are living it!

The practices give everyone a chance to make big strides in this life according to personal desire and commitment, assuming everyone has access to the information. It is about time for that access, yes? It is about time we fully develop all of this in an open and systematic way.

So here we are, having these experiences of human spiritual transformation and these amazing conversations...

The guru is in you.

2006/01/05 14:46:26
Kundalini - Inner Energy Ecstasy
http://www.aypsite.org/forum/topic.asp?TOPIC_ID=686&REPLY_ID=2362&whichpage=-1
Move over Tesla, here she comes ("K" reminders)

Hi Weaver and David:

Weaver: Yoni mudra won't go away. Recall what I mentioned about the purification process continuing far beyond any particular opening. All of the practices continue to be important in promoting a full and balanced opening, within the limits of good self-pacing. The way to handle yoni mudra is to lighten it up (or stop it) during periods of release. Then come back very gradually after the release clears up, looking for that stable balance between practices and purification experiences. "Kundalini symptoms" are symptoms of purification -- energy causing friction in nerves that are not fully purified. Once the nerves are purified, the friction will be much less and much more energy will flow with much less fanfare. In the end, the energy flow is vast and the symptoms minimal. That is the outpouring of divine love mentioned above, in a nervous system that has been adequately purified and stabilized via well-managed practices.

Kundalini experiences can happen to anyone with or without practices. They are a sign of evolution, and we are all evolving -- with practices or not. With practices we can go much faster and further, and with much better balance. That is the difference. If "normal" practices seem to be associated with an aggravated kundalini, then we should self-pace them like we would at any other level of practices.

****

David: Good question about where I am answering questions. Everywhere they come it seems! :-)

Originally, I was concerned that I would be bombarded with so many questions in the forum that the forum would become about me, which I do not want. I want it to be a community where everyone is helping each other at increasingly higher levels. I think this is a healthy path of evolution for the AYP community -- and we all know it will go higher and higher as everyone advances. This will open the door for many more seekers to find assistance, with less reliance on me for the answers. Many of you are answering questions on a very high level already, based on your own experiences. Bravo for that!

So here is the deal. Anyone can ask anything they want here of me or the community. If others can cover the questions, I will not say much (even if it is addressed to me). If there seems to be a gap, I'll jump in. Whatever makes sense. But let's make it a community, not a Yogani Q&A. I think we are doing so, and I hope it will continue to grow like that. The theory is that by the time there are too many questions for me to answer here, there will be many others who can answer them. Let's see if it works.

Given the above community-building plan and my commitment to writing more books and online lessons, I have shifted my position on emails to encouraging everyone to bring their questions here to the forums. That way many of you can help with answering questions and more people will benefit immediately from the public discussion. In other words, the quantity of private emails I will be doing will go down as most of it shifts here to the forums. This is how it should be for all the reasons mentioned. It also adds diversity and more opportunities for exploration of ways to optimize the practices.

Neither AYP nor I have all the answers. AYP is a suggested baseline from which many things can be explored and tested. I believe Jim called it a "safe harbor." That is exactly the function AYP should serve, and yoga should move on to increasingly optimized levels of application as research and practical results warrant. As long as we are working with the underlying principles of human spiritual transformation and a basic set of guidelines like AYP, then we have set the stage for tremendous progress both short term and long term. We are giving birth to a new applied science here...

The language in the forum introductions was modified several weeks ago to cover the shift to encouraging everyone to bring their questions to the forums, and it was also covered in the latest lesson #279 -- http://www.aypsite.org/279.html

The guru is in you.

2006/05/09 10:31:24
Kundalini - Inner Energy Ecstasy
http://www.aypsite.org/forum/topic.asp?TOPIC_ID=1120&REPLY_ID=6705&whichpage=-1
Ajna and Crown

Hi Katrine:

Clearly, something in you wants to move on, and your job has become to manage it for comfort and safety. If I understand correctly, your illness 10 years ago was an opening where it all took off. Life crises are prominent causes of spiritual progress. Indeed, that is what they can be for, if we open and let them. It seems you are finding a balance in it, and if the light practices are helping, then that is all the proof you need. Self-pacing it you are...

Obviously, we can't go around struggling to ignore our experiences. On the other hand, we can favor balancing practices. I suggest if the energy is going too fast, then that is a good time to "carry water and chop wood" -- in addition to the light sitting practices, getting involved in the everyday things that can help ground us. I think you are. These can vary from digging holes in the garden to engaging fully in service for the benefit of others. The divine energy knows what it needs to be fulfilled at any given time. We are but a channel for that ... self-pacing evolves to become accommodating the expression of the divine flow through us in every moment.

As for whether you are "trying" to do all this or not. Well, you remind me of our middle son, who, when little (he's 29 now), we might catch with chocolate all over his face and find the lid off the chocolate cookie jar in the kitchen. His response to an inquiry on that? "I didn't do it!"

The truth of the matter is that if we chase spiritual transformation long enough (lifetimes!), we will wake up one lifetime and find it chasing us.

We didn't do it! But the chocolate never lies, you know. Ask John Wilder. He'll tell you. It is cause and effect ... enjoy the ride! :-)

The guru is in you.

2006/05/10 10:42:41
Kundalini - Inner Energy Ecstasy
http://www.aypsite.org/forum/topic.asp?TOPIC_ID=1120&REPLY_ID=6776&whichpage=-1
Ajna and Crown

Hi Katrine:

It goes without saying that inner silence enables us to weather the vast energy movements that can happen in us on our path of purification and opening. With inner silence, we can just watch and know deep within ourselves that this is part of the process. Our witness never moves, does it? no matter how much ecstatic energy is moving. Nevermind that inner silence is a primary cause of such energy movments also. Stillness in action! :-)

This is why deep meditation is first in AYP, for both progress and protection. This is also why it is not a good idea to begin with "energy work" when starting out on our path. If all of this energy stuff is happening without some degree of the witness, a whole lot of catching up with inner silence will be necessary, working from a disadvantage. And that is assuming we even know how to cultivate inner silence. Quite a few have come to AYP with energy issues over the past few years, not knowing how to cultivate inner silence and the witness, or about the basics of managing kundalini excesses. Most have been helped.

Katrine, in case you did not read it between the lines of my last note, your experiences are very beautiful, and you are right on (cautions included - thank you, Jim). It is not always easy for highly driven yoginis and yogis (yes, you are one at the deepest level), but the payoff will be there. It just takes time and prudent pacing in practices and daily living.

So many here are doing so well, and I am very impressed. It is not only a few. It is all of you, managing your own purification and opening with a little help from the AYP writings and each other. Imagine where we all will be in a decade. Lots of sages running around, I bet. Lots of horizontal sharing, with more and more people around the world finding their path. I hope I live to see it.

Bring on the butterflies!

The guru is in you.

2006/05/24 23:11:25
Kundalini - Inner Energy Ecstasy
http://www.aypsite.org/forum/topic.asp?TOPIC_ID=1170&REPLY_ID=7303&whichpage=-1
Vortex

Hi Alan:

Yes, a whirling can happen and is not uncommon in energy movements associated with purification. It can be whirling in both directions at the same time too -- ascending and descending. If there is disorientation or dizziness it usually will pass pretty quickly. If it gets to be too much, you know what to do -- self-pace...

The guru is in you.

2006/05/26 11:05:07
Kundalini - Inner Energy Ecstasy
http://www.aypsite.org/forum/topic.asp?TOPIC_ID=1170&REPLY_ID=7350&whichpage=-1
Vortex

Hi All:

The minty sensation in the spine and elsewhere is a sign of the GI tract getting into the act, with higher digestion occurring in there, producing a refined somatic ("of the body") substance that permeates the entire nervous system. It is essentially the sexual function refining, combined with increasing porousness of the body tissues due to pranayama, mudras and bandhas. Then food, air and sexual essences combine to produce the alchemy of the somatic substance. It happens in the GI tract and can be felt in the spine during spinal breathing, and eventually all the time. It is what is behind other ecstatic sensations occurring from head to toe as well. It is the actualization of the "cool and warm currents" in spinal breathing that we begin priming with the cool and warm sensations of breath. The mint has a glow to it and is the manifestion of the manipura chakra in the belly too, which means "city of gems." It all ties together like that.

Mint (or liniment) is both cool and warm, yes? That is the sensation, with a glow and rising ecstatic quality as well. It is the stuff of ecstatic conductivity and radiance coming alive. It even whirls, and we may notice that before the minty sensations. It can be coming in any order and in any part of the body, depending on the unique course of our purification.

Fortunately, we do not need an in-depth intellectual understanding of the process to conduct this operation. We just do the easy daily practices with dedication, and in time it happens. Bravo for that!

This is why we talk about the option to do the cool and warm current thing in spinal breathing, and everything else associated with awakening ecstatic conductivity. May the mint be with you. :-)

The guru is in you.

2006/08/06 11:11:27
Kundalini - Inner Energy Ecstasy
http://www.aypsite.org/forum/topic.asp?TOPIC_ID=1385&REPLY_ID=10270&whichpage=-1

frist yoga class

Hi Sadhak:

It is the purity of the spinal nerve and nervous system in general that makes the difference in spiritual progress. As spiritual practice, asanas are for aiding in that, as are spinal breathing, deep meditation, mudras, bandhas, and all the rest of yoga.

I believe there has been too much emphasis placed on strong and erect posture, often at the expense of inner development. It is physical development overriding spiritual development, which is so common in yoga everywhere in modern times, and perhaps in all times. The point is driven home by viable paths that do not focus on asanas at all, and by lazy people like us who meditate leaning against a pile of pillows, and still making good progress. :-)

Yoga isn't just for macho-types. It is for everyone, no matter what the physical circumstances may be. In yoga, at least around here, it is "less pain, more gain."

Of course, there is nothing like a gentle set of asanas to loosen us up inwardly before sitting practices. And being upright is generally better than being reclined while doing sitting practices, so we favor that, as comfortable. For the rest, do what works, and forget about the image of the hardened yogi/yogini sitting like a pillar of strength on a rock ... it will not help.

Also, daily physical exercise taken anytime except right before yoga practices is very good for health and spirit. Activity is good between our sitting practices. It stabilizes inner silence gained in sitting practices, and in this way we become "That" in all we do...

The guru is in you.

2006/11/21 11:24:36
Kundalini - Inner Energy Ecstasy
http://www.aypsite.org/forum/topic.asp?TOPIC_ID=1742&REPLY_ID=13570&whichpage=-1
Excessive energy movement in the head

Hi Weaver:

Sorry to hear you are having some difficulties.

Often times, our subconscious intentions (internal bhakti habit) can fuel excessive purification, even outside practices. Then it can help to get involved with other things. I'm sure you are well aware of the grounding methods in lesson 69. If those are not working for you, then it may be a matter of focusing on other things for a while -- your work (which hopefully is fulfilling), family & friends, service in the community, outdoor activities, a vacation. I went through a similar episode many years ago and ended up taking five years worth of Tai C
Hi classes, while continuing yoga practices. It helped a lot to balance the inner energies.

Continue to be mindful of the full range of kundalini remedies available. There are many ways to tone it down until a particular aspect of purification runs its course, and a combination of measures is often the solution.

We each have a somewhat different course of purification occurring, and we have to self-pace accordingly. In time, it will smooth out. As our collective knowledge grows, we will find more ways to navigate these periods, or, even better, regulate them before they become excessive. We have come a long way since the Gopi Krishna days, but still have much to learn about the process of human spiritual transformation.

If you believe there could be a health issue, it will be wise to see a doctor to get things checked out. Health concerns have their own way of weighing on us, so it is good to address them as necessary.

May balance return to you soon. All the best!

The guru is in you.

2006/11/21 11:47:42
Kundalini - Inner Energy Ecstasy
http://www.aypsite.org/forum/topic.asp?TOPIC_ID=1742&REPLY_ID=13574&whichpage=-1
Excessive energy movement in the head
PS -- Regarding inversion, if it helps, it could be a sign not of too much energy in the head, but of not enough. It can happen. If that is the case, light practice of inversion asanas (yoga mudra, shoulder stand, plow, standing toe touch, etc.), uddiyana/nauli and mulabandha can help. But be careful not to overdo any of these -- don't want to go from the frying pan into the fire!
2006/12/20 20:36:53
Kundalini - Inner Energy Ecstasy
http://www.aypsite.org/forum/topic.asp?TOPIC_ID=1829&REPLY_ID=14677&whichpage=-1
Kundalini/Possession Fear

quote:
_____
Originally posted by yoginstar

QUESTION FOR YOGANI: I added a picture on the dutch lesson number 33......... http://www.odysseyofthesoul.de/AYP/033.htm about halfway down... let me know if you wish me to remove it:-):-):-)
All the best!
_____

Hi Yoginstar:

Not able to read Dutch, so not sure what the context of the photo is. I don't think Sri Yukteswar is mentioned in that lesson. We certainly don't want to imply that full lotus (padmasana) is a prerequisite, or goal, for AYP sitting practices. It is a lesson on simple cross-legged sitting. Later on we offer siddhasana. Padmasana is not instructed in AYP.

So, unless you have a good reason, it probably doesn't belong there. Maybe in a lesson where Sri Yukteswar or padmasana is mentioned, if you like. It would be appreciated that if you add anything like that to include a note such as, "photo added by translator," or something similar, so folks won't get confused about what is in the original lessons.

I see you are up to lesson 42 already. Not bad! :-)

Many thanks, and all the best!

The guru is in you.

2006/12/30 10:25:01
Kundalini - Inner Energy Ecstasy
http://www.aypsite.org/forum/topic.asp?TOPIC_ID=1861&REPLY_ID=15104&whichpage=-1
Kirtanman's a Hothead! (Crown Chakra Exp.)

quote:
_____
Originally posted by Athma_Shakti

these days many peoples practicing yoga is having early crown activity. and many of them are natural born psychics or yogis. but no harm and not to worry. its a good sign of spiritual progress :-)

i think, its happening because the total human consciousness is shifting toward the subtle.
_____

Hi All:

I agree with Athma Shakti on this. We are dealing with a moving target as far as human receptivity to spiritual openings is concerned. We have been accelerating gradually over the past century or so, and now there is an exponential effect kicking in. In the short three years since we started AYP, the acceleration has been very noticeable. Not that AYP is the only thing going on -- many teachings are expanding, and acceleration is happening everywhere. In the case of AYP, the effects of the practices are often becoming noticeable much quicker, and in some cases leading to the kind of rapid purification described in this topic and elsewhere in the forums.

From my side, there is concern for the comfort and safety of everyone, so please do self-pace before symptoms become extreme. And please keep in mind the AYP cautions about going to the crown too soon, or in a haphazard way. The fact that core practices like spinal breathing and deep meditation can now lead to rapid crown awakenings, is cause for extra vigilance in self-pacing. With rapid purification, it may not be so much about keeping practice times as keeping on an even keel during daily activity. As you know, our experience in daily activity, outside our yoga routine, is the real test of our practices. So always adjust practices accordingly. Many are doing an excellent job with this. Thank you!

Something wonderful is coming up everywhere. It will be well worth a few bumps in the road along the way. But let's be sure to keep it on the road.

I am always looking for ways to adapt to changing circumstances, and will continue to do so. The new Samyama book, coming out in January, will look into expanded areas of practice that might have been considered "way out there" only a few years ago. Now we find ourselves quickly entering a situation where we can have a much greater impact on the evolution of the entire human race. As this trend accelerates, each one of us will increasingly have the abilty to dissolve mountains of obstructions holding back planetary evolution. It will not necessarily be a 100% orderly transformation, as we are sometimes seeing on the individual level, and also in the physical environment. Something big is happening, we are all part of it, and we are able to affect it for the better.

Meanwhile, as we are speeding along from here to there, let's not blow it out the top too soon or too much. Remember to chop wood and carry water. Savor the ordinary, even as you accomplish the extraordinary. It is all ordinary... :-)

All the best!

The guru is in you.

2007/01/05 10:56:02
Kundalini - Inner Energy Ecstasy
http://www.aypsite.org/forum/topic.asp?TOPIC_ID=1861&REPLY_ID=15414&whichpage=-1
Kirtanman's a Hothead! (Crown Chakra Exp.)

Hi Kirtanman and All:

The main thing we are concerned about when the crown becomes active (more common nowadays) is maintaining comfort and safety. This is not only for health and wellbeing, but for the sustainability of our path (remember, blasting through doesn't work). If we are so undone that we lose motivation and/or the ability to practice because we are being run over by crown-induced energy all the time, this is less than ideal. So, we keep it on the road as best we can. Yes, self-pacing does become automatic within us in time. It becomes intuitive. That, and ever advancing inner purification eventually lead to the "other side" where we find balance amidst the constantly expanding outflow of divine love. It is a birthing process, and like physical birth, it can be a bit chaotic at times.

There is a practice in the Samyama book coming out this month that may offer some balance to those with crown activity, and offer a smoothening for those who are creeping in the direction of crown opening. Imagine the crown as being an energy door with huge pressure on the inside -- or looking at it another way, as having a huge vacuum on the outside. If the door opens a crack, everything wants to rush out all at once, sucking all that is in here out with it. This can lead to the premature crown opening syndrome.

If we begin to work with our practice on both sides of the door, there is an opportunity to equalize the pressure somewhat. That is what we are introducing in the new Samyama book. The practice is called "Cosmic Samyama."

When we tie all of this together, the possibilities become quite remarkable, not only for us individually, but for the entire world. As inner purification leads to the infinite outpouring of divine love, we find ourselves increasingly in a position to apply expanded applications of samyama within that huge outflow. This rapidly expanding phenomenon of *intentional divine flow* (stillness in action) can change the course of humanity, and has already. It is at the heart of the exponential acceleration in spiritual progress we are seeing everywhere around the world today. It is something we desire -- our destiny.

The guru is in you.

2007/01/05 15:36:54
Kundalini - Inner Energy Ecstasy
http://www.aypsite.org/forum/topic.asp?TOPIC_ID=1861&REPLY_ID=15430&whichpage=-1
Kirtanman's a Hothead! (Crown Chakra Exp.)

quote:
_____
Originally posted by Kirtanman

How do we distinguish between "headed for derailment", and "significant but acceptable" practice results?
_____

Hi Kirtanman:

Experience -- giving rise to intuititive self-pacing. We each must make our own discoveries about this.

How do we learn how much to let off the gas when going into a sharp curve with a steep cliff falling off the outside edge? We learn it carefully, right? :-)

The guru is in you.

2007/02/15 09:59:59
Kundalini - Inner Energy Ecstasy
http://www.aypsite.org/forum/topic.asp?TOPIC_ID=2063&REPLY_ID=17556&whichpage=-1
Help!! serious inner energy problems

Hi IcedEarth:

Sorry to hear you are having some trouble there. Presumably you already know the standard remedies (lesson 69), and some of those have been reinforced by others here.

What could be added is that you are about to go through a big change in location and activity, and you are no doubt anticipating the change, perhaps with some trepidation. It is normal.

If the kundalini energies are running, there can be the tendency for our emotions to become amplified, and the energies along with them. This is particularly true if inner silence is not fully permeating our nervous system, thoughts, emotions, etc.

It could be viewed as the equivilent of pre-change jitters, amplified via an active kundalini. This is why doing mundane grounding activities is good for dealing with excess kundalini energy. As the Buddhists say, "Chop wood, carry water." Your trip can be like that too. Just do it, without so much inner fanfare. Try not to anticipate too much. Just do. Your inner silence will take care of it if you let it.

You will get through it. Once you are settled into the new routine in Spain, things will be much better. Just lay as low as you can with spiritual practices until then, and continue to ground as much as possible. Things will look much better when you get to the other side of Friday. You know they will. :-)

Check in here once in a while to let us know how you are doing. But I suggest you do not hang around the forums all the time, as they can be stimulating too. Focus on what is coming up -- your wonderful study program in Spain. Focusing on what is there right in front of us can be very grounding. Consider upcoming events to be an opportunity to integrate all that is happening inside you with a new external adventure.

Your job is to do, let go, and enjoy!

The guru is in you.

2007/02/15 13:28:38
Kundalini - Inner Energy Ecstasy
http://www.aypsite.org/forum/topic.asp?TOPIC_ID=2063&REPLY_ID=17572&whichpage=-1
Help!! serious inner energy problems

quote:
_____
Originally posted by Anthem11

Not sure why it is rarely suggested for excess kundalini symptoms, but I personally find a super quick fix to excess energies is traditional (read *with ejaculation*) sex. A few sessions for a male with or without a partner certainly brings my energy back to manageable levels.
_____

Yes, Anthem, you are absolutely right on that.

Sexual release is most often discussed in a tantric context, but energy is energy, and it is a real pressure release valve. Perhaps it is not mentioned in the context of kundalini energy management much because so much of the time we are working on going the other way with orgasm.

Of course, having our kundalini energies raging is having too much of a good thing, and we should do what is necessary to keep things on an even keel.

For those interested in increasing the inner energies and promoting the rise of ecstatic conductivity, the inverse is also true -- restraining orgasm (engaging in pre-orgasmic sex) is going to increase the inner energies, so the pressure value works in both directions. It works best in conjunction with a daily routine of sitting practices, including deep meditation for cultivating abiding inner silence.

Thanks for the valuable suggestion.

The guru is in you.

2007/02/23 10:44:35
Kundalini - Inner Energy Ecstasy
http://www.aypsite.org/forum/topic.asp?TOPIC_ID=2096&REPLY_ID=17953&whichpage=-1
Ecstatic radiance?

Hi Christi:

Yes, we can regulate how our energy (ecstatic radiance) affects others. Then what happens is mainly a function of their bhakti -- always the case anyway. If there is a warm stove in the room, everyone makes their own choice on how to relate to that. We too can make a choice on how much we radiate in any given circumstance -- the other extreme is that we can choose to become essentially invisible. It is the management of energy on a higher level. Self-pacing for the benefit of everyone. Our practice is not only about us. It is about everyone! This becomes increasingly clear as we move along our path. Unity...

Thanks for chiming in Shanti with the rest of it.

I will be a bit scarce around here in the coming weeks due to a pressing family commitment, so it will be best to ask questions more openly to whoever can answer. That is also the ongoing policy -- these forums are for everyone to be helping each other. I will put in my two cents whenever able. :-)

All the best!

The guru is in you.

2007/03/01 11:30:34
Kundalini - Inner Energy Ecstasy
http://www.aypsite.org/forum/topic.asp?TOPIC_ID=2096&REPLY_ID=18230&whichpage=-1
Ecstatic radiance?

Hi All:

The reason I haven't addressed the energy effect on others question very much yet is because it is largely a matter of experience and intention.

It is like when we learn to walk, at the same time we learn not to walk into walls or over cliffs. So it is less about "technique" than it is about becoming familiar with our own capabilities via direct experience in our environment, and adjusting our intentions and actions accordingly.

Obviously, we don't want to be frying ourselves or anyone else with our spiritual energy, so we develop our intentions in relation to that, let them go, and the rest is samyama. It is a form of self-pacing. At least that is how I have viewed it for a long time. Perhaps we will develop more definitive methods for energy regulation as time goes on, with more people coming into that realm of experience.

But, as I have mentioned before, much of this is organic development that comes naturally from stillness in action. We can trust that process.

What we don't want to be doing is laboring excessively over (or against) the energy scenery, especially if we are not even seeing it fully yet. We are in transition, and it is a natural process, like learning to walk. There will be no abyss of energy (or ego) disaster as long as we are operating from inner silence. Everything will work out just fine as long as we favor our practices over our experiences, and self-pace as needed.

If some find this to be an over-simplification of a complex process, well, I am happy for that, because it opens the door for more folks to unfold their own destiny. That is the whole game around here -- maximizing access for everyone. We can deal with it. Somehow we have managed, for the most part, to master kitchen knives, automobiles, airplanes and nuclear energy. I'm quite sure we can master spiritual energy also. Call me an optimist. :-)

May the research and development of applied spiritual science continue indefinitely. All the answers are within us.

The guru is in you.

2007/03/04 22:41:00
Kundalini - Inner Energy Ecstasy
http://www.aypsite.org/forum/topic.asp?TOPIC_ID=2096&REPLY_ID=18352&whichpage=-1
Ecstatic radiance?

Hi Doc:

I don't think divine power and worldly power can be regarded as synonymous, though both are expressing from the same source. One is born of loving surrender and is unlimited. The other is born of external manipulation and is limited. While it may not always be clear which is manifesting in the moment, we will always find out soon enough ... "Ye shall know each tree by its fruit."

Interestingly, there will always be power manifesting in one way or other, either divinely through loving surrender, or in a worldly way through willful expression. In reality, it is always going to be a blend in each of us.

426 – Advanced Yoga Practices

There has never been a spiritual master who did not willfully express the tiniest bit of worldly power (some have expressed a lot of worldly power). And there has never been a powerful megalomaniac without some trace of a soul (some have had a lot of soul).

So it is not a matter of being one or the other. We are all both, and we each choose which way to go on that scale -- toward divine expression, or toward egoic expression. The manifestation of power is inevitable and unavoidable. Yet, from where that power is manifesting we can choose -- direct from infinite inner silence that is eternal divine love, or through a limited ego that will run us up on the rocks again and again. Is this such a difficult choice? :-)

The guru is in you.

2007/03/05 13:25:25
Kundalini - Inner Energy Ecstasy
http://www.aypsite.org/forum/topic.asp?TOPIC_ID=2096&REPLY_ID=18372&whichpage=-1
Ecstatic radiance?

quote:
──────────
Originally posted by Doc

The fullest potential of all manifestations and expressions of power within us and through us, for the greatest positive good of all, is dependent upon our willingness to accept our calling for its use with complete surrender to God's Will, IMO. This is the ultimate act of devotion, is it not?
──────────

Hi Doc:

Of course, "God's Will" is "ishta," one's chosen ideal in the act of bhakti. For one person it may be the deity and/or master of a religious tradition. For another, it may be the unconditioned stillness present within, and everywhere. For yet another, it may be the whispering spirits of nature.

So, what is "God's Will?" It is that which we are able to surrender to that represents something greater than our limited personal existence. Our longing and devotion to That will take us forward into the unlimited. It does not have to be religious (the concept of "God" is not mandatory). Nor does it have to be non-religious. It is for no one to judge except each of us in our heart. We will know our own tree by its fruit. And we can self-pace accordingly. :-)

The guru is in you.

2007/03/09 14:47:37
Kundalini - Inner Energy Ecstasy
http://www.aypsite.org/forum/topic.asp?TOPIC_ID=2096&REPLY_ID=18576&whichpage=-1
Ecstatic radiance?

quote:
──────────
Originally posted by meg

Also nice depictions Doc, although the middle one seems off topic.

I have no idea what the 'shine' is that is being discussed. I can appreciate it as a gift that comes from a long-time commitment to purification. Is the 'ecstatic radiance' something different than the 'shine'? I understand the radiance to be That which emanates from within, and far from being a product of our own spiritual constructions. As stated so eloquently elsewhere, the radiance has nothing to do with "me". But the 'shine' is more difficult to categorize, as it is externally located and veiled from most of us. Also, I hope this isn't off topic, but is ecstatic radiance in contrast to pratyahara?
──────────

Hi Meg:

Ecstatic conductivity begins within us and radiates outward over time. As it does, it changes our perception of our surroundings. It is a refinement of sensory perception, an introversion occurring in and around us, and this is the progression of pratyahara, an expansion of the senses beyond physical to encompass the subtle celestial (revealing the shine). As it continues, even the shine (the mist of stillness) is transcended and we see we are blissful stillness (our inner silence) interpenetrating everything. The One.

So it is a progression of purification and opening, leading to ever refining grades of perception and experience. It is all one process of unfoldment, with changing scenery along the way. It is essentially the same gig of purification and opening all the way through from start to finish (if there is a finish).

A less-informed definition of pratyahara is "withdrawal from sensory perception," a denial of our sensory gifts, like denying siddhis and all of that -- essentially running away from our inherent capabilities. This is an immature view that has resulted from a long-standing inability to refine natural human capabilities. The truth is that, with sound practices, all of these aspects of our nature gradually refine over time to yield direct experience of the divine radiating within us and everywhere around us. We cannot get there by denying any aspect of our natural neurobiological functioning. Our nervous system is the doorway that joins us with the divine experience, which is our destiny. To walk though, we have to embrace the door and refine it so it may reveal its ultimate capabilities.

The guru is in you.

2007/03/10 10:18:35
Kundalini - Inner Energy Ecstasy
http://www.aypsite.org/forum/topic.asp?TOPIC_ID=2096&REPLY_ID=18629&whichpage=-1

Ecstatic radiance?

quote:
_____
Originally posted by emc

May I ask if the ecstatic radiance that develops is related in any way to the words "inner sensuality" that is used in samyama?

Has ecstatic radiance anything to do with OUTER sensuality and sexual attraction?

Has the samyama inner sensuality anything to do with developing OUTER sensuality and sexual attraction in a "samsara" style?
_____

Hi EMC:

Yes, the samyama sutra "inner sensuality" is for promoting pratyahara, which is merging sensuality (all the senses) with inner silence. This is part of the process of refinement of sensory perception being discussed here.

While there can be some external sexual energy mixed in with this along the way (a transitional experience), sexuality itself is also being refined to divine expression through our practices, which is what is behind the rise of ecstatic conductivity, ecstatic radiance, and eventually the direct perception of the misty luminous character of bliss consciousness emanating from all things (the shine). And we are That.

So none of this really has to do with expressing or exploiting earth-plane sexuality, if that is your question, any more than the lightness sutra has to do with physically flying across the sky.

We have much bigger fish to fry within, and this wonderful discussion topic gives a taste of it. :-)

The guru is in you.

2007/04/02 19:00:17
Kundalini - Inner Energy Ecstasy
http://www.aypsite.org/forum/topic.asp?TOPIC_ID=2374&REPLY_ID=19774&whichpage=-1
Ida strengthening?

Hi Christi:

I am not sure about the ida stimulation (reminds me of Gopi Krishna), but I am quite sure that effectively addressing a serious kundalini imbalance requires a range of measures applied at the same time -- no magic bullet.

Have you introduced her the to the measures in AYP lesson 69? http://www.aypsite.org/69.html

It is not that complicated, but does require some diligence and flexibility to work through it.

Some light spinal breathing is worth trying. It helps in many cases. I just got an email from someone last week who is having great success with spinal breathing after years of kundalini imbalance. I have received many such reports over the past few years. Spinal breathing helped me also to stabilize a serious kundalini imbalance many years ago, not to mention John Wilder's case. :-)

If spinal breathing doesn't help, just back off. It can't do any harm if undertaken gently.

Then there are the grounding methods -- walking, being outdoors, engaging with and helping other people, forgetting about our own spiritual condition for a while.

Finally, excess heat means a pitta imbalance (a common kundalini symptom) and ayurvedic methods can go a long way in aiding that, beginning with a pitta pacifiying diet. No Chilli Peppers...

What it takes is a combination of known effective methods, and time and patience. That is what lesson 69 is about. That is what all of AYP is about.

Kundalini excesses can always be labeled an "ida/pingala imbalance," and it doesn't mean anything, really, because the chances of manipulating the ida and pingala directly with any success are slim. That's like manipulating our chakras directly. Even if we could, it is like Scott says, how to know when it is too much one way or the other way. Gopi Krishna only did it because he didn't have any other way, and stumbled around for years beforehand. He finally got lucky after a dozen years of hanging out the window with kundalini -- a pretty uninformed approach.

It does not have to be like that in this day and age, if one is willing to take an integrated approach, and remain flexible in self-pacing the remedies, meaning not overdoing with anything. We know much more these days, and it can be done.

It goes without saying that daily sadhana engaged in over the period in question is suspect, since the symptoms have gotten worse. Once the situation has been stabilized, any practices considered for the future should be reviewed carefully. Developing good skills in self-pacing should be high up on the list also -- that can start right now in relation to anything that aggravates the condition.

I hope your friend finds some relief soon. Tell her she can find some good company here. Many here have been through it to one degree or other, and lived to tell the tale. Through our collective experiences we are getting smarter all the time and traveling on to much greater horizons, opening ourselves to abiding inner silence, ecstatic bliss and outpouring divine love.

The guru is in you.

2007/04/04 09:32:17
Kundalini - Inner Energy Ecstasy
http://www.aypsite.org/forum/topic.asp?TOPIC_ID=2374&REPLY_ID=19805&whichpage=-1

Ida strengthening?

Hi Christi:

On the other hand, if it works, use it -- nadi manipulation, or whatever. And do let us know. If it doesn't work, better move on. We don't stand on ceremony here. We are just putting results above all else, and building a knowledge base so others can benefit.

18 years and still struggling with kundalini? The arrows point to the practices in use, and/or some really ornery karma. I'd bet on the former, since karma is pretty much a paper tiger when effective (and well integrated) practices are in use with good self-pacing. Of course, it takes clarity to implement a good routine of sadhana. If we get too far behind the curve with kundalini imbalances, it can become difficult. I have only seen a few cases like that (coming from outside AYP), where the experience itself begins to overide good judgment. That does not seem to be the case here. So, hopefully, some time-tested remedies will help turn the tide.

All the best!

The guru is in you.

2007/04/04 12:47:18
Kundalini - Inner Energy Ecstasy
http://www.aypsite.org/forum/topic.asp?TOPIC_ID=2374&REPLY_ID=19816&whichpage=-1
Ida strengthening?

quote:
_____
Originally posted by Anthem11

I'd hesitate to do pranayama without meditation, how long is she doing of the former? she may want to be wary of doing more than 5 minutes of pranayama. Yogani, do you suggest doing only pranayama to alleviate symptoms like these?
_____

Hi Andrew:

Only very light spinal breathing on a test basis for a few days or weeks (5 min or less per twice daily sitting starting out). If there is some relief, this does not mean more spinal breathing will be better right away. Aiming for a steady routine is much more important. If there is some energy stabilization, then we can add a short session of deep meditation right after spinal breathing, also on a test basis, and see if the two practices can be balanced, along with improvements in the inner energy situation. This is to be accompanied by lots of grounding activity, of course, and a pitta pacifying diet. Keep the practice routines short and get out and be busy in everyday living. If all of that can be stabilized, then there can be progress in the direction of stabilization and growth with more comfort and safety.

In cases where kundalini is raging, it is okay to start the practices in reverse order (usually we begin deep meditation before spinal breathing), as spinal breathing is the more energy stabilizing practice, and that is what we need first with everything being out of kilter. It is a hybrid approach for use in kundalini emergencies only, where the practitioner is coming from outside AYP and does not have sufficient energy stability to begin with deep meditation. The energies have to be dealt with first in this case. As mentioned, quite a few have come in this way and managed to get things stabilized.

Keep in mind that kundalini energies (and excesses -- which can be minimized with an effective approach, including self-pacing) are an interim step on the way to the merging of inner silence with ecstatic conductivity (shiva and shakti/kundalini). This is why deep meditation and spinal breathing are so important to utilize in a balanced way. Spinal breathing balances and expands the inner energies while deep meditation cultivates inner silence. As you know, we have many additional methods to work with on both sides of this equation. Deep meditation and spinal breathing pranayama are the core practices that should be stabilized first, before moving on to additional methods.

Under normal circumstance (here in AYP), we will have a good foundation in inner silence via deep meditation before we have awakened kundalini, and we are in much better shape then, with the witness present, which helps us tremendously to ride through any bumpy periods. The witness (our silent self) never feels the bumps, and we can remain steady even as any storms of energy that may come up are raging.

Honestly, we'd like to move beyond the energy stage (symptoms of purification) and into the abiding inner silence and ecstatic bliss/outpouring divine love stage. Kundalini excesses are a detour that we'd like to avoid. If we do end up in that, then we should reroute with the most effective means available as soon as possible. Better late than never!

The guru is in you.

2007/04/04 23:16:02
Kundalini - Inner Energy Ecstasy
http://www.aypsite.org/forum/topic.asp?TOPIC_ID=2374&REPLY_ID=19833&whichpage=-1
Ida strengthening?

quote:
_____
Originally posted by Anthem11

As a whole I recommend Deep Meditation exclusively but on a couple of occasions, where the person in question is particularly clear, I have suggested that they start with 2 to 5 minutes of pranayama as well. Do you think this is a good idea? On one occasion, a friend of mine had an ongoing energy opening from just 1 week of only Deep Meditation, would it be prudent to recommend pranayama in this situation to help smooth things out? Or would just DM be sufficient? It is not an overload, but more of an energy awakening.

I hope you don't mind sharing your experience on this subject. I think there are a few of us here who may be in the same boat and we may be a little thin on practical insight into these matters.
_____

Hi Andrew:

That is great that you are helping folks get started. I recommend using the writings as much as possible for reference material, so those you expose can form their own relationship with the practices going forward.

I would not recommend starting anyone with two practices at the same time. If a person is clear and stable in deep meditation, that's great. Then it is they who should choose if and when they start spinal breathing. It is healthy if they have to make some effort to find out about the next steps. If the bhakti is there, they will.

If there is some energy right after beginning deep meditation, it would be better to stabilize deep meditation practice before moving into spinal breathing. In this case, spinal breathing would not be in the "curative" category and should be started when the person has stabilized deep meditation and has developed the urge to take the next step, like the lessons say.

Step by step -- this also applies to the hybrid situation discussed in this topic, where someone with a severe kundalini imbalance coming from outside AYP may try some light spinal breathing first. Deep meditation should not be undertaken until spinal breathing and the over all situation has been stabilized.

Some may wish to try deep meditation first in a severe kundalini situation. That is okay on a test basis, though the chances are less for it to calm a serious imbalance. But it could be tried instead of spinal breathing if the practiitioner is so inclined. But not both practices starting at the same time. That would be adding too many variables at the same time, for anyone ... it is the same for any practice we undertake on our journey. If we take on two or more practices at once, and symptoms of excess appear, how will we know what to self pace? It can get messy in a hurry.

The time delayed effect from practices we have discussed from time to time is another factor to consider. All the more reason to be conservative and take on practices one at at time months apart, rather than days or weeks apart, and never two or more at the same time. The guideline is: Always take the time necessary to stabilize one practice before moving on to the next one. Being sure that we have a stable routine is far more important than loading up with practices. That applies at all levels of practice from beginning to advanced.

I am aware of no further shortcuts on this -- not beyond the self-directed practice and self-pacing that AYP already offers, which is pretty fast. Beyond that it is the purification and opening each nervous sytem can withstand with safety. No one is better qualified to assess that than the well-educated individual practitioner.

Applied knowledge is the key. The AYP approach does not lend itself to spoon-feeding beyond an initial jump-start.

The guru is in you.

2007/04/09 11:36:02
Kundalini - Inner Energy Ecstasy
http://www.aypsite.org/forum/topic.asp?TOPIC_ID–2388&REPLY_ID–20070&whichpage=-1
energy overload

Hi Meg:

The good news is that the overload is purification -- creative energy producing friction through our not yet fully purified nervous system. As this process advances, our manifested creativity will become much greater. The trick is to maintain stability during the growth process. So we self-pace and ground.

Isn't it the challenge of all artists -- to be the best channel possible for the infinite creative potential within? It is rarely a smooth ride, as the chaotic lives of so many artists illustrates. Expanding creativity isn't always a comfortable bedfellow. It takes some adjustment, and that takes time.

The means we are utilizing both stimulate our creative opening while buying us the time necessary to adjust. That is what we are aiming for. And, yes, our work is also our practice. The merging is inevitable.

Here's to art -- stillness in action! :-)

The guru is in you.

2007/05/04 11:03:10
Kundalini - Inner Energy Ecstasy
http://www.aypsite.org/forum/topic.asp?TOPIC_ID=2516&REPLY_ID=21429&whichpage=-1
When the fire is too hot...

Hi Kadak, and welcome!

Thank you for the fascinating look at Tibetan yoga. While the terminology is different, it sounds similar to what we are doing here. We are all dealing with the same nervous system, yes?

If I read you correctly, going to the crown is prescribed when a balanced blending of the "red and white drops" can be achieved, which is a process of purification and opening in the spinal nerve.

In AYP, we achieve this via root to brow (ajna) spinal breathing pranayama, which is very stabilizing in most people, plus judicious application of certain mudras and bandhas. All the while, the crown is being purified and opened by proxy, so it can be accessed directly and safely as a gradual merging of ajna (third eye) and crown occurs over time. Ajna (third eye) means "command," and this approach is a well-used and relatively safe one in yoga for managing the energy aspects of purification and opening.

What we are trying to do here is make it an accessible and safe process for everyone, avoiding the calamities that have been so common in many schools of yoga, as you have recognized. Most of these problems can be attributed to premature crown openings, and the practices that are promoted in the name of progress. Ironically, such approaches are often a formula for delay rather than progress, as it can take months or years to sort out the resulting energy imbalances.

The AYP Spinal Breathing Pranayama book recently received a <u>bad review on Amazon</u> from a long time root to crown practitioner, who stated that root to brow route is a diversion and does not work (even though there is strong evidence to the contrary). In the same review he says (apparently removed later) that the medical establishment needs to gain a much better understanding of kundalini excesses so as to deal with them better. These excesses are often created and/or exacerbated by the approach he is promoting!

So, yes, you are right that yoga has some wrong ideas, and continues to promote them strongly.

Even more importantly, and virtually absent from many of the energy oriented schools of yoga, is the cultivation of inner silence in the aspirant. Here in AYP, we regard this to be the foundation of all spiritual progress, including the merging of ecstatic energy with stillness to become outpouring divine love -- unitary stillness in action in the world, expanding Oneness, which is enlightenment on the move throughout humanity.

Accordingly, AYP crosses traditional lines to join some of the best methods of energy cultivation with some of the best methods of inner silence cultivation -- the latter including deep meditation, samyama and other practices. We continue to evolve on all fronts on the basis of practices in relation to real experiences -- cause, effect, and self-pacing of this ever-unfolding dynamic in each of us, and in all of us in interconnected ways.

How does Tibetan yoga address the inner silence aspect? Is there deep meditation or an equivalent in that system? Where do you see improvements being necessary in the Tibetan approach?

All points of view are welcome. All the best!

The guru is in you.

2007/05/04 12:18:38
Kundalini - Inner Energy Ecstasy
http://www.aypsite.org/forum/topic.asp?TOPIC_ID=2516&REPLY_ID=21437&whichpage=-1
When the fire is too hot...

quote:
_____
Originally posted by kadak

Do you moderate the fire with ajna chakra ? Because, as I experienced it, the problem is not the opening of the crown chakra, but the heat coming from under. When the fire is too hot, it burns the head. What I experience as an "opening" of the crown chakra doesn't seem to be dangerous, because I feel it as a "fresh fire" (like breathing the air of the mountains) opening all the little channels + central channel in the head, clearing the mind and giving bliss.
_____

Hi Kadak:

Yes, ajna (third eye) does provide the necessary balance and regulation of ascending and descending energies, while opening the crown gradually. This is built into the spinal breathing pranayama technique we use. The excessive heat in kundalini awakening comes from too much energy moving before the nervous system has achieved adequate purification. Heat and many other kundalini symptoms are the "friction" of too much energy passing through not yet fully purified nerves. This can be caused by activating the crown too early, which draws up too much energy too soon -- a common problem in many kundalini energy oriented schools.

We see a lot of folks coming here from those approaches, and some spontaneous kundalini awakenings too. That is why you see so much kundalini remedy talk going on here. We are doing our best to help.

For those who have been using AYP from the start, the cases of energy excess seem to be fewer and less extreme, and we do have means for dealing with it, the most important being prudent "self-pacing" of practices to prevent things getting out of hand. It works pretty well -- finding a good balance between "enough" and "too much." :-)

If I understand, it appears in Tummo, energy is regulated by staying out of the lower centers instead. Interesting. How does that relate to tantric methods, dealing with sexuality, etc?

On cultivating the "clear light," take a look at deep meditation and see if it fits in. Lots of clear light to be found there.

All the best!

The guru is in you.

2007/06/25 12:06:45
Kundalini - Inner Energy Ecstasy
http://www.aypsite.org/forum/topic.asp?TOPIC_ID=2702&REPLY_ID=23513&whichpage=-1
Kundalini Sneak-peak
...and a reply from email. :-)
Others, please do chime in...

Hi Anthony:

Glad to hear things are moving along for you.

Only to remind that drugs do not produce lasting spiritual change beyond initial glimpses and inspiration to engage in spiritual practices. Beyond that, they can be obstructions, both psychological and biological. Our nervous system knows this inside, and that is why the desire for chemical additives goes down as purification goes up with effective practices.

All the best on your path. It takes time, and you have it all in front of you. Practice wisely, and enjoy!

The guru is in you.

2007/07/12 10:45:22
Kundalini - Inner Energy Ecstasy
http://www.aypsite.org/forum/topic.asp?TOPIC_ID=2751&REPLY_ID=24138&whichpage=-1
24hr ecstatic conductivity

Hi All:

When the resistance (friction) is gone, or even becoming much less, ecstasy is revealed to be the unending outpouring of divine love. This is also stillness in action.

The guru is in you.

2007/07/12 13:20:19
Kundalini - Inner Energy Ecstasy
http://www.aypsite.org/forum/topic.asp?TOPIC_ID=2751&REPLY_ID=24144&whichpage=-1
24hr ecstatic conductivity

quote:
_____
Originally posted by gentlep

quote:
_____
Originally posted by yogani

Hi All:

When the resistance (friction) is gone, or even becoming much less, ecstasy is revealed to be the unending outpouring of divine love.

_____

Is the ecstasy mentioned here is a physical sensation or not?

_____

Hi Gentlep:

Yes, physical, but by decreasing degrees over time (see the lessons on "automatic yoga and physical movements" in the topic index, which are analogous).

Maybe when the energy moved before, we jumped in our chair with a surge of pleasure. Later on, when the energy moves, we may not jump, and the love just pours out. So instead of lurching in ecstasy, we will go help someone, which feels even better. :-)

Expansion of ecstatic divine love feels good (an understatement), and it never ends, reaching far beyond the confines of our body. We are emerging channels for that.

The sensations of physicality with inner energy moving can be compared to water moving through a partially obstructed pipe, which is gradually becoming clear. The degree of obstruction will determine the nature of the sensation. Same water, different levels of obstruction (resistance/friction) yielding different flows. Same divine love, different degrees of sensation and manifestation as purification and opening advance.

The guru is in you.

2007/11/01 12:37:42
Kundalini - Inner Energy Ecstasy
http://www.aypsite.org/forum/topic.asp?TOPIC_ID=3022&REPLY_ID=26601&whichpage=-1
Burning Sensation while meditating

Hi SeekingShiva:

It is a fairly common symptom of purification and opening in that area. It should smooth out and transform over time, becoming more energetic and ecstatic in its nature, corresponding with openings higher up and the rise of ecstatic conductivity in the body.

If the symptom becomes excessive and uncomfortable, then self-pace practices accordingly, particularly mudras, bandhas and any kumbhaka (breath retention) you may be doing. For more on dealing with energy imbalances, see: http://www.aypsite.org/69.html

All the best!

The guru is in you.

2007/11/01 11:48:41
Kundalini - Inner Energy Ecstasy
http://www.aypsite.org/forum/topic.asp?TOPIC_ID=3069&REPLY_ID=26597&whichpage=-1
I want a promotion

Hi mr.regular, and welcome!

The best way to get that "promotion" is to continue with effective daily practices, and favor those over experiences that may come up along the way.

Then human spiritual transformation will be steadily progressing, and life will become increasingly a miracle of abiding inner silence, ecstatic bliss and outpouring divine love -- a continuum of promotions to the infinite. :-)

All the best on your chosen path. Enjoy!

The guru is in you.

PS: See this lesson on "getting reconditioned": http://www.aypsite.org/138.html

2007/12/10 15:52:51
Kundalini - Inner Energy Ecstasy
http://www.aypsite.org/forum/topic.asp?TOPIC_ID=3236&REPLY_ID=27828&whichpage=-1
overwhelming symptoms forehead left side

Hi Mariej and All:

Great assistance being offered above. Thanks!

Here is a copy of an email reply I sent earlier on this same topic (prior practices have since been clarified in a PS to first post above):

Hi:

Yes, it sounds like a kundalini event. Classic really, though a bit on the heavy and imbalanced side. You did not mention what your practices have been. The keys to safely initiating and managing the kundalini process over time (it is a long term scenario) are balance of effective practices through ongoing "self-pacing," and also effective "grounding" in daily life.

Here are a couple of lessons that provide some suggestions:
Kundalini symptoms and remedies -- http://www.aypsite.org/69.html
Left or right side imbalances -- http://www.aypsite.org/207.html

Additional lessons can be found in the Topic Index under "kundalini."

Regarding the medical side of it, I am not a physician, so cannot not advise much there. One thing to be aware of though is that doctors are prone to misdiagnose or be stumped by kundalini related symptoms, as they are not trained in this area. Which is not to say you don't have a medical condition for which a doctor's attention is needed. This sort of medical/spiritual confusion does happen however. There are many examples of it discussed by practitioners in the AYP Support Forums. You are welcome to join in there. The community offers a lot of help and invaluable spiritual networking. The ever-increasing knowledge base is very helpful to the many who are reading along there.

In any case, if you are concerned about numbness (a common kundalini symptom that usually resolves itself), it would be more appropriate to see a neurologist than a dermatologist. Before running off to more doctors (which can get messy), you might take a closer look at the spiritual side of it, try some measures, and see what happens. It is your call, of course.

Wishing you all the best in health and on your spiritual path. Practice wisely and enjoy!

The guru is in you.

2007/12/10 17:06:47
Kundalini - Inner Energy Ecstasy
http://www.aypsite.org/forum/topic.asp?TOPIC_ID=3236&REPLY_ID=27833&whichpage=-1
overwhelming symptoms forehead left side
PS: It should be added that combining practices from more than one system (like TM and AOL) can be tricky, especially the "doubling up" effect that can occur if same-in-class practices (pranayama, meditation, etc.) are done in the same session or day. That can lead to excessive purification and/or too much kundalini stimulation.

What makes this even trickier is the delayed effects that can happen when inadvertently overdoing in practices. Everything can be going along just fine after we have made a big addition to our practices. Then, all of a sudden a few weeks later -- Wham!

That is why we take small steps when adding on to our practice routine within AYP, and especially when combining practices from elsewhere across traditional lines where there may be no track record to guide us. In the latter case, it is our experiment, and all the more reason to be very measured and gradual in our approach.

Not sure if any of this applies in your case, Mariej. It all depends on what practices you were doing when. It is mentioned here as a reminder to all. It is not the first time the subject of combining practices from different teachings has come up around here. It always boils down to -- yep -- self-pacing.

None of this is to say we should not press on in developing more effective integrations of practice. There is much good that can come from prudent experimentation -- the never-ending evolution of applied knowledge. It is the frontier of the quest for achieving human enlightenment on a wide scale in the world. AYP is the result of this kind of research and development, and it is ongoing.

If we are going to test a new airplane for the first time (while sitting in it), we'll be much better off doing it with low flights on a long beach, rather than off a steep cliff. That way we can keep coming back for more tests and fine-tuning until we get it right. :-)

The guru is in you.

2008/01/28 14:28:15
Kundalini - Inner Energy Ecstasy
http://www.aypsite.org/forum/topic.asp?TOPIC_ID=3296&REPLY_ID=29372&whichpage=-1
Kundalini Overload: Grounding/Front Channel Block

Hi Jim and EMC:

The discussion on "front and back" in spinal breathing does not originate in yoga and is not mentioned in the AYP writings either, except when Taoist approaches are being considered.

It has been mentioned that spinal breathing like presented in AYP is "up and down the back." This is not true. The spinal nerve is more in the center of the body than in the back, and in the throat area it is right behind the back of the throat and esophagus (gullet). As ecstatic energy awakens and expands, it is found to be even more in the middle, and less following the physical anatomy of the spine, passing through the entire region of the throat instead. That is what happens as the spinal nerve awakens -- it expands from the center to become a large column of energy, eventually reaching far beyond the body itself. That is ecstatic radiance.

So all this up the back and down the front discussion does not resonate much with the yogic view, particularly as kundalini advances and covers a much broader swath through the body -- becoming one thing, not two things. Spinal breathing follows suit in this, working more or less from the center, and the front and back stuff is dissolved in it. From the yogic point of view, the front and back stuff was never there much in the first place and, in fact, drawing the distinction in mind and practices could become an obstacle to the natural expansion of the internal energies, much the way hanging on to a specific mantra pronunciation can become an obstacle to deep meditation. Spinal breathing works between the two poles of root and brow, and can be much less defined in-between as the energies evolve. In that situation, there is no front or back.

Which is not to say that the front channel symptoms are not real. Certainly they are. But I am not sure the answer will be found in continuing to define and manage the energies in front and back categories. As we know, attempts to categorize and manage the details of internal energy flows can lead to more problems than solutions. A more holistic approach may yield better fruit. A middle way? :-)

Just some thoughts.

The guru is in you.

2008/01/28 18:10:14
Kundalini - Inner Energy Ecstasy
http://www.aypsite.org/forum/topic.asp?TOPIC_ID=3296&REPLY_ID=29383&whichpage=-1
Kundalini Overload: Grounding/Front Channel Block

Hi Jim:

If it is working, facilitating balance and forward progress, then by all means go with it. I was not sure that was the case, given all the back and forth.

I do believe in the long run we have to let go of the mental categorizations though, and allow the process to unfold naturally. Whatever practice regimen we are using will morph accordingly. We will still use the same procedures of practice, but with much less deliberateness -- meaning in stillness with less mental baggage attached. I'm sure you know what I mean -- letting the cosmic barber do his thing. All we have to do is show up, assuming we are visiting the barber best suited for our needs. :-)

As for Lesson 133 (http://www.aypsite.org/133.html), that is about the evolving neurobiology (the yogic view of it), which is refined and transcended in awareness as the process of spiritual transformation proceeds. Our practices refine along with it, including mudras, bandhas, pranayamas, etc. -- some of which facilitate frontal openings, as you know. The expansion of inner silence and the associated energetics, while emanating from the neurobiology, move beyond it. So, while we can talk about up the back and down the front on the physical plane, it all eventually dissolves as we move into identification with the product of that, which is *Oneness*.

Taoist approaches tend to hold on to the categorization and focus on physical components longer than yoga methods do. But in the end, both will dissolve into the same destination.

Well, none of this removes the issues at hand, and I understand that they have to be dealt with, using whatever practical means that are available. Just trying to add a little perspective.

Onward!

The guru is in you.

2008/03/07 11:05:40
Kundalini - Inner Energy Ecstasy
http://www.aypsite.org/forum/topic.asp?TOPIC_ID=3296&REPLY_ID=30984&whichpage=-1
Kundalini Overload: Grounding/Front Channel Block

quote:
_____
Originally posted by Amaargi

Example: A fear of the landlord surfaced and within 2 weeks I was evicted. A belief in lack of money and 'life is hard' cleared and circumstances arose where my bank account was emptied and I lost my job.

This is why people who meditate and affirm positive events for themselves believe they can attract prosperity, new cars, loving relationships etc don't realise that negative thought patterns will also manifest as well. And what many don't realise that buried deep deep in the subconscious is many negative thought patterns instilled from childhood, religious teachings, broken relationships etc.

————

Hi Amaargi:

Good to see you again. :-)

You might consider adding a light routine of samyama right after deep meditation, as this gradually moves the cause and effect of our desires and fears beyond the karmic mechanisms in the subconscious mind. The effect will shift to be coming from within our inner silence instead. Then those negative subconscious backlashes will become much less. It will not happen overnight, but it will happen gradually as we practice samyama as part of our balanced daily routine.

By "light routine" I mean one repetition of the sutras in lesson 150. If that goes well after a few months, then you might consider going to two repetitions. Later on, you may also consider adding cosmic samyama (from the AYP Samyama book) while lying down for rest after core samyama practice. Between these two samyama routines, negative subconscious mechanisms can be neutralized in an accelerated fashion, and we will no longer be subject to negative backlashes from our own thoughts. More than that -- we find ourselves becoming an ever-expanding channel of divine love and positive influence radiating from inner silence wherever we go. Abiding inner silence is the prerequisite for all this, so daily deep meditation continues to be the core practice.

And, of course, if there is any difficulty with samyama or any other practice, we self-pace accordingly. Any changes in our practice routine we do in baby steps, allowing plenty of time for the effects to become known before adding anything else new.

Wishing you all the best!

The guru is in you.

2008/01/03 11:51:17
Kundalini - Inner Energy Ecstasy
http://www.aypsite.org/forum/topic.asp?TOPIC_ID=3320&REPLY_ID=28494&whichpage=-1
Chakra location

Hi All:

In the AYP approach, we regard kundalini awakening to be a whole body event from the very beginning, not specific to any individual chakra. We take the fewest possible incremental steps in practices to facilitate whole body kundalini awakening, and thereby avoid getting hung up in trying to manage the details of the inner machinery (chakras, etc.), which is impossible.

Cultivating a foundation of inner silence is the first step in this process of fewest incremental steps, with the next step being the awakening of ecstatic conductivity in the spinal nerve between root to brow. Whole body ecstatic conductivity on the cellular level occurs simultaneously when the spinal nerve awakens. If we attend to inner silence and awakening of the spinal nerve, the rest will take care of itself. It is a natural process.

This is why the AYP practices begin with deep meditation for cultivating inner silence, and then expand to spinal breathing and other energy related methods (mudras, bandhas, additional pranayama techniques, etc.)

Symptoms occurring in any particular area of the body indicate purification and opening there. This is not where kundalini is beginning to awaken. Awakening kundalini flows everywhere simultaneously, and localized symptoms we are able to perceive are where it happens to be meeting resistance at the moment. While we may be tempted to focus intently on localized symptoms, we will be wise to favor our broad practice regimen over developing complex strategies aimed at localized symptoms.

The symptoms will eventually pass (evolve to ever more refined levels of ecstatic bliss) as whole body purification and opening advance. If we become obsessed with localized symptoms, we may delay the opening of the whole in favor of the part. This is why "energy work" is not encouraged much in AYP. The human nervous system is much smarter than we are for attending to localized functioning. That is why we attend to the whole in the best ways we know, to enable the divine intelligence within us to attend to all the parts, which it can do very well if we will be patient.

Having said that, we will all respond to our symptoms in ways that will bring us a smoother path and a sense of progress. This is certainly legitimate, and it is what self-pacing is all about. At the same time, we should be mindful about our tendency to become obsessed about our perceived symptoms.

It is self-inquiry really -- discriminating and easily favoring the whole over the parts. That is, favoring the subject (our inner silence/witness and whole body awakening) even as we are interacting with and within the objects (our multifarious experiences in life).

In the end, the subject merges with the objects, and only the *One* that has always been remains. Stillness in action and outpouring divine love!

The guru is in you.

2008/01/06 13:17:17
Kundalini - Inner Energy Ecstasy
http://www.aypsite.org/forum/topic.asp?TOPIC_ID=3320&REPLY_ID=28569&whichpage=-1
Chakra location

Hi Albert, and a belated welcome! :-)

There have been discussions in the forums on unique experiential factors noticed in the lower centers for women practitioners. I can't put my finger on the link(s) at the moment, but perhaps the ladies who were involved in those discussions can point you to them.

Generally, in the AYP approach we do not focus too much on the inner mechanics, either intellectually or experientially, as the practices we use are sufficient to cultivate the necessary awakening in both sexes, which is the expansion of inner silence no matter where we happen to be looking in the neurobiology. There is a potential cost in focusing on the detailed mapping -- it can distract us from the whole of human spiritual transformation. This was also discussed in my previous post in this topic, regarding localized kundalini/energy symptoms.

All the best!

The guru is in you.

2008/01/10 08:03:35
Kundalini - Inner Energy Ecstasy
http://www.aypsite.org/forum/topic.asp?TOPIC_ID=3320&REPLY_ID=28697&whichpage=-1
Chakra location

quote:
_____
Originally posted by selfonlypath

I have two other questions about AYP system:
- is it necessary to see chakras and nadis to practice correctly AYP
- what reference lesson provides a detailed solution for grounding
_____

Hi Albert:

No, it is not necessary to see what is happening "under the hood" while driving the yoga car we call AYP. We use the main controls and do our best not to micro-manage the details. :-)

Lesson 69 introduces the subject of grounding. It is further developed in lessons listed in the Topic Index under "kundalini" and "self-pacing." And it is much further developed here in the forums. Check the FAQ on Grounding, and try a "subject only" forum search on "grounding." If you do a full text forum search, an eight page list of topics will come up mentioning grounding.

The "AYP Easy Lessons - Volume 2" book (due out in a year or so) will provide a more organized approach to grounding, as will the "Eight Limbs of Yoga" Enlightenment Series book due out this summer. It is somewhat personal -- some folks like to dig in the dirt, while others prefer to take long hikes. Both are grounding, as are many "down-to-earth" activities.

The guru is in you.

2008/01/06 11:20:31
Kundalini - Inner Energy Ecstasy
http://www.aypsite.org/forum/topic.asp?TOPIC_ID=3324&REPLY_ID=28565&whichpage=-1
Hindus versus Tibetan awakening

quote:
_____
Originally posted by Scott
I also research other systems. There's no sense in throwing our researching and thinking brains away. They are good for making sense out of spirituality. We can turn it into more of a science this way, instead of a mystery like it is to most people. I do think this is what AYP is all about!
_____

Hi Scott:

Yes, this is the crux of it. It is the move from closed to open systems, and continual research and development on the level of the individual practitioner. Eventually this will reach the large research and educational institutions, and I am all for it. That will be when integrated spiritual practices become permanently established in the mainsteam, and AYP can be a stepping stone in that overall process. Not the end -- only a beginning for a new paradigm of ongoing development and practical applications of spiritual knowledge.

See here: http://www.aypsite.org/forum/topic.asp?TOPIC_ID=3267

Interdisciplinary (multi-tradition) studies and effective integrations of practice are central in the migration to open *Applied Spiritual Science*. That is why we encourage such discussions in the corresponding forum categories here -- exploring the full scope of practices and experiences (causes and effects) associated with the process of *human spiritual transformation*.

Many thanks to everyone for contributing!

The guru is in you.

2008/01/11 08:19:52
Kundalini - Inner Energy Ecstasy
http://www.aypsite.org/forum/topic.asp?TOPIC_ID=3324&REPLY_ID=28742&whichpage=-1
Hindus versus Tibetan awakening

quote:
_____

Which lesson on AYP proposes a solution and practice to develop this ego-free vision which is necessary once high levels of kundalini start to manifest unlocking very deep core inconcious blockages ?

_____

Hi Albert:

That is an easy one. Deep Meditation -- Lesson 13, and all related writings, including on Samyama and Self-Inquiry (new book).

This is the cultivation and expansion of inner silence/witness, which transcends and illuminates all energy experiences. Ideally, it is undertaken before kundalini awakens, but any time after will be okay too. The awakening of *Silent Self* is the essential ingredient on any spiritual path. Natural kundalini awakening is both facilitated by and secondary to *That*.

All the best!

The guru is in you.

2008/01/11 12:15:44
Kundalini - Inner Energy Ecstasy
http://www.aypsite.org/forum/topic.asp?TOPIC_ID=3324&REPLY_ID=28745&whichpage=-1
Hindus versus Tibetan awakening

Hi YB:

Silent Self (inner silence, witness), once cultivated, is abiding whether there are thoughts or not. So it is not only a condition of no-thinking, though it does give the mind a foundation in stillness, which tends to calm the mind. It is also the prerequisite for self-inquiry as described in the new AYP book on that subject.

But, no, Silent Self does not mean a condition of no thinking. Rather, it is the ground state of inspired and illuminated thinking, which is what perhaps the others are describing. Same condition, different words.

However, it is misleading to present Silent Self as a condition of "no thinking." Then people get the idea that enlightenment is about killing thinking (and desires). This is not true. Not any more true than yoga being about sitting in a yoga pose. The field of play is beyond such external things, including our thoughts and feelings. Effective yoga practices cultivate the witness without getting into a wrestling match with the mind, emotions or body. It is about going beyond all that and coming back in as Silent Self, even as all the external stuff is continuing.

Yes, once we have been meditating for a while, abiding inner silence will be there even as purification and opening are underway. At some point we begin to see our thoughts as objects separate from our Silent Self, and this is where real self-inquiry begins. It is the beginning of being able to discriminate between Self and all objects, including our thoughts, emotions, the physical environment, and the ongoing purification and opening that are occurring within us. From this point on, kundalini becomes a cakewalk, along with the rest of life.

Silence with noise -- not "noisy silence." :-)

This is why Silent Self (the witness) is at the heart of all spiritual progress. Until we cultivate that, we will continue to be identified with external objects, beginning with our own thoughts. But it isn't our thoughts we have to get rid of. It is abiding Silent Self (witness) that we want to add. That is the result the sages are describing in one way or other, depending on their current experience and personal perspective on how they got to that condition themselves (if they know).

The real question is: How can everyone bring about this condition in themselves quickly and safely?

It is one thing to talk about enlightenment. And something else entirely to be cultivating it by effective means. Then all the answers will be coming from within, and we can give our own description. I am looking forward to hearing about it from more and more people. Bring it on! :-)

The guru is in you.

2008/01/11 13:58:44
Kundalini - Inner Energy Ecstasy
http://www.aypsite.org/forum/topic.asp?TOPIC_ID=3324&REPLY_ID=28748&whichpage=-1
Hindus versus Tibetan awakening

quote:
_____
Originally posted by selfonlypath

Hi Yogani,

After reading your last answer, it makes me think of what tibetan sects calls rigpa or Nature of the Mind" via Dzogchen system which is considered as a secret practice as opposed to shamanism (external practice) and tantrism (internal practice).

Does AYP system provides at a certain yogic level the equivalent of Dzogchen teachings and if yes, what specific lessons adresses the self introduction to rigpa ?

Namaste, Albert

_____

Hi Albert:

That I can't tell you, not being well-versed in the Tibetan systems. Perhaps others can shed some light?

One thing I can say is that the awakening is the same regardless of the system that is being used to approach it, assuming effective means are being applied. There is only one human nervous system with its inherent profound spiritual capabilities, and once things are set in motion via practices, the process will go to the same fruition. The experiences will be of the same nature, with the descriptions colored by background, culture and religion.

A rose is still a rose when called by any other name. :-)

So I don't agree that there are Hindu, Buddhist, Christian, etc. awakenings. All are the same process of *human spiritual transformation*, stimulated by one systematic approach or another, or an evolving integration of approaches (something new) which is where all of this is going in the information age. Modern *Applied Spiritual Science*.

All the best!

The guru is in you.

2008/01/11 22:45:17
Kundalini - Inner Energy Ecstasy
http://www.aypsite.org/forum/topic.asp?TOPIC_ID=3324&REPLY_ID=28756&whichpage=-1
Hindus versus Tibetan awakening

Hi YB:

There is only One. Yet, perceptions change within the One as our vehicle of awareness (the nervous system) purifies and opens. During this process, the witness is first noticed as static, and later on as dynamic, within and synonymous with all that is happening -- stillness in action. Paradox ... and more...

The Silent Self is both the noise and is untouched by the noise. It is perception without identification...

The going out and coming back is the journey from pre-witnessing to witnessing, to discrimination, to dispassion, to outpouring divine love, to unity/Oneness. It is a journey from here to here. No place to go.

The word "realization" conveys what it is. Effective meditation is the primary means for cultivating realization. Samyama and self-inquiry move and reveal living stillness.

Silent Self is not primarily a mental habit. It is a whole body neurobiological awakening. This is why self-inquiry cannot do it alone, except in rare cases.

The energy techniques (pranayama, mudras, bandhas, tantra, etc.) give wings to stillness, facilitating realization of the dynamic nature of Silent Self. This is the natural role of kundalini -- the ecstatic radiation of Silent Self from within us.

The new Self-Inquiry book attempts to present all of this in a practical, usable way. I'm not sure if it succeeds. Let me know. :-)

The guru is in you.

2008/01/12 11:33:44
Kundalini - Inner Energy Ecstasy
http://www.aypsite.org/forum/topic.asp?TOPIC_ID=3324&REPLY_ID=28784&whichpage=-1
Hindus versus Tibetan awakening

quote:
_____
Originally posted by selfonlypath

Dear Yogani,

I hope you realize that i'm totally in the same line.

There is the map to explore the territory. Map is the system or the method and territory is the human spiritual experience. A good system or method can work for someone and not work for another person but this does not mean the system is bad.

In other words, the map is not the territory so at some point, one might need to not attach anymore to the system who provided the initial awakening because attaching is an ego trap but also gives lots of unnecessary arguments (my system is better than yours).

I've studied different systems to realize that they all take you to the same place but the method might be different as well as the speed and associated safety.

The spirit of my posts here is really trans-system integration where I'm looking for certain subsets, techniques so I can recover missing information from *no name system* I practice.

From what you've shared plus the fact i'm totally new to AYP, i suspect the book (self-inquiry) you are about to publish is really connected to Dzogchen. If it is the case, this would mean it is above sutras, tantras and AYP itself.

I would be also very interested to know your views or experiences with authentic shamanism.

In Shakti, Albert

_____

Hi Albert:

We are on the same page, even though coming from different backgrounds. :-)

The ongoing integration of knowledge is surely the way to go. So many fields have advanced tremendously in recent centuries with this approach. Applied spiritual knowledge has not advanced much, except when rare prodigies (avatars, etc.) came along. Once ongoing research, development and optimization of applied knowledge are baked into the system, then there will be no stopping the widespread advancement of human spiritual transformation.

Well, may your high expectations for the new Self-Inquiry book come true -- hopefully not to the point abstraction. :-)
I'll be happy if it succeeds in providing practical suggestions that will help folks better assess what is out there in the field of self-inquiry, and make intelligent choices on how they approach it in relation to their over all spiritual path. Nothing is "All or nothing." It is about the intelligent integration of effective means applied over time, and making adjustments as necessary along the way -- "self-pacing."

Regarding shamanism, I know it isn't primarily about etheogens, as so many believe. It is another approach to the everywhere present process of human spiritual transformation, with important contributions to share, and we are happy to see it explored here along with all other approaches.

The guru is in you.

2008/01/08 14:46:36
Kundalini - Inner Energy Ecstasy
http://www.aypsite.org/forum/topic.asp?TOPIC_ID=3342&REPLY_ID=28627&whichpage=-1
Four q lifting energy in spine

Hi Lookatmynavelnow, and welcome!

The way we do spinal breathing pranayama in AYP, it is not an exploration with energy/experience driven options we follow while doing it. It is a simple procedure that is done the same way every time, no matter what is happening experientially. As Scott and Christi mentioned, the procedure of the practice is in the lead, not the vagaries of the inner energies.

The exception would be if energy symptoms become excessive and uncomfortable, and then we would respond by cutting our daily practice time back temporarily until things stabilize.

There are some enhancements to spinal breathing available that can improve its effectiveness. These are discussed in the Spinal Breathing Pranayama book, and include full yogic breathing, opening the throat on inhalation and restricting it slightly on exhalation (ujjayi), gentle lifting of the eyes (sambhavi), and tracing cool and warm currents up and down respectively. It is not recommended to take all of these on at once -- only one at at time when drawn to do so, allowing stabilization time (weeks or months) in daily practice for each.

Kumbhaka (breath retention) is another matter, and should be approached carefully. In AYP, this is in conjunction with certain practices (yoni mudra and chin pump in particular). Regular spinal breathing is not recommended as a time to do deliberate kumbhaka. The breath may spontaneously suspend at times during spinal breathing and/or deep meditation (pretty common). We regard that the same as any other experience, and easily favor the practice we are doing when we realize we are off it. You are wise not to be rushing into kumbhaka, as you have plenty going on already. Time to stabilize. The key is to stabilize daily practices and inch them to more advanced versions over the long term, not chase or manipulate the energies over the short term. That is the approach here. You have been at this a long time too, so I am sure you know best what you need. A word to the wise is usually sufficient. :-)

As for "raising kundalini," spinal breathing goes both ways. "Grounding" kundalini energies is at least as important as raising them, as many here can attest. Spinal breathing is up and down for good reasons. If the energy wants to go the other way, it doesn't matter -- we gently favor the procedure of our practice.

Btw, there have been extensive discussions in the forums on "grounding." There are many ways to go about it. If you are not thinking much about grounding at this point, you surely will be somewhere down the road.

The path to enlightenment is not primarily about "raising kundalini," which is an intermediate step in the process. Once ecstatic conductivity awakens, it is about balancing and blending, and that takes time of stable daily practice, including getting out in the world for integrating inner silence and the ecstatic energies in everyday living.

In the end, it is a marriage of abiding inner silence and ecstatic conductivity (kundalini) within us, leading to ongoing outpouring divine love and unity. Then we are called to do much more, because we can.

Don't know if that helps with your "plumbing question." It's about the best we can do, given the fact that we do not engage the energies extensively here during practices, and with good reasons. We focus on the main controls, and leave the rest going on inside to natural processes. It seems to be working well for a lot of folks here, and hangups in energy tangents are greatly reduced (I hope). Getting caught up in energy dramas is one of the greatest risks of delay on the path that intermediate and advanced practitioners face.

Another one is getting infatuated with "non-dual self-inquiry" to the exclusion of everything else. But that's another story. It is mentioned because I have finally finished the Self-Inquiry book. Hooray! :-)

All the best on your path. Enjoy!

The guru is in you.

2008/01/09 00:26:35
Kundalini - Inner Energy Ecstasy
http://www.aypsite.org/forum/topic.asp?TOPIC_ID=3342&REPLY_ID=28637&whichpage=-1
Four q lifting energy in spine

quote:

Hi LAMNN:

Sure, the more kicking of the tires the better. But you might try asking them one or two at a time. They will receive more focused attention that way. It's up to you. :-)

One point I can add that might help with some of your in-between, directional and/or increasing/decreasing energy questions is that if there are blockages or energies going hither and yon, making smooth travel up and down the spinal nerve challenging, then we can just skip through to the pole we are heading for in spinal breathing as necessary on inhalation and exhalation. In doing that we will always end up at the brow at the end of inhalation and at the root at the end of exhalation, no matter what. That bypasses the in-between "what if's" that may come up and enables us to conduct complete spinal breathing cycles for our full session while clearing out obstructions in-between at the same time, without getting stuck or taking a ride with the energy in some other direction. Over time, the whole thing becomes much smoother, and not about any particular energy event at all. It never was.

Many people have issues in spinal breathing in the early stages with getting stuck at some level in the spinal nerve or having the energy going off this way or that way. With time in practice, the symptoms clear up and the full spinal nerve becomes accessible, ecstatic, and expansive. We want to stay with the practice that is the cause the purification and opening in the entire spinal nerve. The energy sensations are only temporary side effects -- the friction of energy passing through the yet to be fully purified neurobiology.

Recognizing that it is not about the energy (even as we are stimulating it) and proceeding accordingly is how self-inquiry enters into the conduct of our practice. We make choices in every practice session to follow the procedure, or not, whatever it may be we have committed ourselves to practice. If we do not consistently follow the procedure we have chosen, we are lost. How consistently we choose over the long term makes all the difference. The choices are little ones made daily, which add up to large changes over time.

As you no doubt know, the path of yoga is like building a mountain day by day with a teaspoon, or maybe with a shovel if the practices are highly effective. All the fireworks have little to do with what is being built underneath. This is why developing consistent habits in effective practices is so important.

All the best!

The guru is in you.

2008/02/23 13:06:16
Kundalini - Inner Energy Ecstasy
http://www.aypsite.org/forum/topic.asp?TOPIC_ID=3466&REPLY_ID=30457&whichpage=1
Is this kundalini

Hi TI:

Just to clarify, addressing the crown is not completely avoided in the AYP approach. It is only delayed in focus until the nervous system has been purified and opened enough to support the large body-wide energy flows associated with crown opening. The crown is addressed in a more gradual way. It isn't about the crown so much. It is about attending to the rest of the neurobiology, during which the crown will participate naturally in a balanced way.

This is especially relevant in the natural development of sambhavi mudra to broader scope with the awakening and advancement of ecstatic conductivity, which includes the crown.

The main lessons contain testing procedures and methods for addressing the crown. And Cosmic Samyama (from the Samyama book) utilizes the crown in a balanced way in relation to our cosmic unfoldment.

The over all plan is for progressive and smooth development for as many people as possible. Otherwise, who will want to bother with it?

The Gopi Krishna story is the classic account of the extremes of a premature crown opening. It is pretty old news these days, but still relevant, as many have found, including quite a few in these forums who have taken measures to avoid the excesses that can occur.

Not sure what you mean by crown opening being a possible hazard if kundalini is already active, and not so much before. A premature crown opening and a premature kundalini awakening are essentially the same thing, so to court one is to court the other. In the case of intensive crown practices, there can be delayed reactions that can take a long time to unwind while the rest of the nervous system catches up. Self-pacing in real time with crown practices is difficult, because of the long delays between cause and effect that can occur.

This is why intense crown practices are not recommended in AYP, certainly not in the beginning. Sooner or later that will lead to trouble if not preceded and balanced with other practices providing for whole body purification and opening.

So, while you may be having a good time with the crown now without a full blown kundalini awaking in play, you will not likely be having a good time further down the road, unless you are attending to the rest of your neurobiology.

I realize that many traditions take the top down approach, and perhaps they provide the necessary prerequisite practices to avoid the potential difficulties. But I must say, we have seen quite a few refugees from top down schools here seeking help for kundalini overloads. Many schools seem happy to get people started down this road, but few seem willing to provide the resources to clean up the messes that can result.

It isn't about me. It is about everyone else, and what can be done to provide a progressive and safe path for the greatest number of people. What may seem like the quickest and most direct route now can turn out to be a very slow and difficult route if the potential excesses are ignored.

So, while no one should be fearful of their own awakening, everyone should be aware of the logical steps involved to make it as smooth and enjoyable as possible. It is like learning to drive a car. There are good ways to go about it, and not so good ways. AYP does not claim to be perfect in this. But we are doing our best, including attending to accidents when they occur. The goal is to limit mishaps to minor fender-benders, while avoiding the all out disasters. It's the least we can do, and I think the record speaks for itself. :-)

Practice wisely, and enjoy!

The guru is in you.

2008/03/06 10:02:40
Kundalini - Inner Energy Ecstasy
http://www.aypsite.org/forum/topic.asp?TOPIC_ID=3551&REPLY_ID=30918&whichpage=-1
kundalini rash?

quote:
―――――
Originally posted by emc

Tibetan Ice,

I'll just state what I notice now: You have lately written about many spectacular experiences, which involve very much high frequent energies. At the same time you are now reporting on lots of ringing in the ears and rashes.

My interpretation:

Those are clear signs of energy overload, see for example this topic

http://www.aypsite.org/forum/topic.asp?TOPIC_ID=2884

and if I were you I'd seriously consider if there might be time for some self-pacing - grounding. The kundalini energy has a sleeping effect... It builds up over time and then suddenly can hit with great force, causing great inconvenience and strange uncomfortable symptoms. When you start to get the symptoms it's definitely time to cut back on practices that stimulate energies.

Please, check these links out if you haven't already!

Kundalini excess symptoms: http://www.aypsite.org/forum/topic.asp?TOPIC_ID=2146

Grounding: http://www.aypsite.org/forum/topic.asp?TOPIC_ID=2165

Self-pacing: http://www.aypsite.org/forum/topic.asp?TOPIC_ID=2139

Personally, I'm always on the verge of overdoing, and have to self-pace a lot. Ringing in the ears and rashes are among my first symptoms and what may come after... Phew... I'd rather not tell about!

This is just my interpretation from what I recognize in your posts. You will discover yourself whether it's relevant for you or not.
―――――

Hi EMC:

Good observations and list of references. Thanks!

Hi TI:

Don't forget this one, posted to you a week or so ago: http://www.aypsite.org/forum/topic.asp?TOPIC_ID=3466#30457

From there:
"...A premature crown opening and a premature kundalini awakening are essentially the same thing, so to court one is to court the other. In the case of intensive crown practices, there can be delayed reactions that can take a long time to unwind while the rest of the nervous system catches up. Self-pacing in real time with crown practices is difficult, because of the long delays between cause and effect that can occur.

This is why intense crown practices are not recommended in AYP, certainly not in the beginning. Sooner or later that will lead to trouble if not preceded and balanced with other practices providing for whole body purification and opening.

So, while you may be having a good time with the crown now without a full blown kundalini awaking in play, you will not likely be having a good time further down the road, unless you are attending to the rest of your neurobiology."

This also applies to your recent post on ringing, heat, voices, etc. over here: http://www.aypsite.org/forum/topic.asp?TOPIC_ID=3554

Balance and self-pacing in practices and daily living are very important, especially now. I do not imagine you want things to go further to the extreme -- "cruising for a bruising." It is a much slower and more difficult path, because so much time is spent dealing with symptoms of excess. It is up to you, of course.

Suggestion: Practice wisely within your limits, live a full life, and enjoy!

The guru is in you.

2008/03/06 14:40:25
Kundalini - Inner Energy Ecstasy
http://www.aypsite.org/forum/topic.asp?TOPIC_ID=3551&REPLY_ID=30942&whichpage=-1

kundalini rash?

quote:
───────
Originally posted by John C

So, assuming the gentleman above doesn't have ring worm, and his rash is due to kundalini overload, are there certain features of "kundalini rash" that point to that diagnosis, like whether it is generally itchy or not, where on the body it pops up, and whether it happens only at certain times of kundalini symptoms, and so on? A lot of things can cause a rash.
───────

Hi John:

I agree that rashes can have many different causes. But in this case it is a familiar scenario -- symmetrical/systemic rash combined with a host of other symptoms, all preceded by an aggressive and unbalanced approach to practices (see other posts linked in my previous post). So it has "kundalini excess" written all over it.

A kundalini rash will be symmetrical (both sides of the body), can be poison ivy-like (itchy and oozing in more serious cases), and can occur symmetrically just about anywhere on the body -- arms, legs, abdomen, back, neck, and even face. It can become quite a major thing, as was dramatized to the extreme in the Secrets of Wilder novel. Or it can just be some symmetrical reddening, or even just a flushed feeling (most common). Extreme rashes are pretty rare, usually found only in those who press practices (particularly crown and/or kumbhaka with mudras & bandhas) way beyond what is prudent.

Kundalini rash is caused by excessive inner energy flowing through neurobiological obstructions. That is why we call such events "premature." The nervous system is not ready to handle that degree of inner flow radiating from the center (hence the symmetry). Later on, after the appropriate purification, the nervous system will handle it just fine, and it will be known as an endless flow of ecstatic bliss.

See Katrine's post today for a good later stage description: http://www.aypsite.org/forum/topic.asp?TOPIC_ID=3530#30941 Her practice is very sparing, because it takes very little to keep that huge divine flywheel going once it is approaching infinite velocity, which is infinite stillness, or "the shine," as she calls it. It is interesting that her description is in a topic on "healing," which is indicative of the vast outflow of divine love, and the entrainment that naturally occurs in others, leading to healing.

We have seen rash and energy scenarios of one degree or other many times before, so it is pretty clear what is going on in TI's case. Hopefully it is clear to him, because he will have to make some decisive adjustments in practice to smooth this out.

It should also be mentioned that if anyone feels their health is being compromised, they should go and see a doctor. If it is kundalini, then going to a doctor will not likely turn up anything conclusive (most doctors are stumped by kundalini symptoms), and the lack of a medical answer may point to it being an underlying kundalini event. Unfortunately, it may take a number of costly and inconvenient tests to rule out the usual medical suspects, and unnecessary treatments may be prescribed along the way as well.

The medical versus spiritual symptoms discussion has occurred quite a few times here in the forums, and most of the cases I recall led to kundalini by process of elimination. Sometimes people come here looking for answers after they have exhausted their medical options. So, we speak from experience in offering these suggestions. Still, if health becomes a concern, then we should go to a doctor. It is better to be safe than sorry.

It will be wonderful when the medical profession gets on board with excessive symptoms relating to human spiritual transformation. The prescription can read, "Self-pace your practices, and call me in the morning." :-)

The guru is in you.

PS: In Ayurveda, rash is considered to be pitta imbalance, and there are a variety of natural therapies available for helping restore internal energy balance, beginning with basic diet and lifestyle considerations -- avoid those chili peppers and keep cool and calm. Of course, if the underlying cause (imbalance in practices) is not addressed, Ayurvedic remedies will not solve it.

2008/03/06 16:31:30
Kundalini - Inner Energy Ecstasy
http://www.aypsite.org/forum/topic.asp?TOPIC_ID=3551&REPLY_ID=30947&whichpage=-1
kundalini rash?

quote:
───────
Originally posted by John C

Thankyou Yogani. It's interesting how things can go wrong. Gopi Krishna sure suffered alot back in the old days, and didn't seem to know what to do about it. Maybe some people who are thought to be psychotic are actually having disordered kundalinis instead. Maybe some people who think they are having kundalini visions and voices are psychotic instead. Could that be true as well?
───────

Hi John:

With good education and support, things don't have to go so wrong. We are learning. The old way was to sweep it all under the rug, and nobody benefited much from that. So it is time to face our full possibilities head on, and provide the means for good progress with safety. The technology of the information age makes it much more feasible to do this.

Oh sure, mental illness and kundalini can be confused also. That has been discussed quite a lot in the forums as well. Try a few searches.

The good news is that all these things are going to be addressed in the years ahead, so confusion in these matters will be steadily on the decline. By necessity, the accelerating phenomenon of human spiritual transformation is bringing on a new era in the medical field. Lots of opportunity for research and support. These are exciting times.

The guru is in you.

2008/03/06 17:17:22
Kundalini - Inner Energy Ecstasy
http://www.aypsite.org/forum/topic.asp?TOPIC_ID=3551&REPLY_ID=30950&whichpage=-1
kundalini rash?

quote:
_____
Originally posted by Jim and His Karma

quote:
_____
Originally posted by yogani
A kundalini rash will be symmetrical (both sides of the body),
_____

Yogani, just a data point for you. Mine is on left side exclusively, near coccyx. I'm informed that in Chinese medicine, that's a spot for "fire channel" excesses to manifest. I've lately realized that I had a kundalini awakening at age 12 or so, and I remember having what they called eczema on my left ankle at the time. That's apparently another point on the fire channel route. Sorry to get Taoist about it, you can ignore that part. But this is definitely K rash, and quite assymetrical.
_____

Hi Jim:

Ah, very interesting. I wonder if your rash is the exception that proves the rule. :-)

Do you think there is a consistent symtomatic difference between a left-side or right-side imbalance (non-symmetrical), versus a broad overload (symmetrical/systemic)?

It would be interesting to see the stats on it for a large group of kundalini rash cases. Another scientific study to add to the list!

Well, I hope it doesn't come to that. We should be heading off overloads before they happen. It's kind of hard to do in spontaneous awakening cases (like yours may have been), but certainly doable for those who come to learn practices, because the self-pacing guidelines come in the same box with the practices. We can only hope that everyone reads the directions and takes them to heart.

The guru is in you.

2008/03/07 10:29:21
Kundalini - Inner Energy Ecstasy
http://www.aypsite.org/forum/topic.asp?TOPIC_ID=3551&REPLY_ID=30980&whichpage=-1
kundalini rash?

quote:
_____
Originally posted by Anthem11

Hi Jim,

We all have to manage our practices as we feel are best for ourselves, but since you put it out there, couldn't help notice your pranayama to meditation ratio.

Jim wrote:

quote:
_____
10 mins med once per day, and 10 mins pranayama, and no asana due to a hip injury
_____

Seems like a lot of pranayama for someone who has repeatedly mentioned that he is running on the "high" side in the energy department. From reading the lessons, I always got the impression that staying on a 2 to 1 ratio of meditation to pranayama might be in our best interests in order to progress most quickly and with as little turbulence as possible.

Of course this is all inference on my part from what Yogani has written, but I currently do 2.5 minutes of pranayama, 1 yoni mudra kumbhaka and 8 minutes of meditation followed by 3 minutes or so of samyama. No energy imbalances here to report about as long as I stick to this formula, but we all know how seductive the energy side of the equation can be!:-)An extra 1 minute on any of these practices can be enough to put me a wee bit over.

There aren't any right answers and we all have to manage our practices to the best of our abilities, but interested to see how others balance these practices out or as we shrink our routines, what Yogani recommends in terms of ratios?
_____

Hi Anthem and Jim:

A 1:1 ratio between spinal breathing pranayama and deep meditation may be a bit front end loaded, but everyone is different. I would not say that 1:2 is the ideal SBP/DM ratio, because it could be too much SBP in some cases and a 1:4 ratio could work better for some (as in 5 min SBP and 20 min DM). I think we can say with some certainty that more SBP than DM could be courting energy overloads, but those with a long background in kriya yoga (an SBP path) might disagree.

It is hard to say what the ideal balance will be between spinal breathing and deep meditation. It really depends on individual purification and opening, and on where a person is on their path. It is all over the lot among the many practitioners here. So the right answer is what works best for the practitioner, and that puts it squarely in the hands of self-pacing.

We offer basic guidelines in the lessons (ratios somewhere between 1:4 and 1:2), and after that we each must find our own balance. If there are energy difficulties, then different ratios and times should be tried, keeping in mind the probable delay in effects for several days or weeks with any new configuration. So baby steps are recommended when making changes in any aspect of our routine. Unless, of course, we are dealing with a major overload -- then we should cut back immediately, regroup and ground for a while, and come back with baby steps later on according to our bhakti.

What we know for sure is that spinal breathing pranayama and deep meditation together in sequence are far more powerful than either one is as a stand alone. If we consider that kriya yoga practitioners are trained to do spinal breathing for hours every day, often with limited results after years of practice, it is pretty amazing that a few minutes of spinal breathing becomes industrial strength yoga when followed by 15-20 minutes of deep meditation. It goes the other way too. Deep meditation becomes much more effective when preceded by spinal breathing. Judiciously add on samyama, asanas, mudras, bandhas, kumbhaka, chin pump, bastrika, etc ... and hang on to your hat (while self-pacing). So it goes in the new world of open source integrated yoga practices.

Wish I could be more specific, but I think the variations on ratios and times mentioned by practitioners in this topic alone tell the tale. We each are doing whatever is necessary with the tools we have available.

Hence...

The guru is in you.

2008/03/07 16:31:39
Kundalini - Inner Energy Ecstasy
http://www.aypsite.org/forum/topic.asp?TOPIC_ID=3551&REPLY_ID=30996&whichpage=-1
kundalini rash?

quote:
_____
Originally posted by Jim and His Karma

...what do you mean by "hang on to your hat"? Are you refering to the whiz-bang energetic/ecstatic experience of kundalini arousal?

I guess what I'm asking is this: once spiritual energy is up and running, is there meaningful reason to do further energy work via these other practices? Or are they a toolset for getting that energy moving, period?
_____

Hi Jim:

By "Hang on to your hat," I mean accelerated progress on all fronts within us -- both energetic and in cultivating stillness. Both of these are multi-dimensional. Obviously, no one can do it all at once. Hence the proviso, "while self-pacing."

Each practice has its own particular angle and influence on the whole, and the whole is greater than the sum of the parts. So just because we are getting a boost out of one practice, it does not mean the other practices are not going to add new momentum with balance. Not all energy practices are the same. On the other hand, there is only so much purification and opening the nervous system can accommodate in any given time frame, so it all has to be regulated for that.

In the AYP lessons, the practices are put more or less in the order of influence and importance. But there can be some shuffling according to individual need. For example, samyama can be moved up the list with good effect. Other things are best left in the order given for undertaking them, like deep meditation, spinal breathing, and the mantra enhancements.

It is not expected that everyone will be doing all the practices in every sitting beyond the core practices of spinal breathing and deep meditation. Beginners may tend to strive for a "full boat" more than advanced practitioners. The more seasoned we become, the more we are able to accomplish with less -- the momentum/flywheel effect. Even so, advanced practitioners can benefit from new angles of practice from time to time. It keeps it interesting. There are always new openings. The trick is to find them within the context of our own unwinding karmic matrix, without going off the deep end. The full range of available practices are a tool kit for that.

So, no -- one energy practice leading to an active kundalini does not rule out the other energy practices. But self-pacing might, at least for a while. And then it is baby steps... :-)

The guru is in you.

2008/03/06 10:05:20
Kundalini - Inner Energy Ecstasy
http://www.aypsite.org/forum/topic.asp?TOPIC_ID=3554&REPLY_ID=30919&whichpage=-1
Voice in the head

Hi TI:

See here: http://www.aypsite.org/forum/topic.asp?TOPIC_ID=3551#30918

The guru is in you.

2008/04/01 23:19:37
Kundalini - Inner Energy Ecstasy
http://www.aypsite.org/forum/topic.asp?TOPIC_ID=3702&REPLY_ID=32070&whichpage=-1
Imagination and Breath

quote:
_____
Originally posted by tadeas

I believe Yogani mentioned somewhere that in the beginning the direction wouldn't make much difference, but it's better to keep it simple and convenient for later expansion of your practice.
_____

Yes, thank you, Tadeas.

The lesson on this is aptly called "Which way is up?"
It is here: http://www.aypsite.org/46.html

Tadeas, your advice on the crown is helpful also. Andreas, if you check the references given, you will see where the advice is coming from -- many hard-earned lessons over the years.

As for what others may advise differently in these areas, it will be good to ask them about the long term documented results. If someone knows a verifiable better way, we will all flock to it. We are not proud. Only systematic. :-)

All the best!

The guru is in you.

2008/04/05 11:12:29
Kundalini - Inner Energy Ecstasy
http://www.aypsite.org/forum/topic.asp?TOPIC_ID=3702&REPLY_ID=32231&whichpage=-1
Imagination and Breath

Hi Andreas:

Spiritual integration is found in balancing polarities, and this is why spinal breathing goes up and then down. If we don't do this, the imbalance will become apparent sooner or later in the form of excessive kundalini symptoms.

As the old saying goes, "What goes up must come down." :-)

You may find the "heart breathing" technique helpful for expelling impurities and healing. It can be adapted for the eyes or any other organ. Hopefully not to confuse, but this one goes in the opposite direction of AYP spinal breathing, having a different purpose.
http://www.aypsite.org/220.html
(also see the following lesson)

The guru is in you.

2008/06/06 19:25:15
Kundalini - Inner Energy Ecstasy
http://www.aypsite.org/forum/topic.asp?TOPIC_ID=4007&REPLY_ID=34415&whichpage=-1
Shakti-Shiva and the gifts.

Hi Neli, and welcome!

In the AYP approach, we cultivate inner silence (shiva) and ecstatic conductivity (kundalini/shakti) with a range of practices (see the main lessons). The merging of these two qualities within us occurs naturally, so we don't have to force the marriage. It does not have to be a certain way every day. We just do our practices and go out into normal daily activity, which stabilizes what we have cultivated in practices. It is a process of development with many ups and downs corresponding to our transformation. As inner silence and ecstatic conductivity are cultivated, the inner marriage will happen, and become a full time experience over time. The end result is abiding inner silence, ecstatic bliss and outpouring divine love leading to unity, which is duality becoming non-duality, even while remaining dual. Or, put more simply, ongoing *stillness in action* ... we are *That*.

So we are cultivating the underlying conditions of union every day in our practices, and not too worried about the joining, or which chakra is doing what. It happens naturally by degrees. Like the changes you have experienced over the past ten years, the changes will continue over the next ten years, and so on. Nothing to do but keep going with effective practices, as I am sure you will. :-)

Your symptoms of ecstasy are natural and beautiful, and appear to be stable, so that is good. As you may know, ecstasy results from a flow of inner energy, and is actually a symptom of the process of purification and opening occurring within us. Bliss is an inherent quality of inner silence and does not change, while ecstasy will refine over time as purification and opening advance. Eventually ecstasy and bliss become intimately intertwined, and that is the joining everywhere within and around us -- the emergence of stillness in action. It is also sometimes called *divine radiance*.

Speaking of radiance, the physical symptoms you are experiencing in and around you are also a reflection of ongoing purification and opening, and the ever-increasing outward radiation of divine energy. We all go through the process a little differently, and whatever happens is normal for us. If visible siddhis are occurring, this is a confirmation, but obviously not our destination. If the symptoms become too much, then the practice routine can be shortened a bit to pace the process, something you may not be inclined to do, given your strong devotion to your practice. Strong devotion is good, as long as it does not lead us into excesses we can't handle. Then we can end up going slower while recovering from overdoing. It is up to each practitioner to determine what is the best application of practices, while balancing progress with comfort and safety. In AYP, we call this *self-pacing*. It is as important for advanced practitioners as it is for beginners.

Regarding the levitation and things moving around in the room while you are meditating, if you don't wish to self-pace your practice, then consider taking physical measures to prevent distractions or accidents. In time it will all smooth out and you will have much more conscious control, and can prevent external phenomena from occurring at will. The same goes for causing energy surges in others. In time, we learn how to manage such things, just the way a child learns to walk without falling or knocking the furniture over. Until then, it is good to take measures to minimize the disruptions in our environment, and in others. For a few tips from the AYP perspective, see lesson 155.

Others have come here with similar symptoms over the past few years, and it is not so unusual. What is more notable and important is your strong devotion to your practice and your ability to regard all the hub-bub as a sideshow, which is all it is. So it bodes well for you, and for all the rest of us. Your enlightenment is our enlightenment, and vice versa. We're all in it together. :-)

Speaking of that, another way to reduce random energy surges, bouncing off the walls and ceiling, etc., is to put the divine energy to good use during daily activity. Get out and ground it. Exercise is good. See lesson 69 for more pointers. Another good way to reduce wayward energies is to help others, not necessarily in miraculous ways, but through simple helping and service in whatever ways we may be inclined. There are opportunities for that all around us. This will lead to a more balanced flow that is beneficial for everyone, and enhance our own development in a balanced way also. See lesson 120.

As the Buddhists say: "Before enlightenment, chop wood and carry water. After enlightenment, chop wood and carry water."

Thanks much for sharing. Feel free to chime in anytime. Wishing you all the best on your path. Enjoy!

The guru is in you.

2008/06/09 17:37:55
Kundalini - Inner Energy Ecstasy
http://www.aypsite.org/forum/topic.asp?TOPIC_ID=4021&REPLY_ID=34491&whichpage=-1
kundalini rash?

quote:
_____
Originally posted by Neptune

But is this kundalini rash?
_____

Hi Neptune, and welcome!

It would seem so, unless you have been tramping through the underbrush recently.

Check this topic for a pretty thorough discussion on kundalini rash, and some measures to consider:
http://www.aypsite.org/forum/topic.asp?TOPIC_ID=3551

If you do a forum search on "kundalini rash," you will find quite a lot of information on it here. It is not uncommon when too much inner energy is flowing or if there is an imbalance, and there are a variety of ways to deal with it, beginning with *self-pacing* of our practices. See lesson 69 for more measures.

If you are not engaged in spiritual practices and do not consider yourself to be experiencing an "awakening" of some kind, then it may be something else. In that case, if it persists, then consider taking a medical path.

All the best!

The guru is in you.

PS: Also check this kundalini FAQ.

2008/06/09 18:13:09
Kundalini - Inner Energy Ecstasy
http://www.aypsite.org/forum/topic.asp?TOPIC_ID=4021&REPLY_ID=34494&whichpage=-1
kundalini rash?

Hi Neptune:

Yes, sounds like a self-pacing issue.

In the Secrets of Wilder novel, there is an extreme case of kundalini rash covered. It is learning self-pacing (and grounding) the hard way.

The guru is in you.

2008/06/12 09:54:32
Kundalini - Inner Energy Ecstasy
http://www.aypsite.org/forum/topic.asp?TOPIC_ID=4021&REPLY_ID=34551&whichpage=-1
kundalini rash?

Hi Neptune:

Great to hear things are clearing up.

AYP chin pump is a variation on "thokar," which comes from kriya yoga.

Keep in mind that practices do not have to be all or nothing. A few rotations of chin pump should not be excessive, but do wait until you have stabilized the current condition before resuming, and then it is suggested to go slow and self-pace.

All the best!

The guru is in you.

2008/08/26 13:58:56
Kundalini - Inner Energy Ecstasy
http://www.aypsite.org/forum/topic.asp?TOPIC_ID=4021&REPLY_ID=36804&whichpage=-1
kundalini rash?

Hi Tadeas:

Like with poison ivy and other rashes, once the initial cause of a kundalini rash has been reduced or removed, it can take a few weeks or more for the rash to clear up, depending on the severity. There are exceptions, of course, like catching it early with self-pacing, but that is tricky, due to the delayed effects of overdoing in practices. That is why we should aim for moderation in our practices at all times, and balance them with plenty of activity in-between sittings.

Make sure to engage in grounding activities now, and review other kundalini measures here: http://www.aypsite.org/69.html

Also reduce excessive stress in the daily routine, if there is any, which can also be a factor.

If it persists, consider seeing a doctor, though if it is kundalini there will not be much a doctor can do beyond treating symptoms.

This too shall pass. Wishing you speedy stabilization.

The guru is in you.

2008/07/28 15:03:17
Kundalini - Inner Energy Ecstasy
http://www.aypsite.org/forum/topic.asp?TOPIC_ID=4187&REPLY_ID=35835&whichpage=-1
Enlightenment without Kundalini?

Hi YogaIsLife:

What we call "kundalini" is stillness in the form of energy (prana) moving through us, also called "ecstatic conductivity" here in AYP. The more dramatic manifestions of it that get the publicity are only symptoms of purification and opening occurring within us as we move toward a radiating expression of stillness in all aspects of our life. Later on, kundalini becomes very refined and is known as a blissful outpouring, much as is described by Eckhart Tolle, Byron Katie and others. So we are all heading for the same condition.

Can this end state be accomplished without the extreme symptoms of kundalini? With self-pacing of practices on our path, we have a pretty good chance. Everyone arrives here on earth in a slightly different condition, and therefore our process of purification and opening will be somewhat unique. On the other hand, with sound management of practices, there is the opportunity for us to promote our evolution with the least amount of disruption.

Speaking of disruption, both Tolle and Katie went through extreme anguish and pain before and during their awakenings, and neither recommends that sort of extreme scenario for their students. So we could say that even the so-called spontaneous instances of enlightenment come with energy challenges. The names for these occurrences may be changed to protect the innocent. :-)

No matter who is undergoing spiritual transformation, the same inner neurobiological processes and events will be involved in one way or another. It may come hard or soft, slow or fast, but it will come. There is much we can do to influence it for the better.

Our job here in AYP is to do all we can to make it as progressive and comfortable as possible, and hopefully with reliable results for everyone.

While teachers like Tolle and Katie have a lot to offer to those who have been meditating for a few years, they tend to skip over much of the ground work that is necessary -- things like daily deep meditation, spinal breathing pranayama, and so on. Maybe they don't want us to suffer the way they did, so they tell us to "allow" whatever is happening (don't buy in mentally), and all will be well in stillness. That is their experience, and all they want to do is share the end result with their students right now. Fair enough...

However, for most, that approach will be what we here call "non-relational self-inquiry," the mind left to struggle with itself with limited grounding in inner silence (the witness). All it takes is a little deep meditation, and the mental processes of allowing and self-inquiry become "relational," alive in stillness. Then, away we go with Tolle, Katie, Adyashanti, Ramana Maharishi, Nisargadatta, Krishnamurti, and all the rest of them.

And maybe we can avoid the crisis stages many of them went through by gently addressing the energy component of enlightenment from early on. In fact, with prudent practice, the energy aspect can be experienced as steadily rising ecstasy in the body, as many have reported. This is why in AYP we generally refer to it as "ecstatic kundalini" rather than "crisis kundalini." :-)

There are more and more practitioners here in the AYP forums who are experiencing the ever-present stillness beyond the body/mind, and living it in practical ways in everyday life. We are gradually moving beyond fascination with energy experiences to the kind of enlightenment that has been expounded by the wise for centuries. Bravo!

But, as we advance in our experience and come to live the reality of *stillness in action*, let us always remember from where we have come (the systematic cultivation of inner silence), or we will be teaching non-relational self-inquiry to our successors, and that won't do.

Just as we have taken important lessons from the "spontaneously awakened" teachers of our day, they too can take some important lessons from us. Then everyone wins.

All the best!

The guru is in you.

2008/07/29 10:48:42
Kundalini - Inner Energy Ecstasy
http://www.aypsite.org/forum/topic.asp?TOPIC_ID=4187&REPLY_ID=35856&whichpage=-1
Enlightenment without Kundalini?

Hi All:

I have added this to the above post to affirm the ecstatic quality of the journey. The intention is not to deny or eliminate the lovely scenery along the way. Only to present it within the context of the overall process of human spiritual transformation:

quote:
_____
And maybe we can avoid the crisis stages many of them went through by gently addressing the energy component of enlightenment from early on. In fact, with prudent practice, the energy aspect can be experienced as steadily rising ecstasy in the body, as many have reported. This is why in AYP we generally refer to it as "ecstatic kundalini" rather than "crisis kundalini." :-)
_____

All the best!

The guru is in you.

2008/08/07 10:33:41
Kundalini - Inner Energy Ecstasy
http://www.aypsite.org/forum/topic.asp?TOPIC_ID=4253&REPLY_ID=36108&whichpage=-1
How do I get out of this illusional zone?

Hi arzkiyahai:

Getting beyond the illusion is very simple. It is done by relying first on our own spiritual intuition, rather than on anyone else's, no matter what their status may be. This does not mean we shun all gurus and teachers. That would be as foolish as blindly following one without our inner resonance being constantly consulted for reality checks. All teachers have something to offer, and we can also count on them having qualities we do not wish to indulge in. See this lesson on "enlightenment and perfection" http://www.aypsite.org/260.html

The best way to increase our spiritual intuition is by increasing our abiding inner silence. Here in AYP, that is accomplished through twice-daily deep meditation. Then we gradually become much better able to separate the wheat from the chaff, and we can graze almost anywhere in the vast assemblage of gurus, spiritual teachers and spiritual writings and come away unscathed with something worthwhile. It works!

You know, we are pretty careful around here about drifting into what we call "guru bashing," and, in fact, outright guru bashing is not permitted in the forums, though we can bash ourselves if we like. :-)

Nevertheless, I think it is important that we understand why so much good can be accompanied by so much harm in the spiritual teaching profession. And, more importantly, how we can move forward in ways that will increase the good while minimizing the mishaps.

In this regard, the articles you have linked above on the "intermediate zone" are very informative and helpful, even though some of the guru assessments included are biased.

Of particular interest here is the observation that spiritual teaching in the West is evolving to move beyond the pitfalls of the past to what one author calls a Peer-to-Peer teaching model (see summary below).

Here in AYP, we call it the "horizontal transmission model," where spiritual resources are developed, shared, applied and optimized through the cooperative efforts of many. This way, no one person is able to drag the crowd too far in the wrong direction. Will this work? Time will tell...

To date, the spiritual progress many are unfolding has exceeded expectations. That is to everyone's credit.

So, rather than carrying on the unending search for the perfect external guru/avatar, we can make the best of what we have and go forward from where we are. Everything we need is within us already. There is sufficient spiritual enlivenment in the air now to support this approach anywhere on Earth. These days, a little spiritual desire (bhakti) goes a long way toward attracting the help we need.

Plus, in this information age it is becoming much easier, because accessing real spiritual knowledge and powerful practices is no longer the problem it used to be. We can now create "safe harbors" of effective knowledge that can be applied for ongoing purification and opening of ourselves and used as a base for exploration of additional sources of knowledge. In fact, in this scenario, accessing gurus and teachers is not a problem at all. We can take what has value and move on as necessary, avoiding the common pitfalls of hierarchal systems that we have come to know so well.

All the best on your continuing path. Enjoy!

The guru is in you.

Evolution through four phases of guru phenomenon in the West
(Credited to John Heron: see half way down the page here)

1. In the late decades of the nineteenth century and early decades of the twentieth century, there was just a small guru-invasion from the East with key players like Vivekananda and the spread of the Vedanta movement in the West.

2. Then post-war from 1945 with the publication of Huxley's The Perennial Philosophy, there started a major guru-invasion from the East including the dramatic spread through the 60s and the 70s of Zen and Tibetan Buddhism in the USA and Europe.

3. In the third phase, over the last thirty years or so, alongside the guru-invasion from the East there has been the growing phenomenon of homegrown Western gurus and spiritual teachers claiming the special status of 'enlightenment'.

4. The fourth phase is just getting under way. It seems to be distinguished by four features:

----a. The erosion of guru status as a result of sexual and financial abuse and bullying scandals among both Eastern and homegrown Western gurus and spiritual teachers.

----b. The erosion of 'enlightenment' claims by the proliferation of the number of people, especially in the West, making the claim: the more people who make the claim, the more its narcissistic inflation stands revealed. For the 'enlightenment' claim is also an authority-claim to have followers, a recruiting drive; and the more claims that are made, the stronger the competition among claimants in the market-place for attention.

----c. A growing awareness that spiritual authority is within and that to project it outward onto teacher, tradition or text is an early, adolescent phase of spiritual development in the one projecting, and counter-spiritual manipulative abuse in any guru/teacher who seeks to elicit, to appropriate and to sustain the projection.

----d. The emergence of peer to peer spirituality, which democratizes charismatic, enlightened leadership, and realizes that it is a role which different persons assume at different times, either in the initiation of a peer group or in the continuous unfolding of its process.

PS: Here is an AYP lesson that also traces the rise of Eastern spiritual teachings in the West, including extensive linking to the associated literature/booklist: http://www.aypsite.org/253.html

2008/08/07 13:29:34
Kundalini - Inner Energy Ecstasy
http://www.aypsite.org/forum/topic.asp?TOPIC_ID=4253&REPLY_ID=36110&whichpage=-1
How do I get out of this illusional zone?

Hi again arzkiyahai:

Regarding your personal situation, the suggestion is to favor daily spiritual practices over the easily expandable mental drama of experiences.

Like the many gurus who go astray, getting caught up in the "scenery" of their journey, so too can we go astray when we become overly enamored or fearful about the scenery we encounter along our path. The illusion is our own projection occurring through the mechanics of our perception. We always have a choice about how to regard this, though it might not seem so.

With the prudent application of spiritual practices over time, our perception can be expanded beyond limited illusory projections, and we can move decisively toward greater freedom, even if the same scenery continues to occur within and around us.

One of the best uses for "self-inquiry" is found in allowing experiences to happen without becoming embroiled in them. It is our own burgeoning mind stuff we are interacting with. Abiding inner silence (the witness) is the key in getting beyond this. To the degree we have inner silence, it can be used in this way. It is a natural development that comes with the rise of the witness. As mentioned in the above post, we can increase our inner silence through daily deep meditation.

There are other means that have been discussed extensively in the AYP writings and here in the forums for dealing with excessive energy and other discomforts that may come up. It will depend on your history and spiritual practices what other measures may be applicable. The best place to start in AYP is at the beginning, taking it one step at a time: http://www.aypsite.org/MainDirectory.html

All the best!

The guru is in you.

2008/08/08 09:49:50
Kundalini - Inner Energy Ecstasy
http://www.aypsite.org/forum/topic.asp?TOPIC_ID=4253&REPLY_ID=36132&whichpage=-1
How do I get out of this illusional zone?

quote:
_____
Originally posted by arzkiyahai

Hello Yogani, thankyou for your priceless and very helpful reply.

I am doing spinal breathing pranayama for some time now.

I have couple of questions in regard to daily practices:

1. I talked to someone and he suggested me that at this moment the best thing for me to is grounded and he told me that meditation is very ungrounding, it leaves us ungrounded. That was the main reason for me not doing meditation at the moment. Please suggest me on this.

2. I have started eating chicken. Hoping it is good for grounding.

thanks again.

kindest regards from my heart

Hi arzkiyahai:

Spinal breathing will usually be calming and balancing, but there are exceptions, so be moderate. If energy is increasing in uncomfortable ways, scale back on spinal breathing.

It can be just the other way with deep meditation, depending on the nature of your nervous system and events occurring. Deep meditation cultivates inner silence, which is the ground state of the cosmos and everything in it. So to say deep meditation is not grounding is not recognizing what it is about. On the other hand, in order to cultivate inner silence, purification and opening will occur in the nervous system. This process is stimulated by deep meditation, and may not feel very grounding, depending on the condition of the nervous system. It will depend on your constitution, history and other factors.

There is one easy way to find out if deep meditation will be helpful, and that is to try a light twice daily routine and see what happens. Only about 10 minutes of deep meditation per session starting out, morning and afternoon, after spinal breathing, which should also be light (5 min or so). See the AYP lessons for detailed instructions. If this aggravates the situation, then scale back. No harm done.

Yes, a heavier diet will help quell an overactive kundalini -- your choice on what to eat. An ayurveda vata and/or pitta pacifying diet can also help a kundalini excess. But it is not clear that this is an overactive kundalini, so there are unknowns. This is why it is good to know the long term history of practices (if any) and experiences.

Also check this FAQ for more on grounding: http://www.aypsite.org/forum/topic.asp?TOPIC_ID=2165

All the best!

The guru is in you.

2008/08/14 10:48:01
Kundalini - Inner Energy Ecstasy
http://www.aypsite.org/forum/topic.asp?TOPIC_ID=4253&REPLY_ID=36370&whichpage=-1
How do I get out of this illusional zone?

HI Arzkiyahai:

Thank you for sharing your background. It sheds a lot of light.

Yours is a textbook case of premature kundalini (and crown) awakening taken to the extreme by unknowing excesses in practice, particularly long pranayama sessions and other practices using *breath suspension* (kumbhaka -- a powerful kundalini stimulator), leading to delayed reactions of too much energy flowing. It is common for euphoric experiences to turn unpleasant and unhealthy in cases like this where the practices that have caused them are taken to excess again and again. It is a massive overload.

Using Aum/OM as a stand alone mantra in meditation likely hasn't helped either. See here for comments on this from the AYP perspective. OM is utilized in a more balanced way in a mantra enhancement later on in the lessons.

It is hard to say whether this ongoing kundalini situation is behind all of your health problems, but it is likely that it is a major contributor. It is good that you have gone to doctors (you had no choice, right?). Now it is time to engage in a more prudent course from your side. It will take time, but the situation can be recovered.

For some orientation on what you are into, it is suggested to read these two books, if you have not already:

Kundalini - The Evolutionary Energy in Man, by Gopi Krishna
The Secrets of Wilder novel, an AYP book

From these two, you will see many parallels with your experience, and how the situation can be remedied in time, while restoring good spiritual progress. Of particular importance is the development of abiding inner silence, which, through the stabilizing power of the witness, enables us to weather the ups and downs we will encounter along our path.

Note to others reading along here: The extreme kind of experiences described here are not a prerequisite for spiritual progress, and will in fact delay it, due to the recovery time involved. The Secrets of Wilder novel explores excesses of this kind specifically so they can be resolved in the story through adjustments in practices and living habits, with the solutions then passed on so others are able to avoid the same excesses. It is a big part of what we are doing in AYP -- optimizing practices for maximum progress with minimum mishaps. Gopi Krishna went through his own adjustments over a long period of time, with far fewer knowledge resources available to him than we have today.

Arzkiyahai, it is interesting that this topic started off discussing the so-called "intermediate zone" of spiritual experiences, where practitioners (and gurus) become prone to infatuation and distorted views of their progress and condition. While some practitioners/gurus having ongoing divine experiences may slip into narcissism and declare themselves to be the *avatar* (incarnation of God) of the age, others with ongoing negative experiences (like yours) can edge into obsessive paranoia about being stuck in a dark realm full of malevolent entities who are working to destroy them. There are certainly plenty of people out there who will be happy to support either extreme view -- the avatar infatuation, or the dark forces paranoia. The truth is that neither one of these represent reality. Anyone who has focused on cultivating abiding inner silence will know this, because no such things exist within the light of pure consciousness. It is all in the labeling our mind engages in -- the objectivization of energy experiences by the mind.

Consider this: There is no "entity" (real or imagined) that could ever do as much damage to you as you have done to yourself through uninformed spiritual practices. The solution to the problem is not about managing dark forces, balancing chakras, or getting out of a place you think you are

450 – Advanced Yoga Practices

stuck in. What you have is a hellacious kundalini overload that you have been unknowingly feeding for 12 years, off and on.

So what's next? Moderation in all things (especially spiritual practices), self-pacing, and favoring steadfast rational solutions over infatuations or obsessive paranoia and fear. Following the latter can lead much deeper into a labyrinth of mental confusion. The advice is to favor a sound course of action over the experiences that are coming up. If you can do that, much better times lie ahead.

Here are a few specific suggestions to consider:

1. Don't do intentional breath suspension (kumbhaka) in any practice until your health is fully recovered. That could be years from now. Don't do intentional mudras, bandhas or siddhasana for the same reason (energy stimulation). Maybe some very light sambhavi mudra, which can help stabilize an unruly kundalini. If it doesn't, don't do it. If automatic kumbhaka or mudras/bandhas occur during meditation or at any other time, easily favor whatever practice or activity you are doing over them. In other words, don't intentionally favor any of these practices, even if they are occurring as automatic yoga.

2. Be moderate to light in all practices you undertake, and self-pace at the first sign of excess, including any ecstatic energy flowing. As you have found out, more can easily become less if we are not ready in our abiding inner silence. Self-pacing does not mean quitting practices. It means adjusting the durations of practices in ways that will minimize excesses in experience. Practices are the gas pedal. Experiences are your journey along the road. Manage the gas pedal so you will not drive off the road. You have been driving off the road a lot. :-)
Always remember that there can be a delay between practices and their effects, so it is best to err on the side of caution, especially in your case. It is suggested to read everything you can find on self-pacing in the AYP lessons and forums. If you become an expert in self-pacing, you will greatly reduce your risk of repeating the problems of the past. Here is a starting point: http://www.aypsite.org/forum/topic.asp?TOPIC_ID=2139

3. Find your balance in twice daily practices. That is your balance, not what anyone else thinks it is, including me. It will be what you discover it is. It is important that you find a way to regularly cultivate inner silence, for the reasons mentioned previously. The advice still holds to try twice daily 5 min spinal breathing and 10 min deep meditation. It can be a starting point. If it is too much, do less. If less is too much, then shift to a few minutes of alternate nostril breathing with a few minutes of deep meditation right after. Find a balance in your practices that you can sustain twice daily indefinitely, even if it is only 5 minutes of total practice per session. This is very important, because your spiritual progress does not depend on what you do for three weeks and stop, and then three weeks later on and stop again. You have been through that on a grand scale, yes? Spiritual progress depends on what we can do in practices with stability every single day for the rest of our life. So it is imperative to find a balance that works for you, no matter how modest it may be. You will have the option to consider enhancements in daily practice over time, once you have established a stable routine. A balanced long term daily routine is the key. Before that, we are just flailing around in the wind, and always at risk.

4. Continue with grounding activities. Having an active life is very important to stabilize our inner silence and energies cultivated in practices each day, including healthy activity, exercise, social engagement, good company, good humor, etc. Along these lines, you may wish to add a very light set of asanas before pranayama and meditation (a few minutes of stretching), which help provide a smooth transition from activity to sitting practices. Likewise, make sure to take plenty of rest at the end of sitting practices, which aids a smooth transition from sitting practices to daily activity -- 5 minutes or more lying down at the end of practices is good. If there is roughness or irritability in activity, the first thing to check is our rest period at the end of practices. If you can find a balance between asanas, pranayama, deep meditation, rest, and healthy activity in daily living that you can sustain day in and day out for the long term, without overdoing, then you will be on the way to full recovery with good spiritual progress.

Wishing you all the best!

The guru is in you.

PS: This topic has been moved to the kundalini forum category, where it is a much better fit.

2008/08/07 11:36:57
Kundalini - Inner Energy Ecstasy
http://www.aypsite.org/forum/topic.asp?TOPIC_ID=4254
Kundalini During Sleep

Hi All:

An interesting recent interchange. Comments welcome. :-)

The guru is in you.

Q: From memeggings: Can the kundalini arise when asleep at night?

A very surprising thing happened around 4 or 5 this morning as I slept. A part of my mind noted that the noise in my ears had escalated and was now very high and loud, then energy clamped onto the top and back of my head and within seconds I felt the electric flames rise and dance over my skin, through me, up, and my body felt mild shaking.

Then the part of my mind that noted the loud noise in my ears just prior to this, began calling to archangels and beings of Light and I felt myself thrown up high, then all was oblivion as my body slept and my singing mind went off somewhere, leaving no memory on waking of where I went. (At times I remember my "split" mind's travels into "realms of light" – for want of a better term.)

On awaking in the morning I remembed this and immediately felt energy "clamp" onto the top and back of my head, but very mildly.

Can kundalini arise in sleep spontaneously? I have many times had it arise over the years while awake, or just prior to going to sleep, but never in sleep.

A: Sure, with an active kundalini, those kinds of experiences can happen any time, even during sleep.

The important thing to remember is that kundalini experiences are symptoms of purification and opening occurring in the nervous system. As we continue with daily practices over time, purification and opening become gradually more refined and experiences naturally move toward a steady state of abiding inner silence, ecstatic bliss and outpouring divine love. This is the destination of practices and kundalini.

So when the visions and energy experiences come, it is suggested to favor our routine of practices over following a big drama. The practices will surely move us ahead in our development. The drama will not.

If experiences become too intense, then it is suggested to self-pace (scale back a bit) on practices for a while, and engage in more grounding activities in daily life.

All the best!

The guru is in you.

2008/12/18 09:38:44
Kundalini - Inner Energy Ecstasy
http://www.aypsite.org/forum/topic.asp?TOPIC_ID=4323&REPLY_ID=42541&whichpage=-1
New here! Progress Questions

Hi Michaelangelo:

Etherfish has suggested to you just right. That, and stay busy in your life. Favoring self-paced practice of deep meditation and an active life will balance things out in time. The more we obsess over energy symptoms, the more uncertain our path will be. Just live and enjoy. The answers will be there as you engage in normal activity. You will find it is all stillness in action...

The guru is in you.

2008/08/29 11:25:51
Kundalini - Inner Energy Ecstasy
http://www.aypsite.org/forum/topic.asp?TOPIC_ID=4370&REPLY_ID=36943&whichpage=-1
Kundalini

quote:
_____
Originally posted by madhuheal

Dear Yagani,

In India,there are some yogis/persons are offering 3 day course of Kundalini awakening, it is on the net already, How? and is it something can believable?
_____

Hi madhuheal:

It is good to be skeptical about claims of that sort, while not ignoring them either. We will find the truth by paying attention and releasing. It is within us.

Kundalini is not "all or nothing." There are a thousand levels of energy awakening, beginning with the first stirrings in us that occur with our bhakti (divine desire). In a real sense, anyone who feels spiritual inspiration has kundalini moving already. It is moving here now, yes?

Surely "shaktipat" can have a role in this overall unfoldment. But that is only a jump start. The rest is up to the practitioner and the effectiveness of daily practices in use over time.

The mechanical means for awakening kundalini (pranayama, mudras and bandhas) are well-known these days. It is not so complicated. However, if these means are used prematurely in relation to other practices it can lead to difficulties.

Kundalini (shakti energy) awakening is only half of the equation. The other half is the cultivation of inner silence, which is very important. A major kundalini awaking will be difficult to manage without the presence of abiding inner silence (the witness). It is the long way around on the road to enlightenment. Putting kundalini first is putting the cart in front of the horse. Is there a claim there for stabilizing abiding inner silence? That will be the greater accomplishment over any amount of time. Better to use effective means day in and day out, and be patient. Rome was not built in a day, or in three days...

With claims like that, I think "marketing." Which isn't to say there is nothing of value there. All teachings have some value, even if it is learning what not to do. Unfortunately, most who resort to lavish claims will come up short. The real question is, what system of practices do they offer? Are all the bases of human spiritual transformation covered? What is the long term scenario and support system?

Let your divine intuition be your guide. As time goes on you can rely on it much more than claims others might make. Investigate, inquire and abide in stillness. Then you will know where your path is, and where it is not.

All the best!

The guru is in you.

2008/09/11 23:23:55
Kundalini - Inner Energy Ecstasy
http://www.aypsite.org/forum/topic.asp?TOPIC_ID=4392&REPLY_ID=37611&whichpage=-1
Crown Opening

Hi All:

Enlightenment, traditionally and experientially, is the merging of abiding inner silence with ecstasy, to yield stillness in action, which is outpouring divine love and *Oneness* in everyday living.

So both abiding inner silence (samadhi) and ecstatic awakening (kundalini) are necessary for the whole thing. In the classical Eastern metaphor it is the union of shiva and shakti.

In AYP we cultivate them in that order for more stable development. As many here know, it can be messy to begin with kundalini without having some inner silence established first. Inner silence is our center (our *Self*), and ecstatic conductivity and radiance provide for the expansion of that center to infinite expression. If the energetic side is cultivated in a balanced way from the spinal nerve (sushumna), the potential difficulties of ecstatic awakening can be minimized. It is a matter of keeping things in the right order and proportion, and self-pacing practices along the way. Reliable results come with a systematic approach.

The guru is in you.

2008/09/13 11:23:58
Kundalini - Inner Energy Ecstasy
http://www.aypsite.org/forum/topic.asp?TOPIC_ID=4392&REPLY_ID=37667&whichpage=-1
Crown Opening

Hi Neli:

Samad
Hi is always going to be the product of meditation. By that, I do not mean one particular style of meditation. It is not a sectarian thing. Rather, it the universal principle of attention dissolving in an object. The possibilities are unlimited in that. If one is devoted to ecstatic shiva-shakti union and makes it an object of meditation, then samad
Hi will come. If one is devoted to self-inquiry, then that can lead to samadhi. It is the underlying principle of meditation that leads to the rise of stillness in any activity.

As you know, in AYP we use a systematic process of meditation with mantra, so the cultivation of inner silence (samadhi) is not left to chance. It is very efficient. It is a much longer process in styles of meditation where there is not an effective procedure for handling the many diversions of the mind.

Samad
Hi can happen in any devoted activity -- re: "Zen and the art of motorcycle maintenance." :-) It is a matter of where one's heart is and how efficient the practice is, if it is even called "practice." There is no reason an efficient form of meditation like we use in AYP cannot be used to enhance less structured forms of "meditation" that will occur as we pursue the things we love in life. The more inner silence we have, the more will our life naturally become meditation, and ultimately *stillness in action*.

The guru is in you.

2008/09/14 10:35:00
Kundalini - Inner Energy Ecstasy
http://www.aypsite.org/forum/topic.asp?TOPIC_ID=4392&REPLY_ID=37684&whichpage=-1
Crown Opening

quote:
_____
Originally posted by schtroumpsolis

iwould like to ask yogani ;how can we prepare ourself to withstand all that outpouring of love , vital ans psy energie? Our couciousness is far from ready to withstand all the forces during the process and to maintain it going.
when we do live this enlightment process with the flowing light ,love etc.

f.
_____

Hi f:

The human nervous system is capable of conducting vast divine energy as it becomes purified and opened. This does not happen overnight, and depends largely on an effective daily routine of practices conducted over the long term, with self-pacing so as not to get too far ahead of ourselves. By far the most important aspect of this is the cultivation of abiding inner silence, which enables us to remain steady in the face of any storm. It is the proverbial rock.

The guru is in you.

2008/10/26 15:52:36
Kundalini - Inner Energy Ecstasy
http://www.aypsite.org/forum/topic.asp?TOPIC_ID=4564&REPLY_ID=39513&whichpage=-1
I AM mantra

quote:
_____
Originally posted by riptiz

quote:

it doesn't matter how long we sit in meditation, what matters is that we give our nervous system the necessary time and tools to purify itself otherwise if we step over the edge and overload then we are holding back our spiritual evolution

----

What justification have you for saying that overloading holds back spiritual evolution? Just curious thats all as I've never read that anywhere else.
L&L
Dave

Hi Riptiz:

The simple answer is that if we overdo, we can get to a degree of discomfort with symptoms that we can't practice anymore for a time, maybe a long time if symptoms become severe. It takes time to recover from excesses. That is why I say overdoing can delay our progress, and that less can be more in spiritual practice. I think many have had this experience to one degree or other. It is part of the learning curve we climb to develop our skill in self-pacing.

It is the same with anything, and that is what is behind the saying that we can have too much of a good thing. It never happened to you? :-)

The guru is in you.

2008/10/27 14:34:50
Kundalini - Inner Energy Ecstasy
http://www.aypsite.org/forum/topic.asp?TOPIC_ID=4564&REPLY_ID=39544&whichpage=-1
I AM mantra

Hi Riptiz:

Having energy excesses with normal durations of practice is one thing, and having them by greatly exceeding suggested durations of practice is something else. The first may not be so obvious (requiring gradual fine-tuning in practices), but the other of blatant overdoing is obvious and should be pretty clear to anyone who is paying attention. Both will require self-pacing, and if that is ignored in either case, it can be a tough slog.

The idea that we can "blast through" rough periods by maintaining or increasing practice durations is not valid, and this has been demonstrated time and time again. That is mainly what should be warned about here, because it is not a viable long term approach. Many have fallen off the path of practices for extended periods due to not understanding this. The rise of prudent self-pacing among more and more spiritual practitioners promises to greatly reduce the dropout rate.

As for "pandering to the masses," I had not thought of it quite like that before. The point of view here is that if people have useful information that can help them unfold their divine possibilities, they will be more likely to do something about it. We as a species can no longer afford to do this in small ways ... favoring the few over the many, placing conduct barriers in front of everyone else. That is just teachers dodging their responsibility to provide effective spiritual practices that can be widely utilized. The days of esoteric teaching are coming to an end. It is time for all of humanity to move on, with many more "oars in the water" than in the past...

This does not mean we are throwing laws against harmful conduct out the window. Of course, not. But it is a fact that there are many in prison who can benefit from spiritual practices as much as anyone. Maybe more. Historically, it is well known that "bad conduct" has often been a prerequisite for real spiritual practice and progress.

We learn and grow by our mistakes (and by studying the mistakes of others), not by blindly towing someone else's line.

Right, Neli? :-)

Neli, I think the only reason you are being given some strong advice is because you have mentioned some roughness in daily activity. Maybe you did not have this before doing AYP methods, and that might be because your practices before have not gone as deep. Who knows? We can only go by our experience in daily life and the cause and effect related to our practices. That is all that is being pointed out.

No one will tell you exactly what you must do with your practice. That is your choice. But if things are overloading, or whatever concerns there might be in daily activity, there are some procedures related to our practices that are known to help.

On the other hand, if you are mixing a batch of practices from different sources and doing them all more than is recommended, then it is your own research. We are interested in that here too, but you should be advised that there are risks. Your choice. Please keep us posted.

I would also remind you that in the natural scheme of things stillness comes first and ecstatic energy comes second. With a limitation on stillness, energy will be limited too, though we might tend to think otherwise with so many fireworks being stimulated in our nervous system by our focus on doing that. It is normal to get attached to this sort of thing. It is a stage in our development, and is not the end game. The best kind of ecstatic fireworks are the ones rooted in abiding inner silence -- stillness in action! Then we are free. :-)

The guru is in you.

2008/10/28 11:29:37
Kundalini - Inner Energy Ecstasy
http://www.aypsite.org/forum/topic.asp?TOPIC_ID=4564&REPLY_ID=39561&whichpage=-1
I AM mantra

Hi Neli:

"Towing someone else's line" means living by someone else's rules instead of our own natural inclinations. I was attempting to tie in the yama/niyama discussion with Riptiz with your situation of forced conduct in your youth.

No one should be forced to "tow someone else's line," not in yoga, and not in life. Of course, this challenges traditional yogic teachings, which insist on certain kinds of conduct before powerful practices are given. Times have changed, and so must the application of yoga methods. Nowadays, deep practices bring good conduct much more-so than the other way around. Many practitioners have experienced this in life, so it is not a philosophical speculation.

As I have said in the past, "Experience in daily life is the ultimate measure of our practice." Not anyone's pronouncements about it, or even the scriptures themselves. And experiences inside practices are not the measure of progress either. It is in how our normal everyday life is affected. This is how we know if our practices are doing their job.

That is what we want -- experience-based practice. Neli, your experiences are very good inside practices, and hopefully as good outside practices. That is the acid test. Your living shakti is your ishta, your chosen ideal. This is very good. As discussed in the Bhakti and Karma Yoga book, our ishta will refine over time as we become more purified and more in blissful stillness. Then every movement in life will be a very refined ecstasy -- stillness in action. All of life becomes an extension of our ever-refining ishta.

Surely you know that for many people, kundalini brings strong symptoms of purification and opening, and that if there is no regulation of practices, there can be serious problems. Loving surrender to that process is very good, and will help a lot. But if one is getting ill, then the causes in practice (and in life) should be regulated for a smoother unfoldment. It is common sense, yes?

Your case may not need regulation so much, which is wonderful, but we can't forget about everyone else. It is natural to measure everyone else by our own experience. It is actually a common failing among advanced teachers -- telling others that there is no need to go through the process, and to just jump to the end right now. This disconnect between advanced practitioners and others is very common, and is to be guarded against, for it can lead to a fracturing of the path for many. So, we tell others from where we have come, how we have gotten here, and what systematic methods can be applied to help bring everyone along. That is all we are doing here in AYP.

It seems the reason we got into this discussion is because you felt the I AM mantra was not working energetically. As several have said, the I AM mantra is not for an energetic experience. It is for cultivating abiding inner silence. So, nothing happening is not nothing happening in deep meditation. It is everything happening. :-)

The other part of this discussion on symptoms happened I think because you mentioned roughness in activity. The first thing we say in AYP when that is going on is, "Rest before getting up from practices to smooth the transition back into activity." And second we say, "Self-pace your practices." Maybe the advice came after the symptom passed, so you felt a bit put upon. We all know by now how enthusiastic you are about your practices. Bravo for that!

All intentions are good here, and all are working from where they are. We are not so different. All are on the same road, in slightly different places. It is still one road -- the road of human spiritual transformation.

The guru is in you.

2008/10/29 12:20:27
Kundalini - Inner Energy Ecstasy
http://www.aypsite.org/forum/topic.asp?TOPIC_ID=4630&REPLY_ID=39616&whichpage=-1
Kundalini

Hi krcqimpro1, and welcome! :-)

There are some elements of practice from kriya yoga in AYP, and also elements of practice integrated from many other sources, plus ongoing refinements and optimizations for self-directed practice that are unique to AYP.

It is the natural capabilities found within the human nervous system that support the process of human spiritual transformation, of which ecstatic kundalini is a part. What is within us already defines the journey, not any particular tradition.

If you review the AYP lessons and compare them with what is in kriya yoga, the similarities and differences will be apparent. In case you are not familiar with the details of kriya yoga, if you do a "subject only" search on "kriya yoga" here in the forums, you will find discussions and links to resources on that.

Wishing you all the best on your path. Enjoy!

The guru is in you.

PS: A primary difference is that AYP utilizes a proactive form of deep meditation with mantra, and kriya yoga does not. It is a big difference.

2008/11/12 12:21:11
Kundalini - Inner Energy Ecstasy
http://www.aypsite.org/forum/topic.asp?TOPIC_ID=4667&REPLY_ID=40375&whichpage=-1
Ramtha

quote:
_____
Originally posted by mikkiji

Ah, yes, just what in the world IS this "kundalini" anyway? I studied personally in ashram for several years with one of the spiritual lights of the 20th century, the late Maharis
Hi Mahesh Yogi. He never once, in all the time I studied with him, mentioned the word kundalini. I never heard the term, and we studied many ancient yogic texts with him. I did the yoga practices he taught me (basically, many of Yogani's AYP things) for 30 yeas, period, nothing more or less. In my early fifties, after several months of enforced celibacy (due to family medical circumstances), I too had a spontaneous kundalini awakening, never even having heard of kundalini! I came to gradually understand what was happening, and I did conclude a few things that are mistakenly believed about kundalini. I now understand that the breathing stuff--the so-called "breath of fire", all of that nonsense, is NOT cause but effect! I HAD all of the breathing things take hold of my physical body and just sort of happen to me, during the initial few hours of rising. It's not something you DO to make it happen, it's something that HAPPENS after it's begun. But since people have witnessed this effect, it has

gotten associated as a way to make kundalini rise, rather than merely a side-effect of the rising. The other important misconception involves the relationship between kundalini and enlightenment. They are not necessarily related too directly. One can be enlightened without having kundalini awkwakened, and one can have kundalini awakened without being enlightened. One need not experience kundalini to experience god.
Michael

_____

Hi Michael:

Each of the limbs of yoga are both cause and effect, and all of the limbs of yoga are interconnected within us. So one person's structured practice may be another person's symptom. Personally, I'd rather rely mainly on practices than on symptoms. That's why in AYP we favor the practice over the symptoms. And, as you know, we have plenty of practices. :-)

I agree with you that kundalini of the dramatic symptomatic kind is not a prerequisite or ongoing feature of enlightenment. The drama of kundalini is purification (the friction of awakening energy passing through obstructions) and not the end result. However, the subtle characteristics of kundalini that evolve to permeate the neurobiology as ecstasy and the refinement of sensory perception are essential to enlightenment, as Christi points out. You may not call that kundalini. But it is, in fact, the eventual refinement of the flashy versions of kundalini that some people experience along their path. It is the emergence of our ecstatic nature, ultimately to be dissolved in stillness. In AYP we call it the rise of ecstatic conductivity. That and abiding inner silence (stillness, the witness) are the two pillars of enlightenment. The equation looks like this:

Stillness + Ecstasy = Unity (enlightenment)

In AYP, we use deep meditation for cultivating abiding inner silence (stillness).

Ecstasy (ecstatic conductivity/kundalini) is cultivated with spinal breathing and other pranayama methods (including kumbhaka), plus asanas, mudras, bandhas, and tantric sexual methods.

Rising stillness and ecstasy are blended together (in the equal sign), with samyama, karma yoga, and self-inquiry. Each of these finds its fruition when performed in stillness (presence of witness), which we call "relational" in AYP. The result is "divine radiance."

Bhakti (divine desire) plays an over-arching role in all of this. Bhakti is the fuel of all spiritual progress. Even the tiniest desire for growth contains all of these elements of unfoldment within it, and stimulates them directly.

Now, some will say that stillness is enlightenment, and others will say that ecstatic kundalini is enlightenment. The truth is that both together form enlightenment. It is the union of stillness (shiva) and ecstasy (shakti) which brings an unending outpouring of divine love and the unity experience in daily living, i.e., *Oneness*. In AYP we also call it "stillness in action."

This process is inherent in the human nervous system and is universal. Different paths emphasize different aspects of its development. In the end, all the bases will be covered. It is a natural process, once it gets going. Our job in daily yoga practices is to get it going and keep it going, without overdoing it (self-pacing). Then we come to know what it is by direct experience, right? :)

The guru is in you.

2009/01/28 13:10:40
Kundalini - Inner Energy Ecstasy
http://www.aypsite.org/forum/topic.asp?TOPIC_ID=5089&REPLY_ID=44377&whichpage=-1
Amrita Question

Hi Carson:

When the source of the sweet flowery aroma can't be located, it is likely a hint of amrita (nectar) in the sinuses and nasal passages.

Enjoy, and carry on. Favoring practices over experiences, of course. :-)

The guru is in you.

2009/02/23 11:01:13
Kundalini - Inner Energy Ecstasy
http://www.aypsite.org/forum/topic.asp?TOPIC_ID=5219&REPLY_ID=45790&whichpage=-1
hello-new to the forum

Hi Orient, and welcome!

There can be many causes for what you are experiencing. Since we do not know what your practices are, it is difficult to diagnose specifics in that area. Overloads (and congestion) can be caused by too much practice, particularly pranayama and/or kumbhaka (breath suspension). Even overdoing with asanas alone can do it. You are wise to back off on practices until you find stability. In AYP, we call this "self-pacing," and there is a lot about developing that skill in the AYP lessons and forums.

While there are many places to look in the lessons (see the topic index as Katrine suggested), perhaps this FAQ can serve as a starting point for you, particularly Lesson 69 on symptoms and remedies linked there:

http://www.aypsite.org/forum/topic.asp?TOPIC_ID=2169

If you stick around, keep sharing and interacting, I am sure you will get to the bottom of it. These are just a few bumps in the road, and it will get better as you develop some navigation skills.

It is not necessary to suffer for years with kundalini excesses anymore. There are many means available for dealing with it to maintain good progress with safety on the road of human spiritual transformation.

Wishing you all the best on your path. Practice wisely, and enjoy!

The guru is in you.

2009/02/23 14:03:14
Kundalini - Inner Energy Ecstasy
http://www.aypsite.org/forum/topic.asp?TOPIC_ID=5219&REPLY_ID=45814&whichpage=-1
hello-new to the forum

quote:
_____
Originally posted by orient

Actually my kundalini awakened with mantra and prayer but mostly I would do mantra.I was doing asana and little bit pranayaam too at that time. The mantra does make me calm and silent if done sincerely for a couple of hours or so but it gives me tremendous energy.As already I have too much energies I fall ill with congestion.I have been avoiding yoga asanas bcos it would give me problems.So really presently I dont think I will be able to carry out any practice which releases any energy though I understand that practice is most important. :(its a complication for me
_____

Hi Orient:

Two hour sessions of AYP deep meditation (with mantra) would lead to needing a spatula to scrape the practitioner off the ceiling. :-)

We use two 20 minute meditation sessions per day. Many practitioners use shorter sessions due to rapid openings (self-pacing). You may wish to review the AYP lessons on deep meditation. They are the first lessons here: http://www.aypsite.org/MainDirectory.html

You may wish to self-pace prayer also (and other spiritual influences in your life), until things smooth out. Then you can build back a little bit at a time to find a stable routine that can work for you over the long term. It is our long term routine in practices that will make the difference in unfolding our full spiritual potential, not what we do in any given day, week, or month. For most, the journey to enlightenment is a marathon, not a sprint. The AYP system is geared for that, for cultivating maximum progress while maintaining comfort and safety over the long term.

All the best!

The guru is in you.

2009/03/10 12:28:40
Kundalini - Inner Energy Ecstasy
http://www.aypsite.org/forum/topic.asp?TOPIC_ID=5292&REPLY_ID=46908&whichpage=-1
Why does kundalini rise at some times?

Hi Ampontan, and welcome!

Part of the kundalini experience is a refinement of sensory perception, which corresponds with the rise of ecstatic conductivity. In traditional yoga, this is called "pratyahara," meaning introversion of sensory perception. Along with this refinement we begin to experience our inner dimensions more clearly, AND, at the same time, external environmental events will begin to affect us more deeply also, because our inside and outside are only different aspects of the one reality that we are.

This is how we become more empathetic as we advance spiritually. We "feel" what others feel, and are drawn more to "do unto others" as we would have others do unto us. Eventually we go beyond involvement in sensory perception altogether, to a constant divine outpouring, and that is true pratyahara.

The refinement of sensory perception also results in an increasing ability to perceive the finer vibratory quality of places, people, groups, etc. Like the situations you described.

It is important not to get too carried away with these experiences, and continue to favor our routine of daily practice over our rising sensitivities and other "siddhis" that may occur.

So, carry on and enjoy the ride, but not to the point of being too distracted from the cause of your growth, which is practices. :-)

All the best!

The guru is in you.

2009/03/18 10:26:08
Kundalini - Inner Energy Ecstasy
http://www.aypsite.org/forum/topic.asp?TOPIC_ID=5348&REPLY_ID=47493&whichpage=-1
Kundalini related symptoms?

quote:
_____
Originally posted by Jo-self

Of course, you have ruled out a medical or environmental condition.

One drawback of accelerated evolution is the possibility of 'masking' actual medical problems (or causing them) and not addressing them. Since the allopathic medical profession is not aware of esoteric stuff, you can't really talk to your doctor about them. My wife and I have similar symptoms, yet our doctor looks at us like we're from outer space if we talk about it.

I wonder if their has been some study about this "masking" effect. Or am I just making this up?

jo-self

_____

Hi Jo-Self:

The "masking effect," as you call it, could become an issue with so many having kundalini symptoms these days. This is why it is recommended to get things checked out medically if there are health concerns. In the case of spiritual practitioners, the tests may come up negative. But better to be safe than sorry.

As you point out, there is the matter of members of the medical profession not knowing what they are looking at when kundalini symptoms are present, and in that case there is a risk of receiving treatments for ailments that do not exist. It happens sometimes, particularly in fields where diagnosis may lean toward being subjective, like in psychiatry. And we all know how the pharmaceutical industry has a drug for every imaginable symptom we might have. It is a constant temptation for the doctor to prescribe the heavily marketed salve or pill based on symptoms only, rather than a known underlying cause.

The medical profession as a whole will catch on to kundalini eventually, but there is still quite a lot of denial about what is going on -- human spiritual transformation accelerating on a mass scale. The lag in grasping what is happening is understandable. We are entering a new paradigm where the advanced capabilities of the human neurobiology will become the center of massive research and development in many fields of science.

See my two recent posts here for additional thoughts on this:
http://www.aypsite.org/forum/topic.asp?TOPIC_ID=5282#46901

Meanwhile, don't forget to self-pace and ground. :-)

All the best!

The guru is in you.

2009/04/29 11:04:59
Kundalini - Inner Energy Ecstasy
http://www.aypsite.org/forum/topic.asp?TOPIC_ID=5472&REPLY_ID=49644&whichpage=-1
What is Kundalini awakening?

quote:
_____
Originally posted by Emil

Thanks Krish,
People, can we please have some comments on Krish's note. Is it correct that before K awakening prana only goes up through Ida and Pingala and not through Sushumna?
_____

Hi Emil:

It is not a matter of energy being "off" or "on" in the several channels. It is flowing in all the channels to one degree or other at all times, both before and after kundalini awakening, as Christi points out.

A balanced kundalini (ecstatic conductivity) awakening will be in the center (sushumna), with ida and pingala experiencing increased flow as natural expansion from the center occurs (see Lesson 52 and Lesson 90). It can be gradual, or with sudden jumps from time to time, depending on mode of practice and past karmic factors.

It is also possible for an unbalanced awakening to occur (excess on one side or the other, or between top and bottom), due to unbalanced practice, karmic factors and/or lifestyle. Gopi Krishna is a famous example of a left/right (pingala) imbalance.

So it is not all of one channel and none of the others. The three main yogic channels (sushumna, ida and pingala) are a connected continuum in our subtle neurobiology, with a vast array of channels expanding out from these.

With effective practices, purification and opening will occur simultaneously across the board. It is best to work from the center, meaning from inner silence and from the spinal nerve. From those two all the rest will unfold naturally. This way we can spend our time driving the car with the main controls and enjoying the ride in daily living, rather than getting our head stuck under the hood trying to micro-manage what can take care of itself. :-)

The guru is in you.

2009/05/19 13:20:01
Kundalini - Inner Energy Ecstasy
http://www.aypsite.org/forum/topic.asp?TOPIC_ID=5623&REPLY_ID=51075&whichpage=-1
Head, troath, and hearth...a little.

quote:
_____

Hi all,

After some days with pressure whit heat at some spots in my head,it dissapered two days ago...but know since yesterday im very suprised because i have FACIAL PARALISIS in some areas of my face.
I cant blink whit my right aye along the day (but i can close it for sleeping for example),I cant use the muscles of the rigt side of my mouth.When im eating or drinking the food and water come out from my mouth.When i try to laugh,only half of my mouth can does it.And i look like an person with facial paralisis.And all this paralisis i know is related to a big pressure and heat and pain in a spot back of my head,near oblangata medulla that i have now since yesterday.
Im a little scared,bcause i dont know whats happening.All i know is that its related to my yoga practices.Today i think i have more paralisis that yesterday.Today i cant blink my right eye,and yesterday i could.

Anybody could help me with this???im a little scared...

—————

Hi Miguel:

See a doctor right away to check if this is medically related.

If it is a product of spiritual purification and opening, it should clear up soon. Reduce practices until then.

But better to be safe than sorry. See a doctor.

The guru is in you.

2009/06/04 10:35:50
Kundalini - Inner Energy Ecstasy
http://www.aypsite.org/forum/topic.asp?TOPIC_ID=5736&REPLY_ID=51905&whichpage=-1
Topic disappeared?

Hi Grihastha:

It was a tech glitch, and it is back now:

http://www.aypsite.org/forum/topic.asp?TOPIC_ID=5716

Sorry for the inconvenience.

The guru is in you.

2009/09/16 12:57:07
Kundalini - Inner Energy Ecstasy
http://www.aypsite.org/forum/topic.asp?TOPIC_ID=6345&REPLY_ID=57028&whichpage=-1
Impatient

quote:

—————

Hi Shanti

I tried to follow your steps this morning. Here is the result:

1) Spinal Breathing: I sat on a chair instead of my regular cushion. I kept my eyes open. With the first breath in I imagined the awareness moving up like a thread from the root to third eye. Then back from the eye to root with breath out.

At second breath my eyes became wide open. My forehead became heavy and the third eye spot (where I have the sunken dent) began to throb. I was at the verge of becoming the witness.

So I had to stop the process. Because once I am in witness state, there is no possibilty to imagine anything. Then I just perceive/watch... my thoughts/mind/envoirnment etc.

I began to cry. Don't know why. Its the same when I hear a mantra sometimes. I was not sad or in pain. It was like crying for no reason. Like wailing in missing someone you love so much. I really don't know how to explain... its like having an unbearable orgasm. You are crying with overjoy. But there was no orgasm.

2) Well I pulled myself together and tried the next method. Again, while sitting on the chair I closed my eyes and in my mind said I AM... once... at the second I could say just I..... and my second chakra point near the end of the spine heated up. I was again at the verge of becoming witness. I stopped immediately and opened my eyes.

My back (at the second chakra point) was hurting. It was a clear sign that the energy wanted me to sit in siddhasana so further process can be carried forward.

But I was getting late for work so I suffered the pain for a while and it went away itself. Otherwise I had to sit and complete the daily meditation that takes about an hour.

What shall do then?

I know Energy is a wild horse. Its in me all the time 24 hrs. But for 1 hour in the morning I let this horse do what it likes. The process is smooth to me because I have super strength in me that allows me to do all the asanas without any pain. Once you are a witness there is no pain or overload. I am just impatient.

———————

Hi Manig:

It seems you already have your own style of practice which is more free-form than structured (see Lesson 202), and along with this you are running into some excessive purification.

As Shanti suggested, some structured practice can help balance things out and bring good long term results, but only if you are willing to give the procedures of practice a chance for a pre-set duration of time. Your first attempts at AYP spinal breathing pranayama and deep meditation indicate you are sensitive and in the habit of letting things go wherever they will go. In the case of using AYP practices, the time durations you have been using in your previous practice are much too long. Stabilizing 5 minutes of spinal breathing and 10 minutes of deep meditation (staying with the procedures as described in the lessons), resting, and then going out into normal activity would be an accomplishment. You might find that to be a real eye-opener in daily living. :-)

Neither spinal breathing nor deep meditation require you to do anything if you are in "witness state," as you call it. Both involve favoring the procedure of practice when we become aware that we are off it, coming back into awareness of objects: Favoring tracing the path of the spinal nerve in spinal breathing, or favoring the mantra in deep meditation. It means favoring the procedure when we realize we are off into thought streams, chakra energy things, or any other kind of experience. If energy experiences become too much to favor tracing the spinal nerve, or the mantra, there is an AYP procedure for that also. Check the lessons on deep meditation and spinal breathing at the top of the list here:
http://www.aypsite.org/MainDirectory.html
For further instructions, see the AYP books.

The reactions you had with both AYP practices indicates you have a lot of purification going on, and according to past habit you are inclined to go with it in a free form fashion for long periods. There is nothing wrong with free form if it is your practice. But this is your own thing and is not compatible with structured practices like AYP. There may be a limit to how far you can go with an unstructured approach. It is not an easy path. The drama of free form can sometimes be mistaken for progress. It is only energy after all -- in AYP we call it "scenery." When does the scenery end? Never. That is why we use structured practice to gradually move beyond the scenery to enlightenment.

Important: It is not recommended to be doing both approaches at the same time: AYP, and then slipping into your open-ended free form practice. It will only lead you into more excessive purification. Do one or the other. Not both. There will always be time later for looking at combinations and overlaps between modes of practice. It is not a good place to start.

In the case of starting the AYP practices, it is not recommended to take on both spinal breathing and deep meditation at the same time. For most, it is best to take on deep meditation first, stabilize a daily routine with it for a month or two, and then add spinal breathing right before deep meditation. In your case, maybe starting with spinal breathing is an alternative, since you need some stabilization of energy, and training of attention to the route of stabilization in the spinal nerve (sushumna), root to brow. If you take on spinal breathing first, do not attempt deep meditation until spinal breathing is stable in your routine.

No matter what approach you follow, AYP or other, there is one AYP procedure you can benefit from greatly: Self-pacing. Of course, that requires some patience, a willingness to back off on practice durations when there is too much purification going on. Remember, Rome was not built in a day. :-)

All the best!

The guru is in you.

PS: There is plenty of evidence around here indicating that a patient (self-paced bhakti) path with an effective integrated practice routine is much faster than an impatient path with less attention on incorporating effective structured practices. It seems to me you have the capacity to follow a structured practice if you put your mind to it.

2009/09/17 12:20:59
Kundalini - Inner Energy Ecstasy
http://www.aypsite.org/forum/topic.asp?TOPIC_ID=6345&REPLY_ID=57082&whichpage=-1
Impatient

Hi Manig:

Yes, there are many ways to approach this, and you are not alone in the experiences you are having. Each will choose the particulars of their own path. That is the emerging 21st century paradigm. AYP is an open resource for that.

That said, there are certain underlying principles that are in play, as you can see in Lesson 204. The Eight Limbs of Yoga book updates this list to reflect evolving experiences in the community of practitioners.

If it is your choice to double up the old practice regime with a new one, it will be your experiment, and no one can predict the outcome. All that can be said is that the odds for overdoing will be increased, and this may come as a delayed reaction, so it may be difficult to know what is causing what. That may not be such a problem for you.

Your fortitude for weathering energy experiences seems considerable, and that is a good thing. However, if you are using that to take a random approach to daily practice, results will be less than optimum over time. Some days you will feel like practicing, and other days you will not, sort of an all or nothing approach according to the inner winds. The phrase "Leaf in the wind" comes to mind, but it comes lovingly.

In the AYP approach, we do not take that approach. Practice is structured twice daily. Period. And we have a strategy for maintaining that through the ins and outs and ups and downs of life. There is plenty of flexibility in-between our sittings. It is the structured time in sitting practices that keeps the whole thing moving forward. Experiences come and go. If you rely on experiences for primary guidance in what you will practice each day, it will be an inconsistent path.

If you are asking for recommendations on what to practice, I point you to the AYP lessons and books. The rest is up to you. I cannot advise much on other systems of practice. The possibilities are endless.

These are your choices to make. I am sure you will find an ecology that works for you, a balance between structure and free form, and a balance between effective practices and "gee whiz" experiences.

Remember, it is not the whims of this week or next week that will make the difference. It is what you are doing consistently over years and decades that will produce the result. Not that you must look that far ahead, but each day you set the course that will determine the long term result. There are plenty of ways to apply your impatience to that with good effect. I have been "impatient" about this for nearly 40 years, and still am (for everyone else). It is a matter of applying the most effective tools in a systematic manner, according to individual need, whether the scenery is looming large at the moment or not. It ain't about the scenery. It's about "waking up" beyond the scenery and living *That* continuously and naturally in the here and now. Where else can we live it? :-)

The guru is in you.

PS: On the erection, see here: http://www.aypsite.org/forum/topic.asp?TOPIC_ID=6326&whichpage=2#56835

It is scenery too. :-)

2009/09/18 13:39:56
Kundalini - Inner Energy Ecstasy
http://www.aypsite.org/forum/topic.asp?TOPIC_ID=6345&REPLY_ID=57139&whichpage=-1
Impatient

Hi Manig:

Your bhakti (spiritual desire) is flowing and beautiful. If you combine that with some effective structured practice there will be no stopping the unfoldment. Even bhakti alone is unstoppable, but it can be a rather rough trip that way.

On the impatience, that is the heart of bhakti, so you are blessed. As it leads you to individual liberation, it will also expand to encompass the liberation of all beings. It never ends, but it does become infinitely more joyful. :-)

You have been born in bhakti already, and you shall never die, for this is beyond the body/mind. It flows into the world as divine love.

The guru is in you.

2009/09/19 22:22:02
Kundalini - Inner Energy Ecstasy
http://www.aypsite.org/forum/topic.asp?TOPIC_ID=6361&REPLY_ID=57202&whichpage=-1
Pressure in throat?

Hi BellaMente:

You might find this topic to be of interest, calling for more university-level integrated research on the process of human spiritual transformation, or applied spiritual science:
http://www.aypsite.org/forum/topic.asp?TOPIC_ID=3267

Research in theoretical physics is not mentioned much in there, only because the focus so far has been more in human potential and health, which is where there has been growing funding coming from healthcare-related foundations.

That is not taking into consideration the considerable research in theoretical physics, which is well-funded in its own right, but not to the extent of tying in with research on consciousness ... yet.

In any case, you can count on AYP for moral support in your cause, if not much in the way of tangible resources. We are here, and that is about it. It isn't a small thing. Where else in the world can you find a diverse and fast-growing non-sectarian community dedicated to the practical application of full scope self-directed spiritual practices, with the primary emphasis being on flexible application of methods for developing repeatable results that anyone can achieve? Some may not call that applied science, but I do. It is only the beginning. Educational and research institutions are welcome to join in the far-flung project. We can all support the research while becoming enlightened.

Not to worry, if you have a passion for the work, the work will get done. The more inner purification and opening you cultivate, the easier it will be to observe the nature of reality first hand (in stillness) and explain it to others in the language of your chosen field.

Go for it!

The guru is in you.

2009/09/20 11:22:51
Kundalini - Inner Energy Ecstasy
http://www.aypsite.org/forum/topic.asp?TOPIC_ID=6361&REPLY_ID=57227&whichpage=-1
Pressure in throat?

quote:
_____
Originally posted by BellaMente

I read through the thread and think that an applied spiritual science department will definitely be a hit and I would love to help in any way I can.

Do you have anything specific in mind - specific schools, classes, teachers?

_____

Hi BellaMente:

It might be better to continue this discussion in the research topic, so it won't get lost. I will copy your post and my reply over there. See here:
http://www.aypsite.org/forum/topic.asp?TOPIC_ID=3267&whichpage=2#57226

All the best!

The guru is in you.

2009/09/20 17:54:02
Kundalini - Inner Energy Ecstasy
http://www.aypsite.org/forum/topic.asp?TOPIC_ID=6361&REPLY_ID=57253&whichpage=-1
Pressure in throat?

quote:
_____
Originally posted by BellaMente

I still have the pressure in my throat coming and going. Does it take a while to be fully activated or is it getting blocked then activated, blocked then activated??

_____

Hi BellaMente:

Yes, any symptom like that can come and go, until the neurobiology becomes purified in that area. It can take some time. Then it will become quite blissful.

There are a number things you can do:

1. Carry on with practices, and keep an eye on it.

2. If there is ongoing discomfort, self-pace practices and engage in grounding activity.

3. Try some light chin pump and see if it brings some relief.
Also, see here: http://www.aypsite.org/forum/topic.asp?TOPIC_ID=3414

A subject line search in the forums on "throat" will bring up a few more topics on this.

There are other things that can be done if the blockage becomes chronic, involving the head and other areas. Not common, but it happens sometimes.

Let us know how it goes.

All the best!

The guru is in you.

2009/11/09 14:13:32
Kundalini - Inner Energy Ecstasy
http://www.aypsite.org/forum/topic.asp?TOPIC_ID=6661&REPLY_ID=59518&whichpage=-1
Ida, Pingala and Kundalini Awakening

Hi Krish:

In AYP, balancing the side nadis (ida and pingala) is regarded more as effect than cause with the all-encompassing practices we are using -- deep meditation and spinal breathing pranayama especially.

Focusing on managing particular energy relationships in the neurobiology is not much a part of AYP. We do it in big (global) ways that cultivate natural awakening.

Ecstatic conductivity will come when it is time. With the cultivation of abiding inner silence, it too is effect.

The more important measurement of your practice is in how you are feeling in everyday activity. Is there more peace, happiness, productivity, inclination to inquire and serve others? These are far more important indicators than energy symptoms. The symptoms of energy movement are only signs of friction (from remaining obstructions), after all. When the obstructions become much less, there is just unending happiness and outpouring divine love, no matter what may be happening around us in the temporal world.

The guru is in you.

2009/11/09 22:08:00
Kundalini - Inner Energy Ecstasy
http://www.aypsite.org/forum/topic.asp?TOPIC_ID=6661&REPLY_ID=59542&whichpage=-1

Ida, Pingala and Kundalini Awakening

quote:
_____
Originally posted by krcqimpro1

Thanks for the response, Yogani.I have not seen any noticeable difference in "happiness", peace, etc. Inclination to serve others has always been there, and continues. I suppose I shall have to look keenly for signs of change in these aspects. Since I live alone, there is no one to notice any changes and tell me.However, I have taken this "spiritual" project as the last and most important project of my life and am applying myself diligently. I am certain the results will come.

Krish
_____

Hi Krish:

Have you reviewed Lessons 365, 366 and 367? 366 in particular to address possible under-sensitivity issues.

And there is more on the way!

The guru is in you.

2009/11/10 10:35:06
Kundalini - Inner Energy Ecstasy
http://www.aypsite.org/forum/topic.asp?TOPIC_ID=6661&REPLY_ID=59561&whichpage=-1
Ida, Pingala and Kundalini Awakening

quote:
_____
Originally posted by krcqimpro1

The reason why I am asking this is : for as long as I can remember before starting AYP, one of my nostrils used to be blocked all the time (alternately). However, probably due to the intensity and regularity of practice, I notice that both nostrils are clear most of the time now.
_____

Hi Krish:

It sounds like a good sign, a symptom of balance. An effect. :-)
Not that we should be monitoring our nostrils all the time, or anything else. Just practice and go out and live fully. That is the ticket.

The thing about enlightenment is that it is not something we can acquire or manage. It is something that happens as we let go in stillness as we keep doing. In active surrender mode, it is something we are constantly giving away.

Letting go does not mean we drop our practices or our activities. In fact, we may be doing more of both as the flow of bhakti and divine love increase. It gradually becomes less about our doing (even while doing) and more about our surrender to the process occurring within and through us.

So, perhaps release a bit on wanting a particular outcome, and let go more into the doing. It is a paradox ... a complete loss of control is the gaining of everything. This is where our practices are leading. It is okay to relax with it. Let it go and enjoy...

The guru is in you.

PS: Don't forget to self-pace as necessary. :-)

2009/11/10 12:51:04
Kundalini - Inner Energy Ecstasy
http://www.aypsite.org/forum/topic.asp?TOPIC_ID=6661&REPLY_ID=59564&whichpage=-1
Ida, Pingala and Kundalini Awakening

quote:
_____
Originally posted by krcqimpro1

But my question still is: in all cases of K rising through the sushumna, is the balance of nadis a pre-requisite. It does appear to be so, from all the posts I have read.
_____

Hi Krish:

My experience has been that, like most things in life, it is not all or none. It is a matter of degrees. Progress depends on a willingness to proceed on that basis without a guarantee of the perfect awakening.

Kundalini can be active to one degree or other whether ida and pingala are balanced or not. On one extreme, kundalini can be much more in one of the side channels than sushumna -- the case of Gopi Krishna (a pingala imbalance) is a notable example. On the other extreme, there can be perfect balance between ida and pingala and it is all seamlessly flowing in the sushumna. The vast majority of kundalini awakenings fall somewhere in-between, with things gradually finding balance over time in relation to our activities in life. No one starts with a perfectly balanced kundalini awakening. At least I am not aware of it. Rather, it evolves gradually from wherever it starts, as we integrate our inner developments into our outer life.

So when a teacher says, you must balance your ida and pingala before raising kundalini, or you must do it in order to raise kundalini, they are talking about an idealized path that does not exist. It simply doesn't work like that.

First of all, we cannot manually manage the minute details of our inner energies. If anyone ever tells you they can do that for you, run! Second of all, we do not decide when kundalini will become active. When it is ready to happen, it happens, ida and pingala fully balanced or not.

What we can do is attend to the overall purification and opening of the inner neurobiology from the deepest levels within us in a balanced way, which will facilitate all of these things to occur naturally over time. In this case, the degree of overall purification, opening and balance in the nervous system (including ida and pingala) will be sufficient to support a progressive and safe kundalini awakening.

Here is a lesson that discusses ida and pingala from the AYP point of view -- more about their role in the natural emergence of ecstatic radiance than about trying to manage them. Ida and pingala play a key role in manifesting the fruit (effects) of the natural evolutionary process that we call human spiritual transformation.

The guru is in you.

2009/11/18 17:03:32
Kundalini - Inner Energy Ecstasy
http://www.aypsite.org/forum/topic.asp?TOPIC_ID=6694&REPLY_ID=59889&whichpage=-1
Problems with Throat - Part II

quote:
_____
Originally posted by BellaMente

Yogani are you out there?

Sorry if you are busy but can you clarify on what parts of the head rotation I inhale and exhale for the jalandhara lite? And does the head rest down at the chest in the lite version? Sorry if I missed this somewhere but I can't seem to find the details of the breath anywhere and I am confused...
_____

Hi BellaMente:

It is best to be well-established in spinal breathing before attempting chin pump lite, so there will be no question about the spinal breathing aspect of it. Then chin pump lite can be undertaken for the last minute or two of our spinal breathing session.

For chin pump, we rotate the head steadily, dropping the chin down in a swooping motion toward the hollow of the throat (or upper chest) on the front side of each rotation. We reverse the direction of rotation each time our spinal breathing cycle reaches the brow. See these lessons on details of procedure and effects: 139, 140, 143, 144.

Keep in mind that chin pump is an advanced practice, introduced in the lessons after asanas, mudras and bandhas have been covered. This does not mean it cannot be used earlier, but it is not recommended before we have become stable in spinal breathing pranayama, which will take months or years, not days or weeks.

Christi has given good overall advice on blockages.

Take it easy, and be sure to self-pace practices if symptoms become excessive.

All the best!

The guru is in you.

2010/01/17 12:37:42
Kundalini - Inner Energy Ecstasy
http://www.aypsite.org/forum/topic.asp?TOPIC_ID=7057&REPLY_ID=63052&whichpage=-1
Kundalini/Discomfort/Fear/Surrender

Hi JDH:

This is the process of purification and opening, which we gradually learn to surrender to. With self-pacing of practices in play to keep things on an even keel.

First it is only about us. Then it becomes a partnership between us and the process of awakening. Finally, there is only the awakening, and the divine outpouring.

Fear evaporates along the way ... what remains is stillness in action.

The guru is in you.

2010/01/18 11:19:48
Kundalini - Inner Energy Ecstasy
http://www.aypsite.org/forum/topic.asp?TOPIC_ID=7057&REPLY_ID=63127&whichpage=-1
Kundalini/Discomfort/Fear/Surrender

Hi JDH and Arim:

The "danger" of kundalini is in our mind.

Physical and psychological symptoms will come and go. There is much we can do to mitigate them. If we are meditating daily, we come to know it all as a play in stillness. No fear in that.

Ultimately, we find there is no "other." We are That.

The guru is in you.

2010/02/28 15:52:19
Kundalini - Inner Energy Ecstasy
http://www.aypsite.org/forum/topic.asp?TOPIC_ID=7358&REPLY_ID=65478&whichpage=-1
Ecstatic dissolution! How about the theory?

Hi Bruno:

Theories and philosophies are pretty easy to come by, all devised from particular points of view based on someone's experience. Not necessarily yours, which will be the same in some respects and unique in others.

For this reason, in AYP, we try to keep theory to a minimum, providing basic milestones indicating the emergence of the abiding inner silence and energetic components of spiritual development, and the joining of these in unity. How these components may be experienced along the way on each of our paths may vary.

The experiential maps are pretty easy once practices are underway and symptoms of purification and opening are occurring. Theories will either be confirmed or set aside based on our direct experience. The ultimate scripture is in us.

What is less simple is mapping practices in a way that will be useful for many practitioners. That has been the main focus in AYP.

The assumption is that if the experience can be delivered through effective practices, then the theories will be self-evident, and they will vary somewhat depending on the pattern of unfoldment each of us is undergoing. That is why AYP does not present a precise experiential map. My map and your map may be a little different. Recognizing that is step #1 in providing something useful for a wide range of practitioners.

If there is something theoretical in AYP (and perhaps a bit revolutionary), it is that the human nervous system is regarded to be the center of all spiritual development, and all systems, philosophies, theories and maps are derived from that single truth. Absolutely no one is left out. The systems, philosophies, theories and maps may vary depending on culture, religion, and the particular process of unfoldment occurring, but the human nervous system remains at the center always. In recognizing this and taking it to heart, the practitioner can be freed from a lot of unnecessary baggage that may be taken on in the form of, you guessed it, systems, philosophies, theories and maps!

Sounds like good things are happening there, and in relatively short order. Continue to self-pace as needed to maintain steady progress over time. Remember, practices are not all or nothing. Practice times can be adjusted incrementally to find your balance. That is putting practice in front of theory for best results. :-)

All the best!

The guru is in you.

2010/03/03 11:47:20
Kundalini - Inner Energy Ecstasy
http://www.aypsite.org/forum/topic.asp?TOPIC_ID=7358&REPLY_ID=65583&whichpage=-1
Ecstatic dissolution! How about the theory?

quote:
_____
Originally posted by brunoloff

So Yogani, if you would indulge me, after such a long and carefully written post: Would you reconsider writing such a book? Do you see value in it, either way, and if not why not? And now that I've explained what I mean by "theory" and why I want more of it, could you provide references for such theoretical knowledge?
_____

Hi Bruno:

Yes, I certainly see the value in building a framework of theoretical knowledge on human spiritual transformation. But it is not a one person job. Not even close. It would be like asking the Wright Brothers to document the theory of aeronautics, clearly an impossibility. But they did demonstrate that airplanes can fly, and it was more than enough. That work started the revolution in aviation. This is what I hope AYP can help do in applied spiritual science.

Building an evolving and ongoing science with a solid theoretical foundation is a job for the worldwide scientific community. This is actually addressed with some clarity here: http://www.aypsite.org/forum/topic.asp?TOPIC_ID=3267
There is quite a lot of research work going on already, albeit, not very focused or organized at this time. It is evolving, and accelerating...

No one person could devise a comprehensive theory of medicine, or aeronautics, or electronics. Invariably, a few demonstrated key principles in practice, and then many were inspired to build on that, both theoretically and practically. And it keeps going on indefinitely. This is the way of science.

So if you are interested in applied spiritual science, the topic link above offers some interesting pathways to follow up on, hopefully not at the expense of your daily practice. :-)

Further suggestions on how to inspire and activate the scientific community could be posted there. All suggestions are welcome, especially those that are followed up with <u>action</u>. Don't expect me to do it all. I am only one researcher and author in the vast field of human spiritual transformation. It will take a concerted effort by the scientific community to carry it forward.

All the best!

The guru is in you.

2010/04/22 15:06:09
Kundalini - Inner Energy Ecstasy
http://www.aypsite.org/forum/topic.asp?TOPIC_ID=7442&REPLY_ID=67627&whichpage=-1
Kundalini Heat

Hi Corinna and Carson:

You are both right. :-)

There is a distinction to be made between breathing practices (and breath suspension) without deep meditation, and breathing practices with deep meditation. That is not with the two performed at the same time, but in sequence in the same sittings, with the greatest spiritual results found through consistent daily practice over time.

This distinction may account for the relaxation effects of breathing techniques (with or without suspension) when practiced alone, versus the powerful kundalini awakening affects of similar methods when used (with mudras, bandhas, etc.) in a routine that includes deep meditation. It also may account for why breathing techniques used alone, while helpful for relaxation, are not very progressive as spiritual practice.

As we have discussed in the lessons, pranayama prepares (relaxes) the inner soil of the nervous system so the seed of inner silence may sprout from it. Obviously, both the cultivated soil and the seed must be present for this to occur. Likewise, when inner silence is rising as a result of deep meditation, the soil of the nervous system becomes much more porous (activated), giving rise to the prana-compensating-for-oxygen-deficit dynamic in pranayama referred to by Carson, which is at the heart of the systematic cultivation of ecstatic conductivity (kundalini) through the breath. In the case where pranayama and deep meditation are well-integrated in the practice routine, excessive pranayama (especially with breath suspension) can lead to energy overloads, often coming as a delayed effect, days or weeks after the overdoing occurred.

There are many here who can verify this dynamic. It is part of why we put so much emphasis on self-pacing of practices in the AYP approach, and also why we have relatively few kundalini crises occurring here. Hence Carson's sensitivity on breath suspension practice. Breath suspension for some may not be the same as breath suspension for others, depending on the degree of resident sensitivity (conductivity) cultivated in the nervous system.

The idea is to stimulate maximum progress with minimum discomfort. It seems to be working. :-)

The guru is in you.

2010/04/22 10:34:50
Kundalini - Inner Energy Ecstasy
http://www.aypsite.org/forum/topic.asp?TOPIC_ID=7653&REPLY_ID=67612&whichpage=-1
question for yogani and others

Hi tonightsthenight:

Beyond the principles and practices of self-pacing discussed in the lessons, it has never been much about the symptoms of kundalini here, though there have been plenty over the years.

First and foremost, it has always been about cultivating abiding inner silence in deep meditation and samyama. With that, the energetic aspects find fruition sooner rather than later, and with much less disruption. Certainly much less angst.

Sometimes we may tend to think of our kundalini situation as a spiritual badge, or something like that. We might even be inclined to hang on to it. It can be that all-consuming, particularly with limited presence of the witness (inner silence). But it is only a transitional stage, one that we'd like to bring to its refined condition of loving ecstatic bliss as soon as possible. Then we can get on with the real business of enlightenment, which is the unending outpouring of divine love. That is stillness in action, our inner silence flying on the wings of mature ecstatic conductivity and radiance (kundalini) for the benefit of all. This is a condition of rising unity -- non-duality.

The energetics are not the primary source of this fruition. Abiding inner silence is. This is because self-awareness (Self-knowledge) can never be found through identification with the objects of perception. Only in the rise of pure bliss consciousness and its expression in (as) the world. Kundalini is a facilitator of this, not the underlying cause.

So, rather than focusing on symptoms (energy), I suggest focusing on having a well-rounded routine of practices and daily activity, with self-pacing applied as necessary. It isn't about the symptoms, or the "scenery" -- physical, mental or emotional. It is about favoring a sound meditation-centered practice routine over the long term. This will greatly shorten the interim stage of kundalini awakening, and make for a much smoother ride.

Many have come here with pre-awakened kundalini symptoms like yours. Those who have been able to settle in with this sort of broad-scope approach to practices have found some good progress with less chaos. That's why you will find few panicky kundalini discussions in the AYP support forums. Most have it pretty well in hand here. The panicky discussions there are usually are started by folks coming here with aggravated symptoms originating somewhere else.

Hopefully we can be of some assistance.

Wishing you all the best on your continuing path. Enjoy!

The guru is in you.

466 –   Advanced Yoga Practices

2010/04/23 11:37:37
Kundalini - Inner Energy Ecstasy
http://www.aypsite.org/forum/topic.asp?TOPIC_ID=7653&REPLY_ID=67678&whichpage=-1
question for yogani and others

Hi tonightsthenight:

The symptoms you mention are related to energy accumulating in the head and throat. There are components in AYP that can mitigate this, but they are part of the whole of our practice, and not necessarily magic bullets in themselves for dealing with specific symptoms. That is why I generally offer a broad view, because symptoms are seldom resolved by focusing on the symptoms. If we push in one place, it will often pop out somewhere else. :-)

That said, self-pacing any causative practices and grounding in daily activity are the first orders of business with too much energy in the head.

If there are no known "causative practices," then just ceasing spiritual attention in general can help. That means keeping busy doing other things entirely for a while. This is assuming the symptoms are excessive and not desired to be at that level. And if they are desired, we can cling to them and enjoy them. Our choice. :-)

If you want to know exactly what these particular symptoms mean, neither I, nor anyone, can tell you for sure. The symptoms of purification and opening in each of us are as unfathomable as the karma behind them. Sure, we can talk all day about what this or that sensation means. In the end, it isn't about the symptom. It is about dissolving and transcending the resistance, which leads us forward into unending ecstatic bliss. This is what practices are for.

As far as additional specific measures AYP can offer, chin pump is good for balancing/integrating energy between the head and the rest of the body. If we are meditating with mantra, solar centering can help a lot. Under certain circumstances, targeted bastrika can help, but that one has to be approached carefully, because it can take us in the opposite direction toward more energy.

All of these things overlay on the core AYP practices of spinal breathing pranayama and deep meditation. So no specific method mentioned is guaranteed to produce the same kind of results it can when taken as part of the whole.

Regarding "concepts or obstacles," that is what I was referring to with the "badge of spirituality" phrase. Certainly not a put-down. It refers to the fact that we all tend to identify with our experience, and that identification can perpetuate the situation. It is, after all, identification of awareness with thoughts, feelings and physical sensations that keep us bound up in the first place. All spiritual practice is about unwinding identification of self with the objects of perception, including with an ongoing kundalini situation.

The cultivation of abiding inner silence is the best way I know to do the unwinding, followed by an intelligent approach to ecstatic energy awakening (the wings of stillness in action), samyama (enlivening stillness outward), self-inquiry (when we can do so in stillness), and so on.

So if you are looking for a progressive approach through all this, there is one here. But it cannot be done easily in bits and pieces. It takes an embracing of the whole, and methods that address the whole. Along the way, the specifics are taken care of by the awakening of the whole.

The guru is in you.

2010/04/23 23:33:23
Kundalini - Inner Energy Ecstasy
http://www.aypsite.org/forum/topic.asp?TOPIC_ID=7653&REPLY_ID=67714&whichpage=-1
question for yogani and others

Hi tonightsthenight:

Being established in inner silence is not about "distancing" ourselves from objects of perception and our identification with them. It is about allowing them. In stillness our contraction around these perceptions loosens and then the energy can move with less friction. It is the contraction/friction that causes the discomfort. As long as we are personally trying to control something there will be resistance and discomfort. "Distancing" is a form of controlling.

There isn't an instant way to get to the point of abiding inner silence capable of loosening such contractions. It requires cultivation over time, which leads to abiding witness, which is not touched by physical, mental or emotional symptoms, even while being in them and of them. When we can allow our attention to simply be with symptoms in this penetrating way, without having to do something with them, this is when releases can come.

The self-pacing, grounding, etc., are in a different category, more on the level of energy management, or at least tempering its intensity.

Ultimately, it is our inner silence that carries us through. All the other things are interim measures to smooth external symptoms of the underlying unfoldment, which is why I say that the real work is in engaging in and pacing practices that deal with the whole rather than the parts.

But like I said earlier, if things are going off the scale, then it would probably be best to not even be considering spiritual matters, and go off and do other things for a while, until there is some stabilization. Then you will be in a better position to take a fresh look at all of this.

The guru is in you.

2010/04/24 11:05:48
Kundalini - Inner Energy Ecstasy
http://www.aypsite.org/forum/topic.asp?TOPIC_ID=7653&REPLY_ID=67740&whichpage=-1
question for yogani and others

Hi tonightsthenight:

Perhaps a few pointed questions should be asked (maybe we should have done this first):

1. Kundalini awakening is a partnership between ourselves and the divine. Have you taken ownership of your role in this partnership, or do you consider yourself to be a victim in it?

2. Do you consider yourself responsible to take the lead in navigating through the kundalini aspects of your spiritual journey?

3. Have you redirected your attention from excessive focus on kundalini symptoms into productive activities in daily living to whatever degree you can?

4. What were your practices and daily activity during initial kundalini awakening, and what are they now?

5. Are you engaged in daily physical work and/or exercise?

6. Have you tried a twice-daily routine of AYP spinal breathing pranayama as per Lesson 69?

7. Have you tried a twice-daily routine of AYP deep meditation?

8. Have you tried chin pump and/or any other AYP methods?

9. Are you favoring a vata/pitta pacifying diet?

10. Have you tried Taoist grounding practices, like Tai Chi?

11. What other measures have you tried over the years to find a balance with kundalini?

12. Of all the things you have tried, what has helped, and what has not?

13. What are you inclined to be doing next?

If you can answer these questions, it will give a better idea of what is going on. Right now it is not really clear where you stand in relation to these key areas of consideration.

Thanks!

The guru is in you.

2010/04/25 12:10:29
Kundalini - Inner Energy Ecstasy
http://www.aypsite.org/forum/topic.asp?TOPIC_ID=7653&REPLY_ID=67792&whichpage=-1
question for yogani and others

Hi tonightsthenight:

Thanks for the rundown. That helps.

A key point that has been alluded to several times is the relationship between current practices and symptoms. Self-pacing of practices is a primary control mechanism we have on excessive symptoms, which are essentially too much energy running through as yet not fully purified subtle nerves. Your answers point to you not having a clear handle on self-pacing yet.

What is not always obvious is the "cause and effect" between practices and symptoms because, 1) there can be a time delay between practices and energetic effects, and 2) what we may not consider to be formal practice, per say, like being "meditative" all day, or stoking our bhakti all day, or intensely studying and engaging in activities like this forum, can be highly stimulating to the energies.

Given all of these factors, it is necessary to anticipate and self-pace before the fact in the case of delayed reactions, and regard seemingly innocent desires/bhakti or associations as energy-stimulating practice as well. This is why the suggestion has been made to simply disengage from all spiritual intentions and activities for a while if symptoms are running off the scale. This is the price we may have to pay sometimes for overdoing. There is an extreme example of this scenario in the Secrets of Wilder novel. I'm not saying you are into that, but if you don't take appropriate action, you may end up there.

If we don't self-pace in a structured way, and decide to keep pressing ahead instead, eventually we will be forced to self-pace in an unstructured way that may involve serious health issues. Due to the recovery time involved, the latter is a much slower path, so it makes sense to slow things down now, before you are forced to stop everything for much longer later.

There is the analogy of driving the fast sports car, and allowing for the sharp curves in the road along the edge of a cliff. We can slow down for the curves, and navigate them with relative safety, or ignore them and sooner or later go flying over the edge. Which do you think will bring us to our destination sooner?

Your painful right side imbalance symptom is a clear indication of overdoing, and perhaps even wrong practice. Light sessions of spinal breathing can help (see here on left or right side imbalances). This should be coupled with a general relaxation of all other spiritual endeavors until things even out. These actions can help. But you really have to want the balance. It will not happen as long as you are being a kundalini hero.

You have studied and found out a lot over the years, but your current situation is a clear indication that you are ignoring some of the basics. Your symptoms are not coming out of nowhere. You have caused them. If we do not learn to apply the basics relatively easily, then we will be sure to be learning them the hard way. The easier way is preferred by most. It's your call. If you are a John Wilder type hero, I can sympathize. But there was no AYP around when he was doing his daredevil thing. His journey (and mine) is what led to AYP. :-)

The guru is in you.

2010/04/25 23:26:36
Kundalini - Inner Energy Ecstasy

http://www.aypsite.org/forum/topic.asp?TOPIC_ID=7653&REPLY_ID=67805&whichpage=-1
question for yogani and others

quote:
_____
Originally posted by tonightsthenight

Following this profound suffering, I've kind of had an experience of being "reborn from the ashes" concomitant with some of these intense purifying symptoms, and i have an intense desire to reach a new level, because i cannot conceive of more suffering of the same type at this point. The suffering is purifying, yes, but i simply cannot keep walking through broken glass.
_____

Hi tonightsthenight:

From my experience, this would usually not be a good time to act aggressively on an "intense desire to reach a new level." It is counter-intuitive, in that what we have learned in our culture is to press ahead at all costs to reach our goal. But it is not applicable in this sort of situation. In yoga, pressing ahead, attempting to "break through," particularly when we are energy challenged, will usually land us in more trouble. In situations like this, we find that less is more. A lot more. As we learn to let go, then the openings will happen without the stresses and strains caused by human striving. There is a time to strive and there is a time to let go.

It's your call of course. Just sharing a hard-earned lesson. Others here have been through similar scenarios, and you will find the "less is more" slogan coming up fairly frequently in this community. We all need a reminder on that from time to time, because it is counter-intuitive, especially when the bhakti is surging and we are on fire for that final dash. There is no such thing in yoga. The final dash is not a dash at all. It is a letting go. When the urgency and symptoms have reached a seemingly unbearable peak, that is when less can be more, and when it is good to slow down and let go. We might be amazed by the result. Enlightenment is not a doing. It is an undoing. :-)

The guru is in you.

2010/09/11 22:07:30
Kundalini - Inner Energy Ecstasy
http://www.aypsite.org/forum/topic.asp?TOPIC_ID=8419&REPLY_ID=72823&whichpage=-1
What are Yantras?

Hi Natan:

Here is an AYP online lesson that provides some introductory information on yantras -- specifically "Sri Yantra," with links to illustrations:

http://www.aypsite.org/T25.html

More information is provided in the corresponding lesson in the AYP Easy Lessons book, and in the last chapter of the Tantra book.

All the best!

The guru is in you.

2010/12/19 15:21:27
Kundalini - Inner Energy Ecstasy
http://www.aypsite.org/forum/topic.asp?TOPIC_ID=8868&REPLY_ID=77161&whichpage=-1
"KUNDALINI" documentary feature film

Hi All:

I had the opportunity to watch this documentary recently, and it is very informative.

This is a good introduction to Kundalini, the energetic side of the enlightenment equation, with good coverage of causes, symptoms, and the profound implications for the individual and society. In particular, anyone interested in the influence of Gopi Krishna and current activities in Kundalini-based paths will find this well worth watching.

While the approaches to Kundalini awakening covered are not the same that we take in AYP, the overall information presented is very complementary.

The guru is in you.

Forum 12 – Healthcare – Holistic and Modern

Ayurveda, Acupuncture, Reiki, etc., balanced with modern healthcare methods.
http://www.aypsite.org/forum/forum.asp?FORUM_ID=38

2005/07/12 13:35:01
Healthcare - Holistic and Modern
http://www.aypsite.org/forum/topic.asp?TOPIC_ID=282
Neuro-Energy-Based Healthcare

What is neuro-energy?

Anyone who has been helped by an Ayurvedic diet, an Accupuncture treatment, a Reiki healing or a Chiropractor has some idea about what neuro-energy is. It has other names: prana, chi, life-force, neuro-biological energy, vital essence...

Whatever we call it, it is real. When it is blocked or out of balance, we become ill. When it is in balance, we are on top of the world. The body has an ability to balance its own inner energies, and we call that our natural ability to heal. While modern western medicine uses many amazing technologies, in the end, they too rely on the body's natural healing powers to accomplish their cures. Every system of medicine and healing does. The human body is its own doctor, pharmacy and hospital. All we have to do is give it the best opportunity to function -- to do its thing.

Alternative modalities of healthcare do just that. Their main focus is on promoting energy balance, preferably with lifestyle recommendations that can serve as a preventive measure, enabling our bodies to keep themselves healthy, rather than from the position of dealing with a body with inner energies being way out of balance.

Neuro-energy approaches to healthcare can also be helpful to those on the path of yoga. While yoga promotes balance in the nervous system, it also expands the role of the inner energies in support of the enlightenment process. Sometimes there can be some excess energy, or an imbalance. That is when we apply the principles of self-pacing in our practice, so as not to aggravate what is usually just a temporary bumpy place in the road on the way to enlightenment. If we come to yoga with deep-rooted imbalances, then it can take some extra measures to smooth things out. That is where the energy-based healthcare systems can provide some support.

Ayurveda is particularly strong in support of yoga, because it subscribes to the same core principles and practices, and offers sound means for promoting energy balance in the nervous system. Some Ayurvada resources can be found in the AYP links section at http://www.aypsite.org/ayurveda.html

This forum is for discussing the many alternative healthcare modalities, and how they can support our continuing spiritual progress.

The guru is in you.

2010/11/17 11.04.49
Healthcare - Holistic and Modern
http://www.aypsite.org/forum/topic.asp?TOPIC_ID=282&REPLY_ID=75393&whichpage=-1
Neuro-Energy-Based Healthcare

Hi Krish:

Sounds like a typical result from practices you are having there.

Bravo! :-)

The guru is in you.

PS: Pass it on.

2010/11/18 10:10:32
Healthcare - Holistic and Modern
http://www.aypsite.org/forum/topic.asp?TOPIC_ID=282&REPLY_ID=75441&whichpage=-1
Neuro-Energy-Based Healthcare

Hi Krish:

If you have health concerns, it will be best to ask a doctor. But it seems all you have is a number that confirms that your bodily functions are getting younger than your age. This is quite normal for consistent yoga practitioners. How are you feeling?

If it is a case of going to the doctor to ask, "How come I am getting younger so fast?" then we will all cheer. :-)

The guru is in you.

2006/01/21 11:37:09
Healthcare - Holistic and Modern
http://www.aypsite.org/forum/topic.asp?TOPIC_ID=409&REPLY_ID=2702&whichpage=-1
amaroli -- dosage and concentration

quote:
_____
Patrick wrote here: hello, it is nice to read about people doing amaroli, I have been doing it for 6 years now and I feel better all the time, I am 56 years old and I look like a healthy 40 years old, never sick not like before, I had psoriasis, flu, shingles, pain in my body, now no pain and joy. I am a raw foodist which give a good tasting urine. I drink 90% of my urine and I massage my body with it which is the second half of the therapy.

Cheers, patrick PS: I truly beleive that amaroli is the answer to the problems of this world, political, economical, psychological, environmental and social.

Hi Patrick, and welcome!

Amaroli is an important aspect of yoga for sure. But it is not all of yoga. Its effects are greatly enhanced when combined with a daily routine including deep meditation, spinal breathing pranayama and other yogic methods. Likewise, amaroli improves the effectiveness of the other yoga practices. It is a balanced integration of practices that brings the greatest enhancement in all aspects of life -- physical, mental, emotional and spiritual.

There is a tendency we all have to go for the "magic bullet," i.e., the one thing that we hope (believe) will solve all things. Some folks go very deep into one thing looking for that, only to find later that they missed out on what a broader approach to self-improvement and spiritual development can yield.

Which is not to say that your path is too much of one thing. Only that there are other practices to consider that can enhance your excellent results even further. Perhaps you are well aware of this already, and are showing us only one aspect of your practice routine.

All the best!

The guru is in you.

2006/03/08 13:19:45
Healthcare - Holistic and Modern
http://www.aypsite.org/forum/topic.asp?TOPIC_ID=409&REPLY_ID=4248&whichpage=-1
amaroli -- dosage and concentration

Hi Richard:

There is the possibility of a gradual internalization of amaroli to become an automatic recycling within, which would result in less outflow.

This also happens with vajroli (constant upward processing of sexual essences in the body) as progress in yoga and its tantric elements advances.

I can verify a reduced urine flow, though can offer no scientific evidence on what it is, or if it is from the same cause you are experiencing. If it is yoga-related, amaroli practice itself would not necessarily be the only stimulator of it. It would also be connected with a full range of practices over the long term. At least that has been the observation here.

The ideas of hydration and dehydration take on new meaning if amaroli does internalize over time. The yoga scientists will sort this out eventually. Meanwhile, we pioneers proceed based on our intuition, inner seeing, some trial and error, and prudent self-pacing.

The guru is in you.

2005/08/29 13:17:12
Healthcare - Holistic and Modern
http://www.aypsite.org/forum/topic.asp?TOPIC_ID=443&REPLY_ID=477&whichpage=-1
JALA NETI

Hello Victor & Frank:

Salt content is the main determinant of comfort in neti. Too much salt like in seawater or mutra/urine can cause discomfort. So does too little salt like in tap water. So watering down on too much salt or adding some salt if there isn't enough is the formula. Everyone has their own ideal salt level that is comfortable in the delicate nasal passages.

As for thoughts on jala neti (salted tap water based), it is a good general cleanser of the nasal passages and sinuses, but it and all the other shatkarmas can take a lot of time. There was a time on my path many years ago when there was a strong inner call for all the shatkarmas -- neti/nasal wash, basti/enema, dhauti/intestinal wash, etc. At that time there was more involved than hygienic body cleansing (something much deeper was going on), so I did a lot of shatkarmas then. In recent years the inner call for shatkarmas has been much less, so I spend very little time doing them now -- typing instead!

That is one way to approach the shatkarmas -- if you feel called to them from within, do them. If not, then you will not be shortchanging yourself spiritually by not doing them. Meditation, spinal breathing and the other AYP practices are far more important factors in our spiritual transformation. The interconnectedness of yoga will natually call us to shatkarmas and the other yamas and niyamas, as necessary, along the way. See lesson #149 for more on the interconnectedness of the limbs of yoga. http://www.aypsite.org/149.html

By the way, the shatkarmas are niyamas, and I suppose ayurveda claims them too. So they can be discussed either here in healthcare or in the yama/niyama forum. If the discussion moves beyond cleansing techniques to other yamas and niyamas, it is suggested to switch over to the yama/niyama forum. There is overlap between the forums, just like there is overlap between the limbs of yoga. The One is the many and the many are the One!

The guru is in you.

2005/11/29 19:07:12
Healthcare - Holistic and Modern
http://www.aypsite.org/forum/topic.asp?TOPIC_ID=443&REPLY_ID=1708&whichpage=-1
JALA NETI

Hi Folks:

Nice topic here. For whatever it is worth, it can be a pretty short trip from the neti pot to sucking the lightly salted warm water up from a bowl with both nostrils and expelling it out of the mouth. The bowl can be emptied in a few cycles this way. It can also be expelled through the nose, but that is messier. The nasal pharynx is a natural vessel for this operation, and even has a "dam" in the form of the soft palate to keep the water from running down into the lungs while inhaling it up through the nose (same effect when using the neti pot).

This approach is fast and effective. The longest part of it is waiting for the sinuses to drain, which can take a few minutes. That is true of any form of jala neti, but especially the big kahuna of doing a whole bowl. If you don't wait for the sinuses to drain, you can walk out of the bathroom and suddenly drop a shot or two of water on whomever you might be standing over.

If this jala neti procedure sounds risky, it isn't. I can't remember one time in the last 20 years when I actually inhaled water. We seem to have a natural ability to handle water in this way. But if the salt content is too much or too little, not so pleasant...

The guru is in you.

2005/12/20 12:19:26
Healthcare - Holistic and Modern
http://www.aypsite.org/forum/topic.asp?TOPIC_ID=660
Spiritual or Medical Symptoms?

Hi All:

This is from my email:

Q:
Thanks for all the information you have been giving out. To say that it has changed my life would be an understatement.

I have a question for you. I hope you can refer me to where in your book I can find answer to this.

In your lessons you have talked about blockages manifesting themselves in different physical forms. In some other lessons you have talked about seeing lights in your eyes during early steps towards enlightenment.

Where do you draw the line, and decide to see if this is actually a physical ailment, or is caused by yoga practices?

Here is my scenario - I started practices I learned in your lessons, seriously about a year ago. I have been increasing duration. I have also had a mild neck ache problem. For the past few months it has been severe. At first I wrote it off as energy blockages, and adjusted, but the problem did not go away. I finally went to a doctor, and with his help, discovered that the problem was due to an external cause. Addressing that has provided some relief.

I also started seeing some flashes in my eyes. This normally would be encouraging, but I saw a doctor. The doctor told me that this is a condition known as posterior vitreous detachment, and the flashes are a bad thing. He told me to not try to make the flashes appear. I did some internet research, and discovered that the symptoms match. Had I not consulted the doctor, I could have harmed my eyes tremendously.

I don't want to run to the doctor every time I see something. However, I also do not want to attribute physical symptoms to yoga practices only. So, I am trying to figure out some simple ways to determine when it is appropriate to go to the doctor, and when to take it as an effect (good or bad) of yoga practices.

Thanks.

A:
The simplest way to avoid spiritual symptoms being confused with medical symptoms is to be diligent in applying self-pacing. This means not overdoing in practices, and making adjustments as necessary. Then we will always have reasonable control over results from practices, and if something is happening that is medical, we will have a much better chance of spotting it.

So, do not overdo with sambhavi, yoni mudra, chin pump or other practices that can strain the eyes or neck. The goal is not to see flashing lights. The goal is to gradually cultivate inner silence and ecstatic conductivity. Gradually. If we are doing that, we will not have extreme symptoms. Then if we do have symptoms, we will know better to go see a health care professional.

Of course, I am idealizing things a bit, because there will be times when spiritual symptoms will be strong even with light to moderate practices, so there will be times when the line between spiritual and medical symptoms will be blurred. In those times, we are best to go for safety first with self-pacing and medical advice as we deem necessary, as you have wisely done. The other side of this is the fact that practices like chin pump and sambhavi can aid in clearing up symptoms if these are related to spiritual energy blockages. So, there can be some trial and error in practices during these times. When there are symptoms that seem to be energy related, we can test lightly with practices, and if there is no relief, we back off. I am thinking of chin pump here, and numerous cases we have seen where blockages of energy in the neck have been relieved. But in your case, this apparently was not so, which points to the need for always keeping the medical aspect in mind, and always treading carefully with our practices.

Then again, it is also possible for medical professionals to diagnose spiritual symptoms as medical. It happens all the time in the psychology field with visions, kundalini experiences, etc. So, we always have to use our common sense before being led off into drug treatments and other things that may or may not be treating real illnesses.

As time goes on, the medical profession will gain better understandings of these matters, as will we as practitioners. The AYP forums are a good place to network on these things, so I am going to put this one in there (anonymously) for the group to consider. It is a fascinating subject -- one that I am sure will receive increasing attention in both the medical and yoga communities as we see more and more individuals exhibiting the signs of human spiritual transformation. Society is going to have adapt to the reality of spiritual awakening rising everywhere. There is lots of evidence of it in the neurobiology, yes?

The good news is that we are forging ahead and plowing new ground in the field of applied yoga science. If nothing were happening, we would have much more to worry about. :-)

Btw, the business of flashing lights is also covered in lesson #194, assuming a spiritual symptom in that case. But the warning is always there to

472 – Advanced Yoga Practices

be prudent and not ignore symptoms that could be medical.

Wishing you the best on your chosen path. Enjoy!

The guru is in you.

2006/01/26 10:25:37
Healthcare - Holistic and Modern
http://www.aypsite.org/forum/topic.asp?TOPIC_ID=770&REPLY_ID=2799&whichpage=-1
Practice for Messed-Up Friend

Hi Jim:

I agree with David. Send him the Deep Meditation book, and let him decide. There are plenty of instructions in the book on regulating (or even stopping) practice if there is imbalance. The upside far exceeds the downside.

The guru is in you.

2006/01/26 14:37:31
Healthcare - Holistic and Modern
http://www.aypsite.org/forum/topic.asp?TOPIC_ID=770&REPLY_ID=2809&whichpage=-1
Practice for Messed-Up Friend

Hi Jim:

Voices or not, it is still the person's choice to listen to one source of information or the other. Case in point: The true story and movie, "A Beautiful Mind," about the journey of Nobel Prize winner, John Nash, through life with schizophrenia.

There have been about a half dozen who have written to me over the past couple of years with this problem to varying degrees. I suggested meditation to all of them with the normal advice about favoring the mantra over the scenery, self-pacing, etc. Half were able to continue with meditation and were helped. I don't know what happened to the other half. Have not heard from them.

If the situation is so degraded that no rational choice is possible, then it probably belongs in the medical system. But, as long as there is some rational communication between people, indicating the ability to choose, then meditation has a chance. The only prerequisite for deep meditation is that one can choose in a procedural way -- use the technique, and regulate as necessary. If that ability is not there, then I agree, all bets are off. Not only for meditation, but probably for everything. Then it should be in the doctors' hands. It is unlikely you would have heard from this person at all if things were that degraded.

All of this is another way of saying that deep meditation is so easy that almost anyone can do it if they decide to. Deciding to or not deciding to is a choice that everyone is entitled to make. Of course, people need information to make decisions, and that is what AYP is about -- information. We can't really take responsibility for all the other information that someone is considering, real or imagined. All we can do is share what we know. The rest is up to them, or those who are caring for them.

The guru is in you.

2006/01/26 18:21:27
Healthcare - Holistic and Modern
http://www.aypsite.org/forum/topic.asp?TOPIC_ID=770&REPLY_ID=2816&whichpage=-1
Practice for Messed-Up Friend

Hi Jim:

I also recommended seeking medical help to the same six people. Several had been already and were looking for a different angle, so I gave it. There is also mental illness in my family which I deal with on a regular basis, so I have seen a little and know something about the application of light meditation and breathing techniques in that realm. Success is mixed, and risks are minimal, mainly because people with serious mental illness do not have the ability to practice steadily. It is self-regulating in that respect. In serious cases, the practice is more likely to be colored by the illness rather than the other way around. It just fizzles. So, why bother trying? Well, in my book every single person is worth trying for.

There is no claim here to know how to solve chronic mental health issues, or even physical health issues. That is why you read in AYP fairly often, "If you are sick, go see a doctor." In addition to that, anyone can choose as they wish from AYP. It is an "open source." In a very real sense, nothing here is "recommended." It is information that is available that can be applied, or not. Freedom of the press, you know.

The fact is, the AYP methods can and do help people with many sorts of health problems -- physical and mental. Indeed, the majority who come to AYP are looking for some kind of physical and/or mental relief. Those benefits are aside from the primary purpose of human spiritual transformation, which is what "health" is about anyway. In truth, there is no such thing as an ideal health situation short of enlightenment.

This does not mean AYP is offered as a cure all, though some would like for it to be. Maybe you were hoping too by bringing this thorny question in here? It isn't a cure all. AYP is for people with bhakti (spiritual desire) who are seeking to do something to promote their well-being and spiritual progress. Very often that bhakti is expressed as a desire for healing. I get asked about that every single day. Who am I to say, "No, you are not ready for this information." Instead, I say, "Here it is. Use it wisely. Or don't use it. It's up to you."

The reason why spiritual teachers run away from thorny mental health issues is the same reason why they run away from kundalini issues -- fear for their own prestige and survival. It is not out of concern for the aspirant's well-being. Most who have had kundalini sickness and gone to a "guru" will tell you that. It is too messy. No one likes messes. Well, we can tell them to go to the doctor (ship them off) and leave it alone. It is the easy option. Or we can suggest some gentle spiritual measures that might help, even as we are suggesting an intelligent medical approach at the same time. That's what I try and do.

The guru is in you.

2006/01/28 21:11:16
Healthcare - Holistic and Modern
http://www.aypsite.org/forum/topic.asp?TOPIC_ID=770&REPLY_ID=2841&whichpage=-1
Practice for Messed-Up Friend

Hi Jim:

Don't worry about it. Sometimes we just have to let go when we feel strongly about something. It's all part of the process.

The guru is in you.

2006/03/02 11:20:37
Healthcare - Holistic and Modern
http://www.aypsite.org/forum/topic.asp?TOPIC_ID=861&REPLY_ID=4006&whichpage=-1
Ayurveda diet

Hi Alvin:

Those broken links were to the Transcendental Meditation (TM) organization's free Ayurveda site -- a great resource, now apparently shut down. I'll update the AYP Ayurveda Resources page one of these days.

As for Hong Kong and China ayurvedic diets, maybe best to find a local or regional Ayurveda resource which could address that. If you find one, let us know. Or if anyone reading here knows, kindly speak up.

The guru is in you.

2006/04/10 12:58:46
Healthcare - Holistic and Modern
http://www.aypsite.org/forum/topic.asp?TOPIC_ID=1030&REPLY_ID=5820&whichpage=-1
hormesis and Kumbhak

Hi David:

Excellent observations. 'Yoga and Hormesis' is an area where science can dig in and find some of the mechanics of human spiritual transformation.

The guru is in you.

PS -- Fasting is another one which is being explored elsewhere here. It is also a case where gentle challenging of the system brings out hidden capabilities for transformation in the human neurobiology. That is why we find fasting in many of the spiritual traditions.

2006/04/10 15:36:51
Healthcare - Holistic and Modern
http://www.aypsite.org/forum/topic.asp?TOPIC_ID=1030&REPLY_ID=5822&whichpage=-1
hormesis and Kumbhak

Hi David:

And holdback in tantric sex too ...

"Yama" (restraint) is all over the place in yoga as stimulus, with the response coming from the inner machinery of purification and opening. Not exactly the same as hormesis, but along similar lines of "challenging" the neurobiology in particular ways. If yama is measured (self-paced) in daily practices, then the purification and opening can be sustained over the long term. That is where the real benefit is found in the principle of restraint, in long term cultivation. Then the inner functioning we are cultivating becomes self-sustaining, and we become it -- moving beyond our previous level of functioning to a broader view of our existance and relationship with our surroundings.

The guru is in you.

2006/04/10 17:49:03
Healthcare - Holistic and Modern
http://www.aypsite.org/forum/topic.asp?TOPIC_ID=1030&REPLY_ID=5831&whichpage=-1
hormesis and Kumbhak

Hi David:

There are extremists in every branch of spiritual practice. Maybe it works for a few, but not for many.

It would be like driving 100 miles-per-hour to work every day. It would save time, if one managed to get there. If everyone did it, how many would arrive?

There is no doubt that any of us can go much faster with AYP if we choose to, with extreme discomfort (mortification) being the price for the extra progress. How many would fall off the path along the way? A lot. And most would be very unhappy with me for suggesting such an approach, which I am not!

You know, I have seen some extremists along the way here. They usually have a wild look in their cyber-eyes, a narrow focus on one do-or-die practice, and have a tendency to drop in and drop back out.

474 – Advanced Yoga Practices

Could "mortification of the flesh" be done in a systematic way for spiritual purposes? I suppose so, but that is not what we are into in AYP. Somewhere between doing nothing and mortifying the flesh is the middle road of consistently and gently challenging the neurobiology to evolve over a long period of time. And evolve it will.

I'm not Judas, and am not looking for his help. These temples will disintegrate soon enough without any extra help. In the meantime, let's make the most of our opportunity. :-)

The guru is in you.

2006/07/11 08:22:33
Healthcare - Holistic and Modern
http://www.aypsite.org/forum/topic.asp?TOPIC_ID=1310&REPLY_ID=9234&whichpage=-1
Heal ! Body, mind
Moved to the healthcare forum for better placement.

Be well... :-)

The guru is in you.

2006/07/12 10:18:13
Healthcare - Holistic and Modern
http://www.aypsite.org/forum/topic.asp?TOPIC_ID=1310&REPLY_ID=9268&whichpage=-1
Heal ! Body, mind

Hi Sadhak:

It is an interesting question: Why pranic healing methods mixed in with spiritual practices?

There is a dilemma in it which I have faced many times over in the past few years. Seeking healing and seeking enlightenment/God are not necessarily the same thing, though they certainly can be.

About half the emails that have been coming here over the past few years have been requests for healing of one sort or other. I always stick with the yoga, and if that doesn't help (it often does), I suggest they see a doctor or healer.

The way I see it, if healing is part of our spiritual path, it is fair game in AYP. If it is for its own sake, then it probably belongs in another discussion somewhere else, because our primary interest here is in applying the most effective methods for cultivating spiritual progress.

Of course, the dilemma is that we'd like for everyone to be beyond suffering. But can we accomplish that by healings alone? I think not. Transcendence of illness (and everything else) via the rise of inner silence is the only way to permanently overcome suffering.

So, here in AYP we favor transcendence over the endless energy manipulations of the healing arts. Within that framework, the dilemma is resolved. And that is how I have managed it amidst the barrage of healing requests over the past few years.

The legendary healings of Jesus are an interesting case in point. He attracted many followers in this way, but was it for the right reasons? Were the people looking for more than physical health? Did Jesus actually put people on their spiritual path that way? Of course, in the healings, he made the essential scriptural clarification: "Your faith has made you whole." (i.e. - the healer/guru is in you) It is what we want to be saying here too.

So, has energy work coming from an external source got anything to do with real healing? Ultimately, I think not -- it comes from within. Still, when chronically sick, go see a doctor!

In the meantime, spiritual practices are the best preventive medicine anyone can take -- and often times they can cure illnesses, or, more correctly, they enable us to be cured from within.

We all have the divine instinct to wish others well. If we do so and let it go into God/inner silence, it is healing samyama -- the essence of true prayer -- honest, true and transcendent. It's how real healers work without injury to themselves or anyone else. It is the outpouring of divine love. That kind of healing modality is heartily recommended for everyone, wholly consistent with our aims for spiritual growth and good health, and coming from the right place.

The guru is in you.

2006/07/13 00:20:52
Healthcare - Holistic and Modern
http://www.aypsite.org/forum/topic.asp?TOPIC_ID=1310&REPLY_ID=9305&whichpage=-1
Heal ! Body, mind

quote:
_____
Originally posted by sadhak

But still, I get the feeling that these arts must have their place somewhere. Maybe not here, where everybody is moving out blockages gently enough, without getting hurt. But :-) there *could* be people here, too, who out of enthusiasm, or not paying attention, or lack of proper observation, *do* hurt themselves... and then they end up dropping practices altogether. After all, not everyone has the same level of cognition or right application for various reasons. And that may not mean that they do not have the right intention to begin with either.
_____

Hi Sadhak:

People overdoing with practices was a concern I had when starting out with AYP, and to the degree people reported problems (most often due to pre-existing tendencies), we went immediately into Kundalini management using measures from a range of sources, including ayurveda and basic energy management methods -- grounding mainly. That is what is introduced in <u>lesson 69</u>. As it turned out, spinal breathing is one of the best energy balancers in the whole tool kit, something that was not well known outside the esoteric world before now. It is high level energy work without the distractions of the human intellect, assuming the procedure is followed as instructed.

So, while I kept waiting for all "H" to break loose with so many people taking up the practices, it never did. Why? Because if you give people the tools with good instructions and the means for self-pacing, they will be responsible with the power placed in their hands. While we have had some practice-related energy over-loads from time to time, it has been far less than anticipated. For that I wrote <u>lesson 217</u> about two years ago, and I am happy to say we have gotten even better at managing all of this since then, and we will get better still.

So the naysayers who have preached about the dangers of giving people open access to powerful practices have been dead wrong. With good education, it will work just like in any other field of knowledge. In contrast, fragmented knowledge of practices can be much more dangerous, as many of us have seen over the years. Yoga is not voodoo. It is cause and effect, and we can manage it systematically like any other cause and effect. It is the way of applied science.

In any case, I'm sure there will be instances of people getting ill now and then, for whatever reason, and I am certainly not opposed to doing whatever we can to help.

However, we do not want to become "tent healers." :-) I think most serious practitioners around here would agree on that point.

The guru is in you.

2006/07/28 17:13:22
Healthcare - Holistic and Modern
http://www.aypsite.org/forum/topic.asp?TOPIC_ID=1365&REPLY_ID=9958&whichpage=-1
Can someone shed some light on Kaya Kalpa?

quote:
_____
*Originally posted by bliss_*

Kaya Kalpa is the yogic technique to attain immortality or at least longevity of the physical body. From my limited research there are 2 trends of Kaya Kalpa:

- One uses medicine like herbs, metals, mercury etc... to prepare the pill of longevity.

- The other seems to use yogic like exercises and techniques, one that seems very important is kechari mudra. However I can't find any specifics regarding these techniques.

Could anyone point me to some useful info.

_____

A <u>long time</u> practitioner:

Maharaj: A Biography of Shriman Tapasviji Maharaj, a Mahatma Who Lived for 185 Years -- by T. S. Anantha Murthy

http://www.amazon.com/gp/product/091392217X/ref=ase_advancedyogap-20/103-4923313-7675054?s=books&v=glance&n=283155&tagActionCode=advancedyogap-20

The guru is in you.

2006/10/31 11:32:21
Healthcare - Holistic and Modern
http://www.aypsite.org/forum/topic.asp?TOPIC_ID=1365&REPLY_ID=12761&whichpage=-1
Can someone shed some light on Kaya Kalpa?

Topic moved for better placement. Great discussion on Kaya Kalpa. Please continue. Thank you.

The guru is in you.

2006/11/01 13:10:32
Healthcare - Holistic and Modern
http://www.aypsite.org/forum/topic.asp?TOPIC_ID=1365&REPLY_ID=12789&whichpage=-1
Can someone shed some light on Kaya Kalpa?

quote:
_____
Originally posted by Athma_Shakti

...for many reasons i cannot tell the technique (of kaya kalpa) here, because it may be unsafe if its done without the guru.

_____

Hi Kumar:

This has been said in the past about many of the practices in AYP, and we have found that with good instructions (including self-pacing), the warnings have been unfounded and untrue. In fact, there has been <u>much more</u> progress by many with open availability of knowledge on practices, and fewer mishaps <u>because</u> of the open availability -- meaning, good information on dealing with excesses and pitfalls, which is an ongoing development of information based on the causes and effects in thousands of practitioners.

Conversely, secret teachings tend to be static, and have led to guesswork and poor application of practices by eager self-directed practitioners -- resulting in <u>more mishaps</u> and less progress. This is what we have learned over the past 40 years. With so many stepping up to take on practices of all kinds, the need for better information on all practices is great. Times are changing.

So if you know something and are free to share it, you don't have to worry about us. We will figure out how to make it safe and useable. It will be a matter of toning it down to a simple, effective and safe practice that anyone can use. Perhaps you have some thoughts on this already.

Surely there must be something useful about kaya kalpa that can be shared "open source." What is not openly available is <u>essentially useless</u> on the global scale of things. If a few are benefitting, good for them. How about the millions more who can benefit? It can only happen through good instructions, openly available to all. Then the process of refinement and improvement can be working constantly. This is applied yoga science...

On the other hand, if you have made a promise to keep a secret, then you are bound by your promise, of course, and it is respected.

The word will get out one way or another. It is time for all to be revealed, and be applied in practical ways for the benefit of everyone... :-)

The guru is in you.

2006/11/01 13:38:18
Healthcare - Holistic and Modern
http://www.aypsite.org/forum/topic.asp?TOPIC_ID=1365&REPLY_ID=12791&whichpage=-1
Can someone shed some light on Kaya Kalpa?

quote:
_____
Originally posted by david_obsidian

Yogani said:
On the other hand, if you have made a promise to keep a secret, then you are bound by your promise, of course.

On the other hand, I have made promises I no longer feel morally bound to keep. An example is a promise I made when I was 18 years old, to the TM organization not to reveal anything about the technique they taught me. As I see it now, I made the promise under false understandings, many of those false understandings cultivated by those who required the promise.
_____

Hi David:

Okay, then how about: "...if you have made a promise to keep a secret, <u>and feel obligated to keep it</u>, it will be respected, of course. On the other hand, if you don't, then fire away! We can make good use of the information..." :-)

The guru is in you.

2006/11/02 10:42:44
Healthcare - Holistic and Modern
http://www.aypsite.org/forum/topic.asp?TOPIC_ID=1365&REPLY_ID=12829&whichpage=-1
Can someone shed some light on Kaya Kalpa?

Hi Kumar:

Well said, and thank you for sharing. :-)

Of course, it remains to be seen whether the open source approach in AYP will stand the test of time, and none of us should take the ancient traditional approaches too lightly. Collectively, they are the foundation of all current spiritual progress in the world.

Meanwhile, we have a planet full of people who need practical spiritual knowledge which cannot be served in total using the traditional methods of knowledge transmission, so we continue to press for a solution.

Thank goodness for the internet.

The guru is in you.

2006/08/17 08:54:02
Healthcare - Holistic and Modern
http://www.aypsite.org/forum/topic.asp?TOPIC_ID=1436&REPLY_ID=10626&whichpage=-1
Amaroli on trial
Moved this topic for better placement. :-)

The guru is in you.

2006/10/22 12:35:54
Healthcare - Holistic and Modern
http://www.aypsite.org/forum/topic.asp?TOPIC_ID=1625&REPLY_ID=12497&whichpage=-1
Laying on hands

quote:

...I am most curious if there is an "official AYP view" ... on the whole healing (of others) topic.

_____

Hi Mike:

No, there isn't an offical AYP position on the activity of healing others. It is like any other activity we may be inclined to undertake in our life. The AYP view is that the prerequisite for spiritually elevating our activity in the world is taking care of business at home first by cultivating inner silence and ecstatic conductivity, which leads to the marriage of the two in the form of outpouring divine love. The latter is facilitated by our activities in the world, which are of our choosing. If one is inclined to be a healer, then it can be that. It can be any other kind of activity also. Whatever fulfills us. If we take it in that order, we will be healing ourselves and others at the same time. Obviously, if an activity we we are drawn to is destabilizing our spiritual progress, it will be wise to be measured in our approach -- the principle of self-pacing strikes again. :-)

Regarding what the "other" receives, as has been pointed out above already, it is more up to the other than us. The end of the Jesus story about energy going out is that he said, "Your faith has made you whole." So, whatever we give in this world will be received according to the receptivity of others. The sources of divine energy are unlimited -- present everywhere. It is always the recipient who will initiate and allow the exchange. That is where this phrase comes from: "When the student is ready, the teacher will appear." Likewise, "When the patient is ready, the healer will appear."

Of course, "receiving" is not always benign. It can "taking." It is usually a mixture of both receiving and taking, and that is where the "energy" complications of being in a serving profession crop up. The best preparation for whatever we encounter in life will be found in addressing our own development. Then we will be in a much better position to help others as we may be naturally inclined. So, from the AYP point of view, taking care of our own business with yoga practices comes first. Then the rest will follow naturally...

"Seek first the kingdom of heaven (within) and all else will be added to you..."

The guru is in you.

2007/01/09 08:31:28
Healthcare - Holistic and Modern
http://www.aypsite.org/forum/topic.asp?TOPIC_ID=1904&REPLY_ID=15622&whichpage=-1
Ayurvedic question...

Hi Chard, and welcome!

Ayurveda and AYP are generally compatible, assuming techniques are self-paced and balanced. The main way we use ayurvedic principles in AYP is for balancing the inner energies in relation to kundalini awakening, primarily with diet, though any ayurvedic measures undertaken will be in support of balancing the inner energies (all of ayurveda is about balancing the three aspects/doshas of our inner constitution -- vatta, pitta and kapha).

Ayurveda in AYP is used in conjunction with a range of energy balancing and grounding methods which are discussed in this lesson:
http://www.aypsite.org/69.html
There is a link covering some ayurveda resources there too: http://www.aypsite.org/ayurveda.html

Pursuing ayruvedic methods for health reasons is likely to be consistent with using it for spiritual reasons, as ayurveda is always about cultivating inner balance. Of course, you must be the judge of the effectiveness of any approach or technique, based on your own experience.

Wishing you all the best on your chosen path. Enjoy!

The guru is in you.

PS -- This topic has been moved for better placement.

2007/01/16 10:15:07
Healthcare - Holistic and Modern
http://www.aypsite.org/forum/topic.asp?TOPIC_ID=1957
Serious Mental Health Issues and AYP

quote:

I am suffering from violent impulses , and obsessive thoughts and compulsions accompanic with anxiety neurosis.
Can anyone please guide me with what type of breathing excercises and asanas will help me out.

_____

Hi ag_dwh:

This, or any resource that offers yoga practices to the public, is not really the best place to be seeking this kind of advice.

While yoga practices can aid in stabilizing serious emotional and psychological difficulties, they need to be applied carefully under the supervision of mental health professionals. Most people here, myself included, are not trained or equipped to do that, and certainly not in a public forum.

So the suggestion is to seek professional help with these issues.

Once the psychology is settled down and interest turns to matters of enlightenment from a more positive perspective, then there is much more we can help with here.

Your sincerity in coming here seeking answers is much appreciated, and shows that you can work through this with the right kind of help. People who sincerely want to get better can get better. The good that we persistently intend for ourselves is the greatest power in our life. I wish we could do more to assist. Unfortunately, it is beyond the scope of what we are doing here, and that is our shortcoming, not yours.

Perhaps someone here knows reputable mental health professionals who include yogic techniques in their treatment regimen. That would be the best kind of advice you might find here.

Wishing you all the best on your path.

The guru is in you.

2007/01/22 23:28:49
Healthcare - Holistic and Modern
http://www.aypsite.org/forum/topic.asp?TOPIC_ID=1977&REPLY_ID=16377&whichpage=-1
High Blood Pressure and Kundalini and Medication

Hi Jim:

The "DASH Diet" is a well-researched reliable way reduce blood pressure:
http://www.nhlbi.nih.gov/health/public/heart/hbp/dash
http://dashdiet.org
For a more articles, Google "DASH Diet."

It is a low fat, low salt diet, leaning toward fruits and vegetables. When combined with regular aerobic exercise, it is highly effective.

As for the AYP practices skewing the results in a stress test, it can vary, but over time it tends toward more relaxed body functions rather than hypertensive, due to the rise of inner silence. Even so, the formative stages of kundalini awakening can be very energizing, as many of us know, so hiccups in the body's parameters may happen. So, at any point in time the influence on biological functioning may vary, depending on where we are in our over all development (and also time of day in relation to our practice routine can make a difference).

It will probably take many years of research by the scientific community to determine the full metrics of human spiritual transformation. Of course, with or without the science, we have to use our common sense and self-pace as needed, which includes doing what is necessary to preserve our health for the long haul. We'd like to be practicing as long as possible in this lifetime. :-)

All the best!

The guru is in you.

2007/01/23 11:16:49
Healthcare - Holistic and Modern
http://www.aypsite.org/forum/topic.asp?TOPIC_ID=1977&REPLY_ID=16400&whichpage=-1
High Blood Pressure and Kundalini and Medication

quote:
_____
Originally posted by Jim and His Karma

If you were me, would you avoid this drug? It's a pretty non-invasive one, with few side effects. Though adding drugs to a semi-spiritualized system is always, I guess, a gamble.
_____

Hi Jim:

I would not avoid it indefinitely. If natural methods don't work decisively within a few weeks or months (they can work quickly), you may not have a choice, because walking around with high blood pressure indefinitely is an invitation for a health disaster.

I was in a similar situation about 10 years ago and the approach mentioned worked well for me, so medication was avoided. I also lost 20 pounds without even thinking about it. What has been little known about blood pressure until recent years is the role that a high fat diet plays in it. Fat in the diet is at least as much a contributor to hypertension as salt. This is the significance of the DASH diet -- it reduces both, and the results have been verified to the point that government health organizations now recommend it.

In any case, it is well worth a try, but if it isn't working pretty soon, better do what is necessary medically to get the BP within acceptable limits.

The nice thing about health alarms like high blood pressure, is that they call us back to better habits that can improve our over all health, and spiritual progress too. From adversity comes progress, if we are listening and act. Abiding inner silence cultivated in deep meditation helps a lot in that. :-)

The guru is in you.

2007/03/05 09:25:38
Healthcare - Holistic and Modern
http://www.aypsite.org/forum/topic.asp?TOPIC_ID=2189&REPLY_ID=18367&whichpage=-1
Chelation info

Hi Alvin:

While environmental factors, such as heavy metals, have long been suspected to play a significant role in autism, there are also underlying genetic factors involved, and this is where the hunt for a cure for autism has been going in recent years. See this recent research article: http://www.newsday.com/news/health/ny-hsaut0301,0,966760.story?coll=ny-leadhealthnews-headlines

Like with so many things in life (and in yoga too) -- there is no "magic bullet." Balanced integrated approaches will often produce better results.

Just some food for thought.

All the best!

The guru is in you.

2007/04/16 10:45:30
Healthcare - Holistic and Modern
http://www.aypsite.org/forum/topic.asp?TOPIC_ID=2431&REPLY_ID=20492&whichpage=-1
Throat chakra problem?

Hi Anthony:

You have come a long way in AYP in one short week, with your experiences in deep meditation, spinal breathing, etc. Hopefully it is all confirming for you that "something is happening." With steady practice, so much more will be there for you in a month, a year, and a decade. It is a blessing for you to be moving into core spiritual practices while you are so young. For most it comes much later. Perhaps your health vulnerability has been a cloud with a silver lining. Would you be making so many strides if you were wearing the illusion of indestructibility as so many of us have in this life?

A taste of our mortality now and then is not a bad thing. It has a purpose. It spurs us to action in ways that can be very beneficial.

Regarding your throat and ear condition, I suggest that no one thing will solve it, but an integration of things will. Your attention to healthful diet and lifestyle is wise and will certainly help. Deep meditation will help a lot also, especially over the long term as the process of purification and opening goes deep. Once you are stable in deep meditation practice, having developed a good feel for it, spinal breathing and other energy-related methods can help too, but be sure to take things gradually, one step at a time, so as not to overdo and get out of balance. Your nervous system will let you know. If your condition is deep-rooted (so it seems), these practices will eventually balance it. Patience over time with a gradually developed integrated approach to daily practice will be the key.

Along with the diet and lifestyle measures you are taking, you might consider amaroli, which is urine therapy. While it is not covered in detail in the online lessons, there are plenty of links, and it is covered in the AYP Easy Lessons book. The upcoming AYP book on Diet, Shatkarmas and Amaroli will cover it too.

Besides its long-known role as a spiritual technique, Amaroli is receiving more attention in modern healthcare, with research revealing medical benefits in many areas, including with allergies and reducing susceptibility to infection. Check some of the links in the FAQ here: http://www.aypsite.org/forum/topic.asp?TOPIC_ID=2365

If you decide to take up amaroli, make sure to treat it like any other yoga practice -- being stable in previous practices before beginning, and starting off slow. If adverse symptoms occur, back off until they subside and then creep back up in practice again. Remember, in all things yogic, sometimes more can be less and less can be more. The real results will accumulate gradually over time with prudent self-pacing in daily practice -- that is how permanent progress is achieved.

All the best!

The guru is in you.

2007/04/18 16:02:54
Healthcare - Holistic and Modern
http://www.aypsite.org/forum/topic.asp?TOPIC_ID=2442&REPLY_ID=20599&whichpage=-1
Burning eyes and ringing ears

Hi IcedEarth:

Wish I had a clear answer for you. Have you looked at all the options in lesson 69? Have you been on a heavier diet? A pitta (heat) pacifying diet? (important in this case) http://www.aypsite.org/ayurveda-diets.html

What was it that kicked this off for you originally?

Have you considered doing daily tai c
Hi or marital arts? I know you are in school in another country, so time and access to these things may be limited. It may be that the school routine you are following right now is too much, given what is going on inside. Once you finish this term, a break may be in order, with as few responsibilities as possible. Your choice, of course. Just the prospect of a simpler routine in a month or two can be a comfort.

During peak kundalini periods, a much simpler lifestyle can help a lot. In fact, too much energy can compel us to simplify our lifestyle. It happened to me many years ago. It turned out to be a good thing that actually accelerated my progress with fewer difficulties. I tried to reflect this experience to a degree in the Wilder story.

It isn't forever -- my life is as complicated now as it has ever been. The energy is fine with it, gone long since to ecstatic, mainly because there is much more inner silence and a constant blending of the energy with inner silence, so both become one in all that we do ... that is where it is heading.

Also see this lesson on left and right side imbalances: http://www.aypsite.com/207.html

Not sure if it will help, as it is practice-oriented, and you are not in a position to experiment with practices much right now. One point in there that might help is to not focus on the energies, as this can increase them. This is why "doing other things" can be an effective kundalini remedy.

Taking up deep meditation, as you are thinking, is worth a try, but be sure back off at the first sign of trouble. Deep meditation is not normally much of a kundalini remedy, and spinal breathing is. Maybe in your case, it will be the opposite. If deep meditation feels good, don't ramp up quickly on time. All yoga practices have delayed effects, so start very slow and don't do sudden large increases in practice time. The fruit of deep meditation will be in daily activity, not in the meditation session itself. That goes for any yoga practice we add. It takes some time to see the effects...

Wishing you all the best, and most especially peace and happiness. I think in time it will be okay. Those with the greatest challenges often end up with the greatest gifts. Not that we would necessarily go through all that on purpose. :-)

The guru is in you.

2007/04/19 16:54:45
Healthcare - Holistic and Modern
http://www.aypsite.org/forum/topic.asp?TOPIC_ID=2442&REPLY_ID=20638&whichpage=-1
Burning eyes and ringing ears

Hi IcedEarth:

Your practices early on sound like a litany of the things we are cautious about in AYP -- energy awakening before inner silence cultivation, premature crown practice and opening, overdoing in general, and all of that. Well, live and learn.

It is good confirmation for many of the lessons here, but I would be happier if you could have avoided the rough ride. Here's to a smoother journey from now on. Smoother is much faster. :-)

The guru is in you.

2007/08/31 16:18:35
Healthcare - Holistic and Modern
http://www.aypsite.org/forum/topic.asp?TOPIC_ID=2883&REPLY_ID=25182&whichpage=-1
Urinary Malady

Hi Jim:

There is a relationship between kundalini awakening, urination patterns, and the natural internal evolution of amaroli (recycling of urine in the body) and vajroli (drawing up of sexual essences). It is discussed in the Diet, Shatkarmas and Amaroli book.

Someday science will gets its arms around this.

I am not saying that this is your issue -- only a possible connection. An FYI...

The guru is in you.

2007/09/25 10:00:21
Healthcare - Holistic and Modern
http://www.aypsite.org/forum/topic.asp?TOPIC_ID=2940
Acupuncture for Back Pain

Hi All:

An interesting article called "Acupuncture provides twice the pain relief of standard medicine," with an added twist -- an apparent "belief" component.

http://www.dailymail.co.uk/pages/live/articles/health/healthmain.html?in_article_id=483772&in_page_id=1774

The guru is in you.

2007/10/23 13:21:51
Healthcare - Holistic and Modern
http://www.aypsite.org/forum/topic.asp?TOPIC_ID=3023&REPLY_ID=26273&whichpage=-1
bandha and hypertension

Hi Indian Seeker:

Here is a topic that reviews yoga and hypertension from several angles, including natural preventive means:

http://www.aypsite.org/forum/topic.asp?TOPIC_ID=1977

With regard to shoulder stand and uddiyana bandha, and asanas in general, if the blood pressure is running high, better to go easy, especially with inversion postures. That doesn't mean stop physical practices. It only means not to overdo them. Self-pace as necessary.

All the best!

The guru is in you.

2008/01/15 12:02:09
Healthcare - Holistic and Modern
http://www.aypsite.org/forum/topic.asp?TOPIC_ID=3300&REPLY_ID=28948&whichpage=-1
Anyone Get (non-spiritual) Migraines?

quote:
_____
Originally posted by Jim and His Karma

I need to hasten to add that once you get the knack of this dilation, there's no semblence of actual yawning. Much like after you learn to clear ear pressure, you don't need to actually swallow or yawn. You refine the action to its essence. It's the sensation of temporarily pulling back on a big rubber band that's been constricting at the base of your neck (I "spread out" the dilation slightly, to just below my collarbone, too).

And once you can do that, first, it's a great move to hold in AYP pranayama (and it's in keeping with Yogani's suggestion to be "open" in the throat in pranayama....this is just a much more specific way of attaining that) and second it's much easier to maintain during the day. Though, once again, the jury's out as to how enduring the effects are. My intuition says it's not doing much to diminish the block, it's just routing around it. But who knows....
_____

Hi Jim:

Yes, this is what we mean by opening the throat on inhalation during spinal breathing pranayama. Nice discussion here on some of the underlying reasons. Similarly, there are underlying reasons why we gently restrict the epiglottis on exhalation (ujjayi) during spinal breathing. And we self-pace as always, of course.

Like the old saying goes: "One pill will cure us, and two pills will make us sicker." :-)

The guru is in you.

2008/03/26 12:00:38
Healthcare - Holistic and Modern
http://www.aypsite.org/forum/topic.asp?TOPIC_ID=3511&REPLY_ID=31786&whichpage=-1
Published research?

quote:
_____
Originally posted by Christi

Hi all,

Well, I've had a look through the various sources on the internet, and it looks like we are a long way from proving the effectiveness, or otherwise, of pretty much any alternative therapy. As you said, emc, it looks like there are lots of problems involved in carrying out research that can actually be considered as scientific proof, even if someone had the will, and the money.

So it looks like a book available to the general public outlining the results of the research is still quite a long way away. Thanks for your help guys (and gals).

Christi
_____

Hi Christi:

Yes, this kind of research is still a "can of worms" with many tangents occurring. In time, I believe there will be more focus on the underlying principles, and the development of more reliable research methods. Therefore, what the institutions are doing now is very important. It is a beginning, and it will continue to evolve.

In the meantime, we are doing our small part here. What we lack in resources, we make up for in focus on the underlying principles of human spiritual transformation, which form the foundation of good health. We should continue to encourage those with tangible resources to follow that line. Hence this topic: http://www.aypsite.org/forum/topic.asp?TOPIC_ID=3267

Increased understanding will lead to a sea change in healthcare. We are seeing a glimmer of it now. The tide is turning.

The guru is in you.

2008/03/26 13:52:35
Healthcare - Holistic and Modern
http://www.aypsite.org/forum/topic.asp?TOPIC_ID=3511&REPLY_ID=31791&whichpage=-1
Published research?
PS: By the way, no one here has yet mentioned the extensive research on Transcendental Meditation (over 600 studies), which is alleged to be "scientific," is on the web, and also available in book form: http://tm.org/discover/research/index.html

The TM organization is also a prominent provider of Ayurveda healthcare treatments.

2008/04/02 11:18:18
Healthcare - Holistic and Modern
http://www.aypsite.org/forum/topic.asp?TOPIC_ID=3511&REPLY_ID=32096&whichpage=-1

Published research?

quote:
_____
Originally posted by Christi

I have noticed that the TM research uses timescales of years rather than weeks or months, which could be why they are getting much better results than many other research methods.
_____

Hi Christi:

Yes, I agree.

While the TM organization has unabashedly used scientific research as a marketing tool since the 1970s, stigmatizing themselves along the way, it does not take away from the fact that they have paved a lot of new ground that the scientific community at large will eventually catch on to.

As we unabashedly say in AYP, take what works and leave the rest behind. :-)

The guru is in you.

2008/08/26 11:05:58
Healthcare - Holistic and Modern
http://www.aypsite.org/forum/topic.asp?TOPIC_ID=4356&REPLY_ID=36793&whichpage=-1
Asthma - pranayama?

quote:
_____
Originally posted by Lili

Hi folks!

Do you know if people with asthma can do pranayama and which kind? Is our spinal breathing OK for them?

Lili:-)
_____

Hi Lili:

Light spinal breathing (5 min or less per session) with self-pacing should not be harmful. It can help a respiratory condition.

There is also research indicating that deep meditation can reduce asthma symptoms related to stress.

All the best!

The guru is in you.

2009/03/04 09:27:33
Healthcare - Holistic and Modern
http://www.aypsite.org/forum/topic.asp?TOPIC_ID=5264&REPLY_ID=46389&whichpage=-1
reiki group.what do you think yogani??

Hi Miguel:

Thanks much for sharing your inspiring ideas.

I encourage you to pursue your passion. Discussions and networking for Reiki are certainly welcome here.

However, starting an AYP managed regularly scheduled Reiki event would not be practical right now. We have just rolled out the weekly AYP global meditation and healing samyama sessions for public participation, after three years of gradual evolution. So, you see, these things do not happen overnight. Reiki is not part of the core AYP lessons (or competency) either, so direct management of Reiki events as an AYP function would be a bit presumptuous, I think.

Even so, you should continue with gusto here and everywhere on your path, and I am sure it will evolve into something very beneficial for many. It will take time and persistence. We are here to help everyone do that in ways that are empowering on the individual level, and supporting the worldwide spiritual awakening that is well underway.

Carry on! :-)

The guru is in you.

2009/03/10 11:52:45
Healthcare - Holistic and Modern
http://www.aypsite.org/forum/topic.asp?TOPIC_ID=5282&REPLY_ID=46901&whichpage=-1
Fungus and jock itch

Hi Neptune and All:

Over the years, it has become apparent that a wide range of kundalini symptoms are not able to be diagnosed by modern medicine, so far. Time and again, we hear that "the doctor was stumped" when presented with kundalini symptoms that may be similar to diagnosable ailments, but do not show up in the normal tests.

This doesn't mean we should not go to the doctor when such things occur that may cause us concern. But if the medical tests come back negative, then a kundalini symptom may be present. For that, we should make sure we are not overdoing in our practices, and keeping balance in our lifestyle with good activity and rest.

Meanwhile, the medical profession is going to have to step up to the plate on this as more and more people are appearing with these kinds of symptoms. Hopefully not too many -- we should self-pace, and be especially careful about doubling up with similar practices from different systems. Much can be done to moderate the symptoms of excessive energy flows.

Nevertheless, there can be no doubt that doctors are going to be seeing more kundalini symptoms, and it will be their responsibility to change with the times, and find efficient ways to determine what are kundalini symptoms and what are not. Of course, the medical profession first has to accept the fact that kundalini symptoms do exist. It may take a while, but, by now, the handwriting is on the wall. At least here it is. :-)

Science has a lot to do in the field of human spiritual transformation, and as time rolls on it will become much more obvious.

All the best!

The guru is in you.

2009/03/10 14:03:19
Healthcare - Holistic and Modern
http://www.aypsite.org/forum/topic.asp?TOPIC_ID=5282&REPLY_ID=46944&whichpage=-1
Fungus and jock itch

quote:

Originally posted by Neptune

Hi Yogani,
You are generalizing the discussion here from the groin into the gamut of kundalini related phenomena. That's OK if you wish to do that.

Hi Neptune

Absolutely, because that is what this discussion is ultimately about -- all those mysterious symptoms that do not come up positive for anything in medical tests. I believe that may be the case in this specific instance too, with at least one case that tested negative. So then, what is it?

It is a worthy discussion to be having here, not only for the medical aspect, but also for what to do when it is kundalini related.

There have been a number of discussions on rashes in the forums, and some of them seemed to be kundalini related. Or, at least, no medical diagnosis could be found. So that is the question, isn't it?

There are many other things that can come up that can send people to the neurologist, cardiologist, endocrinologist, etc. Where there are concerns, people should go get checked. That has always been the recommendation in AYP.

At the same time, we don't want the medical profession treating for everything but kundalini symptoms, which can happen. In that case, the cure can be worse than the ailment. There is a process of discovery going on across all the sciences, and we are all in it together. No one expects the medical profession to immediately adapt to something it has not seen much of in the past. But everyone expects the medical profession to adapt in due course. That is what applied science is about.

The guru is in you.

2010/01/18 11:25:31
Healthcare - Holistic and Modern
http://www.aypsite.org/forum/topic.asp?TOPIC_ID=7075&REPLY_ID=63128&whichpage=-1
To Yogani, your healing experiences

Hi Arim:

The body may get sick, but abiding inner silence (the witness) never does.

There is no doubt that yoga often leads to better physical health, and that a nervous system in divine flow (stillness in action) can be an aid to others. Energy flows where it is needed, where there is bhakti.

Healing has to do mainly with the faith of the one who is healing. With that, the energy for healing will come from somewhere, from everywhere.

The guru is in you.

2010/02/23 12:53:59
Healthcare - Holistic and Modern
http://www.aypsite.org/forum/topic.asp?TOPIC_ID=7326&REPLY_ID=65266&whichpage=-1

Anyone have any experience with monoatomic gold?

Hi wakeupneo:

This has been discussed in the forums before.
See here: http://www.aypsite.org/forum/topic.asp?TOPIC_ID=3168
Looks like you were already there. Just providing the link for continuity.

No comment pro or con from here.

All the best!

The guru is in you.

2010/04/23 12:18:42
Healthcare - Holistic and Modern
http://www.aypsite.org/forum/topic.asp?TOPIC_ID=7658&REPLY_ID=67685&whichpage=-1
Can Yoga cure High blood pressure ? / Alt remedies

Hi 11jono11:

For high blood pressure, I suggest three things, all to be done:

1. Twice-daily deep meditation.

2. The DASH diet, which is low salt, low fat, and proven to reduce hypertension (high blood pressure).

3. Moderate cardiovascular (aerobic) exercise at least three times per week. That is 20+ minutes of walking, light jogging, biking, swimming ... anything that elevates heart rate for 10-20 minutes.

Be sure to keep in touch with the doctor on all this, and for adjustments in medication when results occur.

All the best!

The guru is in you.

Forum 13 – Yoga, Science and Philosophy

Seeing yoga through the lense of logic.
http://www.aypsite.org/forum/forum.asp?FORUM_ID=43

2005/07/12 12:06:22
Yoga, Science and Philosophy
http://www.aypsite.org/forum/topic.asp?TOPIC_ID=281
Yoga, Science and Philosophy

For many decades, western science has been looking for objective, measurable evidence of spiritual experience and the so-called "super-normal powers" that are said to exist within human beings. (Eastern science has been looking much longer, so its point of view ought not be ignored by western scientists.)

There has been quite a lot of progress over the years in numerous studies done on meditation, psychic phenomena, near death experiences, UFOs and other kinds of extraordinary human experiences. Yet, questions remain, and the debate rages on. What better place to continue it than here in this forum?

And what about the collected systems of yoga practice being regarded as a science in its own right? Where there is cause and effect, there can be science. If a particular cause (say, a systematic method of meditation) causes a particular effect (like feelings of peace, or rising intelligence), and this is a repeatable "experiment," then doesn't that make yoga itself a science? This is especially true if the many causes and effects involved in a full range of daily yoga practices can be optimized to be highly effective and safe for anyone to use. Isn't this the same process we have gone through in developing all of the wonderful technologies we often take for granted today? A science is most useful when it can be applied successfully to a practical endeavor -- such as promoting human wellfare, or, say, promoting human spiritual transformation and the resulting "enlightened" condition that comes with it. Then it can be called "applied science." That is what we'd like to see happen with yoga -- see it come out of the shadows of ignorance and superstition, and into the full sunlight of practical applied science.

Looking further out on the mental plane, there is also the question of the many philosophies that have evolved in every culture to explain the nature of existence and the role of humanity in it. This forum can also be useful for those who are inclined toward examining philosophical systems, with the goal of utilizing calm and measured reason and logic to answer the question, "What on earth are we doing here?!!"

Some food for thought...

The guru is in you.

2005/12/20 17:13:21
Yoga, Science and Philosophy
http://www.aypsite.org/forum/topic.asp?TOPIC_ID=367&REPLY_ID=2044&whichpage=-1
Siddhis

Hi Alvin and David:

Very interesting discussion. On the E-science side there are quite a few parameters which can be measured that verify something going on during and after deep meditation. And this kind of research has been done by many in a variety of traditions over the last 40 years or so.

One of the most obvious parameters is reduction of breath rate -- reduction of oxygen consumption due to reduced metabolism. Most anyone who does deep meditation will at some point experience a reduction in breath rate, or even a complete stoppage. The thing to do with this when noticed is easily come back to the mantra.

Because the slowing or stoppage of breathing can be an attention grabber, it is covered in some detail in the new *Deep Meditation* book. I mention it here because it is an easy-to-spot E-science thing that verifies something is happening in deep meditation. It is completely automatic during certain stages of inner purification. In the kriya yoga lines a lot of attention is given to breath suspension. It becomes a goal, because it is considered to be analogous with samadhi. Maybe so, but we can be in samad
Hi while breathing and walking around too. That is a more advanced stage -- in samad
Hi and being active in the world. I call it "stillness in action" -- it is inner life pouring out into the world in the form of divine love. In AYP deep meditation, breath suspension is not the goal. It is a by-product of natural spiritual evolution. It is also an E-science indicator of inner developments occurring.

There are many other E-science parameters like this that can be measured, and I expect this will be the course of continuing scientific investigations on yoga practitioners in the years to come.

As for kundalini -- that one has even more E-science parameters. However, many of these "symptoms" can be confused with mental and physical pathologies that have been catalogued in the medical profession (see recent posting touching on this). So the measurements on states involving energy movement in the nervous system and the many internal and external effects associated with this will require a lot of sorting out before the E-science and I-science aspects of advancing enlightenment in the ecstatic realms can be fully understood.

But there is no need to lament this fact. It is the way of science -- application of means, resulting effects, refinement of means, more application, better effects, etc. Like that, round and round goes the optimization process to ever higher levels of useful application...

The Wright brothers managed to get that flimsy first airplane off the ground and fly quite well, even though they knew little of aeronautical engineering. The fact that the airplane flew was enough to get the scientists working on understanding the natural principles involved and refine the application of them to the point where we can now walk onto a jet and go anywhere in the world in a few hours at will. Yoga will go through a similar evolution. Pretty exciting.

You are right David. Though yoga and other systems of spiritual development have been around a long time, we are engaged in a fledgling science here, with much yet to be learned. It is a science that has vast potential to improve the quality of life of all human beings, as much or more than any applied science humankind has availed itself of so far.

The guru is in you.

2005/12/11 23:32:49
Yoga, Science and Philosophy
http://www.aypsite.org/forum/topic.asp?TOPIC_ID=637&REPLY_ID=1903&whichpage=-1
What clears out the energy debris?

Hi Anthem:

The detailed inner workings of spiritual purification and opening are probably best left to be unraveled by scientists in the years to come. We (inside and outside) are the drivers using the simplest controls we can find to operate the complex spiritual machinery that is "under the hood."

The process of purification obviously has to do with stillness -- deep rest of a different kind than sleep, brought on by systematic stilling of the mind and nervous system which enables our body/mind to normalize itself by dissolving inner obstructions. Then there is the activation of the inner energies and the ecstatic component via the suspension of breath, bodily manipulations, and all the rest of yoga that emerges. We can say that the inner energies moving are part of the purification process more as symptom than as cause -- an aftermath of purification, or at least coincident with it. Of course, everything is cause and effect in yoga. But we do know that some causes (energy work) are better placed in a subsidiary role to others (deep meditation).

Where does all the energy go when obstructions are released? Where does a knot go when it is untied? Obviously, the rope is longer, more flexible and can be used for other things than it could when it was tied in knots. It is not so much where the knots went that matters. It is more about what we can do with the liberated rope. In the case of the human nervous system, spiritual energy will flow more smoothly with less friction and upheaval as the obstructions dissolve. It is the flow of love. So we can reasonably say that the energy resistance experienced in the obstructions (and in life in general) becomes a smooth flow of divine love. We are designed to be conductors of that. So that is where the energy goes -- though us as ecstatic bliss and out into the world to transform it to higher expression. As Jim says, it is instinct -- the entire process is wired into the system.

What was an obstruction, a cramp in our life, becomes a flower of ecstatic bliss and divine love. The same energy is still there. Before purification it was angst. After purification it is expressing freely and divinely. The experiences you all have been recording so beautifully in the "Changes in personal life" topic are a testament to this very process. http://www.aypsite.org/forum/topic.asp?TOPIC_ID=545

Bravo!

The guru is in you.

2006/03/29 11:21:23
Yoga, Science and Philosophy
http://www.aypsite.org/forum/topic.asp?TOPIC_ID=647&REPLY_ID=5327&whichpage=-1
What "truth" encompass

Hi Alvin and Katrine:

I have put it a bit more bluntly somewhere else around here.

It is not the job of human spirituality to adapt itself to science. It is the job of science to adapt itself to human spirituality. Since when have the inner workings of nature been accountable to science?

As Katrine points out, it can be science within each of us, and in our honest sharings -- experiencing the causes and effects that are our practices and experiences, and dutifully recording what that is from the perspective of many individuals. That is the essence of yoga science. Whether that fits someone's particular definition of "science" or not, still, what we see here in these discussions is yoga science. Or the beginnings of it at the very least. It is the recording of events that are related to cause and effect. And from the look of it, there is plenty being recorded around here, over and over again, which is the "repeatable experiment" aspect of science.

Do we collectively not know here what the effects of deep meditation are? Do we collectively not know here what the effects of spinal breathing are? Of course we know, because there are many accounts. And the number of accounts will only increase. Are the results always clearly perceptible and right on the beam? Not always. The vehicles of experience (individual nervous systems) do vary. But somewhere under the bell curve of personal accounts there is a commonality of experience, and we can all see that easily enough if we are paying attention. This is far preferable to spending our time trying to squeeze yoga into a scientific model that is not suitable for investigating this particular kind of cause and effect -- practices yielding experiences.

With or without the blessing of traditional science, the work will advance. The way I see it, traditional science has some catching up to do, and none of us are obliged to sit around and wait. So let's get on with it! :-)

The guru is in you.

2006/03/29 13:18:35
Yoga, Science and Philosophy
http://www.aypsite.org/forum/topic.asp?TOPIC_ID=647&REPLY_ID=5336&whichpage=-1
What "truth" encompass

quote:

Therefore, even if a person is 'enlightened', we should look with great skepticism on their claim, explicit or cultivated, that they have a good or great ability to lead us to enlightenment; because this is a claim in the realm of cause and effect.

Hi David:

That is a very good point, and I do hope you develop it.

For sure, we are all accountable to the verifications of cause and effect in whatever we present to others as a truth or a way. The question is, how to put a fair measure on that without getting terribly bogged down? The measurements ought not distort the experiment (Heisenberg principle).

I do not mean to pick on you, Alvin, but it is a fact that over-intellectualizing can disrupt our progress. We will be wise to always make a distinction between the practice and the scenery. It is a letting go. If we are faithfully doing our practices (Oh, there is that word, "faith!"), it will eventually bring us into a perception of things as they are, and then the need for third party verifications will drop away. I know that is a scary proposition for a scientist, but it is not so bad, really. Then the matter of objectively verifying cause and effect melts into a subjective experience that is self-evident, not to mention extremely satisfying.

Of course, demonstrating that to others, and, particularly, offering something that can bring others into a similar experience is another matter, as David points out. In that case, we could say that verifying the cause and effect of "the path" is far more important than the experience of the individual practitioner. Of course, they are the same. It is only a matter of the how many practitioners (a statistical measure) we can bring forward to provide a useful verification of the causes and effects involved in a particular path.

You are right, David, if this had been do-able in the past, we'd have avoided a lot of difficulties. On the other hand, even flawed teachers bring knowledge, sometimes a lot, so the science might have failed us on that score, maybe for all the teachers we have seen in the past century!

But that was then and this is now. At least here in AYP it is all hanging out, so if there are some shortcomings (surely there are), they will be there for all of us to see, and hopefully correct. That sort of transparency has not existed in the past, so this is yet another benefit of an open source approach to spiritual practices. If a spiritual path can be verified, and/or be adjusted to be verifiable, then it will eventually become a paradise for serious practitioners.

On the other side of your question, does a person have to be "enlightened" to offer a verifiable path? Well, that is a tricky one that can lead to accusations of "the blind leading the blind." Nevertheless, it ought to be considered. The spiritual condition of the teacher has always been the primary criteria for measuring the path, and it has rarely been the ideal solution. Does it have to be this way? Personally, I am much more in favor of a collective effort, where no one has the ultimate responsibility for verifying everything. Much better to get the verification from a large group that is experiencing cause and effect in common. That we can take to the bank. See, Alvin? I do believe in science. I think it is essential for getting people like me off the pedestal and off the hook. And so much healthier for everyone too. :-)

On the subject of an individual having strong intellectual tendencies and how that can be a benefit on the path, perhaps some consideration of intellectual methods designed for dissolving "the illusion" would be appropriate. For that, tune in to the new discussion on self-inquiry over here: http://www.aypsite.org/forum/topic.asp?TOPIC_ID=968
The discovery and verification of cause and effect is not nearly so straightforward there, because that class of practice (self-inquiry) is dependent on the presence of inner silence, the witness, for results. So the cause and effect is very tricky in that realm of practice. Nevertheless, if the intellect is hungering to do something to find out what the truth is, then self-inquiry is a supplementary route to examine, beyond our essential sitting practices. At least then our search for truth will be happening in the right place, within our own experience of our daily activities.

The guru is in you.

PS -- And yes, I also agree that just because someone is good at some things, it does not mean they are good at everything. This is a myth that is created by the public, and often the "mythee" begins to believe it too. There is the classic case of the movie star believing the inflated headlines about them in the newspaper. It has happened with many gurus too, as the scope of their knowledge has been "misconstrued" (magically expanded to infinity) by their followers. Many of us have seen what that leads to -- sooner or later it leads to a fall, because it is not real.

2006/01/23 11:31:03
Yoga, Science and Philosophy
http://www.aypsite.org/forum/topic.asp?TOPIC_ID=753&REPLY_ID=2740&whichpage=-1
An under the hood question

Hi Bill, and thanks Anthem. Good question and good answer.

I can add that if we are experiencing symptoms of heat or coolness (maybe both at the same time) in particular areas of the body, we regard them as scenery and easily go back to our practice. I mention this because the machinery is there (chakras, nadis, etc.) and we will notice its purification going on at some point. But the machinery itself is not necessarily the control mechanism. We use the shift lever to control the gears, not the gears to control the gears. Like that, we have our hands on the main controls in our practices, and need not be managing the detailed inner workings.

There is more on this from a different angle (chin pump discussion) just posted here: http://www.aypsite.org/forum/topic.asp?TOPIC_ID=763

Of course, if symptoms of purification become excessive and uncomfortable, then we apply the principle of self-pacing in our practices to keep things in balance for progress and comfort, just as we would ease up on the gas pedal temporarily when going into a sharp curve in the road.

All the best!

The guru is in you.

2006/02/21 09:45:33
Yoga, Science and Philosophy
http://www.aypsite.org/forum/topic.asp?TOPIC_ID=754&REPLY_ID=3651&whichpage=-1
This whole 'desire' thing...

Hi All:

Desires can be redirected, taken higher to divine purpose. It can be done with every desire we have. This is what bhakti is about -- refining the desire process to be effective spiritual practice. See: http://www.aypsite.org/67.html

The guru is in you.

2006/02/05 12:53:02
Yoga, Science and Philosophy
http://www.aypsite.org/forum/topic.asp?TOPIC_ID=790&REPLY_ID=3075&whichpage=-1
Auto suggestion and creative visualization

Hi Thundu, and welcome!

Your step-by-step approach to the AYP practices sounds very good. The only suggestion would be to review lesson #59 and lesson #188 with regard to using OM as a starting mantra, and how we handle the incorporation of OM as an enhancement component later on in AYP deep meditation. It is your choice how to proceed, of course.

It is also your choice on what additional practices to undertake. The suggestion here is to follow your own inclinations in ways that are consistent with maintaining the stability of your sitting practices and balance in daily life. In other words, use the principles of "self-pacing" wisely. Most of us have careers to follow and families to care for, and following our commitments with the best intentions to do good will be more than enough to stabilize and make permanent our inner silence and ecstatic conductivity gained in sitting practices.

Because of this, I have not ventured too far in suggesting a lot of additional practices to be doing in our daily life. It could easily become a burden for many, and then it will not work. The ability to visualize and manifest a more positive reality within and around us will come naturally as we sit twice-daily in our practices and then go out and pursue our heart's longings in the world, having been colored so deeply by the divine. Then it is the divine vision coming from within that we are actualizing.

This does not mean that additional practices should not be done. It just leaves it in your hands, which is where it belongs. AYP aims to cover the essentials. After that, it is all a great and wonderful play. So, do enjoy yourself! :-)

The guru is in you.

PS --
Hi Anthem. Good reply. I posted before seeing it, so this is an echo of your thoughts. :-)

2006/02/06 12:25:20
Yoga, Science and Philosophy
http://www.aypsite.org/forum/topic.asp?TOPIC_ID=790&REPLY_ID=3107&whichpage=-1
Auto suggestion and creative visualization

quote:
_____
Originally posted by thundu

i tried practising I AM first. It wasnt comfortable for me as my mother tongue is actually an indian language. And i was already comfortable with OM to some extent.. thats why i continued OM instead of I AM. As far as pranayama and asasnas are considered i am very comfortable..but meditation 10 min itself looks to me as 1 hr session.. i am not enjoying meditation ... but i really enjoy pranayama... Any suggestion to improve meditation it....or am i suffering because of OM?
_____

Hi Thudu:

You can spell I AM as AYAM, or any other way that has the same sound. It is not about language at all. Just consider it to be a sound that has certain beneficial effects in the nervous system. As mentioned in the referenced lessons, OM is tough for beginners because it is single pole and highly energetic. This might seem good in theory. Afterall, they chant OM in the streets everywhere in India, yes? But for deep meditation it is a lot more to digest. There is 1,000 times more energy when we go deep -- not to mention what direction we are going in the subtle nerves with a particular sound. That is the tuning fork resonance aspect discussed in lessons. There is a method to all of this mantra stuff.

That's why we save OM for later. Your choice...

Btw, there is no reason we can't continue to use OM, or anything else we are familiar with, in the ways we have been taught in our cultural/religious background. Just keep in mind that deep meditation is something entirely different -- and the rules are not the same. With right practice of deep meditation (including right sequencing of mantra), we will find the deep resonant truth in our cultural/religious roots as inner silence comes up. Then OM (or our cultural/religious equivalent) will really shine for us. And if we do not have a cultural/religious equivalent, it will shine anyway. :-)

The guru is in you.

2006/02/07 10:22:31
Yoga, Science and Philosophy
http://www.aypsite.org/forum/topic.asp?TOPIC_ID=790&REPLY_ID=3135&whichpage=-1
Auto suggestion and creative visualization

Hi Thundu:

Yes, that is correct siddhasana, and there is nothing wrong with you.

It is all a process of purification and opening. If we continue with deep meditation and add practices on when we know we are ready, the openings will occur in due course. It is not about expecting any particular outcome on a given day. It is about applying the means daily to purify and open the channels. The rest is up to our natural inner processes. When you notice some quietness, some new clarity dawning during the day after your meditations, then you will know that something good is happening. All the rest will flow from that.

The guru is in you.

2006/03/08 11:16:29
Yoga, Science and Philosophy
http://www.aypsite.org/forum/topic.asp?TOPIC_ID=884&REPLY_ID=4239&whichpage=-1
the misuse of scientific concepts

Hi Alvin and David:

On the other hand, without symbols, parables, analogies and metaphors we would not be able to explain much about spiritual life to those who have not experienced it, or even to those who are advancing in it and needing recognizable sign posts.

In fact, all of the world's scriptures and mythologies rely on these tools. Even Taoism in its matter-of-factness relies on symbol and metaphor. The work of Joseph Campbell goes a long way in exploring and explaining the use of symbols and mythological structures in many cultures (past and present) around the world. This is science too!

But, like any tool, it can be abused, and is, particularly in claiming (going beyond symbol and metaphor) that one thing is the same as another similar looking thing. Hopefully not by present company. :-)

Question: Are some quantum physicists wrong in stating that the unified field and sat-chit-ananda (eternal bliss consciousness) are the same? Have they proved it yet? Are we proving it yet in our practices? Or is it only an inspirational analogy? Does it matter? The proof of the pudding is in the eating -- not in the chemical analysis.

Btw, I am a degreed and licensed professional engineer, and have no credentials whatsoever in the use of symbol and metaphor. But I could not be writing anything here without them!

All of this is somewhat aside from the real science of yoga, which is still in its infancy. It can only be based on the direct observation of cause and effect ... and probably <u>still</u> explained by analogy for a long time to come, just as all science is.

The guru is in you.

PS -- Are the dual helical phenomena found in pranic currents, DNA and string theory demonstrating a principle in common? Someday the scientists will tell us. In the meantime, we are allowed to notice the similarities, aren't we? If we do not notice, how can we ever explore?

2006/03/10 09:37:06
Yoga, Science and Philosophy
http://www.aypsite.org/forum/topic.asp?TOPIC_ID=884&REPLY_ID=4334&whichpage=-1
the misuse of scientific concepts

Hi All:

Of course, there are plenty of measurable "E-science" spiritual events -- a wide range of external and internal physical automatic yogas being an example. Plus lots of worldly performance measures. This is not new.

But that aside, if there is a case to be made for the incompatibility of science and spirituality, then it cuts both ways. Not only should yoga not misuse science, but neither should science misuse yoga. Analysis during yoga practices does a great disservice to yoga. The analogy is the Heisenberg principle, where the measurements disrupt that which is being measured.

Personally, I think yoga and science are very compatible. It is only a matter of adapting science to the task. Since when does nature owe science anything? It is the job of science to exercise flexibility in finding the truth about nature, not the other way around.

Science and analytical methods should respect the delicacies and unique attributes of yoga and the rise of human spirituality. Some have been arguing here for that in reverse -- yoga should respect the delicacies of science. Well, it is a two-way street. With an understanding of this essential point, yoga will work much better. In yoga, the fruit is in the letting go ... including letting go of science, at least during our sitting practices. We can analyze later, and we should!

Presented herewith in the true spirit of science. :-)

The guru is in you.

2006/06/15 12:46:17
Yoga, Science and Philosophy
http://www.aypsite.org/forum/topic.asp?TOPIC_ID=1182&REPLY_ID=8082&whichpage=-1
Kali or Dwapara?

Hi Frank:

From the standpoint of our yoga practices, does it really matter what age we are in? If ever-increasing numbers of people are engaged in spiritual practices (who can deny it?) and progressing on their path, that is a much better metric to gauge the condition (and future) of humanity by. Not only that, it is a metric we can directly influence with our real-time choices and actions.

I tend to favor the practical, and believe that astrological discussions, while sometimes interesting, are academic at best. And, if astrology is being used to make our everyday decisions, it can be downright degenerative and destructive, even in an enlightened age!

Inner silence within each of us knows much better than any star chart.

While we'd like to be in harmony with the stars, and everything else, what we are transcends the stars. In a real sense, we control the stars. When push comes to shove, the influence of pure bliss consciousness will far surpass even the galactic forces. Therefore, the whole issue of what to do with astrology is resolved in <u>deep meditation</u>. Then it boils down to using astrology when it inspires the cause of evolution, and ignoring it when it doesn't!

Based on that rational assessment, I'll go with Yukteswar's assertion that we are into Dwapara and rising fast. When given a choice, why not take the evolutionary one? Much better that the calculations (if any) should serve our needs than the other way around. And, if the need is to justify a negative point of view, well, maybe the point of view needs some adjustment rather than the calculation.

What I mean is, in the end, the numbers really don't matter. What matters is our ongoing commitment (bhakti!) to our journey of human spiritual transformation, and consistently acting on that utilizing the most effective tools we can find. I submit that following the stars into a black hole (real or imagined) is not an effective tool.

Just some food for thought -- from beyond the stars, of course... :-)

The guru is in you.

2006/06/15 23:29:25
Yoga, Science and Philosophy
http://www.aypsite.org/forum/topic.asp?TOPIC_ID=1182&REPLY_ID=8091&whichpage=-1
Kali or Dwapara?

Hi Frank:

Kali yuga or Dwapara yuga? That is macro jyotish/astrology, isn't it?

I believe it to be Dwapara, and thought it appropriate to give the reasons why. If it's not entirely objective, at least it's practical.

The macro is usually much easier to predict than the micro -- predicting the season as opposed to the daily weather. With major disagreements on the macro, where does that leave jyotish with the micro? Are there then two systems of jyotish -- one for an age of ignorance, and one for an age of enlightenment?

In any case, anyone who makes a case for an age of ignorance around here is going to get a rise out of me. It is a POV you are certainly entitled to, but don't look for any sympathy from practitioners who have discovered beyond any doubt that spiritual destiny lies solely within. From that POV, the stars are seen as a reflection of inner space, not the other way around.

If jyotish figures into that sort of evolutionary development in some way, in the here and now (not the next yuga/age, please), I'd be happy to hear about it, and perhaps others would too. Exactly what is the "spiritual technique" of jyotish anyway? Can it be stated simply, and applied equally simply?

In all fairness, on the advice of a jyotis
Hi many years ago, I have been sleeping with a gemstone under the mattress for over 20 years. Ah, the secret is out! Maybe without that stone under there, AYP would never have happened, but I doubt it. That gemstone has been more than canceled out by the fact that we have (according to sthapatya veda, a jyotish-based system of building design) been walking in and out of the wrong side of our house for even longer. And we will continue to, because that is the easiest way in and out. :-)

So where does real spiritual progress come from? Bhakti, deep meditation, spinal breathing, asanas/mudras/bandhas, tantric methods, etc. In other words, daily practices deep in the trenches of the nervous system. That is where the dance is. Then we can walk through the gates of what some might consider hell and only notice the ecstatic bliss. Stars? What stars? Kali what?

Question: Does being in an age of ignorance mean we all will be inspired to redouble our efforts along our path to compensate? If so, I am all for it. And wouldn't that really be an age of enlightenment?

That is what I meant about "controlling the stars." Whatever energy the stars can deliver (positive or negative) we can turn it into blazing bhakti and illusion-shattering spiritual progress. And when we leave this place, we will take that momentum and progress with us wherever we go. That is how we all got here. The vibes aren't so bad compared to last time, are they? Everything is relative. And how quickly we forget. This world is paradise compared to what it was!

But, I suppose it is in the eye of the beholder, which is the whole point, isn't it? Turn on the windshield wipers so those eyes can see that we are already in heaven.

The guru is in you.

2006/06/16 14:03:09
Yoga, Science and Philosophy
http://www.aypsite.org/forum/topic.asp?TOPIC_ID=1182&REPLY_ID=8127&whichpage=-1
Kali or Dwapara?

Hi All:

The passion here is for human spiritual transformation. As far as I can tell after 30 some odd years of looking at it, jyotish/astrology doesn't deserve much credit or blame, either way. The good or bad of jyotish is in each person's view of it, which raises an interesting question: What the heck is it? To the extent jyotish is used by people to justify a negative and unevolutionary point of view, I think it should be thrown out. Period. In that case, it is not helping anyone. That is the reason for my "rise."

Frank, you started it by saying the world is falling apart, and Kali yuga is the reason why. Well, I think that is an irresponsible statement that can perpetuate itself, and suck the life out of people's motivation to practice. Thank you, Lily, for chiming in on that important point. It is not a casual examination of jyotish principles. It is casting a world-view on everyone, and using the ancient "authority" of jyotish to back it up. It must be challenged.

On the other hand, if all predictions and events can be used for spiritual evolution, then jyotish can be useful, challenging us to reach ever higher. In that case, jyotish can be an asset, like anything we encounter in life. But it requires an important element of yoga for this to happen – an ongoing commitment to the spirit and methods of bhakti. With that, we can do "spiritual judo" on any sort of energy that comes (even Kali yuga) and convert it to support our divine destiny of spiritual transformation.

So, to answer your question, Frank, if jyotish can be made to work for our evolution, then we should use it. And if it can't, then the time is not right and it should be put aside. Just like that, samyama is not necessarily the best thing for everyone to be doing until inner silence has been stabilized to a degree through daily deep meditation. In the case of samyama, there are many who indicate some benefit. It is a matter of degree. Some do not experience anything. That's fine. It does not mean they still ought to be doing samyama. They can put it aside and wait until later. No harm done.

Likewise, I don't think jyotish should be used until the necessary ongoing bhakti has been stabilized. If it can't be converted to be an evolutionary force, why on earth use it? Just because a body of knowledge has been developed by sages thousands of years ago, it is not proof of its value today. It is only a hint, a clue in the puzzle. Like anything else, jyotish has to prove its value as spiritual method in the present, in modern terms, to be worth anything. Otherwise, it is just looking backwards – an escape into superstition. It is convenient to raise ancient knowledge up on a pedestal. It is like having an "infallible" guru or church. We don't have to do anything except parrot the party line. Well, we all know about the pitfalls in that.

So, I have to ask, what is the "expected result" of jyotish, and who is benefiting by it in the here and now? Jyotish is not like samyama or any other sitting practice because it cannot be easily put on the back shelf. For those who practice jyotish and are not benefiting spiritually (lots), they will not necessarily know they are not benefiting, and it can become an endless quagmire of superstition, confusion and fear that can become woven into the culture, and very hard to get rid of. It's not like a stalled practice we can easily put on the back shelf until later. Jyotish professes to define the course of our lives. It demands our attention, whether worthy of it or not, and can be like quicksand for those who are not ready with loads of bhakti. It can become a destructive addiction.

It is said that having the "right" jyotishi/astrologer is the key. The key to what? And even the best jyoti
Hi (if honest) will tell you that he/she will be right only a little more than half the time. 70% right would be spectacular, but still a crap shoot. So jyotish is a statistical game, like (pardon me) the stock market. Under the best of circumstances, it is still hit or miss.

The only reason I am making a big deal of this is because, if we are going to look at jyotish/astrology as serious spiritual practice, then it requires the same scrutiny as any other practice -- a thorough examination of cause and effect in relation to real spiritual progress.

If it is just a pastime, a hobby, a glance in the paper at our horoscope, or playing with it on the computer for enjoyment, well then, fine, who cares? But I don't think you regard jyotish in that way, Frank. So, naturally, the question comes up: What is this good for on the path of serious practitioners? How can it help us advance spiritually? Any reasonable explanation will be greeted with open arms. I have no desire to sabotage the field of jyotish, and certainly not any discussion of it here. But it has to stand up, you know, especially when making dire claims that can affect us all. If it is just an interesting hobby and pastime, that is fine. But you can't have it both ways. It is either serious spiritual practice (with observable results), or it is not. Which is it?

This is a serious forum on spiritual practices, and anything that professes to have value in that realm is subject to verification by direct experience.

Only trying to get to the bottom of it, you know. :-)

The guru is in you.

PS   David, now you know the real reason why I am anonymous. The Hope Diamond is under my mattress. The one in the Smithsonian is a fake. To all you burglars out there: Only kidding! The stone is synthetic. Honest ... it is not even worth pawning to help support AYP. So it stays under the mattress...

2006/06/18 00:27:37
Yoga, Science and Philosophy
http://www.aypsite.org/forum/topic.asp?TOPIC_ID=1182&REPLY_ID=8174&whichpage=-1
Kali or Dwapara?

Hi All:

"Yuga busters." Now that is a good one, Alan. :-) Interesting point of view from Yukteswar that we can zoom through the yugas on an accelerated individual level with practices. He is a sage after my own heart!

I was thinking of the phrase, "Beyond the Veda." It is not so outrageous, because inner silence (pure bliss consciousness) is beyond all expressions of knowledge. The vedas are one of those expressions, and a human one, like all others.

Melissa, perhaps the darkness we see is a symptom of purification on a global scale, leading ultimately to a profusion of light. We will find out in time.

David, it is very interesting about the relative value of old knowledge versus new knowledge. I don't think it has to be one or the other. Old knowledge has certain advantages -- particularly a resilience ("the truth lasts"), but it also can have distortions that creep in over time, especially in oral traditions, which can be like playing "telephone."

New knowledge has the advantage of being in the present and not "frozen in time" so to speak. It deals with things as they are developing and can adjust itself to current conditions. On the other hand, new knowledge can be naive and filled with errors without a solid grounding in prior knowledge. Probably the biggest advantage of new knowledge is that it can draw on all that has been recorded before, and move to the next level. In other words, the knowledge we have today is not only new, it is also a preservation and adaptation of the old knowledge to suit present conditions. At least it can be like that if the developers of new knowledge take advantage of previous efforts in the field.

An important phenomenon that straddles both old and new knowledge is progress over the centuries in the development of information preservation systems. It is the ongoing accumulation of knowledge and increasing access to it by more and more people that has been the single greatest contributor to the advancement of human civilization. As information preservation systems have advanced over the centuries from oral, to written, to printed, and now to electronic, the progress of humanity has accelerated exponentially.

When it comes to scripture, there have tended to be interruptions in the multi-generational evolution of information development, even as other fields like the sciences have grown and flourished, perhaps because so few sages have come along over the centuries who could take spiritual knowledge to more usable levels of development. So, what we have had in many cases is rigid hierarchies built around old "frozen" scriptures, and dogmatic interpretations rather than advancements in the knowledge. India may be an exception in this, because many generations seem to have developed their own scriptures there, leading to less rigidity in the spiritual knowledge base. Even so, we still run into the issues of blind acceptance and limited flexibility in many of the Indian traditions. So there is a need for more modern sages to keep the great spiritual heritage of India growing, rather than ending up frozen in the past. Of course, we need that in the West too, where we are just getting restarted after a couple of thousand years of no significant growth in our spiritual knowledge base. We owe a lot to India for helping us out with a jump start. May we return the favor sometime in the future with practical spiritual methodologies incorporating Western creativity and know-how.

I hope that AYP can make a small contribution to the growing base of spiritual knowledge being integrated and refined in the West. With the advent of electronic communications and instant worldwide information availability, we don't have to think of knowledge as being East or West anymore. It is just knowledge for everyone to use and expand upon.

With regard to the Kali yuga discussion, I do think we have to step back and see if the old template fits anymore. As mentioned in my last post, what has been happening for some time now with worldwide spiritual trends does not seem to add up to a new age of ignorance. Just the opposite. I suppose a serious enough cataclysm could send us back to the stone age, or do away with us completely. On the other hand, in a short few thousand years, humanity will be spreading out across the galaxy, and we will no longer be solely dependent on this single small ball whirling through space. Either way, we are obliged to do the best we can with the advancement of spiritual knowledge in the here and now, taking it as far as we can. If there is a tomorrow, there will be many who can benefit from our recorded progress. And if there isn't a tomorrow, well, we will move on from here all the richer in spirit. We will have really lived!

Certainly the positions of the stars will continue to be quantitatively predictable in the present, and far into the future. But will the qualitative interpretations of those positions by the ancient sages still hold true far into the future? That is the question. I guess our descendents will find out. In the meantime, I encourage everyone to make their own decisions about their spiritual practices rather than leaving it to interpretations of the stars. That keeps us squarely in the driver's seat and properly motivated to do something about our spiritual progress.

Btw, I had a very strong reaction in above posts to the idea of our fate being sealed in a Kali yuga style scenario. I believe strongly in self-determination, and will fight tooth and nail for that, as you all know by now. Frank undeservedly ended up in the barrage, and I owe him an apology for that. Sorry, Frank! You were just passing on useful information, as you always do, and I flew off the handle. The intent was not to shoot the messenger, but to say "no" to the message. I believe there is a better way. After all, in our essence, we are beyond both the vedas and the stars!

The guru is in you.

2006/07/05 18:15:43
Yoga, Science and Philosophy
http://www.aypsite.org/forum/topic.asp?TOPIC_ID=1292&REPLY_ID=9015&whichpage=-1
God, Enlightenment...and After

Hi Billeejak, and welcome aboard!

You are getting good answers already, and I'm sure you will get more.

Check the AYP site search for the word "God" on the three sites and you will come up with about 60 lessons and 200 forum pages.

Shhh, don't tell anyone. :-)

All the best!

The guru is in you.

2006/08/03 09:52:47
Yoga, Science and Philosophy
http://www.aypsite.org/forum/topic.asp?TOPIC_ID=1382&REPLY_ID=10192&whichpage=-1
Controlling and limiting spiritual teachings

Hi David and Trip:

Perhaps relating the integrated open source evolution of spiritual knowledge to the applied sciences would be more appropriate, as the methods for cultivating the known characteristics of human spiritual transformation are refined to become increasingly efficient over time.

Of course there is art in this too. We might call it "style," seeking a positive outcome like science does.

However we look at the open source evolution of spiritual knowledge, as art or as science, it is very different from the rigid approach in the closed source systems.

The guru is in you.

2006/09/08 12:00:38
Yoga, Science and Philosophy
http://www.aypsite.org/forum/topic.asp?TOPIC_ID=1479&REPLY_ID=11177&whichpage=-1
The notion of faith...

quote:
_____
Originally posted by Wolfgang

A very philosophical topic ...
_____

...and practical too.

If we have an object or ideal that resonates in us, we can find faith in that. The resonance is key. That will attract us, and heeding that call is the cultivation of devotion/bhakti, which is the engine of all spiritual practice. It is the divine calling us from within.

So listen to what resonates inside, and go for that with increasing persistence. The heart calls us home.

And remember to self-pace...

The guru is in you.

2006/09/22 14:39:28
Yoga, Science and Philosophy
http://www.aypsite.org/forum/topic.asp?TOPIC_ID=1534&REPLY_ID=11474&whichpage=-1
Kechari Mudra - Scriptures and History

Hi Jim:

Welcome aboard! It is always good to have a Sanskrit scholar in our midst to keep us honest. Of course, I know you are here for more than scholarship. Aren't we all? We are the nuts and bolts yoga folks here ... also sometimes referred to as "in the trenches." :-)

Since one of the moderators split this off the original "Kechari Mudra" topic as a new topic (didn't know you were that important, did you?), I took the liberty of adding "scriptures and history" to the title to clarify the potential subject matter. Feel free to change it if it is not suitable. I assume you can, since you are the post on top. If not, let us know.

Looking forward very much to your perspectives on kechari mudra, and everything else yogic.

It is interesting how history delivers science to our door -- from ancient murky wanderings and scribblings, evolving over thousands of years to modern applied science. Of course, those who think the ancients knew more than we do now might take issue with that statement. So, apologies in advance for that. We'd be nowhere without the ancients, that's for sure. But we don't have to change our culture and beliefs to reap the rewards of all the hard work that has gone before. All we have to do is adapt what is verifiably true in the recorded knowledge to our present circumstances, and voila! we've got interconnected spiritual openings happening all over the place. It is a joy to see...

The guru is in you.

2008/05/14 14:28:18
Yoga, Science and Philosophy
http://www.aypsite.org/forum/topic.asp?TOPIC_ID=1534&REPLY_ID=33762&whichpage=-1
Kechari Mudra - Scriptures and History

Hi John:

You may want to write Jim directly with your question. He hasn't been around here for a while. It would be great if you could lure him back for an encore. See if you can get him to lower the price on his book too, so a few of us can afford it. :-)

It stands to reason that kechari and other spiritual methods have evolved over the centuries from their roots in ancient cults and rites. It all had to start somewhere.

There is evidence that the ancient vedic tradition was rooted in shaman-style culture. For example, "soma," which we today understand to be a naturally occurring product of digestion related to the rise of ecstatic conductivity in the neurobiology, is clearly referred to in the vedas as an hallucinogenic plant. So we conveniently have turned it into a metaphor for our internal process. Why make excuses for what has been a gradual evolution of knowledge over time? The evolution continues. In fact, it is accelerating dramatically these days, thanks to the rise of the information age.

There is a tendency we have to think that our ancestors (who may well have been us!) knew more in the good old days than we do today. No doubt the vast spiritual knowledge that has been handed down to us is a treasure beyond all reckoning. However, I think it is much better to use recorded knowledge as a springboard rather than a destination. That is how science works, yes? If not, then it will be time to hand in our computers, cell phones, and ever-expanding real-time knowledge of applied spiritual practices.

We have seen the future, and it is happening now... :-)

The guru is in you.

2007/01/03 08:33:38
Yoga, Science and Philosophy
http://www.aypsite.org/forum/topic.asp?TOPIC_ID=1874&REPLY_ID=15324&whichpage=-1
Akasha the space element?

Hi Bill:

Akasha means inner space (in us and everywhere). Regarding it as the realm/element between materiality and inner silence is pretty accurate.

Akasha is what is manifest out of stillness before anything else is manifest. It is the emptiness that is behind the appearance of all things (verified by modern physics). When we come to know this via human spiritual transformation (the neurobiological process leading to refined inner sensory perception), the solidity of all things is perceived to be porous and luminous with the outflowing of divine love from omnipresent inner silence, which is our Self.

We can use akasha in samyama to help promote this awakening. See lesson 150 and beyond. The Samyama book coming out this month will delve further into practical applications of this, well beyond what we have discussed so far.

All the best!

The guru is in you.

2007/06/05 10:49:36
Yoga, Science and Philosophy
http://www.aypsite.org/forum/topic.asp?TOPIC_ID=2598&REPLY_ID=22794&whichpage=-1
The Ego

quote:
_____
Originally posted by david_obsidian

Well Weaver, I agree with all of that. I have no issues with it when it is put this way. In practice though, as a matter of language, when you say someone is on a higher level of consciousness, it's very strongly mythologizing. When people hear it, according to the way it tends to be interpreted, if they believe it, they have put the guy up on the pedestal in their minds.

_____

Hi David:

This issue is not limited to those who have made some spiritual progress. It happens in all walks of life. Someone puts in the effort to become good at something (anything), and they are automatically judged by a portion of society to be good at everything. It is part of the trappings of fame -- the myth. When taken to extreme, it has been called a "cartoon version" of the person in question. Completely unreal. Sometimes the person themself begins to believe the cartoon. It is an entanglement for all concerned -- part of the drama of life.

Okay, we know about that. Everyone has been warned, and warned again. It will still happen. That's life. The mincing of words will not change it, because it is human nature on both sides in the fame game.

This does not lessen the fact that spiritual progress is real. Abiding inner silence, ecstatic bliss and outpouring divine love are real. And we can all move steadily toward that condition if we apply known causes and effects.

Anyone can choose to move to the "higher" inner ground. The great spiritual icons serve as benchmarks for what is possible, and they are important for that, just as great athletes are important benchmarks for all who seek to excel in sports. It is the same in any field. Desire directed toward an ideal is the fuel of progress in all things -- it is the magic of bhakti. We all need our heroes. So let's not knock down the spiritual icons too much. If they lose their inspirational meaning, so will our own possibilities, and that serves no one.

Regarding "ego," it is only a word describing a condition of consciousness. Weaver's description of consciousness gradually shifting from separateness to unity depicts the journey very well. Ego does not dissolve, since it never existed as a real thing. What ego describes dissolves. That is, the perception of separateness.

So-called "strong ego" is an expression of strong vitality. It can be limited (separate) or spiritually expanded (unifying). When the latter is fully expressing, the concept of ego as separateness drops away, and the vitality is still there in the unity condition. So big ego becomes big unity.

Consciousness expresses according our inner purification and opening. Same consciousness, expanding view. Nothing is lost, except obstructions to our inner nature, and the experience of separateness and limitation. Goodbye separateness. Hello unity.

There is nothing to get rid of. Just open the door and let the inner light shine through. When that happens the words we have used to label previous limitations evaporate along with the conditions they described.

Let's meditate. ... :-)

The guru is in you.

2007/06/06 09:33:17
Yoga, Science and Philosophy
http://www.aypsite.org/forum/topic.asp?TOPIC_ID=2598&REPLY_ID=22835&whichpage=-1
The Ego

Hi David:

I think history will record that a dozen or so great sages collectively turned the tide of understanding about human spiritual transformation in the west (and worldwide) during the 20th century. Most of them are dead now. All had their personal issues, and these will be duly noted.

In the end, it will be about what has been gained on balance, not what dark shadows might have lurked. Humanity needs the positive for its inspiration and future progress. It is up to us to make the most of the opportunities we have inherited. It's good science too. :-)

All the best!

The guru is is you.

2007/06/08 10:51:25
Yoga, Science and Philosophy
http://www.aypsite.org/forum/topic.asp?TOPIC_ID=2598&REPLY_ID=22916&whichpage=-1
The Ego

quote:
_____
Originally posted by david_obsidian

We shouldn't lose sight of the fact that yogic development is not the only important kind of development for ourselves and the world around us.

Amen to that -- stillness in action! Too often, yoga means separating these two, which is a contradiction. :-)

It has also been called "emptiness dancing" by someone we know (Adyashanti). Whatever we choose to call it, the sage is as accountable for his or her actions in the world as anyone. More so, actually, because authority brings responsibility. Ultimately, we are all measured by our deeds, not by our so-called inner state, which is an abstraction. This point is often lost in the culture, in the philosophy, in the spiritual quest, and, of course, in the fame game.

The whole thing is way closer to home than most people think. Before and after, it is about "chop wood, carry water," and how well we do that from both the inner and outer perspective.

Somewhere in there, the thing we have called "ego" becomes much more, and that is the draw for all of us -- expansion of our consciousness and joy in everyday living.

The guru is in you.

2007/06/10 19:49:40
Yoga, Science and Philosophy
http://www.aypsite.org/forum/topic.asp?TOPIC_ID=2660&REPLY_ID=22998&whichpage=-1
Yoga is one of six... what?

Hi EMC:

Maybe he was talking about the "six systems of Indian philosophy," covered nicely here: http://en.wikipedia.org/wiki/Indian_philosophy (the six orthodox schools)

Yoga is one of those systems. Within yoga there are innumerable systems of practice, as many as there are teachers/traditions, each utilizing the Yoga Sutras of Patanjali in their own way.

All systems of yoga practice are interpretations and applications of yoga philosphy. No one has a corner on the market. The AYP approach is summarized here. Taking the eight limbs of yoga strictly in order is a very slow way to go. To each their own. Just don't force it on the rest of us. :-)

Progress with the yamas and niyamas (yogic conduct) will be limited without samad
Hi (inner silence) in the picture. And it is not possible to cultivate samad
Hi without meditation. It is very simple really. It is results we want, not the endless delay that so often accompanies orthodoxy.

The guru is in you.

2007/06/11 08:39:16
Yoga, Science and Philosophy
http://www.aypsite.org/forum/topic.asp?TOPIC_ID=2660&REPLY_ID=23016&whichpage=-1
Yoga is one of six... what?

quote:
───────────
Originally posted by Etherfish

If you look at the website, it looks like he may be talking about doing the eight branches in order each day.
───────────

Hi Ether:

If that is the case, it would be more reasonable.

It should also be noted that there are millions of people around the world doing asanas (yoga postures) these days, for a variety of reasons. Every person doing asanas has the option to expand their practice and experience to pranayama, meditation, abiding inner silence (samadhi) and ecstatic bliss. It can happen naturally through the connectedness of yoga existing in all of us. That is where the operative principles of yoga live as an integrated whole -- in us. The yoga sutras only record what we are already inside.

Many who are utilizing AYP have come to sitting practices from asanas. There is no issue here with anyone undertaking the limbs of yoga in any order that leads them home to the joy of unity in everyday living. Whatever works! :-)

The guru is in you.

2007/12/15 15:35:43
Yoga, Science and Philosophy
http://www.aypsite.org/forum/topic.asp?TOPIC_ID=3267
Seeking Universities for Applied Spiritual Science

Hi All:

Looking out into the future, it becomes clear that creating a long term institutional home for the new field of **Applied Spiritual Science** is a priority. Major universities appear to be the best candidates for this.

In AYP we are helping lay some of the ground work for this new science by addressing the following key points through experiential analysis:

1. There is such a thing as Human Spiritual Transformation, and its characteristics can be mapped.

2. There are known practices (ancient and modern) which advance spiritual development in any individual who undertakes them.

3. Practices can be integrated and optimized in a variety of ways to enhance the process of *cause and effect* in promoting Human Spiritual Transformation.

Where Applied Spiritual Science goes from here will depend largely on the public continuing to come on board, both individually in the form of practitioners, and collectively in the institutions.

We do not need another religion or sect. What we need is continuing non-sectarian research and development on the remarkable capabilities inherent within every one of us. The above three points offer a lot of territory for exploration and discovery.

While AYP will continue to be an open resource for use by pioneering spiritual practitioners, in order to reach the public at large it will be necessary to find a permanent home for this kind of approach to spiritual practice and investigation. It obviously works, so we have every reason to be optimistic that this kind of knowledge will continue to find an increasing presence in the public awareness. As it does, programs will eventually be established on the university level. We'd like to help this process along in any way we can.

So, as a long term plan, I'd like to move toward establishing a department at a major university for the sole purpose of researching and teaching the subject of **Human Spiritual Transformation**. If such a department could be created and funded, then AYP and similar forms of spiritual teaching would find a long term ally, and perhaps even a permanent home.

Obviously, such a university department would be multi-disciplinary, intersecting with neurology, biology, psychology, all the spiritual traditions, and a range of other disciplines. This is why a major university would be ideal, since the many supporting disciplines are already present.

Funding will be a key element. If the money can be found, universities will certainly have interest. There are currently several hundred million dollars in USA grant funds being spent at universities each year on "Complementary and Alternative Medicine" (CAM). So there is precedence for the funding of non-sectarian spiritual research. (Research methodologies for this field have been developed also.) It is only a matter of expanding it from healthcare to also cover the subject of human spiritual transformation.

Only a tiny percentage of present CAM grant money would be needed to launch a Department of Applied Spiritual Science at the university level. Within that institutional structure, course and degree programs could be created, along with a comprehensive research program leading to the publication of many studies on human spiritual transformation. If successfully launched, interest in such a program could become contagious, leading to the formation of Applied Spiritual Science departments at other universities. And then we are on our way. :-)

Getting this together is obviously a very long term project, one that reaches far beyond my lifetime. However, it is certainly worth getting started on. Our successors will thank us. Once the AYP writings and community have achieved a stronger critical mass, this is where I hope to be focusing attention.

It is being broached here now mainly for information, mulling over, discussion, and for identifying possible resources going forward.

All ideas and support leading in this direction are welcome. Thanks!

The guru is in you.

2007/12/15 16:53:39
Yoga, Science and Philosophy
http://www.aypsite.org/forum/topic.asp?TOPIC_ID=3267&REPLY_ID=27970&whichpage=-1
Seeking Universities for Applied Spiritual Science

Hi EMC:

Yes, the Osher Foundation looks like a major player in funding Complementary and Alternative Medicine (CAM) around the world.
http://www.osherfoundation.org/index.php?foundation

One of their big projects here in the USA is the Osher Center at U of California San Francisco School of Medicine. http://www.osher.ucsf.edu/

San Francisco is also where the Osher Foundation is headquartered.

Two other major institutions who fund CAM and spiritual-related research are the US National Institute of Health, and John Templeton Foundation.
http://nccam.nih.gov/
http://www.templeton.org/

The grants and projects are all over the map, as you say. However, other than the oddities, the money goes pretty much for major ailments of society, as it should: HIV, cancer, neurological and psychological diseases, etc.

The real question is: Is any anyone taking the step beyond healthcare, and funding research and education on a large scale covering the process of human spiritual transformation? That is who we are looking for, and, of course, anyone who is actually doing that kind of research and education in non-sectarian mode already.

The more we can hook up with people and organizations doing that, the better. Eventually it can crystalize into something that is primarily about human spiritual transformation. Of course, there are many health benefits (physical and psychological) spinning off from that.

It is getting the horse of spiritual development in front of the cart of body/mind health. There is a lot of cart repair effort going on out there, which is fine. The horse needs attention too, or the cart will never be right. :-)

Thanks much for the feedback. This is a very important subject, because if we are going to help facilitate a major shift in world consciousness, large scale institutional programs will have to be addressed.

The guru is in you.

2007/12/15 18:49:21
Yoga, Science and Philosophy
http://www.aypsite.org/forum/topic.asp?TOPIC_ID=3267&REPLY_ID=27972&whichpage=-1
Seeking Universities for Applied Spiritual Science
PS: Harvard has an Osher Institute also: http://www.osher.hms.harvard.edu

Both U of California-SF and Harvard Osher institutes are linked on the Karolinska Osher Institutet (Sweden) main menu, so they must be affiliated.

EMC, would you be comfortable introducing AYP to Mats Lekander, Director of Karolinska Osher Institutet? It would be a start, and might filter back this way eventually through Harvard and UCSF. We will find ways to work it from this end also. These are the kinds of universities we are interested in for this project, since they already have their feet wet to some degree in studying spiritual practices.

I'd love to do something in Florida (U of FL is close by), but these others seem to be much further along, and have the prestige as well.

It should be pointed out that many universities are doing grant-funded research in Complementary and Alternative Medicine (CAM) these days, but few have formed entire colleges for the purpose. Those that have gone that far seem the logical places that will eventually move beyond CAM studies only to add direct research on the processes of human spiritual transformation.

Of course, a nudge from the funding foundations will help a lot, so they have to be approached also.

If we keep doing our homework here, AYP will be in a position somewhere down the road to make a favorable impression on the institutions, and hopefully help inspire them to develop a broader view on spiritual practices and their far-reaching consequences in all fields of human endeavor.

The guru is in you.

2007/12/16 13:28:08
Yoga, Science and Philosophy
http://www.aypsite.org/forum/topic.asp?TOPIC_ID=3267&REPLY_ID=27988&whichpage=-1
Seeking Universities for Applied Spiritual Science

quote:
_____
Originally posted by emc

I could give it a try. Actually, I have thought of approaching him, since the only thing that could drag me back into science is doing research in this area. Or better up, perhaps I could voluntere and they could use me as a case study!?

I just got an idea - I know about a well known quantum physicist who gets published in journals like Science, who also is a potential healer. What if I could create a meeting with them both and do something cross disciplines? Ah... exciting! :-)
_____

Whatever works! :-)

Thanks much.

The guru is in you.

2007/12/21 10:19:14
Yoga, Science and Philosophy
http://www.aypsite.org/forum/topic.asp?TOPIC_ID=3267&REPLY_ID=28118&whichpage=-1
Seeking Universities for Applied Spiritual Science

Hi Scott:

Your thoughts on this are much appreciated.

The main motivation here is to expand the effort of developing and promoting *applied spiritual science* to the large research and educational institutions, i.e., major universities. Essentially, this is leveraging the concept of our little AYP research and education project into the mainstream of the academic world, where so much more can be accomplished.

We are not able to do it ourselves with the present limited resources of time and money. Neither would an existing online university be able to take it on. A lot of preexisting talent, prestige and financial resources are necessary to pull it off.

That is why I think the leading Universities already doing grant-funded research and coursework in Complimentary and Alternative Medicine (CAM) are the best place to focus. Expanding beyond CAM to research and education in *human spiritual transformation* is the logical next step for them. This would have far-reaching consequences in healthcare and many other fields. Because of the many positive spin-offs, I think ongoing grant funding would be possible.

It is a paradigm shift in the field of spiritual knowledge that is inevitable -- going from from esoteric teachings to wide open applied science. If we don't do anything, it will happen eventually. If we do something, it will happen sooner.

Regarding radio, while doing a show would be great, there just isn't time available here now to support ongoing broadcasts. However, I am available to do occasional phone interviews anytime for radio or print media. So bring it on! :-)

What we really need is an "AYP PR Manager" who can arrange interviews with radio and print media outlets, and much more ambitious PR undertakings later on. Any volunteers?

Once the writing is better in hand (a year from now), I hope to be able to spend more time on PR activities.

The guru is in you.

2008/01/13 10:07:28
Yoga, Science and Philosophy
http://www.aypsite.org/forum/topic.asp?TOPIC_ID=3267&REPLY_ID=28828&whichpage=-1
Seeking Universities for Applied Spiritual Science

Hi Juliet:

Thanks much for that.

Are you (or anyone here) in a position to introduce AYP (and the gist of this forum topic in particular) to Dr. Tiller?

Increasing awareness in the academic community (and funding foundations) on the concept of *Applied Spiritual Science for Human Spiritual Transformation* is the first step in the process of moving it into the mainstream of institutional research and education.

All the best!

The guru is in you.

2008/01/13 12:40:39
Yoga, Science and Philosophy
http://www.aypsite.org/forum/topic.asp?TOPIC_ID=3267&REPLY_ID=28839&whichpage=-1
Seeking Universities for Applied Spiritual Science

quote:
―――――
Originally posted by Juliet

I don't currently know anyone directly connected with Tiller--but I will keep my ears open.

The Institute of Noetic Sciences is another one that's local here:
http://www.noetic.org/

I do know someone with some sort of connection there, which I can explore if there's an interest.

Juliet
―――――

Hi Juliet:

Please do, and thank you.

Ultimately, we are aiming much larger than the Insitute of Noetic Sciences (to major university programs), but entrees at every level in the research infrastructure are desired. All are stepping stones to mainstream research and education. AYP is a stepping stone too. :-)

All the best!

The guru is in you.

2008/01/15 11:35:27
Yoga, Science and Philosophy
http://www.aypsite.org/forum/topic.asp?TOPIC_ID=3267&REPLY_ID=28944&whichpage=-1
Seeking Universities for Applied Spiritual Science

Hi Alvin:

Great suggestions. These stike me as the kinds of discussions that would be occurring every day within a universtiy department devoted to *Applied Spiritual Science*.

Obviously, such a department in a major university does not exist yet (that we know of), and how it eventually forms may be by baby steps through individual research projects (like you are suggesting), or by a big leap through foundation funding and a commitment by a major university to get into it. Probably a combination of both.

From our persepctive in the AYP community, all we have to do is keep doing what we are doing -- facilitating maximum safe progress for the process of human spiritual transformation on the individual practitioner level, and build a community of such individuals able to provide ongoing support for the same process in many others.

In other words, if we can demonstrate the process of human spiritual transformation through causes and effects in a repeatable way, then that demonstrates the essential charactereistics of science, yes? My hope is that our efforts will eventually be noticed by large research/educational institutions, who will then pick up on it and run with the ball.

I don't think we want to be designing the research projects as a central activity here in AYP -- it could be a distraction. It is best left to professional scientists and full time students, and the institutions that can support that kind of work. We'd like to stay focused here on optimizing individual practices and results and, in doing that, hopefully inspire the institutions to take a closer look. The idea is to expand the discussion on human spiritual transformation into the mainstream.

We are not starting from scratch in this, because many universities are already doing research on "Complimentary and Alternative Medicine (CAM)," i.e., researching spiritual methods in healthcare. We know of three major universities that have formed entire departments devoted to that -- Harvard, U of Calif/San Francisco, and Karolinska Institutet (Sweden) -- all supported by the Osher Foundation -- see links in early posts above. So there are some pretty big guns involved in spiritual research already. It only needs to be expanding to the broader frontier of human spiritual transformation. It will happen with or without an AYP in the picture. But I think we can add resources and many datapoints that can help hasten the process when considering any institutional undertaking in *Applied Spiritual Science*.

So we will just keep doing what we are doing, and making connections into the research and education mainstream wherever we can. Any help you can provide for that on any level will be all for the good.

All the best!

The guru is in you.

2008/03/03 14:53:49
Yoga, Science and Philosophy
http://www.aypsite.org/forum/topic.asp?TOPIC_ID=3267&REPLY_ID=30803&whichpage=-1
Seeking Universities for Applied Spiritual Science

Hi Joe:

Thanks much. It is an interesting site and inter-faith organization doing important work in the community.

However, it is not exactly what I mean by "Applied Spiritual Science."

I mean more the kind of experimental science that will gain attention and acceptance in the mainstream scientific community, and society in general, through large institutions. For that reason, the more well-known the institutions the better. That is why we are targeting existing related programs at Harvard, U Of Calif, the National Institutes of Health (Federal funding), and other large institutions and foundations.

Smaller organizations we approach in this endeavor must have the ability (and goal) to boot-strap non-sectarian spiritual R&D to the large national institutions, including bringing the funding to pursue the necessary research. The highly regarded Institute of Noetic Sciences, founded by astronaut Edgar Mitchell, is an example of a non-university organization that can increase the visibility of applied spiritual science to universities and funding organizations.

Btw, this is <u>not</u> about directly funding and expanding AYP. We'd prefer to maintain our independence as a dynamically evolving open resource on spiritual practices, and not be beholding to any large research institution or funding foundation. But it sure will be nice to have some big mainstream collaborators out there. I am for anything we can do to help that along, <u>except</u> sacrificing our independence... :-)

All the best!

The guru is in you.

2008/03/04 00:21:14
Yoga, Science and Philosophy
http://www.aypsite.org/forum/topic.asp?TOPIC_ID=3267&REPLY_ID=30826&whichpage=-1
Seeking Universities for Applied Spiritual Science

Hi Joe:

I don't expect AYP classes to be taught at the university level any time soon. Outside the AYP writings themselves, what little planning has been done for AYP classes has been with yoga studios in mind. That is where it appears we will have our first structured classes. And we can expand from there.

As you know, there is a large amount of written source material on integrated practices being prepared here, which can be useful for both individuals and classes over the long term, including in university programs at all levels. But that is for much later. The materials will be ready long before the university programs are. That is okay. Writings can wait a very long time.

Note: The AYP books have managed to find their way into prisons, university bookstores and libraries, and other interesting places, but it all takes time, and needs a lot of help from many who are interested in making the materials widely available. It can't be done by only a few people, and certainly not by one person.

What I do think we can help with in the near term is to inspire more mainstream research on spiritual practices at the university level -- not do the research ourselves. To accomplish this, we only have to become more visible in our present activities. That's all.

If the Universtiy of Vermont has anything going on in research on spiritual methods, we'd certainly like to know about it, and make the appropriate parties aware of the AYP open source materials and community. I see they have a medical school, which is important because most of the grant-funded research on spiritual methods these days is going on in healthcare.

I believe the fast-growing field of reseach in "Complimentary and Alternative Medicine" (CAM) will become one of the main springboards leading to scientific research on Human Spiritual Transformation, because this is where the resources are already substantial, and increasing every year. As soon as we step outside the medical/scientific community, the resources for research shrink to near zero.

Conclusion: The "glass ceiling" has to be broken from the inside. Or, to put it another way, appied spiritual science has to follow the money. For that, it means informing the university programs that have the most funding for research (and education) on spiritual methods.

Several large universities are already into it to the point of having established departments for Complimentary and Alternative Medicine. This is a big deal. Bigger still, full-blown Applied Spiritual Science is the next logical step for them, which covers health and all aspects of human potential.

One look at what is going on in the the AYP community can offer enough evidence on the possibilities to inspire more scientific research. That is what I hope we can contribute, simply by continuing to do what we are doing here, steadily expanding the open source knowledge-base, and making sure those who are in positions to take the next steps in the scientific community are kept informed.

So, if you can point to anyone in the field, please do so. It is about each of us taking the initiative in our own sphere of influence, and reaching beyond. That is what independent practitioners do. :-)

Thanks!

The guru is in you.

2008/03/06 10:17:27
Yoga, Science and Philosophy
http://www.aypsite.org/forum/topic.asp?TOPIC_ID=3267&REPLY_ID=30922&whichpage=-1
Seeking Universities for Applied Spiritual Science

quote:
_____
Originally posted by Lili

Maybe the AYP program can also be connected to existing applied anthropology programs. I mean anthropology is by now mainstream discipline to be found in most places. At Jonhns Hopkins uni there is also a program called neural science that sounds quite close also. Quite likely there is neural science elswhere too. Perhaps we can write someone about AYP as a promising research subject the only question is what is the research question going to be
_____

Hi Lili:

Good suggestion. Does anyone have contacts in these fields?

The question can be: "What do you think about the phenomenon of *Human Spiritual Transformation*, as discussed here?" -- http://www.aypsite.org

Well, a bit more than that, but you get the idea. They will know it when they see it, and will want to research it. Who wouldn't? :-)

Thanks!

The guru is in you.

2008/03/29 09:16:50
Yoga, Science and Philosophy
http://www.aypsite.org/forum/topic.asp?TOPIC_ID=3267&REPLY_ID=31889&whichpage=-1
Seeking Universities for Applied Spiritual Science

Hi Nancy and Hannah:

Thanks much for those leads. Any follow up by you or others will be much appreciated. The network is still a bit thin, but growing steadily.

We'll get there. :-)

The guru is in you.

2008/07/11 21:30:40
Yoga, Science and Philosophy
http://www.aypsite.org/forum/topic.asp?TOPIC_ID=3267&REPLY_ID=35395&whichpage=-1
Seeking Universities for Applied Spiritual Science

Hi YogaIsLife:

It is probably best to read the lessons and hang around the forums for a while to get a feel for what human spiritual transformation is. And keep practicing daily. Then you will be sure to find out. :-)

Here is a lesson with some basic milestones: http://www.aypsite.org/35.html
Why would anyone want to do this? It is first for the reason you gave: Happiness. But beyond fleeting happiness, transcending everything that could ever go wrong, up to and including death. So it is permanent happiness that the transformation offers, regardless of our external circumstances.

More basically we should ask, why do we do anything in life? Why does nature do anything? Obviously there is a lot of evolution and growth going on everywhere. It is inherent in all living things. We do it because it is in our nature. Why do we climb the mountain? Why do we fly into outer space? Because these things are there, and it is in our nature to do and know more. Or maybe we do it for more selfish reasons -- self-defense. Whatever. The point is that spiritual development gradually frees us from the burdens of this life, while we are still here. Wouldn't we all like to have that? It cannot be achieved by tangible means alone. So we must travel to inner space to have it, into spirit.

Is this for everyone? Well, who wants to be left off the train of evolution, especially if the conductor is calling, "All aboard!" The conductor is that voice inside all of us. :-)

This is also where research comes in, to make the call more clear. It will reveal to us with more certainty the truth about the process of spiritual transformation that lives in all of us. And then we will know. As Jesus said, "You will know the truth and the truth will set you free." This is the purpose of science, yes?

I have a scientific background also, having spent more years in universities than I care to remember, so I know this is where the scientific battles about human spiritual transformation will be fought. These will be the penetrating inquiries and eventual conclusions that will really matter to the public. It is happening already in healthcare at prestigious universities, as described above. There is also some more discussion on research over here, touching on the tangible aspects of measuring results from meditation, etc: http://www.aypsite.org/forum/topic.asp?TOPIC_ID=3511 (see the link to scientific research on Transcendental Meditation in particular -- getting measurable results from intangible practices)

It is an ongoing discussion and evolution in knowledge. I don't see AYP becoming part of a university program. We'd like to maintain our independence. However, we can hopefully inspire those who are in that world to look beyond the physical outcomes of spiritual practices (there are plenty in the health field), to psychological wellbeing and further beyond to how spiritual development can produce tangible positive influences in the world around us. It is a long slow process, but it is happening nevertheless. Awareness of it in the academic and research communities is rising gradually. And more funding is coming for this kind of research every year, spring-boarding from the field of healthcare.

Eventually this kind of research will be recognized for what it is -- applied spiritual science. Maybe not in our lifetime, but in time. We are planting seeds that will sprout and grow to maturity in time. The more self-directed practitioners we have producing perceptible results in their lives, the more seeds will be sprouting. That is what we can keep doing in AYP -- keep planting seeds and helping them sprout. The proof of the pudding is in the eating. :-)

The guru is in you.

2008/07/12 04:07:29
Yoga, Science and Philosophy
http://www.aypsite.org/forum/topic.asp?TOPIC_ID=3267&REPLY_ID=35406&whichpage=-1
Seeking Universities for Applied Spiritual Science

Hi YogaIsLife:

Becoming "stillness in action" is the most natural thing in the world. Not a separation at all, and definitely not passive as far as doing things in the world is concerned. We can do so much more in loving stillness. That is why we call it an "outpouring of divine love." Human beings are designed for that. It is our destiny.

Yoga means "union," and that says it all. The perception of separation is what we are before enlightenment. The thing we are afraid of is the thing we have been already -- divided. Yoga goes a very long way to resolving that. And the fear dissolves...

You said it yourself: "Yoga is life." Pretty exciting, huh? :-)

The guru is in you.

2008/07/28 11:14:13
Yoga, Science and Philosophy
http://www.aypsite.org/forum/topic.asp?TOPIC_ID=3267&REPLY_ID=35826&whichpage=-1
Seeking Universities for Applied Spiritual Science

Hi All:

See the recent email correspondence below for some additional comments on AYP, yoga and science. More comments welcome. :-)

All the best!

The guru is in you.

Q: I was directed to your AYP web site by a friend and was confused by this quote:

"It is a flexible, scientific approach rather than a rigid, arbitrary one."

What's the science behind your approach to yoga?

Thanks!

A: Thank you for your note.

The "science" of AYP is in the fact that only "cause and effect" count. Each person is invited to judge the effectiveness of the practices on the basis of results in their own life. No one is asked to take anything on faith, or on the basis of "arbitrary" proclamations. Furthermore, open communication among practitioners is encouraged in the AYP Support Forums, which is leading to clear identification of the repetition of results in many areas of practice, and also the detailed comparative scrutiny of practices from many traditions, etc.

This may not sound like science in the sense of statistically controlled experiments, and so on, but it is the best we can do at this time. I come from a scientific background and have a desire to see the academic science of it become more systematic and organized.

There has been quite a lot of formal research on various spiritual methods over the past 40 years, but it remains scattered. What limited focus there has been is centered in the healthcare field (alternative medicine). We hope to see that eventually move beyond to a more focused approach for examining the processes of human spiritual transformation. See here: http://www.aypsite.org/forum/topic.asp?TOPIC_ID=3267

http://www.aypsite.org/forum/topic.asp?TOPIC_ID=3511#31786
(and next post on TM research)

Admittedly, there is still a long way to go in ferreting out the deep science of human spiritual transformation, but we have to start somewhere. So here we are.

The most important thing is that we are working with an integration of time-tested methods in open and flexible ways that enable us to optimize causes and effects, while leaving rigid "by-rote" approaches of the past behind when they do not work as well as they should. Results in daily life are what rule. No longer blind faith in knowledge that is handed to us with assured sanctimony.

Hope that helps. Btw, the best place to start in AYP is at the beginning. If you take it in order from here, you will see how the practices are built up step-by-step: http://www.aypsite.org/MainDirectory.html

You are also invited to join in the discussions in the support forums anywhere you like.

AYP is a blend of ancient knowledge with a modern flexible approach of applying knowledge in ways that yield best results. The focus is on applying the simplest possible "control levers" for stimulating the complex processes of spiritual transformation available within us. This is how modern science has yielded so many wonderful advances in many fields of endeavor in recent centuries -- developing simple effective control levers for complex processes that anyone can use with good benefits. The knowledge of yoga and spiritual practices is no different. We are breaking out from the limited thinking of the past, even as we take full advantage of all that has gone before.

Wishing you all the best on your path. Enjoy!

The guru is in you.

2008/07/28 15:56:46
Yoga, Science and Philosophy
http://www.aypsite.org/forum/topic.asp?TOPIC_ID=3267&REPLY_ID=35839&whichpage=-1
Seeking Universities for Applied Spiritual Science

quote:
_____
Originally posted by Eitherway

Dear Yogani,

Please check out http://www.andrewnewberg.com

From his website:

Dr. Andrew Newberg is an Associate Professor in the Department of Radiology and Psychiatry and Adjunct Assistant Professor in the Department of Religious Studies at the University of Pennsylvania. He is Board-certified in Internal Medicine, Nuclear Medicine, and Nuclear Cardiology. He is the director and co-founder of the Center for Spirituality and the Neurosciences, also at the University of Pennsylvania.

He might be interested at advancing the agenda discussed in this thread. Ok, gotta go but will be reading his book soon.

_____

Hi Eitherway:

An excellent potential connection. Thank you!

Here is another neuroscientist -- Jill Bolte Taylor -- who had a serious stroke and lived to tell about it, from the point of view of its spiritual content: http://mystrokeofinsight.com

She has become very well-known from her TED talk earlier this year and subsequent visit with Oprah, and has recently come out with a book. (She was originally introduced in the AYP forums here.)

Dissolving the barriers between science and systems of spiritual practice and their resulting experiences is a high priority in our time, because it is science that will inform humanity about its inherent potential for enlightenment on a wide scale.

All the best!

The guru is in you.

PS: It would be wonderful if we could attract several knowledgeable scientists to come and "talk" with us here. In fact, Jill Bolte Taylor already has an open invitation from us. Anyone with contacts in the scientific community, please let me know.

2008/10/15 13:40:27
Yoga, Science and Philosophy
http://www.aypsite.org/forum/topic.asp?TOPIC_ID=3267&REPLY_ID=38938&whichpage=-1
Seeking Universities for Applied Spiritual Science

Hi Markern:

Many thanks for the ideas. See here for some related thoughts on helping:
http://www.aypsite.org/forum/topic.asp?TOPIC_ID=1154#38937

In the case of research and education, it is a matter of inspired practitioners directly approaching all possible channels.

Thanks, and all the best!

The guru is in you.

2009/03/10 11:40:33
Yoga, Science and Philosophy
http://www.aypsite.org/forum/topic.asp?TOPIC_ID=3267&REPLY_ID=46899&whichpage=-1
Seeking Universities for Applied Spiritual Science

Hi Divinefurball and Krish:

Great stuff. Others are bound to pick up on these things and the synergies will continue to occur. The more we can reveal the rising trend of spiritual science here, the better.

Thank you for sharing!

The guru is in you.

2009/09/20 11:22:11
Yoga, Science and Philosophy
http://www.aypsite.org/forum/topic.asp?TOPIC_ID=3267&REPLY_ID=57226&whichpage=-1
Seeking Universities for Applied Spiritual Science

quote:
_____
Originally posted by BellaMente from here

Thanks Yogani! I read through the thread and think that an applied spiritual science department will definitely be a hit and I would love to help in any way I can. I know the funding will be more difficult but I can get some connections and find out what would have to be done for this. I do not know about the funding coming from healthcare related agencies (the pharmaceutical companies I know are the main funders for health care, at least for medical schools and departments, and I think they would rather continue making their drugs rather than competing with self-healing geared techniques.) I do agree it would have to be at a bigger university with more resources and more publicity. Whether everyone believes in it or not I don't think will matter (people get degrees in theology while most people do not even acknowledge a god.) And there are so many unusual and rare degrees nowadays it is surprising - and at major accredited universities - most of them don't even serve any purpose. At least applied spiritual science is geared towards research and has a scientific purpose - meaning there will be work - while there are popular college degrees that don't really have promising career outlooks (e.g. philosophy). I've read many studies on the effects of meditation published in journals with positive results so I know there is interest out there. (Also, there is a psychiatrist, Lee Sannella, that has worked on kundalini awakenings and would probably support this also.) I really am excited about the idea (I can even see some of the courses and material: scientific research methods, different religions/spiritual texts, quantum mechanics, AYP core principles/practices, maybe certain classes specializing in certain techniques, psychology classes on how the mind effects the body (my last college had that class) and another psychology class that studies in depth accounts of spiritual awakening (Gopi Krishna, Krishnamurti, etc.) It would be similar research to the reasearch done in psychology. I think there should be a lot of advertising and publicity once it starts going though.... I will talk to some people and let you know more information...

Do you have anything specific in mind - specific schools, classes, teachers?
_____

Hi BellaMente:

That's great. All in good time. It is a marathon, not a sprint.

We are going to have to work on the acronym though:
"Applied Spiritual Science" = ASS.

A better one:
"Department of Applied Spiritual Science" = DASS
Much more respectable. :-)

It doesn't matter what it is called, as long as the work gets done.

As for what it turns out to be structurally in the academic/research community, I don't have preconceived notions other than the fact that it will likely follow normal university protocols, which is fine.

What will make this significant is the fact that increasing numbers of people around the world are going though the process of human spiritual transformation. So, rather than only looking back, we are looking at what is happening now, how it can be optimized, and its implications for the whole of humanity. It is what AYP is about, and as the phenomenon grows, so too will interest in the research institutions.

Machart raised a good point earlier: Why attempt to measure the unmeasurable? Why not just let the divine love flow? My reason is a simple one. The more embedded this kind of knowledge becomes in our society, the greater will be its long term relevance. It takes a certain amount of structured knowledge to facilitate a spiritual awakening on a mass scale. For millennia, it has been the job of religion to develop and preserve the knowledge. Now we are in a position to see it migrate into the scientific institutions, which offers important advantages.

All the best!

The guru is in you.

2009/09/20 17:22:57
Yoga, Science and Philosophy
http://www.aypsite.org/forum/topic.asp?TOPIC_ID=3267&REPLY_ID=57246&whichpage=-1
Seeking Universities for Applied Spiritual Science

Hi BellaMente:

Thanks much for your interest in this. It needs dedicated "fire starters" and "implementers" before much can happen. It will take a sustained effort to build the necessary momentum.

It can be either the gradual evolution of classes you suggest, or a big fat grant (most likely CAM-related) on the front end to undertake extensive research on human spiritual transformation. One would eventually lead to the other. Both occurring at the same time would be even better.

As for curriculum, the AYP lessons and books are very much that. After independent practitioner support, it has always been an objective that the two AYP Easy Lessons textbooks (#2 coming next year) and the nine (maybe to become 10) small Enlightenment Series books could support classroom instruction in just about any environment, including university at the undergraduate and post graduate levels. So the AYP writings can be used for that. The curriculum is already there, at least from this author's point of view.

This forum is also a model for how open source communications on spiritual research in a multi-national academic environment can flourish. It is happening here "non-academically" on a high level already, and there is no reason why it could not happen in a similar fashion in the academic community as well. All it will take is more practitioners in the research field, gathering together online for that purpose. It is common in many other fields of research.

quote:
Also, I might be wrong, but I can see this happening a lot faster than you think....
————

The sooner the better. :-)

The guru is in you.

2009/09/21 10:09:08
Yoga, Science and Philosophy
http://www.aypsite.org/forum/topic.asp?TOPIC_ID=3267&REPLY_ID=57292&whichpage=-1
Seeking Universities for Applied Spiritual Science

Thank you, Krish. :-)

2009/10/28 12:53:53
Yoga, Science and Philosophy
http://www.aypsite.org/forum/topic.asp?TOPIC_ID=3267&REPLY_ID=59078&whichpage=-1
Seeking Universities for Applied Spiritual Science

Hi BellaMente:

Your interest in promoting spiritual science in the academic community is much appreciated.

The universities you mentioned sound like suitable candidates. As much as we would like to choose one (Harvard is my first choice), it will ultimately be a university that chooses to pursue applied spiritual science on both the teaching and research sides. So, we should inquire with as many as we practically can, and look for one to grab hold.

Eventually, we will see many universities involved in this, because it is the next great frontier of human scientific knowledge. But not likely in the near future. So we are looking for the few pioneers in research and education for human spiritual development, those who can see beyond the limits of traditional approaches and into the emerging wide-open science of human spiritual transformation -- that which is verifiable cause and effect, applicable within any cultural or religious framework.

Preferred university components for supporting applied spiritual science include:

1. A medical school with research capability in neuroscience and related fields.

2. Interest/background in complimentary and alternative medicine (CAM), with interest/ability to obtain grant funding. This growing area of research funding can be applied potentially to spiritual science.

3. Schools of philosophy and religion (non-sectarian).

4. Schools of psychology and social sciences.

5. Schools of physics and physical sciences.

Ideally, a department of applied spiritual science would draw on all of these, and provide course curricula and degrees of its own. Obviously, this will not all happen overnight. It will start somewhere, perhaps with one class or one research grant, likely with one person in the lead, and evolve from there. It is a long term project.

A journey of 1000 miles begins with a single step. :-)

Thanks!

The guru is in you.

2009/12/01 12:27:12
Yoga, Science and Philosophy
http://www.aypsite.org/forum/topic.asp?TOPIC_ID=3267&REPLY_ID=60466&whichpage=-1
Seeking Universities for Applied Spiritual Science

quote:
_____
Originally posted by msd

Yogani and others, just got up to speed on this thread and recognize the challenge of creating interest in a research grant or other vehicle for creating a class(es)in Applied Spiritual Science. I have racked my brain on how to create an opening at the **University of Florida**. Has anyone approached them yet and who is the point of contact? I have worked in the nuclear division at Florida Power & Light for just over 30 years and a number of our employees are Florida graduates. Most significant is our current President, a Florida alumni who is poised to retire in March 2010, has always provided funding to the university and is a strong advocate of the university. I'm certainly willing to talk with him and see if there is a potential opening. My sense is that we would draft a letter with his concurrence (or a reference to his standing) and send it to the right location for consideration. I would draft the letter with Yogani's final approval and provide a copy to our FPL President to show him our intention. The relationship of nuclear science and Applied Spiritual Science starts with the sanskrit work "anu"(atom),and as a pefix denotes together or similar. What better way to introduce the university to this relationship. Please let me know what everyone thinks and I will move forward with a draft, if agreed.

Thank you,
Mark
_____

Hi Mark:

The University of Florida would be great.

They have nearly all of the pieces suggested here (not sure about CAM). The question is, do they have the inclination yet to expand into this kind of research?

It is the "final frontier" of human exploration, and belongs in all of the large mainstream universities.

Thanks much, and go for it! :-)

The guru is in you.

2009/12/01 12:52:00
Yoga, Science and Philosophy
http://www.aypsite.org/forum/topic.asp?TOPIC_ID=3267&REPLY_ID=60467&whichpage=-1
Seeking Universities for Applied Spiritual Science

quote:
_____
Originally posted by markern

How about Yogani aproaching Yogajournal and asking them to interview him about aplied spiritual science and the wish for it to get established at conventional universities? I think they would like the idea of promoting such an idea and interview Yogani. The what is enlightenment magazine would love the idea I think.
_____

Hi Markern:

Ready here whenever they are. But the approach is best to be by others. Go for it. No time to waste. :-)

The guru is in you.

2008/02/12 12:38:09
Yoga, Science and Philosophy
http://www.aypsite.org/forum/topic.asp?TOPIC_ID=3451&REPLY_ID=29994&whichpage=-1
Enlightenment/Realization/Mental Illness

quote:
_____
Originally posted by david_obsidian

Ramakrishna was a kick-ass phenomenon of a spiritual teacher in India and partly crazy, that's what I say. One up for India! One up for Ramakrishna! One up for crazy people everywhere! :-)
_____

Hi All:

In the avadhuta tradition, a philosophy of non-duality (see Avadhuta Gita), sages are referred to as being "crazy wise." It is a term of endearment.

It is a term that certainly applied to Ramakrishna, in a beautiful way. More than a century later, the West owes its budding yoga to him.

May we become naturally crazy wise like that, and all of humanity will be transformed for the better. :-)

This is not mental illness, of course. It is spiritual genius, and it longs to be awakened in all of us.

The guru is in you.

2008/02/12 14:09:34
Yoga, Science and Philosophy
http://www.aypsite.org/forum/topic.asp?TOPIC_ID=3451&REPLY_ID=29996&whichpage=-1
Enlightenment/Realization/Mental Illness

Hi David:

"Mental illness" is a man made thing, defined by certain measures -- usually in terms of disability, anti-social behavior, or tendency to do self-harm. It depends on who is doing the measuring and with what parameters, doesn't it?

While some would judge a Ramakrishna to be at least part mentally ill, I would not. I would call him "crazy wise." It is just a way of acknowledging the eccentricities of a spiritual condition that is beyond measurement.

Many geniuses have been regarded as crazy (or mentally ill), at least in some measure. But were they? Only to the extent society could not tolerate their behavior, sometimes rightly so, and sometimes not.

It is sort of like asking, when is ahimsa (non-harming) really ahimsa? Is swatting a fly not ahimsa? There is a spectrum of views on this, just as there is for what constitutes mental illness. Obviously, the extremes in either case are not in question. It is the vast middle ground that gets constantly debated.

With enlightenment becoming more common in the years ahead (we hope), the parameters for what constitutes mental illness will have to be redefined. We don't want to be measuring 21st (or 19th) century sages by 20th century standards. We could end up locking up the wrong people!

The guru is in you.

2008/07/11 12:35:18
Yoga, Science and Philosophy
http://www.aypsite.org/forum/topic.asp?TOPIC_ID=4130&REPLY_ID=35367&whichpage=-1
Regarding breathing

Hi Gumpi:

Just to clarify, kumbhaka (breath suspension) is not part of the AYP instructions for spinal breathing pranayama, which is not to say it won't happen naturally sometimes, just as it can in deep meditation. Then we just easily favor the procedure of our practice as given.

The only practices in AYP where kumbhaka is intentionally engaged in are yoni mudra, chin pump, uddiyana/nauli and maha mudra, and then sparingly. A little bit goes a long way, particularly with a full boat of practices in play.

Wherever you learned kumbhaka as part of the procedure of spinal breathing is probably where you should be asking for clarification.

If you are looking to follow AYP methodology, then reviewing the lessons is suggested.

It never ceases to amaze me how many renditions of practice there are out there, with many being invented on the fly right here in front of us, and how often we are asked to justify and/or explain them in the AYP forums.

I guess it goes with the territory of being "open source." Or should we say "open season" on yoga practices? :-)

It is okay to experiment, but it is suggested to be sure to keep one foot in the "safe harbor" of an established knowledge-base. The AYP lessons can serve that purpose.

For those whose path consists of "anything and everything goes," all I can say is, good luck. We have a few practitioners around here like that, some who even offer people off-the-cuff advice on this or that practice de jour (for today only, and a new one for tomorrow). Jeepers!

Newcomers, please be advised that, when in doubt, it is best to check the lessons.

The forums are not the best place to learn a yoga practice routine, but a good place to share and receive clarifications on existing practices, with an eye toward stabilizing an effective long term daily practice routine.

Not picking on you, Gumpi. Just taking the opportunity to offer some general info on what these forums are, and what they are not.

All the best!

The guru is in you.

2008/07/11 17:41:40
Yoga, Science and Philosophy
http://www.aypsite.org/forum/topic.asp?TOPIC_ID=4130&REPLY_ID=35385&whichpage=-1

Regarding breathing

Hi Gumpi:

Spinal breathing with intentional kumbhaka is acknowledged as a common non-AYP practice in a few places in the lessons. There is some tolerance for it, since people often arrive in AYP doing it from other teachings (some I have great respect for, like the late Norman Paulsen). However, kumbhaka in spinal breathing is not instructed in AYP, and for good reason.

I have a lot of experience with kumbhaka in the early years, and this is reflected in John Wilder's "journey of discovery" in the Secrets of Wilder novel, where some serious excesses were experienced. John's system of practices as finally presented does not include intentional breath suspension in spinal breathing, for the same reasons AYP does not. It is a practice that is very difficult to keep stable over the long term. The absence of intentional kumbhaka from spinal breathing is more than made up for by a broad integration of practices that can be kept stable over the long term with prudent self-pacing. It is a much easier path, and more progressive too, because it does not involve the health hazards and long breaks from practice necessitated by the excesses that can be caused by too much kumbhaka.

As for CO_2 and O_2, I don't see the relevance of tracking these in yoga. Maybe for scientific research, but not for regulating our practice. Paramahansa Yogananda made many great contributions in the field of yoga in his day, but his focus on CO_2 and carbon in the blood was not one of them. The truth of the matter is that pranayama (even without kumbhaka) places a slight challenge on the pranic needs of the body that are usually provided for by oxygen through normal breathing. Gentle "restraint of breath" (the meaning of the word "pranayama") thereby stimulates an awakening of the vast pranic storehouse of sexual energy in the pelvic region. This is similar to fasting, which causes the body to draw on fat and other tissues with a purifying effect when deprived of nutrition in the form of food.

So, pranayama is for awakening our internal storehouse of prana, which we call ecstatic energy, or kundalini. As purification advances, the entire nervous system comes alive with this vibrant energy, and we call this the rise of "ecstatic conductivity."

Maybe this explanation of pranayama would not have gone over so well in 1925, so Yogananda came up with the CO_2 and blood cleansing thing to appease the scientific minds of the day. Nowadays, in the face of rapidly rising experiential knowledge of both pranayama and kundalini, the CO_2/pranayama rationale is seen to be irrelevant. At least that has been the experience here. If someone can point to the relevance of CO_2 in regulating yoga practices I'd love to hear about it. I do agree that all of this should be thoroughly studied by the scientific community, but that is another thing -- see here.

In the meantime, just practice daily with good common sense, self-pace as necessary, and enjoy the results in daily life. If you want to get the most out of your spinal breathing, be sure to engage in deep meditation right after. Then you will be cultivating both ecstatic conductivity and inner silence, the two pillars of enlightenment, which gradually merge to yield abiding inner silence, ecstatic bliss and outpouring divine love -- stillness in action! :-)

The guru is in you.

2008/07/11 20:46:35
Yoga, Science and Philosophy
http://www.aypsite.org/forum/topic.asp?TOPIC_ID=4130&REPLY_ID=35392&whichpage=-1
Regarding breathing

Hi Tadeas:

The health hazards are those related to excessive kundalini energy, which can be extreme if kumbhaka is pursued without restraint. Take any of the kundalini symtoms described around here (or in lesson 69) and multiply them several-fold. In the Secrets of Wilder novel there was extreme rash, making the practitioner very ill and unable to do any practices for months. It can happen.

A light amount of kumbhaka during spinal breathing is not likely to be harmful, but it is sometimes hard to tell, due to delayed reactions in the nervous system that may not show up for weeks, months, or even years.

This is not to say everyone who does kumbhaka during spinal breathing will have these issues. Ironically, it is probably more likely to be an issue for an AYP practitioner, because deep meditation greatly enhances the effect of all other practices. The combination of practices produces a whole greater than the sum of the parts.

There are some in kriya yoga who have been doing extensive pranayama (sometimes with kumbhaka) for hours every day for years without significant effects, much to their disappointment. This is probably because they do not have an effective method of meditation to put with their pranayama. But then maybe later after a little deep meditation, boom!

It happens sometimes with asana practitioners too, which is a sort of pranayama (restraint of prana) of the body. One day, boom, kundalini breaks loose, from asanas alone. It is not common, but it does happen. This is why a balanced and self-paced integration of practices is best. It reduces the possibility of sudden overflow, since everything is being purified and opened simultaneously.

We have less room for excess in any single practice in AYP, because the combination of what we are using is much more powerful. That is why self-pacing is so important. It is a blessing really. It is like any powerful technology. We have to learn how to navigate with it safely to get the full benefit, while minimizing mishaps.

To do kumbhaka in spinal breathing or not? It is really your choice. As mentioned, a modest amount should not be harmful. The suggestion if you do it is to go light and self-pace as necessary, keeping in mind that there can be a delayed effect in pranayama practices. Or maybe don't do kumbhaka at all in spinal breathing (except some automatic as it comes), knowing that you have more than enough practices in hand already to get the job done with less risk. Slow spinal breathing by itself is "restraint of breath" also. There are many ways to produce the effect without risking too much overdoing.

The guru is in you.

2008/07/12 13:10:04
Yoga, Science and Philosophy
http://www.aypsite.org/forum/topic.asp?TOPIC_ID=4130&REPLY_ID=35419&whichpage=-1

Regarding breathing

Hi Gumpi:

quote:
Regarding kundalini, you say it is the sexual essences rising up through the body. Also, i think you said once that it is also prana.

Yes, prana, sexual essences and kundalini are different deliniations of the same thing. It is all energy.

quote:
I had been of the understanding that kumbhaka that is unforced actually makes the kundalini stir and rise. I'm not sure where i read that.

Yes, that is right. Kumbhaka is a form of pranayama, restraint of life force taken to the limit. It can happen automatically with the rise of inner silence -- but not to overdo it! See my other posts on this above.

quote:
In my meditations i am finding that it isn't too hard to keep my mind on the mantra and i think i must be doing it wrong because you say the effectiveness comes by way of forgetting the mantra and gently bringing back attention to it - forgetting, going back, forgetting etc etc. So either my concentration is too strong or there is nothing wrong with that?

The procedure is very simple. When you realize you are off the mantra, just easily favor it at whatever level of clarity or fuzziness is comfortable in the moment. It will be different at different times. No forcing. Deep meditation is not about "concentrating" on the mantra. It is about picking it up as a faint mental repetition (dharana), letting it refine (dhyana), and then off somewhere forgetting (samadhi), followed by noticing and then picking the mantra up again. If the mantra is there the whole time, fine. If it comes and goes, fine. If it is hardly there at all, with or without other thoughts, fine. It doesn't matter. Though what is happening can change a lot due to the process of purification and opening going on inside, the procedure of meditation never changes. Very simple.

quote:
Do you consider samad
Hi to be a goal of practice?

The goal in practice is to do the procedure. Nothing else. The goal outside practice is to live life fully according to our inclinations, and enjoy! Meditation enlivens our life with inner silence. That is why we do it. Samad
Hi and inner silence are the same thing. As mentioned in an earlier post, pranayama works on the energetic side, awakening ecstatic conductivity, which enables inner silence (samadhi) to radiate outward into our everyday life as ecstatic bliss and outpouring divine love.

quote:
What do you think about the idea that samad
Hi has to become permanent so that we escape reincarnation?

Samad
Hi does become permanent. That I know. Enjoying freedom from suffering and expressing divine love in this life are reasons enough for it. Whether it ends reincarnation or not, I will have to let you know in the next life, if there is one. :-)

Enjoy the present. It is all we have.

The guru is in you.

2009/05/05 10:28:33
Yoga, Science and Philosophy
http://www.aypsite.org/forum/topic.asp?TOPIC_ID=5567&REPLY_ID=50024&whichpage=-1
The Singularity is Near?

Hi All:

From a spiritual perspective, the question is, if/when machines become self-aware (the singularity), will they eventually be able to become enlightened? Will they be endowed with (or evolve) the necessary internal capabilities? And what are those capabilities?

This is being addressed by the human species (for itself) on an ever-growing scale. Will the machines be far behind?

I Robot: "Who am I? ... I am *That*." :-)

The guru is in you.

PS: It is theoretical, of course. If we can hypothesize (and create?) an "enlightenable" machine, we will likely come to understand our own inner process of spiritual transformation much better. :-)

2009/06/18 11:44:17
Yoga, Science and Philosophy
http://www.aypsite.org/forum/topic.asp?TOPIC_ID=5805&REPLY_ID=52499&whichpage=-1
Who can be more doomed than a withered old man

Hi Maximus:

Your story is not very realistic because the desires of an elderly person are not the same as the desires of a younger person. Not even close. They have been cultured by long experience and by present circumstances. This is why the elderly are generally regarded to be wise, in spite of apparent difficulties.

We can try and project our current state of mind into an old age mode, and make a bad or good story out of it. But the truth is we will not know what it is like until we have made the journey ourselves.

All of which is to say, better to focus on our own life in the present and do what we can to open it to the truth that is beyond all stories. If we have the opportunity to help the elderly, much wisdom can be gained by empathizing with their situation, rather than projecting a story onto it from our limited point of view. It is your choice, of course -- to suffer or not with a self-made reality.

But I have to tell you, we are here to learn from life in every moment, not to decide anything about what it is or is not supposed to be. The mind makes a good servant, but a terrible master. From the perspective of abiding inner silence (the witness) this becomes crystal clear.

Therefore, build your house on the rock of stillness within you that is beyond the mind. Then you will find some peace.

There is far greater power in listening than in deciding. So be still and listen...

The guru is in you.

PS: And, yes, by all means, live life fully as you see fit. :-)

2009/06/20 11:48:38
Yoga, Science and Philosophy
http://www.aypsite.org/forum/topic.asp?TOPIC_ID=5805&REPLY_ID=52575&whichpage=-1
Who can be more doomed than a withered old man

Hi Maximus:

Pursuing desires is part of the mechanics of going beyond them, but since desires are endless, the pursuit will be endless if an additional element is not brought in. That element is abiding inner silence, and with that the nature of desire and its fulfillment is fundamentally changed.

So, while you are making a lot of mental logic about life, death, karma and reincarnation, you are missing the essential point. A five dimensional puzzle cannot be solved in four dimensions. See here: http://www.aypsite.org/36.html

We cannot know the mystery until we become the mystery. It is very simple. Meditate!

The guru is in you.

2009/06/20 18:31:20
Yoga, Science and Philosophy
http://www.aypsite.org/forum/topic.asp?TOPIC_ID=5805&REPLY_ID=52585&whichpage=-1
Who can be more doomed than a withered old man

Hi Maximus:

I'm not sure what point you are trying to make. That someone is doomed? Many someones? What to do about it? There is an eternal evolutionary force in the universe and it lives in us. It is us. So who is actually doomed? Yet, we would like to reduce suffering. It is a valid concern.

Forms come and go. Spirit lives on -- that is what does not change. What we are cannot be created, destroyed, or doomed. What we may assume ourselves to be (identification with the body/mind) can be created, destroyed, doomed, saved and doomed again -- the roller coaster of temporal life.

These mental projections to old age you are making convey a need for practice now, and living fully each day. Yet, your arguments seem to ignore the present, which is where we are living. Are you drawing conclusions about what to do in the present? If so, what?

In any case, in the present we are perpetually dead already, so it is not necessary to project far into the future to learn the lessons of desire and choice.

The Maximus of two minutes ago is dead. Gone forever. He no longer exists. It is only conventional thinking that keeps the illusion of him going. Was he doomed because he did not wear out all his desires before he died two minutes ago? Of course not. Life continues eternally, so no one is doomed. Your awareness is still here, isn't it? So how can you be doomed, even though you have just died unfulfilled?

If we are dying in each moment, is it necessary to be lamenting a hypothetical old age? It isn't about then. It is about now.

As I said back when, leave judgments about old age for the elderly. Serve them if you have the opportunity (they are our teachers), while continuing to live in the present.

The real question is, what is the constant awareness (5th dimension) underneath all these stories? It is suggested to get in touch with that.

If you would rather be right than find the truth about yourself, then keep on exercising mental logic and debate. Maybe it is a desire you are trying to wear out before ... oops, you are dead again... :-)

Glad to hear you are meditating twice daily. Are you noticing more inner presence beyond the ramblings of the mind? That is the real you, the One who lives on (and loves) through all this dying. Consider choosing more from *There*.

All the best!

The guru is in you.

2009/06/21 09:30:35
Yoga, Science and Philosophy
http://www.aypsite.org/forum/topic.asp?TOPIC_ID=5805&REPLY_ID=52610&whichpage=-1
Who can be more doomed than a withered old man

quote:
_____
Originally posted by Maximus

Actually, divinefurball, I'm genuinely trying to know what options the old man have. His incessant crying melts the hearts of the onlookers. Is there some way he can be consoled? Like I was speculating before can he do some kind of control over the process of death? Compassionate religious people have made religious rites for helping the journey of departed souls, it makes more logical to do something in the little time he has left. I have vaguely heard about some Buddhist techniqe called po-wa for doing this.
_____

Hi Maximus:

I receive email from elderly folks quite often, too stiff for doing much physical yoga, and too delicate for aggressive pranayama, mudras, bandhas, etc. I always advise them to meditate in their comfortable chair, and they nearly always feel rising stillness and peace, sometimes profound.

So it is never too late. If thinking is there, so can be deep meditation. We will take the results with us, and pick up where we left off, just as we do each morning when we are reborn in this dream world again. Nothing is lost. The important thing is to make the most of this moment, no matter what our circumstances.

On death and dying, it is suggested to read Kubler Ross, Ram Dass and Stephen Levine. Better yet, be around the dying. It will add much perspective.

The guru is in you.

2010/02/24 11:29:00
Yoga, Science and Philosophy
http://www.aypsite.org/forum/topic.asp?TOPIC_ID=7313&REPLY_ID=65310&whichpage=-1
What is faster than Mind?

quote:
_____
Originally posted by Balance

This oneness itself has been named countless names, including original mind. Because all that is already is this oneness itself, then there is nothing that could ever be a movement beyond it. If there is a movement of mind then it is the movement that is the all-pervading stillness, being this oneness itself, that is all that is. So no, there is nothing faster than mind, because mind is always being the absolute oneness that this is. Knowing this is being this and is the movement that already always is.
_____

Hi Balance:

Agreed, assuming thought, our experience of mind, is "relational" (occurring in stillness). This takes us from theory to practice.

From the perspective and experience of the individual, thoughts are only omnipresent when consciously released in omnipresent abiding inner silence. Before that, thoughts are only objects of perception with which we are identified locally. It is the samyama effect (release in stillness) that enables thought to become omnipresent, and therefore infinite in speed.

Before the samyama effect, a thought is like a picture. After the samyama effect, a thought is the thing itself, and much more via the infinite creative energy of divine outpouring.

The AYP practice of Cosmic Samyama cultivates the omnipresent condition experientially in the individual. Is a thought of the cosmos the cosmos? Released in abiding inner silence it is, instantly. The speed of light is a "slow boat to China" by comparison.

One hundred thousand years to cross the galaxy at the speed of light? How about we meet on the other side, right now. :-)

The guru is in you.

Forum 14 – Gurus, Sages and Higher Beings

Those who help us - mirrors of our inner light.
http://www.aypsite.org/forum/forum.asp?FORUM_ID=21

2005/07/13 11:08:35
Gurus, Sages and Higher Beings
http://www.aypsite.org/forum/topic.asp?TOPIC_ID=286
Gurus, Sages and Higher Beings

It has been said that it is not possible to achieve liberated enlightenment without the aid of a guru. This is true.

But who is the guru and where is the guru? Is he or she a savior who comes to the world to save all of us from our follies? Not really. The guru is a reflection of our own inner cry for liberation. This is clearly stated in the old adage:

"When the student is ready the teacher will appear."

This is not a figure of speech. It is the literal truth. The teacher comes when we are ready. The truth is that all teachers, gurus and spiritual guides are but mirrors of our own inner light.

And where does our inner light come from? From nowhere but our own desire. The phenomenon of the guru is an inner dynamic before it can be an outer one. With the inner fire of longing, we are sure to find an outer teacher or guru. The angels and all the ascended masters will come running to help us if we are longing intensely for God. It is bhakti that brings the guru to us, and us to the guru.

When we do find an outer guru or teacher, we should keep this in mind. The perfection is to be found in us, and not necessarily in anyone we meet. Of course, there are good teachers, bad teachers and in-between teachers. There are even enlightened teachers. As we progress along the path we will know the differences. But there are no perfect teachers. Better get used to that, or you are bound to be disappointed. Expecting perfection from a guru, even an enlightened one, is a sure way to lose out. Why? Because all gurus have faults, and we will either be doubting and running away from them or wasting our time defending them. If we take them at face value and gratefully accept what they have to offer, we will be much better off. Remember, it is the inner guru who is always leading us, and that one is alive in us by virtue of our bhakti. That is the most perfect guru we will ever find.

See lesson #260 for more on the difference between enlightenment and perfection in a guru, at http://www.aypsite.org/260.html

See Lesson #57 for more on the inner guru and outer guru, at http://www.aypsite.org/57.html

This forum is for discussing the in's and out's of gurus, sages and higher beings. There have been and are many great ones, and they deserve to be discussed. They are there for us in the flesh or in spirit as soon as we are there for them. They are the mirrors of our rising inner light. When we recognize this fact, and are constantly calling out and communing with God in our heart, the guru will be everywhere.

Quite a few spiritual masters are mentioned in the lessons. You can find them listed with direct lesson links throughout the topic index at http://www.aypsite.org/TopicIndex.html

Also, in Lesson #253, there is an overview of the procession of gurus who came to the West from India (or influenced the world by other means) over the last hundred years or so. See http://www.aypsite.org/253.html

As always, The guru is in you.

2006/04/28 10:29:27
Gurus, Sages and Higher Beings
http://www.aypsite.org/forum/topic.asp?TOPIC_ID=1081&REPLY_ID=6455&whichpage=-1
Higher and Lower Beings...

quote:
_____
Katrine wrote: I wonder.....the presence you talk about that is a "full" sense (in heart?....head?) - it could be your own silence. It is often perceived as "something other than ourselves". Just a thought. It might also be both - a higher being touching you in the space of your silence.
_____

Hi Katrine, Yoda & Shanti:

It is our inner silence, and it is the expression of our inner silence through our chosen ideal, our ishta. It is both, just as you say. And both are One, just as we are One in the rising unity of our unbounded pure bliss consciousness.

Whatever our ideal or object of devotion may be, the enlivenment of our inner silence via practices will bring our ideal into manifestation. This is related to the process of samyama, where a slight intention initiated and released in the depths of our inner silence can manifest outward with great power.

Fortunately, and by divine design, the degree of power (and moral depth) is in proportion to our presence in inner silence.

This is why Jesus said, "Seek first the Kingdom of Heaven..."

With sound spiritual practices we naturally bypass all the lower planes in favor of something far greater -- that place in us where we, God and the cosmos are One Great Dance of ecstatic bliss and outpouring divine love!

In the Deep Meditation and Spinal Breathing books, I felt it was important to touch on this topic of lower and higher beings, not because it is a primary consideration in AYP (it is scenery), but because many people have experiences of "beings" at one level or another, and I wanted to recognize this and relate it to practices from the AYP point of view.

Shanti, your sharing is very beautiful, and is the experience of "higher being" manifestation discussed in the Spinal Breathing book -- the experience of your inner silence manifesting divinity in a way that expresses your own devotional inclination and interpretation. That is beautiful. We all do the same in our own way as we expand in inner silence and ecstatic conductivity -- find our God or Truth within ourselves in a way that is most intimate and fulfilling for us. Then we can express that unique flow of Grace coming through us in all that we do. It is our marriage with our higher nature, which can be seen as Lover and Beloved, or as Oneness, or as both.

The guru is in you.

2007/02/14 10:58:27
Gurus, Sages and Higher Beings
http://www.aypsite.org/forum/topic.asp?TOPIC_ID=1081&REPLY_ID=17438&whichpage=-1
Higher and Lower Beings...

Hi Mike:

Good question. To my mind it has to do with our bhakti -- and our chosen ideal, which comes from deep within us. While we may choose an external structure/tradition on our path in the beginning, our emerging spiritual experience will be colored by our deeper beliefs. This can explain why a Buddhist might see Mary in a divine experience.

So, yes, our experience will be colored by our expectations -- we will ultimately see things in a way that is most deeply familiar and dear to us. This is why the principles and manifestions of spiritual experience have different names in different cultures. But I do not think the names and concepts determine the experience. It is the other way around.

While the end result may be "unconditioned," the description of that will always be on our own terms, or on terms we have borrowed from a tradition. It doesn't matter, really, as long as we have the experience to be describing.

In intellect-based systems, which all are until real spiritual experience emerges in the form of inner silence and ecstatic conductivity, etc., it might seem that the ideas are creating an expected reality. But, once real experiences arise, they can be explained using any of the intellectual systems or mythologies, assuming these are based on real experiences in the first place. And if they are not, they will be clarified and/or corrected according to what is "seen."

Ramakrisha was particularly interesting in this regard, as he made a point of practicing and achieving spiritual experience via many of the major systems (some quite diverse in approach), and living the mythologies of each in full bhakti mode.

Well, not sure if that answers your question, but it is a point of view -- another set of concepts. To be honest, it always makes me feel good when people come on here and describe their experiences in their own words and concepts, because that is a good indication of the experiences being real, and not necessarily dependent on anyone else's definition or point of view, including mine. :-)

All the best!

The guru is in you.

2006/05/26 23:27:21
Gurus, Sages and Higher Beings
http://www.aypsite.org/forum/topic.asp?TOPIC_ID=1125&REPLY_ID=7372&whichpage=-1
Gurus Gone Wrong

Hi David and Dave:

Thanks for keeping it in balance. I think the time when surrender to another has substantial spiritual benefit is when the other refuses it. Then there is a tension created that is to the benefit of the one who is trying to surrender, and they have only one place to go with it -- within, which is where all the action is.

Unfortunately, this dynamic is rare, and there are many who go astray on both sides of the equation, as David points out. As soon as the business wanders from where it belongs, within the aspirant, it tends to get squandered in co-dependent relationships, entangling both the aspirant and the teacher. It is very hard to have productive interactions on the nuts and bolts of practices in that situation. The whole thing tends to get lost in the fog of the myth.

Still, it can go right sometimes, and, Dave, you seem to be in that kind of relationship. Bravo for that!

Oh, and thanks David for not mythologizing AYP or me. Now, excuse me while I climb back up on my pedestal.

But seriously, as you all know, AYP is a work in progress (literally) as a whole and in every application by each person, and there is lots of room for new understandings and improvements. I expect it will always be that way. It is an unending process of unfoldment of self-knowledge for each of us, yes?

Yet, there is a basic structure we all operate within, defined by the very nature of our nervous system, and there are known principles involved which we can utilize for the purpose of spiritual transformation. There are numerous approaches and nuances within that structure, and each journey is unique to the individual. So there is always a lot to talk about...

The guru is in you.

2006/09/13 12:34:31
Gurus, Sages and Higher Beings
http://www.aypsite.org/forum/topic.asp?TOPIC_ID=1502&REPLY_ID=11299&whichpage=-1
American Guru Tradition, Non-Guru - Adyashanti

Hi Kirtanman:

Yes, I agree that the process of enlightenment is the same everywhere, determined by the inherent capabilities in the human nervous system, rather than by any particular approach.

Of course, different approaches may "bring it on" in different orders of manifestation (some easier to traverse than others), but eventually all the steps have to be gone through, leading to the integration of inner silence and ecstatic energy awakening we talk about so much here.

Your comments on Adyashanti point to the presence of an energy awakening in conjunction with the rise of stillness/Oneness/no-thingness. Not having traveled the Zen path, I can't offer further corroboration, but do find a kinship and loving affection for his condition. I believe we stand on the threshold of many thousands entering this same condition. Won't that be something?

I'm currently finishing up the next AYP Enlightenment Series book on Asanas, Mudras, Bandhas & Kundalini, and have been describing all of this from the other side this time around -- weaving physical methods into an overall routine centered on sitting practices, including spinal breathing, deep meditation, samyama, etc. And then looking at the energy awakening from the neurobiological side, and tracing it back into the emergence of Oneness/Unity. Hopefully this will be helpful to the many out there these days practicing mainly physical yoga.

No matter what our path, "experiences" will be a two-edged sword. To move forward we will have them. Yet, to engage in experiences as "the enlightenment" at the expense of our practices will tend to stall our progress. Spiritual progress does not come from experiences. It comes from practices reaching beyond experiences. A very important point that is not lost on the Zen folks, or on anyone who is engaged in effective spiritual practices.

Paradoxically, enlightenment is not an experience. It is becoming that which is beyond all experience, and thereby becoming the experience itself, which then manifests as outpouring divine love in the world.

The different traditions deal with the inevitable rise of energy experiences in different ways. How they deal with this phenomenon has a large impact on how successful they may be in shepherding folks on through to enlightenment.

Unlike the few people who come into this life more or less ready for enlightenment (I agree with you on that, Weaver), many of us may have a longer road to travel with energy experiences associated with the purification and opening occurring in our nervous system. So it is good if we can understand what these experiences are ("scenery") so we can stay the course, preferably while enjoying ourselves along the way. Ultimately, experiences are transcended, and integrated into the divine purpose, which is stillness in action.

This is what we see in realized people from any tradition. Bring them on! :-)

The guru is in you.

2007/03/14 11:43:15
Gurus, Sages and Higher Beings
http://www.aypsite.org/forum/topic.asp?TOPIC_ID=1502&REPLY_ID=18815&whichpage=-1
American Guru Tradition, Non-Guru - Adyashanti

quote:
_____
Originally posted by david_obsidian

There are many reasons why it is very difficult to keep your self-image mature and in order if you are a successful spiritual teacher. One big reason is that your student's image of you is almost always immature and out-of-order -- it's very difficult to be surrounded by that and not be affected adversely.
_____

Hi David:

Yes, I would agree that Adyashanti is at risk, just as all adored teachers have been. All it takes is a few wayward desires on the part of the teacher (who doesn't have them?) and it can run astray in a hurry.

I once knew an old Indian guru (not famous) who was so lost in his imagined grandeur that he had one of his disciples assigned to peel his grapes for him at meal time, along with many other "personal service" jobs. The poor woman eventually had a nervous breakdown. That is when I knew there was something seriously amiss in the guru system. Nevermind the big scandals. For every big one, there are thousands of small ones. That is the system. It is not so different from the Catholic Church, or any other non-democratic hierarchical system.

The problem arises when a teaching becomes teacher-based, rather than knowledge and aspirant-experience based. Of course, most traditions are about the teacher more so than the knowledge, thanks to the benefits human beings can find within their own bhakti. As so many gurus have said: "Worship me and I will give you salvation."

Due to the power of bhakti in the aspirant, it does work, so we can't completely reject the model out of hand. That is human history.

In all honesty, what gurus who can't avoid seeking adoration should say is: "Worship me and you will give yourself salvation."

That is the truth of it. Ironically, self-serving gurus can help true bhaktis, because the bhakti practitioner will benefit no matter how imperfect the object of their devotion may be. Ramakrishna managed it quite well with only a statue.

On the other side of the coin, some have left detailed writings behind, and these documents alone have formed the basis of accurate spiritual knowledge transmission throughout the ages, as much as is possible in this earth realm. That is why I have placed my bet almost entirely on creating writings. It dampens mythologizing (hopefully) and will last for a long time with minimal distortion (if the writing is true).

These forums are for that too. Did you all know you are writing the ancient scrolls of the future? Not to worry, we will be long gone before anyone realizes we should all be mythologized. :-)

The guru is in you.

2007/03/15 10:47:05
Gurs, Sages and Higher Beings
http://www.aypsite.org/forum/topic.asp?TOPIC_ID=1502&REPLY_ID=18861&whichpage=-1
American Guru Tradition, Non-Guru - Adyashanti

Hi All:

We don't have to make a big thing out of mythologizing, or anti-mythologizing. If we do, we are just creating another ideology.

Ideologizing?! :-)

It is suggested to just be aware of the pitfalls on both teacher and aspirant sides, without becoming obsessed with them, and take the appropriate measures when necessary. It is not necessary to run away from anything.

As it says in the lessons and in the first radio interview, "Take what works for you, and leave the rest behind." That is probably the best advice we can give on moving ahead while avoiding holding ourselves back. It is never going to be all or nothing. We don't have to make that choice. We can harvest the truth wherever we happen to be, especially if we have been cultivating inner silence in deep meditation.

Strong bhakti can operate in this way also. Do you think Ramakrishna was worried about the blemishes on the Kali statue? No. All he saw was the divine outpouring, and it was in him!

The guru is in you.

2007/03/16 09:46:28
Gurs, Sages and Higher Beings
http://www.aypsite.org/forum/topic.asp?TOPIC_ID=1502&REPLY_ID=18878&whichpage=-1
American Guru Tradition, Non-Guru - Adyashanti

quote:
_____
Originally posted by Christi

Hi Yogani,

quote:
_____
Yes, I would agree that Adyashanti is at risk, just as all adored teachers have been. All it takes is a few wayward desires on the part of the teacher (who doesn't have them?) and it can run astray in a hurry.
_____

I am really confused now. Surely Adyashanti doesn't have any wayward desires? I thought that was the whole point? That's why he's an enlightened teacher. If someone is residing in the transcendent glory of their Divine nature and see the All as their true Self, who, or what is going to have wayward desires?

And how can you mythologise someone who has merged eternally with the Divine consciousness? What could be greater than that? Anything else you could say about them would be like so much chaff.
I must be missing something (again).

Christi
_____

Hi Christi:

Time will tell. Adyashanti's condition cannot be conclusively decided to be permanent at this early stage. To assume such would be premature, no matter what appears to be. Which is not to say many cannot benefit. It is only a matter of separating the myth from the reality, until the myth becomes reality, or not. It really doesn't matter as long as there is wheat, because we can always let go of chaff. Likely there will some of both.

Ask again in 10 years, and again 10 years after that. Applied knowledge must be verified over and over again, forever. The same goes for AYP. In the meantime, make hay while the sun is shining, or seems to be! :-)

To do that, there is no need to draw permanent conclusions about anyone else. Our enlightenment does not depend on anyone else's guarantees, successes, or failures. It depends on us. Even the sages are illusions on this earth plane. But our abiding, unshakable inner silence is not an illusion. It just is. No myth there. Go for That undoing, and all else will be done...

The guru is in you.

2007/03/18 11:06:22
Gurs, Sages and Higher Beings
http://www.aypsite.org/forum/topic.asp?TOPIC_ID=1502&REPLY_ID=18950&whichpage=-1
American Guru Tradition, Non-Guru - Adyashanti

Hi Kirtanman:

The essential point in all of this (and your Adyashanti paraphrases cover it well) is that it isn't about the teacher. It is about the aspirant!

Isn't it odd that the teachers keep telling the students, "It is about you!" while at the same time the students keep telling the teacher, "It is about you!"

So what's the answer?

The guru is in all of us! :-)

2007/03/20 11:09:27
Gurus, Sages and Higher Beings
http://www.aypsite.org/forum/topic.asp?TOPIC_ID=1502&REPLY_ID=19060&whichpage=-1
American Guru Tradition, Non-Guru - Adyashanti

quote:
_____
Originally posted by Jim and His Karma

Question: Adya is a rare non-dualist who admits to energy being an issue (e.g. he says he's screwed up some people via something akin to shaktipat, and won't give energy now even if people "beg"). I find that interesting. Has he written or spoken on the issue of energy (I don't mean just shakti) anywhere that can be seen or downloaded? it's of acute interest to me, as every time I let go an iota more, I become much more awash in energy, and I'm always banging right up against the amount I can maximally handle. And not being interested in magic tricks and personal power, it's nothing but hindrance to me. But I do recognize that opening to What Is involves opening to flavors and intensities of energy we usually insulate ourselves against.

Anyway, I'd like to hear his take on it, because, again, it's so unusual to hear about a non-dualist talking about this (I think many advaitans open their minds but not their hearts and bodies - which is why they tend to be a bit cranky and arrogant - and stop there. But I'm digressing).
_____

Hi Jim:

A great question that gets at the practical aspects of non-dualism versus dualism. Kirtanman gave a good answer, and in it we can see both the line and the overlap between non-dual and dual approaches.

Whereas Adyashanti (the non-dualist) says, "Open to it," AYP will say, "Open to it, self-pace, ground, and call me in the morning." :-)

It is the same thing on both sides -- it is the same nervous system and same process of purification and opening going on. The difference is that in dual mode we take more specific actions to mitigate the effects for progress and safety. At the same time, we can agree with Adyashanti 100% in his saying, "Open to it." There is a big difference between opening to the essence of energy (which is stillness) versus projecting energy. This point comes out in the AYP Samyama book, where we are engaged in the paradox of "moving stillness" without projecting it. We allow it, which is exactly the same as opening to it. When we release a sutra in samyama (and, ultimately, all the intentions in our life), we are opening to IT.

So, I see no disagreement between the non-dual and dual approaches here. It is only a matter of "finesse," an idea that an aspiring/fledgling non-dualist might pooh pooh. But I suspect a real non-dualist (as in one experiencing IT) would not argue with any sort of finesse which brings on the "opening to IT." Non-dualists have plenty of finesse of their own. They talk about the experience of non-dualism a lot, going to great lengths to convince incarnated consciousness of its true nature. Non-dual teachers are valued not only for their perceived condition, but also for their ability to convey to others how to unfold it. That is finesse, yes?

For all concerned, it is a matter of "crossing over" from the dual experience of life to fully and naturally live our inherent non-dual nature (oneness/unity), which most agree is "enlightenment." Inevitably this will involve dealing with the kundalini (ecstatic energy) experience as well, because it is a phase (or bridge) everyone must pass through, and that brings us back to your question again, Jim. How to do that?

I think it will depend on the person, and their bhakti especially. Bhakti in this case means devotion to our highest ideal. Successful jnanis (non-dualists) are great bhaktis, because they have placed (chosen) their ideal above all else, and opened completely to it. It is the essence of devotion, which is a condition of constant (active) surrender to our ideal. Enlightened people are constantly engaged in disengaging in this way, and it does not matter by which route they have come -- non-dual or dual. It is pure bhakti they have in common -- the constant flow of self awareness back into IT, always "Open to IT."

Katrine has been an interesting case of crossing over, documented right here in the forums over the past year. As I recall, she came here with energy overload after years of practice and personal trials, seeking to make some sense of it. She learned self-pacing, and the energy continued to expand in a classical kundalini way. Then she moved into a non-dual/bhakti mode, favoring what she calls "staying home." This seems analogous to "Opening to IT." Perhaps she can clarify that. So here is a case of deep meditation and severe traumas in life leading to rising inner silence accompanied by an extreme ecstatic energy awakening, and then to huge bhakti and what is now essentially a non-dual approach. It covers the gamut -- an instructive straddle of dual and non-dual approaches, including a crossover occurring right before our eyes.

Note: It should be mentioned that all who are engaged in effective practices are in crossover from dual to non-dual, with steadily progressing degrees of experience of the transformation. Katrine happens to be one who has gone on the record with a fairly broad view of it, so we can use her experience as a data point. I am sure over time we will see many vivid descriptions of the crossover phenomenon from many more practitioners. Indeed, there are similar accounts from others here in the forums already.

It is bhakti that enables the crossover -- an ascension of our ideal from dual to non-dual, based on real inner experience -- the joining of inner silence (IT) with our inner ecstatic energy flow (kundalini).

In other words, it is we who will choose to "Open to IT" when we are ready with the requisite inner condition cultivated through our own intention. What could be more perfect than that? :-)

The guru is in you.

2007/03/21 11:50:30
Gurus, Sages and Higher Beings
http://www.aypsite.org/forum/topic.asp?TOPIC_ID=1502&REPLY_ID=19135&whichpage=-1
American Guru Tradition, Non-Guru - Adyashanti

quote:
_____

Originally posted by Mike

...As to the absolute 100.00% gold standard then my feeling is that with Vedanta (rather like Taoism) - there are plenty of schools and competing explanations but concensus never was historically reached and certainly wont be at this rate :-)...

...on the other hand I guess in AYP then (unless I have yet to come across it) its up to Yogani to (at some point) define what the Gold Standard is (ie perfection of result of application of AYP techniques)?? Or maybe as such a finely focused practical set of tools such as AYP will ultimately just kind of imply an asymptotic approach to 'the speed of light'...?

More questions than answers.

yrs curiously
_____

Hi Mike:

Here are several AYP lessons on enlightenment:
http://www.aypsite.org/35.html
http://www.aypsite.org/85.html
http://www.aypsite.org/100.html
http://www.aypsite.org/120.html
http://www.aypsite.org/274.html

The lessons attempt to map out cause and effect related to practices, so the phrase "enlightenment milestones" is used to discuss the development of experience as effect. The milestones are not intended to be targets -- merely points of reference for everyone to use as confirmation. Enlightenment is not defined in words. It is defined by experience. In AYP we take the position that none of this will happen with any reliability without utilizing practices as cause.

This is in opposition to the non-dual approach, of course, which claims instant enlightenment to be both the cause and the effect. In AYP, we say that the neurobiology has to "catch up" with any sort of instant realization, and that takes both skill to manage and time. The non-dualists use skill and time too, though it may be denied. Is there any evidence to the contrary? Are lots of folks experiencing "instant enlightenment" out there?

Regarding a so-called gold standard, a condition of "Oneness," defined with a myriad of terms in the traditions, seems to be it. But, I believe there is more, and this is where non-duality blends back into duality -- non-dual duality, the paradox of Oneness.

While a person may reach a condition of "Oneness," what we call "Unity" in AYP, this can be regarded as final enlightenment only by those sages who choose to rest on their laurels. Good for them. It is enlightenment in isolation.

No. There is much more. Enlightenment will not be complete until all of humanity (and the entire cosmos) is self-aware in Oneness. A seemingly impossible task, yes? Nevertheless, Oneness cannot truly be Oneness until all have been brought home to That. The urge for this is what drives sages forward. It is the power of divine love, and we see it in all who serve for the benefit of others.

The lonely sage who holds up his or her Oneness as separate from everyone else (contending that nothing else exists) is an incomplete being. Only in giving it all away for the benefit of others can the sage be said to be enlightened. It is only in pouring out divine love that the enlightenment process can continue, encompassing all that exists (apparently) in the field of duality.

This scenario of true enlightenment residing in sacrifice for others does not sit easily with most people, so it doesn't get much press. Who would choose that from an unenlightened point of view? It is directly opposed to our sense of self-preservation. Or is it? For the person who has achieved Oneness, doing for others is self-preservation, and comes naturally. This is why we hold Christ, Buddha and others who gave all they had for the spiritual progress of others as the highest measure of enlightenment. They are the gold standard.

Anyone who is moved from within to aid others on the path is manifesting Oneness. Much better to manifest Oneness than not. Stillness in action!

And where does it end? It never does. Therefore, real enlightenment is an unending continuum of outpouring divine love. It is not something we can take home and lock in the closet. :-)

The guru is in you.

2007/02/13 11:51:29
Gurus, Sages and Higher Beings
http://www.aypsite.org/forum/topic.asp?TOPIC_ID=2054
Those gurus -- wheat and chaff

quote:
_____
Originally posted by Swami Vajra

Check out http://www.strippingthegurus.com and read some disturbing truths about some of the big name Gurus. No one is perfect, we must keep our balance at all levels of knowledge.
_____

Hi Swami Vajra:

Wow. Thanks for that. The table of contents made me laugh until I cried.

But no need to cry anything but happy tears. The secret is out...

The guru is in all of us. :-)

And for the benefit of all those spiritual teachers and gurus -- without them we would not be where we are today, and where we are today is a vast improvement over where we were a century ago. To a large degree, they were victims as much as anyone. We gave them the power over us, and as the old saying goes, "Absolute power corrupts absolutely" ... at least in worldly affairs it can.

AYP is bound and determined to be something different ... an entirely written teaching that cannot abuse its readers (hopefully). An exciting experiment!

PS: Also see this lesson called, "The Difference Between Enlightenment and Perfection": http://www.aypsite.org/260.html

2007/02/13 17:41:34
Gurus, Sages and Higher Beings
http://www.aypsite.org/forum/topic.asp?TOPIC_ID=2054&REPLY_ID=17412&whichpage=-1
Those gurus -- wheat and chaff

quote:
_____
Originally posted by david_obsidian

Yogani said:
We gave them the power over us, and as the old saying goes, "Absolute power corrupts absolutely" ... at least in worldly affairs it can.

Yip! And That's why I'm watching your back for you, Yogani, not letting people give you too much power over them, however well-intentioned they may be. :-):-)

_____

Thank you, David.

I don't want to end up like those poor blokes in the book. :-)

The guru is in you! And you! And you! And...

2007/02/14 12:15:04
Gurus, Sages and Higher Beings
http://www.aypsite.org/forum/topic.asp?TOPIC_ID=2054&REPLY_ID=17447&whichpage=-1
Those gurus -- wheat and chaff

Hi All:

Just to clarify, any constructive criticism of spiritual methods and approaches is welcome here, no matter who has taught them. That includes questioning any part of AYP -- plenty of discussions of this kind have occurred, and they will continue. We'd like to get at the truth of human spiritual transformation, and be refining the methods indefinitely. It is the purpose of AYP and this forum.

Debates on transgressions in the personal lives of spiritual teachers are not welcome here, because they distract from the business at hand -- the examination of spiritual practices and experiences.

On the other hand, I am not opposed to anyone going to any other literature or forum to learn about or discuss the relative merits or demerits of any spiritual teacher or tradition. So there is no censorship in that sense -- anyone who wants to dig in the dirt of any teacher or tradition is welcome go do it somewhere else. We just don't want it going on here for practical reasons. It is an endless quagmire that will undermine the mission of this forum.

Is it inappropriate to be posting links to such literature or forums here? If it is done constructively within the context of our discussions on practices (as is the case above), I don't see a problem with it. We don't live in a vacuum here. On the other hand, if it becomes someone's mission here to redirect traffic to such sites on an ongoing basis, it will not be welcome, of course.

As you can probably tell, I find some humor in the machinations over this or that guru scandal. It is such old news. It is well known by now that there has been plenty of in-the-dirt chaff coming along with the wonderful spiritual wheat over the past century. I am a wheat man myself, and prefer to leave the chaff to others -- the defeatists who will eventually realize that what they have been looking for so angrily they already have within them.

And I do understand that those who are devoted to a particular spiritual teacher or guru (living or not), and to the concept of the sanctity of the guru/disciple relationship, will be upset. For that, I hope the notable lack of guru bashing in this forum will be a relief, and I do apologize for the occasional fun-poking that might occur by me on this subject.

I deeply love all who have brought spiritual teachings to us in all times and places. Had it been otherwise, we would not be able to be here doing this work now ... that is a thought I find truly depressing. Thank goodness it is not our reality. We are so fortunate to have been blessed by the spiritual teachers and gurus. So I say, let go of the chaff and enjoy the wheat!

The guru is in you.

2007/02/14 13:37:58
Gurus, Sages and Higher Beings
http://www.aypsite.org/forum/topic.asp?TOPIC_ID=2054&REPLY_ID=17463&whichpage=-1
Those gurus -- wheat and chaff

quote:
_____

Originally posted by shivakm

quote:
_____
Originally posted by Swami Vajra

Check out http://www.strippingthegurus.com and read some disturbing truths about some of the big name Gurus. No one is perfect, we must keep our balance at all levels of knowledge.
_____

Swami Vajra: The first part of your comment about your experience giving and receiving mantras and how the practice makes the difference was very useful. However about strippingthegurus, I don't take it as lightly as Yogani did. I don't venture into the personal life to gurus. I only want to look at their teaching. For that matter I do not care how where or what Yogani is and only care deeply about the lessons that he has given us with such earnestness and dedication. I personally think that it is repulsive to get into the personal life of gurus or any one else for that matter and give so much importance and discuss about it. When I questioned about the guru/disciple discipline and the passing of "mantra" the question was just about that and not how the gurus who passed on the mantras lived their personal life. Their personal life is none of my business. I briefly looked at how this book tried to smear some of the well known teachers like Vivekananda and Ramakrihsna Paramahansa and I should only state that it is sad that some one would venture into this kind of attempt at putting the personal life of teachers under microscope. I also do not know how true the statements made on their website are. I feel that it is also unfortunate that you quoted such a site on AYP where we discuss and respect all traditions. Of course you are entitled to your own beliefs and opinions, but why smear others. By reading briefly on the book that you quoted, on the chapter about J.Krishanmurthy, I can say that it is a gross misrepresentation of Krishamurthi's teachings (I should not even say teachings because he never claimed that he was teaching anything). Any one who has read the notes/books of J.Krishnamurthy (commentaries on living series or other books) and has listened to his talks will know that he never claimed any teacher or guru status. In fact he admonished such things repeatedly and asked us to just inquire into our own nature and live in a state of "beingness". He never advocated any one path to enlightenment. He was always adamant that no other person or guru can take us to enlightenment and we have to find it ourselves.

Shiva.

_____

2007/02/14 13:38:29
Gurus, Sages and Higher Beings
http://www.aypsite.org/forum/topic.asp?TOPIC_ID=2054&REPLY_ID=17464&whichpage=-1
Those gurus -- wheat and chaff

quote:
_____
Originally posted by david_obsidian

Shivakm said:
I don't venture into the personal life to gurus. I only want to look at their teaching. For that matter I do not care how where or what Yogani is and only care deeply about the lessons that he has given us with such earnestness and dedication.

Shiva, if you only want to look at their teachings, and are prepared to listen to critiques of their teachings at times, I think you have an appropriate view of the guru.

The problem is when a person has a mythological, magical view of the guru and believes it <u>literally</u>. That's guru-mythologization, as I'm using the term here. In that case, the real guru-person is falling short of what they are believed to be and it can be good for a 'disciple' to know it.

If a person has a mythological view of the guru, but does not believe it literally, they are all set. In such a way, you can use your guru as a symbol for god, and love the guru as you would love god, while knowing that the person is a limited person with shortcomings. Can you keep your bhakti without guru-mythologization? One is useful, the other can be harmful.

Can you have guru-bhakti without guru-mythologization?

You tell me.

_____

2007/02/14 13:57:40
Gurus, Sages and Higher Beings
http://www.aypsite.org/forum/topic.asp?TOPIC_ID=2054&REPLY_ID=17465&whichpage=-1
Those gurus -- wheat and chaff

Hi All:

This discussion on gurus was split off from a mantra/meditation discussion here:
http://www.aypsite.org/forum/topic.asp?whichpage=1&TOPIC_ID=2049

Please keep in mind that the same moderating guidelines apply in this topic as in any other in the AYP forums, so be kind to those gurus. They are always a reflection of our own aspirations. :-)

The guru is in you.

2008/06/24 14:42:20
Gurus, Sages and Higher Beings
http://www.aypsite.org/forum/topic.asp?TOPIC_ID=2287&REPLY_ID=34841&whichpage=-1

Extraterrestrials?

Hi All:

From a recent email interchange, pointing to our role in all of this:

Q: Have i made progress? I am desparate to know. :(

A: From your own previous reports it is pretty obvious that you are making progress -- some stillness coming up, more tolerance, happiness, etc. Opening occurs from our core in stillness in thousands of ways that cannot be measured, but we can sense them over time, yes?

Our awakening is the awakening of the cosmos, and we know how long the cosmos takes to do anything. Fortunately, we human beings can come along pretty quickly in our natural role as portals to the infinite. The ocean becoming self-aware of its whole in each tiny drop. :-)

See here for a cosmic view of you (and the Samyama book on "cosmic samyama"):
http://www.aypsite.org/forum/topic.asp?TOPIC_ID=2287&whichpage=2#34832

Carry on!

The guru is in you.

2007/08/06 11:17:16
Gurus, Sages and Higher Beings
http://www.aypsite.org/forum/topic.asp?TOPIC_ID=2808&REPLY_ID=24575&whichpage=-1
guru and donation?

Hi All:

Here is what is in the AYP lessons on shaktipat--
http://www.aypsite.org/146.html
Check the topic index for other references.

The guru is in you.

2008/02/05 10:54:59
Gurus, Sages and Higher Beings
http://www.aypsite.org/forum/topic.asp?TOPIC_ID=3425&REPLY_ID=29694&whichpage=-1
Adyashanti Interview in The Sun

Hi Jim & VIL:

To put it in bhakti terms, is our ishta (chosen ideal) a non-existent illusion? If so, it is one we need. Likewise with the emergence of divine love and its associated actions, which dissolve the perception of all objects in *Oneness*.

True advaitists (practitioners/experiencers of non-duality) are the greatest bhaktis of all. So they often speak with forked tongue. :-)

It is true that spiritual disciplines (including self-inquiry) can be used to avoid the issue. But if they are effective well-integrated disciplines, the issue will be upon us sooner rather than later. Way better than doing nothing. Adyashanti knows this, but tends to make light of it, which is misleading, because it encourages non-relational self-inquiry -- a slow boat to China.

The guru is in you.

2008/02/05 15:01:31
Gurus, Sages and Higher Beings
http://www.aypsite.org/forum/topic.asp?TOPIC_ID=3425&REPLY_ID=29703&whichpage=-1
Adyashanti Interview in The Sun

Hi All:

There is a certain irony here.

Is is less realistic to imagine a better future and work in incremental steps toward it than to attempt to unwind our strategies of non-relationship to reality in the present? Is there really a difference? Both will take time. Both are being unrealistic if they claim instant results. Both will be avoidance (non-relational) if engaged in for their own sake.

Expectations for either the future or the now are still expectations. And what is so bad about that? Without some vision and enthusiasm, whether it be for now or for later (which is also now), we will not be inclined to be doing much to transcend our perception of objects to *Oneness*.

Obviously, it is not a good idea to proclaim an enlightened age (or "the end") is just around the corner, unless we happen to be wearing a sandwich board sign. Promises of individual enlightenment by such-and-such a time are not a good idea either. It is equally unrealistic to promise that enlightenment is here with us already, even if it seems to be so for the person who is proclaiming it. Each person has their own experience to contend with, their own reality, their own time line, and that is the truth for each of us. It certainly can be unwound and opened with the aid of systematic means, but not in an instant. The prospect of instant enlightenment is one of the greater illusions along the path, causing many people all sorts of trouble.

Rather than go on empty promises about now or later, much better we all do the best we can in practices each day, and what will happen will happen. There is a progression we can go through, with identifiable milestones along the way. Here we call it the process of *human spiritual transformation*.

I don't share the treadmill view of the future (or the past) that Adyshanti seems to have. It is pretty obvious that humanity is advancing in spiritual knowledge and experience, especially over the past century. It has been going on for much longer than that. The dark ages ended around 1000 AD and we have been slowly climbing ever since, albeit not without big setbacks from time to time. It is also clear that progress is accelerating, concurrent with the growth of the practical application of knowledge of all kinds, including spiritual. So what's not to be optimistic about? Is this progress irrelevant to individual enlightenment? I think not, since it bodes well for many millions of individuals who want to live the truth that is constantly tingling inside.

It all comes back to what we are doing to better ourselves today, and that is a function of what inspires us from the past, present or future. Why should we care from where our inspiration comes? It is all in the heart and mind anyway, and ultimately transcended. Any stairway of desire used for that purpose will do. It's a personal choice.

As long as we are not setting ourselves up for a fall with unrealistic expectations. That is a risk in all of this, no matter what ideal or teaching we are using. A major setback in motivation can happen when considering the now just as easily as when considering the then and the when. And, as we well know, a setback can happen when fixating on a "who" too.

It is about taking personal responsibility, using whatever motivation and tools we have, and doing whatever is necessary to fulfill our destiny. It is both spectacular and ordinary. In the Self-Inquiry book, it is called *spectacular ordinariness*.

We will know all aspects of it as we move along, and can describe it in our own words. No need to focus too much on teachers who ramble on about their own experience. Each person's process of unfoldment is much more important than that. Anyone who has a handle on it will agree.

For the record, and if it matters, I don't think Adyashanti and I are very far apart on any of these points. It is only a matter of individual background and perspective on the very same thing. If it is the same thing, how could it be different? :-)

All the best!

The guru is in you.

2008/02/06 09:05:45
Gurus, Sages and Higher Beings
http://www.aypsite.org/forum/topic.asp?TOPIC_ID=3425&REPLY_ID=29720&whichpage=-1
Adyashanti Interview in The Sun

quote:
_____
Originally posted by Jim and His Karma

Lots to drop. You've just got to get damned sick of the seeking, be it inner or outer. You only abandon effort (not the practice....the effort BEHIND the practice!) after seeing through to its futility, and that comes after a whole lot of effort. So it's pretty much required! We exhaust the outer world before seeking, and exhaust the inner world before awakening.
_____

Hi Jim:

The only issue I have with this is the presumption in advaita self-inquiry that realization is of the mind only. Wear down the mind and associated expectations, and there is realization. Voilla!

Well, maybe, but a whole lot of neurobiology has to come along to support that end. Hence the "...so much energy and spiritual by-product" Adyashanti refers to. Stand alone jnana, the path of knowledge, skips all that, and the methodologies for dealing with it. It can make for a rough trip, or no trip at all.

In yoga, the neurobiology is the thing, with the mind being one part of that larger playing field. Hence, many more angles are taken, which I think is an advantage. In yoga, the mental component (jnana) is one of the many angles. In a pure advaita approach, the mental component is the only angle, which is sort of like trying to kill an elephant with a pea shooter. :-)

There is really no way to defend that as a viable approach, with so much more being available these days, and with so little success in stand alone approaches for anything, whether it be self-inquiry, physical practices, pranayama, or even meditation without integration of the many other useful practices we have available.

I agree with David that Adyashanti's conclusion about "practices" is rather superficial and parochial, looking at it from an advaita point of view with too much focus on mental algorithms. On the plus side, he is among the more eclectic of the advaitists and, as I understand it, does support the use of meditation to aid in cultivating the witness. That is to his credit and is pretty good news for his students, and for advaita in general. I suppose his Buddhist background is to be thanked for that.

The guru is in you.

PS: It occurs after-the-fact that the perceived limitations of practice (and over-reliance on the mind) may be part of Adyashanti's pessimism about humanity's spiritual prospects. I have many more reasons to be optimistic! :-)

2008/02/06 11:57:21
Gurus, Sages and Higher Beings
http://www.aypsite.org/forum/topic.asp?TOPIC_ID=3425&REPLY_ID=29735&whichpage=-1
Adyashanti Interview in The Sun

quote:
_____
Originally posted by Jim and His Karma

I'm pretty sure you'll agree with this: the mind be transcended. And that generally can only happen after it's noticed the ever-growing number of dead ends in worldly seeking and in spiritual seeking. One does not surrender if one still believes divine satisfaction can come from a winning lottery ticket. And, after lots of meditation, one does not surrender if one still believes enlightenment awaits as a future stop in one's route of spiritual experiences. Once exhaustion occurs re: the outer world, one turns inward. Once exhaustion occurs re: the inner world, one lets go into What Is.

———————

Hi Jim:

Yes, mind is transcended. But don't you see it is the mind you are putting at the center of the process? A tough slog, because the mind is not at the center. Inner silence is.

"Exhausting the mind" is not part of my vocabulary. "Illuminating the mind" is the way I see the process. Nothing has to be exhausted. Everything becomes awakened from within stillness. Maybe it is symantics, but I think the attitudes we are talking about here are significantly different, and with far-reaching consequences.

I can assure you that with the rise of the witness, the awakening will occur whether one considers themself to be exhausting or illuminating the mind, which will be a relief to many, I'm sure. It was a relief to me. :-)

Much better to be considering adding something than subtracting everything, even if it is the same process occurring. Point of view makes a big difference in this, because who will want to add useful supporting practices while engaged in the never-ending process of trying to exhaust the mind? It is a contradiction.

By Adyashanti's own admission, the path/mental attitude he prescribes is not for the masses (he does not expect much of humanity). The simple path of deep meditation leading to self-inquiry and all other aspects of yoga and fullness in living is for the masses. That is the difference. Exhaustion versus illumination. I'll take the latter, thank you very much. :-)

The guru is in you.

2008/02/06 12:07:55
Gurus, Sages and Higher Beings
http://www.aypsite.org/forum/topic.asp?TOPIC_ID=3425&REPLY_ID=29738&whichpage=-1
Adyashanti Interview in The Sun

quote:
———————
Originally posted by Jim and His Karma

quote:
———————
Originally posted by yogani
But don't you see it is the mind you are putting at the center of the process

———————

No. I see the non-dualists with whom you quarrel putting the mind at the center of the process. They are the straw men in your postings in this thread.

I see Adyashanti putting the mind as part of the process. And that's what I'm saying, too.

———————

Hi Jim:

All these points of view are useful, tickling our awareness.

Thank you Adyashanti, and Jim, and David, and VIL, and Eitherway. :-)

The guru is in you.

2008/02/08 12:12:01
Gurus, Sages and Higher Beings
http://www.aypsite.org/forum/topic.asp?TOPIC_ID=3425&REPLY_ID=29821&whichpage=-1
Adyashanti Interview in The Sun

Hi Eitherway and All:

I don't think it has to be all one approach or the other. No doubt students of Adyashanti can gain some benefit from AYP. And no doubt we are gaining from the teachings of Adyashanti, even as we write.

Certain elements of teaching will not be compatible, and others will be. They use a wall, and we use a mantra -- probably not a good idea to use both, especially at the same time.

It is a logical strategy to keep an open mind and choose what is in the best interest of our progress from wherever we can find it. AYP was built that way, and continues to expand in its scope and integration of knowledge and methods. These kinds of discussions are part of the process.

Seeing Adyashanti as the eclectic Zen Buddhist teacher he is helps with understanding his perspective and statements. Thanks for adding that,

Christi. It is good to be comparing apples with apples, and not apples with oranges, even though both are fruit.

I don't doubt Adyashanti's state of consciousness or sincerity. And I can accept what he teaches as "practice," including the way he defines it -- exhausting the seeker -- essentially a Zen Buddhist approach. On the other hand, I do not see the approach he teaches as being particularly easy or effective for most people. Can his considerable charisma and crowd appeal make up for the difficulties inherent in the approach he teaches? Not likely. Zen Buddhism is not going to bring enlightenment to the whole of humanity. It was never intended to. He knows that, and we know that.

This isn't to say there are not other ways to reach the whole of humanity with effective spiritual methods. We can hope for that, and work toward it. The proof of the pudding will be in the eating.

Incidently, there is considerable hazard in Adyashanti's celebrity, for both him and his followers. I made this point about him some time back, and I hope we don't see the downside of it come to fruition. Time and again it has been demonstrated that a spiritual path revolving around a single person leads to instability (exception - sometimes it works if the person is dead). The bigger it gets, the more unstable it becomes. That is one reason why AYP is a different approach -- about the knowledge and the practitioners' relationship to it, while minimizing the role of a "figurehead" as much as possible. If the knowledge is effective and verifiable by every practitioner, it can continue for a long time as a big wide flat thing that is very stable, instead of a tall narrow thing that is bound to fall over, with everyone left to pick up the pieces.

This is not a reflection on Adyashanti's character or anything. It is just a difficult teaching model to move forward with. Sooner or later, celebrity breeds contempt. That's just how it is.

Well, everyone is doing what they can. Each will put their best foot forward. We are all obliged to do that. Let's just make sure it is our own best foot we are putting forward and not someone else's. :-)

The guru is in you.

2008/02/06 11:21:28
Gurus, Sages and Higher Beings
http://www.aypsite.org/forum/topic.asp?TOPIC_ID=3434&REPLY_ID=29732&whichpage=-1
Maharis
Hi Mahesh Yogi

Hi All:

One of the great spiritual teachers of the 20th century.

Without him, and a few others like him, we would not be here now doing what we are doing.

When it is all said and done, what to say?

Thank you, Maharishi, from the fullness of inner silence that you wished for all humankind, and spent a lifetime sharing.

The guru is in you.

2008/02/10 14:02:41
Gurus, Sages and Higher Beings
http://www.aypsite.org/forum/topic.asp?TOPIC_ID=3473&REPLY_ID=29911&whichpage=-1
Krishnamurti, Meditation and Mantras

quote:
_____
Originally posted by Eitherway

I remember saying Krishnamurti's got it but how do I get it? Of course truth is so much simpler and complicated than that.
_____

Hi Eitherway:

This is the central question and topic of discussion in the AYP Self-Inquiry book. How to travel from Inspiration to Realization?

It is about so much more than simply saying it. And, at the same time, so much less if systematic means are applied.

It is my hope that the little Self-Inquiry book will be a useful companion to self-inquirers of every persuasion, and also be a reasonably practical introduction to the subject for just about anyone. More clarity in this field is much needed.

quote:
_____
Originally posted by Christi

One thing we do know is that Krishnamurti said that humanity would not be ready to understand his teachings for another 50 years. I don't remember the exact date that he said that, but it was probably about 49 years ago.
_____

Our 50 years are up! :-)

The guru is in you.

2008/02/13 09:13:24

quote:

_____
Originally posted by Christi

I don't know what Yogani's stance is on the practice, but I have noticed that continuous mantra repetition (japa) has not made it into the top 20 advanced yoga practices in AYP.
_____

Hi Christi:

That's right, and there is a reason for it. There is a big difference between a "meditation habit" and a "mantra habit." One naturally enlivens our normal daily activity with abiding inner silence, while the other divides our thought process between constant mantra repetition and normal activity (which limits the mantra as a vehicle for cultivating inner silence). People with a mantra habit sometimes have difficulty learning the simple procedure of deep meditation because they are so used to mechanically droning on with mantra during all other activity, giving attention to both (dividing the mind), which is not meditation. This is discussed in the deep meditation book.

Which is not to say continuous japa is not useful for some, but it seems to be a small minority of those who use it.

It boils down to the statistics. We aim for reliable results. :-)

The guru is in you.

2008/02/15 13:11:16

Hi David:

This lesson covers the influences of the AYP mantra syllables, including the enhancements: http://www.aypsite.org/188.html

The "I" thought (in I AM) naturally resonates the brow, while the "EE" thought (in the SHREE enhancement) naturally resonates the crown. This is not done by physically locating the mantra, just as enliving a tuning fork with another resonant one is not done by pointing the tuning fork at the other. It is accomplished simply by general proximity and natural radiation of resonant vibration, which is how the mantra syllables work also. We don't have to think about it. If we do, then that is off the mantra, and we easily come back. :-)

The guru is in you.

PS: And, oh, the AYP mantra system is not the same as the TM mantra system, though it employs the same underlying principles. Any effective mantra system will, because the principles are universal in all of us. I don't claim AYP to be the last word on this. Mantra technology is subtle and complex, and I am sure deeper understandings for more efficient application will develop in the decades ahead, as more people develop the refined perception necessary to directly perceive "cause and effect" with mantra. In the meantime, we are doing our best to make good use of the technology we have.

We can rely somewhat on ancient traditions and scriptures for mantra technology, but all is subject to verification by direct experience for both effectiveness and practicality in modern times. That is the difference between theory and practice.

2008/02/16 16:54:01

quote:

_____
Originally posted by Christi

You mention in the main lessons that OM is not a suitable mantra for beginners. I was just wondering... why isn't it? Is it also a crown mantra?
_____

Hi Christi:

There is some discussion on this here: http://www.aypsite.org/59.html

In the language of the lesson, OM is "circular" and expansive in the energetic sense, and can lead to premature energy awakening if used in deep meditation by beginners. It is not a crown mantra (it activates the medulla oblongata/brain stem), but can contribute to crown activation as part of whole body energy awakening. This is why it is used in the second mantra enhancement in AYP, after initial purification and opening have been achieved with the I AM mantra and the first enhancement. It takes some time to shift to that higher gear.

This does not mean that OM is not appropriate for the traditional uses we are all familiar with.

However, deep meditation is a whole different thing, where mantra influences are multiplied many times over, so the initial mantra used and the way in which the enhancements are added over time are pretty important. Obviously, self-pacing in this long term process is important too. This is discussed in detail in the mantra enhancement lessons -- see "Mantra" in the topic index: http://www.aypsite.org/TopicIndex.html

In the AYP Easy Lessons book, the mantra enhancements are taken a little further.

All the best!

The guru is in you.

2009/02/24 15:57:29
Gurus, Sages and Higher Beings
http://www.aypsite.org/forum/topic.asp?TOPIC_ID=3621&REPLY_ID=45921&whichpage=-1
Krisnamurti

Hi David:

In spiritual teachings, there is also the principle and practice of bhakti (spiritual devotion), which relies on the aspirant's ishta, or chosen ideal. It is the primary inspiration for all spiritual practices that may follow. Indeed, bhakti by itself is a transforming technique. It is the primary (and sometimes only) technique utilized in the world's religions.

So, yes, everyone loves a good story. But, more importantly, everyone loves their chosen ideal, whatever it may be, and we should always be mindful about that.

In spiritual matters, we cannot divorce anyone's story from the "professional" aspects of practice. To do so would be to deny someone their chosen ideal, and the primary inspiration for their path. There is no accounting for the power of bhakti, or a person's chosen ideal. It is theirs alone.

We can certainly offer helpful suggestions, but as soon as we demand a replacement, ideological or otherwise, we will be sectarian. As we know, many of the world's troubles throughout history have been caused by this.

It should also be added that if someone makes a physical guru their chosen ideal, the integrity of the guru is not the primary determining factor in the outcome. It is what is occurring in the aspirant. However we may view a particular teacher, the spiritual dynamic occurring in the student is sacred, and deserves at least a modicum of respect. No one can decide what another person's inner process will be, regardless of external circumstances that might lead us to believe we know better.

Interestingly, that applies to non-duality teachers and their dedicated students as much anyone.

The guru is in you.

2009/02/25 13:00:37
Gurus, Sages and Higher Beings
http://www.aypsite.org/forum/topic.asp?TOPIC_ID=3621&REPLY_ID=45966&whichpage=-1
Krisnamurti

Hi David:

You did not mention bhakti or one's chosen ideal, which are largely emotional, not informational, and carry great evolutionary power. Do these fit into your view? Do you see bhakti as a spiritual practice/phenomenon? If so, how would you reconcile it with your views about sacro-mythology?

The guru is in you.

2009/02/26 13:01:18
Gurus, Sages and Higher Beings
http://www.aypsite.org/forum/topic.asp?TOPIC_ID=3621&REPLY_ID=46053&whichpage=-1
Krisnamurti

Hi TMS:

From the AYP point of view, ishta (meaning, chosen ideal) is whatever inspires us to unfold spiritually and become more. It can be a formal traditional one, but of far greater importance is what resonates within us and inspires us. That can be our practices, our inner process, our possibilities, our lover, child, friend, artistic inspiration, our work, our health, or something we saw on the evening news. It is whatever inspires us to act, and it (our chosen ideal) will evolve to increasingly refined and expanded forms as we purify and open from within. This is because as our experience refines, our perception does also, and we "see" more. Ultimately, our ishta is found everywhere in everything. It is a never-ending unfoldment!

So, as long as you have been practicing, you have had an ishta. It is not possible to practice without a chosen ideal. This is true of non-duality teachings as well, which are very dependent on the principle of ishta, and bhakti! :-)

The guru is in you.

2008/03/19 14:22:56
Gurus, Sages and Higher Beings
http://www.aypsite.org/forum/topic.asp?TOPIC_ID=3635&REPLY_ID=31502&whichpage=-1
Samyama Guru?

quote:
───────
Originally posted by Emil

Hi All,
This is something that has been on my mind for a while.
I've heard that Samyama technique was not taught for hundreds of years (at least not in large scale) and Maharis
Hi was the man who brought it back on the yogic agenda with his TM-Sid
Hi course.
Just wondering is that the case or does anyone know other gurus who taught Samyama in the past few centuries?

_____

Hi Emil:

While many have written and taught "samyama" over the years, I think it is true that Maharis
Hi Mahesh Yogi revived its essence in modern times, which is systematically cultivating the ability to act from within abiding inner silence, leading to the experience of ongoing *stillness in action*.

There is more to be done...

The next step is taking the operative principle of samyama into every avenue of daily living. For that, flexible expansions in the application of samyama are needed, in addition to our structured core sitting practice of samyama after deep meditation. That is what the AYP Samyama book attempts to do -- lay out the essentials of structured practice, and then expand practical applications of samyama from there.

The principles of samyama can also be integrated with other aspects of our practice, such as self-inquiry. Self-inquiry based on releasing intentions in stillness is very effective. We call self-inquiry of this kind "relational," which means inner silence (the witness) and the principles of samyama are present in our self-inquiry practice.

The principles of samyama can be found operating with profound results in every part of our life. It is an ability well worth developing. But inner silence first -- which brings us back to daily deep meditation. :-)

All the best!

The guru is in you.

2008/06/06 18:11:30
Gurus, Sages and Higher Beings
http://www.aypsite.org/forum/topic.asp?TOPIC_ID=3943&REPLY_ID=34409&whichpage=-1
"Higher" Beings

quote:
_____
Originally posted by Proton

Hmmmm....my last comment to Tony appears to have been deleted here.

_____

Hi Proton:

Neither the moderators nor I recall deleting a post of yours here. If you can provide some information about the post (date and content), we can try and retrieve it. Or, if you have a copy, feel free to repost it.

Sorry about the missing post, and all the best!

The guru is in you.

2008/10/16 15:49:20
Gurus, Sages and Higher Beings
http://www.aypsite.org/forum/topic.asp?TOPIC_ID=4483&REPLY_ID=39008&whichpage=-1
Guru Kaliuttamananda Giri Swami Ganga Puri -SwamiG

Hi Carson:

Enlightened people can fall flat on their face like anyone else. The good news is that it leaves little lasting impression (limited identification), and that is why calamities befalling the enlightened are often accompanied by infectious laughter. :-)

There is additional good news. Because enlightenment is not some distant imaginary perfection, we each will find it to be much closer to what we are experiencing right now. It is very near, and with daily practices, getting nearer all the time. It is ... *Now*.

For some additional perspective, see this lesson on "enlightenment and perfection": http://www.aypsite.org/260.html

Does this mean an enlightened person can be grumpy? Sure. It also means that they will attract mainly those people who need (or are willing to put up with) a grumpy teacher. Everyone has a choice on how they conduct their life -- both teachers and students. The enlightened and the nearly enlightened. :-)

No one has a corner on the market.

The guru is in you.

2008/10/16 16:33:07
Gurus, Sages and Higher Beings

http://www.aypsite.org/forum/topic.asp?TOPIC_ID=4483&REPLY_ID=39013&whichpage=-1
Guru Kaliuttamananda Giri Swami Ganga Puri -SwamiG

Hi Carson:

Ah, but enlightenment is not what we think it is. It is what it is, and that is a paradox -- stillness in action.

As mentioned, that is good news, because as long as we hold enlightenment in mind as this or that, it will be out of reach. It is only in letting go that we become it by degrees. The rise of inner silence within us is the essence of this process.

If someone is abusive, it does not matter whether they are enlightened or not. People will ultimately be judged by their actions, not by what we have imagined them to be, or by what we think they will give us in exchange for putting up with their abuse. It is also questionable whether a "friendly" teacher should be held high up on a pedestal. In either case, we will be stuck in co-dependence.

Ideally, an external teacher will be relatively easy to transcend to something much more that is *within us*, with no external co-dependence. That is the real challenge in spiritual teaching -- helping others release into direct relationship with their divine *Self*.

The guru is in you.

2008/10/17 13:28:26
Gurus, Sages and Higher Beings
http://www.aypsite.org/forum/topic.asp?TOPIC_ID=4483&REPLY_ID=39066&whichpage=-1
Guru Kaliuttamananda Giri Swami Ganga Puri -SwamiG

Hi All:

Being of a practical type, I prefer to view definitions of enlightenment in terms of its essential observable constituents that can be cultivated within us in practices. Otherwise, and pardon me for saying so, it is just a lot of talk.

By "essential observable constituents," I mean stillness, ecstatic conductivity, and the blending of these two in outpouring divine love and unity. In AYP, we have focused on developing an effective integration of practices that can cultivate all three of these over time. The proof of the pudding will be in the eating, not in the speculation about it.

As for enlightenment without bliss, well, I suppose if stillness did not move one iota, there would be no sensation of anything, but that is hard to imagine for anyone who is alive and experiencing stillness moving naturally into action. Then we know ourselves to be blissful silence, and the movement is an ecstatic outpouring of love. In my opinion, these are qualities of enlightenment, paradox and all.

So, no, I don't think enlightenment can be known without an inherent sense of joy, because *That* is what we are. One may be able to throw lightning bolts all around, and zing people's inner energy too. But without joy, it doesn't mean much, does it?

Even the stodgiest of saints can agree on that point. Enlightenment is stillness, which naturally emanates as joy, even though nothing is really moving at all. :-)

The guru is in you.

2008/10/17 15:05:07
Gurus, Sages and Higher Beings
http://www.aypsite.org/forum/topic.asp?TOPIC_ID=4483&REPLY_ID=39075&whichpage=-1
Guru Kaliuttamananda Giri Swami Ganga Puri -SwamiG

Hi Mufad:

Personality (there will always be some) is going to shade the presentation one way or the other. But negativity cannot reside in stillness. The question is, does the person have the student's best interest at heart? Yogananda used to rant and rave at certain of his students, and then turn and wink at the others. In other words, his stillness was expressing in a certain way for the benefit of the student, with joy still radiating within and through. The video you just linked looks joyful, but I'd hesitate to call it "enlightenment." How about a nice boost for the lady? Her own surrender was the far greater part of it. :-)

As for the right side of the heart thing, it is under the hood, which does not mean we won't notice something happening there as part of our overall unfoldment. Certain teachers may focus more there than others. It is a part of the whole. If we do not address the whole, the part will not be enough. I suspect the lady in the video found this out later on. There is no magic bullet for instant enlightenment, as much as we'd like to believe it. Boosts are available (plentiful!), if we are able to allow them. But then it takes more time in practices...

Hi Carson:

I think an enlightened person has all knowledge in seed form, as we all do. Perhaps an enlightened person can study less to pass a test (not guaranteed). They do have to open their eyes and look at the information to make the inner connection with the objective world. It is all inside us, but the objective expression of knowledge requires an outside connection. This is what karma yoga is about. Doing and letting go. If we are not willing to let go, it will not work. Spiritual practices gradually put us in a much better position for this. Spirit has its own agenda -- maybe even to fail the test! There is knowledge in this also.

By its very nature, the search for perfect knowledge or a perfect being is an obstacle to our enlightenment. When we can let go of that, we will begin to find the real thing. That goes for seeking the "perfect guru" too. There is no such thing, except in our imagination.

The perfection comes from accepting the imperfections and carrying on. Then the truth flows through us like a tidal wave.

The guru is in you ... and everywhere outside too. :-)

2008/12/05 07:22:12
Gurus, Sages and Higher Beings
http://www.aypsite.org/forum/topic.asp?TOPIC_ID=4864
Adi Da (Da Free John) 1939-2008
Received in email:

In the early evening of Thursday, November 27, His Divine Presence, Avatar Adi Da Samraj, Departed from the Body. He was in His Fijian Hermitage, Adi Da Samrajashram (the Island of Naitauba). His Passing was entirely peaceful and free of any struggle. He Passed of natural causes. At the time of His Passing, He was Working in His Art Studio, surrounded by devotees who were engaged in serving His Artwork. On November 30, His Body was interred in the most sacred Place of Adidam - the secluded Temple which Avatar Adi Da established in 1993 (at Adi Da Samrajashram) as His burial place. On the morning of His Passing, He had completed His Writing of The Aletheon, the book which He designated as "first and foremost" among all of His Writings. Avatar Adi Da worked on The Aletheon intensively for the last two years, bringing all of His most essential Spiritual and philosophical communications into a final form. The Aletheon is scheduled for publication by The Dawn Horse Press in 2009. His Divine Presence Bequeathed to humankind a Legacy of Inexhaustible Profundity and Limitless Blessing-Power.

For more information on Adi Da, see: http://en.wikipedia.org/wiki/Adidam

2009/09/26 11:33:42
Gurus, Sages and Higher Beings
http://www.aypsite.org/forum/topic.asp?TOPIC_ID=6421&REPLY_ID=57664&whichpage=-1
Who are you?

Hi Manig:

I agree with the earlier advice that this is a relationship that is for you to explore and develop. I would only suggest to favor a balance, because wide open automatic yoga can lead to injury and delay on our path, as discussed in the Eight Limbs book, and many other places in the AYP writings. It is really at the core of self-pacing for maximum progress with safety.

Regarding Shirsasana (head stand), do be careful, because improper alignment and/or overdoing can lead to physical injury. Here are my 2 cents on it, along with thoughts from others: http://www.aypsite.org/forum/topic.asp?TOPIC_ID=833#3459

All the best!

The guru is in you.

2009/12/08 14:53:58
Gurus, Sages and Higher Beings
http://www.aypsite.org/forum/topic.asp?TOPIC_ID=6811&REPLY_ID=60934&whichpage=-1
Swami Satyananda Saraswati took mahasamadhi

Hi All:

A leading 20th century teacher and author on spiritual practices. A major contributor in moving yoga writings from obscure theory to clear practical instruction for everyone, a trend that is discussed in this lesson: http://www.aypsite.org/253.html

Without the work of great ones such as this, there could be no AYP.

Thank you, Satyananda. You will live with us always.

The guru is in you.

2010/03/05 16:44:05
Gurus, Sages and Higher Beings
http://www.aypsite.org/forum/topic.asp?TOPIC_ID=7380&REPLY_ID=65671&whichpage=-1
UG Krishnamurti ?

Hi Karl and All:

It is amazing how much attention UG Krishnamurti got by saying, "Don't listen to me." And, quite obviously, through past associations and conspicuous confrontations with popular spiritual teachers of the time (see here).

He spent many years engaged in spiritual practices and pursuits. But never mind all that, so he advises. He claimed that where he ended up had nothing to do with any of that background. Really? No cause and effect? Is that what we see going on around here?

Was this another forgetful (enlightened) mountain climber?

Does it matter? Only to the degree it could divert sincere seekers into non-relational self-inquiry, and the kind of chaos UG's life exemplified. On the other hand, if he helps, by all means partake. You may be "ripe".

It is your call. :-)

The guru is in you.

PS: Karl, regarding your difficulties with meditation, perhaps we can address that if you can be more specific.

2010/03/06 10:14:21
Gurus, Sages and Higher Beings
http://www.aypsite.org/forum/topic.asp?TOPIC_ID=7380&REPLY_ID=65690&whichpage=-1
UG Krishnamurti ?

quote:
_____
Originally posted by karl

Meditation might be veiling the truth and allowing me to stumble blindly and passively towards something that feels uncomfortably like the death of this body. Maybe if I stop then I return to the surface.
_____

Hi Karl:

Are you sure you are not over-intellectualizing the process? Where is this drama coming from? Deep meditation is not a veiling. It is an unveiling. While that is the gradual death of identified awareness (not the body), it is the birth of liberation -- the dawn of abiding inner silence (witness) and the end of suffering. Nothing to fear in this. The end result is natural. The drama we create about it is not natural. Better to just practice and go out and live. Be sure to self-pace practices as needed, which you are doing. Practices are not all or nothing. They can be calibrated to benefit any situation.

The realities of cause and effect in practices cannot be suspended after-the-fact by UG Krishnamurti, or anyone.

quote:
_____
What I hear is that those who really do meditate end up with serious mental problems and it seems to me that someone who is considered insane would be functioning on another level which has similar consequences to the splitting of awareness from the body (the body goes on functioning without awareness).
_____

I have heard that too, but there is no clear evidence of it, especially not around here. There is evidence of people over-doing practices sometimes and going through difficulties as a result, but we have that well-covered in AYP with self-pacing guidelines and support.

Yoga is not a splitting. It is a joining, which is the most sane thing in the world. Before that we are split in the drama of life -- duality. With deep meditation we are on our way to union -- non-duality, which (paradoxically) is an endless outpouring of divine love.

The guru is in you.

2010/03/07 09:32:27
Gurus, Sages and Higher Beings
http://www.aypsite.org/forum/topic.asp?TOPIC_ID=7380&REPLY_ID=65740&whichpage=-1
UG Krishnamurti ?

quote:
_____
Originally posted by karl

Dear Yogani has anyone gone completely crazy doing this stuff ??? Where the hell is the door ?:-)
_____

Hi Karl:

Ask around and I think you will find many here coming to grips with their spiritual destiny, which is a letting go. For most it is a gradual process.

Is any of this true? It doesn't matter what I think. It is suggested to check out the landscape of the community, study the AYP writings, and keep up a balanced (self-paced) routine of daily practice and activity. Then you will find out for yourself. It is not about thinking. It is about doing.

The guru is in you.

Forum 15 – Books, Web Sites, Audio, Video, etc.

Resources for inspiration and spiritual study.
http://www.aypsite.org/forum/forum.asp?FORUM_ID=24

2005/07/13 12:00:28
Books, Web Sites, Audio, Video, etc.
http://www.aypsite.org/forum/topic.asp?TOPIC_ID=287
Books, Web Sites, Audio, Video, etc.

One of the Niyamas (observances) is svadhyaya, which means spiritual study.

An interesting thing happens with many people when they begin to meditate. They become voracious readers of spiritual literature. It is one of the many examples of how the limbs of yoga are connected in us. Do one aspect of yoga, and the other aspects are stimulated.

There is plenty out there to read and study. In AYP, we try and point to as many resources as possible.

Of particular interest are the "Yoga Texts" near the bottom of the list in the AYP links section, at http://www.aypsite.org/Links.html

There is also a book list on this web site with over 400 yoga and spiritual titles, with direct links to Amazon.com. See http://www.aypsite.org/booklist.html

Increasingly, web sites, audio recordings, and videos are becoming available that can add new dimensions to our spiritual study.

Finally, there is the growing family of AYP books, ebooks and audiobooks (coming soon), which can be found at http://www.aypsite.org/books.html

This forum is the place to discuss all those great books, web sites, audios, and videos you have run across in your travels.

The guru is in you.

2005/10/17 09:12:53
Books, Web Sites, Audio, Video, etc.
http://www.aypsite.org/forum/topic.asp?TOPIC_ID=302&REPLY_ID=995&whichpage=-1
The Secrets of Wilder

Hi Trip:

Thanks for sharing your Secrets of Wilder reading experience.

Keep in mind that John Wilder's journey is a process of discovery that is not perfect. This shows the human side of the spiritual adventure as many of us might experience it if we traveled a similar road, including some of the wrong turns and blind alleys that can happen. Fortunately, after a rough and tumble ride, our "every man," John Wilder, finally does get it together (big time), and along the way he is increasingly in a position to transmit the knowledge of human spiritual transformation to many others, beginning with his dear lovemate, Devi Duran.

As for consistency with AYP, it is as much as possible given the evolving nature of the knowledge in the story. The "practice chart" on page 209 is the best place to make such a comparison, and you will find at that late stage in the story, the correspondence is there -- consistent with the late stage sequencing of AYP practices, which is a bit different from early stage sequencing.

One way to view the AYP lessons is as being where the Secrets of Wilder knowledge arrive in the end ... or even beyond the Secrets of Wilder story, which is, in fact, the truth. The first drafts of the novel were written before the AYP lessons were written. In some ways, the Secrets of Wilder is a history of how the AYP lessons came to be. That is to say, the AYP lessons are the more advanced and complete rendition of the knowledge. The Secrets of Wilder is, in part, about how we got here -- to a comprehensive open system of practices. In other ways, it is about where we are going.

Welcome to the new paradigm! :-)

The guru is in you.

2005/11/04 22:32:08
Books, Web Sites, Audio, Video, etc.
http://www.aypsite.org/forum/topic.asp?TOPIC_ID=302&REPLY_ID=1389&whichpage=-1
The Secrets of Wilder

Hi Meg:

The dissent is welcome. Not everyone wants to be around for the messy business of growing a tree. It's perfectly fine (and smart) to come and enjoy the fruit. Pass the sweet oranges, please. :-)

More fruit coming soon!

The guru is in you.

2006/05/24 00:09:46
Books, Web Sites, Audio, Video, etc.
http://www.aypsite.org/forum/topic.asp?TOPIC_ID=329&REPLY_ID=7286&whichpage=-1
Reply Topic - Books, Web Sites, Audio, Video, etc.

Hi Sadhak:

The best "book" is a nervous system awakening with inner silence and ecstatic conductivity. It tells all. Before that, the best books are those that help provide the means to cultivate that awakening. Also good are books that inspire the quest and the desire to practice daily.

While there are plenty of books that inspire, those that offer effective and organized practices are few and far between. Satyananda did a fine job with his, as did Swami Rama and a few others. AYP has been developed, in part, to help fill the void in books on practices, in the hope that then we will have many more of the living books -- awakening human nervous systems. Can't have too many of those!

So I agree with you 100% about reading priorities on the path. On the other hand, there is no telling from where we will find our next inspiration -- it can come from the most unexpected place. With strong bhakti, everything in life becomes "the book." The target keeps getting bigger and bigger, or so it seems as the love pours out. Fullness pouring into fullness...

The guru is in you.

2006/05/25 22:37:54
Books, Web Sites, Audio, Video, etc.
http://www.aypsite.org/forum/topic.asp?TOPIC_ID=329&REPLY_ID=7332&whichpage=-1
Reply Topic - Books, Web Sites, Audio, Video, etc.

Hi Sadhak:

Only you can know whether to pursue a particular course of practice. It will resonate in your heart and in your bhakti if it is a means that will help bring you good progress. If it is, then you will find the resources and teacher necessary to fulfill it. Rather, they will find you!

The guru is in you.

2007/01/03 11:56:31
Books, Web Sites, Audio, Video, etc.
http://www.aypsite.org/forum/topic.asp?TOPIC_ID=425&REPLY_ID=15339&whichpage=-1
Movies Anyone?
Movie: East Of Eden -- (based on John Steinbeck's novel) -- James Dean's first Hollywood picture, 1955. A useful study on good and evil, and how the labels can mask the opposite. Moral of the story -- The heart and free choice reveal a higher path than rules of conduct and labels.
2007/06/29 09:19:46
Books, Web Sites, Audio, Video, etc.
http://www.aypsite.org/forum/topic.asp?TOPIC_ID=425&REPLY_ID=23636&whichpage=-1
Movies Anyone?

Hi All:

"Peaceful Warrior" is out on DVD now. They did a pretty good job with it. 25 years from book to movie.

The focus is on personal spiritual choices in relation to athletics (gymnastics), and day-to-day living.

http://www.amazon.com/Peaceful-Warrior-Widescreen-Scott-Mechlowicz/dp/B000QEIOSU/ref=pd_bbs_sr_1/103-4409649-9630267?ie=UTF8&s=dvd&qid=1183122767&sr=1-1

http://www.blockbuster.com/catalog/movieDetails/278546

The guru is in you.

2007/08/15 15:46:29
Books, Web Sites, Audio, Video, etc.
http://www.aypsite.org/forum/topic.asp?TOPIC_ID=425&REPLY_ID=24825&whichpage=-1
Movies Anyone?

Hi All:

DVD -- **The Last Mimzy** -- A fun mainstream kids/family fantasy/sci fi adventure with sri yantra/mandala (really!), worm-hole time travel, nano-technology, human DNA key, Alice in Wonderland connection, miracles galore, and saving the planet (of course).

Something for almost everyone ... I especially liked the introduction of Sri Yantra (see AYP illustrations) into the mainstream, and not a bad job of it either. It will lead to broader awareness of spiritual practices. :-)

The guru is in you.

2007/12/23 00:04:00
Books, Web Sites, Audio, Video, etc.
http://www.aypsite.org/forum/topic.asp?TOPIC_ID=425&REPLY_ID=28152&whichpage=-1
Movies Anyone?

Hi All:

Harvey, (1950), with Jimmy Stewart (one of his personal favorites)

The story of a man who has a friend named Harvey, who is an invisible 6 foot 4 inch rabbit.

A clever and humorous story about sanity/insanity and (ultimately) spirituality.

It starts out slow and keeps getting better and better, with surprises along the way. Wonderful ending.

All the best!

The guru is in you.

2008/10/29 16:25:09
Books, Web Sites, Audio, Video, etc.
http://www.aypsite.org/forum/topic.asp?TOPIC_ID=425&REPLY_ID=39628&whichpage=-1
Movies Anyone?
Yogis of Tibet: A Film for Posterity
(Available on Netflix)

A rare up-close look at the few remaining Tibetan ascetic yogis and their practices, made possible by 50 years of Chinese oppression in Tibet. I would have felt better if it came to us by another route, but am thankful for the valuable perspectives all the same. You will see bits and pieces of AYP sprinkled through here, plus other elements of practice that have been discussed in these forums. Pretty illuminating stuff.

The guru is in you.

PS: Some clips from this film can also be found on YouTube.

2005/12/08 23:21:42
Books, Web Sites, Audio, Video, etc.
http://www.aypsite.org/forum/topic.asp?TOPIC_ID=631
Deep Meditation - Pathway to Personal Freedom

Hi All:

The new AYP *Deep Meditation* book is up on Amazon. The cover image and description should be up there soon.

I have modified the books page on all three websites to include the new book and also upcoming *AYP Enlightenment Series* books on Spinal Breathing, Tantra and more. So the books page is now both an ordering links center and a road map for anyone who is interested in current AYP books or future ones scheduled for publication. And it is an open challenge for me to keep to the schedule too. I always like a challenge. :-)

You can find the revised books page here: http://www.aypsite.org/books.html

The web site side bar has also been updated to include the *Deep Meditation* cover image with a built-in link to its Amazon USA page. Also, a brief announcement is included on the top line of the home page. Soon there will be announcements in the AYP Yahoo groups as well.

So *Deep Meditation* is officially launched. Many of you already have copies on the way via the free offer for handing the books out, which I greatly appreciate your help on (and the offer is still open). I look forward to receiving your feedback on the book, and to your reviews on Amazon.

The guru is in you.

2005/12/09 11:28:09
Books, Web Sites, Audio, Video, etc.
http://www.aypsite.org/forum/topic.asp?TOPIC_ID=631&REPLY_ID=1852&whichpage=-1
Deep Meditation - Pathway to Personal Freedom

Hi Near:

The eBook version of *Deep Meditation* should be out within a few days. You will know either by checking on Amazon or when the eBook links on the AYP books page go "live."

If you want to hand some books out, I will send you some for free. Just respond to the offer. :-)

The guru is in you.

2005/12/11 00:04:47
Books, Web Sites, Audio, Video, etc.
http://www.aypsite.org/forum/topic.asp?TOPIC_ID=631&REPLY_ID=1884&whichpage=-1
Deep Meditation - Pathway to Personal Freedom
Near and others:

The *Deep Meditation* ebook just showed up on Diesel ebooks, it is all there and ready to download. It shows as not printable, but it is.

I expect we will see it on Amazon very soon.

The guru is in you.

2005/12/11 09:40:59
Books, Web Sites, Audio, Video, etc.
http://www.aypsite.org/forum/topic.asp?TOPIC_ID=631&REPLY_ID=1888&whichpage=-1
Deep Meditation - Pathway to Personal Freedom

Okay, both Amazon and Diesel **ebook links** for "Deep Meditation" will be working shortly on the AYP books page -- http://www.aypsite.org/books.html

As some of you may have noticed, I opened the free book offer up to the AYP Yahoo readership, and have 30 requests so far, and growing. That is in addition to the 15 or so we have done here in the forums. Lots of books going out, which is just as it should be for this one, because it is for the mainstream.

Thanks all!

The guru is in you.

2005/12/13 15:08:25
Books, Web Sites, Audio, Video, etc.
http://www.aypsite.org/forum/topic.asp?TOPIC_ID=631&REPLY_ID=1934&whichpage=-1
Deep Meditation - Pathway to Personal Freedom

Hi Alvin:

The *Deep Meditation* table of contents is copied below. Also see the first Amazon review here. I hope the first of many. It is a small book and will easily fit in your room. The *AYP Easy Lessons* book is much bigger, but you should squeeze that one in there too. And don't forget the *Secrets of Wilder*. They can all be downloaded in ebook form, which takes no room at all beyond the computer space. :-)

The guru is in you.

Table of Contents

Chapter 1 – "Who Am I?" 1

Chapter 2 – Deep Meditation 7
How to Meditate 7
When and Where to Meditate 11
Questions On Your First Meditation 14
The Possibilities 19

Chapter 3 – Steps of Progress 23
Navigating the Path of Inner Purification 23
Visions and Energy Experiences 69
The Rise of Inner Silence – The Witness 82
Stillness in Action 86

Chapter 4 – Freedom 90
Unshakable Inner Silence and Ecstasy 91
Refinement to Ecstatic Bliss 95
Expansion of Divine Love in the World 97

Further Reading and Support 103

2006/01/31 11:47:32
Books, Web Sites, Audio, Video, etc.
http://www.aypsite.org/forum/topic.asp?TOPIC_ID=776&REPLY_ID=2921&whichpage=-1
questions/suggestions on the AYP books

Hi Alvin:

The AYP ebooks have exactly the same content as the physical books, are not changing, and are sold separately. I am not set up to sell (or give) them to anyone -- it is quite involved to become an e-tailer/downloader of ebooks. I'd prefer to be a writer rather than a book seller. The ebooks go through the worldwide distribution channels and can be bought anywhere through many retailers at about half the price of the physical books. The physical books are distributed worldwide too, though it is not as easy to obtain them everywhere around the world due to shipping costs. Where did you order from? Amazon Japan is closest to you, but not all Amazon sites discount the same or have the books immediately available. Larger discounts can sometimes offset higher shipping costs, and if the books are immediately available (like at Amazon USA) the wait can be less even though the distance is more.

There could be other book sellers close by, including e-tailers. It depends on who is interested in selling the books. See the Google links near the bottom of the books page for many more sources for the AYP books and ebooks around the world: http://www.aypsite.org/books.html

It takes time to develop fluid distribution of physical books. Once the initial broad distribution ordering channels have been set up, which has been done, the greatest single factor in retail availability is **customer demand**. Think about it. If you owned a bookstore, would you carry a book that no one was coming in and asking for? Only if you made it your project to sell that book to the public. For the rest, you'd have to go with what people were coming in looking for, or go broke. That is why retailers can't afford to stock books for purely idealistic reasons. Their survival is at stake. A lot is being done to inform retailers everywhere about the AYP books. They will be in at least four big trade shows this year with huge international attendance by book sellers. But if the public is not asking for the books, the stores will not be doing much to promote them. Bookstore walk-ins by readers are a great way to increase awareness, and getting the books on the shelves can be achieved that way. But it will take more people walking in buying them to fuel the process. It is the same with e-tailers. They will stock the books in their warehouse only if there is demand. Amazon does stock the AYP books in the USA, and on a limited basis in the UK, but not in Canada, the rest of Europe or Japan. That is another reason why you have to wait. They are ordering the books after you are ordering them. It takes 48 hours for the printer to ship an order from the USA or UK to the retail seller. That all has to happen before the retailer can ship the books to you. Once it is stocked in the e-tailer's warehouse, then it is out the door to you within 24 hours when you order on the web.

The best thing we can do to promote the AYP books and increase distribution is to increase public demand. If public demand increases, more booksellers will carry them in stock. Also, with increasing public demand, it will be much easier to publish the books locally in India, China, Australia, and other places that are far from the current sources in the USA and UK. Every publisher, distributor and bookstore wants a book that the public is asking for. Customer demand. It will take time. Years. Maybe many years. AYP is not going out of style any time soon. In the meantime, the best primary focus for me to have is on completing the writings, which will take a few more years, at least. Then maybe I will have more time to be a salesman.

I am hoping all of you will help fill in before then. :-)

Thanks so much for your support. Sorry you have to wait. Hopefully someday no one will have to wait for spiritual knowledge. I am doing the best I can. I hope you understand I cannot give it all away online without going broke myself -- which would stop AYP dead in its tracks. Plus, I think it is very important to have the books out there, independent of the Internet. We need to find a balance, with support coming from all sides. It cannot be from one side only. That will not work in the long run. The process of spreading this kind of knowledge needs many supporters willing to take appropriate actions over a long period of time.

It is a long term process -- like practices -- gradually dissolving obstructions so the divine can flow through us and out into the world. We'll get there, in every way...

The guru is in you.

2006/02/01 12:31:09
Books, Web Sites, Audio, Video, etc.
http://www.aypsite.org/forum/topic.asp?TOPIC_ID=776&REPLY_ID=2946&whichpage=-1
questions/suggestions on the AYP books

Hi Alvin:

If you suggest to http://www.yogamatters.com that they list and carry the AYP books, they can do it. Simple as that. As mentioned, the AYP books are available to retailers (including online ones) through major distributors in the USA and UK -- http://www.aypsite.org/books.html

Just as we can do physical walk-ins requesting our local bookstores consider carrying the AYP books, we can also do online walk-ins. It is the same thing.

All the best!

The guru is in you.

2006/02/01 12:39:06
Books, Web Sites, Audio, Video, etc.
http://www.aypsite.org/forum/topic.asp?TOPIC_ID=776&REPLY_ID=2947&whichpage=-1
questions/suggestions on the AYP books
PS -- Oh, guess what?
http://www.yogamatters.com does have the AYP Easy Lessons book -- Here. Good price too. But they have not listed the other AYP books yet. Looks like they need recommendations on the Secrets of Wilder and Deep Meditation. Apparently that is how they select their offerings -- by recomendations from yogis/yoginis.

They also have a yoga store in **North London**. A place for somebody to do an AYP walk-in! Pick up a yoga mat and a leotard while you are there. :-)

2006/02/02 12:43:16
Books, Web Sites, Audio, Video, etc.
http://www.aypsite.org/forum/topic.asp?TOPIC_ID=778&REPLY_ID=2987&whichpage=-1
Yoga Nidra

Hi Riptiz and All:

I don't know the author of the subject CD, Swami Janakananda. Perhaps you are referring to Swami Jnaneshvara ("Swami J"), with whom I have had some contact in the past. We do not agree on all things, but there is no rating going on that I am aware of. All teachers are respected here. Everyone has an oar (or two) in the water and is rowing the boat forward the best they know how.

If you want guru ratings, go to Sarlo's Guru Rating Service, where you can see every guru under the sun rated, often with tongue in cheek. He even rated me, sort of. Sarlo comes from an Osho/Rajneesh background, which explains in part his whimsical approach, plus a slight bias toward you-know-who. :-)

On yoga nidra, I will get to it in more detail someday. It is a bit of a fad at the moment -- a bit overrated. In AYP, we view it mainly as effect rather than cause -- the natural rise of inner silence (the witness) around the clock, including during sleep, as a result of sitting practices, particularly deep meditation and samyama. Is listening to yoga nidra CDs okay? Sure, as long as it is not done at the expense of sitting practices, or our rest.

The guru is in you.

2006/03/01 11:28:04
Books, Web Sites, Audio, Video, etc.
http://www.aypsite.org/forum/topic.asp?TOPIC_ID=858
AYP eBook Prices Reduced

Hi All:

Effective today, the eBook prices for the *AYP - Easy Lessons for Ecstatic Living* book and *The Secrets of Wilder* novel have been reduced 13% and 10%, respectively.

This, combined with retailer discounts, will help make them more affordable for download around the world.

The *Deep Meditation - Pathway to Personal Freedom* eBook price remains the same.

With these changes, all of the AYP eBook prices are now one-half the paperback prices, before retailer discounts are applied.

For details, see the eBook and paperback links here: http://www.aypsite.org/books.html

The guru is in you.

2006/03/03 11:48:29
Books, Web Sites, Audio, Video, etc.
http://www.aypsite.org/forum/topic.asp?TOPIC_ID=858&REPLY_ID=4065&whichpage=-1
AYP eBook Prices Reduced

Hi All:

Thanks for the words of support.

Any tangible help is much appreciated. Donations or purchases of books at <u>deep</u> discount (5 or more - write for details) are both welcome. So far, donations and book sales are running neck and neck as far as financial help for AYP goes, like two turtles in a horse race. :-)

Of course we'd prefer for the books to be winning in the broad marketplace. It is a primary goal to distribute the AYP writings far and wide. The books are also intended to support AYP financially over the long term. So far this has not been happening. So we will have to see how it goes, and make financial decisions over the next year as necessary.

For those not wanting to use Paypal, please write me for a snail mail address.

All financial contributions are being used to help make the AYP writings more available around the world.

All the best!

The guru is in you.

2006/03/10 19:00:32
Books, Web Sites, Audio, Video, etc.
http://www.aypsite.org/forum/topic.asp?TOPIC_ID=890&REPLY_ID=4359&whichpage=-1
Practice in Secrets of Wilder

Hi Weaver:

Yoni Mudra Kumbhaka -- <u>Lesson 91</u>.

The guru is in you.

2006/03/28 10:00:23
Books, Web Sites, Audio, Video, etc.
http://www.aypsite.org/forum/topic.asp?TOPIC_ID=907&REPLY_ID=5274&whichpage=-1
Secrets of Wilder

Hi Bewell:

It is great to hear of your integration of these vital principles on the path. And with you coming from your own unique background too. It is a lesson for us all.

As it has been said, "A word to the wise is sufficient." :-)

The credit goes to you. May the honeymoon blossom into long term fulfillment. Carry on!

The guru is in you.

2007/03/12 11:31:02
Books, Web Sites, Audio, Video, etc.
http://www.aypsite.org/forum/topic.asp?TOPIC_ID=907&REPLY_ID=18727&whichpage=-1
Secrets of Wilder

Hi Maximus:

The Secrets of Wilder is a modern allegory (symbolic representation) of the Christian Gospels -- a relentless quest for ultimate truth and the sharing of that truth, which involves several people (not only John Wilder) sacrificing for the many. That is the central theme of a classic hero's journey, and it is happening around us in real life all the time. None of us would be sitting here today if someone had not sacrificed something for us.

The Secrets of Wilder is more specific about spiritual practices than previous books of this kind, which is the aspect of the story that traces causes and effects in practices and how they can play out in the individual, in relationships, and, ultimately, in the flowering of a broader spiritual awareness in our society.

If none of this sits well with you, well, it raises the question of whether anything is more important than the survival of our individual material selves. Surely there must be more to life than that, even if it is just caring about someone else enough to value their wellbeing. I suggest you consider who you might be willing to sacrifice something for -- a loved one, a neighbor, or all of society. As soon as we can care about someone or something beyond our physical self, even for a minute, we are becoming more. That is the whole point you know -- to aim for something higher, and, in doing so, become something more than we were before. It takes a surrender to accept that the "something more" is beyond the reach of our current ideas and prejudices.

We also must be willing to act within the context of our surrender, engaging in our unfoldment. This is "active surrender."

Could a caterpillar become a butterfly without surrender and engagement in its process of transformation? (a metaphor in the Wilder story) It is just the same with us. To become more, we must be willing to surrender to becoming more, and act. It can happen in many baby steps, and sometimes in big leaps. In the case of human beings, there is conscious choice involved.

The themes in the Secrets of Wilder story are universal, with many of the specifics of spiritual methodology and experience added for good measure.

The Secrets of Wilder isn't Ayn Rand, who was the queen of seeking only personal self interest. On the other hand, the ultimate pursuit of personal self-interest will inevitably lead us to the interest of all others, for we are One. All seekers come to that sooner or later. This is represented dramatically to an extreme in the Kurt Wilder (John's brother) subplot in the story.

All roads lead home...

The guru is in you.

2006/03/24 22:44:43
Books, Web Sites, Audio, Video, etc.
http://www.aypsite.org/forum/topic.asp?TOPIC_ID=970&REPLY_ID=5057&whichpage=-1
Digital Version of AYP Book

Hi Jim:

If it won't download from your Amazon digital locker (did you try again?) then better contact Amazon. I can go back to the ebook publisher to see if there is problem at the source, but they are gone until Monday. If it is a problem at the source, I expect I'd have heard by now, but will check anyway if you do not have it soon. Let me know.

Sorry about the difficulty.

The guru is in you.

2006/03/25 07.10.20
Books, Web Sites, Audio, Video, etc.
http://www.aypsite.org/forum/topic.asp?TOPIC_ID=970&REPLY_ID=5064&whichpage=-1
Digital Version of AYP Book

Hi Jim:

I am reporting it to the ebook publisher.

Did you try it on another computer? I know that does not help you on your laptop. The reason I suggest this is that I had a similar download problem on one of my computers when the ebook first came out (not with other ebooks), and it did download on another computer. I reported it to the ebook publisher then and we never did find out why it happened. Since then, I have not heard of anyone else having this problem, so assumed it was a quirk on my machine. But now you have it.

The guru is in you.

2006/03/26 21:51:01
Books, Web Sites, Audio, Video, etc.
http://www.aypsite.org/forum/topic.asp?TOPIC_ID=970&REPLY_ID=5189&whichpage=-1
Digital Version of AYP Book

Hi Etherfish:

The paperbacks and ebooks for all the AYP books are the same. Of course, each has its inherent advantages and disadvantages unique to the medium. But the content is the same.

The guru is in you.

2006/03/27 11:03:57
Books, Web Sites, Audio, Video, etc.
http://www.aypsite.org/forum/topic.asp?TOPIC_ID=970&REPLY_ID=5220&whichpage=-1
Digital Version of AYP Book
Here is the note back from the ebook publisher, Lightning Source, on the problem:

Hi Yogani,
We will work with Amazon through this issue. This could fail for a number of reasons - incorrect reader, reader not activated, etc.

Thank you.

536 –   Advanced Yoga Practices

I also informed them of your problem downloading Deep Meditation, Near.

Thanks for your patience.

The guru is in you.

2006/03/27 17:34:03
Books, Web Sites, Audio, Video, etc.
http://www.aypsite.org/forum/topic.asp?TOPIC_ID=970&REPLY_ID=5237&whichpage=-1
Digital Version of AYP Book

Hi Yoda:

Hopefully the book is better than the cover. :-)

The guru is in you.

2006/05/27 19:02:35
Books, Web Sites, Audio, Video, etc.
http://www.aypsite.org/forum/topic.asp?TOPIC_ID=1178
Tantra - Discovering the Power Of Pre-Orgasmic Sex

Hi All:

I just noticed the new AYP Tantra ebook is up on Diesel. See here:
http://www.diesel-ebooks.com/cgi-bin/item/0976465590

The paperback version should be in the channels within a few of weeks. Paper moves slower. :-)

All the best!

The guru is in you.

2006/05/28 11:42:40
Books, Web Sites, Audio, Video, etc.
http://www.aypsite.org/forum/topic.asp?TOPIC_ID=1178&REPLY_ID=7433&whichpage=-1
Tantra - Discovering the Power Of Pre-Orgasmic Sex

Hi All:

Yes, Melissa, the book is left-handed, "giving sex its due" in support of right-handed sitting practices, which are mentioned from time to time in the book with referrals to the other AYP writings.

Jim, the idea that spawned these small inexpensive AYP Enlightenment Series books was that the original AYP Easy Lessons book is a bit much for many to swallow all at once -- in size, in content, and in price. So these E-Series books are designed to provide easy doorways into the knowledge.

Also, different people have initial interest in different aspects of practice, and these little books make it easy for anyone to individually approach deep meditation, spinal breathing pranayama, tantric sexual practices, etc., and then move on to the broad picture of yoga, as desired. So the E-Series books can be recommended to people according to their interests in a more targeted way than can be achieved by handing them the two-pound AYP Easy Lessons book. Much less expensive too. If a small AYP book resonates, then the aspirant can move on to the big book, or to other small books. It can go however the aspirant likes. That's the idea.

The same is true of the Secrets of Wilder novel, which is for those who would like to read about the discovery and application of the practices in a modern story. The novel is another kind of doorway into the broad field of spiritual practices.

As for the "more thorough treatment" of the practices in the E-Series books, it is true. That is because these have been written later in time and reflect the fourth time through the practices in published writings (original Yahoo lessons, AYP book, Wilder...), plus the ongoing interactions that have been occurring in private emails and here in the forum. In that sense, everyone has been chipping in on the writing effort. So, as far as they go, the E-Series books are more refined. But they are still entry level into each category of practice, and the AYP Easy Lessons book continues to be the whole course, with additional material like mantra enhancements, more advanced applications of spinal breathing and the other practices, weaving all the pieces together with self-pacing, etc.

Btw, the last book in the E-Series is planned to tie the whole thing together in an introductory way also. It is tentatively called: "Eight Limbs of Yoga - The structure and Pacing of Self-Directed Spiritual Practice." Like the other E-Series books, it will have refinements reflecting the evolution of the writing over time. All of which goes to reinforce the point that there is no last word in AYP. I am sure others will be adding many more words long after this keyboard has gone silent. Let's hope so...

On selling the nine E-Series books as a set, perhaps that can be addressed once they are all finished. Right now, it is about the writing, and getting the books out there as quickly and easily as possible. We have the formula for that in the USA and Europe. India remains a challenge for having the books available there, though I did get a little bit of good news on that today.

The AYP books page will be updated in the next week or so to cover the titles and release schedule for all nine E-Series books -- the goal is to have them done by the end of next year, and we're on schedule so far. I'd also like to release the nine E-Series books in audio-book format, and hopefully we can start seeing those by next year also.

Near, I hope you are right about the Tantra book drawing a larger audience to AYP. While the work goes on here, we are yet to hit the "big cosmic nerve" that will draw broad public awareness to AYP. Maybe the Tantra book will help with that?

Jim, you must forgive me for not following your advice put nude photos of Paris Hilton in to create a huge audience for AYP, though I did give it some serious consideration. :-)
No pictures in this Tantra book, except for the Sri Yantra. It is a practical yoga book, one of the few on tantric sexual practices that does not sell out to obsessive attitudes. Will that help draw a wider audience to AYP? Time will tell...

The guru is in you

2006/06/02 18:54:54
Books, Web Sites, Audio, Video, etc.
http://www.aypsite.org/forum/topic.asp?TOPIC_ID=1178&REPLY_ID=7710&whichpage=-1
Tantra - Discovering the Power Of Pre-Orgasmic Sex

Hi All:

Amazon now has the AYP Tantra ebook up and running. You can find links to it on both Amazon and Diesel on the books page here:
http://www.aypsite.org/books.html

The paperback version should be up on Amazon, and everywhere else, in about 10 days. The links will be activated on the books page as soon as it shows up.

The guru is in you.

2006/06/07 23:39:39
Books, Web Sites, Audio, Video, etc.
http://www.aypsite.org/forum/topic.asp?TOPIC_ID=1178&REPLY_ID=7824&whichpage=-1
Tantra - Discovering the Power Of Pre-Orgasmic Sex

Hi All:

The paperback version of *Tantra* is up on Amazon USA now -- shipping within 24 hours. The cover image and description will be there soon. It should not be long before the book shows up on all the other sites.

The AYP websites are being updated and announcements are going out accordingly. See the books page for links -- http://www.aypsite.org/books.html, or the cover image can be clicked on any AYP website page to find it on Amazon USA.

As always, Amazon reviews are welcome!

The guru is in you.

2006/06/09 17:03:57
Books, Web Sites, Audio, Video, etc.
http://www.aypsite.org/forum/topic.asp?TOPIC_ID=1178&REPLY_ID=7904&whichpage=-1
Tantra - Discovering the Power Of Pre-Orgasmic Sex

Hi All:

We have all the Tantra book Amazon links up now, except Canada and Japan, which I expect will be along shortly. The cover image and description have been uploaded to the sites, and ought to be up soon too. The book is also up on Barnes and Noble -- that link, along with the other USA book chains, is at the end of the listings on the books page.

Part of the Tantra book title has been **CENSORED ON AMAZON SITES IN EUROPE**. That is amazing, since we are supposed to be the prudes over here in the USA, and it did not happen here. The title is listed like this:

USA (correct) -- "Tantra - Discovering the Power of Pre-Orgasmic Sex"

Europe (censored) -- "Tantra - Discovering the Power of Preorga"

And no, they did not run out of room, as many titles are longer and don't get cut off like that.

Now, what we need is a good book burning. That will bring in some readers for sure. :-)

The guru is in you.

2006/06/10 18:57:13
Books, Web Sites, Audio, Video, etc.
http://www.aypsite.org/forum/topic.asp?TOPIC_ID=1178&REPLY_ID=7929&whichpage=-1
Tantra - Discovering the Power Of Pre-Orgasmic Sex

Thanks Lavazza. I'll report it. I believe all Amazon sites in Europe and Japan feed from the UK site. So the curtailed AYP Tantra title has gone far and wide.

The guru is in you.

2006/06/25 08:47:10
Books, Web Sites, Audio, Video, etc.
http://www.aypsite.org/forum/topic.asp?TOPIC_ID=1247

Assistance for Yoga in Romania

Hi All:

There is a small group of yoga practitioners in Romania building a spiritual library for the public, and seeking spiritual book donations, old and new. See their website and email contact here: http://www.sundari.way2web.ro

The guru is in you.

2009/05/21 14:15:21
Books, Web Sites, Audio, Video, etc.
http://www.aypsite.org/forum/topic.asp?TOPIC_ID=1380&REPLY_ID=51242&whichpage=-1
What are you reading?

Hi All:

"The End of Your World" by Adyashanti (new book)

Practical advice for those dipping in and out of unity/non-duality experiences.

The advice is specific to "Adya-Zen-style" awakenings, which can be a little (or very) rough. We avoid much of that (or hope to) in AYP with the pre-cultivation of abiding inner silence -- the witness. Even so, Adyashanti offers a lot of practical information here for anyone who is involved in self-inquiry and non-duality. Good stuff!

The guru is in you.

2009/09/11 11:31:30
Books, Web Sites, Audio, Video, etc.
http://www.aypsite.org/forum/topic.asp?TOPIC_ID=1380&REPLY_ID=56715&whichpage=-1
What are you reading?

quote:
_____
Originally posted by emc

Reading Adyashanti's "The end of your world" and the devilish, evil design of this journey is exactly what I was afraid of and sort of already knew... and even worse in some parts that I hadn't thought of... he's just pointing it out very clearly! Shit bad news. But a good book. Read it and drop your illusions about the beautiful spiritual journey!
_____

Hi emc:

I may have recommended this book to you some time back. It should be pointed out that Adyashanti is speaking to an audience he is familiar with: his students and others who come to enlightenment being strong on self-inquiry and weak on meditation. Throw in a few strong doses of guru shaktipat for good measure. The result can be quite a lot of chaos, often with little abiding inner silence to absorb it with.

So I would not say that "The End of Your World" is representative of what people will experience with the AYP approach. Rather, it is the kind of unfoldment one might experience if the cart gets in front of the horse. It is an excellent book for that, and I highly recommend it to anyone who feels that they are getting ahead of themselves, for any reason whatsoever. It can serve as a reminder of the importance of daily deep meditation, and a more self-paced approach in general.

Keep in mind that real enlightenment is unending ecstatic bliss and unifying outpouring divine love. All the rest is scenery, as is the enlightenment itself. Nothing going on here at all, but love. :-)

The guru is in you.

2006/08/07 10:51:49
Books, Web Sites, Audio, Video, etc.
http://www.aypsite.org/forum/topic.asp?TOPIC_ID=1394
The Spiritual Cinema Circle -- DVD Club

Hi All:

Received an email on this today -- a DVD club for spiritual movies:

http://www.spiritualcinemacircle.com

Also see links on the bottom of the page on spiritual cinema genre.

The guru is in you.

2006/08/13 13:00:11
Books, Web Sites, Audio, Video, etc.
http://www.aypsite.org/forum/topic.asp?TOPIC_ID=1419
AYP and changes in the eBook market

Hi All:

If you have gone to get an AYP ebook (or any ebook) from Amazon lately, you will have noticed that Adobe and Microsoft ebooks are no longer available on Amazon (AYP ebooks are in Adobe format). Amazon discontinued carrying both formats near the end of July (without any warning), and they will be coming out with their own ebook format through a wholly owned subsidiary called http://www.mobipocket.com. Amazon has implied in an email reply received here that the Mobipocket format will be expanded from current PDA/handheld platforms to desktop/laptop computers and offered on the Amazon website. But when this will happen is unknown.

The AYP books page has been edited to reflect Amazon's exit from Adobe and Microsoft ebooks, and alternate reliable ebook vendor links are provided for all of the AYP ebooks.

When Amazon has ebooks available on their site again, the AYP books will most likely be offered in that format also. I will keep you posted.

Just to make things interesting, Google is planning to expand the capabilities of its fast-growing book database to cover paid online reading, to be available maybe next year, which will no doubt present a challenge to the ebook market. The AYP books will be there too.

As the changes in the online world continue to occur, we will keep up. Thanks for your patience in all of this.

All the best!

The guru is in you.

2006/09/20 20:56:49
Books, Web Sites, Audio, Video, etc.
http://www.aypsite.org/forum/topic.asp?TOPIC_ID=1526
AYP Asanas, Mudras & Bandhas book is out!

Hi All:

The new book is out: **Asanas, Mudras and Bandhas - Awakening Ecstatic Kundalini.**
As the title implies, this one is jam-packed with information on physical practices (with updates on many, including kechari mudra), and gives new meaning to the phrase "yoga postures" in relation to the rest of the limbs of yoga.

The book and ebook versions have appeared in the retail distribution channels, and the AYP Books Page links have been updated.

It is also available for quantity deep discount ordering and shipping direct from the printer -- see here for quantity discount ordering information.

Here is an excerpt from the introduction to give you a flavor:

"Like much we may encounter as we travel along our chosen spiritual path, this small volume on Asanas, Mudras and Bandhas presents a paradox.

In contrast to the huge, nearly exclusive emphasis on yoga asanas (postures) seen around the world today, we intentionally go lightly on them here, instead presenting a compact and efficient asana routine as preparation for sitting practices, including spinal breathing pranayama and deep meditation.

Once a balanced relationship between asanas and sitting practices is established, we move into instructions for advanced mudras and bandhas (inner physical maneuvers), which are woven into the tapestry of our daily practice routine like golden threads.

Then we cover the awakening and management of our inner ecstatic energy – Kundalini – and its ultimate consequences. Ecstatic awakening and its steady expansion outward through our nervous system to full divine expression is, after all, what asanas, mudras and bandhas are for.

In short, this book puts a wide range of yoga practices into perspective, moving decidedly away from the *magic bullet* single solution syndrome, and offering a clear, balanced road map for those who seek to achieve the ultimate aims of yoga. In this, asanas, mudras and bandhas have an important role to play..."

The guru is in you.

2006/09/30 18:53:11
Books, Web Sites, Audio, Video, etc.
http://www.aypsite.org/forum/topic.asp?TOPIC_ID=1526&REPLY_ID=11770&whichpage=-1
AYP Asanas, Mudras & Bandhas book is out!

Hi Bill:

Glad to hear the new book is helping on the front end of your practice routine.

It was written with two audiences in mind-- Folks like you looking for a compact routine of asanas (postures) to put in front of spinal breathing pranayama and deep meditation, and for those who have been mainly into asanas (maybe extensively) who are looking for ways to integrate their practice into a more balanced routine of asanas, spinal breathing pranayama, deep meditation, mudras and bandhas, and other practices covering all the limbs of yoga.

After all, asanas represent only one of the eight limbs of yoga. Why not put all the limbs together? That is what yoga is in its full application, and leading to full results of unshakable inner silence, ecstatic bliss and outpouring divine love.

And ... it can be done efficiently, without overloading a busy lifestyle...

The guru is in you.

2006/10/02 08:07:22
Books, Web Sites, Audio, Video, etc.
http://www.aypsite.org/forum/topic.asp?TOPIC_ID=1566&REPLY_ID=11846&whichpage=-1
Spiritual movies - Fight Club
This topic moved for better placement.

Also see this topic called, "Movies Anyone?"
http://www.aypsite.org/forum/topic.asp?TOPIC_ID=425

The guru is in you.

2006/10/06 10:40:52
Books, Web Sites, Audio, Video, etc.
http://www.aypsite.org/forum/topic.asp?TOPIC_ID=1571&REPLY_ID=11972&whichpage=-1
Tantra Book review

Hi Anthem:

Thank you for the very nice review. And also for reminding others about the importance of reviews on Amazon. Yes, they are very important -- perhaps the single most important factor in helping the AYP books reach more people.

What the readers think about the AYP writings is what matters the most, and if it is shared, then others will know. Otherwise, no one will know. So please do speak up, everyone.

There is a new book out, "Asanas, Mudras and Bandhas - Awakening Ecstatic Kundalini," awaiting reviews. :-)

Wishing you all the best on your chosen path. Enjoy!

The guru is in you.

2006/10/22 14:12:39
Books, Web Sites, Audio, Video, etc.
http://www.aypsite.org/forum/topic.asp?TOPIC_ID=1628&REPLY_ID=12501&whichpage=-1
God Without Religion

quote:

Originally posted by Sparkle
For those (both students and teachers) who understand what works - some combination of pranayama, meditation, bhakti and inquiry tend to be the pillars of the given system of practices [we don't discuss the latter all that much in AYP, but the tendency toward inquiry* is an obvious effect of the other two activities --- just read through our forum posts, for evidence of that!).

Originally posted by Kirtanman
*Using the term [inquiry] somewhat loosely - though I think most of us involved with AYP would say that inquiry (i.e. Who am I? What is God? Is there a "God"? Where does the Self begin? Or End?, Etc. Etc.) both drives our practices, and AYP forum participation, to a degree --- and/or is an effect of them.

Hi Sparkle and Kirtanman:

Good perspectives. Yes, in AYP we are getting around to self-inquiry as *effect*, and then using it to add further *cause* to our development. It will be the topic of an e-series book next year. The title hints at the order of development we aim for here, with inner silence (witness) coming first:

"Self-Inquiry - Dawn of the Witness and the End of Suffering"

And, interestingly, self-inquiry is a close cousin of bhakti, which is the next book after that. I know you are happy about the connection, Kirtanman. There are no walls in yoga ... only overlapping principles of human spiritual transformation... :-)

Regarding Sankara Saranam, he has done a good job of bringing the gift of practical pranayama techniques to many, as far as he has gone. As far as I know, he stops shy of open source access to full-scope spiritual practices.

Not sure I agree with his geo-political confrontation with organized religion. Promoting such conflict is a hot button for a lot of people, but of no real consequence in the overall scheme of individual spiritual practice, which is what will cultivate human evolution ever forward. As long as we forge ahead with practices, organized religion (and every other institution) will be compelled to reinvent itself and play its role in bringing self-directed spiritual practices to the masses. It is happening already in many religious organizations. They must change to avoid being left behind. The institutions will do whatever is necessary to maintain their following. In the past, the institutions led their uninformed members (the blind leading the blind), and we know the long history of disastrous results. Times are different now. With an increasingly better educated and spiritually evolving public, the institutions will be compelled to follow the people, or lose their relevance.

Therefore, I'm for moving ahead with an internal renaissance rather than an external conflict with organized religion. That does not exclude being resolute in letting go of what is untrue in organized religion, which is the message in the Secrets of Wilder novel. In the end, it is not about religion. It is about what the people choose for themselves. The religions will follow that, because they must. They have no power except what is given them by the people. Organized religion is not the culprit. We are. The mayhem of the religions and all institutions is our mayhem, and we can turn it around by systematically opening ourselves to the divine within. Maybe Sankara comes to this logical and empowering conclusion also. Don't know -- have not read his book yet.

The guru is in you.

2006/10/26 13:01:00
Books, Web Sites, Audio, Video, etc.
http://www.aypsite.org/forum/topic.asp?TOPIC_ID=1628&REPLY_ID=12589&whichpage=-1
God Without Religion

Hi Kirtanman:

David illustrates the point more clearly and forcefully than I did. As soon as we begin to use a non-sectarian teaching on yoga practices as a soapbox to express our political views, something important is lost. Walls go up right away. It becomes sectarian -- the very thing we may be railing against.

It is not that social causes are not important, or that wrongs should not be righted in the world. It is a matter of what level we choose to act from. Will it be from the level of ideology, or from the level of inner silence?

Inner silence has no ideology -- it just is, and all that is good springs naturally from that infinitely blissful foundation within us. Inner silence is, by its nature, infinite power for positive transformation. On the other hand, promoting ideology leads to conflict, endless debate, and worse. The only salvation to be found in ideology will be if it can be transcended with real spiritual practices. Without that, it is only a distraction to spiritual progress -- part of the ubiquitous and neverending scenery of life. In AYP we'd like to favor practices over all of that.

This is why political and social action discussions are not allowed in the AYP forums. They quickly lead to endless ideological debates and a kind of spiritual oblivion.

It is my understanding that Sankara Saranam comes from an intellectual middle eastern heritage, with a background in debate. He has obvious scruples with how political power flows in the world. That's fine. We all have our scruples. But what has it got to do with yoga?

It is certainly not the approach that Sankara's preceptor took. Paramahansa Yogananda spent his 30+ year career reconciling the eastern and western religions in totally positive ways, using yoga as a bridge. Thanks largely to him, we have the application of the principles and practices of hatha and kriya yoga expanding in both the east and west today. I doubt we would have progressed to this stage if Yogananda had spent his time focusing on the miserable history of the religions. He went beyond all that in everything he did, straight to the source, our divine inner being. That is an example we can all be inspired by.

The negative is so obvious, and no lasting solution will ever be found within its inherent structure. A new element is needed. That "fifth dimension" mentioned in AYP lesson 36 -- tapping into our inner silence, pure bliss consciousness. The way to solve the puzzle is to go beyond it.

If Sankara's argument is for doing that, I am all for it -- and the more directly to it the better.

The guru is in you.

2006/10/26 17:17:01
Books, Web Sites, Audio, Video, etc.
http://www.aypsite.org/forum/topic.asp?TOPIC_ID=1628&REPLY_ID=12597&whichpage=-1
God Without Religion

Hi Kirtanman:

It is good that you brought the book up here. Some very useful lessons for all of us. Many thanks. It is good to look at everything in the spiritual arena, as long as we don't end up going on an extended detour from ourselves. Not likely with inner silence coming up.

As for where the "AYP fold" is, when you find it, let me know. Hopefully there is none. :-)

Keep on dancing in the light!

The guru is in you.

2006/10/28 10:07:15
Books, Web Sites, Audio, Video, etc.
http://www.aypsite.org/forum/topic.asp?TOPIC_ID=1628&REPLY_ID=12635&whichpage=-1
God Without Religion

Hi Kirtanman:

I am certainly willing to give Sankara the benefit of the doubt, and do plan to read his book.

If he has repaired his prior grumpy "non-sequitur" ways enough to make a credible case in his book for deconstructing dogma, then it can be worthwhile. Maybe he is the Don Quixote of the yoga world, jousting with all those institutional windmills, and he could succeed in some measure. He is marketing his cause very hard.

Whether or not he offers a viable "reconstruction" in the form of full-scope self-directed spiritual practices is another matter. In that sense, he may end up being a help to AYP, cutting folks loose from dogma with his sword so they can become free to seek their divine inner destiny. Just what you said in your first posts here. So we have come full circle. :-)

There is a new breed of spiritual innovators rising out of the stodginess of the old traditions. It is happening all over and is a fascinating thing to watch. It bodes well for the future. We are all on the same team.

The guru is in you.

2007/10/27 11:13:53
Books, Web Sites, Audio, Video, etc.

God Without Religion

Hi Joshua, and welcome!

And isn't it interesting that we probably never would have heard of the grumpy Sri Yukteswar had it not been for the dedicated bridge-building and constant outpouring divine love of his disciple, Paramahansa Yogananda? And also interesting that Sankara Saranam, man of many scruples, considers Yogananda to be his guru.

It just goes to show that we each will carry our own torch, regardless of who may have inspired us. Some will use their torch as a light, while others may go about setting fires. It all works out in the end. :-)

The guru is in you.

2008/12/08 18:01:21
Books, Web Sites, Audio, Video, etc.
God Without Religion

Hi Carson:

Institutions, religious or otherwise, can only survive if people are buying what they are selling. The ones that adapt to the changing needs of the people will survive and thrive, and the ones that don't won't.

The place where change originates is with the people. In spiritual matters it is pretty obvious what must be done: The people should have access to effective tools to purify and open themselves according to their own desire, individually and collectively. As the process of inner divine unfoldment advances, the institutions that support the global transformation that is underway will continue to have relevance.

It does not happen overnight, but it does happen.

Clearly, it is happening. Power to the people!

The guru is in you.

2008/12/09 13:19:37
Books, Web Sites, Audio, Video, etc.
God Without Religion

Hi Carson.

Human need becomes purified as consciousness expands, and that changes everything. It happens on meditation seats, and naturally moves out from there. It is stillness in action. Nothing can resist, because it is the source of all.

The guru is in you.

2008/12/09 14:47:30
Books, Web Sites, Audio, Video, etc.
God Without Religion

quote:
_____
Originally posted by CarsonZi

Hi Yogani,

I understand that human needs change as consciousness changes, but what I am saying is that until human need reaches a breaking point, nothing is going to change. When it DOES change it will happen VERY fast and will most likely be catastrophic for the majority of humanity. And organized religion will be opposed to the changes, not for them, if organized religion even lasts long enough to see the changes we are talking about.

Love,
Carson
_____

Hi Carson:

It is changing, right before our eyes. The suggestion is to keep practicing (everyone!), and be patient. :-)

The guru is in you.

2006/11/04 16:56:16
Books, Web Sites, Audio, Video, etc.

Amazon "Search Inside" added for all AYP Books

Hi All:

Amazon's "Search Inside" feature has been turned on for all of the AYP books on all of the Amazon websites -- USA, Canada, UK, France, Germany and Japan.

This is the electronic equivalent of being able to thumb through a book in a bookstore, viewing the table of contents, searching and browsing pages. You can find links to all of the AYP books on Amazon here: http://www.aypsite.org/books.html

The AYP books currently include:

*Advanced Yoga Practices - Easy Lessons for Ecstatic Living
*The Secrets of Wilder Novel
*Deep Meditation - Pathway to Personal Freedom
*Spinal Breathing Pranayama - Journey to Inner Space
*Tantra - Discovering the Power of Pre-Orgasmic Sex
*Asanas, Mudras and Bandhas - Awakening Ecstatic Kundalini (NEW!)

Also, five additional books on practices coming out over the next year are shown at the above web link.

Wishing you all the best on your chosen path. Enjoy!

The guru is in you.

2006/11/15 08:34:22
Books, Web Sites, Audio, Video, etc.
http://www.aypsite.org/forum/topic.asp?TOPIC_ID=1714&REPLY_ID=13296&whichpage=-1
Some questions regarding Secrets of Wilder

Hi ckdCosmo, and welcome!

Very happy to hear you are enjoying the Secrets of Wilder -- a story near and dear to my heart.

The practice is called "kechari mudra." It is covered in the AYP Easy Lessons book, and the Asanas, Mudras and Bandhas book.

You can also read about it online, beginning here: http://www.aypsite.org/108.html
It is discussed a lot here in the forums too.

All the best on your path. Enjoy!

The guru is in you.

2006/12/06 16:16:00
Books, Web Sites, Audio, Video, etc.
http://www.aypsite.org/forum/topic.asp?TOPIC_ID=1798
The Guru ... (is in who?)

Hi All:

"The Guru" -- Fun "East meets West" movie, with a message.
(adults only)

http://www.imdb.com/title/tt0280720/

The guru is in you.
 Yes, you! :-)

2006/12/18 10:46:25
Books, Web Sites, Audio, Video, etc.
http://www.aypsite.org/forum/topic.asp?TOPIC_ID=1821&REPLY_ID=14578&whichpage=-1
Per Request - Kirtanman's Top 10 Kirtan Artists

Hi Kirtanman:

Thanks much for this marvelous contribution to the knowledge base.

May the dance continue! :-)

The guru is in you.

2006/12/17 12:59:57
Books, Web Sites, Audio, Video, etc.
http://www.aypsite.org/forum/topic.asp?TOPIC_ID=1827
India Editions for AYP Books Now Available!

Hi All:

Thanks to the efforts of Grasroutes in New Delhi, several of the AYP books have been published in **India Editions** and are now available:

Advanced Yoga Practices - Easy Lessons for Ecstatic Living, Retail - Rs. 490

Deep Meditation - Pathway to Personal Freedom, Retail - Rs. 95

Spinal Breathing Pranayama - Journey to Inner Space, Retail - Rs. 95

Note: Discounts may be offered at the discretion of booksellers. Shipping charges may apply.

The books can be obtained through the Grasroutes website and online through Grasroutes on eBay.in. Direct links by book have been added on the AYP Books page for purchase of the **India Editions** through **eBay.in**. The remaining "F&S India" links on the books page are for USA editions.

The books are also available at the following **New Del**
Hi bookstore. More bookstores throughout India will be listed soon:

The Variety Book Depot
AVG Bhavan, M3 Connaught circus
PO Box 505, New Delhi-110001, India
email: varietybookdepot@rediffmail.com ; artmesh@yahoo.com
tel: 23417175, 23412567

It is hoped that the response to these offerings will enable us to have all of the AYP books published in India Editions and available on an ongoing basis.

Wishing you all the best on your chosen path. Enjoy!

The guru is in you.

2007/01/12 10:53:06
Books, Web Sites, Audio, Video, etc.
http://www.aypsite.org/forum/topic.asp?TOPIC_ID=1827&REPLY_ID=15890&whichpage=-1
India Editions for AYP Books Now Available!
PS: Please note the updates to the above post. We are making good progress in India! :-)
2006/12/18 23:40:09
Books, Web Sites, Audio, Video, etc.
http://www.aypsite.org/forum/topic.asp?TOPIC_ID=1830&REPLY_ID=14599&whichpage=-1
AYP book vs. Enlightenment Series

Hi Insideout, and welcome!

Weaver has given you a pretty good answer.

Maybe some additional perspective from here will help. The AYP Easy Lessons book is a preservation and expansion (about +20%) on the original online lessons, which were madly written from Nov 2003 until Sept 2004. That is through lesson 235 (plus the same period for the Tantra lessons), which is as far as the first big volume goes -- there will be a volume 2 someday to pick up the writing that has been put online since, plus offline additions.

The big AYP volume is by its fluid nature less organized than the AYP Enlightenment Series books, but does contain practices that are not in the E-Series (mantra enhancements, bastrika methods, more on kechari, and other add-ons). The big book is broader in scope in that sense, covering quite a few advanced nuances. That is also true of the more recent online lessons (eventually to become volume 2), which also cover material that will not be found in the E-Series books (like hybrid yoni mudra applications, for example.) Those kinds of advanced refinements would be out of place in an E-Series book.

The purpose of the E-Series is to provide clear entrees into individual (or classes of) practices in digestible bites, easy to absorb and apply, less expensive per book, and much less daunting than wading through a 500 page nuance-packed textbook (though a friendly one by most accounts :-)).

Because the E-Series books were written "as books" offline, they are better organized. And since they have been and are being written later in time than the first big book, they have clarifications that make them more complete at present in terms of presenting the essential practices.

The E-Series books also are designed to appeal to particular interests people might have, and to lead them naturally from that particular focus into the broader scope of yoga practices.

So there are some ironies working here:

1. The big book has more "stuff" practice-wise, but is somewhat less refined due to its primary source material being generated in the online lessons.

2. The E-Series is very focused in terms of specific practices, and does a better job of presenting those. It should also be mentioned that the E-Series has been in the process of "breaking out" in terms of covering more and more "stuff" that has not been documented in the online lessons, nor in AYP Easy Lessons Volume 1. The upcoming Samyama book is a case in point. It will cover several samyama techniques that are brand new in the AYP writings. There will be more new material in future E-Series books as well.

This shift of the E-Series to presenting new practices not in the online lessons is partly out of financial necessity, and partly due to the fact that I can only write one set of instructions at a time. Having to choose, I have chosen the books. It is my hope that all of the new material will find its way into the online lessons eventually -- worldwide public access is at the center of the AYP mission. When and how that happens going forward will depend on both the time available to do it and on AYP becoming self-supporting, which will hopefully happen somewhere down the line.

Some have asked, "Why didn't you just write one big book and be done with it?"

It is part of the fate of being a "spiritual scientist," rather than a stuck-in-the-mud guru, I guess.

While I think we have done a pretty good job so far of nailing down the essential principles and basic methods of human spiritual transformation, the writing that is occurring at any point in time is not the last word.

AYP is an ongoing evolution that will continue to depend on causes and effects found to be occurring in practitioners everywhere. So we don't shy away from difficulties encountered or any new information that comes in. Refinements are being made all the time, and I expect this will continue indefinitely. Eventually we will get it to a highly refined state (maybe), but I do not see that happening entirely on my watch. It is an ongoing research project.

These forums are also an important part of it, because communication on these matters among practitioners at all levels of experience is essential to carry the process of knowledge development forward.

So, which AYP books to read? I'd say the E-Series for getting the core practices down, and the big book for the advanced whistles and bells, if interested. It can be a pretty fruitful journey using either one or the other. As Weaver points out, both is even better, but that is a matter of how gung-ho one is about studying and implementing yoga practices.

When the AYP writing is all said and done (my part of it, anyway), it might be a dozen or so books. If done well, it will be a very condensed body of work on the ins and outs of human spiritual transformation, which others can use to take it to the next level in the decades to come. It sure beats reading 400+ books to pull it together, though anyone is welcome to. A list is provided with lesson 253. :-)

However you decide to approach it, by all means, enjoy!

The guru is in you.

2006/12/19 10:35:57
Books, Web Sites, Audio, Video, etc.
http://www.aypsite.org/forum/topic.asp?TOPIC_ID=1830&REPLY_ID=14610&whichpage=-1
AYP book vs. Enlightenment Series
PS: It should be added that the Secrets of Wilder novel looks at the discovery of the practices and their effects through the eyes of the seeker, and the circle of friends and family (who are not always supportive). The reader can take the journey of spiritual transformation vicariously, warts and all. From that point of view, there are quite a few lessons in the novel that are not necessarily emphasized elsewhere in the AYP writings.
2007/01/10 16:01:03
Books, Web Sites, Audio, Video, etc.
http://www.aypsite.org/forum/topic.asp?TOPIC_ID=1915
New Book! Samyama - Stillness, Siddhis & Miracles

Hi All:

The newest AYP book is now in the distribution channels, available in paperback and ebook worldwide. The full title is:

Samyama - Cultivating Stillness in Action, Siddhis and Miracles

Check the AYP Books Page for bookseller links: http://www.aypsite.org/books.html

The Samyama book is also available for shipment as part of any quantity discount order. For details on the quantity discount program, see:
http://www.aypsite.org/forum/topic.asp?TOPIC_ID=1248

Note: A Radio Interview on the new Samyama book was conducted on January 28, 2007. A recording can be listened to here:
http://www.aypsite.com/audio.html

This volume of the *AYP Enlightenment Series* goes significantly beyond previous AYP writings on Samyama. Here is the **Table of Contents** to give a flavor:

Table of Contents

Chapter 1 – The Making of Miracles
--How Our World is Manifested
--Discovering Our Vast Inner Potential
--Becoming a Channel of Infinite Expression

Chapter 2 – Samyama
--The Yoga Sutras of Patanjali
--The Technique of Samyama
--Questions and Answers on Daily Practice
--Symptoms of Purification and Opening
--Self-Pacing
--Rise of the Active Witness

Chapter 3 – Expanded Applications
--Cosmic Samyama and Yoga Nidra
--Samyama and Yoga Postures (Asanas)
--Prayer and the Principles of Samyama
--Samyama in Daily Living
--Siddhis – Super-Normal Powers
--The Importance of a Methodical Approach

Chapter 4 – Stillness in Action
--Relationship of Inner Silence and Ecstasy
--Flying on the Wings of Ecstatic Bliss

--Let Go and Let God

Appendix – The Samyama Sutras of Patanjali
(Interpreted and simplified for optional research)

Further Reading and Support

Wishing you all the best on your path. Enjoy!

The guru is in you.

2007/01/24 14:07:11
Books, Web Sites, Audio, Video, etc.
http://www.aypsite.org/forum/topic.asp?TOPIC_ID=1915&REPLY_ID=16464&whichpage=-1
New Book! Samyama - Stillness, Siddhis & Miracles

Hi All:

Nearly all of the Samyama bookseller links are up and running now -- http://www.aypsite.org/books.html

The "search inside" feature will be added for this book on all Amazon sites worldwide within a few weeks. This will greatly improve visibility on the Amazon sites and in the web search engines. Even now, a book search for "samyama" on any Amazon site pulls it up at or near the top of the list, and on Google it currently comes up on pages 2 & 3.

Amazon reviews on the Samyama book are greatly appreciated, as these have a large impact on visitors to the book page, and are also included in the web search engines.

It appears Barnes and Noble online is now carrying all of the AYP books in stock with 24 hour shipping. That is a great new development.

All the best!

The guru is in you.

2007/01/26 10:45:21
Books, Web Sites, Audio, Video, etc.
http://www.aypsite.org/forum/topic.asp?TOPIC_ID=1915&REPLY_ID=16594&whichpage=-1
New Book! Samyama - Stillness, Siddhis & Miracles

Thanks much, Mike.

Sometimes it takes a few days or weeks for Amazon to update an author listing of books when a new one is added, but eventually they do.

Yes, there are very few books on "Samyama" out there, so searching on that will invariably bring it up. We seem to be plowing new ground here. :-)

In any case, the AYP books page has direct links to all the books.

The guru is in you.

2007/02/11 18:21:46
Books, Web Sites, Audio, Video, etc.
http://www.aypsite.org/forum/topic.asp?TOPIC_ID=2046
AYP eBooks with Audio Introductions by Yogani

Hi All:

We have installed download capability direct through the AYP website in preparation for the Enlightenment Series **AudioBooks** that will begin coming out in a few months.

In setting up for direct downloads, we are now also able to offer all of the **AYP eBooks** through the AYP website. Not only that. Since the PDF eBook downloads from AYP are in zip files, it was decided to add a several-minute MP3 **Audio Introduction** by me to each of the eBooks, without changing any prices. So, by downloading an AYP eBook directly through the AYP website, there is a little bonus -- me speaking to you! :-)

You can find these "special edition" eBooks on the AYP Books Page under each book through the link called "**eBook w/Audio Intro**."

Or, you can go directly to the eBooks with Audio Introductions via these links:

Advanced Yoga Practices - Easy Lessons for Ecstatic Living
The Secrets of Wilder - A Novel
Deep Meditation - Pathway to Personal Freedom
Spinal Breathing - Journey to Inner Space
Tantra - Discovering the Power of Pre-Orgasmic Sex
Asanas, Mudras & Bandhas - Awakening Ecstatic Kundalini
Samyama - Cultivating Stillness in Action, Siddhis & Miracles

Important Note: Another advantage of downloading eBooks directly through AYP, is that if there is any difficulty at all, you can write me and the issue will be resolved immediately. In fact, if you have any problem with any AYP eBook from any vendor, just write me, and we will take care of it. We did not have the ability to directly resolve Adobe eBook reliability issues in the past, and this is another reason why I wanted to add the capability to deliver the AYP eBooks ourselves via download to anyone anywhere. Now we can, and **eBook reliability is guaranteed**.

Wishing you all the best on your path. Practice wisely, and enjoy!

The guru is in you.

2007/05/02 19:02:42
Books, Web Sites, Audio, Video, etc.
http://www.aypsite.org/forum/topic.asp?TOPIC_ID=2512
AudioBooks - AYP Enlightenment Series

Hi All:

Thanks to the audio processing expertise of Trip (Brett), we now have the **Deep Meditation** book available for download in MP3/iPod AudioBook format.

It can be accessed from the AYP Books Page through a link under the Deep Meditation book, or by going to this direct link:

http://www.aypsite.org/books-dmaudiobook.html

We hope to have the **Spinal Breathing Pranayama** book out in AudioBook format in a month or so, and the rest of the **Enlightenment Series** books by the end of the year.

Thank you, Brett, for all your hard work on this project.

Wishing everyone all the best on your path. Enjoy!

The guru is in you.

2007/05/09 16:10:58
Books, Web Sites, Audio, Video, etc.
http://www.aypsite.org/forum/topic.asp?TOPIC_ID=2512&REPLY_ID=21660&whichpage=-1
AudioBooks - AYP Enlightenment Series
PS: A press release has gone out on the Deep Meditation AudioBook. See here:
http://www.aypsite.org/pressrelease10.html

2007/05/17 09:24:25
Books, Web Sites, Audio, Video, etc.
http://www.aypsite.org/forum/topic.asp?TOPIC_ID=2512&REPLY_ID=22014&whichpage=-1
AudioBooks - AYP Enlightenment Series

quote:
_____
Originally posted by Sparkle

Not being well versed in MP3 and iPod stuff, can someone enlighten me about whether I can download this onto a CD or DVD. Or do I need an MP3 player or iPod ?

Thanks :-)
_____

Hi Louis:

No, you don't need an iPod. MP3 files can be played on any computer on standard audio players, with MS Media Player being the most common (default in Windows), or on any portable MP3 player.

Many CD burners have software to make standard format audio CDs out of MP3s, and many of the newer CD players and DVD players also play MP3 format without conversion.

The audiobook download is zipped into a single file (75 MB) in EasyZip format, which is not a problem for most systems to unzip automatically. If you do not have zip software built into your operating system, you can get free EasyZip here, and many other places:
http://www.thefreesite.com/easyzip111.htm

The zipped audiobook file contains 43 MP3 files/tracks adding up to 2 hr 45 min of listening, plus one PDF text file with a welcome message.

All the best!

The guru is in you.

2007/06/25 11:10:13
Books, Web Sites, Audio, Video, etc.
http://www.aypsite.org/forum/topic.asp?TOPIC_ID=2512&REPLY_ID=23511&whichpage=-1
AudioBooks - AYP Enlightenment Series

Hi All:

The **Spinal Breathing Pranayama Audiobook** is up on the website now. It is available in MP3 download, and will be available in CD format soon. All of the Enlightenment Series audiobooks will be available in both MP3 and CD formats. See these links:

Spinal Breathing: http://www.aypsite.org/books-sbpaudiobook.html
Deep Meditation: http://www.aypsite.org/books-dmaudiobook.html
Books Page (E-Series): http://www.aypsite.org/books.html#es

We have added **audio track lists** for the Spinal Breathing and Deep Meditation audiobooks on the above web pages, which provide much more detailed information on the subjects covered. There are **streaming audio sample tracks** available on the book pages too.

It will not be long before Tantra, Asanas/Mudras/Bandhas, and Samyama will be up there in audiobook format also.

Brett is the one responsible for all the audio editing and production. Many thanks, Brett! I only did the reading, which is the easy part. :-)

Happy listening, everyone, and all the best in your practices. I hope the audiobooks will be helpful to you.

The guru is in you.

2007/07/01 13:39:50
Books, Web Sites, Audio, Video, etc.
http://www.aypsite.org/forum/topic.asp?TOPIC_ID=2512&REPLY_ID=23693&whichpage=-1
AudioBooks - AYP Enlightenment Series

Hi All:

The **Tantra AudioBook** has been added to the website today, including a streaming audio preview:
http://www.aypsite.org/books.html#tantra

Enjoy!

The guru is in you.

2007/07/14 23:13:38
Books, Web Sites, Audio, Video, etc.
http://www.aypsite.org/forum/topic.asp?TOPIC_ID=2512&REPLY_ID=24201&whichpage=-1
AudioBooks - AYP Enlightenment Series

Hi All:

The **Asanas, Mudras and Bandhas AudioBook** has been added to the website today, including a streaming audio preview:
http://www.aypsite.org/books.html#amb

Enjoy!

The guru is in you.

2007/09/19 11:00:51
Books, Web Sites, Audio, Video, etc.
http://www.aypsite.org/forum/topic.asp?TOPIC_ID=2512&REPLY_ID=25579&whichpage=-1
AudioBooks - AYP Enlightenment Series

Hi All:

The Samyama AudioBook is now available for download in MP3 format here: http://www.aypsite.org/books.html#sam

A streaming audio preview is available there also.

It is planned to have the Deep Meditation and Spinal Breathing Pranayama AudioBooks available in CD format soon through CD Baby (USA) -- these are three CD sets with very nice packaging.

All of the Enlightenment Series books are available in MP3 AudioBook download, up through Samyama -- five so far.

Diet, Shatkarmas and Amaroli will be the next MP3 AudioBook, and I will let you know here when it is ready.

Many thanks to Trip (Brett) for making the AudioBooks possible!

The guru is in you.

2007/09/19 22:55:35
Books, Web Sites, Audio, Video, etc.
http://www.aypsite.org/forum/topic.asp?TOPIC_ID=2512&REPLY_ID=25594&whichpage=-1
AudioBooks - AYP Enlightenment Series

Hi All:

For those who are interested in clarifications on Samyama practice, a second streaming audio preview track has been added to the Samyama audiobook page. There are 11 questions on practice with detailed answers. It is about 30 minutes long.

See track #12 (Questions and Answers) here:
http://www.aypsite.org/books-samyamaaudiobook.html

All the best!

The guru is in you.

2007/10/26 18:16:18
Books, Web Sites, Audio, Video, etc.
http://www.aypsite.org/forum/topic.asp?TOPIC_ID=2512&REPLY_ID=26388&whichpage=-1
AudioBooks - AYP Enlightenment Series

Hi All:

The **Diet, Shatkarmas and Amaroli AudioBook** is now available for download in MP3 format here: http://www.aypsite.org/books.html#dsa

A streaming audio preview is available there also, about 18 minutes worth.

Now we are caught up with the MP3 audiobooks for all of the AYP Enlightenment Series books that have been published to date. Hooray!:-)

For all of the AYP direct downloads listed on one page (audiobooks and ebooks with audio introductions), see: http://www.aypsite.org/books-xdirdownload.html

CDs for all of the audiobooks will also begin appearing in the weeks and months ahead.

The next new Enlightenment Series book is coming out in a month or two:
Self-Inquiry - Dawn of the Witness and the End of Suffering

Many thanks to Trip (Brett) for making all of the AudioBooks possible!

The guru is in you.

2007/11/17 14:42:02
Books, Web Sites, Audio, Video, etc.
http://www.aypsite.org/forum/topic.asp?TOPIC_ID=2512&REPLY_ID=27087&whichpage=-1
AudioBooks - AYP Enlightenment Series

Hi All:

The **Deep Meditation Audiobook** is now available in **CD format**.

The **Spinal Breathing Pranayama Audiobook CD version** is in preparation and will be available soon.

Each Audiobook CD version consist of a 3 disc set packaged in a case with insert materials. It is a very nice presentation suitable for gift-giving.

All of the AYP Enlightenment Series Books are available in **MP3 download format** through multiple channels worldwide. We are gradually catching up in making the CD versions available.

All the best!

The guru is in you.

2007/11/26 23:13:41
Books, Web Sites, Audio, Video, etc.
http://www.aypsite.org/forum/topic.asp?TOPIC_ID=2512&REPLY_ID=27323&whichpage=-1
AudioBooks - AYP Enlightenment Series

Hi All:

The Spinal Breathing Pranayama CD AudioBook is up on CD Baby now. You can find the link for it (and the Deep Meditation CD AudioBook) here:

http://www.aypsite.com/books.html#dm

The guru is in you.

2008/03/09 17:18:12
Books, Web Sites, Audio, Video, etc.
http://www.aypsite.org/forum/topic.asp?TOPIC_ID=2512&REPLY_ID=31074&whichpage=-1
AudioBooks - AYP Enlightenment Series

Hi All:

The **Deep Meditation AudioBook** is now available on the **Amazon.com MP3 Download Site** here:
http://www.amazon.com/gp/product/B00153S666/ref=dm_sp_adp?ie=UTF8&qid=1205091056&sr=8-10

... including previews for the 43 sound tracks in the audiobook.

Not sure when the rest of the audiobooks will show up on Amazon. We are working on it. Most of them are available on **iTunes** now, but that may change due to changes occurring in the audiobook download industry. It is a very fluid situation.

All of the AYP AudioBooks (seven to date) can be downloaded directly through the AYP website here: http://www.aypsite.org/books-xdirdownload.html

That local availability will not be changing. :-)

All the best!

The guru is in you.

2007/05/31 16:27:50
Books, Web Sites, Audio, Video, etc.
http://www.aypsite.org/forum/topic.asp?TOPIC_ID=2616&REPLY_ID=22605&whichpage=-1
Great pointers

Hi Alan:

From the AYP point of view, it does not have to be all one thing or the other. In fact, becoming polarized in a single practice greatly increases the risks. Yoga is forever multi-dimensional, reflecting the broad inherent capabilities within our nervous system, a fact that can sometimes be forgotten in our enthusiasm for an exciting new angle on human spiritual transformation.

While some advaitists promoting non-dual self inquiry to the exclusion of all else might not like to hear it, self inquiry is aided tremendously when integrated with a daily routine of deep meditation, spinal breathing pranayama, etc. The whole of integrated practice is much greater than the sum of the parts.

Cultivating inner silence via deep meditation is especially important for advancing in self inquiry, or in any other yoga practice. This is consistent with non-dualism. Our inner silence is the non-dual nature of life itself.

While non-dual self inquiry is very appealing to the intellect, it can also lead to great personal difficulty (and getting very stuck) if not balanced with other practices and normal everyday living. This is true of any practice that is taken to excess to the exclusion of everything else.

Balance is the key. Hey, that's your name, isn't it? :-)

Wishing you all the best on your chosen path. Practice wisely, and enjoy!

The guru is in you.

PS: Abiding inner silence always leads to self inquiry, but self inquiry does not always lead to abiding inner silence.

2007/05/31 17:16:33
Books, Web Sites, Audio, Video, etc.
http://www.aypsite.org/forum/topic.asp?TOPIC_ID=2616&REPLY_ID=22607&whichpage=-1
Great pointers

quote:

Originally posted by Balance

From my understanding the approach I'm investigating isn't an intellectual practice. There are fundamental thoughts (questions) that arise and are released. This is a process that occurs naturally. the answers are not found in thought.

Yes, agreed, and that process finds its source in inner silence -- the witness. Lacking some abiding inner silence, the intellect has a tendency to get tangled up in the details, because where stillness is not present there will be endless discrimination. This is what makes self inquiry a two-edged sword. If it isn't helping release the mind, it will be further entangling the mind (24/7!). It is a very difficult practice for those without at least some abiding inner silence.

The impeccable logic of non-dual self inquiry is very seductive. Perhaps we have had a glimpse, and feel drawn. Even so, maintaining a stable effective practice is a very different thing.

That is one reason why we have not covered self inquiry in depth in AYP so far. But times are changing. Stillness is on the move. :-)

The guru is in you.

2007/06/08 10:13:24
Books, Web Sites, Audio, Video, etc.
http://www.aypsite.org/forum/topic.asp?TOPIC_ID=2651&REPLY_ID=22912&whichpage=-1
Osho - The Book of Secrets

Hi theglock:

Yes, I've read it. Excellent book. Osho's "opus magnum." It is mentioned in the lessons here: http://www.aypsite.org/T21.html

It (tantra) is about much more than sex, of course. So is the Book of Secrets, and the ancient scripture it is commenting on -- mainly the Vigyan Bhairava.

Osho (Rajneesh) was the most eclectic of the 20th century gurus, in stark contrast to other greats who placed their bets on one or two primary techniques. Osho took it the other way, to the extreme, discussing so many methods, that providing a practical daily routine out if it all turned out to be the greatest weakness in his approach. From the beginning, this left his followers to "indulge" in ways that threw the application of his teachings out of balance. So it goes. We learn from these things. :-)

As for mind "not being good," not sure what you mean. Mind is mind, heart is heart, feet are feet. If we systematically illuminate from inside with deep meditation and other well-integrated practices in the routine, all is illuminated and brought to higher external expression, including mind.

We shouldn't blame the hammer if the carpenter has not learned to use it correctly. I'd be surprised if Osho blamed the hammer for the carpenter's shortcomings. He was wiser than that. I know he liked to rant about human foibles sometimes. That's okay. We all have our rants. :-)

In the end, what matters is how useful the information is. Osho made a good contribution, as did many others. Now it is up to us to take it forward from here.

Wishing you all the best in that. Practice wisely, and enjoy!

The guru is in you.

2007/06/08 12:17:44
Books, Web Sites, Audio, Video, etc.
http://www.aypsite.org/forum/topic.asp?TOPIC_ID=2651&REPLY_ID=22920&whichpage=-1
Osho - The Book of Secrets

quote:
_____
Originally posted by theglock

That the mind is not good in that it is always attempting to calculate and divide and thinks with logic. It sets up barriers. From what I understand he feels that you don't slowly escalade to enlightment, it just hits you with a bang and you will no longer recognize yourself.
_____

Well if the big "bang" happens, it happens -- watch out for the aftershocks. We have seen more than a few big bangs around here, and the cleanup continues... :-)

In the meantime, deep meditation will be delivering us surely and safely. Even with all of his talk about "meditation," Osho may have missed this important point. He was moving around so much, and maybe he forgot that the way to strike water is to keep digging in one place. That is his weak point. He is more of an encyclopedia on spiritual methods than an instruction manual. While the former can be very inspiring and helpful, the latter is more practical.

It is an evolution of knowledge. We are all stepping stones to the next stage of better application and results. It is the way of applied science.

The guru is in you.

2007/08/06 13:36:29
Books, Web Sites, Audio, Video, etc.
http://www.aypsite.org/forum/topic.asp?TOPIC_ID=2819&REPLY_ID=24578&whichpage=-1
Diet Shatkarmas Book Release Date?

Hi Michael:

The **Diet, Shatkarmas and Amaroli** paperback should available on Amazon and other channels within one to two weeks. The links will be updated here as it becomes available in the various channels:
http://www.aypsite.org/books.html#dsa
(Reading sample and Table of Contents links are available here also)

As you say, it is available in ebook format now. It is also available now for direct ordering through me as part of any quantity discount order.
http://www.aypsite.org/forum/topic.asp?TOPIC_ID=1248

We hope to have it out in audiobook format in one or two months.

All the best!

The guru is in you.

2007/08/09 09:52:45
Books, Web Sites, Audio, Video, etc.
http://www.aypsite.org/forum/topic.asp?TOPIC_ID=2819&REPLY_ID=24635&whichpage=-1
Diet Shatkarmas Book Release Date?

Hi All:

The **Diet, Shatkarmas and Amaroli** book showed up on **Amazon USA** today. See link here: http://www.aypsite.org/books.html#dsa

The cover image and "search inside" will be added soon.

Book reviews on Amazon are greatly appreciated -- one of the best ways to help AYP reach more people. That is assuming the book is any good, of course. :-)

It should not be long before the book appears on the rest of the book seller sites.

The guru is in you.

2007/08/09 12:38:30
Books, Web Sites, Audio, Video, etc.
http://www.aypsite.org/forum/topic.asp?TOPIC_ID=2819&REPLY_ID=24641&whichpage=-1
Diet Shatkarmas Book Release Date?

Thanks YB.

It's up on Amazon UK now too.

The guru is in you.

2007/08/08 22:54:53
Books, Web Sites, Audio, Video, etc.
http://www.aypsite.org/forum/topic.asp?TOPIC_ID=2825&REPLY_ID=24622&whichpage=-1
self-inquiry book release date?

quote:
_____
Originally posted by clk1710

i'm looking forward to reading the new Self-Inquiry book. when's the release date? thanks!
_____

Hi Clk1710:

It's out there a couple of months. I hope in October. There have been some unavoidable delays here.

It will be a different kind of self-inquiry book for sure. :-)

The guru is in you.

2007/08/26 13:40:20
Books, Web Sites, Audio, Video, etc.
http://www.aypsite.org/forum/topic.asp?TOPIC_ID=2873
"Mother Teresa: Come Be My Light"

Hi All:

New Book -- **"Mother Teresa: Come Be My Light"** ... Letters of Mother Teresa.

http://www.reuters.com/article/topNews/idUSN2435506020070824

Mother Teresa's life is a good example of how deeds speak louder than words, even her own words.

If someone says they are enlightened, or not, or is called enlightened by others, or not, it matters little. It is deeds that will tell the tale of divine love flowing in the world.

No doubt that daily deep meditation would have made Mother Teresa's wonderful karma yoga even more effective.

The guru is in you.

2007/11/06 12:56:22
Books, Web Sites, Audio, Video, etc.
http://www.aypsite.org/forum/topic.asp?TOPIC_ID=3104
DSA Book gets a Kudo in New Age Retailer Magazine

Hi All:

The Diet, Shatkarmas and Amaroli (DSA) book has received an honorable mention in the New Age Retailer Magazine holiday issue. See below.

In spite of some efforts, AYP has attracted little attention in the "New Age" community so far. This certainly won't hurt.

The guru is in you.

From New Age Retailer:

Good news! Your product was reviewed in the Holiday issue of New Age Retailer, the No. 1 trade magazine in the spiritual marketplace for more than 21 years. A PDF copy of the review is attached for use in your marketing materials or for posting on your website.

http://www.aypsite.com/NewAgeRetailer-DSA-review.pdf

2008/09/02 10:58:54
Books, Web Sites, Audio, Video, etc.
http://www.aypsite.org/forum/topic.asp?TOPIC_ID=3175&REPLY_ID=37127&whichpage=-1
Yogani books at India-Chennai?

quote:
_____
Originally posted by sushman

The 'Self Inquiry' and 'Bhakti & Karma yoga' books are not available in http://www.Firstandsecond.com website.

Any reason?
_____

Hi Sushman:

The India edition of Bhakti and Karma Yoga is in the process of being printed. For more information, contact the publisher, Grasroutes, here: http://www.grasroutes.com/html/yoga.html

All the best!

The guru is in you.

2007/11/29 11:08:23
Books, Web Sites, Audio, Video, etc.
http://www.aypsite.org/forum/topic.asp?TOPIC_ID=3198&REPLY_ID=27456&whichpage=-1
Napster

Hi Mac:

Thanks for the heads up on "Spinal Breathing Pranayama" on Napster.

Look for the "Tantra" and "Asanas, Mudras and Bandhas" audiobooks in the digital distribution channels very soon. Napster and iTunes are currently the largest channels (with many more smaller ones out there). We are able to reach most of the digital distribution channels through CD Baby, in addition to having the CD audiobook versions there. We are working to have the MP3 audiobooks available on the new Amazon MP3 download service also.

We plan to have all of the completed Enlightenment Series audiobooks in all those digital distribution channels in the next month or two, and keep adding as new AYP books are completed.

Note: For those who are concerned about illustrations for the MP3 download audiobooks, internet links to PDF files are provided in the audio. The AYP direct download versions of the audiobooks include the PDFs right in the download zip file.

All the best!

The guru is in you.

2007/12/06 08:46:00
Books, Web Sites, Audio, Video, etc.
http://www.aypsite.org/forum/topic.asp?TOPIC_ID=3227&REPLY_ID=27705&whichpage=-1
Which book has all the online lessons?

Hi Rkishan:

The AYP Easy Lessons book you refer to covers the online lessons up to main lesson 235 and tantra lesson 35, plus about 20% new material in the form of "lesson additions and illustrations" that are not currently available online. This is the most complete version of the lessons up to that point, covering the core practices of AYP, including mantra enhancements and advanced forms of pranayama (spinal bastrika, etc.), asanas, mudras and bandhas, and tantric methods. The online lessons beyond main lesson 235 and tantra lesson 35 have not been put into book form yet, and this will be done later in AYP Easy Lessons Volume 2, which will include a lot of new material. When Volume 2 is complete, these two large volumes will constitute the full AYP teachings, as much as can be done up to that point in time.

Meanwhile, the small AYP Enlightenment Series books, being written after AYP Easy Lessons Volume 1, are concise and clear approaches to the core practices of AYP, and are designed to offer many easy entry points into the over all body of knowledge. Substantial new material not covered in AYP Easy Lessons Volume 1 or in the online lessons (yet) is included in the Enlightenment Series from the Samyama book onward. This is material that will be included and expanded upon in AYP Easy Lessons Volume 2.

AYP continues to be a work in progress. Hopefully in a few years it will all be there in detailed lesson form (two volumes), and also in the enlightenment series, providing many points of entry.

The "whole enchilada" will be in the AYP Easy Lessons volumes, so you are focusing on the right one for that. Add on the enlightenment series books at least from Samyama onward as they come out, and you will be up to date.

These forums are also an ever-evolving discussion on practices, filled with much useful information. Once the enlightenment series is done, I hope to return to posting online lessons again, leading to AYP Easy Lessons Vol 2.

For those who are interested in vicariously experiencing the journey of human spiritual transformation in story form, practices and all, there is the Secrets of Wilder novel. We are working to cover it from all angles, so there will be no mistaking the infinite potential that exists in everyone, and a practical approach to daily practice for realizing It. :-)

All the best on your path. Enjoy!

The guru is in you.

2007/12/06 15:12:11
Books, Web Sites, Audio, Video, etc.
http://www.aypsite.org/forum/topic.asp?TOPIC_ID=3227&REPLY_ID=27715&whichpage=-1
Which book has all the online lessons?

quote:
_____
Originally posted by rkishan

Yogani,

Thanks. So, if I get AYP Easy Lessons book, Samyama and Diet, Shatkarmas and Amaroli, I should have all the lessons written so far. Am I right? Does this include all the lessons for Asanas, Mudras and Bandhas?

I already have The Secrets of the Wilder and enjoyed the book!

Thanks,
Ram.
_____

Hi Ram:

Yes, that's right. The additional online lessons beyond main 235 and tantra 35 are mostly about nuances of experience and combinations of practices that are already covered in the AYP Easy Lessons book. The Enlightenment Series books you mentioned have new material in them not found anywhere else in the AYP writings. The same will be true of the next Enlightenment Series book on Self-Inquiry.

All the best!

The guru is in you.

2007/12/16 09:29:58
Books, Web Sites, Audio, Video, etc.
http://www.aypsite.org/forum/topic.asp?TOPIC_ID=3227&REPLY_ID=27979&whichpage=-1
Which book has all the online lessons?

Hi Julied:

Glad to hear the Deep Meditation books were happily shared.

No, have not done that again, and am not able to. Over 2000 books were given away worldwide at that time, and it nearly broke the bank here. However, anyone can do it using the quantity discount offer here: http://www.aypsite.org/forum/forum.asp?FORUM_ID=34

Many have taken advantage, and so the free books are still flowing via AYP community members.

All the best!

The guru is in you.

2008/01/09 18:11:22
Books, Web Sites, Audio, Video, etc.
http://www.aypsite.org/forum/topic.asp?TOPIC_ID=3350
AYP Self-Inquiry Book Becoming Available

Hi All:

The new Self-Inquiry book is beginning to move into the channels. The full title is:

Self-Inquiry - Dawn of the Witness and the End of Suffering

The direct download eBook version (with audio introduction) is available now. The physical book and audiobook versions should be available later this month.

See here for description, contents, previews, and purchase links: http://www.aypsite.org/books.html#si

This little book goes a long way toward putting some clear metrics (measuring rods) on self-inquiry in relation to the rise of inner silence (the witness) and enlightenment -- information that has been much needed in this sometimes confusing area of spiritual practice.

I hope it will be a useful road map for those who find themselves drawn to self-inquiry. Most everyone is as practices advance and the witness and ecstatic conductivity are coming up. The mind loves to get into the act, and under the right circumstances it can be a big help. :-)

Wishing you all the best on your path. Enjoy!

The guru is in you.

2008/01/10 08:53:55
Books, Web Sites, Audio, Video, etc.
http://www.aypsite.org/forum/topic.asp?TOPIC_ID=3350&REPLY_ID=28699&whichpage=-1
AYP Self-Inquiry Book Becoming Available

Hi Mac:

Glad to hear you are finding the book helpful.

It is funny, you know. Yoga and spiritual development are so much not about mind. Yet, we humans are all about mind. So, for that reason, self-inquiry seems to be a very logical approach to spiritual development. It is down right seductive. :-)

Recognizing and accepting that, this little book attempts to map out a "middle way" that will hopefully lead to a tempering of the mental flights of fancy we are all prone to. Self-inquiry will only work when released in stillness (the witness), which is an ongoing marriage of energy with inner silence -- the foundation of enlightenment. In the book it is called *relational self-inquiry*.

When the book shows up on Amazon in a couple of weeks, I hope anyone who finds it beneficial will put a review there. It helps a lot for spreading the word. Thanks!

The guru is in you.

2008/01/16 12:58:36
Books, Web Sites, Audio, Video, etc.
http://www.aypsite.org/forum/topic.asp?TOPIC_ID=3350&REPLY_ID=29004&whichpage=-1
AYP Self-Inquiry Book Becoming Available

Hi All:

The Self-Inquiry paperback book is now available for Quantity Discount orders, which are placed through me and are shipped directly from the printer in Tennessee, USA or London, UK.

The paperback book should begin showing up on Amazon worldwide and in other channels within a week or so. The respective links on the Books Page will be updated as soon as the book appears.

We also have the India paperback edition and MP3 AudioBook in the works.

All the best!

The guru is in you.

2008/01/20 10:41:33
Books, Web Sites, Audio, Video, etc.
http://www.aypsite.org/forum/topic.asp?TOPIC_ID=3350&REPLY_ID=29103&whichpage=-1
AYP Self-Inquiry Book Becoming Available

Hi YB:

Thank you. Yes, the Self-Inquiry book has shown up on Amazon USA, UK and other international sites. They do not have inventory yet, so the delivery times are still showing to be quite long. That will change as the books move into the physical channels. The more orders they get, the quicker that will happen. The title is showing incorrectly on the European sites, and a correction has been submitted. "Search Inside" should be appearing soon, and hopefully some reviews from all of you. :-)

Thanks, and all the best!

The guru is in you.

2008/01/25 00:15:40
Books, Web Sites, Audio, Video, etc.
http://www.aypsite.org/forum/topic.asp?TOPIC_ID=3350&REPLY_ID=29253&whichpage=-1
AYP Self-Inquiry Book Becoming Available

Hi All:

The **Self-Inquiry MP3 AudioBook Download** version is now available, including a streaming audio preview you can listen to on the website: http://www.aypsite.org/books.html#si

Enjoy! :-)

The guru is in you.

2008/02/07 23:27:52
Books, Web Sites, Audio, Video, etc.
http://www.aypsite.org/forum/topic.asp?TOPIC_ID=3350&REPLY_ID=29804&whichpage=-1

AYP Self-Inquiry Book Becoming Available

Hi All:

The Self-Inquiry book is now in stock at Amazon USA, available for immediate shipping. It took a while, but it is there now. We are working to complete listings and reduce ship times from the other sources shown on the AYP books page.

This one has been a bit slower setting up in the distribution channels than previous books. We are getting there.

Thanks for your patience.

The guru is in you.

PS: Amazon reviews are much appreciated by anyone who has read the book. Only a few reviews so far, but they are good ones. Thank you! :-)

2008/02/26 13:10:52
Books, Web Sites, Audio, Video, etc.
http://www.aypsite.org/forum/topic.asp?TOPIC_ID=3504&REPLY_ID=30564&whichpage=-1
A New Earth - Tolle's Free Online Classes

quote:
_____
Originally posted by Shanti

Wonder if re-sending the books will help?
_____

Hi Shweta and Kathy:

It couldn't hurt. It has been a couple of years since I have sent anything to Oprah. I only send a few out to yoga publications with each new book published now. It got to be too expensive to send to a long list, and the response was very small.

I have a mailing list of about 70 publications and reviewers here if anyone would like to send any of the AYP books out in quantity, or even target (or retarget, like Oprah) some of the key ones.

Thanks!

The guru is in you.

PS: Bless Eckhart Tolle. He is helping bring non-sectarian spirituality to the masses. Much needed. Bless Oprah too. :-)

2008/03/01 09:41:27
Books, Web Sites, Audio, Video, etc.
http://www.aypsite.org/forum/topic.asp?TOPIC_ID=3523&REPLY_ID=30678&whichpage=-1
Yogani's Writing

quote:
_____
Originally posted by Jim and His Karma

I bounce between thinking that 1. his books go through endless revision and massaging and 2. thinking he's simply in a flow state when he writes and doesn't need to do more than a couple drafts. Lately I'm leaning more toward the latter. Just out of intuition, but also I don't think there's a level of massaging and revision that can yield that particular result. I don't think....

But let's see what Yogani says (if he doesn't mind chiming in, that is!).
_____

Hi Jim and All:

Yes, it is #2. This is especially true of the E-Series books, which are not written incrementally over time like the AYP lessons are. For the E-Series books, there is a formation stage when the content is being gathered and organized inside with practically nothing being written beyond an evolving table of contents. And then it all pours out in a few weeks. The internal formation stage can take much longer than the actual writing.

Once the writing happens and there is a complete draft, it is only a matter of cleaning up my poor typing, spelling, and removing distortions I added to the process. None of this affects the original flow very much, except to hopefully make it more readable. When editing, the first priority is always to put myself in the reader's shoes, but I think the flow has taken that into account already. There are also several others who read the draft, which is a big help in cleaning up the messes I add to the flow. I am a very imperfect channel for this, and most of the work that is done on the draft is to compensate for that.

As for how it affects people, I think that comes from both sides, with the reader side being the dynamic aspect over the long term. Once completed, the writing is the writing, and it is the reader who then becomes the channel. With spiritual practices in the picture, every reading experience is certain to be more insightful than the last.

Which just goes to show...

The guru is in you.
:-)

2008/03/01 09:45:45
Books, Web Sites, Audio, Video, etc.
http://www.aypsite.org/forum/topic.asp?TOPIC_ID=3523&REPLY_ID=30679&whichpage=-1
Yogani's Writing
PS: It is stillness speaking to stillness.

2008/03/01 12:04:05
Books, Web Sites, Audio, Video, etc.
http://www.aypsite.org/forum/topic.asp?TOPIC_ID=3523&REPLY_ID=30690&whichpage=-1
Yogani's Writing

quote:
_____
Originally posted by Jim and His Karma

I've always had a lot of writing projects in semi-dormancy (especially when there's no deadline forcing their production!). For years, I thought this was a sign of laziness on my part. And maybe it was, a little. But since meditation has increased my self-insight, I understand that what I'm doing is allowing stuff to "bake"...the internal formulation you're talking about. The laziness enters the equation when baking/formulation has happened yet I don't actually start typing! :-)

I guess a lot of the angst famously experienced by artists (re: the fickleness of Muse) is due to the ineffable fact that external output only really flows when the idea is fully embraced by silence, which pushes it outward (it's all samyama!). You can't force it...in fact, forcing kills it!
_____

Hi Jim:

Deadlines help, especially ones that are advertised, since a promise made is a promise to be kept. And necessity is the mother of invention.

Publicly stated deadlines require us to prioritize things, and our inner processes will follow the lead, or compel us to rearrange our commitments. Either way, the entire process is expedited, usually at a cost to the person who is in the deadline cross-hairs.

Creativity would like to take its sweet time within us. The truth of the matter is that the expression of creativity (art) will not happen much without a perceived need for it. At the same time, what few of us realize is that we are all on a deadline. It is called our lifespan. So there's not a minute to waste, or is there?

To quote the immortal words of Joe Walsh (again). "People tell me I'm lazy, but it takes all my time."
I can relate to that when the internal formation process is going on. :-)

As most know, I have used published deadlines to help keep the AYP books flowing. Constant deadlines get tiring after a while though, so I'm looking forward to loosening them once the E-Series is caught up this summer. The intention is to move ahead at a more relaxed pace after that, with a return to online lesson posting, etc. That can be a pretty crazy life too, with all the email that is generated, but I am betting that much of it can be diverted to the forums where so much wonderful support is available now. Thank you!

Yes, the writing and its external trappings (work, deadlines, etc.) are very much samyama. As with our yoga practices, or anything else, it takes time to clear the channels and become fluent in whatever it is we are doing in life. It is the rise of stillness in action.

The guru is in you.

2008/03/01 12:38:10
Books, Web Sites, Audio, Video, etc.
http://www.aypsite.org/forum/topic.asp?TOPIC_ID=3523&REPLY_ID=30694&whichpage=-1
Yogani's Writing

quote:
_____
Originally posted by Jim and His Karma

My only confusion is the word "perceived"...is that the optimal term? I don't "perceive" where the sutra goes, or where it needs to go. It innately flows to need in a way that seems apart from perception (though I guess perception may sometimes inform the process).
_____

Ah, but who is perceiving? Something is using all the external faculties to make these things happen, even in our conscious choices. Where is the separation in this? Why should we look for a separation? It only gets in the way.

Just because I perceive a need to add 1 + 1 = 2, that doesn't mean a cosmic process isn't involved.

Just so, internal creative process + perceived need + action = art. Deadlines and work are part of that, so we do what must be done. Who care's who is doing it? In its fully developed state, it is doing itself. But we can't experience that if we keep second guessing the process. That is why the suggestion is to engage in spiritual practices and go out and do, using all the tools we have been blessed with, including our ability to perceive a need and choose to engage in effective action to fill it. That is what service is.

Where does all that come from? Inside. But the inside is outside and the outside is inside, you know. It is all one thing, until we separate it. :-)

The guru is in you.

2008/03/01 15:49:01
Books, Web Sites, Audio, Video, etc.
http://www.aypsite.org/forum/topic.asp?TOPIC_ID=3523&REPLY_ID=30701&whichpage=-1
Yogani's Writing

quote:
_____
Originally posted by Jim and His Karma

quote:
_____
Originally posted by yogani
Ah, but who is perceiving?
_____

Oh, no...you've turned into Sailor Bob Adamson! :-)
_____

Hi Jim:

That kind of inquiry by itself is "non-duality dodgeball." I can say that, being the one who just threw it at you. :-)

It is the follow-up that really counts, as in what to do to realize *That* without getting the mind wrapped around the axle 300 times. It is what the Self-Inquiry book is about.

The guru is in you.

PS: Thank you, VIL. Yes, everything we have done has led to this convergent moment.
2008/04/03 10:42:19
Books, Web Sites, Audio, Video, etc.
http://www.aypsite.org/forum/topic.asp?TOPIC_ID=3707&REPLY_ID=32138&whichpage=-1
Kriya Yoga

Hi John:

Since AYP started being published back in 2003, it has often been associated with this or that tradition. I guess it is part of the never-ending human quest to apply labels to everything. While it is true that the integrated approach to practices utilized in AYP considers methods found in many traditions, it is not an off-shoot or clone of any tradition. So the labels do not apply.

Kriya Yoga gets singled out pretty often as being a more hefty path of which AYP is but a shadow. Actually, I think the reverse is true, in the sense that Kriya Yoga has become a shadow of what it was in the distant past. That is what happens to spiritual paths as they travel the dusty corridors of time, particularly secret paths, which most paths have been until now. They tend to become ingrown and fractured, with the remains becoming over-embellished and diluted in their effectiveness.

For example, there is evidence that the "advanced" versions of spinal breathing found in modern Kriya Yoga, involving chakra visualizations and mantra recitations, are actually degradations in the basic no-frills, highly effective practice of spinal breathing that we use in AYP. It is telling that the loaded-down Kriya Yoga version of spinal breathing requires much longer sittings while producing fewer results.

And there is really no comparison between Kriya Yoga "passive listening" omkar meditation and the "active favoring" of mantra in deep meditation as used in AYP. They are completely different practices, producing very different results.

These two comparisons alone place Kriya Yoga and AYP in different universes, so it is misleading to equate them.

Other practices which might seem to be shared between Kriya Yoga and AYP are also applied in fundamentally different ways. Plus, there are important elements of practice in AYP that are not part of Kriya Yoga -- such as tantric sexual methods and samyama.

It is really about optimizing results. While we see people "busting out all over" in the AYP community, we don't hear much from the stodgy environs of Kriya Yoga. Maybe they are just more modest and less enthusiastic about spiritual openings than we are? :-)

Much more can be learned about the origins of AYP by studying John Wilder than by studying Babaji and Lahiri Mahasaya. Which is to say, AYP is based more on the natural neurobiology of human spiritual transformation found in all of us than on any handed down tradition. It is good to study the traditions, but not so good to get stuck in them. A viable spiritual path should reflect causes and effects occurring within us in the present, not clinging to by-rote methods that have been handed down. If it works in the present, then use it. And if it doesn't, then better keep looking. That should apply when considering any system of practice, including AYP.

So, while there may appear to be similarities between Kriya Yoga and AYP, such comparisons are only skin deep. I have great respect for the venerable tradition of Kriya Yoga, but what we are doing here is not a clone of it, and certainly not a less powerful version of it. Let the results speak for themselves.

All the best!

The guru is in you.

2008/04/18 12:11:06
Books, Web Sites, Audio, Video, etc.
http://www.aypsite.org/forum/topic.asp?TOPIC_ID=3791&REPLY_ID=32788&whichpage=-1
Yoga Nidra

Hi Snake:

I can't answer your question specifically, but can say that AYP Cosmic Samyama is a powerful form of Yoga Nidra. We look at Yoga Nidra as a high octane practice further down the line in the over all scheme of AYP, coming after deep meditation and core samyama practice are well-established.

Which is not to say those who begin with another style of Yoga Nidra elsewhere and come to AYP later are on a wrong track. Surely not. It is a great place to be coming to AYP from. Anyplace is. :-)

The main differences between Cosmic Samyama and most styles of Yoga Nidra practice are:

1. From the beginning, Cosmic Samyama is inner-guided rather than guided by an external CD or other person.

2. Samyama technique is used in the practice sequence of touching 16 realms (in sutra form) within and outside the physical body, which systematically cultivates the process of dynamically expanding stillness on the individual and cosmic levels -- the two being the same.

Cosmic Samyama is covered in the AYP Samyama book.

The guru is in you.

2008/05/28 12:22:39
Books, Web Sites, Audio, Video, etc.
http://www.aypsite.org/forum/topic.asp?TOPIC_ID=3970
Tips on Secrets of Wilder Practice Chart

Hi All:

From an email exchange:

Q: In the Secrets of Wilder book it has a chart on how to go about the practices. Would it be possible to put page number in relation to the master manual (AYP Easy Lessons book) of where we could find each practice? I tried to cross reference and some of them I could not find in the manual.

A: If you check the topic index in the back of the AYP Easy Lessons book (or here), you will find corresponding lessons for the practices. Of course, some of the practices have different names than in the Wilder book.

Looking at the chart, "breath suspension" is kumbhaka, "nine prayers" is samyama, "spiritual eye purge" is yoni mudra kumbhaka, "root seat" is siddhasana, "root lift" is mulabandha, "eye lift" is sambhavi mudra, "medulla pull" is slightly furrowed brow (part of sambhavi), "palate lift" and the two subsequent stages ("altar of bliss" and "upper passages") are stages of kechari mudra, and "*i am's* embrace" is whole body mudra (see "micro-movements" in the topic index).

You can also find most of the practices covered concisely in the small Enlightenment Series books -- the titles and book descriptions tell the tale.

I am working on the ninth Enlightenment Series volume now -- "Eight Limbs of Yoga". It has an expanded version of the practice chart in it, more description with it, and cross-referencing to AYP instructional materials on practices. The new practice chart also brings the terminology back to the yogic versions, tying in with the rest of the AYP writings. The Eight Limbs book should be out in July. "Bhakti and Karma Yoga" (Enlightenment Series book #8) will be out in a few weeks. So, we will be caught up with scheduled books pretty soon. Then it is on to adding more online lessons, leading eventually to AYP Easy Lessons Volume 2.

The Secrets of Wilder was the first book I wrote (first drafted back in 2003), with the mission of making the practices more accessible for westerners. Hence, no yogic terminology in there. It is about experiencing the journey in story form in a western cultural setting. Hope you enjoyed it. :-)

The guru is in you.

2008/06/11 11:33:28
Books, Web Sites, Audio, Video, etc.
http://www.aypsite.org/forum/topic.asp?TOPIC_ID=4026
AYP Bhakti and Karma Yoga Book

Hi All:

The **Bhakti and Karma Yoga** book is out. You can find it here: http://www.aypsite.org/books.html#bky

The book is now available in the Amazon paperback and third party ebook channels. It can also be ordered through the quantity discount program.

It will be mid to late July before the AYP Direct Download ebook (w/audio intro) and MP3 audiobook versions will be available, because I will be out of town for the next couple of weeks.

As always, candid Amazon reviews are much needed and appreciated. It is one of the best ways to help pass the word on AYP. Amazon is where AYP receives much of its first time public exposure.

Thanks much, and all the best!

The guru is in you.

PS: It is expected that the last scheduled Enlightenment Series book, **Eight Limbs of Yoga**, will be coming out by the end of July also.

2008/07/16 10:53:17
Books, Web Sites, Audio, Video, etc.

AYP Bhakti and Karma Yoga Book

Hi All:

The "eBook with Audio Introduction" version of **Bhakti and Karma Yoga** (BKY), directly downloadable through AYP, is now available.

These are the PDF ebooks with mimimal security (password only), which are easily portable, and do not have the reliability and portability issues of Adobe secured ebooks. And if there is ever a problem (with any AYP ebook), just write me and we will fix it up quickly.

In addition, the MP3 AudioBook version of BKY should be out in about a week, also a direct download.

You can find them both (and all BKY editions) here: http://www.aypsite.org/books.html#bky

The direct download editions (eBooks and AudioBooks) for all the AYP books are listed here: http://www.aypsite.org/books-xdirdownload.html

Happy reading and listening! :-)

The guru is in you.

2008/07/26 14:40:29
Books, Web Sites, Audio, Video, etc.
AYP Bhakti and Karma Yoga Book

Hi All:

The Bhakti and Karma Yoga MP3 AudioBook is up on the books page now and available for download.

There is a streaming audio preview available there too. See the track list here: http://www.aypsite.org/books-bkyaudiobook.html

Enjoy! :-)

The guru is in you.

2008/06/21 15:03:41
Books, Web Sites, Audio, Video, etc.
books similar to wilder

Hi Tubeseeker:

Four "personal journey" predecessors to the Secrets of Wilder are Siddartha, Jonathan Livingston Seagull, the Way of the Peaceful Warrior, and the Celestine Prophesy.

While none of these go as far as the Secrets of Wilder in terms of actual practices and mapping the process of human spiritual transformation, they do provide helpful frameworks of spiritual knowledge and good inspiration.

Also check out Life and Teaching of the Masters of the Far East by BT Spalding, a rousting series of spiritual adventures written nearly a century ago.

The Secrets of Wilder is intended to be a step forward in spiritual fiction, an attempt to bring this kind of writing closer to the actual practices and experiences on the journey. Time will tell if it succeeds. I hope we will see more story telling of this type in the future.

Autobiography of a Yogi and the Gospel of Ramakrishna are terrific spiritual books -- the first for inspiration and the second for a detailed chronicle of the journey itself. However, I would put both of these in a different class than the books mentioned above, since neither is a novel (though perhaps embellished a bit), and both are presented from the point of view of traditional Indian spiritual culture. Nothing wrong with that. Two others in this category are Swami Rama's Living with the Himalayan Masters, and Muktananda's Play of Consciousness.

For more spiritual stories and biographies, see here:
http://www.aypsite.org/booklist11.html
and here:
http://www.aypsite.org/booklist10.html

All the best!

The guru is in you.

2008/07/13 00:22:27
Books, Web Sites, Audio, Video, etc.
The Book on the Taboo Against Knowing Who You Are
Amen to that. :-)

It has been said that it is good to be born in a religion,
but not so good to die in one.

The guru is in you.

2008/09/18 14:52:37
Books, Web Sites, Audio, Video, etc.
http://www.aypsite.org/forum/topic.asp?TOPIC_ID=4461
AYP Eight Limbs of Yoga Book

Hi All:

The **Eight Limbs of Yoga** book is finished. This is the ninth AYP Enlightenment Series book, and ties it all together. The book includes a practice chart like the one in the Secrets of Wilder novel, only more comprehensive and fully explained.

The AYP direct download PDF eBook version (with audio introduction) is available now, with other eBook versions soon to follow. Over the next few weeks the Paperback and MP3 AudioBook versions will become available.

See here for information and availability: http://www.aypsite.org/books.html#8lim
Or click on the "Eight Limbs" cover image in the right-side margin on any page of the forum or website.

All the best!

The guru is in you.

2008/09/25 22:51:14
Books, Web Sites, Audio, Video, etc.
http://www.aypsite.org/forum/topic.asp?TOPIC_ID=4461&REPLY_ID=38132&whichpage=-1
AYP Eight Limbs of Yoga Book

Thanks much, All.

Looks like the Eight Limbs paperback version will be ready and submitted to Amazon and other retailers next week, with listings probably showing up the following week. The audiobook version will not be far behind.

Amazon reviews are always much appreciated. It is one of the best places to share thoughts on any or all of the books, where many who do not know about AYP can get a first taste.

Will be taking a short break here, and then diving back into the online lessons, after a two year absence while doing the e-series. Still a lot of ground to cover in the online lessons. It's good to be coming back to where it all began. :-)

All the best!

The guru is in you.

2008/10/04 10:41:13
Books, Web Sites, Audio, Video, etc.
http://www.aypsite.org/forum/topic.asp?TOPIC_ID=4461&REPLY_ID=38563&whichpage=-1
AYP Eight Limbs of Yoga Book

Hi All:

The **Eight Limbs of Yoga** paperback book is now on Amazon USA (cover image, description and "search inside" to be added soon). It is also on Barnes and Noble USA. The book is expected to be on the rest of the Amazon sites (Canada, UK, Europe, Japan) in a few days. See here for all links: http://www.aypsite.org/books.html#8lim (or click the book cover image in the right side margin)

The book is also now available for **Quantity Discount** orders direct through AYP, by itself or in combination with any other AYP books. See here on that: http://www.aypsite.org/forum/topic.asp?TOPIC_ID=1248

The **AudioBook** version has been recorded and is in editing. We should see that one out soon also.

All the best!

The guru is in you.

PS: For those who have read the **Eight Limbs of Yoga** book already, a candid review on Amazon USA (or anywhere) will be much appreciated. The same goes for the **Bhakti and Karma Yoga** book that came out this summer, which has only 4 reviews on Amazon USA so far. Thanks!

2008/10/25 00:09:30
Books, Web Sites, Audio, Video, etc.
http://www.aypsite.org/forum/topic.asp?TOPIC_ID=4461&REPLY_ID=39448&whichpage=-1
AYP Eight Limbs of Yoga Book

Hi All:

The **Eight Limbs of Yoga MP3 AudioBook** is out and now available for download direct from AYP and from Payloadz. Over the next month or two it will show up on Amazon, iTunes and CD Baby.

Links for the MP3 AudioBook (as well as Paperback and eBook editions) can be found here: http://www.aypsite.org/books.html#8lim

There is an audio preview there too.

All the best!

The guru is in you.

2008/10/29 22:59:49
Books, Web Sites, Audio, Video, etc.
http://www.aypsite.org/forum/topic.asp?TOPIC_ID=4461&REPLY_ID=39644&whichpage=-1
AYP Eight Limbs of Yoga Book

quote:
_____
Originally posted by x.j.

I looked on Google and there are 91,000 entries there already on "The Eight Limbs Of Yoga". And how many books have already been written as commentaries on Patanjali's original treatise of this same title? I seem to remember there are something like 66 books already written on that. So Yogani, before I order your skinny book on this subject, could you tell me right up front: Have you found something left to say that hasn't been said before? (I have atleast three books on the same topic, and with the same title, gathering dust on a book shelf.)
I hope it's OK to make such an impertinent though candid comment. I imagine others have had the same question in their mind though not spoken. I guess I am a bull in the china shop. Uh Oh.
x.j.
_____

Hi x.j.:

The AYP Eight Limbs of Yoga book is not a commentary on the the Yoga Sutras or the Eight Limbs. It uses these as a touch stone and jumping off point to tie together the practices covered in the eight previous Enlightenment Series books, which, taken all together, constitute a practical approach to applying the essentials of the ancient knowledge for modern self-directed practitioners.

The subtitle of the book is, "The Structure and Pacing of Self-Directed Spiritual Practice," which is a pretty good description of what it is about. If you'd like more detail on what is in it, check the table of contents and the more detailed audio track list here:
http://www.aypsite.org/books-8limbsebook.html
...and here:
http://www.aypsite.org/books-8limbsaudiobook.html

The book also contains a "practice chart" for the AYP system, with supporting description. It is an updated version of the early chart found in the Secrets of Wilder novel.

So, for anyone interested in reviewing the whole AYP system, why it is what it is, how it fits together, and how it can be built into a daily practice routine over time, this is the best we have so far. We will elaborate further in AYP Easy Lessons Volume 2, whenever that happens.

The guru is in you.

2008/10/07 10:28:53
Books, Web Sites, Audio, Video, etc.
http://www.aypsite.org/forum/topic.asp?TOPIC_ID=4547&REPLY_ID=38659&whichpage=-1
New AYP book?

quote:
_____
Originally posted by Magne

Hi
I'm just wondering if the main AYP book will come out in a new edition soon? I would like to have ALL the lessons (-288)in the book..
Yogani, are you planning to release more lessons before printing a new edition containg the rest? I have a complete collection of the books, including all audiobooks on my iPhone:-), so it would be nice to have a complete main lessons book also, not just a computerprint of lessons not contained in the book
Keep up the great work!
_____

Hi Magne:

Thank you. Very happy to hear you are finding the AYP writings helpful.

Now that the nine Enlightenment Series books are complete, the plan is to go back to online lesson posting soon, which will eventually lead to another large AYP Easy Lessons book -- Volume 2. I can't say exactly when that book will come out, but would think not more than two years away. Believe it or not, it only took one year to write and publish the first one, but I may be slowing down a little now. Then again, who knows how it will all come out once we get going in that mode of writing again? :-)

There is quite a lot of new material to cover in the lessons (much of it is introduced in concise form in the last five books of the Enlightenment Series), plus covering the ongoing discussions on experiences. So much has happened in the community of practitioners that has led to refinements in the AYP system. It has always been an integration of one person's experience with the experiences of many, and the lessons will continue along those lines, with new material being presented and mixed with Q&As (shifting from email to these forums). It is expected that about 200 new lessons will be added before AYP Easy Lessons Volume 2 is realized. It will pick up where the first volume left off, at Main Lesson #235 and Tantra Lesson #35.

In the meantime, 70-80% of Volume 2 will be showing up online as we go (as you mentioned, some is there already), so we can read and discuss while we wait for the new book. I like that approach. Doing online lessons is much more fun than being locked away to write hundreds of pages at a time with a publishing deadline hanging over it. No more deadlines for a while. :-)

All the best!

The guru is in you.

2008/10/16 13:08:34
Books, Web Sites, Audio, Video, etc.
http://www.aypsite.org/forum/topic.asp?TOPIC_ID=4563&REPLY_ID=38993&whichpage=-1
Must read on kriya yoga practice

Hi x.j.:

I am not aware of any video on AYP chin pump, but that may be addressed eventually here:
http://www.aypsite.org/forum/topic.asp?TOPIC_ID=4578#38988

AYP chin pump (an adaption of Kriya Thokar) is quite gentle, using only gravity to swing the head down toward the hollow of the throat in the swooping portion of rotating the head. It should be prudently self-paced according to individual need, so as not to become a strain. With the rise and stabilization of ecstatic conductivity, it can be effective as a very small movement -- part of "whole body mudra."

Here are two original lessons on chin pump:
Chin Pump: http://www.aypsite.org/139.html
Chin Pump Lite: http://www.aypsite.org/144.html
(see related nearby lessons also)

All the best!

The guru is in you.

2009/04/14 06:13:30
Books, Web Sites, Audio, Video, etc.
http://www.aypsite.org/forum/topic.asp?TOPIC_ID=5454&REPLY_ID=48667&whichpage=-1
Purchased AYP ebooks no longer accessible

Hi Polycue:

Sorry you are having difficulty with the Adobe secured ebooks. In part because of this, AYP offers ebooks (as well as MP3 audiobooks) for direct download here: http://www.aypsite.org/books-xdirdownload.html
These ebooks are zipped PDF files with an MP3 audio introduction included, and no onerous security.

Anyone who is having problems with AYP Adobe secured ebooks can receive direct download replacements at no cost by writing me here.

All the best!

The guru is in you.

Note: The AYP ebooks are also available on the Amazon Kindle reader. The Amazon conversion for Kindle alters book format, especially pages with illustrations. Just a heads up on that.

The AYP direct download PDF ebooks mentioned above can be viewed on the Sony Reader, or any other device that can handle PDFs. The PDF ebooks used to be password-protected, but that was removed a few months ago to facilitate the Sony and other readers.

2009/04/26 21:40:07
Books, Web Sites, Audio, Video, etc.
http://www.aypsite.org/forum/topic.asp?TOPIC_ID=5527&REPLY_ID=49434&whichpage=-1
Material overlap between AYP texts

Hi Luke, and welcome!

While this post was written over a year ago, it is still a good summary of what the AYP books cover:
http://www.aypsite.org/forum/topic.asp?TOPIC_ID=3227#27705

Update: The 9 Enlightenment Series books were completed in Sept 2008, online lesson posting resumed in Nov 2008, and AYP Easy Lessons Volume 2 is looking like 2010 or 2011 at this stage.

All the best!

The guru is in you.

2009/05/13 12:09:59
Books, Web Sites, Audio, Video, etc.
http://www.aypsite.org/forum/topic.asp?TOPIC_ID=5598&REPLY_ID=50681&whichpage=-1
Bodhisattva on the metro
:-)
2009/06/17 11:18:28
Books, Web Sites, Audio, Video, etc.
http://www.aypsite.org/forum/topic.asp?TOPIC_ID=5802&REPLY_ID=52450&whichpage=-1

One Day

quote:
_____
Originally posted by Shanti

...Maybe we need to find a way to put Yogani's audio recordings from YouTube and/or Yogani's radio interviews out there? Yogani? Trip?
_____

Will check into it. Thanks! :-)

2009/08/12 10:26:26
Books, Web Sites, Audio, Video, etc.
http://www.aypsite.org/forum/topic.asp?TOPIC_ID=6109&REPLY_ID=54997&whichpage=-1
Need books

Hi Anandatandava:

The number of books out there is endless. For promoting whole body ecstatic conductivity, the AYP lessons and books aim to reveal the underlying principles, and practical methods for activating them. That includes the full range of practices. An integrated approach is recommended over focussing on any one part to the exclusion of other parts. In the AYP approach, that means daily deep meditation established first before pranayama, mudras, bandhas, tantric sexual methods, etc. Without the rise of abiding inner silence, ecstatic conductivity will be limited in its reach. That prerequisite also applies to kechari mudra, which I know you are very interested in.

For those who would like to help out with books, anyone can provide an Amazon gift certificate sent to your email, and the books can be sent direct to you from Amazon. I assume the email address attached to your member ID here goes to a family member and contact and implementation of Amazon gift purchases can be achieved in that way. If someone needs an email address for sending an Amazon gift certificate to you, it can be obtained from me. Not positive, but I believe Amazon gift certificates can be sent anonymously.

Btw, elsewhere here you expressed interest in Ramakrishna. The "Gospel of Ramakrishna" by "M" is the definitive work on his life and teaching. It is about 1000 pages. It comes in an abridged version also. Ramakrishna was not primarily a tantrika, regarded mainly as a bhakta (devotional yogi), though overlap can certainly be found. His relationship with his ishta deva (goddess Kali) was both devotional and romantic -- divine romance! :-)

All the best!

The guru is in you.

2009/11/09 10:52:29
Books, Web Sites, Audio, Video, etc.
http://www.aypsite.org/forum/topic.asp?TOPIC_ID=6655&REPLY_ID=59501&whichpage=-1
Yogani Books

Hi Raja:

If you go to the AYP books page, you will see several links under each title for India paperback editions available through online retailers. There may also be a bookstore carrying them in Bangalore. Check with the publisher for that at chandrikark@gmail.com. That is Grasroutes in New Delhi. The quantity discount for AYP books may also be used with them.

Miguel is right, the ebooks (and audiobooks) can be downloaded anywhere in the world. On the books page, there are multiple links under each title for that also. For direct downloads from AYP, see here: http://www.aypsite.org/books-xdirdownload.html

Thanks much for your interest in the AYP books. All the best!

The guru in you.

2009/11/09 14:23:29
Books, Web Sites, Audio, Video, etc.
http://www.aypsite.org/forum/topic.asp?TOPIC_ID=6655&REPLY_ID=59519&whichpage=-1
Yogani Books

quote:
_____
Originally posted by krcqimpro1

Hi Yogani, After the "AYP" book containing 235 lessons, when is the next paperback coming out containing all the new lessons you have added in the last 3 or 4 years ?
Krish
_____

Hi Krish:

Hoping to have AYP Volume 2 (another big one) out by the end of 2010. That will cover the online lessons (with additions) from main 235 and tantra 35 onward. Right now, we are at main 367 and tantra 70. I expect we will end up somewhere around main 450 and tantra 80 for Volume 2.

All the best!

The guru is in you.

2009/11/25 09:22:33
Books, Web Sites, Audio, Video, etc.
http://www.aypsite.org/forum/topic.asp?TOPIC_ID=6746
eBook Reading Devices and AYP Books

Hi All:

As you may know, all of the AYP books are available for the Amazon Kindle here. This is Amazon's proprietary format ebook reader, which alters book format, moving some of the illustrations around on the pages. Other than that inconvenience, the Kindle formatted ebooks are fine.

There has been an announcement recently that all Kindles will receive a software upgrade soon so they can also read standard PDF documents. This is good news, because all of the AYP ebooks are available for download in standard PDF format here.

As far as I know, all the ebook readers that are out now cover PDF format -- Sony, Barnes & Noble, etc., so we are covered for all devices as ebook readers become more popular. Amazon Kindle is expanding to cover PDF reading to keep up with the competition.

Speaking of competition, Google Book Partners has announced they will be rolling out paid online reading of ebooks in 2010, so any device with an internet browser can become an ebook reader. All of the AYP books will be available through that source also.

Of course, the AYP ebooks can be read on your computer in PDF format, which is where it all started. And the AYP ebooks continue to be available through the original Adobe-secured format channels, like Diesel. Additional sources for the AYP ebooks can be found on the books page.

Just an update on the evolving state of affairs for ebooks. We are doing our best to keep up. :-)

Enjoy!

The guru is in you.

2009/12/11 23:32:20
Books, Web Sites, Audio, Video, etc.
http://www.aypsite.org/forum/topic.asp?TOPIC_ID=6841&REPLY_ID=61187&whichpage=-1
Question re: AYP Book

Hi Jivaakabhasana_Yogi:

The big AYP book has about 20% more material in it than the online lessons. It goes to Main Lesson 235 and Tantra Lesson 35. The online lessons are now up to Main 374 and Tantra 71. In about a year the online lessons (plus additions) beyond the big AYP yellow book will be put into an another big AYP Vol 2, and the two volumes together will have all the lessons -- about 500 altogether. So you will need both volumes to cover all the lessons.

Here is something I wrote about it a couple of years ago:
http://www.aypsite.org/forum/topic.asp?TOPIC_ID=3227#27705
(The nine Enlightenment Series books were completed since then)

And something more recent:
http://www.aypsite.org/forum/topic.asp?TOPIC_ID=6655#59519

All the best!

The guru is in you.

2010/01/09 10:15:37
Books, Web Sites, Audio, Video, etc.
http://www.aypsite.org/forum/topic.asp?TOPIC_ID=6998&REPLY_ID=62441&whichpage=-1
Secrets Of Wilder

Hi Krish:

Happy to hear you enjoyed the Secrets of Wilder (SOW). You know, it was the first book written, before AYP started, and inspired me to do AYP. That John Wilder is an inspiring fellow.

Because SOW came first, and AYP after, the practice discussions in AYP should be taken as the priority over SOW. And the writings continue to evolve, driven mainly these days by experiences in the community of practitioners. When it gets to the point where the writing is going totally in circles, I will stop. :-)

Keeping all of that in mind, here are a few comments on your questions:

1. "I AM" and "*i am*" (etc.) are literary devices that were used to denote the refinement (inward going) characteristics of the mantra. That's all.

2. AYP instructions on chin pump take precedence.

3. Medulla pull is sambhavi (it actually pulls far below the medulla, at the root). I am's embrace is ecstatic whole body mudra in AYP (which is a mixture of intentional and automatic, beginning with a raising of the eyes).

4. Breath suspension is kumbhaka, which is used in chin pump and yoni mudra in AYP. Yes, palate lift is kechari.

5. Yes, SOW is fiction. Like all fiction, it is a story constructed with a mixture of real and fictional events. Obviously, the practices and many of the experiences are real, as many here can verify. Where reality and fiction meet in the novel is best left to the reader's imagination, and bhakti. :-)

All the best!

The guru is in you.

2010/02/13 12:47:19
Books, Web Sites, Audio, Video, etc.
http://www.aypsite.org/forum/topic.asp?TOPIC_ID=7273&REPLY_ID=64830&whichpage=-1
New AYP-Inspired Website: LivingUnbound.Net
Bravo! :-)

2010/03/11 08:46:11
Books, Web Sites, Audio, Video, etc.
http://www.aypsite.org/forum/topic.asp?TOPIC_ID=7401&REPLY_ID=65958&whichpage=-1
Khecari Vidya PhD Thesis by James Mallinson

Hi Alwayson:

Upon inquiry, Jim Mallinson ("flying fakir" in the forums) replied with this:

Thanks for alerting me to this. I had in fact come across the thesis on scribd a while ago. I'm happy for people to download it, but I'd like to alert them to the fact that there are significant improvements in the published book - hundreds of corrections/changes, improvements to the typesetting, Sanskrit in Devanagari, and, perhaps most usefully, an index. At £85 or whatever it was for sale for, I didn't expect anyone other than libraries to buy it, but I've just discovered that Routledge are about to release a paperback edition for £22.50. Indica books in Varanasi are also about to publish an Indian paperback edition, which should retail for about 500 Rs. Khecari-mudra-practising insomniacs might find it easier to take a book to bed with them to help them sleep rather than a pdf!

All the best,

Jim

2010/05/12 23:28:21
Books, Web Sites, Audio, Video, etc.
http://www.aypsite.org/forum/topic.asp?TOPIC_ID=7774
Enlighten Up!

Hi All:

Documentary film: Enlighten Up!

An informative, sometimes hilarious, and sometimes touching 6 month journey of "a skeptic" through the many incarnations of yoga, West and East.

Here it is on Amazon. It is available on Netflix instant watch also.

Enjoy! :-)

The guru is in you.

2010/07/20 17:54:07
Books, Web Sites, Audio, Video, etc.
http://www.aypsite.org/forum/topic.asp?TOPIC_ID=8132
AYP eBooks - New Formats and Price Reductions

Hi All:

With the help of a fantastic programmer, whom we will call "J" for now, AYP is moving into a position to participate in the ebook revolution that is finally getting underway with the new e-readers and tablet computers coming out now. This has required adding EPUB and MOBI ebook formats in addition to the PDF ebook format we have been using since the beginning. It has been a major technical project, and is now nearly done.

In addition to the technical restructuring, there is a commercial restructuring going on in the ebook industry, which is enabling us to lower AYP ebook list prices.

Here is what it all means for AYP ebook reading and pricing:

With the new MOBI files, reading AYP ebooks on the Amazon Kindle is much improved.

The new EPUB files will enable the AYP ebooks to be in the Apple iBookstore for iPad, iPod and iPhone reading, It will take a few months to get it set up, but it is coming.

EPUB also covers Barnes and Noble Nook, the Sony reader, and a host of other e-readers and tablet computers. Many e-readers and tablet computers also read PDF files, so PDF is not becoming obsolete -- it remain the highest quality/resolution ebook file to use, reflecting the exact format of the physical book. EPUB and MOBI files reformat the book to fit the reading device being used.

Direct downloads of ebooks through the AYP website **now include PDF, EPUB and MOBI files in the Zip File you download**, and also the short MP3 introduction. It is three for the price of one, and the price of one is now less also. These are non-DRM (non-digital rights management) files, giving the reader maximum flexibility for all reading devices in the household.

Price Reductions
With the large players now vying for publishers to sign up with them, the share of ebook revenues going to publishers has increased. To share that with readers, all AYP ebook list prices have been reduced as follows:

AYP Easy Lessons -- was $14.95, is now $9.99
Secrets of Wilder Novel -- was $7.95, is now $5.99
Enlightenment Series eBooks (9 of those) -- were $5.99, are now $4.99

These list prices are effective immediately for AYP Direct Downloads, and will show up in all the distribution channels as their systems are updated.

Keep in mind that AYP Direct Downloads now provide PDF, EPUB and MOBI formats for the price of one ebook, so chances are good that whatever reading device you are using, we have you covered. If not, non-DRM EPUB files can be converted to additional formats using the free Calibre ebook management software.

eBook format and price changes above are reflected on the corresponding AYP book pages.

On top of all of this, the Google eBookstore is opening sometime this summer (or winter down-under), which will enable ebook reading and downloading on any device with an internet browser. Google has signed up the independent brick-and-mortar bookstore industry in the USA, so we will soon see Google ebooks offered on hundreds of independent bookstore websites. The AYP books have been on Google for years, and will now be available through the new Google eBookstore. Links to the AYP ebooks on Google will be added to the AYP Books Page as soon as they are available. The list prices will be the same as above.

Happy e-reading, and, as always, wishing you all the best on your path! :-)

The guru is in you.

2010/07/29 12:56:01
Books, Web Sites, Audio, Video, etc.
http://www.aypsite.org/forum/topic.asp?TOPIC_ID=8132&REPLY_ID=71414&whichpage=-1
AYP eBooks - New Formats and Price Reductions

Hi All:

The AYP Easy Lessons book conversion (the last one) is done now, with the ebook available via direct download, including PDF, EPUB and MOBI (Kindle) formats in the same zip file.

Additional bundling of the ebook files has been done with the audiobooks, and multiple ebook ("box set") downloads. Links to these direct download offers can be found in the top left border on any page of the forums and main website.

The Amazon Kindle Store has been brought completely up to date with the new ebook files also.

Down the road a bit, look for AYP in the Apple iBookstore, Barnes and Noble (Nook) eBooks, Google eBookstore, and more.

Happy reading, practice wisely, and enjoy! :-)

The guru is in you.

2010/07/29 14:03:05
Books, Web Sites, Audio, Video, etc.
http://www.aypsite.org/forum/topic.asp?TOPIC_ID=8132&REPLY_ID=71418&whichpage=-1
AYP eBooks - New Formats and Price Reductions

quote:
─────────
Originally posted by Panthau

Any plans on translations? (not that i´d think about doing that, that´d need a lot more skill then i have)

─────────

Hi Pan:

The approach has been for translators of the AYP books to take responsibility for publishing and distribution, including paperback and/or ebook, with a simple sales royalty coming back to AYP.

There has been some discussion about direct downloads from the AYP website. But this is an English site, so not sure if that makes sense. Probably better to follow what is customary in-country. Translated AYP book offerings would be a logical add-on to a translation website for the AYP online lessons, plus standard book and ebook distribution channels for that language. All in good time.

The epicenter of the ebook revolution is the USA, where paper books are plunging in favor of ebooks on hand-held reading devices (Kindle, iPad, Nook, Sony, etc,). That is why we have been upgrading and restructuring the AYP ebook offerings.

The revolution has not arrived in other parts of the world yet, but it will. :-)

The guru is in you.

PS: AYP book translations (mainly the DM book so far) have been occurring in Czech, Norwegian, Spanish, and possibly German (check with kashiraja).

2010/09/09 14:16:11
Books, Web Sites, Audio, Video, etc.
http://www.aypsite.org/forum/topic.asp?TOPIC_ID=8132&REPLY_ID=72762&whichpage=-1
AYP eBooks - New Formats and Price Reductions

Hi All:

Last month, we took the new eBook formats (discussed above - covering all reading devices) and started bundling them into Zip files for substantial savings on multiple eBook downloads.

Then we figured out a way to do it for all of the 9 AudioBooks (with free eBooks included), without anyone having to do a 600 MB download. :-)

Finally, bundling of three of the E-Series books (DM, SBP & AMB) has been done for those wanting concise instructions for starting up an AYP practice routine for very little cost.

All of these bundles can be found here: http://www.aypsite.org/books-xdirdownload.html#bund

Enjoy!

The guru is in you.

2010/09/23 19:14:56
Books, Web Sites, Audio, Video, etc.
http://www.aypsite.org/forum/topic.asp?TOPIC_ID=8132&REPLY_ID=73155&whichpage=-1
AYP eBooks - New Formats and Price Reductions

Hi All:

Google Checkout has been added as a payment option for all AYP Direct Downloads.

Now both Paypal and Google Checkout show up as payment options when individual or bundled download items are added to the shopping cart.

I believe with these two, we cover every country and territory in the world. If that is not true for where you are, let me know, and we can look into it.

All the best!

The guru is in you.

2010/09/25 14:30:23
Books, Web Sites, Audio, Video, etc.
http://www.aypsite.org/forum/topic.asp?TOPIC_ID=8132&REPLY_ID=73225&whichpage=-1
AYP eBooks - New Formats and Price Reductions

Hi Parallax:

It's a brave new world, with spiritual practitioners doing their thing everywhere. Bravo! :-)

The guru is in you.

2010/11/17 15:21:17
Books, Web Sites, Audio, Video, etc.
http://www.aypsite.org/forum/topic.asp?TOPIC_ID=8756
American Veda - History of Yoga in the West

Hi All:

This is a new book just out. The full title and Amazon link are:

American Veda -
From Emerson and the Beatles to Yoga and Meditation -
How Indian Spirituality Changed the West
By Philip Goldberg

This is the best history on Yoga coming to the West I have seen so far. It is an extensive and scholarly work, and also very easy to read. No stones were left unturned. If you were intrigued by the brief history of Yoga coming to the West in Lesson 253 and want the full course, this is the book to get. (Btw, the AYP Booklist linked in Lesson 253 has recently been expanded from 400 to nearly 500 books.)

It should be mentioned that "American Veda" came here in an unusual way. The author, Phil Goldberg, contacted me over a year ago and we did a phone interview. So AYP is mentioned in the book, and Yogani as "perhaps the most ungurulike of the nongurus" (p221). That sounds about right, and speaks volumes about what we are doing here in AYP.

The guru is in you.

 :-)

PS: Phil Goldberg is currently making the rounds promoting this new book. His schedule and additional information can be found here: http://www.americanveda.com

2010/11/23 22:02:33
Books, Web Sites, Audio, Video, etc.
http://www.aypsite.org/forum/topic.asp?TOPIC_ID=8756&REPLY_ID=75647&whichpage=-1
American Veda - History of Yoga in the West

quote:
_____
Originally posted by tadeas

Finally something about AYP in print... Now you or AYP can get that wikipedia page :)
_____

Hi Tadeas:

I hope someone does it someday, preferably about AYP and the great work all of you are doing with it, rather than that anonymous guy. :-)

The guru is in you.

2010/12/02 12:31:35
Books, Web Sites, Audio, Video, etc.
http://www.aypsite.org/forum/topic.asp?TOPIC_ID=8830
Yoga Body: The Origins of Modern Posture Practice

Hi All:

This is a new book (with Amazon link):

Yoga Body: The Origins of Modern Posture Practice by Mark Singleton

It is a scholarly work that traces the evolution of asana (postures) over the past several hundred years, to become the vast industry it is today. The journey entails ancient knowledge, greatly altered by social, religious and political forces in colonial India, and carried forward by popular western fitness movements since the early 1900s. An interesting read for anyone who seeks to understand how modern hatha yoga is related to spiritual practice, and how it is not.

There is nothing wrong with postures for health and fitness. But for anyone who aspires to spiritual practice, modifications to a postures-dominated practice will be necessary to encompass the full scope of the eight limbs of yoga. This is what the AYP Asanas, Mudras and Bandhas book is about. It is also covered in AYP Easy Lessons - Volume 2 (including an enhanced AYP asana routine), which will be out in a few weeks.

All the best!

The guru is in you.

2010/12/06 22:51:27
Books, Web Sites, Audio, Video, etc.
http://www.aypsite.org/forum/topic.asp?TOPIC_ID=8846
AYP Easy Lessons Volume 2 is Available

Hi All:

The AYP Easy Lessons Volume 2 book showed up on Amazon USA today. In the coming days and weeks the ebook and paperback links will be activated for the many channels listed on the books page.

For status, you can check the links here: http://www.aypsite.org/books.html#ayp2

Volume 2 expands dramatically on the first AYP Easy Lessons volume, with numerous refinements in the application of core practices, and many new practices related to middle and end stage development on the path to enlightenment. As always, the AYP lessons reflect the needs of the ever-advancing community of practitioners, continuing to be an experience-based open resource.

I hope to have direct downloads from the AYP website for Volume 2 available tomorrow (bundled PDF, EPUB & MOBI), and the Amazon Kindle store listing and other channels will not be far behind.

All the best!

The guru is in you.

PS: You may have noticed that Google also opened their mammoth ebookstore today (the AYP ebooks are there). When it rains it pours. :-)

2010/12/08 15:53:47

570 –   Advanced Yoga Practices

Books, Web Sites, Audio, Video, etc.
http://www.aypsite.org/forum/topic.asp?TOPIC_ID=8846&REPLY_ID=76358&whichpage=-1
AYP Easy Lessons Volume 2 is Available

Thanks All. :-)

For an update ... since the first post above, the new AYP Vol 2 eBook has been added to the AYP website direct downloads (includes PDF, EPUB & MOBI formats in the zip file). The eBook has also been added to the applicable discounted bundled offers (some have been waiting for this).

The eBook is now on Amazon Kindle for both USA and UK. It will be several weeks before Barnes&Noble Nook, Apple iBooks and Kobo are set up. Not sure when it will show up in the new Google eBookstore. Maybe soon.

On the paperback side, in addition to Amazon USA, Barnes&Noble is listing the book now. Still waiting for Amazon's international sites to list it. It will take a few weeks to get the cover images, descriptions, "search inside," etc. set up on all the various sites.

Links for the major channels can be found here: http://www.aypsite.org/books.html#ayp2

Book Reviews Requested: One of the best ways to share the AYP writings with others is in the form of book reviews, especially on Amazon. Having just arrived, AYP Vol 2 has no reviews so far. Anyone with an Amazon account can do a book review there. For those who do not have the book yet, it covers the online lessons from Main #236 and Tantra #T36 onward, with 15-20% new material added. If you are familiar with the lessons that have been posted since 2005, you are basically familiar with Volume 2, and can offer your comments in a review. A lot of new stuff since the first AYP Easy Lessons volume came out 6 years ago. We have come a long way, both as practitioners and in the documentation.

As it says in the Volume 2 introduction: "We owe our heartfelt thanks to the many yoga practitioners around the world who have stepped forward and contributed to the development of these lessons through their sincere sharing of experiences and questions. Without them, this second volume of the AYP lessons would not have happened."

Thank you All. The journey continues!

The guru is in you.

2010/12/08 21:20:34
Books, Web Sites, Audio, Video, etc.
http://www.aypsite.org/forum/topic.asp?TOPIC_ID=8846&REPLY_ID=76381&whichpage=-1
AYP Easy Lessons Volume 2 is Available

quote:
_____
Originally posted by Katrine

That's great Yogani :-)
I am very grateful for all your outpouring.

Ordered my first Kindle today - so hopefully when I get home to Oslo end December it will be there waiting :)

That way - with all my travels, some lightness of air will substitute the weight of the matter :-)
_____

Hi Katrine:

I assume you mean the Kindle e-reader gadget will be waiting for you in Oslo. The Amazon ebooks themselves can be read on any computer or mobile device with free downloaded Kindle software. So if you got the AYP Vol 2 Kindle ebook, you will not have to wait to read it wherever you happen to be. And, of course, you can read it on the Kindle e-reader gadget too.

Many thanks! :-)

The guru is in you.

2010/12/08 21:40:40
Books, Web Sites, Audio, Video, etc.
http://www.aypsite.org/forum/topic.asp?TOPIC_ID=8846&REPLY_ID=76385&whichpage=-1
AYP Easy Lessons Volume 2 is Available

quote:
_____
Originally posted by Holy

The bundle again is very nice! Thanks =)

Do you plan to make direct topic links into the second volume too? It is not too hard to type in the site number and scrolld own a little bit more, but the comfort with it was great.

Another hint would be, but all this is up to your ebook-programmer :) to have a hyperlink on the actual subject page back to the main listing. This would increase the overall usage of the pdf-files even more. The other file-types were not tested.

The content is great anyway, thanks again!
_____

Hi Holly:

The PDF and EPUB editions both have a side bar link-driven table of contents (TOC) that can be kept open while reading (in Adobe Reader and Adobe Digital Editions, and some other ereaders). The MOBI/Kindle format from AYP can also support a sidebar link-driven TOC, but most Kindle readers (all?) do not have the ability to show it in the same window with the book text (it has to be called up from the menu). The advantage of a sidebar link-driven TOC is that one can jump anywhere in the book with one click, so following references in the text is easy.

Embedding links in the book text is another way to provide navigation, but it is very labor intensive to include that feature for the many hundreds of lesson references in the big AYP textbooks. Still, we do have it in the AYP Vol 1 EPUB and MOBI editions (not PDF), and will eventually have it in the Vol 2 EPUB and MOBI editions.

It should also be mentioned that quite a few lesson references in Vol 2 are going to Vol 1, because the two books constitute a continuous series of lessons with many interconnections. It goes without saying that AYP Vol 2 does not stand alone. And now that Vol 2 is out, neither does Vol 1, for intermediate and advanced practitioners especially. :-)

Not sure if that covers all of what you are asking, but that is the basic navigation scheme we have in the AYP Easy Lessons ebooks.

All the best!

The guru is in you.

2010/12/08 22:21:35
Books, Web Sites, Audio, Video, etc.
http://www.aypsite.org/forum/topic.asp?TOPIC_ID=8846&REPLY_ID=76390&whichpage=-1
AYP Easy Lessons Volume 2 is Available

quote:
_____
Originally posted by Clear White Light

Good news indeed,

I was wondering, will some sort of discount be available for purchasing hard copies of both volume 1 and 2 together? I'm sure those of us who haven't yet purchased the first edition would find that very appealing. :)
_____

Hi CWL:

The only "direct sales" of paperbacks done from here are through the quantity discount program at 55% off list prices, plus shipping direct from the printer. Due to shipping costs, the savings come with buying roughly 5 or more books. It is preferred to use the quantity discount program for larger orders to support teaching, retreats, etc, because it is time-consuming to process and administer the orders. It has never been the intention to get into retail sales here.

Amazon will be discounting the Vol 2 paperback once the book settles into their system. Volume 1, which also lists at $39.95, goes for under $30 with free shipping, and Volume 2 should end up about the same once it is established. Amazon sometimes offers a further price break with their "frequently bought together" program, which shows up on many of their book pages. These two volumes are likely to end up in that, but a further discount may or may not be there. Unfathomable are the calculations of Amazon. :-)

By far the least expensive way to get the AYP books is in ebook form as bundled direct downloads through the AYP website. You can get AYP Vols 1&2 for $15, with a free Secrets of Wilder novel thrown in. But not everyone wants ebooks. In the case of the two big AYP Easy Lessons volumes, there will be an advantage to have them both available physically. Easier to jump back and forth that way. The ebooks have other advantages -- portability, and especially the ability to do searches, which comes in handy when working with over 1000 pages of instructional material.

All the best!

The guru is in you.

2010/12/09 10:10:11
Books, Web Sites, Audio, Video, etc.
http://www.aypsite.org/forum/topic.asp?TOPIC_ID=8846&REPLY_ID=76405&whichpage=-1
AYP Easy Lessons Volume 2 is Available

quote:
_____
Originally posted by Parallax

quote:
_____
Originally posted by yogani

Having just arrived, AYP Vol 2 has no reviews so far.

_____

I think it does now

:-)

2010/12/09 10:23:41
Books, Web Sites, Audio, Video, etc.
http://www.aypsite.org/forum/topic.asp?TOPIC_ID=8846&REPLY_ID=76406&whichpage=-1
AYP Easy Lessons Volume 2 is Available
PS: I missed responding to a question about AYP on eBay. As far as I know, all listings on eBay must be re-listed every few weeks, and that is not viable to do here. The AYP paperbacks have shown up on eBay from time to time through third party sellers. (here's what's there at the moment).

The AYP ebooks are not currently available through third party sellers, but that is changing with the Google ebookstore roll-out, which can be mirrored by any third party seller. So maybe someone will put the ebooks on eBay.

The AYP audiobooks (MP3 and CD) have always been available to third party sellers through CD Baby. Don't know if any of those have ever been on eBay, but it is possible.

The guru is in you.

2010/12/09 12:39:00
Books, Web Sites, Audio, Video, etc.
http://www.aypsite.org/forum/topic.asp?TOPIC_ID=8846&REPLY_ID=76416&whichpage=-1
AYP Easy Lessons Volume 2 is Available
PPS: There is a press release available on the new book, here: http://www.aypsite.org/pressrelease15.html
Anyone with media contacts, feel free to pass it on.

Thanks!

2010/12/06 22:54:25
Books, Web Sites, Audio, Video, etc.
http://www.aypsite.org/forum/topic.asp?TOPIC_ID=8847
AYP in the New Google eBookstore

Hi All:

Google opened their new eBookstore today, and all the AYP ebooks are in it. Links can be found under each AYP title on the books page here: http://www.aypsite.org/books.html

That will soon include the new AYP Easy Lessons Volume 2 also. See over here on that: http://www.aypsite.org/forum/topic.asp?TOPIC_ID=8846

Google is taking a multi-pronged approach to selling ebooks, offering online reading on any device with an internet browser, and also downloads to standard computers and mobile reading devices (e-readers, tablets and phones). They have PDF and EPUB formats now, and plan to add MOBI for the Kindle. They are also opening it up to a vast network of partners, so anyone with a website can sell ebooks from Google (including bundling of ebooks with paper book sales by any retailer). This is particularly attractive to struggling independent bookstores who have been mostly left out of the digital revolution.

No doubt ebooks are going to be dove-tailed with Google's pervasive web search and advertising capabilities, making ebooks as visible as these core services that Google provides. So it looks like Google aims to be the juggernaut in ebooks that they are in search and online advertising. They have some tough competition, so we'll see. In any case, Google's entry means that ebooks are here to stay.

Happy reading, and all the best! :-)

The guru is in you.

Forum 16 – Enlightenment Milestones

Where is yoga taking us? Reporting experiences along the way.
http://www.aypsite.org/forum/forum.asp?FORUM_ID=27

2005/07/13 09:24:37
Enlightenment Milestones
http://www.aypsite.org/forum/topic.asp?TOPIC_ID=285
Enlightenment Milestones

What is enlightenment, and how can will it unfold as we continue with our daily practices?

There are many AYP lessons that deal with this question in relation to our practices. Here are a few examples:

Enlightenment Milestones - http://www.aypsite.org/35.html
The One is the Many and the Many are the One - http://www.aypsite.org/254.html
Divine Ecstasy and Enlightenment - http://www.aypsite.org/258.html

The question is not so much, what is enlightenment? The question is, what are we doing every day to purify and open to our full inner potential? If we do that, we will begin to get a flavor of what enlightenment is soon enough. Then it is not a theory or a philosophical determination anymore. It is by direct experience, and we can very simply put it in our own words.

The great 19th century yogi, Lahiri Mahasaya put it in his own words this way: "Enlightenment is a merging of emptiness with euphoria."

Many who have been doing deep meditation and spinal breathing pranayama for a while will know that this simple statement is true.

This forum is for sharing experiences on the road to enlightenment. Seeing milestones as we travel along can encourage us to keep up our practices. On the other hand, we may see very few milestones, and one day suddenly find ourselves at the destination. It all depends on how our purification is happening inside. Each person is unique in that. We all go at our own speed and in our own way. There is no set pattern for how it will happen. But if we keep up our practices day in and day out for as long as it takes, it will happen!

The guru is in you.

2005/10/12 12:06:00
Enlightenment Milestones
http://www.aypsite.org/forum/topic.asp?TOPIC_ID=516&REPLY_ID=952&whichpage=-1
Yoga and Yogam/ manifestation & tumo

Hi Nandhi:

Thank you for your kind sharing from the siddhars of South India. It is not often that those with traditional Indian yoga background will embrace an "open source" on practices like AYP, though I think many would like to. But it is non-traditional, yes? Boundaries to cross. That is what we do in America -- cross boundaries. Hopefully with the best possible results. :-)

Your encouragement since the beginning has been much appreciated, and I wish you well in your important spiritual work in Los Angeles -- http://www.nandhi.com

The guru is in you.

Yogani

2005/11/07 11:26:24
Enlightenment Milestones
http://www.aypsite.org/forum/topic.asp?TOPIC_ID=577&REPLY_ID=1438&whichpage=-1
Bliss Goes Dead

Hi All:

There is ecstasy. There is bliss. There is ecstatic bliss. And there are plateaus in experience. Where we are in all of this is far less important (and often unknowable) than our ongoing practices which keep it coming. But here are a few benchmarks that might be helpful:

On the difference between ecstasy, bliss and divine love see lesson #113 - http://www.aypsite.org/113.html

From the lesson you can gather that bliss is unchanging (an aspect of pure bliss consciousness) and ecstasy is changing (pranic energy flow). With ecstasy, there is the element of "friction" in the subtle nerves caused by obstructions that are being flushed out by pranic energy. That is the dynamic aspect of ecstasy. In the end, or during plateaus, more energy will flow with less friction, which brings us into the subtle joining of ecstasy and bliss -- ecstatic bliss. That is where ecstasy (dynamic) is moving in stillness. The divine paradox.

When it gets to that stage, the process is still hankering to go somewhere. Where? Out into the world as outpouring divine love. That is where karma yoga really takes off. Then there is a whole new realm of flow, ecstasy and the friction of energy moving through obstructions leading to ecstatic bliss again in the outer world. That is stillness in action in the world, flowing endlessly out from us. That is why we end up saying, "Your evolution is my evolution." We're all in it together. The One is the many and the many are the One. So yoga ultimately looks far beyond the individual body/mind. It is an organic process that keeps expanding. I mention this because it is the next step after the stillness of ecstatic bliss - the outpouring to unity, which flies on the wings of divine love.

How to know if we are on a plateau or in ecstatic bliss for good? Just ramp up the pranic energy practices a bit - spinal breathing, siddhasana, mudras, bandhas, etc. We will find out soon enough. Either way, we will be flowing outward as divine love in due course. It is our destiny.

The guru is in you.

PS -- Also, we do get used to advancements very fast, and therefore will often feel less contrast with the same experience, and sooner or later wanting more... That is part of what drives us out beyond our individual development to aid in the development of others...

2005/11/07 11:45:11
Enlightenment Milestones
http://www.aypsite.org/forum/topic.asp?TOPIC_ID=577&REPLY_ID=1440&whichpage=-1
Bliss Goes Dead

Hi Jim:

It can happen, and you have the right attitude about it. Just another step on the journey...

The guru is in you.

2006/01/26 10:16:33
Enlightenment Milestones
http://www.aypsite.org/forum/topic.asp?TOPIC_ID=694&REPLY_ID=2797&whichpage=-1
Enlightenment Milestones

quote:
_____
I have reread all the lessons in the AYP index on "the witness" but was wondering if you could define or elaborate on the "the flat witness" outlined in your quote above? Is it similar to living in the here and now 24/7 (or most of the time) and not constantly taking any mental thought trips?
_____

Hi Anthem:

The first emergence of the witness (I used "flat" to emphasize inner stillness) is a duality situation. That is, all the thinking and activity goes on pretty much as usual. The difference is we find that we are effortlessly observing it all. Inner silence is there, and we actually first notice it by the contrast with activity occurring inside and outside us. In time, we develop some skill in operating from stillness and then it moves out into thinking, feeling and the events happening around us in the world. Samyama is a means for promoting this development -- manifesting ourselves from stillness and moving outward. But even so, the activity inside and around us is still going on -- it is only that our relationship with it is changing. We become it on the deepest level of our being, which is not the same as egoic identification. Duality gradually dissolves, and we experience "stillness in action," which is the rise of the unity experience. Our choices in action are changed by this, because our perception is becoming non-dual -- unifying -- which is the essence of divine love operating in the world. All of this corresponds with the neurobiological transformation going on within us via practices.

Interestingly, this evolutionary process resolves the dual versus non-dual nature of existence argument once and for all. Ultimately, it is about the condition of the human nervous system and our perception through it. The perception is the reality (so both arguments are valid), and with practices the perception changes gradually from dual to non-dual.

As for being in "the now" and not taking any thought trips, with the emergence of the witness the thought trips will still be happening, and we will be watching them play on the screen of our silent awareness, so technically we are not taking the trip (and yes, that is in "the now" early on). Later on, the thought trips will become illuminated by the divine channeling through us, and we will be That. The thought trips do not stop. However, their essence does change to divine quality and purpose, and that is the difference.

The guru is in you.

2006/01/29 21:49:51
Enlightenment Milestones
http://www.aypsite.org/forum/topic.asp?TOPIC_ID=694&REPLY_ID=2860&whichpage=-1
Enlightenment Milestones

Hi Anthem:

One explanation is that those who apparently become suddenly enlightened were born close to it. This implies a lot of spiritual work in previous lives, if one subscribes to the reincarnation theory. And, if not, well then, who knows how they arrived in the near enlightened condition? They are here, and that is a good thing.

You know, folks like Tolle are still evolving too, as teachers working to offer something practical to others. Sages who are not doing that are not of much help to the rest of us, or ultimately to themselves. There is no free lunch until everyone is on board.

All aboard! :-)

The guru is in you.

2006/01/30 10:06:10
Enlightenment Milestones
http://www.aypsite.org/forum/topic.asp?TOPIC_ID=694&REPLY_ID=2881&whichpage=-1
Enlightenment Milestones

Hi All:

Anthem, I agree that near death experience (NDE) can have a profound spiritual effect -- but it is rarely the final step -- there is no such thing as a final step really, only ever higher degrees of divine outpouring and illumination. Interestingly, there have been a few who have written in here over the past couple of years looking for practices to expand on (or manage) what their NDE gave them. Not that we should run off and have a NDE. :-)

John Wilder was into pressing the envelope. And he did, in fact, have a NDE that was a confirmation and transition point in his work.

Lavazza, I agree about sages in isolation affecting everyone, but I think it is often over-rated. We can't know for sure about such claims, can we? As it says in the Bible, "By their fruits ye shall know them." Sages who are active in the world have a special role, because they empower the people to act for their own spiritual benefit instead of relying on anonymous invisible forces, which can breed superstition. It is the cultivation of divine presence (pure bliss consciousness) that counts. After that, to each their own. Those who seek to enable people everywhere to reveal it directly in themselves via practical means are meeting the challenge where it lies. My hat is off to Tolle and all who are giving it a go. It is the most important work on the planet.

The guru is in you.

2006/01/30 16:48:38
Enlightenment Milestones
http://www.aypsite.org/forum/topic.asp?TOPIC_ID=694&REPLY_ID=2893&whichpage=-1
Enlightenment Milestones

quote:
_____
Originally posted by Lavazza
Well I certainly do not know, but this was a very advanced guy and he was very generous in sharing and he would not critisize other sages for not sharing. So in his my mind he knew for sure that these sages were already helping people.

_____

Hi Lavazza:

In the old days, they used to call it the "Great White Brotherhood" -- Those anonymous sages meditating behind the scenes, uplifting all of humankind which was in no position to do it for itself. I am sure there must be a "Great White Sisterhood too." My hat is off to all of them. :-)

At least in part thanks to them, we now have thousands teaching in the open, and thousands more are joining in each year. It is a time for stillness in action...

The guru is in you.

2006/02/01 14:28:27
Enlightenment Milestones
http://www.aypsite.org/forum/topic.asp?TOPIC_ID=694&REPLY_ID=2952&whichpage=-1
Enlightenment Milestones

Hi David:

Hey, I've been sliced and diced plenty already. And I'm sure the best is yet to come. Rodney Dangerfield's got nothin' on me.

The guru is in you.
 Go pick on him/her/it. And then just easily come back to the mantra.

It is all purification... :-)
2006/02/02 23:36:33
Enlightenment Milestones
http://www.aypsite.org/forum/topic.asp?TOPIC_ID=694&REPLY_ID=3013&whichpage=-1
Enlightenment Milestones
Elvis has left the building, but Yogani hasn't yet. Word has it that he changed his ID because the old one (database owner one) had so much internet file baggage stuck to it that it died.

Is this indisputable evidence of reincarnation? :-)
2006/01/18 15:11:58
Enlightenment Milestones
http://www.aypsite.org/forum/topic.asp?TOPIC_ID=742&REPLY_ID=2615&whichpage=-1
Samad
Hi in the Produce Aisle

Hi Jim:

Great story. I loved Mystiq's Kerala pilgrimage story too...

Could've been the bag boy. Maybe one of those peaceful warriors? Or an indigo child playing in the aisles? A lot of folks are doing AYP in California these days -- could've been one of those too. Was anyone looking at you bedazzled, like you were the burning bush? :-)

These are interesting times. Much more "inner seeing" happening, and there's much more around to see too. Inner openings and inner perceptions go together on all sides.

We are all living in paradise, and are finally beginning to notice!

The guru is in you.

2006/01/19 08:38:26
Enlightenment Milestones
http://www.aypsite.org/forum/topic.asp?TOPIC_ID=742&REPLY_ID=2629&whichpage=-1
Samad
Hi in the Produce Aisle

Hi Jim:

Who said anything about power? Power is illusion. The real prize is something far greater than power. Joy is the underlying thing. That is real. It is what's left when all the rest is purified and opened up. Inner seeing is not power. It is joy! ... a synonym for pure bliss consciousness.

It is joy that will have us all bedazzled and rolling in the aisles, and it is everywhere. Stillness is its essence. :-)

The guru is in you.

2006/01/19 10:29:00
Enlightenment Milestones
http://www.aypsite.org/forum/topic.asp?TOPIC_ID=742&REPLY_ID=2634&whichpage=-1
Samad
Hi in the Produce Aisle
Very true, David:

The greatest miracle of all is people choosing to do what it takes to tap their own vast potential. Facilitating that choice in others is no small task, but well worth it -- a surrender of its own special kind to what evolution is leading us all to. And you are right. We can all facilitate it. Please do!

The guru is in you.

PS -- Jim, Your California story is a joy. The art of humor is a divine gift. Keep em comin'

2006/01/22 14:43:17
Enlightenment Milestones
http://www.aypsite.org/forum/topic.asp?TOPIC_ID=742&REPLY_ID=2725&whichpage=-1
Samad
Hi in the Produce Aisle

quote:
_____
Originally posted by Etherfish

Thanks David,
"This tendency to 'throw the baby out with the bathwater' is indeed a noteworthy error. It seems to be a sort of bug in the human system. Here's a question: isn't our tendency to halo-ize people the other side of the same coin? Making people all-good, and all-bad is the way of children, isn't it?"

Yes, I totally agree idolizing someone is the other side of the coin to condemning someone. People who do it think there are extenuating circumstances; the person did something *so bad* or *so incredibly good* that they deserve it. But it's the same thing as enlightenment not being a permanent state that guarantees no further mistakes. There are no extenuating circumstances. nobody's worth idolizing, and nobody's bad enough to be condemned. It's fun to do either for a little while though.
Well, it should be the way of children to think black or white like this, but it seems to be the way of a majority of adults from my viewpoint! It isn't helped any by movies portraying people as all good or all bad.
I really appreciate the ones that don't.
_____

Hi David and Etherfish:

This is a very important point you are discussing. It is really at the heart of successfully navigating the spiritual path, and life. As long as we are painting the world "black" and "white" we have little chance of seeing the innumerable shades of gray, and the baby will be thrown out with the bath water again and again. And all the while we will be ricocheting from one extreme to the other.

AYP is a product of "seeing" the shades of gray in the many teachings that are out there, and in myself, over many years. It is about much more than "who" we are considering. The process of seeing what is true also has to do with how we regard our practices and experiences each day. Once we have let go of the idea of this or that guru, practice or experience being all bad or all good, we are well on the to integrating the whole thing together and speeding along on our way home. We then have come to grips with the essential truth that all things in life are a blend of light and shadow playing on the screen of our silent awareness. When we know this to be the case in our practices, we are in a much better position to cull through, separate the wheat from the chaff, add on, self-pace effectively, etc. All of that is dependent on our seeing.

Thankfully, being able to make these distinctions better and better comes with the rise of inner silence. Then, as time in daily practices passes, we find that we are carrying no flag except the flag of the witness, which sees all with no overlay of bias whatsoever. Then we are able to sip the divine nectar from everywhere, while keeping our feet out of the mud at the same time. :-)

Your recognition of this truth is colossal -- an intellectual recognition that is rising to be an everyday "wired-in" direct perception. Practices bring us steadily closer to that.

The guru is in you.

2006/02/06 06:18:09
Enlightenment Milestones
http://www.aypsite.org/forum/topic.asp?TOPIC_ID=791&REPLY_ID=3086&whichpage=-1

Rose-colored glasses

Hi Anthem:

It is a sign of inner silence and ecstatic conductivity being perceived on the outside. It can be viewed as purification expanding outward, which is another form of inner purification.

To borrow a line from an old Beatles song:
"Your outside is in and your inside is out..."

A simpler way of putting it is, we are beginning to see things as they really are -- our world made of and radiating divine light, which is an expression of our own inner Self. It is a taste of second stage enlightenment. When love begins to pour out through that, then that is a taste of third stage unity. http://www.aypsite.org/35.html

Nice experience. Enjoy it, and move on... :-)

The guru is in you.

2006/02/22 15:56:53
Enlightenment Milestones
http://www.aypsite.org/forum/topic.asp?TOPIC_ID=851&REPLY_ID=3742&whichpage=-1
Why I Don't Want to be Enlightened

Hi Jim & Shanti:

Since we can never get rid of desire completely, the way around the enlightenment quest thing is to learn to give it away -- the enlightenment, that is, if that's what we want to call it. After all, enlightenment is a total letting go, so in that sense it is not something we can ever "get." This is part of the bhakti expansion process that goes from redirecting our everyday desires toward our own enlightenment (see lesson 67), and then onward to redirecting our desire for personal enlightenment to serving the enlightenment of others. In this way we end up giving all of our spiritual progress away, and wind up with nothing (actually everything), and that is enlightenment. See this lesson on "getting enlightenment": http://www.aypsite.org/120.html

Of course, we can't easily skip from ordinary personal desires to serving the enlightenment of others. That is what creates proselytizers -- they are takers, not givers. We must have something to give first, and that is what sitting practices are for. If we are experiencing the divine flow within ourselves, it will naturally go to others. That is where it wants to go. That is the so-called outpouring of divine love I mention from time to time. It dissolves the personal enlightenment question, moving it onto a larger stage of endeavor that is no longer personal, but societal.

On the way to that nowhere (everywhere), we can use our desires as stepping stones from one level to the next. Shutting off (or "letting go" of) desires for a while might offer some temporary relief, a band-aid on the unceasing hankerings of this life, but to try and do so indefinitely is to pit ourselves against the forces of nature

Better to go with the flow, yes? This is the great strength of bhakti. We cannot stop the flow of life, but we can direct it into more evolutionary expressions, beginning with brushing our teeth ... oops, I mean doing our spiritual practices. :-)

The guru is in you.

2006/03/23 08:59:57
Enlightenment Milestones
http://www.aypsite.org/forum/topic.asp?TOPIC_ID=959&REPLY_ID=4928&whichpage=-1
Now the discipline of yoga
Oh, Katrine, we are thanking you.

You are an angel amidst angels. Or maybe that 100th monkey Melissa was talking about. :-)

The guru is in you.

2006/04/06 13:57:36
Enlightenment Milestones
http://www.aypsite.org/forum/topic.asp?TOPIC_ID=1009&REPLY_ID=5701&whichpage=-1
The Ride, Destination, and Faith...

Hi All:

Obviously, there are many ways to look at "the witness." As many ways as there are means to cultivate it and people to experience it. It is at one time an occasional revelation, another time an ongoing separation (that untouched feeling), then a permanent state from which both structured and unstructured practice can be conducted, and, finally, a joining back into all of our activity as "stillness in action," that endless outpouring of divine love -- a paradox to end all our paradoxes. Indeed, the universe is that from the beginning, yes? An outpouring from stillness. Who says something can't be made out of nothing? :-)

I don't see the witness itself as "a skill," though I understand how it could be seen that way. It is "a priori" -- self-evident, uncreated and unmoving, even as it moves outward through us. It is arrived at as a natural state of being through skill (yoga) applied beforehand and ongoing. Once it emerges as what we are, the witness is cognized as our state of being -- the effortless foundation of our 24 hour existence. From there, that state of being can be used for further development, but that is not the witness as skill. It is using our state of being as witness to move forward with increasing clarity of empathy and discrimination. In that way, inner silence moves steadily outward into our environment of thoughts, feelings, body and physical surroundings. We could say it is the witness using the witness to achieve the fullness of self-awareness. The witness doesn't move, but it does everything.

And then we know: "I am That, you are That, and all this is That."

It is Love, omnipresent and everlasting in this grand illusion we call time and space...

Well, these are just words. Much better to come to know the real thing via practices, and describe it accordingly, which everyone is doing beautifully here. It can be explained in many ways. It is wonderful to have the thing happening to explain. Of course, like everything else, all skill emanates naturally from the witness. That is why we say, cultivate inner silence in deep meditation and the rest will happen. Bravo for that!

The guru is in you.

2006/04/06 16:28:34
Enlightenment Milestones
http://www.aypsite.org/forum/topic.asp?TOPIC_ID=1009&REPLY_ID=5709&whichpage=-1
The Ride, Destination, and Faith...

quote:
_____
Originally posted by weaver

Those of you who have found more of the witness, do you find that it gives you more control of how you can choose to think or feel in a given situation?
_____

Hi Weaver

Absolutely. That is the beginning of stillness in action. Once we begin to operate from stillness, everything gradually becomes an expression of stillness. That is when samyama works. That is when self-inquiry works. That is when tantra works. That is when everything works. Not only do we gain more control, we also bring more power, empathy and morality into everything we do.

It's the p-p-p-power of love.

Sorry, that's an old Huey Lewis and the News thing. :-)

The guru is in you.

2006/04/29 17:05:41
Enlightenment Milestones
http://www.aypsite.org/forum/topic.asp?TOPIC_ID=1087&REPLY_ID=6476&whichpage=-1
the urge to merge

Hi Anthem and Katrine:

Yes, I agree that it is bhakti -- the eternal love-magnetism that constantly draws us closer to our true nature. The interesting thing about this is that, in the end, the merging goes the opposite way we are seeking from our egoic sense, even though it is our egoic desire that has been stimulating the process from the beginning.

What I mean is that inner silence awakens (or, more correctly, we awaken as inner silence) and comes into our daily life, rather than we leaving daily life to go into inner silence, or however we regard that "great beyond." Our bhakti is not bringing us to It. Our bhakti is bringing It to us!

It might sound like semantics, but it is true. Another way to look at it is from our changing perspectives as we move from egoic point of view to inner witness point of view (just reviewed in Lesson 282). If we are becoming the witness, then where do we need to go? What do we need to merge with? From that inner perspective it is the witness that needs to do the merging back out into daily living, and will do so via the rise of ecstatic bliss (the ego helps with this too, as you say). Before we were seeing as the witness, we were wanting to go the other way, to something beyond our thoughts, feelings and this physical existence. Then it reverses. So it is a sort of two way trip. Going in to become inner silence, and then coming back out as inner silence on the wings of ecstatic bliss and divine love to become all that we see in the world. So it is ultimately a two way merging...

If we are looking at this from both sides -- outside looking in and inside looking out -- we may, in fact, feel like we are going in both directions at once. It can happen. The whole thing is a process that is playing out in the ongoing purification and opening of our nervous system -- the vehicle of our consciousness and sense of self. Our point of view is changing as we advance in practices and experiences, and this question of merging can come at us from different angles at different times, depending on which perspective we are looking from in the moment. The truth is that the whole thing is going on in one place, right where we are now, no matter which point of view we are looking at it from. This body is the temple, and right here and now is where it is happening. There is no place else to go. But, still, there some more traveling to do, yes?

Some traveling music, please... :-)

The guru is in you.

2006/10/06 15:02:31
Enlightenment Milestones
http://www.aypsite.org/forum/topic.asp?TOPIC_ID=1581&REPLY_ID=11994&whichpage=-1
God Realization

quote:
_____
Originally posted by Balance

Does anyone suppose that it is possible to become enlightened without experiencing any kundalini events? Writings of, or by, many enlightened people don't mention such things having been experienced. Is it just a matter of course that being in a body one will have kundalini experiences?

Maybe those people just didn't feel it was necessary to mention. As you say there are as many experiences as there are people, could kundalini experiences be "overlooked" in some cases. It's hard to imagine something of that nature being overlooked.

_____

Hi Balance:

Sure, it is possible. Kundalini symptoms are the experience of purification occuring in the nervous system, and they are specific to the unique matrix of obstructions within us. Purification can occur without much in the way of symptoms, if practices are undertaken in a balanced way. Purification can be occurring steadily underground, deep within us. Then, one day, we will notice that our view has changed. It can happen like that.

There are plenty of accounts of advanced souls in history going through dramatic experiences on the way to enlightenment -- time in the desert, dark night of the soul, fire and brimstone, etc. Which does not mean we all will ... better not to draw too many conclusions about experiences happening or not happening ... just keep going with practices with good self-pacing and we will see whatever "scenery" there is along the way.

Interestingly, the ancients did not have the refined level of yoga technology and understanding we do today, so they may have been exposed to more extremes than we are, not less. We owe them a lot -- those courageous spiritual pioneers who paved the way for all of us. And may those who come after us have even better information on the means and processes of human spiritual transformation.

There are many indications in the historical writings that the enlightenment process is universal, with the human nervous system being the common denominator. Every culture has its own terminology to describe the journey, and they all are describing in one way or other the same things we are talking about here on a daily basis. We can read similar descriptions of transformation from many sages coming from diverse geographies and traditions over the centuries.

As for kundalini going up, or down, or sideways, it is all of these. The neurobiology of kundalini is spread throughout the body (in every cell!) and we will experience sensations wherever purification happens to be occurring in the moment. There is also the phenomenon of "ecstatic conductivity" that arises throughout the body, so experiences in one area will be instantly connected with experiences elsewhere, and everywhere -- this is the neurobiology of rising Oneness. It gradually expands over time, reaching beyond the body, assuming we are continuing with practices. If we are not continuing with practices, then the pattern of purification can stall in a particular area, giving rise to experiences that do not necessarily represent the broad progression of unfoldment.

Experiences do not produce spiritual progress. Practices do.

And "grace" comes to those who cultivate bhakti (desire for God and/or Truth), and subsequently engage in practices. Then the whole cosmos is rushing to promote our spiritual progress. "Grace" can also come (seemingly out of nowhere) to those who have longed for awakening and engaged in practices in the past, perhaps an unremembered past. In that case, it can be called "karma."

Just some food for thought. Welcome aboard VIL! :-)

The guru is in you.

2006/10/06 17:12:08
Enlightenment Milestones
http://www.aypsite.org/forum/topic.asp?TOPIC_ID=1581&REPLY_ID=11999&whichpage=-1
God Realization

quote:
_____
Originally posted by VIL
...do you think that there is an innate wisdom, intelligence [Kundalini] that can unblock certain areas without a particular practice that will produce spiritual progress? The reason that I ask is that I do not practice anything and the Kundalini is moving ever upward on its own accord. Or is it something I do subconsciously or does it have to do with Karma? I dunno.

_____

Hi VIL:

Yes, there is certainly in innate wisdom that is eager to open us with all the force of nature. This is an energy manifestation of our own inner nature. Our essential nature is *inner silence*, also called *pure bliss consciousness.* Before we consciously become "that" through daily deep meditation and other means, we can still be in partnership with the energy manifestations of it, or perhaps feel victim to the energy, depending on the degree of inner silence (our true self) we have stabilized in our nervous system. This is why we place deep meditation first in AYP -- because inner silence is the foundation of all spiritual progress. Kundalini is just energy moving instinctively inside us. We have to transcend it to manage it. Then it becomes relatively easy.

Regarding an active kundalini, it really does not matter how how we got to this point. What matters most is how we manage it from now on. In AYP there are a variety of ways to balance and safely promote the advance of kundalini unfoldment. Spinal breathing pranayama is chief among these.

In the case of Gopi Krishna, who I believe you mentioned, he spent years in arduous yoga practices with intense desire and effort, casting his fate to the wind, and eventually achieved a crown opening. Unfortunately, he did not have the knowledge either before or after his opening to conduct a more orderly transformation, so we have a famous story of kundalini throwing this fellow from pillar to post for 15+ years. Well, it does not have to be that way.

Which is not to say you have been trying to make this happen, at least not in recent memory. But now that it has happened, the question is, how are you going to handle it from now on? You are in a much better position than Gopi Krishna was, thanks to all the work that has been done by many people since his time.

How we proceed will determine whether we have a long drawn out process vascillating between excess and stagnation, or a progressive and smooth awakening that is not getting stuck as we spend more time analyzing the experiences of our purfication than engaging in the means that will move us steadily and safely onward through our opening.

580 – Advanced Yoga Practices

While there is a vast innate intelligence at work, it is also very much a matter of <u>cause and effect</u>. Nothing happens without reason, and in spiritual matters that reason is embodied in our thoughts, feelings and actions.

Btw, quite a few have come to AYP over the past few years with previous spontaneous kundalini awakenings, some very extreme, and in most cases the practices have been useful for stabilizing the inner energies and leading to relatively smooth and steady progress. So there are tested resources here, not only for those who are starting out, but also for those who have found themselves in need of some tools on just about any part of the path.

On the other hand, if you would like to wing it, that is okay too. It is your path and no one here is going to tell you what to do. AYP is an open resource that anyone can use for self-directed practice. You will get plenty of suggestions though. :-)

All the best!

The guru is in you.

2006/11/13 15:55:26
Enlightenment Milestones
http://www.aypsite.org/forum/topic.asp?TOPIC_ID=1707&REPLY_ID=13257&whichpage=-1
Progress in practise.

Hi DhanrajK, and welcome!

Everyone is a little different in how inner purification progresses. If you are following the procedure of deep meditation, the work is being done. If there is no obvious symptom of progress, you can still be sure it is happening underneath, and sooner or later an opening will be happening. If we dig the well in one place long enough, we will strike water. There is plenty of water inside you -- infinite!

No one is lacking in that respect. It is only a matter of methods, gentle persistence, and time.

You may wish to try 5 minutes of spinal breathing right before deep meditation. That will help loosen up the subtle nerves, and enhance the inward reach of your deep meditation. If the routine with both these practices is smooth after a few weeks, and you want to add some more oomph, then add a short asana routine (about 10 min) right before spinal breathing. That will help open up the nervous system also.

Your desire and determination (bhakti), will also be an important factor over time.

All the best!

The guru is in you.

2007/03/26 16:18:53
Enlightenment Milestones
http://www.aypsite.org/forum/topic.asp?TOPIC_ID=2293&REPLY_ID=19428&whichpage=-1
Enlightenment and death cycles
Maximus said:
quote:
_____
What if the lonely sage does so thinking "God helps those who helps themselves" and that everyone has to move forward by themselves by their own spiritual desire, and there is little I can do?
_____

Hi Maximus:

Here is the riddle: What do we do when our nervous system has been purified and opened to the point where we see others as expressions our own dear self?

This is the basis of "Do unto others..."

This is also why I say enlightenment is most identifiable in those who consistently serve for the benefit of others (moved in their own way). In them we can see that the loss of separation is real. Of course, it takes time to know this for sure about anyone, and even about ourselves. The best time to draw a conclusion is after the person is dead, and even then we could be wrong. But perceived spiritual condition doesn't matter one iota if good works are being done and everyone is barreling along by choice on their own road home. That is all that matters.

Your question assumes a separation. It may apply in that arena, but not for the enlightened (or on the way), who will increasingly see their own dear self in everyone else, and act accordingly.

Wasn't it Forrest Gump who said, "Enlightened is as enlightened does." Or am I misquoting him? :-)
He actually said, "Stupid is as stupid does." Same difference. "Ye shall know each tree by its fruit."

Btw, it is absolutely true that "God helps those who help themselves." In fact, it is essential. The ongoing choice (devotion/bhakti) has to be there for anything to happen. As soon as it is, all of creation automatically runs to help. All of the masters and all the energy in the universe are waiting on the ones who are getting up and helping themselves. Yes, absolutely. No true sage is going to be ambivalent about that. Neither will most of the rest of us. We're all in it together...

It does not take years of daily deep meditation to feel this reality coming up in us. It can emerge pretty quickly, especially these days with inner silence stirring everywhere.

The guru is in you.

2007/09/03 11:35:43
Enlightenment Milestones
http://www.aypsite.org/forum/topic.asp?TOPIC_ID=2890&REPLY_ID=25251&whichpage=-1
i am's Embrace

Hi Bewell:

In the AYP lessons we call it "whole body mudra."

http://www.aypsite.org/212.html

Whole body mudra ("*i am's* embrace" in the novel) is a natural part of the advancing experience of ecstatic conductivity and radiance, which keeps refining over time. It is the rise of outpouring divine love, which is inner silence in motion.

Enjoy! :-)

The guru is in you.

2007/09/24 14:49:43
Enlightenment Milestones
http://www.aypsite.org/forum/topic.asp?TOPIC_ID=2897&REPLY_ID=25651&whichpage=-1
Nirvikalpa Samad
Hi & Nirodha?

quote:

Originally posted by thomas

Its a matter of definition and classification and in different traditions it can vary somewhat. However, from my understanding in AYP nirvikalpa samad
Hi would most correspond to that state when the "witness" becomes permanently sustained through all levels of consciousness, ie. waking, dreaming and sleeping. In other words, the nervous system has become sufficiently purified to prevent the clouding over of the witness by experience or whether one is sleeping or awake.

This, of course, is not an end state but really a new beginning. The Heart then begins to play a more dominant role and begins to dissolve the boundaries between in and out ... this and that ... giving rise to increasing levels of Love to be shared with all.

Perhaps, Yogani would clarify or correct ...

Hi Thomas, Kris and Darko:

Yes, that is a reasonable explanation of rising nirvikalpa samadhi, and it would seem to be in the direction of nirodha as well. One nervous system, the same emerging enlightenment experience, and different words to describe it. It is the process of attachment (identification) becoming less and less as inner silence comes up within us, even as we may become more and more engaged in the processes of the world around us, because they are all aspects of our own dear self.

The abiding inactive witness, finding itself awakened amidst activity, could be said to be mid-stage nirvikalpa. In AYP, we call it the first enlightenment milestone.

Inner silence is known in deep meditation, going in and out, due to our process of inner purification and opening driven by seeds (savikalpa). By this process, inner silence becomes gradually more present in daily activity as the abiding witness (impervious to seed). Then, with the awakening of ecstatic conductivity over time, the witness emerges to become one and the same as, and consciously expressing through, all activity. The active witness!

Oddly enough, the highest stage of nirvikalpa is often found to be very active in the world, with inner silence (the witness) fully engaged in action without attachment (seedless).

In the Yoga Sutras, Patanjali calls this "Dharmamegha -- the virtue-pouring cloud" (4-29). In AYP we call it outpouring divine love. Whatever we call it, it is fully engaged disengagement -- the paradox of stillness in action, the state of unity. Some call it sahaja nirvikalpa samadhi. Others, like the Buddhists, simply call it "being awake." We'd like to be in the position to offer our own description based on direct experience resulting from effective daily spiritual practices. And so we shall! :-)

There is some debate among scholars and theorists as to whether the fluctuations "stop" or not in nirvikalpa samadhi. To me, this the same as the argument over whether the nature of existence is non-dual or dual. It is all semantics. It is what it is, no matter which system is used to describe it. When we see for ourselves through our own purifying nervous system and refining perception, we will know what it is, and can call it whatever we wish. The names are derived from the experience, not the other way around.

Seeing is believing. Therefore, much better to practice and find out, than to theorize. It doesn't matter how enlightenment is described. It is still enlightenment, and it is open to everyone.

The guru is in you.

2008/01/14 13:29:13
Enlightenment Milestones
http://www.aypsite.org/forum/topic.asp?TOPIC_ID=3365&REPLY_ID=28879&whichpage=-1
Where is Soul and/or Higher Self?

Hi Crouch55, and welcome!

You might find this post on soul evolution interesting, and the referenced book: http://www.aypsite.org/forum/topic.asp?TOPIC_ID=1261#19744 The book (*The Solar System*, by AE Powell) goes into detail on the evolution (individuation and expansion) of consciousness through the mineral, plant, animal, human and celestial kingdoms.

In AYP, while we don't use the term "Higher Self" often (try a forum search), it is inherent in many other terms we use in the writings: inner silence, the witness, Self (big "S"), Silent Self, Being, pure bliss consciousness, etc. As far as "soul" is concerned, it is the individuation of Higher Self, which survives the advent of the enlightened condition. While we are still in the body, even the personality and ego can be said to survive, in divinely illuminated ways. This is discussed in the new Self-Inquiry book.

I presume that you are interested in "the thing itself," rather than specific terminology. Depending on culture and religion, sages have used many terminologies to describe the identical condition -- which is the end result of the process of human spiritual transformation, cultivated by the application of effective spiritual practices.

Some just call it "*That*," which can also be translated to mean "Higher Self." No matter what name we give, it is the same condition/experience across all the traditions, revealed by the inherent, ever-present, and remarkable spiritual capabilities of the human nervous system.

BTW, Ralph Waldo Emerson, one of the first prominent Americans to study eastern philosophy, called it the "Oversoul."

A rose is still a rose when called by any other name. :-)

All the best!

The guru (Higher Self) is in you.

2008/01/17 09:28:31
Enlightenment Milestones
http://www.aypsite.org/forum/topic.asp?TOPIC_ID=3379&REPLY_ID=29012&whichpage=-1
Strange natural occurances as a result of practice

Hi Scott:

Try Googling "synchronicity." I'm sure we could come up with lots more examples of it here. Just another day in the life of yogis and yoginis ... purification and opening. :-)

All the best!

The guru is in you.

2008/01/17 10:30:50
Enlightenment Milestones
http://www.aypsite.org/forum/topic.asp?TOPIC_ID=3379&REPLY_ID=29019&whichpage=-1
Strange natural occurances as a result of practice

quote:
_____
Originally posted by Scott

Mac,

The birds were all different kinds, which are in the area I'm in. They usually don't mix together like they did.

Yogani and EMC,

It may be synchronicity...it's just that such theories tend to fall into the area of spirituality that I try to avoid: beliefs. I'll look more into it, though.
_____

Hi Scott:

It is just part of the scenery along the way. It's not necessary to believe or disbelieve. Just continue on with practices. :-)

All the best!

The guru is in you.

2008/02/26 07:36:13
Enlightenment Milestones
http://www.aypsite.org/forum/topic.asp?TOPIC_ID=3508&REPLY_ID=30546&whichpage=-1
Pushing through the fear

Hi Scott:

Nice scenery. :-)

The fear doesn't necessarily have a reason. It can be as simple as energy passing through the neurobiology in ways it has not before. In that sense, fear is a symptom of purification and opening, like any other experience. It will pass as all symptoms do -- transforming to much quieter ecstatic bliss. You will get over it. It takes some time. Kundalini is not an overthrow of our life. Those who view it as an overthrow may have difficulty for obvious reasons -- it can breed a victim mentality, and then one is getting dragged from pillar to post. Much better to view it as a partnership, and proceed accordingly. The partnership approach leads to more stability. We have the methods to secure the partnership -- practices, self-pacing, grounding... Of course, it all gets surrendered along the way, but in ways that enable us to live a normal life. That is pretty important.

The key is to not rush out and act on our fear, or even on our ecstatic bliss. Life can go on as it has before, and we will be happier in it...

The Zen folks are very wise about this, saying before enlightenment it is "Chop wood, carry water." And after enlightenment it is "Chop wood, carry water."

In other words, just carry on with normal life.

There is the old idea that when the energy begins to flow, everything has to change on the outside. We should leave the job and the family, run off to the ashram, and all that. Personally, I think it is an over-reaction to something that is ultimately pretty ordinary. In the old days, maybe it was okay when awakenings happened in a tiny percentage of the population. It didn't matter much that a few people were running off when they didn't have to. Maybe isolation made sense back then. The society could afford it.

But what will happen when 10%, 20%, or 50% of the population is awakening? It will happen. With old school solutions it will be chaos -- unnecessary chaos. Sure, we will have more ashrams for those who simply must take off, but everyone else can just continue on where they are, meeting their daily responsibilities like always. Why not? We are all in the same boat. Isn't it wonderful?

It is a bit like winning the lottery. Some people quit their job, get a new house, a new car, a new family, new friends, whatever, and end up miserable. The smart lottery winners stay put and make very gradual changes in their life, if any at all. And they do well with their wealth over the long term, learning to wear it comfortably in ordinary daily living.

Kundalini is like that. We may have a big opening. So what else is new? Hopefully not too much at once on the outside. It can be destabilizing. So, once breakthoughs are occurring, it is all about keeping a steady course. Pacing and grounding -- which are about attending to the mundane things in life. It is about what we are already doing every day right now. Having responsibilities is a blessing in this, keeping us involved in spiritually integrative action, though we may grumble about it in the beginning. "What am I, this sacred divine being, doing sitting in a Dilbert Cube?" Being a sacred divine being, that's what. It is as real in the Dilbert Cube as it is in the ashram. More real, actually, because living in the world is where the rubber of spirituality meets the road. That is where inner life is integrated with outer life.

Incidently, staying with the ordinary during our transformation is how the ordinary becomes extraordinary in its own quiet ways. Stillness in action. Steadily rising happiness, based in equanimity. This is how the society will be illuminated in every nook and cranny, with enlightenment rising in people in every corner of the world. Not primarily in the ashrams, and not primarily by extraordinary acts. If something appears externally extraordinary, it rarely is. Less is more. Much more.

"Chop wood, carry water."

All the best on your wonderful journey from here to here!

The guru is in you.

PS: Looking forward to hearing/seeing your enlightenment commercial. :-)

PPS: Your encounter with the locked door at Cincinnati Yoga School reminded me of this:

"I have lived on the lip of insanity,
wanting to know reasons,
knocking on a door.
It opens.
I have been knocking from the inside!"

Jelaluddin Rumi – 13th Century Sufi Mystic

2008/05/12 13:22:30
Enlightenment Milestones
http://www.aypsite.org/forum/topic.asp?TOPIC_ID=3896&REPLY_ID=33654&whichpage=-1
yogani, enlightenment

Hi Tubeseeker:

I am where I am. The cumulative AYP writings are an effort to share the long-time journey here and the practices used, which hopefully can help others.

It's the best I can do. Beyond that, personal proclamations will only muddy the water. It isn't about me anyway. It is about you.

Take what works, leave the rest behind, and enjoy.
Very simple, yes? :-)

The guru is in you.

PS: While the Secrets of Wilder novel is not my story specifically, it provides a lot of opportunity for personal reflection on the process of human spiritual transformation -- the "What is it like?" part. Everyone has their own story to tell, and I hope all the stories will be told in some way. This is how we collectively move on...

2008/09/20 15:52:56
Enlightenment Milestones
http://www.aypsite.org/forum/topic.asp?TOPIC_ID=4466&REPLY_ID=37890&whichpage=-1
bliss verses tension

Hi Beck, and welcome!

You might find this lesson interesting for some additional perspective on on bliss, ecstasy, their marriage, and the emergence of divine love:
http://www.aypsite.org/113.html

As for purifying the nervous system, it is like a window that requires cleaning to see all that there is to see. As the window becomes clear, the tension and discomfort become much less, because the essence of what we are is flowing much more smoothly -- we come to know ourselves as *stillness in action*. Along the way, we use a systematic self-paced approach for cleansing, so we don't stir up more dust (discomfort) than we can handle at any point in time.

To demonstrate that this is not a new concept, here is what is on the dedication page in the new AYP **Eight Limbs of Yoga** book, quoted from the ancient *Yoga Sutras of Patanjali (2:28)*:

"Through practice of the limbs of Yoga,
whereby impurities are eliminated,
there arises enlightenment..."

Some things never change. All the best on your path! :-)

The guru is in you.

2008/09/20 17:04:33
Enlightenment Milestones
http://www.aypsite.org/forum/topic.asp?TOPIC_ID=4466&REPLY_ID=37896&whichpage=-1
bliss verses tension

quote:
_____
Originally posted by newpov

Yogani,
quote:
_____
you said: we come to know ourselves as stillness in action
_____

Is your "stillness in action" exactly the same as what the Upanishads mean by the Self or the Atman? And, in this state does there still remain a sense of individuality?

newpov
_____

Hi newpov:

Yes, and yes, as far as I know. That is non-duality while making no effort to deny the apparent duality of the world (including our individuality). Engaging in such denial is one of the pitfalls of the mind (see the *Self-Inquiry* book). Much better to accept the paradox for what it is, and let the divine pour out into it. Hence, *stillness in action*. :-)

The guru is in you.

PS: Turiya (4th state of consciousness after waking, dreaming and dreamless deep sleep states) is not stillness in action. It is stillness only -- the witness. When stillness and ecstasy join, that gives rise to stillness in action -- outpouring divine love and unity.

2008/11/23 10:46:44
Enlightenment Milestones
http://www.aypsite.org/forum/topic.asp?TOPIC_ID=4774&REPLY_ID=41072&whichpage=-1
Is this Nirvikalpa Samadhi?

quote:
_____
Originally posted by Ananda

i've experienced turya once, but i don't consider myself to be anywhere close to an avatar:-).

nor do i consider yogani and a lot of the other enlightened out there.

so i don't think it's a necessity to be an avatar to experience ultimate states of conscionsness.

namaste,

Ananda
_____

Hi Ananda:

As the lesson Christi linked points out, turiya is not an ultimate state of consciousness, or an advanced condition we aspire to. It is only inner silence, which everyone touches every time they lose the mantra in deep meditation. It is the ever-present reservoir of stillness within us. As we advance in our practices, it becomes a normal part everyday living. But it is there from the very beginning also. Anyone who has experienced inner silence, a sense of witnessing events from within, knows turiya. Everyone has, yes?

Turiya means, "the fourth state" of consciousness, pointing to an ordinariness, and it is naturally experienced in life along with the other three states: waking, dreaming sleep and deep sleep.

With deep meditation and related practices, we gradually cultivate our nervous system to experience turiya simultaneously with the other three state on an ongoing basis. It is abiding inner silence. So, turiya is not a destination. It is our inner well-spring of peace, energy and creativity that is always available. It is our Self.

A good way to regard turiya is as "living stillness," not as a distant condition of enlightenment. It is only a mantra away, and soon abiding as the witness in all that we do. :-)

The guru is in you.

2008/11/25 12:27:53
Enlightenment Milestones
http://www.aypsite.org/forum/topic.asp?TOPIC_ID=4774&REPLY_ID=41203&whichpage=-1
Is this Nirvikalpa Samadhi?

Hi All:

Here is the paragraph for "avatar" from the AYP Glossary of Sanskrit Terms, which is not guaranteed to be a perfect match with traditional definitions:

quote:
_____
Avatar – Means, "incarnation of God in human form." Also is regarded to mean a spiritual savior of humankind. The birth of an avatar is sometimes foretold beforehand, and he or she typically undergoes the trials of achieving final enlightenment, and then takes on a mission to help many others advance spiritually. Well known avatars in the East include Krishna and Buddha, and in the West, Jesus. Many avatars have come to earth, and most are little known. Everyone has the inherent ability to become an avatar because everyone contains the same divine potential. The primary mission of an avatar is to show us that this is so.
_____

Actually, I thought "avatars" were those little animated figures people pose as in "real-as-life" video games. Incarnations of divine us, right? Are we living in a video game? :-)

The guru is in you.

2009/03/09 12:35:51
Enlightenment Milestones
http://www.aypsite.org/forum/topic.asp?TOPIC_ID=5298&REPLY_ID=46818&whichpage=-1
Finding AYP is a kind of milestone too

Hi Realmystic, and welcome!

Thanks much for your kind sharing. It is always good to have the benefit of those with long experience in this game. :-)

We are in a new era where the journey is becoming much more clearly understood to be centered in every individual. It has always been like that, of course. But we have sometimes been distracted by externals, whether it be a guru or God "out there" somewhere. Having been through so much, now many can observe for themselves that the doorway to the divine is much closer to home, right in here.

Which does not mean we ought to dispense with whatever or whoever "out there" inspires us to open our inner doors. Wherever we have found our inspiration and assistance, it has been good, and continues to be. The divine is everywhere, longing to fly on the wings of our bhakti (divine desire) and rising inner silence. Because of all that has gone before, we are able to see the process of human spiritual transformation much more clearly from the inside now.

With the increasing flow of divine energy occurring through everyone around the world, "peer-to-peer" horizontal transmissions of spiritual knowledge are spontaneously occurring everywhere. AYP is a symptom of that paradigm shift.

What we need are the most effective tools, freely available, continually being optimized on the individual level, on a journey that is self-inspired and self-directed. With that occurring in every culture and community on the planet, there is no limit to what humanity can accomplish in divine unfoldment.

Onward!

The guru is in you.

2009/04/18 09:42:13
Enlightenment Milestones
http://www.aypsite.org/forum/topic.asp?TOPIC_ID=5449&REPLY_ID=48863&whichpage=-1
Beyond Enlightenment

Hi Krish:

Self-realization before transformation? Interesting take on the process of human spiritual transformation. :-)

Since it is essentially the same process everywhere, this can be taken to mean that the "intimate" recognition of our potential to a degree (to any degree?) is "self-realization" in Aurobindo's terminology. And then we continue on with all the rest of it.

I think presenting "self-realization" as a prerequisite to transformation is misleading, since it implies much more than may actually be going on, and could lead to some castles being built in the air. Perhaps Aurobindo seeks to inspire by projecting immediate self-realization? I could buy into the rationale if we replaced the phrase "self-realization" with "abiding inner silence" (witness - 1st stage), as Christi mentions above. Much more "transformation" coming after that.

It is different semantics being used to describe the same process.

If it is not that, then it is getting the cart in front of the horse, as so many non-dual teachings do. After all, in the quote you gave, Aurobindo describes self-realization as "attainment of a certain state of consciousness..."

Isn't an attainment a transformation?

Well, the terminology doesn't matter so much. What matters is that we are becoming it -- the attainment, the transformation, the works! :-)

The guru is in you.

2009/04/18 10:07:46
Enlightenment Milestones
http://www.aypsite.org/forum/topic.asp?TOPIC_ID=5449&REPLY_ID=48865&whichpage=-1
Beyond Enlightenment
PS: Someone recently emailed me asking for a "definition of enlightenment." Here is what I wrote back. Perhaps it has some bearing on this discussion:

Hello:

Every tradition has its own definition of enlightenment. Ultimately, it boils down to the aspirant's growing experience. Without direct experience, all the definitions in the world mean nothing.

As the lesson says (#323), consider it to be an unending journey of unfoldment, rather than a fixed condition or event. In that way, we are able to ask ourselves, "Is my condition better now than last year? Am I happier, more creative, more at peace?" These are the things that matter. We'd like to know we are on the right track. Are we feeling "more enlightened" now than before? If so, good deal. Then keep going with the present program. If not, then maybe consider looking for improvements in practice.

Because people always ask, these milestones were laid out early on in the AYP lessons:
http://www.aypsite.org/35.html
It is a rough template of signature experiences that can occur along the way. Enlightenment has been discussed many times since then, in the lessons, in the books, and in the AYP Support Forum community where you are invited to chime in. Everyone benefits from the open discussions.

Here is one of the more popular lessons on enlightenment, called "Getting Enlightenment:"
http://www.aypsite.org/120.html
Moral of the story: You will know you are getting it when you are able to give it all away - nothing else to do.

Ultimately, enlightenment is becoming "stillness in action," or Oneness, which is an endless outpouring of divine love. We can become permanent channels for That, the thing itself, with the inherent experience of it being Joy.

But none of that means anything until the aspirant finds out through direct experience. And that is why in AYP we focus on effective practices that anyone can use according to their inner inclination ... much better to offer means than definitions. :-)

All the best!

The guru is in you.

Yogani

2009/08/03 15:47:07
Enlightenment Milestones
http://www.aypsite.org/forum/topic.asp?TOPIC_ID=6066&REPLY_ID=54542&whichpage=-1
Losing Self Judgements

Hi Carson:

This is a key realization. But, like self-inquiry, it can only be carried beyond the intellect if it is "relational," if there is enough abiding inner silence to remain increasingly in a condition of letting go, even as we act.

Someone recently asked me in email about this as it relates to errant words or actions by spiritual teachers (examples are abundant). Here is part of what I wrote back, as it might pertain to anyone in considering conduct (edited for this discussion):

quote:
_____
The primary motivation of a spiritual teacher is compassion, and letting that flow with minimum interference. If the teacher is liberated, they will not be much concerned about illuminating the remaining shadows in their own personality, unless it has been a priority for the person prior to enlightenment and carries forward by momentum. So karma has a role to play in what spiritual teachers do -- how they express themselves. It will not be perfect, even if the liberation is. Life in the world and liberation are in different realms, even though the *Self* will radiate much love, joy and healing into the world. This is the natural rise of yama/niyama, which will always be a lesser or greater reflection of the *Self*, never a 100% perfect reflection. Many continue to seek that 100% worldly perfection over their own freedom. It is something of a wild goose chase.

Do I find myself making statements that are incorrect, or biased in ways that are not beneficial to someone? Rarely and all the time, depending on who is judging. I judge it much less than I used to. It is beyond our reckoning. At some point we have to hand responsibility over to the divine and trust the process. That is what liberation is.

_____

The guru is in you.

2009/08/03 22:41:45
Enlightenment Milestones
http://www.aypsite.org/forum/topic.asp?TOPIC_ID=6066&REPLY_ID=54560&whichpage=-1
Losing Self Judgements

Hi Carson:

You will know it is working (relational in stillness) when you feel joyful, child-like, eternally in love with *Self/God*, and not the doer of anything, though much may seem to be going on. :-)

The guru is in you.

2009/12/04 11:34:48
Enlightenment Milestones
http://www.aypsite.org/forum/topic.asp?TOPIC_ID=6788&REPLY_ID=60668&whichpage=-1
Sushumna Nadi

Hi Carson:

Though it sounds like a spiritual purification experience, no one here (including me) can guarantee that it is not a vision health issue.

Many practitioners have had these kinds of experiences with no health issue involved, but you never know until you check with the doctor. Your call.

All the best on your ever-evolving path. A joy to see here. :-)

The guru is in you.

2009/12/12 17:50:43
Enlightenment Milestones
http://www.aypsite.org/forum/topic.asp?TOPIC_ID=6843&REPLY_ID=61225&whichpage=-1
Awakening in real-time

Hi Wayne:

What you are requesting is what has been going on in these forums for years.

I'm not sure how many will want to step forward and say, "Well, I was writing/blogging while practicing for all these years, and now I am enlightened." :-)

Nevertheless, it is all here for you to see.

Everyone here is awakening in their own time and in their own way. So there are plenty of data points for you to compare.

All the best!

The guru is in you.

2010/05/17 12:14:36
Enlightenment Milestones
http://www.aypsite.org/forum/topic.asp?TOPIC_ID=7808&REPLY_ID=68890&whichpage=-1
Samvega

quote:
_____
Originally posted by CarsonZi

Anyone gone through a mid-life crisis and is willing to comment on whether the definition of samvega fits with your experience?
_____

Hi Carson:

It is interesting to see what age demographic has the greatest viewership of AYP Youtube videos -- mid-life:

http://www.aypsite.org/images/AYP-YouTube.jpg

Sooner is obviously preferred, but it is never too late! :-)

The guru is in you.

588 –   Advanced Yoga Practices

2010/05/17 13:41:06
Enlightenment Milestones
http://www.aypsite.org/forum/topic.asp?TOPIC_ID=7808&REPLY_ID=68893&whichpage=-1
Samvega

quote:
_____
Originally posted by Anthem11

HI Yogani,

61000 views seems like a very impressive number?!
_____

Hi Anthem:

That was for 2009. It is over 90,000 views now, with similar age and gender distribution.

The 2009 Youtube demographics link was pulled from here: http://www.aypsite.org/forum/topic.asp?TOPIC_ID=4975

The guru is in you.

2010/08/08 12:19:28
Enlightenment Milestones
http://www.aypsite.org/forum/topic.asp?TOPIC_ID=8232&REPLY_ID=71723&whichpage=-1
Having Second Thoughts...

Hi Ethereal Ecstasy:

The AYP position on this is given here: http://www.aypsite.org/206.html
Some will not agree, and that is what makes the path interesting. :-)

And, yes, the AYP style of spinal breathing pranayama works quite well. The results are well-known, as many have attested.

Of particular importance are the method of meditation and additional practices that are performed in each sitting with spinal breathing pranayama. It is the integration of effective practices that makes the difference, not primarily the style of spinal breathing being used. In AYP, we regard the simplicity of spinal breathing pranayama practice to be important, to avoid watering down its effectiveness. That, combined with additional simplified effective practices, makes the AYP routine a very powerful catalyst for purification and opening.

But talk is cheap you know. The true test will be in your own practice. The proof of the pudding is in the eating. Beyond basic assessments, little can be accomplished through analysis. Much better to do.

So pick an approach, practice daily, and make adjustments as necessary along the way. Your direct experience with these things will be the most reliable and useful feedback you will get on your path. That is the formula, no matter what approach you may follow. It is about your results in practice, not anyone else's.

Everything is going to work out fine. Just do it. :-)

The guru is in you.

PS: On a related point, the variety of spinal breathing that uses the reverse direction of tracing the spinal nerve on inhale and exhale was discussed here from the AYP perspective: http://www.aypsite.org/46.html
Again, some will disagree. That's life. It is suggested to choose your course, and go. Let your experience be your guide. :-)

2010/08/27 11:53:42
Enlightenment Milestones
http://www.aypsite.org/forum/topic.asp?TOPIC_ID=8329&REPLY_ID=72425&whichpage=-1
Increasing amounts of Pratyahara?

Hi Carson:

You might want to review this lesson: http://www.aypsite.org/17.html

The same situation is possible without much awareness being present, or remembered (like you had), due to to the process of inner obstructions being dissolved in deep meditation.

It is not necessary to take special measures to "stay awake," other than meditating comfortably sitting up, with or without back support. What is happening is natural, and clarity of inner awareness will return as purification and opening advance. You may or may not notice outer sensory perceptions during meditation.

In any case, we just follow the easy procedure of meditation, and when time is up we rest adequately before getting up.

The guru is in you.

PS: If you look up "sleep" in the topic index on the main website, you will find several more lessons related to this subject.

2010/08/27 12:47:09
Enlightenment Milestones
http://www.aypsite.org/forum/topic.asp?TOPIC_ID=8329&REPLY_ID=72428&whichpage=-1
Increasing amounts of Pratyahara?

quote:
_____
Originally posted by CarsonZi

Hi Yogani and thanks for chiming in here....had kinda hoped you would :-)

I'm quite familiar with Lesson 17 (and I just read it again) as it is part of the AYP Level 1 lessons in the hands-on AYP classes. This sentence here:
"No sensory experience, no mantra, no thoughts, but still conscious inside – were you asleep? Probably not." almost applies to my situation except for the line about still being "conscious inside".... I had no sensory experience, no mantra, no thoughts, but I wasn't seemingly "conscious".

Does that change the reality of whether or not I was sleeping?

Love!
_____

Hi Carson:

That's why this line was added above:

quote:
_____
The same situation is possible without much awareness being present, or remembered (like you had), due to to the process of inner obstructions being dissolved in deep meditation.
_____

Yes, it can happen like that and not be "sleep" in the normal sense. But it is a normal experience that can happen in deep meditation to one degree or other. It is deep purification going on, with a temporary loss of awareness.

A word to describe this kind of experience in meditation is "blackout." It is distinctly different from regular sleep, and is a direct result of deep meditation. I prefer not to use that word much, because it may be misinterpreted in some way. But that is essentially what it is. It is part of the journey of purification and opening, and like all experiences (or lack of them), it will pass as new openings occur.

We just keep on favoring the procedure of practice, and it all passes by and opens up in the light of pure bliss consciousness. :-)

The guru is in you.

2010/12/02 22:42:20
Enlightenment Milestones
http://www.aypsite.org/forum/topic.asp?TOPIC_ID=8834&REPLY_ID=76081&whichpage=-1
The Joy of being an AYP instructor

Hi Carson:

It is very humbling for me to see what so many are doing with my feeble sharings. Whatever is of value is coming from beyond.

It is obviously awakening in all of us.

The guru is in you.

Forum 17 – Yoga and Relationships

Our relationships with self, partner, family, friends, co-workers, animals, and everything else.
http://www.aypsite.org/forum/forum.asp?FORUM_ID=52

2005/12/07 18:31:07
Yoga and Relationships
http://www.aypsite.org/forum/topic.asp?TOPIC_ID=545&REPLY_ID=1839&whichpage=-1
Changes in personal life

Hi All:

Kundalini is not a beginning or an end really. It is the long process of awakening ecstatic conductivity that never ends, because it keeps going, reaching eventually far beyond our physical body. It is the physical aspect of our infinite pure bliss conscousness unfolding on the material plane. It is both a manifestation and a realization of That. The refining perception (pratyahara) and the ever-expanding neurobiological dynamic go together.

If kundalini is forced, at can be a rough beginning, with big jerks and upheavals -- all that stuff in lesson #69. With less forced methods it can begin very smooth and gentle, like some nice sexual feelings going up from the pelvis into the spine and the rest of the body that keep expanding deliciously over years and years. Either way, kundalini is really felt instantly everywhere, which is why I use the word "conductivity" to describe the underlying phenomenon which is instantly present everywhere in us through the vast wiring in the nervous system. But it starts in the sexual biology. No doubt about that. Once it is underway, the ability to pick up wherever we left off will be there, in this life or in the next one.

Interestingly, the root is awakened and connected via conductivity from many levels in our practices and body, including the head mudras. Later on, especially the head mudras. But in the beginning, it is more involved with siddhasana, kumbhaka, bandhas, and tantric sex too. It starts in the basement, but the main stimulation and control is ultimately from the attic.

Well, however it is in the beginning, it will smooth out over time with good practices and self-pacing, and be much less overbearing as time goes on. You can be sure of that if you are on the path of self-paced yoga practices. Then it will be refining to ecstatic bliss, and pouring out all over the place via our internally illuminated acts. And then we don't see how we ever could have been any other way. It is our natural state coming out. It is a homecoming!

The guru is in you.

2005/12/10 23:36:48
Yoga and Relationships
http://www.aypsite.org/forum/topic.asp?TOPIC_ID=545&REPLY_ID=1883&whichpage=-1
Changes in personal life

quote:
_____
Originally posted by Melissa

In this somewhere else - I WAS everything and everything and everyone was connected. and it was the most awesome experience ever. But I haven't been able to get back there, no matter how much Pink Floyd plays in the background!
_____

Hi Melissa:

It was a peek between the clouds on the path of purification. While it seemed there was a choice, it really depends on finishing the housecleaning project -- clearing the clouds. And we all know how to do that by now. That is the real choice we have.

The guru is in you.

2006/02/26 12:01:55
Yoga and Relationships
http://www.aypsite.org/forum/topic.asp?TOPIC_ID=836&REPLY_ID=3881&whichpage=-1
a painful path and spiritual friends

Hi Jim:

The deep meditation we do here is not introspective. It is the centering of attention in inner silence. It is away from introspection, not toward it. It is toward inner stability -- calming of the restless mind at its root in consciousness, especially between sessions, which is when we all need it.

Other forms of meditation may focus on the content of the thinking process, in which case I would agree with you. But in the case of deep meditation, we are going beyond the thinking process, stabilizing it from within.

As for metabolism, yes, it slows down during deep meditation. Then we get up and go be active in the world, which integrates inner silence with activity. No introspection there either. It is not a path of withdrawal into the mind. This approach is beyond introspection and any tendency for depressive thinking that may exist. It is not involved with the content thinking at all!

The guru is in you.

2006/02/26 13:09:43
Yoga and Relationships
http://www.aypsite.org/forum/topic.asp?TOPIC_ID=836&REPLY_ID=3883&whichpage=-1

a painful path and spiritual friends

Hi Jim:

There is a big difference between going inward to thinking, and going inward <u>beyond thinking</u> to stillness. The two are not even remotely similar. Deep meditation is the latter.

There is no argument on the usefulness of asanas. However, the best approach to resolving problems of any kind is multi-pronged. Most here understand that.

You are saying that deep meditation should not be used to aid in moving beyond dark moods and depressive thinking, and I have to take issue. If you are right, and since no one is exempt from that condition, then we should suspend AYP right now and go back to the traditional approach of going through the limbs of yoga slowly one at a time. And good luck with that -- it does not work for many. That is why we are here utilizing an open and integrated approach -- self-directed.

With the door opening beyond thinking to inner silence, many are clearly seeing beyond the mistakes and gloom of the past. More inner awareness is not a bad thing. It reveals and heals. What right do we have to say someone should not have the option of deep meditation? It is a presumption that is not consistent with this modern approach.

Depression is not a forbidden territory owned by a piecemeal mentality. It is an illusion we all share in. It is time for us to move out of there by illuminating with the infinite light source beyond the labyrinth of darkness...

The guru is in you.

2006/02/26 16:07:44
Yoga and Relationships
http://www.aypsite.org/forum/topic.asp?TOPIC_ID=836&REPLY_ID=3893&whichpage=-1
a painful path and spiritual friends
Points all well taken, David. The question is, who is the best person to figure out whether deep meditation is going to be helpful or not for a particular case of depression? I believe it can only be the practitioner, based on their personal experience. I trust the practitioner's experience over anyone else's advice, including mine! Of course, the practitioner will never find out if we forbid certain measures for what we consider to be a "serious condition."

That is really the only disagreement I have with you, Jim -- I don't think it is for another to decide what is the best course for us to follow in resolving our problems. Possibilities, pro and con, and recommendations? Absolutely. Black and white exhortations? I cannot agree with that.

Who is prone to depression anyway? Depending on the measuring rod, it could be a few of us, or all of us. I don't know where to draw those lines. But nature does. "Severely depressed" people will not likely be able to maintain a routine of deep meditation practice -- so I repeat the contention that the whole process is self-regulating. That goes for any practice, including asanas. So why should we tell people what they must practice and what they must not practice? If it is available with a reasonable track record and good instructions, and they are looking for a solution, they will find out for themselves soon enough, and more than likely within an acceptable level of risk. Let's not unduly bias the information either way. Then it has the best chance for useful application.

Excellent points today from Richard, Kathy and Anthem too ... picking up on some of them here.

Alvin, give it some time. Maybe quit trying so hard, pamper yourself a bit, have a good laugh , and help out a few nearby who are in need. As Kathy says, they are not hard to find ... Gee, so much good advice here. We all should be feeling better pretty soon. :-)

The guru is in you.

2006/02/27 15:51:07
Yoga and Relationships
http://www.aypsite.org/forum/topic.asp?TOPIC_ID=836&REPLY_ID=3922&whichpage=-1
a painful path and spiritual friends

Hi Jim:

I'm grateful that you came back and further expressed your views. That is what the forum is for.

Am I going to change my position on deep meditation and depression? No. That is because self-pacing already addresses the downside for anyone who runs into difficulties with deep meditation, or anything else in AYP. Nowhere in AYP does it say that one size fits all, or that everyone ought to be doing a particular practice regardless of the outcome.

I do not disagree with the cautions and downsides presented by you and others in this topic. Points well taken. But I do not agree on making deep meditation taboo in depression situations. There are also successes mentioned in postings by others here on using deep meditation with depression. With your approach, would they have had the opportunity for that kind of progress? Perhaps with the use of asanas as you recommended and moving to meditation later. It worked for you. While, obviously, I do not oppose it, will everyone have the time and inclination to go through a focused asana program and hold off on meditation? Is waiting to meditate the best thing? Maybe for some (in your case it worked out). But clearly not in all cases. And maybe if you had known about deep meditation "back in the day," it would have been a wonderful complement to your asana strategy, and you'd be even further along than you are now. We'll never know, will we?

I can remember many years ago going through some pretty serious depression a few times. I was doing asanas, pranayama and deep meditation. There were times when I was too depressed to do any of the practices. But every time they all came back, and deep meditation always came back first. It was automatic self-pacing.

If we are in chronic debilitating depression, then seeing a doctor is the thing to do. <u>That I do recommend</u>. Then we can ask the doctor about means for relief, including meditation. AYP is one of the resources for that.

An underlying principle of AYP is that people are entitled to have access to the means for human spiritual transformation, and apply them as they see fit. It is a radical departure from the secretive highly parsed approaches of the past. Until the government decides to regulate the availability of spiritual practices, I'd like to keep the information open to <u>everyone</u>. It gives the most people the best chance to derive some benefit. Does it involve some risks? Yes, all information does. The risks in AYP have proven to be far less than the gloom and doom scenarios that have been preached. And the benefits have been very good, off-setting the risks by a wide margin.

Even for those who have contacted me with severe emotional problems, the benefits have exceeded the risks, so I will not rule out deep meditation as an option to be considered by anyone. Due to the unfathomable nature karma, it is impossible to know who will take to spiritual practices easily and who will not. We never know until we try. Therefore, in my opinion, with self-pacing solidly in the picture, trying deep meditation is worth the risk for anyone.

The guru is in you.

2006/03/19 20:41:38
Yoga and Relationships
http://www.aypsite.org/forum/topic.asp?TOPIC_ID=935&REPLY_ID=4732&whichpage=-1
The passing of a friend
Dear Kathy:

It has been said that every end is a beginning. Change is not easy, yet the river of life keeps flowing. The seasons go round and round. What can we do but go on? I hope you find comfort in the eternal flow, and in celebrating the precious blessings shared by your friend. May those special yesterdays become loving tomorrows. The gift of a life shared is eternal also. He is not gone -- only transformed, and in your heart for always.

The guru is in you.

2006/03/26 14:26:49
Yoga and Relationships
http://www.aypsite.org/forum/topic.asp?TOPIC_ID=979
Self-Pacing for a Roommate or Spouse

quote:
―――――――
Near said: I have a doubt, hope someone can help me out here. When I meditate there is some pain in my roommate's ajna chakra. What do I do about it? self-pace?
―――――――

Hi Near:

Though maybe this was offered in jest in relation to a private discussion :-), it is an interesting question, and not so far-fetched. There have been several couples who have written me over the past few years with this very issue. And, indeed, one person would sometimes end up self-pacing practices for the benefit of the other.

The other alternative is for the roommate to self-pace by putting a safe distance between themselves and the source of the intense spiritual light. That has happened also.

Is yoga tricky, or what? And we are only scratching the surface.

This is a real issue for couples and others in close proximity who are on the path. Anyone with examples, feel free to post...

The guru is in you.

2006/09/26 16:35:51
Yoga and Relationships
http://www.aypsite.org/forum/topic.asp?TOPIC_ID=1546&REPLY_ID=11593&whichpage=-1
Spiritual Soul Mates !

Hi All:

Long term success in marriage is based on surrender -- learning to put the needs of others above our own, while not becoming a doormat in the process. There is great spiritual value in this. Every marriage will be as yogic as one or both partners choose for it to be each day, just as in any other spiritual endeavor.

It may seem like the obvious solution would be to marry a "spiritual" or "unselfish" person. Maybe ... but it will almost never turn out as expected. In fact, holding on to expectations is the number one (and maybe only) cause of unhappy and failed marriages, and every marriage will repeatedly test us on that point, guaranteed.

Therefore, of far greater importance will our own intention to grow in loving service, which can easily look beyond the inevitable ups and downs that will occur in every marriage. Loving service can grow in all sorts of marriages, because it is not based on the marriage itself, but on individual commitment to spiritual growth. So, where we end up with our marriage will ultimately have less to do with where we started out than with what we do with it over the long term.

Of course, romance and finding an ideal "soul mate," get all the press and hoopla. The fact is, any marriage takes a lot of soul-searching and hard work, and the vast majority of that occurs long after the honeymoon is over. The rewards far exceed the sincere sacrifices. Those who give receive a thousandfold.

The guru is in you.

2006/09/27 12:04:22
Yoga and Relationships

http://www.aypsite.org/forum/topic.asp?TOPIC_ID=1546&REPLY_ID=11626&whichpage=-1
Spiritual Soul Mates !

quote:
_____
Originally posted by david_obsidian...However, it may be helpful to believe for a time, that "just one of the partners is enough to build a successful marriage". That could provide critical motivation (and hope)! :-)
_____

Giving does tend to be infectious, though it expects nothing in return. It is its own reward. :-)

The guru is in you.

2008/02/07 12:05:55
Yoga and Relationships
http://www.aypsite.org/forum/topic.asp?TOPIC_ID=3438&REPLY_ID=29783&whichpage=-1
Raising Children

Hi All:

The most important message our children receive from us is in how we live our own life. Even if words are not spoken, our children know what we are up to, and that will be the influence they receive from us over the long term more than anything else.

Putting it in those terms might sound a bit scary. But, you know, our children are very smart. If we give them the opportunity, they will take the best from us, and let the rest go. Therefore, the next most important thing in parenting is to give our children the opportunity to choose as they grow up, in ways that are both progressive and safe. Not recklessly progressive and not suffocatingly safe. Hmmm ... self-pacing. If we can do that, they will bloom according to their own unique purpose.

As adults, it is important for us to know that, no matter how we were raised, we always have a choice for how we live our life and for how we relate to others, including our children. Spiritual practices can play a key role in this, providing for purification and opening to the divine within, from where all love and goodness come.

Marriage and having children is certainly spiritual practice also.

Btw, over here we are looking at children from a new angle. We have three grown sons, two are married, and we just welcomed our first grandchild. A second grandchild is due in a few months. More joy, with less work. :-)

All the best!

The guru is in you

2008/02/07 12:15:46
Yoga and Relationships
http://www.aypsite.org/forum/topic.asp?TOPIC_ID=3438&REPLY_ID=29784&whichpage=-1
Raising Children

quote:
_____
Originally posted by clk1710

I hear that one's life changes so completely and to be honest, my biggest concern is maintaining my sadhana..... any thoughts on that??
_____

Hi CLK:

Yes, having children (and living the modern life-style in general) is a challenge for yogis and yoginis to keep up practices. This lesson is applicable: http://www.aypsite.org/209.html

It is well worth the inconvenience in the long run. Much more is gained than is lost. Actively pursuing our passion in the world (whatever it may be) while keeping up practices is a very fast path. Maybe the fastest. Stillness in action! :-)

The guru is in you.

2008/08/12 14:08:23
Yoga and Relationships
http://www.aypsite.org/forum/topic.asp?TOPIC_ID=4282
New Forum -- Yoga and Relationships

Hi All:

For some time it has been on the agenda to add a forum category on "Yoga and Relationships."

So much of our time and energy in daily life is involved with others in one way or other, and there is no question that our spiritual practices can have a profound effect on all of our relationships. So now we have a place to discuss it. :-)

The plan is to move relevant existing topics into this forum category on relationships that are currently scattered around the forums. If you can think of any, feel free to suggest the links here, so we can consider them for movement.

And, of course, new topics are encouraged. I hope we see many new discussions here on the influence of spiritual practices and experiences in

594 – Advanced Yoga Practices

our relationships -- people, places, creatures, things, etc. And most importantly with our *Self*, which is the underlying relationship that illuminates all others.

Many thanks to all for your thoughtful contributions to the AYP forums over the years!

The guru is in you.

2008/08/12 17:14:06
Yoga and Relationships
http://www.aypsite.org/forum/topic.asp?TOPIC_ID=4282&REPLY_ID=36295&whichpage=-1
New Forum -- Yoga and Relationships

Thanks, Scott.

As you can see, we found quite a few topics to move here. I am sure there are more.

It turns out we have been discussing relationships from many angles for years here in the forums. It has just been spread all over the place.

Now it is in one place. :-)

The guru is in you.

2010/12/07 08:16:12
Yoga and Relationships
http://www.aypsite.org/forum/topic.asp?TOPIC_ID=8647&REPLY_ID=76266&whichpage=-1
forgiveness etc

quote:
_____
Originally posted by Lili

Hi Christi,

Why is holding on to stuff a problem? I don't see anything wrong with holding on to the stuff that you like. What's the problem with this? Cheers, Lili
_____

Hi Lili:

Nothing wrong with enjoying life, while knowing that all things pass. It makes life all the more precious and sacred. But "holding on" to it leads to disappointment, because circumstances will change. As the Buddha taught, "Attachment is the root of all suffering."

To hold on or not to hold on is not a mental exercise. It isn't like that. When it is viewed this way, it is "non-relational" (in the mind, not in stillness), and will lead to even more suffering. The way to have everything and be bound by nothing is to cultivate and come to live in the permanence of abiding inner silence, becoming the essence of stillness in action. Then life is a flow of loving joy in all things, and there is no suffering in the constant comings and goings of life.

The guru is in you.

Forum 18 – Yoga, Career and Money

The relationship of our spiritual path with career and making a living.
http://www.aypsite.org/forum/forum.asp?FORUM_ID=51

2006/12/14 15:52:37
Yoga, Career and Money
http://www.aypsite.org/forum/topic.asp?TOPIC_ID=1817&REPLY_ID=14484&whichpage=-1
Abundance and lack

Hi Maximus, Bill and All:

I can confirm Doc's experience, having traveled a similar path. Family responsibilities can add an anvil of purification to our yoga. The key is in maintaining effective daily sadhana (practices) over the long term (not always easy), while accepting the opportunities for service that rise naturally during the process. It can all be yoga.

Not all of us who have a busy family life or other big responsibilities asked for it, or knew what we were getting into even if we did ask for it. :-) But once we have it, there are big spiritual opportunities.

This is not to disparage the single life. At times, the grass seems greener on the other side of the fence, no matter which side we happen to be on. Whatever our life is, it is a matter of pursuing our desires within that framework, while engaged in daily yoga practices. Whatever we do, for whatever reason, will be elevated in that way. However we approach it, we will be serving the greater good, because that is what is inherent in all of us. It is the essense of our nature, pure bliss consciousness, and this is what yoga cultivates to express outward through us into the world. And the world will teach us from its side, one way or the other.

The one caution in all of this is not to expect anything to happen without our active engagement in the process, whatever we find our process to be. Our progress will not be coming if we sit and wait, or are denying the road before us. No one else will do it for us. God will not do it for us. It will not happen if we are denying our own desires and opportunities to move forward. All roads lead home, as long as the road we are on is our own, and we are actively treading it.

So, whether we are materialistic or not, it is all leading to the same place if we are engaged in spiritual practices. There is no way that inner silence can lead anywhere else. Fulfilling material desires is not in opposition to this. It is part of the journey. In time we come to see the material aspects of life in better perspective. It is not such a big deal. Denial of a road not taken is a much bigger deal, especially if it is our road!

So, meditate, and go out and do what moves you, whether it be fulfilling inner desires or outer commitments -- eventually they will be the same. This is the fruit of persistent yoga. Practices and everyday living will gradually change our view of things, and we will come to know what is real. The truth of life is joy.

The guru is in you.

2007/10/12 16:48:24
Yoga, Career and Money
http://www.aypsite.org/forum/topic.asp?TOPIC_ID=2985
Forum on Yoga, Career and Money

Hi All:

For some time, there has been the thought to add a forum for discussing spirituality, career and money. This comes in part from the many questions on this subject that have come here over the years, and a realization that AYP has more to contribute beyond the simple (and true) maxim, "Meditate daily and all will come."

There has also been the thought to add a few new titles to the **AYP Enlightenment Series**, with **"Yoga and Money"** being one of them, for possible publication in 2008. We'll see.

The same posting guidelines will apply here as for any other AYP forum. No commercial solicitations are permitted. So this is not a place to discuss get rich quick schemes, multi-level marketing, stock recommendations, or things of that nature.

This forum is about fulfilling our **Dharma** (our most spiritually evolutionary activity in life) while fulfilling our financial responsibilities. Finding harmony between our spiritual practices and what we do for a living is an important part of the path. Indeed, both are essential ingredients that cannot be separated.

The apparent incompatibility we may find between our spiritual aspirations, our career, and money can be resolved over time as we advance in our yoga practices.

As inner silence gradually expands within us, it illuminates all of our outer activity. Our career may or may not change. But our relationship with our work certainly will with an opening heart and ever-increasing peace, creativity and joy, as our attention naturally shifts from identification with external objects (including thoughts, feelings and the objects of the world) to become absorbed in stillness and the flow of outpouring divine love.

Business and money then become a flow of consciousness along with everything else, and regulated in accordance with the principles of divine energy flow. The ancient time-tested methods of good money management embody these principles, just as the methods of yoga embody the principles of human spiritual transformation inherent in everyone. We are the doorway to the infinite, limited only by the temporal obstructions lodged within us. The methods of yoga are for dissolving these obstructions in our neurobiology.

As we continue with our practices and are increasingly able to hear the call of our dharma within and around us, we can clearly see beyond the old limitations to a much fuller expression in all aspects of our life.

Wishing you all the best on your chosen path. Practice wisely, and enjoy!

The guru is in you.

2007/10/30 11:38:45
Yoga, Career and Money
http://www.aypsite.org/forum/topic.asp?TOPIC_ID=3063&REPLY_ID=26510&whichpage=-1
Law of Attraction Revisited

Hi Meg:

Gratitude? Yes.
Intention? Certainly.
Letting go/surrender? Absolutely. (from samyama -- see note below)
A willingness to act, often in unfamiliar directions? Essential.

The last one is often missed in the process. The time we spend waiting for something to happen or lamenting our lack is time we could be spending in action fulfilling our destiny.

Stillness cannot be stillness in action unless we are in action. And that often will mean outside our normal pattern of so-called comfort. After all, it is the status quo that is holding us back. Moving in new directions will bring us into levels of fulfillment we have not considered.

That does not mean chucking everything. It means moving from where we are in the direction that is presented to us by the divine flow. As long as we are saying "no" to that, hoping for wished for things to fall in our lap, we will likely stay stuck. The miracle is what happens while we are busy pursuing the life before us with gratitude, intention, and surrender. It can also be called, "active surrender."

There can be no disappointments if we are fully engaged in this process, for each step leads to the next, and every step is an adventure filled with divine purpose and surprise. We need not judge the outcome. The lilies of the field do not, and see how beautiful they are? :-)

The guru is in you.

Note: Our samyama practice itself is not for manifesting specific things. It is for increasing our ability to engage in all of life as "stillness in action," which results in many automatic manifestations of the divine flow that are appropriate to the circumstances we find ourselves in.

2007/10/31 10:03:09
Yoga, Career and Money
http://www.aypsite.org/forum/topic.asp?TOPIC_ID=3063&REPLY_ID=26567&whichpage=-1
Law of Attraction Revisited

Hi All:

While the statement "God helps those who help themselves" might seem incongruent to those attempting to dissolve ego, "Thy will be done" may not resonate with those who have strong desires to get things done in this life.

In fact, both are true. Divine paradox...

Having desire to get things done is not anti-spiritual, and neither is it anti-spiritual to go out and vigorously pursue our desires, including applying the principles for illuminating our desires and actions with divine energy -- samyama and the law of attraction. Whatever works for us.

So, just practice and go out and do! If we do that, the rest will take care of itself.

It is much more difficult to keep second guessing ourselves, our motives, our actions, whether we should have desires, act in the world, etc. It can lead to a kind of paralysis.

The doubt is the downside of self-inquiry when it is overdone. Nowhere in AYP does it say that we ought to be constantly second-guessing our motives and actions, and it will not say that in the AYP Self-Inquiry book either. It is strongly encouraged to go out and live our life freely and fully. :-)

Incidentally, as far as I have been able to determine in this life, after sitting practices, the easiest way to become fulfilled, transcend duality, and make a living too, is to help others feel fulfilled. There are thousands of ways to do this through our intentions, our actions and our art. We don't have to wait or go anywhere to do it. It is right here, right now.

See this lesson: http://www.aypsite.org/120.html

All the best!

The guru is in you.

2008/05/03 10:37:19
Yoga, Career and Money
http://www.aypsite.org/forum/topic.asp?TOPIC_ID=3849
If only I had money. Then I could...

Hi All:

The below is from a recent email interchange. This has been an issue for most of us at one time or other in life. Please feel free to chime in with comments and suggestions based on your own experience.

The guru is in you

Q1: I'm new in meditating but I've experienced some benefits. This made me realise the potential Yoga has for my life.

There is one thing though that feels as an obstacle:

I'm an immigrant in the UK. I came here few years ago from Bulgaria and it has been hard ever after. It is a struggle for survival-working long hours to pay the bills. I was lucky and now I'm studying Dentistry-but the program is hectic and it leaves me hardly any spare time for anything else. The insufficient money and the lack of my own home here is still a great deal of issue for me. I'm eager to concentrate more on spiritual enlightenment, but the hectic busy life stile doesn't leave me with much time.

The reason to e-mail you now is to ask you something probably many people have already asked you. May be you'll think it is a silly question and it has nothing to do with spiritual enlightenment, but I'll ask it anyway.

Is there any method in meditation that when practiced for a long time would increase my intuition?

Being able to intuitively predict future events such as lottery draws, or betting. Although it seems very non-spiritual, such ability would help me sort out my financial status and it would help me buy my own place here in London. Having enough money to cover my expenses would allow me to spare more time for spiritual and meditation exercises. If one is transfixed too much in their physical existence it is hard to turn and be enlightened and spiritual and hence kind and good to other people. Poor men are desperate and can not afford to allow themselves to be kind- may be I'm wrong, but it is how it feels at the moment.

Thank you in advance and I hope my question was not very disturbing!

A1: Hi: The truth is, as we are able to release our desires into stillness without expectations, they will find the best way to manifest in our life, and not usually as we might expect. This is the benefit of long term practice of deep meditation and samyama -- ever refining to become a natural flowing of life in love.

If we pursue money for the sake of money, there will be little joy in it, no matter how much of it we get. Much better to work persistently at the things we love. Then there will be less imbalance and more happiness over the long term.

It sounds like you are building a wonderful future there in the UK. All your hard work and sacrifice will pay off. In the meantime, you may want to review this lesson on keeping practices going within a busy work schedule: http://www.aypsite.org/209.html

Don't worry, everything you need will be there. Just keep following your dream, your highest ideal.

Q2: I just wanted to add something else.

No, I don't pursue money as a solemn goal-I more like need it in terms of means to further enhance my spiritual enlightenment. Having cleared the worries of day-to-day existence would give the freedom to choose my own way, instead of being forced to take a particular way in order to cover the bills. I hope I'm managing to make myself clear to you! That's why in a way I'm looking for a kind of a short cut to stabilise the financial matter quickly so I can get to a more serious spiritual cleaning without being distracted by basic uncertainty.

BTW. I almost forgot,

I meant to ask you one more thing. Does Yoga and meditation in general have and reference to the Law of Attraction? I mean is there a philosophy in Yoga with provisions to the belief that what you are thinking about you bring in existence? I was watching "The Secret" and "What the Bleep do we know" recently and although these two are kinda of simplistic way to explain this law I liked the idea of having positive thoughts would bring more of what we are positive and grateful about. I found some similarities with what you were saying in some of your teachings. What do you think about this law and how do you apply it in your personal life?

A2: Unfortunately, it does not work like that.

"If only I had some money. Then I could go and do what really interests me."

Money is not the cause of anything. It is an effect of how we live our life. It is a manifestation of our energy. To the extent it is not, it will cause problems. That is why "instant riches" are accompanied by unhappiness on balance in so many cases.

I understand your sincerity, but it is a bit misplaced. Keep working toward your goals, be steady in your practices, and all will come.

As for the "law of attraction," if you have not already, check out the AYP Samyama book.

This is a good topic for the support forums. I am sorry no one else is benefiting from our discussion so far. Is there something we can do about that? :-)

See here: http://www.aypsite.org/forum/forum.asp?FORUM_ID=51

Q3: Thank you for taking time to answer my questions!

I've been looking for answers of questions like this for sometime and maybe this is the reason to be able to find your web site (it was given to me by chance from a complete stranger-talking about spookyness:))-so for me The Law of Attraction works (and always has been, but I didn't realise it before). I have bought from Amazon 2 of your books-Deep Meditation and the Samyama book about the miracles. I'm waiting for them to be delivered. On the web site you were talking about practicing Samyama and the chance to achieve levitation as one is getting deeper and deeper in practice-is that really possible. What makes it possible?

Should you like you can publish my questions and your answers on your site if you think that someone else can benefit from it-I don't mind. I'll can register and put them on your site's forums, but it will happen later in the summer-I'm having the end of the year exams next week, and I'm e-mailing you in my breaks between my reading sessions.

Anyway, thank you once again for the time and patience to talk to me!

I've really enjoyed our conversation and I hope to be able to ask you more precise questions about meditation as I go along with practice!

A3: Glad to be able to add some perspective for you from the point of view of yoga.

All the best!

The guru is in you.

2008/08/18 15:49:05
Yoga, Career and Money
http://www.aypsite.org/forum/topic.asp?TOPIC_ID=4311&REPLY_ID=36515&whichpage=-1
flowering of conscioussness and worldly life
...and here is the reply... :-)

Hi YogaIsLife:

The way we can live a purer life in this world is by continuing to work on ourselves from within, which you are doing. This produces profound effects for everyone. You should follow your professional education and career with the intention of integrating your highest ideal into it over the long term. This is the best way to make a better world.

Going away to a so-called simpler life is not likely to be a better solution, because we take ourselves wherever we go. :-)

This would be a good one to bring to the "careers" category of the AYP Forums. I hope you do, for you can get more suggestions there, and everyone will benefit.

The guru is in you.

Hi All:

There have been several yoga and career inquiries coming to my email lately. Inner silence is finding more of a role in such considerations. While this may seem confusing at first, the end result will be more clarity in what we do in our career.

The professions of science need people who are integrating their rising inner silence more than the ashrams do. This is how the world will be made better, by those who are expanding their inner vision and having a greater say in how our institutions move forward.

So, to all who have been drawn to a career, the suggestion is to go for it, while integrating your highest ideal into your ongoing endeavor as you move steadily forward. With practices in play and inner silence rising over the long term, you will find that anything is possible.

The guru is in you.

2008/08/18 17:39:29
Yoga, Career and Money
http://www.aypsite.org/forum/topic.asp?TOPIC_ID=4311&REPLY_ID=36523&whichpage=-1
flowering of conscioussness and worldly life

Hi All:

Here is one I wrote recently to someone in med school, having doubts about the medical profession...

Hi:

Thank you for your kind thoughts and sharing.

You have an interesting background, and great potential to help others for a better life. So often, the struggles of our youth are a search for our vision and our path. We can sense it, and the steps of our awakening can be messy, kind of like childbirth. :-)

While it may not seem like it, this is a great time to be studying medicine. A shift is getting underway in the profession, though it may be barely visible at present. Yet, more is being spent every year on R&D in Complimentary and Alternative Medicine (CAM), and I think this is going to be a major spearhead in the transformation of our society to prevention-based healthcare, and ultimately a shift to a central focus on cultivating the underlying process of human spiritual transformation.

So, where you are is a good place, assuming you want to be part of this long term shift, which it appears you do. The thing to do is get on with it by connecting the dots between where you want to go personally and professionally with what has to be done right now to keep heading in that direction, i.e., pass those exams, do that residency, become fully credentialed, and move on through while favoring the kind of career in medicine you want to have, rather than the kind that past ways would compel you to have. Bringing your ultimate aims in tune with present activities will help you find the motivation to do what is necessary to move ahead. It is the effective application of bhakti!

It is important that more people in the science professions make these connections, and carry forward. People of science have a lot to say about where society is going. The present system is not impregnable. It can evolve, and it will. It must. That is the nature of science.

You are really in a much better position than I was coming through school 40 years ago. My education was in engineering and I felt many of the same frustrations and lack of motivation you have. In my case, there were no fully integrated open source spiritual teachings (it was all closed source and sectarian) and my industry was not one moving into a spiritual transition like yours is. After school, I went into a 30 year technical and business career, and worked quietly underneath all the while to develop for myself what would eventually become AYP. So here I am, reporting on what was discovered, and now your generation can take it to the next level, which is ongoing development and widespread application of this kind of knowledge. It can change the quality of life for all of humanity. We know that from our own experiences.

So, if you get the credentials and some solid experience under your belt, both spiritual and professional, then gradually blending these together can develop into a very rewarding career.

Many of the seemingly mundane traditional skills we develop in our profession can provide a foundation for future innovation. There would be no AYP if the spiritual component in me had not been combined with the technical, writing and relationship skills developed over the years in the professional environments I was in. So, what may seem boring and irrelevant now, will eventually become a part of your overall ability to undertake actions that can fulfill your dreams. Knowing this can bring great relevance into the most mundane of tasks in the present, and we can then do them with more joy and enthusiasm. Of course, rising inner silence plays a major role in this, going far beyond the intellectual part of it. Then we can just happily do what has to be done (stillness in action), and in time we see the openings that our actions have created, and then do what has to be done there. In that way we gradually become instruments of not only our own evolution, but of the evolution of everyone around us. See how that works?

As for specifics, don't expect it all to happen right away. It will take a lifetime. As you continue to find more joy in each day, a great patience will arise also. With expanding stillness and expanding patience, no undertaking will be impossible. If it is CAM you want, then I suggest looking at the major institutions involved in it that are mentioned in the "Applied Spiritual Science" forum topic I started some months ago. If you go to the National Institutes of Health CAM website (in the topic), many other programs are listed. So there are quite a few options for a young physician wanting to gain experience in this field. I am not saying it will be easy. It will be a can of worms, because there is still a lot of confusion out there about what "health" really is and how we can improve it, and little understanding about the spiritual underpinnings of health, which also transcend the condition of the physical body. Some of the "healthiest" people I have known have been terminally ill in the physical sense. So that is the challenge you are laying out as your potential career. Actually, it is really quite exciting to be approaching it in a way that gets to the bottom of things. So I say, go for it! :-)

Regarding your question about a role for open systems like AYP in medicine, definitely! Honestly, I do not know of any other open system that is as fully integrated as AYP. There are no closed systems that are either. But this does not mean that there are not many other knowledge sources in play. There certainly are. In fact, currently, all the CAM research that is occurring out there is with other systems, fragments of the whole for the most part. An integrated approach like AYP is not the subject of a single study that I am aware of. We are still very much below the radar -- an R&D project in our own right. It will change eventually, but that is how it is today. AYP is still primarily a web phenomenon and an ongoing experiment. So the work continues, still largely behind the scenes of the mainstream, though interest is on the rise. Perhaps we are the 1000 gorilla of the future in open source integrated spiritual systems?

Regarding your question about teaching certifications, due to AYP being still early stage, I think certification of teachers is a bit premature. It is still primarily a web-based peer-to-peer transmission of knowledge. If and when AYP begins to enter structured teaching environments in medicine, universities, yoga studies, etc., then I think the need for certifications will become obvious, and someone will do something about it. On the other hand, with the AYP writings being what they are, I think there will always be a sort of self-certification built into it -- people are either following the teachings, or they are not. Even at this early stage, we see a lot of variations in application of the knowledge in the forums, and it is usually pretty clear who is doing something close to AYP, and who is not. Who knows, maybe someday the AYP writings can serve as part of the basis for an academic program with degrees and recognized credentials like in medicine, engineering and other fields. I'd like that, because it would be a permanent implant in our culture that would assure the knowledge for future generations.

I am in favor of the development of any programs that will advance human spiritual evolution over the long term on the basis of verifiable applied knowledge, rather than the charismatic personalities that come and go. It is time to move on to something much more solid in the field of applied spiritual knowledge.

Carry on!

The guru is in you.

2008/08/19 08:28:23
Yoga, Career and Money
http://www.aypsite.org/forum/topic.asp?TOPIC_ID=4311&REPLY_ID=36540&whichpage=-1
flowering of consciousness and worldly life

quote:
_____
Originally posted by YogaIsLife

Actually, about the issue of teacher certification I wanted to ask something as well to yogani. I have thought of teaching the ayp system to other people, on an informal basis. The meditation I am doing is being helpful to me and I thought of sharing it to close friends or relatives that might need something like this. I also thought of giving small workshops maybe to teach this kind of meditation to others, always giving this people the links to the original website for further consultation. This won' be something I will be doing systematically but only when a certain occasion may call for it. Do you agree with this spread of information? I think so, but just checking :-)

I find one problem though, when explaining the meditation to other people, people I know. I cannot really explain them why we say 'AYAM'. First off english is not my language so they think is weird in the first place to say that instead of anything else, and also in general people are not familiar with meditation or any of this 'esoteric stuuf', and although they are willing to try something that will enhance their lifes, they don't understand what they are doing. So I don't want to scare them off by giving a too esoterical explanation (involving subtle bodies and so on) but I would like to tell them something simple that they can understand and apply. Any thoughts?
_____

Hi YogaIsLife:

Starting a meditation group would be great. There are several who have done that, and it can be very fulfilling.

Ether has given you good guidance on the mantra. It is not necessary for you to go into depth to explain everything. Just refer them to the lessons and books. Also, look under "mantra" in the topic index for lessons on mantra, language and meaning.

All the best!

The guru is in you.

600 – Advanced Yoga Practices

2008/08/19 09:10:35
Yoga, Career and Money
http://www.aypsite.org/forum/topic.asp?TOPIC_ID=4311&REPLY_ID=36541&whichpage=-1
flowering of consciousness and worldly life

quote:
_____
Originally posted by YogaIsLife

One last question :-) One thing that puzzled me in Yogani's post. You said : 'Some of the "healthiest" people I have known have been terminally ill in the physical sense.' I had the idea that spiritual development = good health but that seems not to be the case all the time. Why is that? Do you mean that sometimes it takes an illness to make us spiritual healthy (illness as cause)?

_____

Ah, this one has come up before. :-)

Developing spiritually is developing health beyond the body. And the concern is, are we leaving the body? Leaving all of this behind? Well, eventually we have to, right? Or we may be limited physically due to circumstances beyond our control. But even as we are becoming inner silence (the witness) apart from our identification of ourselves with the physical, the paradox of "becoming" (without suffering) all that we are witnessing arises also. I wrote about the practical aspects of this recently over here, in discussing the presence of the witness during a physical crisis: http://www.aypsite.org/forum/topic.asp?TOPIC_ID=4307#36506

And yes, spiritual development brings better physical health, mainly because our inner purification and opening (if conducted in a balanced way with self-pacing) counteracts the influences of stress, strengthens immunity and the body's regenerative processes, etc. These things are fairly well known, and it is where the CAM research dollars have been going. But the body is not forever, and the obsessive quest for physical immortality is illusional thinking, even if we may end up having it someday!

The point is that our freedom and happiness are not bound up in the body, even a healthy one. They are bound up in our state of consciousness. For those who are on the path, the physical challenges we face, including our mortality, can be used to advance our spiritual progress. That is what I meant by some of the "healthiest" people I have known being terminally ill in the physical sense. It is not the case for everyone, but there is a peace and luminous expansion that can rise in some who have a terminal illness. It raises the question, what is health anyway? Is death a failure?...as is the current belief in the medical profession. What does it mean to save someone's life? These are hard questions that the medical profession is beginning to ask itself, and that is good, because the most important part of our "health" has to do with much more than the condition of our body. This does not mean we disregard physical health. It means we look beyond physical health to a much broader landscape that includes physical health, even while transcending it.

Being a responsible science in search of the truth, the medical profession must consider these things. Ultimately, that will be good news for humanity for both physical and spiritual health. :-)

The guru is in you.

Forum 19 – Other Systems and Alternate Approaches

Christian, Jewish, Taoist, Buddhist, Sufi, Shaman, AYP Modifications and more.
http://www.aypsite.org/forum/forum.asp?FORUM_ID=29

2005/07/13 12:39:52
Other Systems and Alternate Approaches
http://www.aypsite.org/forum/topic.asp?TOPIC_ID=288
Other Systems of Spiritual Practice

By now, AYP has been blessed to receive visitors from just about every tradition on the planet. It is an honor to be able to share something that can be useful to people engaged in many different systems of spiritual practice. Likewise, AYP has been enriched in quiet ways by exposure to these many ways of approaching the task of human spiritual transformation.

This forum is for those who are engaged in systems of practice other than AYP. Much can be gained by looking across the lines that separate the various systems. What we will find is common threads, confirmations and, sometimes, revelations that would not be possible otherwise.

All paths, traditional and esoteric, are welcome here -- Christian, Jewish, Taoist, Buddhist, Sufi, Shaman and more...

So please do share your path and practices, if you are permitted to do so, so that all might benefit. Let's compare notes. Whatever our different orientations may be, we all share one thing in common on the spiritual journey -- this marvelous human nervous system, this temple of God, our glorious doorway to divine experience!

The guru is in you.

2005/08/06 15:48:41
Other Systems and Alternate Approaches
http://www.aypsite.org/forum/topic.asp?TOPIC_ID=379&REPLY_ID=314&whichpage=-1
Mantra and Jyotish

Hello Frank:

In AYP, the goal with regard to mantra has been to simplify it down to the level of universality. If that sounds like a contradiction, then we are probably on the right track, as divine expression nearly always involves paradox -- usually involving the simplest and most complex things.

There are whole books sitting here in the library filled with mantras, and, as you say, we can parse the spiritual anatomy down to the finest aspect of chakra and nadi with mantra. And then we can build it all back up again to cover every aspect of our inner vibration. But what for?

Since AYP started, folks have written from India with advice on what specific mantras to use for wealth, health, social standing, marrying off a daughter, anything you want. Long lists of mantras have been sent here. I will need a bigger hard drive soon to store them all.

Invariably, the people who have had the most trouble letting go into native inner silence with AYP deep meditation have been the those who have been using the most mantras for the most purposes for the longest. For them, it is by rote, and the habit of innocence of attention has been corrupted by the cultural overlay of mantra, and so has the science of mantra overall been corrupted by this.

The question that has been asked in AYP is, what is the simplest most practical approach to mantra we can come up with that everyone can use effectively starting right now? And how can this be enhanced periodically to take the process of unfolding permanent inner silence broader and deeper as soon as the nervous system is ready for a mantra gear shift? It is about cultivating inner silence broadly and deeply in the nervous system, and then marrying this with the rise of ecstatic conductivity (cultivated by the other means) to complete the enlightenment circuit. It is not about this or that chakra, ishta deva, tattva, jyotish factors or whatever. These are but aspects of the great wheel of the human spiritual anatomy and its evolutionary transformation which we are directly stimulating with yoga methods.

In AYP, the mantras (the original "I AM," plus two enhancements in the online lessons, and one more in the AYP book), are geared to the overall nervous system. They are called "global" in the lessons. More specifically, they are geared to the observable experiences of resonance in the sushumna (spinal nerve), which controls the unfoldment of the entire nervous system. In taking this approach, we have been able to offer a universal approach to meditation and mantra that anyone who chooses to can use, with immediate and ongoing positive effects occurring in most cases. It is not a "traditional" approach, but that is what we are doing here.

While I have the greatest respect for the accumulated knowledge of yoga over thousands of years, I am also wary of the complexity that tends to creep in whenever human beings focus more on the means than on the end. So that is why AYP is so simple and easy -- and non-traditional. For more particulars, see lesson #188 on AYP mantra design at http://www.aypsite.org/188.html

As for the traditional approaches to mantra, I'm sure we'd all love to hear more, particularly on how the most simple and effective means for our enlightenment can be effectively applied. If we are looking at mantras as an academic study, or as part of a study of Sanskrit, then that is fine. But let us be clear on what is effective practice and easily assimilated by everyone versus what is a fascinating academic study.

We are pretty much "in the trenches of yoga" here, focused on real causes and real effects, so pardon me if this comes across as more utilitarian than scholarly. We can do scholarly too, but it is not nearly as much fun (or consequential) as having Shiva (inner silence) and Shakti (ecstatic conductivity) in a full-blown orgy going on everywhere in the nervous system. :-)

The guru is in you.

2005/08/05 22:57:08
Other Systems and Alternate Approaches
http://www.aypsite.org/forum/topic.asp?TOPIC_ID=382&REPLY_ID=300&whichpage=-1
Night Techniques

Hello All:

Here is a Q&A from my mailbox a few months ago on sleep techniques. Having tried some methods years ago, I am not much for them, for the reasons mentioned. If anyone has something practical to offer that can provide additional stable growth without throwing everything else out of whack, do feel free to post it!

****

Q: I've noticed a number of times that I'd just be on the point of falling asleep and my mind would be doing some yogic thing --- might be my mind is on the base of my spine or some other part of my body --- and whazam! it gets aligned in some sort of energetic way, a connection, a yogic advancement is made. And I wake up.

This doesn't happen regularly for me. But it has happened often enough for me to notice it.... and to speculate, like a scientist....

Is this a known phenomenon? It seems to me to be something *like* the mind going to some state of transcendence, some deep connection in which the desire (activated by a feeling for the particular part of the body which the mind is attending) is realized by an alignment of that part of the body... a little like the theory behind samyama practice, but entirely spontaneous.

Do you know if there is any way to exploit this, yogically? Or is it (for now at least) just a random fruit that is thrown our way every now and then?

A: There's no question that attention, particularly when grounded in inner silence after years of deep meditation, has a purifying effect on the subtle neurology and physical body. That is the natural principle involved in samyama, and also in the practices that involve body-located attention (spinal breathing, yoni mudra, chin pump, spinal bastrika, etc.). These are systematic methods designed to cover the full range of neuro-biological openings. We also know that if a particular purification event becomes so strong in meditation that we cannot easily pick up the mantra, we can allow the attention to go to it to help dissolve that particular unwinding.

The automatic yoga you are experiencing at the sleep boundary involves that natural principle of silence-based attention fostering purification. I experience it regularly too, and also during dreaming and deep sleep, not to mention at all odd times during the day. That is what happens when inner silence becomes a 24 hour experience. It is always at work in one way or another cleaning us up inside. Can it be exploited as additional practice? I think the practices just mentioned do.

Can we do a better job of instigating and supervising a "yoga nidra" (yogic sleep) style of attentive purification? Perhaps. Yoga nidra is a hot item on the yoga circuit these days -- a sort of fad, really. The idea of getting enlightened while sleeping is appealing to the time-efficient mind. Go to sleep ignorant, and wake up enlightened. What could be better? I know that isn't what you are suggesting, but perhaps you are looking for ways to optimize the waking/sleep state boundary to facilitate these kinds of releases. I know some methods, but do not recommend them. My experience with them has led to sleep disruption and deprivation (scientific investigations in any field will lead to some dead ends, and so far that is where I am on sleep techniques), so I really have nothing useful to offer in that department. An expanding list of (market driven?) teachers claim to, however, and the way to find them is by searching on yoga nidra. Also check the methods of the Tibetan Buddhists (a la Evans-Wentz books) and the Toltec (Shaman) traditions. All of these are big into sleep boundary practices.

As you know, the AYP approach is to cultivate inner silence in sitting practices, emerging to be coexistent with waking, dreaming and deep sleep states. It is a bit old-fashioned (very), but it works. If you run across an approach for utilizing the gap state between waking and sleep states that has some practical potential, without turning sleep on its head, do let me know.

We all need our sleep. zzzzzz

The guru is in you.

2005/08/27 09:24:23
Other Systems and Alternate Approaches
http://www.aypsite.org/forum/topic.asp?TOPIC_ID=436&REPLY_ID=452&whichpage=-1
A realized Christain Mystics view on Pranayama.

Hello Adam:

Thank you very much for posting that. It is spinal breathing in Christianity! An excellent example of how practitioners in Christianity, and in all the traditions, are expanding from faith (bhakti) alone into practices that directly address the neuro-biological aspects of human spiritual transformation. It is an important shift that has been slowly coming up over the past 50-100 years, corresponding with the arrival of yoga systems in the West. For some history of this migration of Eastern knowledge, see AYP lesson #253 at http://www.aypsite.org/253.html

What we are seeing is a synthesis of methods crossing traditional lines, which is a very good thing.

Another Judeo/Christian approach that was brought to my attention some time ago is the Essene Nazarean Church of Mount Carmel, which is not shy about making a direct connection with yogic methods from the East. See http://www.essene.com/B'nai-Amen/yoga.htm

Perhaps other readers here know of other Christian applications of the formerly esoteric knowledge. If so, please let us know. I say "formerly esoteric" because we aim to open it all up here for everyone to see, compare, integrate and further refine. It is time for that.

None of this is to say that the mystical practices emerging in the Western traditions these days are all Eastern yoga-based. The nervous system is what it is, and the principles and practices involved in purifying and opening it are universal. So these methods (with variations) can originate with any "seer" in any part of the world. Indeed, all of the world's traditions were started by such individuals. It is only fitting that the traditions should rediscover their mystical roots in modern times and finally share with the public the methods that spawned them in the first place. Mr. Richardson and many others are doing just that. Bravo!

The guru is in you.

2005/09/30 11:45:42
Other Systems and Alternate Approaches
http://www.aypsite.org/forum/topic.asp?TOPIC_ID=500
Mixing Taoist and Yoga Practices

This is a Q&A from my email that is representative of questions I receive from time to time on whether Taoist and Yoga methods can be mixed. If you have any thoughts on this, feel free to post them.

Q: I have some questions I was hoping you can offer some advice or comments on. I am currently learning a taoist practise of self cultivation that largely deals with yin and yang chi. In level 1 of the system we are to make full the yang center which corresponds
to the dan tien and the yin center which corresponds to the perinium. Is there any yoga or taoist practise that you have heard about or read about that has an anology. When one is full in these centers they progress to level 2a which is to compress the yang c
Hi stored in the dan tien into a small ball. Have you heard of any practises in taoist or yoga studies that try to do this. When one has passed this level it is then onto level 2b where the goal is to rotate the dan tien in order to break 5 chakras or nerve plexus that surround the dan tien. Have you heard of any practises in taoist studies or yoga studies that do this. After this, one enters level 3 where the dan tien or this small ball of yang c
Hi is suspended by some ganglia. Level 3 is to break free from the ganglia and unite with the yin c
Hi that is stored in the perinium where one enters level 4.

I was curious if you have heard of any taoist practises or yoga practises that have similar techniques or exercises to accomplish any or all of the steps listed above. Some clarifications or points or analogies would be most helpful.

A: Of course, both taoist and yoga systems are dealing with the same human nervous system and capabilities. While the two approaches are similar in some ways, there are many differences too, and a full marriage does not seem to be easy, or practical.

The taoist approach is much more energy (chi/prana) oriented than yoga, storing it and utilizing it for both worldly and spiritual purposes, perhaps because of its marital arts energy management orientation. Yoga goes for a holistic vertical integration immediately energy-wise in the spinal nerve (sushumna) and therefore does not cover the particular energy manipulations and storage at the dan tien (a point just below the navel) you mention. No marital arts orientation in yoga. Yoga also puts a lot of emphasis on the cultivation of pure bliss consciousness (inner silence) via meditation and related methods, which is a very important difference from most taoist systems.

I am a long time tai c
Hi practitioner myself, and find it to be an excellent "grounding" practice, which can be a benefit in yoga during various stages of inner purification. I have also investigated other taoist methods over the years and have found benefit in the taoist tantric approach, which clarifies the meaning and practical application of brahmacharya (the preservation and cultivation of sexual energy). Beyond a daily tai c
Hi routine and using some of the taoist tantric principles and methods (built into the AYP tantra lessons), I have not pursued the energy management methods you have mentioned very much, so cannot offer additional comparisons with yoga on those. Perhaps others have looked further into those aspects than I have.

Keep in mind that my orientation has been yoga since the beginning 30-some years ago, and I have drawn on other systems, including taoist, to supplement yoga as practical. Maybe your orientation is taoist, and you are looking to supplement it with other systems, like yoga. There is nothing wrong with that. But there will only be so much you can use from other systems, depending on what you regard your core system to be. It is very difficult to equally divide practices between two or more systems, and that I do not recommend. Much better to choose a system having good set of compatible tools and then supplement here and there as necessary. That is what I did with yoga. In my case, a lot of the supplementing came by reaching across the lines dividing the various yoga systems themselves. I call it an integration of advanced yoga practices, as you know. There was a much higher rate of compatibility there. So, if taoism is your core practice, maybe it would be better to be looking across the various lines within taoism first. I know that some taoist lines pay much closer attention to meditation than others. That is what many taoist systems are missing in my opinion. I do not believe that enlightenment can be achieved via chi/prana management alone. It is the same problem we find in kriya yoga, kundalini yoga, and other predominantly prana-based yoga systems. Deep meditation has to be brought in to complete the circuit of polarities. Inner silence and ecstatic (chi) energy must be joined everywhere to complete the process of enlightenment. So we need both sides -- not only one side.

How TAOism became so CHI-oriented is something of a mystery. In chasing the CHI, the TAO itself (undifferentiated pure bliss consciousness) seems to have gotten overlooked. So TAOism has become CHI-ism. From where I sit, the question is not how to do more with CHI. The real question is how to get the TAO (inner silence) back into TAOism. Perhaps this is already covered in the line of taoism you are following. As mentioned, some taoist lines do include meditation. But not many...

Just some food for thought.

I wish you all success on your chosen spiritual path. Enjoy!

The guru is in you.

Postscript -- On the surface, it might appear that navi kriya (just covered in AYP lesson #275) and mulabandha/asvini would address the perineum to dan tien question raised above. I don't believe so, as these practices do not involve the storage and further manipulation of pranic energy at that level in the body. Rather, they are for enlivening and promoting the full integration of ecstatic conductivity body-wide -- cultivating the "whole body mudra." So, while taoist and yoga methods are working in the same areas of the nervous system, the goals and results may be quite different. For more detail on the yoga side of it, see http://www.aypsite.org/275.html

Perhaps those experienced with taoist methods can add more from that perspective.

2005/10/01 00:38:18
Other Systems and Alternate Approaches
http://www.aypsite.org/forum/topic.asp?TOPIC_ID=500&REPLY_ID=798&whichpage=-1
Mixing Taoist and Yoga Practices

Hi Andrew:

There can be little doubt that the original masters of kriya yoga are enlightened beings. Lahiri Mahasaya, the first visible person in the kriya line - late 1800s, said that enlightenment is a "merging of emptiness and euphoria." I have quoted that one in the lessons, because it captures the importance of cultivating both inner silence and ecstatic conductivity in the nervous system as distinct components of the enlightenment process. Metaphorically, these are shiva (silence) and shakti (ecstasy) within us, and each has its own cultivation requirements.

You know, kriya yoga has gone in so many directions since its early days that one has to go through several lines just to find all the original pieces. It has been done as much as possible for AYP. Not only with kriya, but with all the major yoga systems.

It may be that deep meditation played a prominant role in kriya yoga at one time, but evidence of it now is hard to find. My thoughts on combining pranayama and deep meditation are expressed early in the lessons. See http://www.aypsite.org/43.html I don't think it is an effective approach, and have seen evidence of it in those who have gone this way, bringing me to the conclusion a long time ago that it is not possible to do effective pranayama and deep meditation at the same time. Some may disagree.

In fact, in the original system of kriya yoga, a passive form of meditation was specified to be done after spinal breathing. That method is less effective than the pro-active mantra yoga method we use here in AYP. That is why AYP is what it is -- an attempt to improve on what has gone before, or perhaps restore what has been fragmented and eroded would be a better way to put it. If you take the modern forms of kriya yoga, or just about any other tradition, it is a pretty watered down situation these days. Blame it on the foibles of people and the passage of time ... it is no reflection on the great ones.

That is why I think it is so important to collect and integrate all of this precious knowledge and put it in writing as an open source. If we don't, there won't be much left to work with in a few more generations. Hopefully, gifted souls will test the work we are doing now and take it to the next levels of clarity in the decades to come.

The guru is in you.

2005/10/02 17:36:48
Other Systems and Alternate Approaches
http://www.aypsite.org/forum/topic.asp?TOPIC_ID=500&REPLY_ID=807&whichpage=-1
Mixing Taoist and Yoga Practices
Yes, where there is the will, there is a way.

The guru is in you.

2005/12/18 14:31:15
Other Systems and Alternate Approaches
http://www.aypsite.org/forum/topic.asp?TOPIC_ID=500&REPLY_ID=2022&whichpage=-1
Mixing Taoist and Yoga Practices

Hi Chiron:

Here are some Taoist resources from the AYP book list: http://www.aypsite.org/booklist3.html

Some of the clearest writings on Taoist practices are by Mantak Chia. Two more of his books are shown on the sexology list: http://www.aypsite.org/booklist13.html

Useful stuff to know, but you will not find much on deep meditation in any of these books, and that is a major shortcoming.

All the best on your chosen path!

The guru is in you.

2005/12/22 10:41:50
Other Systems and Alternate Approaches
http://www.aypsite.org/forum/topic.asp?TOPIC_ID=500&REPLY_ID=2079&whichpage=-1
Mixing Taoist and Yoga Practices

Hi Sunflower:

Thanks much for chiming in on this one. You have added some nice perspectives.

There can be no doubt that both Yoga and Taoism have wandered somewhat from their roots. That is a combination of market demand and the withering of the message over the centuries of being passed down.

The good news is that the "roots" are in us, and we can rediscover them by testing the means at our disposal and refining our way back to what is true in us. Open communications are the way, so phooey on the esoteric approaches, I say. :-)

As for Taoist versus Yoga methods, there are some significant differences, and thank you, Jim, for reminding us on the breathing techniques especially (spinal breathing versus microcosmic orbit).

Yet, it is not as different as it might seem, at least not in AYP. We do not go up and out the crown. That is regarded as dangerous in the AYP approach, due to risk of premature crown opening (many complications) and other things related to maintaining speed and balance of purification and opening. AYP merges both ascending and descending energies from root to brow (third eye, as we call it) in spinal breathing. Big difference from straight up and out the top. And we start with deep meditation, a separate practice, which is direct merging of our sense of self with inner silence from the very beginning. We keep deep meditation as the central core practice, even as we are adding many other things on. AYP is a dual cultivation of inner silence and what we call "ecstatic conductivity" in the nervous system. Together, these two merge to become the One within and around us. And that is experienced as outpouring divine love. The Tao (stillness) in action!

The cultivation of ecstatic conductivity involves direct application of sexual methods as well, with overlap with Taoist methods in the AYP approach to tantra.

Taoism as you describe it, with the stillness component (the Tao) cultivated, is not so different. Yet the methods are different, in Taoism aiming more for stillness in action (marital) from the beginning, which is something we arrive at in AYP along the way (stillness first, then action). Either way, it is the same nervous system we are dealing with, so the same capabilities will manifest in an order more or less according to the means applied. Assuming optimal application of methods in each system, the end result will be the same. That is why the traditions have so much in common -- all are working with the same human vehicle.

I think it is good for Taoists to have some understanding of Yoga and for Yogis and Yoginis to have some understanding of Taoism. Which is not to say one ought be doing both systems at the same time. Neither can we be driving two cars at the same time. But the more we know about cars in general, the better driver we will be of our own car.

All the best!

The guru is in you.

2005/12/22 19:11:57
Other Systems and Alternate Approaches
http://www.aypsite.org/forum/topic.asp?TOPIC_ID=500&REPLY_ID=2101&whichpage=-1
Mixing Taoist and Yoga Practices
"Why can't i do ayp practices while doing all my other stuff?"

Hi Sunflower:

Well, deep meditation (sitting practice) may be a good addition to your practice. It is the first step in AYP. Beyond that, you may want to be careful not to be overlapping or doing cumulative time in related but different Taoist and Yoga practices. You especially should avoid "doubling up" on breathing practices (doing multiple kinds of pranayama or kumbhaka from different systems in the same session or day), which can lead to excessive energy flows and the unpleasant symptoms that go with that.

I guess we said enough earlier on the challenges of mixing Taoist and Yoga practices. Deep meditation can help a taoist practice. Some of the taoist tantric methods can help yoga. A tai c
Hi routine is very good for grounding wayward energies for yogis and yoginis. Some find the "inner smile" to be a nice addition to yoga. Further mixing becomes increasingly complicated. Beyond the few elements just mentioned it pretty much gets down to choosing one style of practice or the other. Otherwise, you can end up using two systems of practice trying to do the same thing, and overload the nervous system.

I think the key word is "complement." What can we use from other systems to complement what we are already doing? How can we fill in any holes in our practice? We are looking for complementary elements of practice, not necessarily duplicate ones. AYP was built using that sort of logic.

And, lo and behold, we are ending up doing a pretty good job of filling in Patanjali's eight limbs of yoga. And we're not done yet... :-)

The guru is in you.

2005/10/28 23:46:33
Other Systems and Alternate Approaches
http://www.aypsite.org/forum/topic.asp?TOPIC_ID=557&REPLY_ID=1243&whichpage=-1
Vipassana Retreats

Hi Near:

I can't speak for Vipassana, but strongly recommend against doing AYP deep meditation for 11 hours, or even much more than your regular time in a sitting. If you want to take a "retreat" at home with AYP, I suggest the multiple session approach, but not more than three sessions a day starting out. You will be surprised at the additional purification with just one more session in a day. Four sessions in one day is really pouring it on, so take it easy -- self-pacing, you know.

See the following lessons for more detail, or look up "Retreats" in the topic Index:

http://www.aypsite.com/148.html
http://www.aypsite.com/193.html
http://www.aypsite.com/250.html

The guru is in you.

2005/11/01 14:54:00
Other Systems and Alternate Approaches
http://www.aypsite.org/forum/topic.asp?TOPIC_ID=562&REPLY_ID=1315&whichpage=-1
TM

quote:

Originally posted by trip1

While we are on the subject, I purchased Maharishi's book, "The Science of Being and the Art of Living" ... I have been meaning to give it a read (after I complete a few other books) since I noticed that Yogani called this book "a classic" in lesson 253...

Hi Trip:

It is a classic because it is one of the few books written in the 20th century that makes the case for pure bliss consciousness (inner silence or "Being") being the ground state of all existence and the ultimate source of all our progress and happiness. In the West, this was revolutionary at the time (1960s), and paved the way for the entire consciousness movement that went into high gear during that period.

Interestingly, advanced quantum physics has come along and all but verified the ground state consciousness premise in the years since. (Hey, what the bleep do they know? :-))

I think the points of view expressed in this topic about the TM organization are realistic on both sides. It is a great teaching that has suffered due to many missteps in the marketplace.

So the world moves on ... thankfully a much better place because of the hard work and sacrifices of so many.

The guru is in you.

2005/12/10 10:06:15
Other Systems and Alternate Approaches
http://www.aypsite.org/forum/topic.asp?TOPIC_ID=635
Swara Yoga and Helping Patanjali

Hi All:

Here is another one from my email.

Q:
Almost 10 years ago, I picked up a small book called "Breath, Mind and Consciousness" by Harish Johari. It was on an almost forgotten practice called Swara Yoga.

Of late I have have rekindling of interest in this topic and decided to do a search to see if anything came up (10 years back, Breath, Mind and Consciousness was the only book I could find on the subject.) Surprisingly, even today there are perhaps only 2 or 3 books that I could find.

Being presented as a Tantric technique, I was wondering if you had come across it, and if you knew of other resources where more can be learned on the practice?

A:
I believe the late Swami Rama was into swara yoga, among other things, and incorporated it into his writings on practices. Among his best books on practice are *Path of Fire and Light, Vols 1&2*. You can find them on the AYP book list, here: http://www.aypsite.org/booklist1.html

As for swara yoga itself, my understanding of it is that it is a primarily a pranayama system. I do not know if it is a well-rounded path, also covering meditation and other aspects of yoga practice. Of course, as we are finding now, any good path with some missing pieces can be filled in with good results.

Interestingly, I have found in my later years that just about all paths draw from the same practices. Each system usually focuses on a few elements to the exclusion of other elements. Yet, when you review everything that is out there, what emerges is a broad common tool set that all the systems are drawing from.

Where does this tool set come from? It comes from the human nervous system!

By far the best writing on the broad range of elements of practice that we humans have built within us is the Yoga Sutras of Patanjali. He really nailed it. That is why nearly all systems of yoga claim to be doing his "eight limbs." The Yoga Sutras are a document of a few dozen pages that was written some 500 years ago (some say much longer -- ancient Indian texts are not dated). However long people have been reading the Yoga Sutras, it is a pretty amazing document...

The eight limbs are an excellent measuring rod by which all systems of practice can be measured for completeness. This is discussed in AYP lesson #149 http://www.aypsite.org/149.html

The open and integrated approach in AYP is an attempt to get all of the elements of practice down in writing in detail in a logical and usable sequence. What we are finding now is that just about any system that comes forward is much more easily understood when placed up against all these elements of practice we are identifying and utilizing. Gone are the days of mysterious esoteric systems that evoke lots of superstition. At least, I hope those days are gone.

It is time for applied yoga science to prevail. The research you are doing can be to that end also. Please do continue to share in the open "melting pot" of the AYP forums, where we all can continue to integrate the best knowledge available from every possible source. Everyone will benefit accordingly.

Btw, Johari is best known for his excellent books on chakras and yantras. I did not know he had done any books on actual practices. That has always been my main interest -- documented practices. Since I did not find much over the last 30+ years, I decided to write it myself. May many more do the same! Openly published knowledge is what will take us out of the dark ages of spiritual practice and into a much more enlightened era. Patanjali has proven that beyond any doubt. It is time we gave him some help. :-)

The guru is in you.

2005/12/10 19:12:14
Other Systems and Alternate Approaches
http://www.aypsite.org/forum/topic.asp?TOPIC_ID=635&REPLY_ID=1876&whichpage=-1
Swara Yoga and Helping Patanjali

Thanks much, Jim.

You have "nailed it" too. If I have seemed a bit stubborn at times about maintaining the AYP lessons pretty much as thay are, it is because I want to keep that harbor in one place. With that base intact, we can explore the many options you allude to without flinging ourselves to the four winds, so to speak.

It is a thrill to see the AYP lessons being used in this way -- either as a primary teaching, or as a spring board to new understandings. As I have said, I don't see the AYP knowledge as a fixed tradition or the last word in yoga. Rather, it is a baseline, an open source that can be used in many ways as we increase our understanding and the application of means that promote human spiritual transformation.

It's a new approach in yoga. We can always use new ideas. It is important to be looking forward at least as much as we are looking back. :-)

The guru is in you.

2005/12/10 23:28:29
Other Systems and Alternate Approaches
http://www.aypsite.org/forum/topic.asp?TOPIC_ID=635&REPLY_ID=1882&whichpage=-1
Swara Yoga and Helping Patanjali

Hi Melissa:

Sometime in the next year I plan on adding "self-inquiry" to the AYP writings, which is the mind stuff. In yoga parlance it is called "jnana." It has not been covered much so far because it really depends on a stable ground of inner silence to be effective as spiritual practice -- like samyama does, though much more so. Without inner silence, self-inquiry is only intellectualization. Nothing wrong with that for analysis, but it is not a penetrating yoga to the extent we like to focus on around here.

The mind is only good in yoga if it is dancing in stillness, and jnana is for that in later stages. We will know we are ready for jnana when every thought is a wave of bliss. Before then, it can be rather punishing, and none too progressive yogically speaking. That must be where the expression "beating our brains out" comes from. :-)

Better to use deep meditation to soften things up for a few years. Then the mind falls into jnana without even trying. We become it.

It took me a long time to understand what jnana is. At the same time I found out what Ramana Maharis
Hi was talking about. It always comes back to one thing -- inner silence. In That, all can be known.

The guru is in you.

2005/12/11 08:53:30
Other Systems and Alternate Approaches
http://www.aypsite.org/forum/topic.asp?TOPIC_ID=635&REPLY_ID=1887&whichpage=-1
Swara Yoga and Helping Patanjali

Hi Melissa:

The reading is great as you are moved to do it. It is a natural "niyama" -- spiritual study -- springing out of inner silence.

Our reading provides inspiration which, in time, is transformed to realization. Ramana Maharis
Hi certainly qualifies for that.

For a long list of spiritual books, check the AYP book list at: http://www.aypsite.org/booklist.html
Not required reading! :-)

The guru is in you.

2005/12/12 09:51:01
Other Systems and Alternate Approaches
http://www.aypsite.org/forum/topic.asp?TOPIC_ID=635&REPLY_ID=1907&whichpage=-1
Swara Yoga and Helping Patanjali
"please clarify for me the difference between the terms jnana and vedanta"

Hi Anthem & Jim:

The way I look at it is, jnana is a system of yoga practice (self-inquiry is the practice) and vedanta is a philosophy for folks who like to sit around and jawbone about the non-dual nature of reality, while pooh-poohing the value of practices. You can tell I prefer the former over the latter? I'd much rather eat the pudding than analyze it. On the other hand, books on the nature of pudding are okay too -- as long as they are inspiring us to keep up our yoga. :-)

"Where are the AYP lessons on self-inquiry?" you ask.

That is one I am still in the process of simplifying for practical application, and I hope to have a little AYP Enlightenment Series book on it out in 2007, and probably a lesson or two online before then.

Self-inquiry involves developing a skill and habit of questioning our ingrained assumptions about how we perceive and interact in the world, getting behind and systematically dissolving the knee-jerk judgments we constantly make that sustain our separation from the whole and the unhappiness that goes with it. Well, deep meditation gradually does this for us, giving us a base of "self" behind the thinking process, as many here are observing.

When we have "self" (inner silence) it is much easier to do the inquiry. Self-inquiry in an AYP mode will be for taking advantage of that naturally occurring transformation, the rise of inner silence, and building on it. In other words, I don't see self-inquiry as a core practice, and that is why I am in no hurry to trump it up here. More often than not, so-called self-inquiry is a trap for the ego-intellect and can be a major distraction on the path. That is especially so if inner silence is lacking to begin with -- then self-inquiry is nothing but mental masturbation.

When self-inquiry does come out in AYP, you can be sure it will be as simple and practical as possible, and only an add-on to what we are gaining already through existing practices, with inner silence coming up in our lives and doing the very deed we are discussing here -- automatically making us better self-inquirers.

The guru is in you.

2006/01/07 16:14:55
Other Systems and Alternate Approaches
http://www.aypsite.org/forum/topic.asp?TOPIC_ID=701&REPLY_ID=2381&whichpage=-1
kriya yoga board

Hi Snake:

Some prefer a traditional approach. Others are more inclined to a self-directed approach. Both can be viable paths.

AYP is offered as an open resource for the latter. It is not about me. It is about what works for the practitioner. The proof of the pudding for any approach is in the eating.

The only one who is wrong in all of this is the one who thinks their way is the only way. That has nothing to do with the efficacy of either approach. It is something else entirely.

Wishing everyone the best on their chosen path. Practice wisely, and enjoy!

The guru is in you.

2006/01/09 13:58:45
Other Systems and Alternate Approaches
http://www.aypsite.org/forum/topic.asp?TOPIC_ID=701&REPLY_ID=2418&whichpage=-1
kriya yoga board

Hi David & Snake:

Yes, the trick is in knowing what to keep and what to let go. It is not a matter of being "authorized" by someone. It is a matter of "seeing." With the seeing approach, all channels of knowledge become useful resources to build a whole that can be much greater than the sum of the parts. That is the wonder of successful integration, if one can pull it off.

There is something happening in the world today that is working in favor of this kind of approach:

In this time of rising spiritual awareness, the Truth is more easily discerned (seen) by everyone than in years past. With this greater awareness on the rise, the population in general is becoming much more savvy about what works in spiritual practices, and what does not.

So what I have been doing in putting AYP together is only part of the tip of a vast iceberg. We are in the midst of a huge upsurge in public sensitivity to the practical aspects of spiritual practice.

Given the new environment, we can now ask the question:

Does Truth need an external guru, a lineage, or a tradition to be valid?

No. Whether knowledge is coming from an established tradition or from somewhere else, its primary validation will in the practitioner's rising awareness. This has always been so, but the practitioner has been operating with a disadvantage (too many vision-limiting inner obstructions) -- until now.

There is a new dynamic rising (the guru/seer in everyone) that is going to separate the wheat from the chaff in all matters spiritual. The intolerant types may grumble for a while, but this is a new day. A new paradigm is rising up. No one is exempt from the expansion of inner silence and ecstatic conductivity being cultivated by those who are engaged in effective practices around the world.

Something profound is happening in all of us, and it can't be ignored. Seeing is believing, yes?

And, yes, in this wondrous transformation, I am irrelevant! I am a witness to it along with everyone. Ain't it grand? :-)

You are all becoming rishis (seers), and I know you will make the best of it. I believe in you...

The guru is in you.

2006/01/29 10:36:47
Other Systems and Alternate Approaches
http://www.aypsite.org/forum/topic.asp?TOPIC_ID=772&REPLY_ID=2845&whichpage=-1
Tonglen

Hi Yoda:

I have not done this practice with any deliberateness, but do believe in the principle of each of us having the ability to uplift many others according to our inner purification and opening. I see it as a more organic process, whereas, when one is ready, it will happen naturally. Of course, it depends mainly one one's own purification and opening, which brings us back to self-directed practices. We are in the best position to help others when we have developed skill in helping ourselves spiritually. If we have done that, the broader effect around us happens all by itself. Then a technique like you describe may have much greater benefit. Also, the divine flowing through us will find a thousand other ways to uplift everyone. Interestingly, that will manifest according to our own inclinations. When the channel is open, our individuality in everyday life becomes the divine channel.

There is also the principle of service (engaging in dissolving the obstructions in others through giving of one's self) being a path of individual purification -- karma yoga. The degree of effectiveness of karma yoga will be dependent on inner openings achieved so far -- cultivation of inner silence, ecstatic bliss and the resulting outward flow of divine love. At a certain point in the process, service becomes a natural and essential component for the expansion to continue. But service forced at the beginning will not necessarily be the most effective approach. I think the same would apply in utilizing the technique you mention. We all know when it is time for us to serve others, when our heart is ready for that, and the ways will be apparent. Before then, it is mainly an inside job. When we are drawn outward into service, the outside has also become inside (our heart), and it is still an inside job. :-)

The guru is in you.

2006/01/29 12:44:34
Other Systems and Alternate Approaches
http://www.aypsite.org/forum/topic.asp?TOPIC_ID=772&REPLY_ID=2851&whichpage=-1
Tonglen
PS: For something similar, but not geared toward taking in negativity, see the "Heart Breathing" practice in the AYP lessons here: http://www.aypsite.org/220.html

This is different from the tonglen technique you described, in that it brings in divine energy on the in-breath and releases impurities on the out-breath. It is done between the third eye (brow) and the heart space. It is an inverted hybrid of spinal breathing which can be used to purify the heart -- not to be confused with full-scope spinal breathing which goes in the other direction and covers the entire sushumna (spinal nerve) from root to brow, including the heart space. For full-scope spinal breathing, see here: http://www.aypsite.org/41.html

2006/03/05 16:34:55
Other Systems and Alternate Approaches
http://www.aypsite.org/forum/topic.asp?TOPIC_ID=875&REPLY_ID=4136&whichpage=-1
Ajita's Method of Samyama

Hi Ajita:

I have split off your post from here: http://www.aypsite.org/forum/topic.asp?TOPIC_ID=854 to form a new topic on the style of samayama you practice and teach.

Thanks very much for sharing!

The guru is in you.

2006/03/07 10:41:15
Other Systems and Alternate Approaches
http://www.aypsite.org/forum/topic.asp?TOPIC_ID=880&REPLY_ID=4196&whichpage=-1
Ajita's method of Pranayama

Hi Ajita:

I assume you are referring to this booklet you wrote on subtle anatomy: http://www.xs4all.nl/~rajayoga/EN/SubtleAnatomy.pdf

Thank you for sharing your insights on spiritual anatomy. It is a nice exposition on the double helix effect of shiva and shakti energies. It is the DNA helix analog found on more than one level within us, and tying in with super string theory too, yes? We have covered that here in a much simplified way, focusing mainly on the counter-directional swirling of ascending and descending energies around the spinal nerve (ida and pingala around sushumna). It is covered in the AYP lessons too. It only gets a brief mention because it is not part of AYP spinal breathing practice. In AYP we always favor the procedure of the practice over experiences that come up so as not to diverge our attention from causes into the effects, which can defeat the practice and our progress.

That said, I am aware that other systems work outside the spinal nerve (main highway), directly within other energy pathways as practice. Is that the case in your system? If so, I am sure many here will be interested in how you address it in way that is both simple and globally effective. Those are the watchwords here: simplicity and effectiveness. I think the future of yoga for the masses lies in that kind of approach -- finding the primary levers that anyone can use for easily promoting and managing the complex process of human spiritual transformaiton.

It is like what the graphical user interface (GUI) and "point and click" did for the masses in computing. A person no longer needs to be writing complex computer code to reach high levels of productivity on a computer, like all of we non-programmers are doing here right now.

When yoga goes this route, and everyone can master the complex process of human spiritual transformation with an open system of simple practices that can be easily managed (self-paced), then we will truly enter the age of spiritual practices, just like we entered the information age over the past few decades when the controls were simplified and disseminated to everyone. Every age has had this essential characteristic in common -- the ability to utilize complex processes in nature via refinements to the simplest, most effective and universally available methods of application. When it is made simple enough so everyone can do it, the "next age" begins in earnest.

Well, I will get off my soapbox now. :-) Please do share what you can on pranayama practice, keeping in mind that we are a bunch of numbskulls here (especially me), always seeking the holiest of grails -- the simplest and most effective application of the principles of human spiritual transformation.

Many thanks for joining in the discussion!

The guru is in you.

2006/03/10 09:08:06
Other Systems and Alternate Approaches
http://www.aypsite.org/forum/topic.asp?TOPIC_ID=880&REPLY_ID=4333&whichpage=-1
Ajita's method of Pranayama

Hi Ajita:

You are describing natural processes in a very clear way. But what is the practice? That is where the simplicity and effectiveness matter the most.

The guru is in you.

2006/03/13 10:53:40
Other Systems and Alternate Approaches
http://www.aypsite.org/forum/topic.asp?TOPIC_ID=880&REPLY_ID=4436&whichpage=-1
Ajita's method of Pranayama

Hi Ajita:

David is right. On the other hand, no one expects you to change your mode of teaching overnight, which is geared to personal face-to-face instruction, like most teachings traditionally have been. That being the case, the most we can reasonably ask for is an outline of your system, which you have generously given some of, and it is much appreciated. The more you are comfortable sharing on yoga across the board, the better for everyone.

What we are doing here in AYP is a new approach -- a grand experiment, you might say, seeing how much can be conveyed in writing. It is not for everyone. At the same time, the ability of many to pick up and go with detailed written instructions alone has been gratifying.

The biggest revelation has been the high level of responsibility in self-pacing that nearly all practitioners have displayed with wide-open availability of advanced practices leading to many new experiences. This puts to rest once and for all the perennial argument that seekers cannot be trusted with practices without a lot of personal handholding by a guru. It just is not true, not in this time and place. The message of AYP is that most aspirants with a mind to, who have good information, can regulate their own practices.

That is a useful data point for teachers everywhere. If the practices are simple enough, effective enough and well-documented, much more can be conveyed much faster and we can get on with it, instead of staying mired in the inertia of the past.

No matter what the mode of instruction may be, I encourage all teachers to take note of the fact that much more can be done to provide access for the millions who are thirsting for knowledge of practices. It is simply a matter of giving the knowledge in a usable form to all who want it, and bypassing the artificial barriers and hierarchies that limit access. Open systems of practice are the wave of the future. This is how the world will be changed, and it is time.

This change will not put yoga teachers out of business. It will vastly increase the number of students, because direct assistance, follow-up and satsang on practices and the resulting experiences are always going to be necessary. This fledgling forum is an online example. It is only a matter of time before the discussion on self-directed practices overflows into the physical world in a big way.

The guru is in you.

2006/10/31 15:01:22
Other Systems and Alternate Approaches
http://www.aypsite.org/forum/topic.asp?TOPIC_ID=880&REPLY_ID=12773&whichpage=-1
Ajita's method of Pranayama

quote:
_____
Originally posted by Doc

...the mere striving for Union with God through earnest Sadhana allows each of us to be led according to our individual capabilities, by the Grace of God, until we reach Samadhi, regardless of our faults or shortcomings, regardless of our talent or intelligence, regardless of the methods we practice, since all things are possible for God! See you at the top! Hari Om! Doc
_____

Hi Doc:

Agreed 100%. If we are dedicated enough, we can build a house with any set of tools. The principles of human spiritual transformation are fairly generous. At the same time, without enough of them being effectively applied in concert, making progress can be a long grind. Even so, bhakti alone will eventually get us there -- like the little train engine that could, you know: "I think I can ... I think I can ... I think I can..."

Bhakti (devotion to our ideal, put into action) is the fuel for all spiritual progress. Beyond that, it boils down to methods, and the more of those we have access to the better, as far as I'm concerned. Not that we can practice everything without a logical plan -- that won't work. Basic understandings of the efficient integration of the various classes of practice (eight limbs, right?) and self-pacing are necessary. Even without these understandings, the intensely determined aspirant will not fail -- such is the power of bhakti. In the latter case, there may be a considerable frying along the way, but the heart-on-fire bhakti yogi/yogini will not care much (a la the Secrets of Wilder).

Nevertheless, the rest of us will prefer a more stable and bearable journey, while at the same time not getting bogged down in excessive "safety measures" along the way. So, the trick is to be hot with bhakti, use the best tools we can find, and learn to practice within our comfortable limits over the long term. With that, anyone can do this. And finding ways that can make it possible for anyone to do it is a worthy goal, I think.

AYP is not intended to be a final or complete answer in all of this. Just an open source "best shot" at making it as easy, effective and safe as possible. I'm sure improvements and variations will abound in the future, as they have up until now. Let's hope so. The last thing we need is another static system of practices. That is why we keep the discussion as open and flexible as possible. Everyone has a valuable point of view. There is much to be learned from all of the dedicated practitioners, teachers and traditions on the planet. So much good work has been done. It is a joint effort.

Yet, in the end, we each must choose what works best for us. Around here, loyalty to a system will go only as far as its effectiveness. That is how it should be in a scientific approach -- the door is always open for improvement.

Here's to progress, by whatever means we can muster and hammer out for best results. It is by reviewing causes and effects and making the necessary adjustments along the way that we can optimize our momentum.

Thank you again for sharing, Ajita ... I hope we have not scared you off. :-)

The guru is in you.

2006/11/01 17:18:10
Other Systems and Alternate Approaches
http://www.aypsite.org/forum/topic.asp?TOPIC_ID=880&REPLY_ID=12801&whichpage=-1
Ajita's method of Pranayama
It's okay, Alan.

One of the best educations in life can be found at "Foot-in-Mouth University." We are all in that school, you know. :-)

In relation to that, inner silence and the yama/niyama it naturally brings up will not let us off the hook. You have clearly demonstrated your sensitivity in that ... an inspiring lesson for us all.

The guru is in you.

2006/11/02 12:01:51
Other Systems and Alternate Approaches
http://www.aypsite.org/forum/topic.asp?TOPIC_ID=880&REPLY_ID=12834&whichpage=-1
Ajita's method of Pranayama

quote:
_____
Originally posted by david_obsidian

bewell said:
I tried the method of "imagining your sense of taste extending 15 cm above your head" (I had not heard of it before) and immediately, for the second time in my life, I tasted a sweetness like honey.

It seems to me that there is something to this practice. It definitely produces a positive subtle yogic effect when I try it, and the effect may have something in common with Kechari mudra. At the same time though, in and of itself, I doubt it would have been anywhere nearly as powerful for me as my kechari practice is. Another twist on the whole thing is that, whereas I definitely feel the subtle effect from doing that now, I'm not so sure I'd have felt it nearly as well without the kechari background. Every advance in Yoga breaks ground for further advances.

From his writings, I'm inclined to suspect that Ajita is experiencing genuine and profound yogic effects; that is, he is a genuine 'strong yogi'. However, from the perspective of these experiences (and with the background given by tradition), he may be inclined to believe that he can easily transmit these strong subtle practices. But this is not at all easily acheived. The possession of yogic abilities, unfortunately (sadly perhaps), doesn't necessarily make the teaching of them easy, or make the 'advanced' people extremely effective at teaching. That's the reality of it, I believe, and the reality goes counter to the mythology of the 'realized siddha', which can give us unreasonable expectations.

Fair play to anyone for trying though!!
_____

Hi David:

Yes, perhaps it is the "forgetful mountain climber" syndrome -- lesson 84.

There is this guy yelling from the top of the mountain, "Just be here now!" But few may know exactly how he got there, including him! The prerequisites for benefiting fully from the lesson may be missing.

That is why clear trail-blazing all the way from the bottom of the mountain to the very top is essential. The more we know about climbing the mountain from bottom to top, the more we can gain at all levels, including from those who are on top, even if they may not recall how they got there (or how we can get there).

This may be a case in point...

The guru is in you.

2006/03/22 22:20:00
Other Systems and Alternate Approaches
http://www.aypsite.org/forum/topic.asp?TOPIC_ID=909&REPLY_ID=4914&whichpage=-1
Jesus and The Buddha: Closer Then We Think

quote:
_____
Jim Wrote: (in fact, I tend to visualize him more as trimming shrubs)
_____

Actually, been moving a lot of furniture lately. Someone else's, of course. :-)
2006/03/22 23:50:10
Other Systems and Alternate Approaches
http://www.aypsite.org/forum/topic.asp?TOPIC_ID=909&REPLY_ID=4918&whichpage=-1
Jesus and The Buddha: Closer Then We Think

quote:

Jim wrote: My point was that the same flow that brought me to AYP brought Yogani to write it.

_____

That's how I see it too. It would be a blessing if everyone did. The force is with us. :-)

2006/03/23 17:51:22
Other Systems and Alternate Approaches
http://www.aypsite.org/forum/topic.asp?TOPIC_ID=909&REPLY_ID=4988&whichpage=-1
Jesus and The Buddha: Closer Then We Think

Hi Shanti:

In my case, the difficulty is not in your very sweet and much appreciated ways of saying thank you. It is my own ignorance and lack of experience on how to be thanked in this kind of thing. There are certain ways that one is supposed to behave in such situations, which I have limited experience in. However, wherever I see it going on, it seems to be out of control and/or abused in some way, so I have decided to avoid it as much as possible. It is like fame, which I also hope to avoid. So much misery there. Life is so simple here, relatively speaking, and I hope to preserve it. It is very selfish, I know. But that is how I can do the work best, so it is practical too.

Be assured that your thank you's are much appreciated here, and that Yogani continues to muddle through in his own peculiar way. :-)

The guru is in you.

2006/03/23 19:52:30
Other Systems and Alternate Approaches
http://www.aypsite.org/forum/topic.asp?TOPIC_ID=909&REPLY_ID=4996&whichpage=-1
Jesus and The Buddha: Closer Then We Think

Hi Shanti:

Yes, your joy is my joy. That is the payoff. The same with everyone else who finds something good in AYP. The greatest joy is in seeing people becoming self-sufficient on their path and making steady progress. That is real.

That is why I say "thank you" instead of "you are welcome." :-)

The guru is in you.

2007/05/02 14:54:09
Other Systems and Alternate Approaches
http://www.aypsite.org/forum/topic.asp?TOPIC_ID=1074&REPLY_ID=21310&whichpage=-1
Kriya Yoga vs. AYP

Hi Christi and Blackmuladar:

Chin pump (dynamic jalandhara) is similar to thokar, navi kriya is covered in AYP lesson 275, and we use deep meditation after spinal breathing pranayama (similar to "kriya proper") instead of omkar. Omkar is OM nada (listening for OM). In AYP we do not use that due to it's on-again off-again nature. OM does occur in AYP practitioners, as many have experienced. We regard it to be primarily effect from our practices rather than cause, and favor our practices instead. Then we get more ecstatic OM as effect!

OM is the vibration of ecstatic conductivity and radiance rising in our nervous system, giving way over time to merging with inner silence, and becoming outpouring divine love -- stillness in action.

AYP is not kriya yoga, but does use some similar methods, plus other techniques in ways not occurring in kriya yoga which produce more effects in less time, with prudent self-pacing of course.

No long sittings in AYP -- lots more time to go out into daily life and play in our inner silence and ecstatic bliss. :-)

The guru is in you.

2006/06/09 11:40:44
Other Systems and Alternate Approaches
http://www.aypsite.org/forum/topic.asp?TOPIC_ID=1204&REPLY_ID=7884&whichpage=-1
lineage

Hi All:

For the record, I never heard of "Siddhar Tantira Yoga" before Nand
Hi visited AYP a couple of years ago. We were both amazed at the similarity of our knowledge, even though our backgrounds are entirely different.

Which goes to show that the truth of spiritual transformation is the same everywhere, and always derived from the same source -- the human nervous system. So, if you are looking for true lineage, look within! AYP and other systems can provide some useful tools to help with that. The rest is up to you...

Btw, David is correct -- my background is multi-source, which resulted in the integration of practices that became AYP. So AYP is a derivation based on causes and effects (applied yoga science), not a single-source hand-me-down. Those seeking an evolution of knowledge may find that reassuring, while those seeking a traditional approach may be a little nervous. In fact, AYP can be viewed as both -- a common-sense modern integration of traditional elements of practice with their roots in antiquity.

It is what it is, and here we are. Onward and upward! :-)

The guru is in you.

2007/07/05 09:14:46
Other Systems and Alternate Approaches
http://www.aypsite.org/forum/topic.asp?TOPIC_ID=1208&REPLY_ID=23822&whichpage=-1
sun gazing

quote:
_____
Originally posted by Christi

As I remember, Yogani has devoted one of the main lessons in AYP to this very subject, so it could merit some serious attention.
_____

Hi Christi and All:

Yes, here it is: http://www.aypsite.org/167.html

Nothing more to add, except to say that the AYP forums are primarily for support in practices, not for discrediting teachers or practitioners of any persuasion. That belongs in the anti-cult and anti-charlatan forums, which are plentiful elsewhere on the internet. A preoccupation with it here can become a distraction from the main mission of the forums.

Let's take what is useful for our spiritual practice, wherever we may find it, and move on into the light of ecstatic bliss and outpouring divine love. :-)

All the best!

The guru is in you.

2007/07/06 09:48:48
Other Systems and Alternate Approaches
http://www.aypsite.org/forum/topic.asp?TOPIC_ID=1208&REPLY_ID=23915&whichpage=-1
sun gazing
From the dedication page of the Samyama book:

"Life is a Miracle!"

:-)
2006/07/31 14:42:58
Other Systems and Alternate Approaches
http://www.aypsite.org/forum/topic.asp?TOPIC_ID=1375&REPLY_ID=10091&whichpage=-1
Kashmiri Shaivism & Yoga

quote:
_____
Kris said: I'm interested if the highest view in yoga equates to that held in Kashmiri Shaivism.
_____

Hi Kris, and welcome aboard!

Yes, I think so. Both are aiming for the same result ... human spiritual transformation.

I can't say much about Kashmir Shaivism practiced as a religion, but one of their main scriptures, the 4000 year old Vigyan Bhairava (also by other spellings), is up there with the Bhagavad Gita, Yoga Sutras of Patanjali and the Hatha Yoga Pradipika as a valuable ancient recording of practical spiritual knowledge, and much older too. It covers the basic principles of meditation, samyama, spinal breathing pranayama, tantric sexual technique, and other methods.

We touch on the Vigyan Bhairava in a few places in AYP:

http://www.aypsite.org/136.html
http://www.aypsite.org/T21.html

It is also the source for the dedication page quote for the AYP Tantra book that came out in June.

Wishing you the best on your chosen path. Enjoy!

The guru is in you.

2006/11/29 18:54:15
Other Systems and Alternate Approaches
http://www.aypsite.org/forum/topic.asp?TOPIC_ID=1389&REPLY_ID=13884&whichpage=-1
Samyama with planets & stellar formations

Hi Naz, and a belated welcome!

While I am not an astrologer either, I welcome your research here.

Of course, the best way to get at the truth is to find it in ourselves. It is also pretty important to find others who can confirm what we are experiencing to whatever degree is possible and to help advance the research by uncovering new angles, and, most importantly, to help us get beyond our own illusions about what we are doing. Then everyone grows. It seems to be what you are looking for. That is what we are up to here.

Though AYP has come originally from a refinement and integration of ancient practices from the traditions of bhakti, mantra, kriya, hatha, kundalini, tantra and other systems of yoga, there is certainly room for any other resources that can help enhance our progress, and planetary spiritual transformation while we are at it. To my way of thinking, that means knowledge and practices that can be used in practical ways by everyone with less and less hand-holding needed over time. Stars and planets or not, it will take a lot of people getting involved in effective, easy-to-use self-directed practices to make it happen. Perhaps it is written in the stars, because it seems to be happening. :-)

By your own admission, you are one of the only ones on the planet doing this kind of work. So the burden is really on you to convince the rest of us that you know what you are talking about, and that something practical can come from it. You have started doing so by offering some exercises, and a few have nibbled. That's good!

But I have to tell you that referring to experts in related fields as kindergartners in your field is not going to win you much serious attention -- not here, or anywhere. That would be the case even if we didn't know what we are doing here, which is a debatable point. Others might see you in exactly the same way from their own limited perspective. What good is that?

Spiritual communications begin with honoring people where they are right now, no matter where that is. Can we really know where they are? We are all divine beings wearing disguises, yes? That kind of recognition is one of the best measures of real spiritual progress. Not whether or not we have gone beyond whatever cosmic thingy we think we have gone beyond. It is happening right here, right now and that is all there is. How we do it here and now together is all that matters. The rest is all BS. See?

Okay, end of lecture. :-)

If you haven't been miffed and gone off in a huff (caution, this is a test!), I for one would like to hear more about your work. But remember, we are a bunch of dummies here (angels in disguise), and you have to make it so easy that even a kindergartner can get it. Otherwise, who cares? Would you buy a computer that could only be operated by typing in all the code line by line on a black screen? If so, you have come to the wrong place. We all use graphical user interfaces here (I think), and many of us also go for the very powerful and easy-to-use yoga practitioner interfaces. It really does work, and we are making progress day by day. If you have some more of that, bring it on!

The guru is in you.

PS -- It should also be mentioned that in a month or so a new book on samyama is coming out, which will significantly expand on the applications of samyama in AYP. Interestingly, we will be going more cosmic, so your research may be timely, and perhaps even much needed and appreciated as we continue to move forward.

2006/12/05 10:49:37
Other Systems and Alternate Approaches
http://www.aypsite.org/forum/topic.asp?TOPIC_ID=1389&REPLY_ID=14104&whichpage=-1
Samyama with planets & stellar formations

Hi All:

Just a reminder to everyone that personal conflicts are off limits in the AYP forums, and are best taken elsewhere.

On another subject -- this topic :-)

Naz, you have not described the technique of samyama you are using. From the kinds of results you are decribing, it does not sound like the same technique we are using in AYP. The samyama method we use here does not produce negative effects such as sutras conflicting with each other, negative energies, etc. It is not possible, because pure bliss consciousness does not contain these qualities. A sutra, or combination of sutras, no matter how negative externally, or poorly arranged, will not produce a negative result when effectively dissolved in samad
Hi (pure bliss conscousness -- inner silence). There is always the possibility of excess purification going on in the nervous system, but that is simply too much of a good thing happening, and it can be regulated with prudent self-pacing, which is a staple in AYP.

So, the samyama technique itself is of far greater importance than the sutras we choose. Here we choose them for broad-based purification in the nervous system, and it is important to stick with a given set of sutras over time in daily practice, so they can go deep and do their work in stillness. If we keep pulling up and replacing a tree we have planted, it will not be easy to grow a tree. This does not mean we don't make adjustments in sutras once in a while, but we make them sparingly. It is the same with the AYP mantra and its several enhancements. We keep digging the well in one place to create the best opportunity for striking an abundance of water. And we do!

In AYP we are currently using "qualitative" sutras, laying the groundwork for "quantitative" sutras, which we will be adding in the new Samyama book. By "quantitative," I mean "dimensional" in terms of inner space and outer space, which are two aspects of our cosmic nature. In yoga, we are gradually cultivating and joining these in our conscious daily experience. It has far-reaching implications in the quality of our life.

The results you describe, Naz, sound like the effects of projecting consciousness through the sutras external to samadhi/absorption, and producing the various colors of those sutras without sufficient internal qualities of pure bliss consciousness -- so any kind of light or shadow can come out of it and create the kind of conflicts and negative effects you describe. I am sure it all makes sense astrologically with those kinds of projections happening. But that isn't samyama the way we think about it and do it here. Not knowing the specifics of your technique, it is hard to say more.

In AYP style samyama where the sutra is dissolved in inner silence, there is no color or shadow produced. In fact, if there is limited inner silence, little to nothing will be produced. To the extent there is abiding inner silence present in our nervous system (a function of our foundation in deep meditation practice), there will not be a coloring dominated by the sutra, rather a flavoring of pure bliss consciousness itself, which cannot be negative or conflicted by its own nature. For this same reason, we say that samyama of the AYP variety is "morally self-regulating" -- meaning, doing this samyama for the wrong reasons will not work. When there is inner silence present, and the technique is done correctly, easily and naturally, the results are always going to be positive and very powerful. And if inner silence isn't there, nothing much will happen.

From the classical point of view of Patanjali's yoga sutras, samyama encompasses the last three limbs of yoga -- dharana (attention touching the object/sutra), dhyana (the object/sutra released and dissolved), and samad
Hi (absorbed in pure bliss conscousness). All three qualities are necessary for samyama to be occurring. Samyama is not the projection of anything. It is a letting go into stillness. Everything finds its home in stillness and comes out naturally illuminated with divine purpose -- the entire cosmos! That obviously goes for all of our sutras, whether they be qualitative or quantitative/dimensional. No harm can come to us or anyone from any sutra that is used with the correct technique of samyama. Only by deliberately using a sutra _externally_ can harm be produced, and we do not do that here -- that is not samyama.

So, if you are having conflicts and negativity coming from sutras, I'd say it is more likely a red flag on technique than on sutra selection.

For more info on AYP deep meditation and samyama technique, see:
http://www.aypsite.org/13.html
and
http://www.aypsite.org/149.html
...and the subsequent lessons for each.
Or review the appropriate AYP books.

All the best!

The guru is in you.

2006/12/05 16:36:23
Other Systems and Alternate Approaches
http://www.aypsite.org/forum/topic.asp?TOPIC_ID=1389&REPLY_ID=14124&whichpage=-1
Samyama with planets & stellar formations

Hi Naz:

You are free to speak your mind, within limits. We do not permit the bashing of any tradition, guru, or teacher ... or each other, as has already been said. It is counter-productive to our purpose here, which is the ongoing positive integration and refinement of the best methods available, regardless of source. We will do our best not to bash you, but if you want to be welcome, you must return the favor. It is up to you, and the moderators.

They will be tightening the reigns on your posting from here forward.

The guru is in you.

2006/12/12 19:09:44
Other Systems and Alternate Approaches
http://www.aypsite.org/forum/topic.asp?TOPIC_ID=1389&REPLY_ID=14452&whichpage=-1
Samyama with planets & stellar formations

Hi All:

While karma is going to be flowing no matter what, our nervous system will always be the primary vehicle for the expression of karma, and that expression can be greatly altered by our spiritual practices and the resulting rise in our divine inner condition.

For example, if the stars have had us on course to be run over by an armored truck at a certain point in our life, then perhaps after a few years of deep meditation and other yoga practices, the truck would miss us, the back door would fly open, and all the money would fall out at our feet. Well, not a very good example, but you get the idea. :-)

Karma and astrological influences will express in our life according to our spiritual condition, not according to any by-rote formula. One person's bane will be another's boon, even when the influences are exactly the same. We cannot change it significantly by changing our outer circumstances -- our incarnation, natal chart, or whatever. Wherever we end up, we will only pick up where we left off with our spiritual evolution.

However, we can vastly improve the outcome of all influences in our life by changing our inner spiritual condition, which can be addressed with effective yoga practices right here, right now. No need to be throwing the dice when we have a sure thing in hand. The nervous system we are sitting in right now is the doorway to the infinite!

The guru is in you.

2006/09/23 10:13:12
Other Systems and Alternate Approaches
http://www.aypsite.org/forum/topic.asp?TOPIC_ID=1509&REPLY_ID=11493&whichpage=-1
Interview of B K S Iyengar

Hi All:

The new AYP book, "Asanas, Mudras and Bandhas - Awakening Ecstatic Kundalini," attempts to address these issues in full, while honoring all sides which have brought such wonderful contributions. It is not a matter of right or wrong. Only a matter of everyone having the opportunity to find balance across all the limbs of yoga. The necessary adjustments are not as radical as it might seem. But the results are. :-)

The guru is in you.

2006/09/27 11:53:08
Other Systems and Alternate Approaches

http://www.aypsite.org/forum/topic.asp?TOPIC_ID=1509&REPLY_ID=11625&whichpage=-1
Interview of B K S Iyengar

quote:
_____

Victor wrote: I feel that Mr Iyengar seems to be very misunderstood. He absolutely DOES practice meditation in his own practice. It is my impression that he feels that meditation falls under the heading of religion and while he is a bramhin by birth and has always practiced the religious rituals of his tradition he does not teach meditation in his school.

Shanti wrote: In India, we always associate Yoga with asanas. Pranayam falls under yoga too.. but again as a part of asanas. However, meditation, japa, finding God.. its all about religion over there.

_____

Hi All:

To be honest, I have always wondered why meditation is so conspicuously absent from yoga studios in the west, and it is one of the reasons why AYP was started. What Victor and Shanti have said above offers a real reason why things are the way they are, and points to a path for resolving the issue.

Mystic, admittedly, the teachers you have mentioned highlight the value of meditation. Some even teach varieties of it. But none has penetrated the way hatha yoga has in the west. So the real issue is how to integrate all the limbs of yoga into the vast field of hatha schools, so everyone can have the opportunity to find the full benefits. If this will be a help to India, so much the better, for she is certainly the mother of all this knowledge, and no one here is lost on that point. No matter where we hail from, we owe her a lot...

To find a way forward, some shakeup is always necessary. As soon as we are resting on our laurels, red flags should be going up. We can honor the traditions that have given us so much, but hopefully not at the expense of our progress. Too much is at stake. We must do what is necessary to bring the knowledge of human spiritual transformation to everyone.

I am much more interested in pressing for the advance of applied spiritual science than in preserving the status quo, though we cannot move forward without doing some of both. I view the traditions not so much as an absolute, but as a sling-shot that can be used to propel us into a future where rapid spiritual progress for the people will be the norm rather than the exception. Of course, refinement and integration of practices for effective self-directed use are necessary to accomplish this, which is a shakeup.

So I think this is a valuable discussion, disagreements and all. :-)

The guru is in you.

2006/09/27 13:52:06
Other Systems and Alternate Approaches
http://www.aypsite.org/forum/topic.asp?TOPIC_ID=1509&REPLY_ID=11630&whichpage=-1
Interview of B K S Iyengar

quote:
_____

Originally posted by riptiz

Hi Yogani,
I think it's down to peoples perception of yoga. Earlier this year 3 ladies came to my meditation class after hearing there was a yoga class. They came with towels and mats and as soon as I saw them I realised they were going to be disappointed.When I politely informed them we were a meditation class they simply left saying they were hoping for a 'good workout.' Shame they didn't realise their brains would have had a 'good workout.'
L&L
Dave

_____

Hi Dave:

It is "market-driven," and physical practice is the predominant perception of yoga today, as you say.

On the other hand, what would the perception be if all the limbs of yoga were offered under one roof? What would the market be asking for then? We will not find out until all the limbs are offered in an effective usable form, and the perception in the marketplace is gradually expanded to cover all of what yoga is.

It is as much about what is being offered as it is about what the market expectation is. Market expectations will change as the offering is expanded. This is what will happen over time.

Maybe you should add asanas. :-)

The guru is in you.

2006/11/28 11:30:13
Other Systems and Alternate Approaches
http://www.aypsite.org/forum/topic.asp?TOPIC_ID=1514&REPLY_ID=13832&whichpage=-1
Anyone done TM and now AYP?

quote:
_____

I can't seem to get on with mantras in general, even "I AM" keeps me on the level of thinking(aboutthis forum..Yogani..am i doing this right..etc..). To me meditation is going beyond thought, which i can mostly do by just leting go of all thoughts and staying in that space.Not sure if i am progressing spiritually, but it does seem to re-energise me a bit.

Hi Katrina, and welcome!

As you no doubt know, thoughts (regardless of content) in deep meditation are part of the process, and easily favoring the mantra will take us beyond thinking again and again like clockwork. If we come right back into thoughts, that is purification happening, and we easily come back to the mantra again. This is a proactive process of going beyond thinking that gradually leads to permanent inner silence, something that takes much longer to cultivate by passive (non-mantra/mindfulness) meditative means. In fact, mindfulness techniques typically involve much longer sessions. It can be done either way. It is a matter of how much we'd like to accomplish with the time we have available, and also how much time and attention we'd like to have available to move on to additional techniques that can further enhance our rate of progress.

Here in AYP, it is all about effectiveness and efficiency. Of course, our preferences and natural style have to be honored as well. We each have our own road to travel, and we pick our own roadmaps. :-)

All the best!

The guru is in you.

2006/11/29 10:35:15
Other Systems and Alternate Approaches
http://www.aypsite.org/forum/topic.asp?TOPIC_ID=1514&REPLY_ID=13876&whichpage=-1
Anyone done TM and now AYP?

Hi Christi:

Good advice from all, and thank you for finding that old post of mine. It saves me some writing. :-)

I would only reemphasize that picking up the mantra on whatever level we find ourselves is the key to avoiding that disjointed feeling of being settled (in silence) and yanking ourselves out into a clear mental pronuciation of the mantra. As we advance, picking up the mantra becomes more and more virtually in silence itself -- very faint and fuzzy. This phenomenon of being both in and out of inner silence at the same time is also at the heart of samyama practice.

This does not mean trying to begin the mantra as faint and fuzzy when we are on the surface level of our thoughts, or as a beginning practitioner. We pick it up where we are. Over time of daily practice (months and years), the mind and nervous system become more infused with silence all the time -- a natural vehicle for it. As this happens, we find our starting point in deep meditation (and life in general) to be much more in silence. That is the fruit of deep meditation, and it leads to many other benefits in both practices and experiences. I still have not gotten them all written down!

But AYP deep meditation practice itself is pretty solidly documented now. For more perspective and clarity on the practice, try the little Deep Meditation book.

The guru is in you.

2009/05/21 13:48:19
Other Systems and Alternate Approaches
http://www.aypsite.org/forum/topic.asp?TOPIC_ID=1514&REPLY_ID=51241&whichpage=-1
Anyone done TM and now AYP?

quote:

I practiced TM for many years before turning to ayp and i have to say that i do not find the ayp mantra to be as effective. Maybe it's just a personal thing but my TM mantra seems to bring better experiences and inner tranquility into my life so even though i found ayp to be very nice and sincere i am personally refering back to the path i was on before. Why i found the need to change in the first place i will never know but it taught me a lesson i will never forget.... god bless and good luck!

Hi UniversalMind:

If the TM program resonates for you, then go with it. See this lesson from way back in 2003: http://www.aypsite.org/19.html

The advice is still the same today. However, we have come a long way with AYP since then, and it may be good to keep an open mind about some things. It does not have to be all one system or another. There are no absolutes in this world.

For instance, while the TM program is very good for some of the key limbs of yoga, it is lacking in some others. So it may make sense to pick up some of the other pieces of yoga, if so inclined. I am talking about spinal breathing pranayama in particular, which adds a big boost to spiritual progress when added in front of meditation, as Kirtanman has pointed out. Other tools that may be short in the TM program are mudras and bandhas, tantric sexual methods, shatkarmas, ecstatic kundalini considerations, self-inquiry, self-pacing, and so on.

You may not feel you need any of this, and that is fine. Nevertheless, it is all there in a reasonably flexible and integrated form, and that is something we did not have back in the 20th century.

I say "back in the 20th century" because all knowledge that is not evolving will be specific to the time in which it became fixed. This applies to spiritual knowledge as much as any other knowledge, though historically it has not been seen that way, due to the secretive (esoteric) nature of spiritual knowledge (techniques especially) over the centuries. So the knowledge was actually deteriorating over time, and then being "revived" by someone from time to time, only to slowly fade away again. Fixed and fading, fixed and fading. Like that. It has been the pattern of spiritual knowledge over the centuries.

Transcendental Meditation and Kriya Yoga are both revivals that occurred in the 20th century of much older knowledge that had faded over time. So they are 20th century knowledge. We could even say that Kriya Yoga is 19th century knowledge, because what Yogananda popularized in the 20th century was a modified version of the revival brought by Lahiri Mahasaya in the 19th century.

In any case, as soon as these became "fixed," they became dated.

Now we are in the 21st century, and new integrations of methods and understandings of the process of human spiritual transformation are occurring. Spiritual knowledge is evolving.

One of the challenges we face today is to put approaches in place so the knowledge will keep evolving indefinitely. If we don't, it could become fixed knowledge, and then start to fade. I am speaking of AYP, which I hope will be ever-renewed and updated as practitioners are able to bring new perspectives from direct experience.

This open and evolutionary approach to utilizing spiritual knowledge seems to be happening in many quarters across the spectrum these days. It is fueled by the combination of the information age with many more people reaching advanced stages of spiritual awakening and feeding back into it, so many others can leverage from there. I'd like to think it is an exponential growth that is occurring. If so, we may be able to move beyond the fixed and fading repetitive scenario at last. It is no longer about nailing the knowledge down into a fixed philosophy or set of tools. It is about doing whatever is necessary on an ongoing basis to facilitate the emergence of human enlightenment on a global scale.

All of which is to say, if it works for you, use it. And if it doesn't work for you, find something that will. Likewise, if it works, but can work better, then do what is necessary to improve it. This is the formula for constant progress.

That applies to all systems of spiritual knowledge, including AYP. That is how applied science is supposed to work. Nothing is carved in stone like it used to be -- literally. :-)

The guru is in you.

2006/10/30 14:31:22
Other Systems and Alternate Approaches
http://www.aypsite.org/forum/topic.asp?TOPIC_ID=1520&REPLY_ID=12732&whichpage=-1
The Jesus Prayer...
Topic moved for better placement.

Sorry this is being done so late in the discussion. This is a very informative topic on the Christian meditation tradition. Please keep going. Thank you.

The guru is in you.

PS -- Welcome aboard Doc!

2007/08/30 11:59:36
Other Systems and Alternate Approaches
http://www.aypsite.org/forum/topic.asp?TOPIC_ID=1530&REPLY_ID=25149&whichpage=-1
an experience worth reading

Hi SuperTrouper, and welcome to the forums!

Simplification and minimizing the daily duration of practices to be manageable while maximizing the results is definitely the way to go in this busy modern world. I think you will find many here who resonate with that. It is, in fact, a primary objective in the AYP approach -- optimizing "cause and effect" in our practice routine, so everyone has the opportunity to enhance their spiritual progress through self-directed practice.

A key goal is for results-based "applied spiritual science" to become an ongoing and evolving discipline. This is how humanity has progressed dramatically in virtually every other field of knowledge. Now it is time for it to happen in the spiritual arena, where the walls dividing rigid sectarian approaches are dissolving and the best from all quarters is coming together.

In the AYP approach, our regular daily activity in the world is part of the process, naturally stabilizing and expanding the inner silence and ecstatic conductivity we are cultivating in practices. We practice to bring about permanent improvements in our daily life. From this point of view, yoga is not something we do instead of living in the world. It is something we do to enhance living in the world, where all of ordinary life gradually becomes infused with abiding inner silence, ecstatic bliss, and outpouring divine love. It is do-able! :-)

Lahiri Mahasaya was a great pioneer and wellspring for the transmission of advanced spiritual techniques to the public (largely through 2nd generation disciple, Paramahansa Yogananda), and it is wonderful to see his teachings presented with such clarity on the site you are referring to: http://www.kriyayogainfo.net

Your previous source of practices, Swami Satyananda (disciple of Swami Sivananda), has also made wonderful contributions to rising public awareness of the methods of human spiritual transformation, as have many others over the past 150 years (for some history, see http://www.aypsite.org/253.html).

In AYP, we capitalize on the methods of kriya, and also integrate the most effective methods from mantra yoga, hatha yoga, kundalini yoga, tantra and other spiritual disciplines.

"Self-pacing" is at the heart of the AYP approach, enabling us to apply powerful methods of practice in an integrated and manageable way for maximum progress with comfort and safety.

Wishing you all the best on your chosen path. Enjoy!

The guru is in you.

2007/08/31 15:01:05
Other Systems and Alternate Approaches
http://www.aypsite.org/forum/topic.asp?TOPIC_ID=1530&REPLY_ID=25179&whichpage=-1
an experience worth reading

Hi SuperTrouper:

There is a pretty good summary of the main AYP practices in this lesson: http://www.aypsite.org/204.html

The big AYP Easy Lessons book is the most complete layout of the practices (about 20% more material than online). Eventually there will be another big one -- "Volume 2." These volumes will be the master documents for AYP when all is said and done.

Because they were written later, the small AYP Enlightenment Series books (6 out to date) provide additional clarity on the basic practices, and new techniques in the Samyama and Diet/Shatkarmas/Amaroli books. Upcoming E-Series books will include new material as well. The E-Series is designed to provide many doorways into the AYP practices, according to individual interests.

The Secrets of Wilder novel contains a nifty chart (minus the Sanskrit) that summarizes the key AYP practices and how they can be built up in a daily routine.

All the best!

The guru is in you.

2006/10/28 09:32:28
Other Systems and Alternate Approaches
http://www.aypsite.org/forum/topic.asp?TOPIC_ID=1642&REPLY_ID=12634&whichpage=-1
Theosophy

Hi All:

You can find my two cents on Theosophy in lesson 253. It played a significant role in my formative years. There is also a Theosophy section in the AYP booklist. This does not mean everyone has to run out and read Theosophy. It is mainly for those who can't stop studying spiritual philosophy. :-)

Theosophy is long on philosophy and short on actual practices. It was the times, you know. Now we have shifted...

Still, sometimes it is fun to discuss how the cosmos works. It makes for good samyama too -- embodying the cosmos with our own infinite awareness, and vise versa. That's not philosophy anymore. It is practice. More on that later...

The guru is in you.

2006/11/10 11:45:20
Other Systems and Alternate Approaches
http://www.aypsite.org/forum/topic.asp?TOPIC_ID=1695&REPLY_ID=13120&whichpage=-1
Has anyone here learned the TM-Sid
Hi technique ?

Hi RealShon, and welcome!

What you are asking about is the ancient practice of samyama, and that is offered in the AYP lessons beginning here: http://www.aypsite.org/149.html

The AYP practice instructions are fairly informal and rely heavily on the aspirant's ability to engage in self-directed practice over the long term. That is true of formal instruction also. Once you get home from the course, it is just you and your practices. No one can make a good long term practice for you but you. Of course, we all get by with a little help from our friends, which is what these forums are about. :-)

If you are looking for formal instruction in samyama practice, the TM organization is an excellent place to get it, assuming you can afford it.

Wishing you all the best on your chosen path. Enjoy!

The guru is in you.

PS -- The next AYP book (due out at the end of the year) is called "Samyama - Cultivating Stillness in Action." It will look at samyama applications going significantly beyond what is currently in the AYP lessons.

2006/11/11 09:15:15
Other Systems and Alternate Approaches
http://www.aypsite.org/forum/topic.asp?TOPIC_ID=1695&REPLY_ID=13139&whichpage=-1
Has anyone here learned the TM-Sid
Hi technique ?

Hi RealShon:

Here is a long time TM teacher who has posted in the AYP forums a few months back: http://www.aypsite.org/forum/topic.asp?TOPIC_ID=1340

I'm sure he will be happy to give you his perspectives on the TM/Sid
Hi program and the AYP approach to samyama practice.

Being a new member, you may have to post a couple of more times before the member profile direct link email service here will be automatically turned on for you.

All the best!

The guru is in you.

2006/11/11 10:33:35
Other Systems and Alternate Approaches
http://www.aypsite.org/forum/topic.asp?TOPIC_ID=1695&REPLY_ID=13144&whichpage=-1
Has anyone here learned the TM-Sid
Hi technique ?

quote:
_____
Originally posted by yogani

Here is a long time TM teacher who has posted in the AYP forums a few months back: http://www.aypsite.org/forum/topic.asp?TOPIC_ID=1340

I'm sure he will be happy to give you his perspectives on the TM/Sid
Hi program and the AYP approach to samyama practice.
_____

PS -- Also check his July 5, 2006 post in this topic: http://www.aypsite.org/forum/topic.asp?TOPIC_ID=1034

In fact, you may like to read the whole topic. :-)

Have fun moving on to more and more abiding inner silence, ecstatic bliss and outpouring divine love!

The guru is in you.

2006/12/23 16:16:22
Other Systems and Alternate Approaches
http://www.aypsite.org/forum/topic.asp?TOPIC_ID=1848&REPLY_ID=14796&whichpage=-1
Kabbalah, Gnosticism and Christianity
Another take on scripture, copied from this topic: http://www.aypsite.org/forum/topic.asp?TOPIC_ID=1728&whichpage=5

Hi All:

The "truth" of the scriptures is only real if it can be verified in human experience, because human experience is what the scriptures are recording in the first place. The scriptures were written (or orally transmitted) by human beings! They are "absolute" only when mythologized to be so, and this has both pros and cons. The best scriptures are those which can also provide practical means for cultivating the spiritual potential which their authors professed to be resident in all human beings.

Scriptures can be useful when taken on blind faith over the short term, aiding in promoting bhakti and direct spiritual experience, and thus helping dissolve blind faith. But, if taken as absolute truth on blind faith indefinitely, without ongoing spiritual growth via effective practices, scriptures can become the foundation (or excuse) for grossly aberrant conduct in human beings. Any knowledge reduced to the level of an "ideology" and taken on blind faith on an ongoing basis will lead to conflict with other ideologies also taken on blind faith. When a scripture has been reduced to an ideology, beware!

Like any knowledge, scriptures can be well-used or terribly misused.

The real test of any scripture is in whether its highest ideals can be actualized in human experience. That is where the rubber meets the road. For thousands of years many dedicated practitioners have recorded their experiences on the path of human spiritual transformation, and, in some cases, recorded practical means to cultivate the divine outpouring in everyone. We owe them a great deal. How we use the information is up to us -- hopefully for the betterment of all humankind.

Just one person's opinion. :-)

The guru is in you.

2006/12/24 14:47:07
Other Systems and Alternate Approaches
http://www.aypsite.org/forum/topic.asp?TOPIC_ID=1848&REPLY_ID=14819&whichpage=-1
Kabbalah, Gnosticism and Christianity

Hi All:

Yes, please do continue this interesting discussion on Kabbalah, Gnosticism and Christianity (which has just been split off to form a new topic here), and continue the discussion on Immaculate Conception and Tantra over here: http://www.aypsite.org/forum/topic.asp?TOPIC_ID=1820

Admittedly, there is some overlap, but I know everyone will do their best to maintain the appropriate distinctions between topics ... and civility, of course. :-)

The guru is in you.

2006/12/26 15:40:54
Other Systems and Alternate Approaches
http://www.aypsite.org/forum/topic.asp?TOPIC_ID=1848&REPLY_ID=14884&whichpage=-1
Kabbalah, Gnosticism and Christianity

Hi All:

Pardon me for interrupting, but sectarian and/or political debates are not part of what we want to be doing in the AYP forums. There are plenty of other places to engage in such discussions.

We are interested in spiritual practices, their conduct, their effects, and optimization of the process of human spiritual transformation for maximum safe progress.

Please note that the name of this forum is "Other Systems of Spiritual Practice." Discussions on practices are welcome here from any source whatsoever. We can gain a lot from eachother that way. But the sectarian haggling is not welcome at all. We are yogis and yoginis here, and opportunistic ones at that. So we are always looking for useful angles on practice, and not a rehash of the foibles of human history.

As for the dangling discussions on secret codes, inner circles, secret societies and teachings, better to limit those also, because they only reinforce sectarian divides. There is no "us and them" here. Only us.

In AYP we have no secrets! Anyone who wants to mention a secret here, better be prepared to tell it, and in practical terms directly related to the conduct of our daily spiritual practices. That we are very interested in.

Thanks very much for keeping these points in mind. :-)

The guru is in you.

2006/12/26 19:12:22
Other Systems and Alternate Approaches
http://www.aypsite.org/forum/topic.asp?TOPIC_ID=1848&REPLY_ID=14894&whichpage=-1
Kabbalah, Gnosticism and Christianity

Hi Doc:

It isn't about the people or the doctines here. It isn't even about being offended or not. It is about the practices, and what we can do with them here and now for best results. That is what we strive for in AYP.

No moderator here is going to play referee in a sectarian fight, real or imagined, nor try and parse every comment that is made. We do not know whose opinion about doctrine is right. It is the obvious excesses and personal attacks that will be regulated. That we do understand. We owe that to all the practitioners who come here looking for support and useful information.

It is up to the participants in this topic to try and make something useful out of it. If there is a sectarian accusation or argument that has to be made, please take it offline. We have a responsibility to all who are dropping in here every day -- many who are new visitors. The readership is at least 10 times the membership, and growing all the time. Please keep it in mind.

All ideas can be presented in creative ways that serve the needs of everyone involved. There is no need to offend, or take offense in these public forums. Obviously, we can only control our own side of it, and we should do the best we can with that.

Every tree is known by its own fruit, so extra labeling is not necessary. In extreme cases, the moderators will step in. It is rare around here, so if anyone feels like they are being picked on, better take a good look in the mirror.

If contributions that are useful for practices cannot be offered, then it is probably better to stay away, because the conflicted discussions don't really help anyone, and, in fact, drive people away. No one is served by that, so we are not going to let it go on for long. That's just how it is in this kind of environment.

The guru is in you.

2007/01/03 07:53:59
Other Systems and Alternate Approaches
http://www.aypsite.org/forum/topic.asp?TOPIC_ID=1879&REPLY_ID=15317&whichpage=-1
Stellar Triangle Formations
Note: Topic moved for better placement.
2007/02/18 15:28:01
Other Systems and Alternate Approaches
http://www.aypsite.org/forum/topic.asp?TOPIC_ID=2065&REPLY_ID=17775&whichpage=-1
"The Secret" gets out

Hi All:

Inner silence is synonymous with "surrender," and also with "believing," because these involve letting go of our personal expectations. This is where we can find the connection between samyama and the law of attraction to the extent these are operating with results in our life.

This was discussed in the radio interview on samyama, where the radio host and call-in opened up the discussion from samyama to law of attraction and affirmation style systems. They are all stimulating the same principles of samyama within us that Patanjali expounded in the Yoga Sutras centuries ago.

The guru is in you.

2008/08/26 16:21:31
Other Systems and Alternate Approaches
http://www.aypsite.org/forum/topic.asp?TOPIC_ID=2112&REPLY_ID=36813&whichpage=-1
Cannabis

Hi CarsonZi:

That is wonderful. The credit really goes to you for digging in and doing the practices in the face of considerable adversity.

Perhaps you could remind your doctor to report back to his professional association and any research institutions he is affiliated with to encourage research on the role of meditation and pranayama in this situation. Obviously, something is going on here, and maybe many more could benefit.

All the best to you and your lovely bride! :-)

The guru is in you.

2008/08/28 09:00:34
Other Systems and Alternate Approaches
http://www.aypsite.org/forum/topic.asp?TOPIC_ID=2112&REPLY_ID=36894&whichpage=-1
Cannabis

quote:
_____
Originally posted by CarsonZi

What I REALLY hope to do in the near future though is start an AYP meditation group aimed towards helping those at my clinic (and if that goes well at others clinics too) trying to get off of methadone. At least I will see if there is any interest there. The least I can do is lead others to the liberation of being drug free and yoga'd up:-) Thanks again.
CarsonZi
_____

Hi CarsonZi:

Yes, this would be a wonderful thing to do. Something for which you are uniquely qualified.

The guru is in you.

2007/04/07 10:22:00
Other Systems and Alternate Approaches
http://www.aypsite.org/forum/topic.asp?TOPIC_ID=2394&REPLY_ID=19954&whichpage=-1
How to learn TM- Sid
Hi here?

Hi AYP, and welcome!

Very auspicious name you have chosen. :-)

If you purchase the small AYP book called "**Samyama - Cultivating Stillness in Action, Siddhis and Miracles**," you will have the latest and most condensed information on Samyama practice as taught in AYP. It goes significantly beyond what is contained in the online lessons and previous AYP books. The Samyama book is not expensive and is available in both paperback and ebook formats here:
http://www.aypsite.org/books.html
If you decide to get the ebook, the version with the audio introduction is recommended.

As for comparisions with the TM program, sorry, I can't help you with that, except to say that the AYP approach is a lot less expensive (open source) and more flexible in its application. Also, there is no emphasis in AYP on the external performance of siddhis such as yogic flying, though the internal aspects are fully covered.

If it is the TM program you want specifically, then you should go to them for it, as has already been suggested. You will not find a replica of it here. But for mature self-directed practitioners, maybe something better.

Wishing you all the best on your path. Practice wisely, and enjoy!

The guru is in you.

2007/04/13 14:40:18
Other Systems and Alternate Approaches
http://www.aypsite.org/forum/topic.asp?TOPIC_ID=2421&REPLY_ID=20341&whichpage=-1
Yoga and Buddhism?

Hi All:

The distinction I aways try and make is between the belief system and the operative practices that are contained in it.

Debating what works practice-wise is much more fruitful than debating one belief system versus another. Belief systems are a matter of personal preference which we can honor in each other, while practices are much more measureable in terms of cause and effect in daily living. Practices are often found to be complementary (if not directly overlapping) once the lines that divide belief systems have been crossed. Whatever works!

May our beliefs not overshadow what has practical benefit, even if we find it on the other side of an imaginary wall. There is only one nervous system design that is giving rise to all human perceptions, including the many variations in view based on culture and belief. Each point of view is therefore valid from its own perspective.

The practices that are used in all of the traditions have much more in common than is generally known. This makes sense, since we are all working with the same vehicle of experience, and the same process of human spiritual transformation.

So what's to argue about except the relative effectiveness achieved in integrating the many practices which have all been designed for accomplishing the same thing? The whole is greater than the sum of the parts. :-)

The guru is in you.

PS: Personally, I am not much for giving this eclectic approach a name (though we had to), since it only leads to the question, "As opposed to what?!!"

2007/04/13 17:34:57
Other Systems and Alternate Approaches
http://www.aypsite.org/forum/topic.asp?TOPIC_ID=2421&REPLY_ID=20350&whichpage=-1
Yoga and Buddhism?

quote:
_____
Originally posted by Mike

As I say its perhaps more of a problem of human nature than a system... but of course systems are designed to funnel human beings in a certain direction. The same thing applies to Taoist and Tibetan (in particular) practices - folks are not at all keen about doing the dull seemingly non-progress spadework on the unglamorous foundational stuff.
_____

Hi Mike:

It seems to be the same question/argument that comes up among the yoga traditions: Is it necessary to learn "codes of conduct" before we learn meditation and other powerful practices? It is discussed in this lesson on the eight limbs of yoga, after the limbs are listed:
http://www.aypsite.org/149.html

The upshot is that deep meditation enhances spiritual conduct naturally from within, and is therefore a favored approach to enhancing spiritual conduct, rather than an externally enforced approach. Not all yoga schools agree on this point, as is discussed in the lesson. Maybe similar disagreements on where to start with practices occur in Buddhism also?

Additionally, yes, there is some overlap between belief and practice. In yoga it is part of "bhakti" -- devotion to our chosen ideal, which operationally is (by many names) the single most important spiritual practice in all the religions. In most religions, the belief system provides the ideal, but not always. It is the person who chooses this, which is what makes belief systems personal, and deserving our respect. That does not mean someone else can't have a completely different ideal associated with the same belief system. That too is personal, and deserving our respect. A chosen ideal cannot be imposed from outside with effective results. It must be chosen within each person with deep emotion to have the desired effect. Check out the article on bhakti just resurrected recently here: http://www.aypsite.org/forum/topic.asp?TOPIC_ID=1891#20269

Sorry I can't put these concepts into Buddhist terminology. Maybe in the next lifetime, if there is one. :-)

All the best!

The guru is in you.

2007/04/26 10:11:52
Other Systems and Alternate Approaches
http://www.aypsite.org/forum/topic.asp?TOPIC_ID=2421&REPLY_ID=21017&whichpage=-1
Yoga and Buddhism?

Hi All:

I'm enjoying this discussion very much also. Many connection points. Good food for thought and inspiration for practice, regardless of one's chosen path.

Thank you!

The guru is in you.

2007/05/11 13:37:46
Other Systems and Alternate Approaches
http://www.aypsite.org/forum/topic.asp?TOPIC_ID=2426&REPLY_ID=21749&whichpage=-1
Like Yoga, Only With Jesus ...

Hi Doll, and welcome!

Your work with postures incorporating Christian principles is wonderful.

The increasing connection between modern Christianity and the perennial wisdom on human spiritual transformation is of great importance. I view all effective methods of spiritual practice to be part of a great continuum of practical knowledge that can be applied by anyone, regardless of culture or creed.

The spiritual capabilities inherent in every human nervous system form the common denominator in all people.

As Kirtanman points out, the **Secrets of Wilder** novel was written to help open a door to the Judeo/Christian world, demonstrating the possibilities for powerful practices emerging spontaneously from within a modern western cultural framework, and what the global implications of this can be. To provide clarity for western readers, there is no Sanskrit terminology in the book, and the story occurs in a contemporary Christian setting. It is something of an allegory of the New Testament, taking out the cultural overlay of Roman times, and replacing it with the cultural strengths and weaknesses of our modern times. The struggles the main character and his associates go through in discovering and refining real spiritual practices and the resulting experiences are graphically portrayed, perhaps more so than in any previous book of this kind.

The novel was the first writing I did in 2003, before the AYP online lessons began. Brought up Christian in the USA, I have always seen the practical spiritual methods of both west and east to be aspects of the same whole, and have presented AYP from this point of view since the beginning -- non-sectarian. My hope is that people from all backgrounds will find benefit.

Your website and classes are a wonderful effort in this direction. We need many more doors opening to the truth within. :-)

Wishing you all the best in your teaching and on your path. Enjoy!

The guru is in you.

2007/10/30 23:14:10
Other Systems and Alternate Approaches
http://www.aypsite.org/forum/topic.asp?TOPIC_ID=2452&REPLY_ID=26552&whichpage=-1
Reiki Tummo - A Path to the Heart

Hi Steve:

Thanks much for your generous sharing on Reiki Tummo. An interesting path and an inspiring journey! :-)

The guru is in you.

2008/03/19 15:15:11
Other Systems and Alternate Approaches
http://www.aypsite.org/forum/topic.asp?TOPIC_ID=2661&REPLY_ID=31506&whichpage=-1
Could this be from Jesus himself?

quote:
_____
Originally posted by anthony574

I am very interested to know what yogani thinks of realjesus if he has read it. I read some of it and so far I have very mixed feelings. Part is due to a fear of Jesus from the horror of modern Christianity. Another is that realjesus seems to have a more strict and somewhat "absolutist" view of the purpose of life which scares me a bit. But at the same time it is extremely inspiring and although I am skpetical that it is really Jesus - the ability for the articles to explain every successive nuance and question is incredible. It seems that there are no gaps - everything is explained although I feel a resistance to this explanation...which in turn is explained!
_____

Hi Anthony:

I don't think it matters whether this is real Jesus or not. What matters is whether we are clearing our own inner obstructions to open our vision. If studying something or listening to someone helps with that, then it is good. If it does not, and only stirs up doubt and fear, then let that part go. It is the same with any teacher. We will not find our salvation (or demise) in any outside source. We will find it within ourselves. Outside sources can help us open our inside source, as long as we don't let those same outside sources distract us. That is the trick.

See this lesson for a few pointers: http://www.aypsite.org/260.html

Always remember that the color we are seeing is the color we are creating ourselves. What kind of glasses are we wearing? To inquire about this is a good idea, especially if we are being upset too often. Our discomfort is a call to action in a new direction. Maybe time to think about getting a new pair of glasses?

Is all this darkness we are seeing really true, or only our coloring of things? What would it be like if we turned it around inside, switching the color from dark to light? What would it be like to develop the ability to do that on an ongoing basis? Is that the ideal we have? If not, what is our ideal for how we will live our life?

Ultimately, it cannot work if we continually put our ideal in the hands of others. We will be blown about like a leaf on the wind. The solution is to take a stand on what it is we want for ourselves, and steadily move in that direction, regardless of distractions. If Jesus in blazing glory comes to us in deep meditation, what do we do? Easily come back to the mantra ... like that. He will also be there later on for a friendly chat when we have finished with our practice.

It might help to take a look at Byron Katie's "Loving What Is." The AYP Self-Inquiry book can be a useful companion to it. Then the importance of daily deep meditation will become clear in relation to our inquiry into our perceptions (coloring) of the world. The doubt and fear can be penetrated more quickly that way and, in time, be replaced with a radiant inner stillness that knows no doubt or fear. This condition cannot be manipulated by any outside force, because it is beyond all that. It is our *Self*.

So it is logical to favor our inner development over outer influences, yes? Take what helps, and leave the rest behind. That goes for everything you read here too. It is your path and you are in charge. :-)

Practice wisely, and enjoy!

The guru is in you.

2007/08/12 19:39:22
Other Systems and Alternate Approaches
http://www.aypsite.org/forum/topic.asp?TOPIC_ID=2841&REPLY_ID=24766&whichpage=-1
Christian beliefs and reincarnation

quote:
_____
Originally posted by Hannah

Thank you to Wolfgang, Sparkle and Weaver for your input. I detest sticky situations such as this and would really like to handle it gracefully and without offense. You guys are great! :-)
_____

Hi Hannah:

There is also a good reference book on the AYP booklist called **Reincarnation - An East-West Anthology** by Head and Cranston. It's a classic.

http://www.aypsite.org/booklist14.html

"Reviewing reincarnation in the world's religions, including scriptural quotes and essays. Also includes essays on reincarnation from hundreds of prominent Western thinkers from many countries throughout our recorded history. This is an extensive work on the subject."

You can hand them the book, and leave it at that. :-)

The guru is in you.

PS: If you follow the book link to Amazon, you will find related books there too.

If you'd like to take it to the next step, hand them a copy of the **Secrets of Wilder** novel -- it is a Christian story with practices and reincarnation in it.

2008/01/12 15:48:25
Other Systems and Alternate Approaches
http://www.aypsite.org/forum/topic.asp?TOPIC_ID=2972&REPLY_ID=28797&whichpage=-1
Shamanic Yoga

Hi Gnosis:

The "kicking of the tires" is appreciated. It is the best way to distill out the truth. That goes for any approach to spiritual development, with or without an in-the-flesh guru.

AYP is one persons's experience being shared openly and blended with the experiences of many. That is what open source knowledge is -- an evolving integration. It offers some big advantages.

Whether or not it represents a viable path to enlightenment for the many remains to be seen. It is an experiment. So far, the results have been promising. My hope is that many others will join in to help carry it forward to become a true *Applied Science*. Time will tell.

As far as I know, the serious casualties within AYP have been very limited (nil?), far less than most of the traditions I am familiar with, even with many here traveling much faster than on traditional paths. In fact, we have inherited quite a few casualites from some of the traditional guru paths, and been able to help most of them. This is because collectively we take responsibility to make sure those having difficulties receive the best support we can give. I don't know of any traditional guru approach that goes to such lengths. The results here speak for themselves.

If anyone out there considers themselves to be in a spiritual crisis of any kind, please do step forward. Chances are good we can help.

There is strength in numbers, and I'd go so far to say that a savvy community of practitioners can be a stronger support system than an individual guru can be, assuming the community knowledge-base is well-developed, and being applied and refined in practice by many on an ongoing basis. Then there will be few surprises, and support will be comprehensive. This will be especially true when large numbers of people become involved -- more than any single teacher can address. It will "take a village" to get the job done on a worldwide scale. That is where we are heading.

At this point in time, folks are drawing on the AYP approach (in whole or in part) at many stages along the path, from beginner to quite advanced. Given that diversity, we seem to be managing pretty well. So what's the beef?

In theory, I can see why there can be complaints about a non-physical-guru path. It isn't traditional. But what about in practice, where the rubber actually meets the road? Just because there are horror stories out there, both in the guru traditions and outside them, it is not a direct reflection on what is going on here. Rather, it is a testament that we might actually know what we are doing!

As Sparkle suggested, adding some hands-on experience to scholarship can go a long way toward addressing concerns. You might be pleasantly surprised. :-)

I suspect the open source community method could work for any approach to spiritual development (including shamanism), assuming a comprehensive knowledge-base and seasoned community of practitioners can be assembled. It takes time and a lot of work. I am very grateful to all who have helped AYP come to the level it is at today. We still have a long way to go, but we have traveled a great distance in only a few years. The prospects are exciting.

All the best!

The guru is in you.

2008/07/04 16:15:33
Other Systems and Alternate Approaches
http://www.aypsite.org/forum/topic.asp?TOPIC_ID=2972&REPLY_ID=35162&whichpage=-1
Shamanic Yoga

Hi CarsonZi, and welcome!

I think you will find open discussions here on just about every approach to the natural process of human spiritual transformation. There are no taboos really, except perhaps giving in to the *magic bullet syndrome*, which is a tendency we all have toward becoming obsessed about one thing or another. Even obsession for God has it's downside (too much of a good thing). That is why we talk about "self-pacing" a lot in the AYP writings in relation to all spiritual methods. With so many powerful tools available these days, we are now largely driven by the need for practicality in our ongoing management of causes and effects.

Real yoga is about finding a balanced integration of means, leading us surely and safely to our natural unfoldment of abiding inner silence, ecstatic bliss and outpouring divine love. That is what AYP is about. And so, anything goes, as long as it can be demonstrated to work over the long term. :-)

Entheogens are not necessarily excluded from the equation, but they do require an extra caution because they have more to do with initial inspiration and less to do with the final outcome, and the risk of addiction always lurks. No doubt they have played a key role in the earliest spiritual explorations of humankind, as you mentioned (see here also).

There has been a major evolution in spiritual methodologies since ancient times (epitomized in the Yoga Sutras of Patanjali), and we continue to forge ahead in optimizing the application of powerful practices in the present. What remains to be determined is whether entheogens have a significant role to play. That depends on the individual practitioner and where they happen to be on their path. The truth is that spiritual inspiration can come from many sources. We each come to engage in daily spiritual practices by our own route, always from within ourselves.

Below is an excerpt from the AYP "Diet, Shatkarmas and Amaroli" (DSA) book, where the role of entheogens is reviewed. The discussion remains open, with practical cautions stated as necessary.

Wishing you all the best on your path. Enjoy!

The guru is in you.

Halluncinogenics and Yoga

In the native cultures of the world (including in ancient India), spiritual experience has sometimes been associated (and ritualized) with the ingestion of hallucinogenic substances derived from plants. In modern times, the use of such substances for recreational purposes has become common, especially marijuana, certain types of mushrooms, and synthetic substances, particularly LSD, which rose to prominence in the youth counter-culture of the 1960s and 1970s. Many from that era give some credit to their drug experiences in helping launch them on serious and drugless spiritual paths later on. It cannot be denied. This leaves us with two lingering questions.

First, are drug experiences necessary to embark on a spiritual path? The answer is obviously, no, for many pursue spiritual awakening without a drug experience being the initial stimulus. However, it can be said that in many cases, some sort of initial altered state of consciousness led to the inspiration and desire for a more permanent awakening. Such an initial experience can be caused by an accident, an illness, a spontaneous inner awakening, spiritual vision, or other life-altering event. Or maybe the aspirant just knows inside that there is something more to life than the conventional knowledge society is offering. The seed of spiritual desire can germinate from many causes. Ultimately, the call comes from within.

Drugs are only one of many ways people can be inspired to pursue a broader possibility within. In virtually all cases where an initial altered state is experienced, it will only be a preview, and not the onset of permanent spiritual transformation. It is important to recognize that any particular spiritual experience does not constitute a final outcome. For moving toward a final outcome in terms of spiritual progress, a different strategy is necessary, one which will systematically and gradually promote the purification and opening of the nervous system to its full capabilities.

This leads to the second question: Are drugs an aid in ongoing yoga practice? If there is any initial benefit found in the artificial experience produced by drugs, then the repetition of that experience is not likely to take us further. To assume so is yet another flight of fancy – the magic bullet syndrome. In the case of continuing with hallucinogenic drugs to recreate a particular kind of experience, we will be producing the opposite effect underneath – adding to the obstructions lodged deep within our nervous system.

Spiritual development is not primarily about having a temporary peak experience. Rather, it is a natural and permanent awakening, which can be achieved only through ongoing deep inner purification. This is why anyone engaged in daily deep meditation will find urges for substances that produce artificial experiences falling away. This applies to hallucinogenic drugs, alcohol, tobacco, caffeine, and eating habits that retard the natural expression of the divine light emerging from within us.

2008/07/05 05:01:06
Other Systems and Alternate Approaches
http://www.aypsite.org/forum/topic.asp?TOPIC_ID=2972&REPLY_ID=35176&whichpage=-1
Shamanic Yoga

quote:
_____
Originally posted by tadeas

CarsonZi, check out yogani's post over here: http://www.aypsite.org/forum/topic.asp?TOPIC_ID=3138#27015 - another excerpt from one of the books, covering also soma.

———

Thank you, Tadeas, for pointing to that post. Here is another one on soma and the "nectar cycle," looking at it from several points of view: http://www.aypsite.org/forum/topic.asp?TOPIC_ID=3204#27584
(also see related posts in that topic)

All of this is a permanent shift in the neurobiology, reflecting the rise of inner silence and ecstatic conductivity, stimulated by a range of effective daily practices.

It is not a short-lived experience, but a permanent transformation of our inner functioning, which has ongoing profound effects in our everyday life. The rise of "enlightenment" is not dependent on external substances, but is found to be radiating naturally from within us. This is why we say the human nervous system is the doorway to the divine.

Or, as put so eloquently by Rumi, the great Sufi mystic (from the dedication page of the AYP "Bhakti and Karma Yoga" book):

"I have lived on the lip of insanity,
wanting to know reasons,
knocking on a door.
It opens.
I have been knocking from the inside!"

It is a matter of optimizing the process to open the door in a way that is self-sustaining and permanent. I think this is why entheogens do not find a more prominent role in the toolbox of yoga, because the experiences they provide are neither self-sustaining nor permanent. However, there may some inspiration to be found in them under certain circumstances. From there it is up to the practitioner to move on to more lasting measures that enable the neurobiology to do what it can do very well by itself. Once that has been addressed effectively, the high never ends. :-)

Isn't it true that in advanced Shaman traditions (such as Toltec), the use of entheogens is transcended along the way? This would seem to be a logical evolution. It is certainly what happened in most systems of spiritual practice in India since vedic times. As knowledge steadily advances, humankind enjoys greater benefits ... so it goes.

It is good to honor the ways of the past, but not to get stuck in them. Never-ending innovation is the key in all fields of knowledge, including spiritual.

Onward!

The guru is in you.

2007/11/17 13:02:31
Other Systems and Alternate Approaches
http://www.aypsite.org/forum/topic.asp?TOPIC_ID=2974&REPLY_ID=27085&whichpage=-1
the bible

Hi Kingdom, and welcome!

Study of scriptural writings in the tradition(s) that resonate with us is certainly an important part of our spiritual path. Desire/devotion is a key factor in this, as in all matters spiritual. Eventually, spiritual study becomes internalized to be a direct cognition of truth within us, assuming we have been engaged in an effective integration of daily spiritual practices over time.

This is as true for Christians as for anyone, as the ancient monastic orders well know. Now it is time for everyone to know. With daily practice of deep meditation, breathing techniques, physical postures and maneuvers, intelligent management of sexual energy, and other methods, human spiritual transformation is in the cards for everyone. We are wired for it. This is the message of the Bible:

"The kingdom of God is within you..."

You might be surprised how many in this community come from Christian roots, myself included. Of course, sectarian posturing and proselytizing are not part of the discussion here. We are interested in what works for people of all backgrounds, and that is why you can find people from every tradition in the AYP community. The human nervous system is the common denominator in all spiritual matters -- each of us is a doorway to the infinite. No exceptions.

The Secrets of Wilder novel is a story about how life-changing spiritual practices can be undertaken and reach fruition within a Christian cultural framework. It can happen in every cultural framework, and does!

Wishing you all the best on your chosen path. Enjoy!

Christ is in you.

Here we also say, "The guru is in you.
" Same thing.

2007/10/18 12:21:57
Other Systems and Alternate Approaches
http://www.aypsite.org/forum/topic.asp?TOPIC_ID=3005&REPLY_ID=26121&whichpage=-1
On Changing Mantra

Hi John Joe, and welcome!

On changing your mantra, it will all depend on who you ask, and ultimately on your own feelings and choice.

You can guess what a TM teacher might say. :-)

In AYP, the mantra is your choice. Information is provided on the characteristics and strategy of the AYP mantra system. Also, a "heads up" is given on the AYP mantra enhancements and possible inconsistencies between other mantras and the enhancements, which may have a bearing on one's long term mantra strategy.

On the other hand, it is possible to use a mantra and meditation style from another system and take advantage of many of the AYP techniques without running into conflicts. However, it is suggested not to combine similar classes of practice (meditation, pranayama, etc.) from different systems in the same routine. This can result in a "doubling up" effect leading to excessive inner purification and the discomfort that can come with that.

"Self-pacing" of practices is always center stage in AYP, enabling us to undertake a full range of powerful methods in an integrated way, which may not be possible in more rigid systems. AYP is a progressive flexible system based on managing "causes and effects" in our routine on an ongoing basis, an approach that is suited for serious independent practitioners.

From the AYP point of view, it is always your path and your choice. If you are willing to take the responsibility for self-directed integrated practice, you can find a lot of help in the AYP writings, and in this forum.

One thing you will not find in the AYP writings is what to do with other systems of practice. It is best to go to the source of those for that. On the other hand, there are plenty of individuals here in the forum from many different backgrounds who may offer their own opinion on just about any aspect of practice, AYP or other. Maybe others with a TM background will offer a few comments.

Wishing you all the best on your chosen path. Practice wisely, and enjoy!

The guru is in you.

2007/11/08 09:49:33
Other Systems and Alternate Approaches
http://www.aypsite.org/forum/topic.asp?TOPIC_ID=3078&REPLY_ID=26822&whichpage=-1
The Four Aggreements

Hi Eddie:

That is great!

Here is a link for those who might not be familiar with the four agreements: http://www.aypsite.org/forum/topic.asp?TOPIC_ID=466

The guru is in you.

2007/11/29 14:00:04
Other Systems and Alternate Approaches
http://www.aypsite.org/forum/topic.asp?TOPIC_ID=3193&REPLY_ID=27473&whichpage=-1
Gayatri mantra

Hi John, and welcome!

Actually, what you are saying fits with the spirit of AYP, and I am sure will resonate with many who are here also.

We are rebels with a cause here, with endless outpouring divine love being the end game. "Experiences" pale by comparison. That's why everyone is encouraged to favor the practice over the experiences. :-)

All the best!

The guru is in you.

2008/02/17 17:03:57
Other Systems and Alternate Approaches
http://www.aypsite.org/forum/topic.asp?TOPIC_ID=3314&REPLY_ID=30194&whichpage=-1
Kunlun Nei Gung

Hi Scott and Jim:

It is not possible to say what is kundalini and what it is not with such parsing and distinctions. It is a never-ending labyrinth, like trying to categorize all the grains of sand on a beach. We we can say with some assurance that kundalini is all energy related to the rise of ecstatic conductivity, no matter how little or how much. That is, ecstatic conductivity radiating up from the loins, which is the source of kundalini (and even that is disputed sometimes). Beyond that general description, we are getting into all the grains of sand. Who needs it?

If a spigot is dripping slowly, it is water.
If it is running in a steady stream, it is still water.
If the pipe breaks and there is a big deluge, that is water too.

It's all water, isn't it? It is all one thing. Enlivened neurobiological energy in this case, to whatever degree that is (via the spigot). Others may wish to make all sorts of distinctions with great authority, but it doesn't mean much.

Regarding breath suspension, that can happen during deep meditation with little or no energy moving, so breath suspension is not necessarily an indicator of ecstatic conductivity or kundalini. It is an indicator of inner silence and a temporary suspension of metabolism. It is common in deep meditation, and gradually shows itself in our daily activity (safely) along with the rise of inner silence.

Energy movements will be accompanied naturally by breath suspension only if there is inner silence present (it will happen). And, as we know, there can be substantial energy movement without much inner silence present. We may call that "premature kundalini awakening," depending on the severity of the symptoms.

Keep in mind that there is only one human nervous system with a given range of transformative and experiential capabilities, no matter what techniques we may be using. When stimulated, those experiences can be described in different ways, but they will be essentially the same experiences.

So, the chances are pretty good that everything we find out about kunlun will be more or less analogous with what we already know from AYP, or from any tried and true spiritual path. It is only a matter of the effectiveness of the particular practices we may be using, and the mental structure that is being built around perceptions of the internal dynamics that are occurring. We can avoid a lot of unnecessary distraction by regarding it all as, yes, "scenery!"

Well, just a few observations from the AYP perspective. I hope to be reading about kunlun in a few weeks. Will let you know if I see anything significantly different. So far, it looks like a lot of attention on "scenery," but that may not be Mr. Max's doing, unless it is mainly the scenery he is selling. If that is the case, then let the buyer beware. :-)

All the best!

The guru is in you.

2008/02/19 18:50:15
Other Systems and Alternate Approaches
http://www.aypsite.org/forum/topic.asp?TOPIC_ID=3314&REPLY_ID=30277&whichpage=-1
Kunlun Nei Gung

Hi All:

I have had an opportunity to go through the little Kunlun Nei Gung book. It is sincere, and does overlap with most of the AYP energy-related practices, with the possible exception of level 3 kunlun, which is a visualization practice intended for grounding. The prior two levels I'd classify as "kundalini" practices, especially level 2 involving kumbhaka (breath retention) combined with posture and attention.

The central role of sexual energy, including some clear overlaps with AYP, makes it obvious that kunlun is kundalini-related, by whatever other name it may be called. It is an interesting approach, and even speaks to some of the stories of high mountain Asian monks playing "body heat" games in the freezing cold, etc.

It's a nice little book. Clear and concise. We like that around here. The author deserves credit for downplaying the scenery aspect, of which there can be plenty, as has been discussed in this topic already. He also speaks of the reduction of energy friction in the nervous system as the nerves are cleared over time. Energy friction is the primary cause of movements, "automatic yoga" and other energy-related phenomena. The gradual reduction of neurobiological friction leads to smoother practice and more refined experiences. This is the same process of purification and opening we have discussed often in AYP.

It appears that inner silence, to the extent cultivated, is a derivative of kunlun practice, if that. It is not addressed directly. So, deep meditation may be a good complement to kunlun practice. But much of the rest of AYP may be doubling up, including spinal breathing, asanas, mudras, bandhas, kumbhaka, etc. It is back to the same questions about combining Taoist and Yoga practices that were discussed here:
http://www.aypsite.org/forum/topic.asp?TOPIC_ID=500

As is usually the case when comparing Taoist and Yoga practices, the former tends to be energy-based (martial roots), while the latter tends to be consciousness-based (meditation/vedic roots). That seems to be the case here too. That's just how it is.

As for the long term results of Kunlun versus AYP and other systems, we'll have to see what Scott, TopFlight and others have to say down the road. I'm looking forward to feedback whenever it may come.

All the best!

The guru is in you.

2008/04/11 11:31:42
Other Systems and Alternate Approaches
http://www.aypsite.org/forum/topic.asp?TOPIC_ID=3314&REPLY_ID=32541&whichpage=-1
Kunlun Nei Gung

quote:
_____
Originally posted by Eitherway

Ok, I know that it hasn't been very long since ayp was introduced to Max's Kunlun practice but I was wondering what if any conclusions are being drawn about this path. Is it worth pursuing or at this point just continue with the wonderful Ayp practices or better yet is there a way to take the best from Kunlun and add safely to our core ayp practice of deep meditation.

Dear Yogani, what is your advice on this at this point??
_____

Hi Eitherway:

I'm not really the right person to answer this, not being a Kunlun Nei Gung practitioner. Some here have been doing the research, self-pacing their way through it, so their experiences and opinions (some posted above) are the best we have so far. In time, we will know more.

All the best!

The guru is in you.

2008/04/16 12:23:48
Other Systems and Alternate Approaches
http://www.aypsite.org/forum/topic.asp?TOPIC_ID=3314&REPLY_ID=32716&whichpage=-1
Kunlun Nei Gung

quote:

Originally posted by Eitherway

Ok, I know that it hasn't been very long since ayp was introduced to Max's Kunlun practice but I was wondering what if any conclusions are being drawn about this path. Is it worth pursuing or at this point just continue with the wonderful Ayp practices or better yet is there a way to take the best from Kunlun and add safely to our core ayp practice of deep meditation.

Dear Yogani, what is your advice on this at this point??

Hi again Eitherway:

I just recalled this post from earlier in this topic:
http://www.aypsite.org/forum/topic.asp?TOPIC_ID=3314&whichpage=2#30277

A better answer to your question than the last one. The best I can do under the circumstances. :-)

All the best!

The guru is in you.

2008/05/29 10:03:33
Other Systems and Alternate Approaches
http://www.aypsite.org/forum/topic.asp?TOPIC_ID=3314&REPLY_ID=34164&whichpage=-1
Kunlun Nei Gung

Hi All:

I don't see the distinction between kunlun energy and kundalini either. Are c
Hi and prana different? Not likely. Only in the utilization...

The physical movements experienced in kunlun are not unique, except there is more emphasis on them as practice than in yoga. This may be in line with the martial roots of Taoist practices versus the more consciousness oriented roots of Yoga.

Which raises the question again about the long term cultivation of inner silence in kunlun, and in Taoist practices in general. It is addressed in a few Taoist schools (with deep meditation style practice), but not many. The question is whether it is addressed in kunlun. It is an essential point with long term implications for the practitioner.

Here are two previous posts on these matters I did in this topic way back when:

http://www.aypsite.org/forum/topic.asp?TOPIC_ID=3314&whichpage=2#30277
http://www.aypsite.org/forum/topic.asp?TOPIC_ID=3314&whichpage=2#30194

The suggestion is to temper enthusiasm for the dramatic experiences and look for stillness rising in daily activity. The former is mostly a passing show. If the latter is coming, then the path has real merit.

A few more cents from the yogic point of view, for whatever they might be worth. :-)

All the best!

The guru is in you.

2008/02/13 12:27:33
Other Systems and Alternate Approaches
http://www.aypsite.org/forum/topic.asp?TOPIC_ID=3332&REPLY_ID=30021&whichpage=-1
Chanted, and mentally recited Mantras

quote:

Originally posted by emc

And is the witty twist in how Yogani uses the I AM mantra in his book "Secrets of Wilder" only a semantic funny thing? Or do I miss something there? It is repeated so often as if Jesus really said "I AM the way", as if it really would have had something to do with the I AM mantra... but it can't have, can it? It's just a little mind boggle right now...

Hi EMC:

Being a novel, the Secrets of Wilder takes a few liberties in picking up on common themes that can make the story more relevant and inspiring for English speaking (mainly American) Christian readers. While writing it, I did not expect that it would find an international audience.

One of these common themes is picking up on well-known English Biblical phrases like, "I am the way..." and the God of Moses speaking "I am that I am..." and so on.

Another theme that is used, common in Christianity and other religions, is touching as an initiatory action (tapping the breastbone in this case). I can't tell you how many times I have been asked where to go to get that tap. I always say that the first time anyone sits in deep meditation, they are tapped from the inside, and every time thereafter. It is true!

In addition, the Secrets of Wilder story reflects the classic theme of the "hero's journey," so well described in the work of Joseph Campbell. The novel loosely corresponds with the story in the Christian Gospels also.

None of this should have a bearing on the practices themselves, or on how people of different language, religion or culture may wish to approach them. If I were Swedish, the Secrets of Wilder may have presented a different sort of story, like *The Secrets of John the Viking* :-), and the themes unique to language and culture would have been developed for that. But the practices would be the same, including the use of I AM (AYAM) as mantra for vibrational quality only in deep meditation, which I hope is made clear in the Secrets of Wilder novel.

Finally, I should point out that the first draft of the Secrets of Wilder was written in early 2003, before AYP was started, or even conceived of. When the first draft of the novel was done, it became clear that if more people were to be reached more quickly, then the practices should be transmitted directly on the internet in open source lesson format. With that realization, the novel was set aside and AYP was started in late 2003. After the first AYP Easy Lessons book came out in late 2004, the novel was finished up and published as the second book in mid 2005.

So the novel was where it all started. We have come a long way since then.

Hopefully, putting the writings in the context of when and why they were done will help separate language and cultural factors in the novel from the actual practices, as may be needed.

The guru is in you.

PS: I don't know if AYP ever would have happened if the novel had not been drafted first. Apparently, John Wilder inspired me to look far beyond the borders of sleepy "Coquina Island." Funny how things happen. I hope he has done the same for others. :-)

2008/01/12 10:13:54
Other Systems and Alternate Approaches
http://www.aypsite.org/forum/topic.asp?TOPIC_ID=3356&REPLY_ID=28777&whichpage=-1
Polyphasic Sleep

Hi Brett:

Thomas Edison kept a cot in his laboratory and was known to work around the clock for extended periods, taking cat naps every few hours. Not sure if he did this all his life. It must have driven his employees crazy.

Haven't tried it myself. My sleep cycle goes from very short to very long, with naps being rare. It seems to have a life of its own. Good thing I am "retired" ... Ha! :-)

The guru is in you.

2008/01/13 15:50:16
Other Systems and Alternate Approaches
http://www.aypsite.org/forum/topic.asp?TOPIC_ID=3356&REPLY_ID=28853&whichpage=-1
Polyphasic Sleep

Hi Tadeas:

My sleep cycle is normal as far as I can tell, with the variations mentioned above. However, my perception of it is very different than it was years ago. Much more presence of inner silence/witness now.

That is pretty much the message of yoga. Life's experiences will go on. However, our relationship to them will change dramatically over time.

There is an issue with "sleep techniques" which is seldom highlighted by those who promote them. If they are undertaken before there is sufficient inner silence/witness to support them, there can be the hazards of sleep deprivation. It is the same with premature self-inquiry (non-relational - without witness), which also has hazards.

The guru is in you.

2008/02/14 18:20:02
Other Systems and Alternate Approaches
http://www.aypsite.org/forum/topic.asp?TOPIC_ID=3454&REPLY_ID=30072&whichpage=-1
Deep medtiation = vipassana?

Hi John:

There is a fundamental difference between forms of meditation that use breath or mantra as the object. The difference is that when metabolism slows down and breath suspends, breath can no longer be the object of meditation, whereas a mantra can be used far beyond breath suspension deep within the faintest realms of awareness. In that sense, breath meditation will cycle to where metabolism/breath suspends, whereas mantra meditation will cycle to where mind is transcended.

One might argue that suspended metabolism and breath are the same as transcended mind. Maybe, but that is not the experience of mantra meditators, who can keep meditating to deep absorption in pure awareness (samadhi) regardless of the degree of suspension of metabolism and breath.

It seems reasonable to say that vipassana with breath depends on functioning of both body and mind, while deep meditation with mantra depends on mind only.

It is well known that short twice-daily sessions of deep meditation with mantra are more than enough to get the job done (with longer sessions becoming problematic), while vipassana with breath can be practiced for much longer periods without overdoing. This suggests that deep meditation with mantra is a much more potent practice. Hence the need for careful regulation, self-pacing, etc.

I agree that all roads lead to Rome (or home). It is only a matter of the posted speed limit, and how fast we'd like (and can stand) to travel. :-)

The guru is in you.

2008/02/21 11:13:58
Other Systems and Alternate Approaches
http://www.aypsite.org/forum/topic.asp?TOPIC_ID=3489&REPLY_ID=30366&whichpage=-1
Something to try...

Hi Shanti:

Very beautiful.

Yes, it is a version of samyama, and will depend on the initial presence of some inner silence and a basic understanding about its potential, as you say.

The aspect of picking up on negatively charged thoughts as well as positive ones with samyama is covered in the Samyama book in the chapter on expanded applications. There it is pointed out that samyama on negative obstructions produces purification equally well as samyama on thoughts with positive implications.

Inner silence does not care whether objects are colored positive or negative. It will purify and illuminate them all in stillness. This is why the phrase "morally self-regulating" applies to all true samyama practice.

The emotional coloring itself brings in the power of the bhakti element (negative emotions can be used positively), though we should not go out of our way to be emotionally coloring thoughts during samyama, as it can impede the process of releasing. If the emotional charge is there already, this is good, but we should not be trying to create it during samyama practice itself. It will divide the mind.

In the section of the Samyama book on expanded applications it is suggested that those who are inclined to work on "world problems" can do so with samyama on emotionally charged words like: *poverty, hunger, disease, fear, hatred, war, and so on...*

Samyama will not increase the power of these emotionally charged ideas, but dissolve them bit by bit in the light of pure awareness, yielding outpourings of divine love. The more people who are doing this around the world in unstructured or structured ways, the more dissolving of the obstructions (contracted awareness) there will be.

Well, this is looking a bit beyond the insightful individual application you have shared, but I could not resist pointing out the connection. The microcosm is the macrocosm, and our influence within stillness can be expressed accordingly without limits. :-)

Carry on!

The guru is in you.

2008/02/22 12:34:22
Other Systems and Alternate Approaches
http://www.aypsite.org/forum/topic.asp?TOPIC_ID=3489&REPLY_ID=30424&whichpage=-1
Something to try...

quote:
_____
Originally posted by Shanti

"Getting" samyama played a big part in getting this. In Samyama tho.. we pick the word and drop it and rest in the silence and feel the silence move outwards (at least that is what I do).. in this case tho it's slightly reversed.. it is while I pick the thought (word) I stop. It almost feels like.. since I was going to bring up a thought and did not do so.. I feel like I have access to the energy that was going to be used to make that thought (maybe that is why Louis, you felt the energy in your sutra).
_____

Hi Shanti and All:

Recall that the original instruction for picking up a sutra in samyama is to pick it up at a very faint and fuzzy level. This can also be interpreted to mean "the energy before the thought."

Few can do this in the beginning, so we go through the procedure in fairly external and clunky ways in the mind for a while. But, in time, the procedure refines, as is the case in all practices, and then we are touching those sutras before they become objects in the mind, just as you are describing. And, yes, then we have access to much more energy in practice ... and in daily activity as the habit of samyama becomes gradually more prevalent in our everyday life.

The more we are picking up pre-thought, the more powerful samyama is, and the less we are grinding on gross thinking in the body-mind. This is a natural evolution that comes with deep meditation (cultivating the witness) and samyama (cultivating action from within the witness). It can't be forced. It is an evolution in stillness. We just favor less, and less will gradually come. And, as we know, less is more. :-)

Some might ask, what is the difference between samyama and self-inquiry?

There is an intimate relationship between the two practices for sure, and this is pointed out in the Self-Inquiry book. We could say that, in the beginning, self-inquiry is a less structured and more free-ranging practice we can do informally as we go about our business every day, assuming we have enough abiding inner silence to fuel a "relational" practice. There can be much benefit in it.

Samyama, on the other hand, is structured within our twice-daily sitting routine, and creeps out as an inner habit into daily living from there along with abiding inner silence. Perhaps in the long run there is no difference at all between samyama and self-inquiry, as we find ourselves operating more and more from within stillness. When we can experience a sutra before it forms, then we also will have the abilty to experience all thoughts and perceptions before they form, and then can allow action to flow from within stillness all the way out. Stillness in action...

Another way to look at it might be to say that deep meditation and samyama are structured methods for developing the ability to live as stillness in action, while self-inquiry is how we can exercise that growing ability in real life situations.

That is what we are talking about here in a very practical way. Beautiful! :-)

The guru is in you.

2008/03/15 13:52:10
Other Systems and Alternate Approaches
http://www.aypsite.org/forum/topic.asp?TOPIC_ID=3580&REPLY_ID=31338&whichpage=-1
Squatting Bandha

Hi John:

You may find these two lessons to be of interest:
http://www.aypsite.org/92.html
http://www.aypsite.org/179.html

Variations of the tunnel (concentric circles) experience are pretty common among practitioners, with star, stars, or light at the end (or in the center). It is an "effect" of practices -- purification and opening yielding a clearer view of our inner dimensions. In time, it is all seen to be *stillness in action*, inside and outside.

Then geography becomes holography, where one thing (pure awareness -- our *Self*) is realized to be the projected reality in all things. Non-duality and duality rolled into *One*.

All the "looking" in the world will not bring about this realization. Only effective structured practices will. That's why we favor our practices over the lovely scenery encountered along the way.

Look, enjoy, and move on. :-)

All the best!

The guru is in you.

PS: By the way, seeing the inner tunnel and light is not a prerequisite for ongoing spiritual progress, or for enlightenment. Many do just fine without it. Therefore, making this particular (or any) experience a goal of practice will not necessarily be a long term aid on the path. The success of the vision will be found in our moving beyond it. That's what practices are for.

2008/03/16 11:19:40
Other Systems and Alternate Approaches
http://www.aypsite.org/forum/topic.asp?TOPIC_ID=3580&REPLY_ID=31367&whichpage=-1
Squatting Bandha

Hi All:

It should also be added that the real frontier of spiritual progress is found in our daily activities. Are we more at peace, more creative, more joyous, more inclined to help others?

Whiz-bang internal experiences pale in comparison to the improvements in quality of ordinary life that can be cultivated through daily practices.

Extraordinary ordinariness! Why settle for less? :-)

The guru is in you.

2008/07/17 12:16:15
Other Systems and Alternate Approaches
http://www.aypsite.org/forum/topic.asp?TOPIC_ID=3691&REPLY_ID=35582&whichpage=-1
Where am I at now?

Hi TI:

The topic and post links do not change when a topic is moved, and all new posts are highlighted with pink folders and appear in the active topics list where everyone can see, so nothing is lost. It has just been moved to where it belongs.

Your exploration is very interesting and educational for many, but it has little to do with the AYP system of practices, and can be confusing to newcomers looking for support in the AYP practices. That is why we have the "other systems" forum category, for all these other explorations and practice discussions, which are very valuable, but should be clearly distinguished from the AYP system. The "other systems" category accomplishes that. Also, if you are giving advice on practices, it does not hurt to mention whether that advice is consistent with the AYP system or not, if it is not obvious already. It helps minimize the confusion factor for the many who are reading here.

No topic would ever be deleted unless it was grossly offensive to the readership, and then only after multiple efforts by the moderators to address the offenses with those committing them. Your topic does not resemble that kind of scenario at all. It's a great topic, and now it is in the right place. So carry on... :-)

All the best!

The guru is in you.

2008/07/17 16:53:38
Other Systems and Alternate Approaches
http://www.aypsite.org/forum/topic.asp?TOPIC_ID=3691&REPLY_ID=35589&whichpage=-1
Where am I at now?

Hi TI:

The topic and post ID numbers do not change when a topic is moved, and the URL has not changed. This topic is ID=3691, and it will always be that. The forum number is not part of the topic URL. The database knows which forum category to go to by internal means.

If you find any previous links that are not working anymore, let me know. I'd be curious to find out why, since none of the URL info has changed. We have been moving topics for years, and as far as I know we have not lost a link yet.

Your ruminations are an interesting study, if not a clear path that anyone could follow, and I hope you will continue recording your journey. It will be interesting to see where you end up.

Where are we at now? :-)

The guru is in you.

2008/07/17 23:53:10
Other Systems and Alternate Approaches
http://www.aypsite.org/forum/topic.asp?TOPIC_ID=3691&REPLY_ID=35595&whichpage=-1
Where am I at now?

Hi TI:

The first link you gave is for page 4 of the topic. The next one is for page 5. If you copy the one for this page, it will be page 6. Moving right along. :-)

These link variations have nothing to do with the topic moving.

If you want to make a link to a particular post, click the little globe in the top bar of the post and it will give it to you.

The guru is in you.

2008/08/07 18:52:29
Other Systems and Alternate Approaches
http://www.aypsite.org/forum/topic.asp?TOPIC_ID=3691&REPLY_ID=36119&whichpage=-1
Where am I at now?

Hi TI:

I don't think it says anywhere in the AYP writings that we are supposed to "ignore" the scenery of our experiences. What it says is to "favor our practice over the scenery." When we are not practicing, we can enjoy the scenery all we like, or allow it in a self-inquiring way, if we have abiding inner silence (the witness) present.

We are not running away from anything. We are going toward something -- the procedure of our practice when we are sitting, or the routine of our life during everyday activities.

So, it is about favoring our practice, whatever it is. The real issue here is, What is your practice?

If we do not have a well-established practice, what can we favor? The endless confusion of mind stuff, that's what.

The truth is that changing the practice every week, day, or hour is no practice at all, and no one can get very far with that approach. It is just an endless kaleidoscope of mind stuff. If we want to find water, we have to learn to dig in one place for quite a while (for as long as it takes). Until we get that key point, it will just be more of the same. There is no getting around it.

So, it is suggested to pick a practice (any practice!) and stick with it exclusively for at least 6 months. Then you can see what is happening with that, and will have a much better chance for steady progress. Your spiritual progress depends on developing that kind of consistency more than anything else you have brought up here.

It is your choice, of course. All the best! :-)

The guru is in you.

2008/08/08 12:18:02
Other Systems and Alternate Approaches
http://www.aypsite.org/forum/topic.asp?TOPIC_ID=3691&REPLY_ID=36136&whichpage=-1

Where am I at now?

Hi TI:

I am not suggesting you become a practitioner of the AYP system. Only that you stick with one system (any system) for a while. That, and clearing up the "favoring the practice over the scenery" issue, were the only points I hoped to get across.

On the latter, if we are practicing one system and then become attracted to another system during our session (no matter what it is), that is just part of the scenery of that session, and we easily favor what our practice is. If we want to change systems, then we can make that decision in a logical fashion later on outside practices, based on a much broader assessment than a vision we have had somewhere in the foggy depths of our purification process (or the latest book we happened to read). Changing our practice is a big decision that ought not be taken lightly. If we find ourselves making these kinds of assessments and changes daily or weekly, both inside and outside our practice sessions, then we'd better step back and ask ourselves what it is we are doing. What will be the blueprint and support system for our path and our progress? Even the "no-practice" paths have blueprints and support systems.

I can't really advise you on Buddhist practices or other systems, but can say that using visions for objects of meditation is problematic, because sometimes they will be there and sometimes they won't. The payoff in meditation is in using the same object every day over a long period of time. Then we go deep. This is the advantage that a mantra brings. It will always be there at whatever level of consciousness we happen to be, and can serve us over the long term as we cultivate and stabilize inner silence in our life. This kind of stable practice also provides a foundation for additional practices that take advantage of rising inner silence. It is a systematic approach with a long term view.

Regarding your comment about "exploding" a vision, to what end? Inner silence? Well, we don't need pyrotechics for that. But if that is a system that interests you, and it has an established teaching with a track record, and you want to go that way, then do that. And stick with it.

And, yes, this is not about me. It is about you, your choices and your journey. AYP is a toolbox, but not the only toolbox. It is best to be using primarily one toolbox at a time, and use it deeply, _becoming_ its most subtle nuance. It takes time. Jumping from toolbox to toolbox, or trying to use multiple toolboxes at the same time, will not work. There will be no depth or nuance, except the nuance of the mind, which is illusion.

I'm very happy to hear you have gained some benefit from the AYP writings, though I cannot trust that you have given the practices their due, or any non-AYP practice you have been discussing here either. It is not an easy position for a teacher to be in, and that is why I rarely come into this topic. I think a teacher from any other system you have dabbled in would feel the same way. A teacher is obliged to be as clear and straightforward as possible, not too much of a moving target. A student has a similar obligation, to him/herself. Without some consistency on both sides, it will not work. That leaves the student to reinvent the wheel alone. It might seem like fun for a while, but in time it will prove to be the most difficult and unreliable path -- a multi-layered labyrinth that could take lifetimes to find a way out of.

But that is life, isn't it? We are all attempting to cross over -- some in big boats, some in small boats, and some with no boat and swimming in circles. :-)

All the best!

The guru is in you.

2008/08/09 00:55:04
Other Systems and Alternate Approaches
http://www.aypsite.org/forum/topic.asp?TOPIC_ID=3691&REPLY_ID=36154&whichpage=-1
Where am I at now?

Hi TI:

No, you have not been practicing AYP. You have been using the AYP toolbox as a mobile platform to try dozens of other things, constantly modifying, blending, adding, subtracting, etc., and it continues with fundamental alterations in practice mentioned in your last note. It is a constant stream of short-lived experiments. That is fine if it works for you, but it should not be presented as "practicing AYP," because it isn't, and it will be confusing to anyone in the learning stage. Don't forget, there are many new practitioners visiting these forums.

It is one of the reasons why I say the forums are not the place to learn the AYP practices. The forums are a great place for open discussions on practices and experiences, which are very welcome, but it is best to go back to the lessons for the practices themselves.

If it is any consolation, I am honored that you have chosen to use AYP as a loose baseline for your wide-ranging experiments. That is something. But neither I nor anyone can predict the long term results. There is no blueprint and no support system that can affirm what you are doing.

One thing I can tell you is that if you are not using the rise of inner silence in daily living as a primary metric, and doing what is necessary to cultivate it, then you will miss the boat. All the rest of the stuff, as flashy as it may be, is small potatoes. So please do keep that in mind.

The guru is in you.

2008/08/09 13:59:42
Other Systems and Alternate Approaches
http://www.aypsite.org/forum/topic.asp?TOPIC_ID=3691&REPLY_ID=36170&whichpage=-1
Where am I at now?

Hi Dave:

Thanks for chiming in. I thought you might, since your system of practice has been mixed and matched here, along with many others. :-)

TI cannot be faulted for his enthusiasm, or for wanting it all right now via a Muktananda or Krishnamurti-style "spontaneaous awakening." But can this be accomplished by focusing on the extreme symptoms of such an event, or on fragments of practice that may have led to it? Not likely. In fact, many would prefer to avoid the extreme symptoms, and this is possible. See here for more on dramatic spontaneous awakenings.

That is the ongoing issue with the spontaneously enlightened. They (or their symptoms) are often mimicked at the expense of sound practices that will bring about the desired result. If an awakening occurs without significant practices in this lifetime, the teaching by the spontaneously enlightened person will often be limited on effective means, and over-exaggerated on recreating the appearance of the end result.

We are seeing light shades of this more and more often in AYP, with some finding themselves experiencing non-duality in what seems a spontaneous manner. I aways remind those having these experiences to be sure to let people know what practices came before that led them to the experience of non-duality. Good things are happening for sure, and we must not forget how we got here, so many others can follow.

It is not wrong to want it all right now, but an effective systematic approach is going to be necessary for the vast majority of aspirants. With that, anyone can do it.

Even so, a spontaneous awakening may happen for TI, with all the attendant fireworks. He wants that, and we can wish it for him.

But it will not change the underlying fact that the end result is not the path. Hence the great value of reliable systems of practice that cultivate the condition of abiding inner silence (samadhi). With *That*, our awakening is assured.

The guru is in you.

2010/02/16 10:10:54
Other Systems and Alternate Approaches
http://www.aypsite.org/forum/topic.asp?TOPIC_ID=3691&REPLY_ID=64954&whichpage=-1
Where am I at now?

quote:
_____
Originally posted by Tibetan_Ice

To this day I still feel like I have not found the 'inner silence' during mantra meditation. I have found some very quiet spaces but in those quiet spaces there have always existed the visions and/or lights/colors so I still don't know if this would qualify as 'inner silence'.
_____

Hi TI:

It is because for the most part you are not meditating, which is a very simple and consistent procedure. Instead, you are totally into observing the "scenery," analyzing it, endlessly modifying the practice to play in it, reporting on it, etc. That is not meditation. If you just let go of all that and do the simple procedure, no matter what, you will experience inner silence in no time. And, in time, you will become inner silence 24/7. That is worth a million times all the scenery we could ever have. It's not about the scenery. When you get that, you will be meditating like a champ. :-)

All the best!

The guru is in you.

PS: Have you read the AYP Deep Meditation Book? I mean really read it? If you want abiding inner silence (the peace that surpasses all understanding), that will tell you how. The rest is up to you.

2010/02/16 23:54:24
Other Systems and Alternate Approaches
http://www.aypsite.org/forum/topic.asp?TOPIC_ID=3691&REPLY_ID=64971&whichpage=-1
Where am I at now?

quote:
_____
Originally posted by Tibetan_Ice

Are you saying that there are no lights that can be seen during inner silence and that if you see lights you are not in inner silence? Is inner silence black or formless?
_____

Hi TI:

Not saying that at all. Experiences can be anything. Anything at all. Today they are one thing. Tomorrow they will be something else. It does not matter what they are. I am not saying that experiences are to be shunned or condemned. I am saying that the content of experiences is not relevant during the simple procedure of meditation.

So why do you keep asking about content? The fixation on content in meditation is an obstacle. If you can regard that need for content to be like any other thought and easily favor the mantra whenever the "sight-seer" appears in a session, you will have it. As long as you are actively looking for content to evaluate, favoring that, you will not be meditating.

You can be a tourist, or you can be a meditator. But you can't be both at the same time. You do have a choice, you know. Nothing is etched in stone. :-)

The guru is in you.

2010/02/17 10:25:35
Other Systems and Alternate Approaches
http://www.aypsite.org/forum/topic.asp?TOPIC_ID=3691&REPLY_ID=64993&whichpage=-1
Where am I at now?

Hi Ananda and TI:

We can have all the scenery, but should not forget that it is the cultivation of inner silence that produces the scenery, not the other way around. When we are meditating, that is one thing. When we are riding off to Tandraloka, that is something else. We cannot do both at the same time. That is the point.

That's why when we are meditating and that golden chariot rolls up, we will be wise to favor the mantra. The chariot will also be there later, especially if we have been effective in our meditation practice over time. Abiding inner silence is the doorway to everything, not the least of which is the end of suffering.

The guru is in you.

2010/02/18 09:57:21
Other Systems and Alternate Approaches
http://www.aypsite.org/forum/topic.asp?TOPIC_ID=3691&REPLY_ID=65028&whichpage=-1
Where am I at now?

Hi TI:

Any or all of the variations in experience (and mantra) you mentioned above are fine. The particulars are not important. What is important is the intention.

If the intention is to favor the mantra when we realize we are off it, and allow it to go however it will (patterns do not matter), then this will lead to losing (refinement) of the mantra, which is the cultivation of inner silence. This is the process we keep repeating easily for the allotted time of our meditation session.

If the intention is to analyze, control, question, modify, report, etc., this will not be meditation. And it will not matter what system of meditation we may be following. All meditation procedures involve systematically going beyond the object, whether it be mantra, breath, nada, vision, sensation, concept, or whatever.

It is dharana (attention on an object), becoming dhyana (natural dissolving of the object), becoming samad
Hi (absorption in inner silence). These are the last three limbs of the eight limbs of yoga, which gives an indication of how important this process is in the overall scheme of yoga. Samyama also utilizes these three limbs, in a different way.

Obviously, choosing and sticking with a method of meditation is important. We can't cross the vast ocean of samsara (impurity/illusion) in two or more boats at the same time. It is all about developing and maintaining consistency in practice over time.

This is the only question we need to be asking ourselves about meditation: "Am I in a consistent practice with a proven method?" All the rest is diversion.

We can never, ever, ever! put it in a mental bottle. Meditation is about emptying the bottle, and dissolving the bottle. So all this talk is not very relevant - only to get rid of doubts about the simplicity of sitting down and doing it every day. That's all. If it is going to keep going in endless circles of mental analysis, etc., don't expect any serious meditator to take that ride with you for long. It is not about creating complexity. It is about releasing into simplicity. Meditation is for that.

The guru is in you.

2010/04/20 16:25:15
Other Systems and Alternate Approaches
http://www.aypsite.org/forum/topic.asp?TOPIC_ID=3691&REPLY_ID=67504&whichpage=-1
Where am I at now?

Hi TI:

Your experiences are not so unusual. What seems unusual is the tendency to analyze during practice, which can become an obstruction if favored. Therefore, when analysis comes, just ease back to the mantra. That's all that is necessary. It is not a focusing. It is a gentle favoring when we notice we are off into something else. It does not matter what that something else is.

I am sure a "Buddhist map" can tell you exactly where you are with experiences in the overall scheme of things, usually at the expense of continuing progress. Figuring out where we are has absolutely nothing to do with our spiritual progress, and, in fact, can arrest our progress in "analysis paralysis."

Both Buddhists and yogis in the know will tell you the same thing: Keep practicing with consistency, favoring the procedure of your practice over the scenery along the way. This is not a guarantee of consistent experiences of any kind during practice. It will, however, guarantee your progress.

Anything can happen in practice, with thoughts, visions, lights, sounds, and all the rest. The mantra can be big, small, loud, soft, flat, shimmering, clear, fuzzy, irritating, ecstatic, anything. And, yes, it can go on for days, weeks, or months in a particular mode, until purification and opening lead us into more realms of inner stuff that are purifying and opening. None of it matters in relation to the procedure of meditation.

What matters is how we are feeling during the day. Are we more relaxed, energetic, creative, loving, finding more synergies occurring naturally in our life's journey? These are the things that indicate that our practice is working. This is where practices pay off, not in what happens while we are sitting in meditation.

The only reason to discuss experiences that occur in meditation is to coax practitioners back to application of the procedure, and to boost confidence to proceed with consistency. Other than that, there isn't any reason to discuss the scenery. It is yours, and you can enjoy it if you like. Whatever is there is there until it isn't anymore, and there is no point in fretting about anything being there or not being there.

It is your practice. It is suggested to continue with it and see what is happening outside practice in ordinary living. If you keep doing the practice according to procedure, forget about the internals of it, and go out and live fully, the results will be there.

It is your path and your choice. Carry on!

The guru is in you.

PS: Yes, crown practices, taken to excess, can lead to instabilities. That's old news around here. :-)

2008/05/09 00:01:25
Other Systems and Alternate Approaches
http://www.aypsite.org/forum/topic.asp?TOPIC_ID=3851&REPLY_ID=33546&whichpage=-1
Psychicisation

quote:
_____
Originally posted by Gnosis

To be honest, I would like to get Yogani's take on this. I have never heard of meditation being used to predict the future with any precision or accuracy. I don't even think you can compare meditation and divination it's like comparing an apple to a screw driver, two completely different things.
_____

Hi Gnosis:

Well, since you asked... :-)

Nothing that attempts to predict the future in objective terms can be considered to be spiritual practice, regardless of whether it works or not, because all spiritual practice is about living in the continuum of the present. It is fine to read the weather report, but that has little to do with spiritual practices like deep meditation. "Apple versus screw driver," as you say.

Does deep meditation enable us to know the future objectively? No. But deep meditation and related practices do bring the future continuously into our now, meaning, we become harmonized with the flow of karma. Not eliminating karma, but transforming its influence through stillness in action flowing naturally through us. Then there are no threats, no dangers lurking around the corner which we must anticipate. Only the ever-flowing present, and the flow of divine love in the now. In strange (some might say miraculous) ways, seasoned meditators seem to avoid the so-called negatives of life, even when the same things are happening that others may consider negative. The entire perception of life is changed, not able to impinge on who we are -- inner silence. Then we are more able to act in ways that serve the common good, rather than avoid. It is very practical.

A seasoned meditator may lose interest in reading the weather report, because even when it rains the meditator will rarely get wet. And if she does, it will usually be for a good reason, and there will be laughter. That is how it goes. It is a very free life, with minimal calculations. It is also a very responsible approach to life. It takes time in daily sitting practices and in daily activity to gradually cultivate this mode of functioning. It is worth doing.

It is fine to explore divination and such if that is what interests you. Maybe you will tire of it in time. Maybe not. Either way, it has not got much to do with effective spiritual practices, which is what most people are interested in here. To the extent the results of divination distract from spiritual practices and living fully, it can be a liability like any obsession, and that is for you to figure out as you move forward. Time tends to take care of everything, especially for those who meditate.

It is suggested to keep up your daily spiritual practices. That way you get to have your cake and eat it too -- pursuing your present desires, while gradually going beyond them to fulfill your highest ideal. Your spiritual evolution will take care of everything as long as you are cultivating it daily. Do remind yourself every now and then that enlightenment can never be calculated, only cultivated. Enlightenment is the gradual release of calculation, and the natural transcendence of karma.

That is the difference between an apple and a screw driver. Be mindful not to lose one for the sake of the other. :-)

All the best!

The guru is in you.

2008/05/09 15:13:04
Other Systems and Alternate Approaches
http://www.aypsite.org/forum/topic.asp?TOPIC_ID=3851&REPLY_ID=33563&whichpage=-1
Psychicisation

Hi Gnosis:

What you may not know is that some with opinions on divination have formed those opinions based on long experience in the same tracks you are mentioning, and more. So what you think you know exclusively may well have been let go (or is still used) by others after much previous exposure. Don't be so quick to rule out other opinions for convenience. Most people here speak from hard-won experience.

One thing is for sure. A sage (or entire tradition) may offer effective knowledge with one hand and not so effective knowledge with the other. It is always going to be a mixed bag. It is up to us to intuit what is true for us and move ahead, leaving the rest behind. This is most effectively done in stillness, which is an important benefit of deep meditation -- the rise of spiritual discrimination. The more we rely on others to make these choices for us, the more stuck and vulnerable we will become. That is not divination -- it is fact.

We can only become self-reliant by cultivating realization of our silent Self. The same will be true for those who come to us for advice, and we have a responsibility to give clear guidance that will minimize codependent relationships.

Realization is not an over-night event. Those who say it is instant are speaking only for themselves (maybe), and certainly not for anyone else. The answer cannot be found in words, books, or calculated opinions. It is within us, and is known in stillness as we advance in practices. In the end, it is an outpouring of divine love that answers all questions before they are asked, which is life in natural flow, always in the present. That is real divination.

Practice wisely, and enjoy!

The guru is in you.

2008/07/16 14:11:42
Other Systems and Alternate Approaches
http://www.aypsite.org/forum/topic.asp?TOPIC_ID=4120&REPLY_ID=35564&whichpage=-1
Prana Vidya, Anyone?

Hi All:

I too have found the excellent Satyananda and Bihar books to be very helpful over the years, even though they take a somewhat different angle than AYP on unfolding human spiritual transformation -- more hatha and sannyasin oriented and less deep meditation, samyama, hatha and tantra in-the-world oriented.

Whatever works. All paths lead home, as long as we can stay on one. :-)

The guru is in you.

2008/07/23 11:26:14
Other Systems and Alternate Approaches
http://www.aypsite.org/forum/topic.asp?TOPIC_ID=4120&REPLY_ID=35701&whichpage=-1
Prana Vidya, Anyone?

Hi John:

While I agree that spinal breathing may be considered to be part of prana vidya, by whatever definition, I do not agree that any form of pranayama can be rightly called meditation. While some systems take this approach, it is not what we are teaching in AYP, and not consistent with the yoga sutras of Patanjali either, which clearly delineate the practices of pranayama and meditation as two of the eight limbs of yoga. Nevertheless, many systems combine them in practice, at the risk of missing the full benefit of both practices, deep meditation in particular.

This is an important point, and is at the heart of distinguishing paths that tend to be hatha-oriented from those that are broader in approach and address deep meditation as a separate and distinct practice. I'm sure the debate will go on, and all I am saying here is that we should make the distinction between the two approaches, so we might someday know the truth about it, hopefully by the benefit of our own experience. :-)

The discussion about pranayama not being meditation, or visa versa, has occurred several times before in the forums in relation to various Yoga and Buddhist systems of breath awareness. It is covered in the AYP lessons also. The essence of the debate from this side is that, while the breath can provide an object for meditation up to a point, it ceases when the breath naturally suspends, thus curtailing the opportunity for "deep meditation" leading to the full cultivation of abiding inner silence (samadhi). As you know, in AYP deep meditation we use an inward sound as the object (mantra), and the inevitable natural suspension of breath presents no limitation in this. In AYP, we do our spinal breathing pranayama as a separate practice before deep meditation. This provides for the full benefit of both practices.

On a related point, which is often asked about, favoring breath awareness at the same time while using the mantra is not recommended, because it divides the mind and waters down the effect of deep meditation. The breath is treated like any other thought, sensation or experience that may come up during deep meditation -- the mantra is easily favored again when we notice that we are not on it.

Pranayama, depending on the technique used (practiced separate from deep meditation in AYP), can deliver a settling of the nervous system, the balanced awakening of ecstatic conductivity, and the introversion of sensory perception (pratyahara). This is both a preparation for deep meditation and an important component of human spiritual transformation. But it is not samadhi, which requires systematic means to go much deeper to inner silence. In the end, it is the natural joining of these two cultivated qualities (ecstatic conductivity and abiding inner silence) that enable the enlightened condition to flower in ordinary life -- stillness in action, which is an endless outpouring of divine love.

Well, not to belabor the point, but it usually gets me going when pranayama is called meditation, or visa versa, because blurring the lines can blur the practice, and there is no telling how far off we might wander. That is from the AYP point of view, of course, which I am obliged to present. Everyone must make their own distinctions and choices about these things. When in doubt, check the yoga sutras, where the benefits of integrated yoga practice are beautifully expressed. Or maybe check the AYP lessons? And, by all means, continue to explore the possibilities ... rhetorically, or otherwise... :-)

All the best!

The guru is in you.

2008/07/24 12:02:33
Other Systems and Alternate Approaches
http://www.aypsite.org/forum/topic.asp?TOPIC_ID=4120&REPLY_ID=35732&whichpage=-1
Prana Vidya, Anyone?

Hi John:

That is wonderful, and no one can deny your experience, least of all me. :-)

Nevertheless, I think is important to remain clear about the distinctions between pranayama and meditation. The traditions that have smooshed them together into a singular concept and practice have often done so at a cost to their practitioners, which can be seen in results over the long run.

Another way to look at it is to say:

Pranayama is the control and enlivenment of prana.
Meditation is the transcendence of prana.

Is there some overlap? Yes, certainly. But one function cannot replace the other. By whatever means, we need both functions operating in daily practice to move forward toward enlightenment.

The guru is in you.

PS: It might be helpful to look back at your practices over the years and see how much has been meditation and how much has been prana/energy-related practices. I recall you have been very strong on mantra use in the past. Could it be your pranayama is doing so well in transcendence now because of your background in meditation? Often times, present experiences on our path are not so much about what we have been doing lately, but more about what we have been doing over the long term in the past -- laying the groundwork for breakthroughs with minimal additional cultivation required. In other words, we get ripe.

Teachers sometimes make the mistake of focusing too much on the "what I have done lately" (epitomized in the saying, "Be here now!"), rather than the forgotten years/decades of effective practices that have formed the foundation of purification and opening that can now be enjoyed in the present with a little bhakti, pranayama, self-inquiry, whole body mudra, or whatever.

Just some food for thought...

Whatever the case may be, it is suggested to keep things in balance going forward, and enjoy! :-)

2008/11/28 18:25:12
Other Systems and Alternate Approaches
http://www.aypsite.org/forum/topic.asp?TOPIC_ID=4541&REPLY_ID=41429&whichpage=-1
May I introduce the highest Buddhist practice?

quote:
_____
Originally posted by Suryakant

quote:
_____
Originally posted by themysticseeker

What the hell does the rainbow body have to do with leading people out of suffering and into the path of enlightenment?
_____
Unless one is perfectly enlightened, one does not know with absolute metaphysical certainty whether or not any given individual's particular path of enlightenment may or may not require said individual to temporarily engage concepts such as, for example, the Tibetan Buddhist rainbow body.
_____

Hi All:

Yes, isn't it ironic that when we feel we have transcended our intellect, the first thing we do is judge the paths of others with our intellect?

It is a common mistake made by those who profess non-duality (real or imagined). It boils down to an assumption of our exclusive correctness, and then the teaching automatically becomes simplified down to the statement: "Just be, like me."

And to blazes with what everyone else is doing!

There are certainly next steps beyond that narrow view, where we can begin to see that everyone is on a valid path in their own right, and we learn to respect that and share in ways that can help aspirants move forward from where they are, instead of from where we are. The latter is impossible, you know.

Unfortunately, many buy into this kind of faulty teaching, but maybe not so much around these parts, where a broader view tends to prevail. It keeps us all honest. :-)

The guru is in you.

2008/11/28 18:40:33
Other Systems and Alternate Approaches
http://www.aypsite.org/forum/topic.asp?TOPIC_ID=4541&REPLY_ID=41430&whichpage=-1
May I introduce the highest Buddhist practice?
PS: As many here know, the advice in AYP is to favor the practice (whatever our practice is) over the scenery (whatever the scenery may be). If the practice is effective, in time we will know the truth. We will know it by direct experience, not by what anyone else tells us it is, or is not.
2008/11/28 22:20:01
Other Systems and Alternate Approaches
http://www.aypsite.org/forum/topic.asp?TOPIC_ID=4541&REPLY_ID=41444&whichpage=-1
May I introduce the highest Buddhist practice?

Hi TMS:

But what if you are wrong? To whom else (living) can you point for verification of what you are saying? And how can everyone benefit similarly without falling into despair over the life they are now living? Despair is the fruit of a path based on the intellectual gymnastics of nothingness. There are many here who can verify that.

These are legitimate questions that a traveler may ask of one who claims to know the way. All you have shared so far is concepts, criticisms of what others are doing, and some methods that may or may not deliver.

Incidentally, the breath retention method you recommend **here** can be destabilizing or outright dangerous for some practitioners. Perhaps it will be better to work on the system rather than on the beliefs of others.

I am not trying to give you a hard time. Well, maybe a little. It is all for the good. :-)

No one here is obliged to take anyone's word for it, least of all mine. The measure of truth is not in our words. If it is to be found anywhere, it will be in reliable means leading to direct experience of the unending freedom we all have longed for. That is all that matters. The proof of the pudding is in the eating.

Your experience and how you arrived in it are of much greater interest than exhortations about how others ought to think and believe. Thanks for sharing.

The guru is in you.

2008/10/30 10:24:29
Other Systems and Alternate Approaches
http://www.aypsite.org/forum/topic.asp?TOPIC_ID=4625&REPLY_ID=39657&whichpage=-1
Question for Buddhists in this forum

Hi Solo, and welcome!

Sorry for the delayed response. Since my background is not in Buddhist practices, I can only offer a limited perspective. Hopefully others with the background will chime in.

It is generally not a good idea to mix practices from several traditions, particularly for beginners. On the other hand, there is the possibility to fill in missing elements of practice by reaching across traditional lines if we are clear about what we are doing.

A good example of this is considering adding mantra-based deep meditation to paths that are limited to pranayama or breath-based meditation methods. The reason for considering this is because effective meditation with mantra (I AM) will go much deeper than meditation with breath, resulting in more effective cultivation of abiding inner silence, which is the cornerstone of all spiritual progress. This is discussed over here:

http://www.aypsite.org/forum/topic.asp?TOPIC_ID=3454#30072
(Also see the rest of the posts in this linked topic)

While advanced methods of Buddhist meditation do cover meditation "beyond the breath," these methods are more complex and not well known. The method of deep meditation we use in AYP is simple and does not require alterations along the way, though optional mantra enhancements are available for those who are stable in practice and inclined to speed up their progress later on.

You might ask: If I take up AYP deep meditation, what happens to my breath-based meditation? Good question, and maybe some who have come from a Buddhist background and are using AYP deep meditation can comment.

The only advice I will give on that is not to try and do both practices at the same time, as this will water down the effects of both. It will take some time to train the attention to easily favor the mantra rather than observing the breath, but it will happen. It is a normal transition of habit in technique, which we deal with often in the AYP system. I believe some here use AYP deep meditation, and then observe the breath at other times during the day, during activity. This is not an AYP instruction, but something that has been mentioned.

The way breath is used in AYP is in pranayama practice, which is not regarded to be meditation, even though the attention is used in particular ways in relation to the breath. Spinal breathing pranayama is the flagship form of pranayama in AYP. All of these methods are covered in the main lessons, linked at the top of this page -- it is suggested to review the lessons in order.

The caution that is always given with regard to combining different systems of practice, is to be careful not to "double up" on similar forms of practice in the same session or day. This is especially true for pranayama, where the effects of different styles will be cumulative and can lead to an energy overload. Sometimes this will come as a delayed effect, days or weeks after practices have been undertaken, so prudent "self-pacing" of practice durations is recommended, even when using AYP practices only.

Whatever you decide to do in practices will be your choice. AYP is an open resource that can be used as much or as little as desired.

Regarding kundalini, that is also covered in the AYP lessons, and extensively in these forums as well, with many individual histories available for review. Feel free to share more about your experiences and ask questions. There are many here who can help, and everyone benefits from the open discussions.

Wishing you all the best on your chosen path. Enjoy!

The guru is in you.

PS: Newpov, you replied here first. Thanks! :-)

2008/10/28 17:27:25
Other Systems and Alternate Approaches
http://www.aypsite.org/forum/topic.asp?TOPIC_ID=4628&REPLY_ID=39577&whichpage=-1
Biblical Translations.

Hi Carson:

It is a debate that has been going on among Christians for a long time. There are many quotes that can be dug up to support either argument. Just Google "kingdom of heaven within." I'd prefer to avoid the academic debate (the mincing of words), because direct experience is what matters to me.

In other words, the best way to find out where the kingdom of heaven is is to go there. Then we know where it is. Of course, that too can be debated endlessly. It is a question of what one prefers, heaven here and now, or heaven far removed and much later. I will take it here and now, thank you very much. That is putting an experience before the idea of an experience, which is more fulfilling. :-)

Did Jesus actually say it? Since the scriptures were written years after his death, it is hard to say. And not all those writings ended up in the New Testament. Did you check the original Greek? The Roman Church (and all churches since) have edited to suit their purposes. Regardless, what we know about the life of Jesus exemplifies the kingdom of heaven being within him, and within all of us, not to mention what is found in all of the world's religions. There is only one truth about human spiritual potentiality. We are confirming that in modern times.

Someone who does not think the kingdom of heaven is within will gain the same benefits from deep meditation as anyone else. We don't have to call it the kingdom of heaven within, and it will be what it is anyway -- how about "inner silence?" If the kingdom of heaven turns out to be somewhere else, we will be much better able to find it with deep meditation and the infinite expansion of abiding inner silence.

Btw, how does your father read the saying from the Psalm: "Be still and know that I am God."?
Never mind!

The guru is in you.

2008/10/28 17:53:08
Other Systems and Alternate Approaches
http://www.aypsite.org/forum/topic.asp?TOPIC_ID=4628&REPLY_ID=39580&whichpage=-1
Biblical Translations.

Hi Carson:

The best argument you can make is to go on living your life the best you can, walking ahead in your own truth.

It is a bit late to change that quote, since it is in the AYP books also. Well, I am in good company. Many Christians have heard the words (seen the life) of Jesus that way. That is what I heard as a small lad in Sunday school, even if it was never said (it may have been). Some can see that word, "within," and some can't. It will be on the test at the end of the class. :-)

The guru is in you.

2008/10/28 18:08:24
Other Systems and Alternate Approaches
http://www.aypsite.org/forum/topic.asp?TOPIC_ID=4628&REPLY_ID=39581&whichpage=-1
Biblical Translations.
PS: Ironically, the most "fundamental" thing about Christianity is that elusive word and idea, "within." It conveys the essence of all spirituality.

If I were to write a one word scripture, it would say: "Within."

2008/10/28 18:30:14
Other Systems and Alternate Approaches
http://www.aypsite.org/forum/topic.asp?TOPIC_ID=4628&REPLY_ID=39586&whichpage=-1
Biblical Translations.

Hi Carson:

Why compromise later when you can compromise now? You can live your life as you choose, and the rest of your family can live their lives as they choose. There is nothing wrong with a little tolerance. Who knows? If you become more tolerant of them, it might even rub off on those in the family who are prone to judge you. Which is not to say you are responsible for the choices they make in their lives, about you or anything else. You are only responsible for your own choices.

Life really can be that simple and free. :-)

The guru is in you.

2008/10/28 23:52:08
Other Systems and Alternate Approaches
http://www.aypsite.org/forum/topic.asp?TOPIC_ID=4628&REPLY_ID=39599&whichpage=-1
Biblical Translations.

Hi Carson:

We can be tolerant of a noisy neighbor, but if they knock our door down and try to overrun us, we must throw them out ... at least until they develop better manners.

The rose is lovely, but it also has thorns. :-)

The guru is in you.

2008/10/29 11:57:01
Other Systems and Alternate Approaches
http://www.aypsite.org/forum/topic.asp?TOPIC_ID=4628&REPLY_ID=39611&whichpage=-1

Biblical Translations.

Hi Carson:

It always comes back to our own path and our practice. The more steady we become in that, the less others will be able to intrude. And they will know it by our demeanor.

We attract what we get, and the more in abiding stillness we become, the less adversity we will attract, or notice. That is when karma becomes our friend, for all karma is used by stillness in action for an evolutionary outcome. With the family interactions, you are in the early stages of it now. Your urgency and approach will gradually change as you continue forward in being true to yourself. You will know what to do...

Carry on! :-)

The guru is in you.

2008/10/29 12:53:12
Other Systems and Alternate Approaches
http://www.aypsite.org/forum/topic.asp?TOPIC_ID=4628&REPLY_ID=39620&whichpage=-1
Biblical Translations.

Hi Carson:

Your main risk in all of this is bending back to the will of others, which is how you got spun off in the first place. Ironically, it is the rigidity of your family on spiritual matters that led you to the path you are on now, traveling by a difficult route to be sure. But here you are. If you put their will over your path, you could land back in the soup. I don't think that will happen at this late stage, but thought to mention it anyway.

Your youth as described reminds me of a troubling documentary called "Jesus Camp," which is about extremist fundamentalist Christians deliberately brainwashing their children. Most rational people see it as child abuse, but the perpetrators see it as God's will.

I agree with Christi that discussing religion with your family probably has more downside in it than upside. Just live!

Wow Christi. What a beautiful post on Christian roots. Thanks! :-)

The guru is in you.

2008/11/21 09:52:52
Other Systems and Alternate Approaches
http://www.aypsite.org/forum/topic.asp?TOPIC_ID=4776&REPLY_ID=40964&whichpage=-1
witnessing "great happiness" in Vijnana Bhairava

Hi Newpov:

For some additional perspective, here is an AYP lesson on Vigyan Bhairava (spellings of it vary), including a link to the the Paul Reps English translation of the 112 techniques: http://www.aypsite.org/T21.html

It is an amazing scripture for sure, and one of the oldest, covering a range of practices for cultivating human spiritual transformation.

In the case of the linked lesson, the Vigyan Bhairava was quoted to highlight the essential principle in tantric sex. It is technique #43, and that passage was also used as the dedication at the front of the AYP Tantra book.

All the best!

The guru is in you.

2008/12/16 14:06:53
Other Systems and Alternate Approaches
http://www.aypsite.org/forum/topic.asp?TOPIC_ID=4865&REPLY_ID=42457&whichpage=-1
Guided Deep Meditation

quote:
───────
Originally posted by riptiz

Hi Carson,
I don't think anything regarding the distribution of the cd. I don't own the copyright.Perhaps if guruji can find someone with the skills to market it online then he will do.I will ask him at the end of the month when I return to the ashram.Perhaps you might point me in the direction needed for online distribution.
L&L
Dave
───────

Hi Dave:

www.cdbaby.com (in USA) covers CD and MP3 distribution through many major channels -- Amazon, iTunes, CD stores, etc. You can also buy CDs and MP3s on their site. They are one of the largest and most reputable for independent recording artists. It takes time and effort to get set up with them (but not expensive). In the long run it is worth it. All of the AYP audio is there (nine audiobooks). We also do direct MP3 and ebook downloads through http://www.e-junkie.com

644 –   Advanced Yoga Practices

and http://www.payloadz.com

You have to come up with the CDs for CDBaby. They are distribution only. There are also "CD on demand" companies that can do both production and distribution, but I know less about them. In today's market, you can do fine with MP3s only. CDs are in demand less and less.

Good luck!

The guru is in you.

2008/12/16 14:33:11
Other Systems and Alternate Approaches
http://www.aypsite.org/forum/topic.asp?TOPIC_ID=4869&REPLY_ID=42458&whichpage=-1
Holding the breath while walking

Hi All:

There are two sides to this.

For those in good health, holding breath in athletics is not usually harmful, though there are reasonable limits in everything.

For those using daily yoga practices, holding breath can lead to accelerated kundalini awakening, especially if breath retention (kumbhaka) is incorporated into a full routine of practices including deep meditation, several kinds of pranayama, asanas, mudras, bandhas, tantric practices, etc. An energy awakening can happen with delayed effect and much discomfort for a long time if breath retention is taken to excess in yoga practices. A dramatic instance of this is covered in the Secrets of Wilder novel, and it is covered in the AYP lessons also. There are first hand reports on it here in the forums as well. Many email correspondences here over the years have been about kundalini difficulties caused by excessive breath retention.

In yoga, a little bit of breath retention goes a long way. Self-pacing in practice is very important, which may include tempering our bhakti (spiritual desire) a bit at times. We each must find our balance, and take into account the time delayed effects associated with breath retention in yoga.

For some lessons on how breath retention is used in conjunction with AYP practices, see "kumbhaka" in the website topic index.

Where do athletics end and yoga begin? That is for each practitioner to determine by direct experience. :-)

All the best!

The guru is in you.

2008/12/20 10:53:58
Other Systems and Alternate Approaches
http://www.aypsite.org/forum/topic.asp?TOPIC_ID=4894&REPLY_ID=42649&whichpage=-1
osho critical/ against transcendental meditation

Hi YB:

Yes, karma is the answer -- the result of past actions in thought, word and deed, which leave latent impressions on all levels of mental, emotional and physical life.

The primary way of unwinding the latent impressions of karma is not in changing behaviors, nor in dwelling on regret, but in transcending behaviors in stillness through deep meditation. Then both the latent impressions and the behaviors that have caused them become gradually less. We have more freedom to choose (and inquire). Then it is no longer action creating latent impressions, but stillness in action (outpouring divine love) leaving very little impression at all.

Those who are engaged in daily deep meditation notice that actions do not leave the same lingering impressions that they did before. Instead, there is a silent inner witness rising amidst all activities. This is because the latent impressions (impurities) of the past are becoming less, there is more inner silence, and this brings rising freedom. This is the process of human spiritual transformation.

This process can be clearly noticed and is often measurable in improving health and well-being, and the rise of abiding happiness in life. Science is taking note. :-)

The guru is in you.

2009/01/12 12:12:25
Other Systems and Alternate Approaches
http://www.aypsite.org/forum/topic.asp?TOPIC_ID=4910&REPLY_ID=43368&whichpage=-1
The One & Only Way

quote:
_____
Originally posted by david_obsidian

So it is -- the Buddha found reification of a Supreme Self to be a problemmatic aspect of teaching, which it can be -- it can get in the way of enlightenment. So he devised a teaching method to get around that problem, that's all. It's not true that he's talking about a different elephant though. He's talking differently about the same elephant.
_____

Hi David and All:

Yes, and that elephant is the human nervous system, with its inherent spiritual capabilities. There is only one of those, and the destination can only be known by the experiencer.

Discussions of a destination or underlying reality are pure speculation, even when presented by the enlightened, because it will mean little to nearly everyone else. Much better we each engage in sound practices and move forward. Then we will find out what it is in daily living, and can share that in our own words, while wisely acknowledging anyone else's sharing of their experience. In that way, we can develop a profile of human enlightenment and the paths to it, without dividing up into armed camps. There is no such thing as a "one and only way." There is a one and only vehicle for spiritual experience, the human nervous system, and many approaches for enabling its full capabilities.

It is about our journey right now, and what means can facilitate our process of inner purification and opening day by day. It is about cause and effect, and our direct experience as we move forward. That is real. Intellectual presentations of the nature of reality, no matter how profound or pedigreed, are unreal.

Direct experience on the level of each individual is the final arbiter of the value of any path. It is not about debating which is the most authentic ancient knowledge. It is about what practices will work to open us in the present. It is not so difficult. We can readily see what works and what does not by optimizing causes and effects in practice.

So, what is the system of practice being proposed here? Or are there several? That is fine too. Whatever works! :-)

The guru is in you.

2009/01/13 00:46:16
Other Systems and Alternate Approaches
http://www.aypsite.org/forum/topic.asp?TOPIC_ID=4910&REPLY_ID=43408&whichpage=-1
The One & Only Way

quote:
_____
Originally posted by themysticseeker

You can't just get in a car and drive, if you don't know where you are going. The view of ultimate reality is not pure speculation. The Buddha described it.
_____

Hi TMS:

In this case it can be argued that the car (nervous system) knows better where it is going than the mind, and that the mind in all of its cleverness can become an obstacle on the journey. That is, until mind becomes committed through bhakti to effective spiritual practice.

Indeed, for the learned, the path to true knowledge is an unlearning, a surrender into the wisdom of unknowing. Then there can be the transformation of thirst for intellectual knowledge into thirst for direct experience and the means for cultivating it. Not much can happen until this transformation in intention is occurring. Once the intellect has been surrendered to the process, it can be a great help.

There is no such thing as a sure definition of the end state. There is only the experience of it, which can be known and described only after the fact, never before. If an enlightened person (like the Buddha) describes reality or a destination after the fact, it is only valid from his/her point of view. For nearly everyone else it is a mental structure before the fact, and, while inspiring, can also be an obstacle if it becomes an intellectual obsession. What reality is for an enlightened person is speculation for everyone else who has not experienced that condition. This is the gap between teachers and students where so many have gotten stuck. We have to get past it, and that cannot be done with the intellect alone.

Sound practices transcend all this. Self-inquiry methods (including favoring witnessing) are part of it, but are only effective once the abiding witness has emerged, which is a function of meditation, not inquiry. In AYP, we call it "relational self-inquiry," released in abiding stillness, which is samyama.

There can be an overlap between meditation and inquiry. If inquiry is practiced diligently as stand-alone for a long time, it will eventually give way to meditation (transcendence of the object, leading to stillness), but this is a difficult way to go. If it were not, we would have much less talk about emptiness and much more direct experience of the thing itself in expanding radiance, which leads to a very different kind of discussion -- more along the lines of non-stop overflowing ecstatic bliss and laughter, rather than endless ideological posturing. It is pretty easy to tell the difference, yes? :-)

I believe we are all after the same thing. It is only a matter of integrating the methods that will get the job done sooner rather than later. There is still a lot of work to be done in this area. Thanks to the great work of the ancients, open modern communications, and ongoing innovation occurring on many sides, it is gradually getting better. Bravo!

The guru is in you.

PS: So, do you think it is better to argue tooth and nail for emptiness being the absolute end state, or is it better to just practice and let it be empty? :-)

2009/01/13 01:38:32
Other Systems and Alternate Approaches
http://www.aypsite.org/forum/topic.asp?TOPIC_ID=4910&REPLY_ID=43413&whichpage=-1
The One & Only Way

quote:
_____

All things are empty from the beginning, including thoughts.

So emptiness is the basis of the path, not something to achieve Yogani.

————————

Hi Alwayson:

I don't think we disagree on that.

However, who is experiencing emptiness as their everyday reality? For all who are not, it is only a concept. The question is, how does everyone move reliably from concept to direct experience? Without such means, the concept will become a castle in the air, an obstacle.

Sorry, but in these times conceptual proclamations (even from the enlightened) count for nothing without the means for verification by many in the present through direct experience. This is what we mean by "a path" or "a way." Much more is required. Or is it much less? :-)

If you are going to promise that I can get from New York to Los Angeles in a few hours, then you must deliver the airplane along with the promise. Otherwise, it is false.

The guru is in you.

2009/01/13 10:47:30
Other Systems and Alternate Approaches
http://www.aypsite.org/forum/topic.asp?TOPIC_ID=4910&REPLY_ID=43422&whichpage=-1
The One & Only Way

quote:
————————
Originally posted by themysticseeker

The body, the nervous system and the mind are all part of the plane. The whole cosmos is the plane. What is it going to hurt someone to look into the middle way, dependent arising and emptiness? It won't bite you. Take a look at Nagarjuna's Fundamental Wisdom of the Middle Way.

————————

Hi TMS:

In the AYP approach to self-inquiry, the objective is a fruitful blending with all non-dual paths. Care is taken not to exclude any approach, and Nagarjuna's (or any other Buddhist) non-dual teaching is no exception.

However, in the AYP system, red flags are placed wherever there is a risk of slipping into the pitfalls of the mind, and there are quite a few such places. All of this is laid out in the little AYP Self-Inquiry book.

It boils down to cultivating at least some abiding inner silence (witness) <u>before</u> diving head-long into self-inquiry and non-duality. This applies to other areas of spiritual practice as well, such as samyama and karma yoga.

So, your background in meditation is serving you well, opening the door to radiant emptiness. For those of us who are having a taste of non-duality, let us be wise in sharing with others how we got to this point, so they will have the same opportunity. Fair enough?

The guru is in you.

2009/01/14 18:24:25
Other Systems and Alternate Approaches
http://www.aypsite.org/forum/topic.asp?TOPIC_ID=4910&REPLY_ID=43493&whichpage=-1
The One & Only Way

Hi All:

You would think that non-duality teachers would be the first to point out the mental pitfalls in their teachings, since the considerable hazards are part of the journey they propose. Few do.

To his credit, Nagarjuna, the Buddhist sage often referred to in this long belabored topic and a few others, does address the pitfalls in these quotes:

"The Conqueror [Buddha] taught openness [sunyata: emptiness] as the refutation of all [any] views. But those who hold openness as a view are called irremediable [impossible to remedy]."

"Openness [sunyata] wrongly conceived destroys the dimly witted. It is like a snake grasped by the head, or a garbled incantation."

He says it much more strongly than we do <u>here in AYP</u>. But the message is the same. <u>Meditate!</u> This is how all views and concepts are transcended.

I do not recall anyone on the yoga side of this discussion being particularly attached to the concept of Self, non-duality, or any other concept of destination, certainly not as part of core practice. So the whole discussion has been rather trivial so far. We are yet to see any "meat" coming in the form of real practices.

Perhaps these ideas are being projected to counter views of the Divine Self in Hindu culture, which AYP is not. No doubt the Hindus need help, as do all the religions, including the Buddhists. The religions will be naturally illuminated from within by many new practitioners in the 21st century, not by philosophical arguments.

What we do in AYP is practice and go out and live life to the fullest. This provides for a natural integration of inner purification and opening with daily living, which is an observable joyful illumination through the radiance of emptiness. It really has nothing to do with conceptualizations. It is about experiencing the truth rising through direct experience in life.

Ironically, the conceptualizations and rigid views of reality in this discussion are coming from somewhere else. Not from AYP, and certainly not from the Buddha or Nagarjuna. From where then?

Nevertheless, the window on Buddhist ideas is appreciated. The more views we have of human spiritual transformation, the better. And the more it looks like the same elephant. No surprises there. :-)

The guru is in you.

2009/01/14 18:41:05
Other Systems and Alternate Approaches
http://www.aypsite.org/forum/topic.asp?TOPIC_ID=4910&REPLY_ID=43496&whichpage=-1
The One & Only Way

quote:
_____
Originally posted by alwayson

then yogani, you are a buddist
_____

No labels, please. We have too many already. :-)
2009/01/15 11:24:52
Other Systems and Alternate Approaches
http://www.aypsite.org/forum/topic.asp?TOPIC_ID=4910&REPLY_ID=43523&whichpage=-1
The One & Only Way

Hi TMS:

Know that many here are praying in stillness for peaceful resolution of your personal challenges. It is part of what this community is about.

I'd just like to point out that challenges in life can force us to surrender our fixed ideas, and this is meditation (transcendence of the object). Then we are in the peace of emptiness, and everything is resolved in that.

But must we wait for a crisis for meditation to happen? There has to be a better way. What we need is a systematic and efficient method of meditation we can do every day, even when there is no crisis. Then, when the crisis comes, we are already in abiding inner silence and the crisis isn't a crisis. It is just stillness resolving itself in an evolutionary way, as it always does.

It is the Christian principle of building our house upon the rock, rather than on sand. Or the three little pigs building their house of brick, rather than of straw. :-)

Ideas are sand and straw, and abiding inner silence is the rock and the bricks.

This is the value of systematic daily meditation, which I know you know. It is good for all of us to be reminded often, because it is so important.

All the best!

The guru is in you.

2009/01/15 14:56:06
Other Systems and Alternate Approaches
http://www.aypsite.org/forum/topic.asp?TOPIC_ID=4910&REPLY_ID=43534&whichpage=-1
The One & Only Way

quote:
_____
Originally posted by themysticseeker

...The practice I mentioned is based on a practice of meditation. It's really a post-absorption practice, where one uses adverse circumstances to test one's level insight. So in that sense, you are correct. Using the wild emotions on the path is not a beginner's exercise.
_____

Hi TMS:

But who has a choice when the crisis is raging? We will be in it, like it or not. The method you describe may or may not work, according to what practices have gone before.

If it works, it indicates the presence of some pre-cultivated abiding inner silence, what you call "a post-absorption practice." In AYP terms, this is called "relational self-inquiry," which is surrendering an idea, emotion or intention in stillness, whereby further purification and opening occur, which can be expressed in the resolution of a difficult situation. It is an application of samyama, and the resulting resolution is a form of siddhi.

If it doesn't work, it is "non-relational self-inquiry" (without inner silence), and not much will happen. The situation will tend to grind on with minimal inner illumination. That is a signal that the cultivation of abiding inner silence through daily meditation can help. This also applies in the case of ordinary everyday inquiry, which will tend to get stuck in mental concepts without the presence of abiding inner silence. So it is not only about being prepared for a crisis. It is about being prepared for everyday living.

The mechanics in this are the same regardless of the tradition or situation. It is only a matter of terminology and the methods we use to activate the spiritual capabilities that are present within all of us.

The fact that living in stillness is not complicated or out of reach is good news for everyone. It is not a mind thing. It is a beyond the mind thing. That is the key thing. :-)

If we have an idea, feeling or intention, and can let it go in abiding inner silence, then that is the ticket. It isn't about the idea. It is about having the abiding inner silence to release the idea into, which is a product of effective daily meditation. Then we will know emptiness and its radiance in everyday living.

The guru is in you.

2009/01/30 09:58:58
Other Systems and Alternate Approaches
http://www.aypsite.org/forum/topic.asp?TOPIC_ID=5094&REPLY_ID=44449&whichpage=-1
A secret practice from buddhism and hinduism

quote:
_____
Originally posted by NagoyaSea

Ananda, perhaps in time you could look at the Amazon kindle? It costs about 300 up front (more than I can spend right now and plus they're backordered), but you can download many books to it wirelessly. The book you refer to is about 119 via kindle. Anyway, perhaps in future it might be an option. Most books downloaded to kindle are much cheaper and in time could save. Plus you can take thousands of books with you everywhere easily on it....

just a thought.

Kathy
_____

Hi Kathy and All:

The AYP books are available for Kindle also. See here.

But be forewarned. For some (many?) books, the present Amazon conversion process from MS Word or PDF to Kindle alters the formatting, especially if there are illustrations. The books are still readable, but may not be as originally formatted. Given that, a PDF ebook may be a better choice. Not sure if James Mallinson's book has formatting issues on Kindle, or if it is available in PDF ebook. The AYP books are available in both.

I once asked James about the price on his book, and he said that the publisher has control of pricing and he was disappointed with what they did, limiting the book's exposure and sales by pricing it nearly out of the market. No one benefits from that -- not the author, not the publisher, and not the readers. So why do they price it so high? Is it a fancy book with a lot of color printing and a high production cost? If not that, then what? A misguided sense of value? A book (or anything) is worth only what people are willing to pay for it, yes?

This is one of the factors that distinguishes limited-access spiritual teachings from open source spiritual teachings. It is something we are pretty sensitive about around here. :-)

The guru is in you.

PS: What does this say about the value of free teachings?
Well, we pay in other ways, with our bhakti and commitment to daily practice, which are much more valuable than money. For this, the knowledge has to be available first!

2009/01/30 14:24:02
Other Systems and Alternate Approaches
http://www.aypsite.org/forum/topic.asp?TOPIC_ID=5094&REPLY_ID=44456&whichpage=-1
A secret practice from buddhism and hinduism

quote:
_____
Originally posted by divinefurball

Hello, and best wishes to all. The reason - from the publishers point of view, which I am not defending - for the high cost of specialised academic texts like Prof. Mallinson's, is the expectation that only one small run of books will be sufficient to fulfill academic needs. Since the cost of production is about the same as it is for a book expected to have large, or multiple print runs, the consumer end price is proportionally higher for 'low print run books'. Routledge was likly unaware of the rising intrest in Mallinson's topic outside the academy. If they see the demand, it might come out in a cheaper paperback someday - after they have recovered production costs of course!
_____

Hi Divinefurball:

That makes sense, and explains why college textbooks are so outrageously expensive.

While it may be too late for this particular book, there is a way around the pricing issues associated with low unit volume books printed with costly offset plates in the traditional way.

The alternative is modern "print-on-demand" technology, where the cost of producing one book is nearly the same as the cost per book of producing 1000 books, or 10,000 books. They are digitally stored, and printed and shipped (quickly) as they are ordered "on-demand," not piled up in a warehouse. No expensive offset plate setup. It is done with PDFs and advanced printing and binding technology. Very efficient and economical. All of the AYP books are done this way, and it has been a life-saver for making multiple low unit volume titles available at a reasonable cost.

Of course, traditional publishers offer more than warehouses full of books that have to be sold in a way that will recover their large printing setup costs. They also offer distribution channels. So it will take more than print-on-demand alone to unseat the inefficient process that is in place for textbooks. It will also take distribution. As soon a large college textbook publisher/distributor moves to print-on-demand, the entire industry will make a dramatic shift, and students won't have to borrow a fortune to obtain their textbooks anymore.

And we won't have to pay so much for translated Sanskrit scriptures from the academic world either. :-)

The guru is in you.

2009/03/08 12:30:28
Other Systems and Alternate Approaches
http://www.aypsite.org/forum/topic.asp?TOPIC_ID=5249&REPLY_ID=46756&whichpage=-1
Watch-your-Thoughts Meditation

Hi Sushman:

It is the policy of the AYP forums that if a teacher requires aspects of their teachings to be kept confidential, then we want to honor that here. So kindly edit your post to cover the teachings in a way that does not violate the requirements of the tradition in question.

It is fine to describe principles and elements of practice (no one owns those), but we are not really at liberty to reveal the specifics of teachings by others that are private.

It is not necessary for us to cross that ethical line to present an effective well-integrated system of practices here that is open to all.

Thanks!

The guru is in you.

2009/03/15 12:26:44
Other Systems and Alternate Approaches
http://www.aypsite.org/forum/topic.asp?TOPIC_ID=5328&REPLY_ID=47297&whichpage=-1
Recomendations of Hara/Taoist meditation?

Hi Jack:

Recently I was asked about this from the standpoint of "storing" energy in the hara (belly) to improve stability in life. Below is what I wrote back. Hope it is helpful.

Hello:

Yes, in Taoist systems, Hara (or Dan Tien), is about storing energy in the belly and acting from there. This is central in ancient Chinese and Japanese martial arts, which evolved later toward spiritual paths. Yoga began as spiritual in ancient times and continued as spiritual, with more emphasis on cultivating inner silence and radiance outward, divine ecstatic outflow, etc. Under normal circumstances, divine outflow (natural karma yoga) is preferred over storing energy at the naval (marital arts technique). But everyone is different in purification and opening and it is not always going to be a straight line from practices to divine outpouring. So intermediate methods for managing energy are often needed. Self-pacing and grounding are developed for that in AYP. But, as you say, sometimes more is necessary.

An area of development for AYP in the lessons later this year will be more focus on those who are over-sensitive to yoga practices (excess energy flows, imbalances, blockages, etc.), and also on those who are under-sensitive, who seem not to experience much observable effect from yoga practices. So the lessons will be looking at modifications to the baseline AYP system as needed to address these variations in the experience occurring in some practitioners. It has been going on already in the community, with many things being tried by many people (for right reasons or wrong reasons) and it was addressed somewhat officially by me in several posts in this topic:
http://www.aypsite.org/forum/topic.asp?TOPIC_ID=5103

In your case, if you are looking for more stability in the Hara way, then consider Taoist methods. The writings of Mantak Chia are very good for this. His work in Taoism has been similar to what AYP has been doing in Yoga -- bringing to the public over the years many techniques that were not openly presented before. Also see Jim & K's writing on his energy issues and how he has been addressing them by integrating Taoist methods with his yoga practices, here: http://www.aypsite.org/forum/topic.asp?TOPIC_ID=3296

Of course, if you have local support for applying useful methods (of any kind) that can enhance your experience in daily living, go for it. And yes, please do share your experience with the AYP community, so all can benefit.

For the record, for a period of about 10 years during raging kundalini, I used a daily Tai C
Hi routine in addition to yoga practices with good effect (covered in Lesson 69 and elsewhere). Tai C
Hi is a Hara/Dan Tien based practice. Later on (about 10 years ago), nearly all the energy went to outward divine flow (divine outpouring) and the Tai C
Hi became less essential, though I still do practice it occasionally as needed. If the divine outpouring had not occurred (hara evolving from storage mode to pass-through radiance mode), there likely would be no AYP, and I would have a well-stored energy belly instead, constantly ready for the fight (metaphorically speaking). :-)

So that is the trade-off, which characterizes the main difference between Taoist and Yogic methods.

650 –   Advanced Yoga Practices

In both systems, the cultivation of abiding inner silence through meditation is essential. This is generally much better recognized in Yoga than in Taoist systems. So I think both systems have something useful to offer each other.

All the best!

The guru is in you.

2009/03/15 17:40:21
Other Systems and Alternate Approaches
http://www.aypsite.org/forum/topic.asp?TOPIC_ID=5328&REPLY_ID=47321&whichpage=-1
Recomendations of Hara/Taoist meditation?

quote:
_____
Originally posted by YogaIsLife

Hi Yogani,

Thank you for sharing that.

A question came to my mind while reading your post - you said you had about 10 years of a kundalini ride and then the energy accumulated transmutated outwards into outpouring divine love (that is great by the way!). My question is whether all the while, as I suppose you had been meditating for many years prior to all that, you were awake, i.e., had abiding inner silence and was aware of the essence of what you are.

I guess it may correlate with the 3 phases of enlightenment that you identify:

- abiding inner silence (witnessing) cultivated by daily deep meditation
- the rise of ecstatic conductivity
- the merging of the two (=outpouring divine love)

Is this correct?

Do you think one that has only the witnessing state (1st phase) is enlightened? Maybe so, but not "outpouring"? :-)

Thanks!
YIL

P.S.: MAybe I'm being too technical here...:-)
_____

Hi YIL:

Yes, that is correct. I was fortunate to have many years of deep meditation before going through the kundalini stage. On the other hand, I did not have many of the tools we have available today for navigating the kundalini stage, so a lot of "R&D" occurred during those years. Many of the things that are routine now in AYP were ferreted out during those years. The Secrets of Wilder story provides a facsimile for some of those experiences -- a process of learning by trial and error.

As for enlightenment, I do not see it as a fixed absolute thing. The three stages are signature experiences we may notice emerging along the way, and are for general confirmation of progress as we keep moving forward. As many here know, these experiences are real. Yet, there is no end destination where we can say, "I have arrived!" (Be leery of anyone who proclaims that.) When we are there, we will not be exclaiming anything. The greatest enlightenment is the one that does not speak much of itself. It only does for others, continuing the purification and opening in everyone. And that too is an ongoing journey. Where does it end? Let's keep going and find out. :-)

Along the way, what we might be inclined to call "enlightenment" is always going to be relative to what came before and what is to come later. If we feel better than last year, we are relatively more enlightened compared to last year, right? And we will see what it will be next year as we continue to practice. Of course, it is what it is in the now, and that is most important. The rest of it is about keeping up our motivation (bhakti) for continuing on our path. What we think about it doesn't matter all that much. What we do consistently over the long term makes all the difference.

In the AYP Self-Inquiry book, one of the "pitfalls of the mind" that is discussed is the "illusion of attainment," or thinking we have "arrived." Because of the rise of the witness in so many quarters these days, there are quite a few people around who may be inclined to reside in this pitfall. It's time to move on!

While the witness stage is often presented as "enlightenment," it is only the beginning. It is the starting point for illuminating all of the human race, and beyond. This can only happen as we, as the witness, become ecstatically energized and continue to act in the world. That is the divine outpouring, which we also call stillness in action. It is no longer about whether any one person (or few persons) is enlightened or not. It is about everyone becoming enlightened. It is the ongoing evolution of our species.

The guru is in you.

2009/03/16 12:01:47
Other Systems and Alternate Approaches
http://www.aypsite.org/forum/topic.asp?TOPIC_ID=5328&REPLY_ID=47363&whichpage=-1
Recomendations of Hara/Taoist meditation?

quote:
_____

Originally posted by Christi

Hi Yogani,

Thanks for writing about your Taoist experiences. Before the energy was transformed totally into outpouring divine love, did you experience a large build up of energy in your hara/ dan tien? If you did, how many years did that last for? Hope you don't mind me asking.

Christi
_____

Hi Christi:

No, the Tai C
Hi was used here to help ground and stabilize the energies for use in daily life, and this was an ongoing process without a pronounced shift from inner energy storage to natural ecstatic outflow.

In my case, the priority was never for storing energy, though the stabilization of flow that Tai C
Hi assisted with was much appreciated. After consideration, I decided not to go for more in-depth marital arts training (I had a little), which would have put more emphasis on the "energy storage in hara" aspect. It was clear early on that natural outpouring was the way it would go for me, and nurturing and stabilizing that was always the focus. So I did not become deeply involved in "controlling" inner energies, rather, letting them go their natural route toward ecstatic radiance instead. This is reflected in the AYP writings, with focus more on cultivating inner silence and enabling natural ecstatic conductivity and radiance than on personal regulation of the inner energies from either the Yogic (chakras) or Taoist (hara) side. Hence the phrase, "Under the hood." :-)

The resulting experience has been that stillness moving into natural ecstatic outflow becomes increasing service to all according to divine need (karma yoga). We become a channel for that. The more we let go, the more powerful the divine outflow becomes.

I am not suggesting that everyone must go the way I did. The philosophy in AYP is for assisting the natural unfoldment within everyone, however that may occur. It is a process that is bigger than any of us, and bigger than any particular approach for enabling it. Therefore, AYP is a resource where individual choice always comes first, for one's chosen ideal, and for the methods that are applied.

The guru is in you.

2009/03/16 12:57:03
Other Systems and Alternate Approaches
http://www.aypsite.org/forum/topic.asp?TOPIC_ID=5328&REPLY_ID=47372&whichpage=-1
Recomendations of Hara/Taoist meditation?

quote:
_____
Originally posted by Christi

Hi Yogani,

Thanks for the reply.

Whenever you write a post to me these days, you always use the word "service"... have you noticed that? :-) I'm starting to think it's some kind of subtle hint. :-)

* laughing *

Christi
_____

Hi Christi:

Well, service happens to be one of the effects of yoga, and an elixir for the excesses and attachments associated with energy experiences, whether positive or negative. No need to rush it though. Just do whatever comes naturally. You already are. Thank you! :-)

The guru is in you.

2009/03/26 12:01:33
Other Systems and Alternate Approaches
http://www.aypsite.org/forum/topic.asp?TOPIC_ID=5388&REPLY_ID=47998&whichpage=-1
mantra to breath: do I have to change my practice?

quote:
_____
Originally posted by Christi

...I have noticed that although there are many forms of pranayama, kriyas and other techniques in AYP, there is only one form of meditation, which I think is a shame as yoga is rich with meditation techniques.

I have noticed here in the forums that many people find themselves at times unable to practice at all because of increased sensitivity to the practices, and that could be avoided with a broader base of more gentle techniques.

Just as a side note, metta bhavana is another very gentle practice (coming from the same tradition as breathing meditation) and brings you even closer to your heart than breathing meditation does. They compliment each other well, especially for sensitive people.

————

Hi Christi:

I think we are headed in that direction, as per the discussion here on research on modifications to AYP practices, and the "bell curve" spanning the range of practitioner sensitivity and lack of sensitivity to practices:
http://www.aypsite.org/forum/topic.asp?TOPIC_ID=5103

It is only a matter of how and when it becomes formulated, tested by many, and made part of the systematic approach to practices. A broadening of the AYP approach to cover a wider range of practitioner sensitivities is inevitable, is happening already, and is a priority for future writings.

Discussions like this one are very useful, and a key part of the evolution that is constantly occurring in the community. It is the kind of thing that no one person can represent experientially. It takes a village. :-)

Thanks!

The guru is in you.

PS: It is not only meditation being viewed for sensitivities. It happens with other practices too, depending on the individual. There are numerous examples of sensitivity to many practices here in the forums -- many discussions on self-pacing for maintaining progress with comfort and safety. So we are talking about a wide field of ongoing knowledge development, which I expect will be occurring for a long time into the future through the efforts of many researchers.

2009/05/05 15:45:51
Other Systems and Alternate Approaches
http://www.aypsite.org/forum/topic.asp?TOPIC_ID=5538&REPLY_ID=50058&whichpage=-1
Buddhism, The Rainbow Body and Enlightenment

Hi Alwayson:

Enlightenment cannot be known or measured by words or ideology. Only by the thing itself, which is beyond all words and measures.

The question is, do human beings become enlightened in all traditions, and outside the traditions too? Yes, they do, and one enlightenment label cannot be measured against another one by those who have not traveled beyond words and ideology. Those who have will not measure at all.

So go beyond your intellectualizations with spiritual practices, and you will be less inclined to judge others who describe the same human spiritual experiences with different words than you do.

If Hinduism has been a disappointment for you, and Buddhism resonates, then go for it. No one here is opposed to that. Circumstances may be just the opposite for others. It doesn't matter.

What matters is our practice, which enables us to let go of our sectarian views and live the truth/dharma within us. That is the most important thing.

As long as our main concern is for being on the winning team (ideology), we will not be in the game. It isn't about that. Anyone can win on any team. So pick your spot and play with all your heart. These forums are for supporting that, not for quibbling about which tradition is better than another.

The guru is in you.

2009/05/17 20:11:43
Other Systems and Alternate Approaches
http://www.aypsite.org/forum/topic.asp?TOPIC_ID=5648&REPLY_ID=50951&whichpage=-1
noticed

Hi Brother Neil:

If this is spinal breathing you are attempting to do, just go right past the navel and make sure you end up at the brow at the completion of inhalation and at the root at the completion of exhalation. It is not necessary to stop at any point in-between. If we get stuck, we can pass through that place or jump right over it. That way we are covering the full length of the spinal nerve, which is the best way to assure that obstructions everywhere in-between and beyond will become gradually cleared out. In the AYP approach, we do not attempt to "clear chakras" individually. The approach is much more holistic, and so are the results.

Of course, doing deep meditation right after spinal breathing is the other half of the formula. The two practices done in sequence will produce far greater results than either one alone.

The guru is in you.

2009/07/16 12:30:00
Other Systems and Alternate Approaches
http://www.aypsite.org/forum/topic.asp?TOPIC_ID=5943&REPLY_ID=53600&whichpage=-1
Sacred Herbs & Self-Realization

quote:
————

Manipura... any way I could get an e-mail when someone posts replies.

_____

Welcome Godrealized!

We do not use an email post-notification service for the forums, due to the clutter it would create in everyone's mail (and on the forum server). At times this can be a very busy place.

The easiest way to keep track of forum activity is to bookmark the "active topics" link on the top menu. It works very well.

There is also an RSS feature for the forums which can be helpful for keeping track. See the RSS link near the bottom of the list of links in the left border here.

All the best!

The guru is in you.

2009/09/10 17:55:13
Other Systems and Alternate Approaches
http://www.aypsite.org/forum/topic.asp?TOPIC_ID=6316&REPLY_ID=56649&whichpage=-1
Why no Madhyamaka subforum?

quote:
_____
Originally posted by alwayson2

There is an Advaita Vedanta subforum, but there is no Madhyamaka forum?

Considering the fact that 600 years after Nagarjuna, Advaita Vedanta was created as a hybrid between Mahayana and Upanishadic thinking?

"The Essential Vedanta" by Eliot Deutsch, among other works, documents how the Vedantins from the ninth century looked back 600 years to ancient Nagarjuna and borrowed Mahayana ideas.

I thought Yogani was against a partisan belief system? At least Madhyamaka does not make any claims of reality...

_____

Hi Alwayson:

The short answer is because this is a support forum for the AYP system of practices. Forum categories are selected for how they relate to the AYP system and what its practitioners are doing, not according to which tradition should be getting more visibility.

If Buddhist methods can be presented with clarity and relevance, with potential for clarifying or supplementing the scope of the AYP system, they are welcome to be discussed in the "other systems" forum category. You are free to open a topic on Madhyamaka in other systems.

There have been some concerns about the contentiousness and murkiness of some of the Buddhist discussions here in relation to the relative clarity of the AYP approach, so the question isn't whether Buddhist discussions deserve more forum visibility, but whether it might eventually become necessary to limit them so they will not overwhelm the entire forum.

Don't get me wrong, the Buddhist discussions have been welcome, informative and appreciated so far. But this isn't E-Sangha, you know. Buddhist-style discussions are not going to be permitted to dominate the AYP forums.

I think the present setup with the "other systems" category provides a reasonable vehicle for exploring the many systems of practice that are out there. Whether it works out in a balanced way over time in relation to the AYP forums' primary mission, we will have to see.

All the best!

The guru is in you.

2009/09/10 23:30:49
Other Systems and Alternate Approaches
http://www.aypsite.org/forum/topic.asp?TOPIC_ID=6316&REPLY_ID=56667&whichpage=-1
Why no Madhyamaka subforum?

quote:
_____
Originally posted by alwayson2

So just to be clear, you are saying that AYP Practices follows Advaita Vedanta philosophy in the vein of Adi Shankara?

_____

Hi Alwayson:

As Etherfish points out, AYP does not follow a particular philosophy or doctrine. It follows the cause and effect of practices and their results in the human being. The starting point in my case long ago was yoga, so that is the nomenclature that has been used, simplified to plain English as much as possible.

The "Jnana Yoga/Self-Inquiry - Advaita (Non-Duality)" forum category actually used to be combined with the "Bhakti and Karma Yoga" forum category. It was split out into a separate forum category a few months ago, when it became clear that many here are spontaneously moving into self-inquiry practices of various kinds. This is in line with the AYP assertion that the rise of abiding inner silence (the witness) is the primary cause of self-inquiry, not the other way around. See Lesson 322 and the Self Inquiry book.

Does all of this have corresponding cause and effect in the various systems of Buddhist practice? I am quite certain it does, but we are yet to see it simplified for ordinary human beings. While those long terminology-laden Buddhist topics are interesting for those who have the aptitude, simplification of the process of human spiritual transformation they are not. So we should keep working on that for everyone's sake. :-)

Thanks!

The guru is in you.

2009/09/20 12:10:11
Other Systems and Alternate Approaches
http://www.aypsite.org/forum/topic.asp?TOPIC_ID=6316&REPLY_ID=57231&whichpage=-1
Why no Madhyamaka subforum?

quote:
_____
Originally posted by Konchok Ösel Dorje

The fruit is in the looking. Just look...
_____

The quality of the looking is dependent on the clarity of the looking glass. Yoga is first about purifying the looking glass. The fruit in the looking comes after that. :-)

The guru is in you.

2009/09/19 14:14:40
Other Systems and Alternate Approaches
http://www.aypsite.org/forum/topic.asp?TOPIC_ID=6360&REPLY_ID=57190&whichpage=-1
Before Kundalini erupts

Hi TI:

Just chiming in to say your focus (bhakti) has sharpened considerably since the wild and woolly days of "Where am I at now?", and it is a joy to see.

Thanks so much for dropping back in with the update. Everyone benefits.

Carry on! :-)

The guru is in you.

2009/10/13 11:00:50
Other Systems and Alternate Approaches
http://www.aypsite.org/forum/topic.asp?TOPIC_ID=6475&REPLY_ID=58380&whichpage=-1
Havn't we all missed the point of Yoga?

Hi RyanO, and welcome!

Duality and non-duality really depend on one's point of view in the present. As self-identification with projections of mind are gradually dissolved through practices, the truth with a thousand names and philosophies (or no name at all) becomes known first hand.

We use the structure of Patanjali's eight limbs to some degree here because he did such a fine job of integrating the "levers" of human spiritual transformation. It is a great reference, and jumping off point. But we are not obliged to adhere to his philosophical view, or anyone else's. We are obliged to pursue whatever opens our nervous system to its inherent divine capabilities here and now. Philosophy is not the final arbiter of anything. Direct experience is.

All philosophies and spiritual methods, past and present, have been derived from the human being. In AYP, we look back only enough to keep going forward. Better to be mostly looking out the front windshield than the rear view mirror. There is no substitute for transformative action undertaken today. :-)

Onward!

The guru is in you.

PS: "A" becomes "B," and then becomes "A" again, so all can become "B," and so on. It is the natural flow of divine love. No mental structure can contain it, or comprehend it. Yet, we are that eternal becoming. :-)

2009/10/13 17:46:10
Other Systems and Alternate Approaches
http://www.aypsite.org/forum/topic.asp?TOPIC_ID=6475&REPLY_ID=58393&whichpage=-1
Havn't we all missed the point of Yoga?

Hi RyanO:

Thank you. I think you have a healthy way of looking at it. For most of us, a gradual merging of small self with big Self is preferred over the executioner's ax. Many more will be interested in that.

The practices we work with in AYP are for that gradual ripening. Then the fruit falls off the tree in due course. Not that everything is perfect, but we seem to be heading in the right direction, with improvements in methodology being incorporated as we find them. For some, the path may lead to exploring methods outside the field of yoga, which is okay. Everyone is a little different in their process of purification and opening. We are interested in practical results for the most people. The most important scripture resides within each of us, in stillness.

The guru is in you.

2009/10/12 12:10:11
Other Systems and Alternate Approaches
http://www.aypsite.org/forum/topic.asp?TOPIC_ID=6517&REPLY_ID=58326&whichpage=-1
Nada Brahma Sound Current

Hi Hyperspesh:

Many practitioners have experienced inner sounds during meditation and at other times. If you want to explore doing a practice with it, that is your choice. I'd suggest not doing it during your regular meditation with mantra, as you will be replacing the practice that is bringing the experience with the experience itself. It is purification and opening that brings such experiences, and as you know, we always easily favor the mantra over experiences that come up during meditation when we realize we have gone off.

Nada meditation is a common practice in some of the traditions, kriya yoga in particular. They use it instead of mantra meditation, and it is called "omkar."

We do not use nada meditation in AYP for one simple reason. It is not consistent. Sometimes nada is there, and sometimes it isn't. So much of a nada yoga practice can be spent waiting around for something to occur.

This isn't to say you could not use nada as an add-on. If your heart is in it, and the vibration is there, enjoy it, preferably not at the expense of deep mediation and other structured practices you may be doing.

A measured approach is suggested to avoid overdoing, particularly if nada leads you toward the crown. If you begin to get over-done, make sure to self-pace.

Others here with nada experience may have additional input.

All the best! (...and Aloha from Florida) :-)

The guru is in you.

2009/10/17 12:20:25
Other Systems and Alternate Approaches
http://www.aypsite.org/forum/topic.asp?TOPIC_ID=6546
World Community for Christian Meditation

Hi All:

A "Christian Meditation Center" opened recently in our area, and we come to find it is part of a worldwide movement: http://www.wccm.org

It is mantra meditation with some similarity to what we are doing in AYP. May they live long and prosper. :-)

The guru is in you.

PS: This style of meditation, popularized by John Main, has been discussed in a few places in the forums. Here's one:
http://www.aypsite.org/forum/topic.asp?TOPIC_ID=708

2009/12/12 12:54:09
Other Systems and Alternate Approaches
http://www.aypsite.org/forum/topic.asp?TOPIC_ID=6842&REPLY_ID=61211&whichpage=-1
mantra enhancements three or more enhancements ?

quote:
───────
Originally posted by tmer

I would like to know, there are more enhancements ? , it is possible to place more shree before the mantra, or put more NAMAH after the mantra?
───────

Hi Tmer:

No, that's it for now as far as AYP is concerned. But there is no telling what the future might bring.

Of course, anyone is free to try anything, but when it is not covered in the lessons, it will be the practitioner's independent research. We welcome feedback on all such adventures. We learn that way. Best to post it in "other systems," so as not to confuse those seeking support for the AYP practices as instructed in the lessons.

Enjoy!

The guru is in you.

2009/12/13 14:54:11
Other Systems and Alternate Approaches
http://www.aypsite.org/forum/topic.asp?TOPIC_ID=6842&REPLY_ID=61268&whichpage=-1
mantra enhancements three or more enhancements ?

Hi All:

We ended up with two parallel topics of the same name here, so two responses are being copied here to create one topic:

Anthem11 said:

Hi tmer,

Of course it is possible, but it is not recommended or consistent with the AYP lessons.

All the best!

Tmer said:

Hi Anthem11

you think this be possible? I wonder if you can create a problem or danger, I would like to understand whether to make these additions as the nervous system react ? and wy it is not recommended ? very thanks for reply :-)

2010/01/13 09:46:56
Other Systems and Alternate Approaches
http://www.aypsite.org/forum/topic.asp?TOPIC_ID=6921&REPLY_ID=62664&whichpage=-1
What Does Practicing No Path Mean?

Hi All:

I have been tempted to put a few cents into this discussion, but nothing came. So practice continues... :-)

The guru is in you.

2010/01/01 13:37:13
Other Systems and Alternate Approaches
http://www.aypsite.org/forum/topic.asp?TOPIC_ID=6946&REPLY_ID=61995&whichpage=-1
Navi Kriya- Yogananda's version

Hi Krish:

My experience has been that the more we load down energy practices (pranayama, mudras and bandhas) with visualizations and mantras, the less effective these practices are, because they then tend to become complex mental exercises rather than subtle cultivators of ecstatic conductivity.

Coming from the other side (cultivation of abiding inner silence), the same is especially true of deep meditation. If we divide the mind with extra activities while meditating, other than simply favoring the mantra at increasingly refined levels whenever we notice we are off it, then the efficiency of the procedure will be greatly reduced.

This is not to say other approaches are wrong. Each will stand on its results over time. It is up to the practitioners in every approach to make the best of what is being offered. That is one of the main reasons why AYP is "open source."

So using mantras during navi kriya and other energy practices is not taboo. Just not part of the baseline AYP system. The variations from the baseline are endless. :-)

The guru is in you.

2010/01/15 18:02:07
Other Systems and Alternate Approaches
http://www.aypsite.org/forum/topic.asp?TOPIC_ID=7054&REPLY_ID=62946&whichpage=-1
Pranayama/Awakened K. before Meditation

Hi Akasha:

You are talking about two different approaches to practice, and you will have make your own choice on which to follow. Obviously, you can't follow two approaches at once, and you can't expect one approach to redefine itself to suit the needs of another approach.

One thing I can tell you: Many of the people who arrived here with pre-existing kundalini difficulties came from pranayama and kundalini-focused paths, not from meditation-focused paths. I am not saying that those who begin with meditation are not going have energy challenges at one time or other, but from my experience, the incidence of it has been far less, and much more manageable due to the cultivation of abiding inner silence (the witness) in meditation.

So is pranayama more stabilizing than meditation? No, not always.

As you know, AYP represents a balance of methods for cultivating both inner silence and ecstatic conductivity. If that does not work for you as constituted, then try something else.

Probably the best place to find an answer to your question is from those who promote pranayama techniques first and meditation later on. That is not the AYP approach. It is another system.

Thank you for posting about this in the right place. :-)

The guru is in you.

2010/01/16 10:43:37
Other Systems and Alternate Approaches
http://www.aypsite.org/forum/topic.asp?TOPIC_ID=7054&REPLY_ID=62993&whichpage=-1
Pranayama/Awakened K. before Meditation

Hi Akasha:

You are free to experiment. It is your path.

Do keep in mind that overdoing with pranayama may not be immediately apparent due to delays in results, which is pretty common.

This is why we suggest small steps in AYP, especially with energy-related practices. And preferably preceded by the cultivation of abiding inner silence, which is not overthrown by any sort of upheaval. It's your call.

The guru is in you.

2010/01/18 12:34:11
Other Systems and Alternate Approaches
http://www.aypsite.org/forum/topic.asp?TOPIC_ID=7071&REPLY_ID=63129&whichpage=-1
the importance of nadi shodhana pranayam

Hi All:

For the record, I practiced nadi shodhana pranayama (alternate nostril breathing) for nearly 20 years, for 10-15 minutes twice daily before deep meditation. The last 5 years of that, I used kumbhaka, mudras and bandhas extensively, mainly because alternate nostril breathing was not producing an ecstatic awakening -- relaxation only. The result of the aggressive additional measures was an unstable kundalini awakening, which after several years, was finally stabilized with self-pacing, grounding, and spinal breathing pranayama.

For the nearly 20 years since then, I have used spinal breathing (with the additional methods in the lessons) with excellent results for a balanced continuation of kundalini expansion and integration with abiding inner silence.

Throughout this long period, extensive work with the cultivation of inner silence has been ongoing with deep meditation, samyama, self-inquiry and the various enhancements in practice on that side of the equation, which we have covered in the AYP writings.

The Secrets of Wilder novel presents a facsimile of this journey, simplified and compressed in time. It is a much "wilder" journey than what the AYP system has become in terms of its simplicity, balance, and sophistication in self-pacing for maximum progress with comfort and safety. And the evolution continues, based on the experiences of many.

So it should be pointed out that the objective in the AYP forums is for experience-based sharing, rather than spouting theories based on what any particular guru or tradition said or did. If a practice is good, then we'd like first-hand descriptions, pros and cons, and how that can fit into a practical daily routine that can be undertaken in this modern world. We'd like to know about ongoing results, challenges, and solutions that are worked out to address real-time issues that are bound to come up.

Trumpeting platitudes on practice while dropping names of famous gurus and traditions is easy. We are beyond that here. We'd like to know what works based on hard-earned experience over the long term. We'd like for it to be useful and practical. In-the-trenches yoga based on real experience. That is what we are doing here.

Omarkaya, so far, all you have done here is tell everyone what you think they ought to be doing, often at the expense of the clarity of paths other than yours. You quote impressive sources on fragments of knowledge, without offering any sort of integrated systematic approach, or evidence of real experience. I encourage you to take note of the community you are in, the levels of experience that are present, and the depth of research on practice that is going on here. Consider that you have something to learn also. We all do.

Nothing is black or white. There are a thousand shades of gray. There are many viable approaches. Opinions expressed by many here are based on long experience, so not to take them too lightly.

The guru is in you.

2010/01/18 14:36:30
Other Systems and Alternate Approaches
http://www.aypsite.org/forum/topic.asp?TOPIC_ID=7071&REPLY_ID=63142&whichpage=-1
the importance of nadi shodhana pranayam

Hi Omarkaya:

Nadi Shodhana is not an enemy. It is one of many tools that have been explored for the AYP toolkit. In this case, explored extensively for many years, and found to be secondary to other things determined to be more balanced and more effective for cultivating human spiritual transformation.

It is what it is.

This does not mean nadi shodhana will not be a useful practice for those who are energetically sensitive and need a relaxation technique. It is an excellent relaxation technique, and does facilitate meditation afterwards.

For those following the AYP approach, I do not recommend using nadi shodhana with kumbhaka, mudras and bandhas for kundalini awakening. It is not a mixture that will lead to a stable outcome.

This is not to say nadi shodhana is not appropriate as core practice in other paths. I am only saying that its role is limited in the AYP baseline system.

So by all means share your opinions, preferably based on experience, rather than what someone else said or wrote about it. In this community, direct experience trumps scripture and external gurus. The truest scripture we are ever going to find is within us, assuming we are using effective tools to access it.

And...

The guru is in you.

2010/01/18 14:55:38
Other Systems and Alternate Approaches
http://www.aypsite.org/forum/topic.asp?TOPIC_ID=7071&REPLY_ID=63146&whichpage=-1
the importance of nadi shodhana pranayam

quote:
_____
Originally posted by omarkaya

Yogani when you mean you want real experienced results,what do you exactly mean?ive been experiencing the great labour of this nadi shodhana pranayam,for almost 20 years and believe me its incredible good and helpful for mind and body,its an authentic detoxifying and purifiying pranayam tremendously balancing ,very practical for different variations of itself ,thats why it is a complete practice in itself and wonderful to reach deep meditation.
_____

That's great. Go for it. But don't impose it on others as the only way, because it isn't the only way.

The guru is in you.

2010/01/21 10:55:29
Other Systems and Alternate Approaches
http://www.aypsite.org/forum/topic.asp?TOPIC_ID=7092&REPLY_ID=63396&whichpage=-1
How Theravada, Vajrayana and AYP Converge

quote:
_____
Originally posted by Sparkle

quote:
_____
Originally posted by adamantclearlight

Now, AYP has almost all these elements.

Adamant
_____

Hi Adamant
I think you may be neglecting the self-inquiry aspect of AYP, it is possible that this may de-link as you describe, especially inquiry like Byron Katie's and other similar one's.
_____

Hi Adamant:

Sparkle makes good point. The AYP approach to self-inquiry is "baseline," and can support any method of inquiry, including Buddhist dependent origination. So the enhancement you are suggesting for AYP is already there by virtue of you mentioning it. :-)

Whatever works!

The guru is in you.

2010/01/22 16:39:10
Other Systems and Alternate Approaches

on alternate approach to mantra enhancements

Hi All:

Sorry, but I gave up commenting on mantra variations and alternatives a few years ago. I think it was after about the 1000th email asking about an alternate mantra.

The variations are unlimited ... and the choice is yours.

All the best!

The guru is in you.

2010/01/25 17:26:16
Other Systems and Alternate Approaches
Japa Mala

quote:
_____
Originally posted by Victor

So is simply using the beads as a counting device doing japa? Is that a different practice? I simply do the AYP mantra the way that Yogani teaches but each time I do the mantra I move my fingers one bead. At the end of one round I go the other direction. After 2 rounds I am done for that practice as it takes about 20-25 mins. It has felt good to me for several years and not sure what makes it so different.

_____

Hi Victor:

This is not AYP deep meditation according to procedure. It does not allow for spontaneously losing the mantra in stillness and coming back when we realize we have gone off it, unless you are "losing it" very rhythmically according to a mala count and arriving at the right time duration of practice every time, which is highly unlikely.

Some meditations we will pick up the mantra once and be gone in pure bliss consciousness for the whole session. Other times we will be much on the surface with the mantra. And everything in-between. It all depends on the process of purification and opening occurring within us at any point in time. Externally regulating this process will reduce its effectiveness.

It is not for us (or a mala) to say how many times we will return to the mantra. Using a mala to count mantra repetitions to measure a specific time duration will tend to hold us on the surface. Using a clock is a better approach for this kind of meditation. It allows for a more natural process to occur during our meditation session, leading to much deeper penetration in stillness.

This is not to say mala is not useful for other forms of mantra (or prayer) repetition, but not for AYP deep meditation.

Here is what I said about it in Lesson 86:

quote:
_____
Mala beads are for a different kind of approach to meditation, and to pranayama as well. They are for counting. Malas were around long before clocks, and the number of mantra repetitions and breathing cycles were counted to have a measured approach, so as not to overdo or underdo practices. This produces a small restriction, especially in meditation, because it ties the mantra to an outer activity, ticking off the beads one by one with the fingers. It becomes an unconscious habit, yet still we are regulating the mantra with an outer activity. With the clock, we can let the mantra (and the breath in pranayama) go naturally according to the unique purification need of the nervous system. We have talked a lot about this already. Using the clock is a flexible approach to measuring the amount of inner practices. Of course, we will peek at the clock now and then, but in time we find that our automatic inner clock is nearly as good as the outer one. The outer clock then becomes an occasional confirmation of the inner one. There is a lesson (#23) on this in the meditation Q&As called, "Watching the clock."

_____

The guru is in you.

2010/01/27 17:34:44
Other Systems and Alternate Approaches
Japa Mala

Hi Victor:

Don't know if your email has changed in the last few years, but I emailed you on this earlier today. Copied below.

As for a timer, I have never used one. A clock or watch has always been sufficient here.

The guru is in you.

Hi Victor:

I wanted to make sure you saw this:
http://www.aypsite.org/forum/topic.asp?TOPIC_ID=7109#63826

I had to step in there to avoid possible confusion for others on AYP deep meditation procedure.

This is not to imply you have been wasting your time. If you decide to move from mala to clock, you can consider it to have been a useful stepping stone to a deeper practice. Moving to the clock could be considered to be like adding a mantra enhancement. :-)

All the best!

The guru is in you.

Yogani

2010/02/24 12:02:03
Other Systems and Alternate Approaches
http://www.aypsite.org/forum/topic.asp?TOPIC_ID=7338&REPLY_ID=65312&whichpage=-1
John Kabat-Zinn - Mindfulness Meditation

Hi amoux:

Perhaps before you go in an entirely new direction, review this lesson for over-sensitive meditators, and consider trying breath meditation:
http://www.aypsite.org/367.html

It has been helpful to those who have had sensitivity issues with mantra.

Before that, you might try backing off to 10 minutes with the mantra, with a good rest before getting up. It may be as simple as making a time adjustment with adequate rest afterward. It does not have to be all or nothing. This is what self-pacing is about.

Your choice. Wishing you all the best!

The guru is in you.

2010/03/15 11:20:24
Other Systems and Alternate Approaches
http://www.aypsite.org/forum/topic.asp?TOPIC_ID=7427&REPLY_ID=66092&whichpage=-1
Rebirthing / Breathwork - my experience

Hi Harmony:

Sorry, I'm not familiar with that system of practice. I would only suggest being careful not to overdo, or to "double up" on similar practices from more than one system in a given session or day. It can lead to overloads. It should also be mentioned that there can be a delayed reaction when overdoing with pranayama. What feels good now may not feel good later if developing a balanced daily routine for the long term is not the first priority.

Note to All: I am asked every week in email and the forums to comment on at least a dozen "other systems" of practice. It is not possible for me to respond to all of these requests. The suggestion to those who are interested in comparing AYP to other systems of practice is to become familiar with the AYP baseline system through study of the writings and daily practice. Then you will be in the best position to form your own opinion about other systems of practice in relation to AYP, and proceed accordingly.

All the best!

The guru is in you.

2010/03/15 13:32:06
Other Systems and Alternate Approaches
http://www.aypsite.org/forum/topic.asp?TOPIC_ID=7432&REPLY_ID=66105&whichpage=-1
Alternate nostril breathing and root to crown SBP?

quote:
_____

Originally posted by Yogsadhak

Thank you Christi,

Since the 20 kriyas of Swami Satyananda includes both circular and linear practices as well as awakening the chakras intensely,

Is it not giving the benefits of AYP, Taoist microcosmic orbit and ancient Kundalini yoga,which actually place some emphasis on the chakras as is the tradition of yoga itself?
_____

Hi Yogsadhak, and welcome!

It may be so, but why are you seeking verification from elsewhere? Isn't your own daily practice enough verification? It is either working for you or it isn't, and it seems any questions you have about Satyananda's teachings should go back to Bihar or others who are qualified in that system.

AYP is a system also, but that does not mean AYP practitioners are experts on everything else, or that one system is "better" than another. Each will travel their own path, and it is the practitioner's choice. Here is a lesson on the consideration of other paths: http://www.aypsite.org/19.html

Also, you might like to take a look at this, posted today in another topic:
http://www.aypsite.org/forum/topic.asp?TOPIC_ID=7427#66092

quote:
_____
Note to All: I am asked every week in email and the forums to comment on at least a dozen "other systems" of practice. It is not possible for me to respond to all of these requests. The suggestion to those who are interested in comparing AYP to other systems of practice is to become familiar with the AYP baseline system through study of the writings and daily practice. Then you will be in the best position to form your own opinion about other systems of practice in relation to AYP, and proceed accordingly.
_____

It has always seemed odd when people come and ask me or other AYP practitioners to explain or justify another system. Yet, this is exactly what people keep asking over and over again.

If you are attempting to establish a superiority claim of one teaching over another, it will not go far here, because all practitioners are encouraged to find what works best for them, and it is not always going to be the same thing for everyone. We accept that fact in AYP, and do what we can to provide flexibility for the practitioner through extensive application of self-pacing and alternate approaches available within the AYP baseline system.

One size does not fit all. Yet, we all have to pick something, and stick with it for the long term if we expect to find significant results. That applies to any system.

What anyone "thinks" about one system versus another is of little consequence. The question is, are you practicing daily for the long term? If you are, using a time-tested approach, then all the answers will be there for you, and you won't have to be asking others to tell you what you can only find out in yourself through direct experience.

You can be sure that whatever you decide to do on your path will be respected here, and a return of the favor is expected. Share your journey. We'd love to hear about it. Always favor real practice over the "scenery" of endless speculation, and enjoy!

The guru is in you.

PS: A discussion on alternate nostril breathing in relation to AYP spinal breathing pranayama can be found at the end of Lesson 41.

2010/03/15 19:18:59
Other Systems and Alternate Approaches
http://www.aypsite.org/forum/topic.asp?TOPIC_ID=7432&REPLY_ID=66123&whichpage=-1
Alternate nostril breathing and root to crown SBP?

Hi Yogsadhak:

It is great to know about a lot of practices. It is a sign of the times. It is even better to be applying only a few practices with effectiveness, year in and year out. The suggestion is to continue to practice with balance and consistency, learn from your experience, and make adjustments occasionally as needed.

So far, you have only mentioned energy practices. In the AYP approach, deep meditation, the cultivation of abiding inner silence, is regarded to be primary, with energy practices coming after to facilitate the expansion of inner silence through the rise of ecstatic conductivity (kundalini) throughout the neurobiology. But not all systems take that approach.

In AYP, we also cover systematic applications of samyama and various modes of self-inquiry, which are for further cultivating abiding inner silence, and expanding and stabilizing the witness quality in everyday living, leading to unity (Oneness) and the ongoing experience of "stillness in action." This leads naturally to an outpouring of divine love and a tendency toward service to others.

Carry on!

The guru is in you.

2010/03/15 23:00:36
Other Systems and Alternate Approaches
http://www.aypsite.org/forum/topic.asp?TOPIC_ID=7432&REPLY_ID=66128&whichpage=-1
Alternate nostril breathing and root to crown SBP?

Hi Yogsadhak:

AYP deep mediation encompasses dharana, dhyana and samad
Hi in one fell swoop, steadily cultivating permanent abiding samad
Hi through twice-daily practice. Samyama also covers the last three limbs of yoga, going in the reverse direction, "moving stillness" from the inside out. Both of these are specific techniques that can be easily undertaken in an efficient daily routine of practices, which can also be developed to include energy cultivation techniques (pranayama, mudras, bandhas, tantric sexual methods, etc.). Together, these cultivate abiding inner silence and ecstatic conductivity, and the joining of the two, which is the marriage of stillness and ecstasy within us.

You are still talking mostly about energy practices and experiences, which is only half of the enlightenment equation. In the AYP approach, deep meditation and related inner silence cultivation methods play a much more prominent role.

The most important question any spiritual aspirant can ask is, What is my consistent daily practice? If the answer to that changes every week or month, then it is time to take a step back and assess the situation. Spiritual practice is not about the energy experience of the week. It is about the gradual process of human spiritual transformation cultivated over years. For that, it is good to systematically address both sides of the enlightenment equation (inner silence and ecstatic conductivity), which requires consistency over time in the corresponding practices, no matter what system we may be using.

All of this is built up in a logical fashion in the main lessons.

The guru is in you.

2010/03/16 11:15:54
Other Systems and Alternate Approaches
http://www.aypsite.org/forum/topic.asp?TOPIC_ID=7432&REPLY_ID=66133&whichpage=-1
Alternate nostril breathing and root to crown SBP?

Hi Yogsadhak:

Spinal and targeted bastrika are hybrids of bastrika and spinal breathing, found to have some benefit for clearing localized blockages under certain circumstances. These are traditional elements that have been combined for optional use. There are other hybrids available in AYP, such as yoni chin pump and yoni spinal breathing. All of these are optional. Everything in AYP is optional. :-)

Still focusing almost exclusively on energy practices? It is suggested again to balance inner silence and energy practices. Man does not become enlightened by energy practices alone. Why worry so much about finer points in the energy practice department, when there is a huge gaping hole in the meditation department?

Lahiri Mahasaya said, "Enlightenment is the merging of emptiness (inner silence) with euphoria (ecstatic energy)." Somewhere along the way the importance of cultivating the emptiness side became largely forgotten in kriya yoga (and elsewhere). AYP's tools in this area offer an opportunity for enhancement for those who sense that something has been missing. Energy experiences can be very seductive, but are not so spiritually progressive by themselves. It takes two to do the enlightenment tango -- inner silence and ecstatic conductivity.

The guru is in you.

2010/03/16 23:59:56
Other Systems and Alternate Approaches
http://www.aypsite.org/forum/topic.asp?TOPIC_ID=7432&REPLY_ID=66150&whichpage=-1
Alternate nostril breathing and root to crown SBP?

quote:
_____
Originally posted by Yogsadhak

How is the "I AM" mantra more important or powerful than the primordial OM? What are your thoughts on Chidakasha Dharana?
_____

Hi Yogsadhak:

Regarding the I AM mantra versus OM, see here: http://www.aypsite.org/59.html
Also see "Mantra - Enhancements" in the topic index on the main website. We do include OM later in an enhancement.

Regarding Chidakasha Dharana, it will be best if I refrain from commenting on other styles of meditation, because the number of them is unlimited, and the requests for comments keep coming in by the boatload. A line has to be drawn somewhere. This one is covered implicitly in the lessons already anyway. Can you find it?

Others, feel free to put in your two cents.

The guru is in you.

2010/07/17 11:07:17
Other Systems and Alternate Approaches
http://www.aypsite.org/forum/topic.asp?TOPIC_ID=8110&REPLY_ID=71023&whichpage=-1
Spirit Masters

Hi Nayarb:

Belief systems and objects of devotion serve their ultimate purpose by enabling us to go beyond the externals to their (and our) source -- inner silence. Living in inner silence (divine Self) while active in the world is the objective of all systems that lead to the truth.

Our chosen ideal (ishta) can be anything, and its value is not in conceptualizing and sustaining identification with it, but in refining it through prayer, meditation, samyama and other actions we take on behalf of our spiritual progress. This process of refinement is covered in detail in the AYP Bhakti and Karma Yoga book.

"Spirit guides" can serve that purpose just as any other ishta can. In the case of living gurus (or any other interactive teacher), it is incumbent on them to encourage the transcendence of reliance on their presence in time and space.

Yoga is therefore not at odds with religion, but in support of it, always encouraging us to look beyond the surface of objects and doctrine, to the depth of inner silence that is the One supporting us all.

As we have said: "The One is the many and the many are the One."
This is what Lesson 421 on spirits attempts to convey in practical terms.

Sounds like good things are happening there. Deep meditation will fulfill the truth in our beliefs, regardless of our culture or creed. The human nervous system is the doorway, and we each have one of those. :-)

Sorry, not familiar with the kriya yoga system you mentioned. Perhaps others here will have some perspective on that.

Wishing you all the best on your continuing path. Practice wisely, and enjoy!

The guru is in you.

2010/07/26 22:54:59
Other Systems and Alternate Approaches
http://www.aypsite.org/forum/topic.asp?TOPIC_ID=8159&REPLY_ID=71332&whichpage=-1
A Living Kriya Master?

quote:
_____
Originally posted by KriyabanSeeking

Also, in the FAQ section, it says, "To Subscribe or Unsubscribe from any level of subscription, you can use the "My Subscriptions" link, located near the top of each page to manage your subscriptions. Or you can click on the subscribe/unsubscribe icons ( ) for that Category/Forum/Topic you want to subscribe/unsubscribe to/from." however, I dont;t see these anywhere. How do I subscribe to specific posts? Thanks!
_____

Hi KriyabanSeeking, and welcome! :-)

Due to technical and resource factors, we have the subscriptions feature for the forums turned off. That is why you don't see it here.

One of the easiest ways to keep up with what is going on in forum categories and topics of interest is to become familiar with the "active topics" feature on the top menu. This enables you to see the latest posts for a selected period of time, sorted by forum category and topic. To see the last post in a topic, click the blue arrow next to the last poster's name.

The forums also have an RSS feature, which can be found under "communities" near the bottom of the left border menu on any page.

All the best!

The guru is in you.

PS: You can link any forum or topic by bookmarking it in your browser. You can also get a link for any specific post in the forums by clicking on the little globe icon with the arrow in it at the top of any post of interest. There are other ways to navigate that you will discover as you become more familiar with the forums. Those are a few of the basics.

2010/09/17 10:55:32
Other Systems and Alternate Approaches
http://www.aypsite.org/forum/topic.asp?TOPIC_ID=8448&REPLY_ID=72950&whichpage=-1
Meditation for all levels of Spiritual Seekers?

Hi Ram:

Thank you for your sincere sharing.

Sorry you have had such difficulties with meditation over the years. You are wise to self-pace and adjust your practices as necessary for best results with comfort. That is the suggestion for everyone from the beginning.

I would take issue with one comment you made above:

It has not been the experience in the AYP community that the "majority" of people are not ready for deep meditation. While there have been some who have had difficulty, it has been a small minority, based on reports we have received over the years. We have been working to address those who are over-sensitive, as you know, culminating in these three lessons that address both ends of the sensitivity scale:

On the Range of Sensitivities: http://www.aypsite.org/365.html
On Under-Sensitive: http://www.aypsite.org/366.html
On Over-Sensitive: http://www.aypsite.org/367.html

These have been aimed at finding solutions for those who wish to meditate, who may have particular sensitivity issues.

In some cases, meditation of any kind may not be appropriate at all for a time. But this can change in a flash. There are cases here of people who were under or over sensitive, and then it changed suddenly (or in a relatively short time) with a blockage dissolving.

"Unfathomable are the portents of karma."

Since most do derive benefits from deep meditation with minimal disruption, I will continue to suggest it as a starting point, simply because it is a fast path for most, and that is what people want. For those it is disruptive for, self-pacing and alternate approaches will continue to be suggested.

With so many benefiting, I think it would be counter-productive to go back (here in AYP) to the kind of "gated" systems of practice that have contributed to the lack of spiritual progress in humanity over the centuries, including endless frustration for the many who have sought effective paths of practice to move forward according to their bhakti. It has been to address this very situation that AYP was created -- laying all the options on the table, putting the practitioner in charge, and not a third party whose fixed ideas may be wholly inappropriate in any given situation.

Everyone deserves the opportunity to find out for themselves if they are ready for powerful spiritual practices or not. Those who are over-sensitive will find out soon enough, and they should step back according to the advice given in the AYP writings. The risks are minimal if the self-pacing guidelines are followed. There are plenty of alternative approaches available, which you have pointed to in your sharing above.

And as you say, when any practitioner is ready for more, it is here. :-)

We are experiencing a paradigm shift from teacher-directed practice to self-directed practice. It has been new territory with risks and benefits. The risks are associated mainly with each person's ability to take responsibility when using powerful tools. It has been successful beyond what I could have predicted, and that is a testament to the capability of human beings to make good use of tools that are openly available. This lesson provides further thoughts on the matter of responsibility in practices: http://www.aypsite.org/217.html

Wishing you all the best on your path. Continue to practice wisely, and enjoy!

The guru is in you.

2010/09/17 17:37:11
Other Systems and Alternate Approaches
http://www.aypsite.org/forum/topic.asp?TOPIC_ID=8448&REPLY_ID=72962&whichpage=-1
Meditation for all levels of Spiritual Seekers?

Hi Ram:

There are at least as many beginners utilizing the AYP writings as experienced practitioners. I have not noticed more who are sensitive to deep meditation coming from any particular level of experience, or lack of it.

While it is yet to be proven conclusively, I believe that you could teach these practices to any group of people anywhere in the world, and the profile of results (and sensitivities) among the people would be essentially the same. This is what we are seeing so far with a wide sample of practitioners across the world. Time will tell if the results continue that way.

People come to AYP for all sorts of reasons, ranging from purely spiritual, to personal health and happiness issues. There is no one profile that fits everyone who comes here. AYP practitioners represent a cross-section of every kind of personality, level of experience, cultural and religious background. So it is not a good idea to generalize on what kind of person uses AYP, and what spiritual advantage they may have over any other person anywhere else. The human nervous system is what we all have in common.

Btw, sensitivity to meditation and other practices is not a symptom of spiritual underdevelopment. It can be a high conductivity in the nervous system, which is an advanced condition indicating a certain kind of inner purification, but with some imbalance that is lingering from who knows when or why (karma).

All of these things can be worked through with a methodical approach, and with persistence and patience.

Carry on! :-)

The guru is in you.

2010/09/25 13:35:58
Other Systems and Alternate Approaches
http://www.aypsite.org/forum/topic.asp?TOPIC_ID=8448&REPLY_ID=73220&whichpage=-1
Meditation for all levels of Spiritual Seekers?

Hi All:

This is really a debate about who is in the majority -- those who can pick up with deep meditation at the start and experience benefits without major disruptions, versus those who may not. It is also a debate about whether humanity as a whole has been advancing in its receptivity to the causes and effects found in advanced spiritual practices like deep meditation and spinal breathing pranayama.

The modern view is that those who can benefit from these practices are in the majority, and that there is a rising receptivity in the whole of humanity resulting from the increasingly widespread use of spiritual practices around the world over the past century.

The traditional view is that nothing has changed in the evolution of humanity over the centuries, and that everyone must be pre-qualified before receiving advanced practices by passing through the preliminary wickets of yoga (yama, niyama, asana, etc.).

Obviously, AYP represents the modern view. For the perceived minority who may be over-sensitive to deep meditation with mantra (for whatever reason), many measures are offered to balance and protect against potential hazards (primarily energy overloads). So whether sensitivity is an issue in the beginning, or later on (it too can happen), ample means are available for dealing with it in a self-directed manner, and moving ahead. For long-time meditators (perhaps the most sensitive of all, while at the same time largely unfazed by the ups and downs in life), the maxim is "less is more." This has been covered in the later lessons.

The truth is, sensitivity to inner spiritual processes is not the primary issue. Nearly everyone will experience it at one time or other along their path. The real issue is education. With good education, all challenges along the path can be navigated. Without good education, most will shrink from the path, and the journey will be left to the very few, which has been the history of humanity up until now. In this new information age, we find ourselves in a position to change that for future generations.

We must do something to advance along our path. What that something is will depend on the person -- not only their capacity, but also their desire (bhakti). The view in AYP is that how to proceed is an individual choice. For this, many tools have been provided, which, in the vast majority of cases, have been used with responsibility.

This debate about the spiritual readiness of humanity could go on for 100 years (it probably will). Whatever the truth may be, no one can deny that we are living in a time when increasing information about spiritual practices and their effects is changing the face of spiritual teaching everywhere. It is incumbent on all of us to deal with that in a responsible manner. However much humanity may be the same, the information available has expanded dramatically. Like it or not, that is changing the game.

Meanwhile, who will be benefiting as we debate the readiness of humanity for this? Turning it all back to the old ways would be a high price to pay for those in every corner of the world who, however many they may be, are ready to move ahead with advanced practices. We can't go back, because the cat is out of the bag. We can only go forward. The only thing that could stop it would be the demise of the internet.

Clearly, one size in practices does not fit all, even though there is a tendency in humans to impress upon others that what we believe is the best for everyone. Accordingly, I have some concern that the heavy hand of tradition is beginning to over-step itself here.

Keep in mind that AYP is an open system, which means anyone can use it, or not use it, according to personal preference. If it does not work in a particular case, then the seeker is encouraged to keep looking until they find an approach that does work for them, no matter where it may be found. From the AYP point of view, there are no limitations in this. But do not expect the AYP system of practices to throw itself out the window while promoting freedom of choice. It is a baseline teaching, and the baseline will be preserved as best as possible.

In seeking out alternatives, whether they be traditional or not, do not try and redesign the AYP baseline system in the process. That will not work. It will only lead sincere seekers into confusion, and be helping no one.

If alternate approaches are being proposed, such discussions are welcome here, but ought not be at the expense of clarity about what AYP is, and they should be conducted in the "Other Systems" forum category, where it will be clear that they are something different from the AYP baseline system, and not attempting to discredit the ongoing work that is occurring here.

Fair enough?

The guru is in you.

2010/09/26 10:05:51
Other Systems and Alternate Approaches
http://www.aypsite.org/forum/topic.asp?TOPIC_ID=8448&REPLY_ID=73247&whichpage=-1
Meditation for all levels of Spiritual Seekers?

Hi rkishan:

This is a very informative discussion, and can be helpful to many. It is, however, mainly about alternative approaches, so we will move it to the "Other Systems" forum category. The discussion can continue there as desired.

Many thanks to everyone for contributing, and all the best on your chosen path!

The guru is in you.

2010/10/18 15:09:12
Other Systems and Alternate Approaches
http://www.aypsite.org/forum/topic.asp?TOPIC_ID=8597&REPLY_ID=73954&whichpage=-1
Negative energies.

Hi Miguel:

There is a big difference between a gathering where people come to unload their "stuff" externally, versus a gathering where group meditation is occurring using an effective technique for bringing everyone to inner silence. In the second case, "stuff" (karmic baggage) is dissolved mostly internally, and not spread around very much externally.

In the first kind of group, you may well bring someone else's baggage home with you. In the second kind of group (with deep meditation), everyone will more likely bring home less baggage, including less of their own!

Clearly, all groups are not equal in their effects, and it is up to each of us to decide which kind of group is best for our spiritual development.

It is a mistake to categorize all "spiritual" groups under the same heading energetically. Legitimate meditation groups (and retreats) can be very quick in dissolving the very concern you are raising. This is the predominant experience of many who attend real meditation groups and retreats.

Of course, any group or practice that over-stimulates a sensitivity we might have should be "self-paced" as necessary. But let's not throw out the baby with the bathwater. :-)

The guru is in you.

2010/10/18 16:44:41
Other Systems and Alternate Approaches
http://www.aypsite.org/forum/topic.asp?TOPIC_ID=8597&REPLY_ID=73958&whichpage=-1
Negative energies.

quote:
───────
Originally posted by tonightsthenight

Is there any practice you can prescribe to help me fend off this unloading? Or is it enough to simply "not buy into it"?
───────

Hi tonightsthenight:

Twice daily deep meditation.

Abiding inner silence is the best defense for all kinds of mishaps, and it is permanent. It is realizing our essential nature. Mental strategies, psychic structures and shields are temporary, and don't work very well anyway. They will dissolve in abiding inner silence also, along with all the garbage that is stuck to them. :-)

Much better to go immediately beyond all structures to what is real. The unreal cannot harm us when we have become stillness in action.

Until then, we may have little choice but to use less effective strategies, or walk away from unloading. These are reasonable measures, until we have transitioned to a more permanent resilience in stillness, and have much more freedom to be in any environment. At the same time, we will get much better at recognizing the energetic pitfalls in life, and automatically neutralize their negative effects before they can manifest. This occurs in stillness also.

The guru is in you.

2010/11/08 22:38:20
Other Systems and Alternate Approaches
http://www.aypsite.org/forum/topic.asp?TOPIC_ID=8705&REPLY_ID=74958&whichpage=-1
Done For

Hi tonightsthenight:

May it smooth out for you soon.

I don't know what your practice is (you have repeatedly said it is not AYP), so it is difficult to make definitive suggestions from this end, other than to put more focus on consistently cultivating abiding inner silence, if possible. That takes the edge off all adversity, whether it is kundalini or other life challenges.

Wishing you all the best on your continuing path, which clearly must be your own way.

The guru is in you.

2010/12/03 23:11:04
Other Systems and Alternate Approaches
http://www.aypsite.org/forum/topic.asp?TOPIC_ID=8838&REPLY_ID=76133&whichpage=-1
Paarayana

quote:
───────
Originally posted by Saagaram

I'm just saying "hey look what I found." Anyway. Peace out!
───────

Hi Saagaram and welcome!

What you found is an idea, and it is a start. It will take years (maybe decades) of earnest effort to unfold the reality of the actual condition the idea conveys. It is not something you can create (or uncreate) with your mind. It has to be cultivated in your subtle neurobiology and in your bones, and that awakening takes time.

The Buddha spent many years on the path of practices before he found his "instant" enlightenment. Then he formulated the "four noble truths" and the "eight-fold path," and many nuances of it while spending the rest of his life (some 40 years) tirelessly serving others on their spiritual journeys. That is a more realistic view of the Buddha, and a more realistic view of what is involved in human spiritual transformation. It is not much about holding a philosophical view on non-doing, or playing a game about having a non-view, which is nothing but another castle in the air. We are talking about something much more real and lasting than that. Not something we have to remind ourselves (or anyone else) about every five minutes. Enlightenment is something we uncover within us, something that is self-sustaining and ever-lasting. It cannot be argued for or against.

Having an ideal is very important, but if you don't take practical steps to realize it, you will find the going getting tough pretty soon. See how it goes in the coming months. See how it is when you are facing hardship. If you can stand firm in your new-found belief for six months, you will have proved yourself stubborn enough to be worthy of long term practices, if you are able to make a rational connection between cause and effect. And if you get worn out before six months are up (most taking your position do), then you will be ready for practices even sooner. Or maybe you will drop the whole thing for a while. One thing is for sure. You can't sustain the idea or non-idea indefinitely. Something with more staying power will have to be uncovered deep within you. That is what meditation is for. Buddhists do meditate, you know. And so do we here.

Also, you may want to check out this lesson on the art of doing nothing: http://www.aypsite.org/84.html

Wishing you all the best on your (non)path. Good luck, and Enjoy!

The guru is in you.

2010/12/04 11:20:34
Other Systems and Alternate Approaches
http://www.aypsite.org/forum/topic.asp?TOPIC_ID=8838&REPLY_ID=76154&whichpage=-1
Paarayana

Hi Saagaram:

The Buddha disavowed living an extreme ascetic lifestyle, which he had done without any meaningful results. He did not disavow meditation, living a monastic live (optional), or serving others. In other words, he did not disavow effective practices. He did not disavow what you are doing either. He taught a balance between all these elements according to individual need. So if what you are doing fits your need, that's great, but don't expect it to be the same for everyone.

The comments I made about seeing if you can keep up what you are doing (or not doing) for 6 months are based on many who have come around with similar non-duality arguments, which 9 times out of 10 are only intellectual, and unsustainable in practical living. So it is just a heads up in case you are a beginner, which your statement, "Hey, look what I found" seems to imply. Maybe not.

In any case, the approach you are describing works best when entertained in abiding inner silence. In AYP we call that "relational self-inquiry" (in stillness) with the opposite being "non-relational self-inquiry" (in the mind). This is far more than a theory. The terminology actually evolved from the direct experiences of many who have come to it from various directions, including from the same (non)position you are describing. It is discussed in detail in the AYP lessons, starting around here: http://www.aypsite.org/321.html

All of which is to say, meditation of some kind (the primary means for cultivating abiding inner silence) is essential for anyone who aspires to live a non-view, represented by Krishnamurti or anyone like him. The non-view itself can be an object of constant meditation (Krishnamurti's teaching), but that approach has been found by many to not be very efficient. So more efficient and easily applied methods for cultivating abiding inner silence have been developed. It is all for the same purpose.

The awakening of abiding inner silence (the witness) is the key, no matter what approach one is following. Maybe you were born with it. If so, good for you. And if not, then there is work to do. The truth about it is for you to determine, or to ignore as you see fit. There is nothing wrong with affirmation, as long as it is balanced with honest self-inquiry, preferably in stillness, the wellspring of all wisdom.

The goal here at AYP is to help as many as possible find their way forward on their own terms. That does not mean offering nothing. A lot of proven tools are available here, being used in many configurations. That is what AYP focuses on -- the tools, and the many ways they can be applied, depending on individual need. It is a resource that is open to all, to use or not use however each sees fit. That's all.

All the best!

The guru is in you.

PS: Yes, AYP began with basic discoveries on practice here, but has continued to evolve over the years with the collective discoveries of a large community of practitioners, which as a body of knowledge is far more significant than any one person's experience or point of view.

2010/12/04 18:14:41
Other Systems and Alternate Approaches
http://www.aypsite.org/forum/topic.asp?TOPIC_ID=8838&REPLY_ID=76167&whichpage=-1
Paarayana

quote:
_____
Originally posted by Bod
Hi Tree

I'm reminded of a wonderful passage from the novel "Siddhartha" by Herman Hesse, when the main character, a "samana" and eager spiritual seeker, comes across the Gotama Buddha and engages in a metaphysical conversation with him. After a lengthy discourse, the Buddha replies with a loving smile:

"You are clever, O samana. You can speak cleverly, my friend. Beware of too much cleverness!"

I have to remind myself of these hearty words since I myself am fond of debate and playing games with words and concepts!

Namaste.
_____

It could also be said that no one wins in a Buddhist-style debate, least of all the one with the cleverest argument. :-)

The guru is in you.

2010/12/05 00:23:31
Other Systems and Alternate Approaches
http://www.aypsite.org/forum/topic.asp?TOPIC_ID=8838&REPLY_ID=76192&whichpage=-1
Paarayana

quote:
_____
Originally posted by machart

Sometimes these advaita vs practices debates can go on and on and on ... and on.
_____

Hi All:

Just to be clear, there is no argument on advaita vs practices within the AYP approach. One leads to the other going in either direction and the two are 100% complementary. The connection is very clear on the experiential level for quite a few here, and this is what counts.

What I will always challenge is a stand-alone intellectual approach to advaita, because it leads people into non-relational self-inquiry, which is not only ineffective for most, but can be damaging to a person's motivation to engage in everyday living, fulfill their responsibilities, etc. Natural enlightened non-duality (stillness in action and outpouring divine love) is liberation in all circumstances of life, while intellectual non-duality (in mind only) can lead to misery and despair over a falsely assumed meaninglessness of life.

Whether Saagaram is one or the other only he or she can know. But that isn't the point. The point is that telling people in a large public community that practices are not necessary is like telling people they can materialize on the other side of the country without using an airplane to get there. While it may be so for the one saying it, it is a disservice to present that as a practical approach for a broad community of aspirants.

The philosophy of advaita/non-duality can provide useful inspiration (an ideal), but there is little practical value beyond that for a large number of seekers representing many levels of unfoldment. Most will be unable to take the leap. They simply are not ripe and ready for it. For that reason, I will always challenge stand-alone intellectual approaches to realization, even if the person offering it is legitimate in their own experience.

It isn't about any particular person, or their spiritual condition. It is about what will work for the community, and the whole of humanity. Toward that end, the AYP approach to self-inquiry, and letting go into non-duality when ripe and ready for it, is presented in a way that is approachable by anyone, with clear experiential markers along the way. Many of the common pitfalls can be avoided this way.

The guru is in you.

Forum 20 – Illuminated Poetry, Quotations and Stories

Put your own writing here, and your favorite quotes and stories.
http://www.aypsite.org/forum/forum.asp?FORUM_ID=25

2005/07/13 12:54:36
Illuminated Poetry, Quotations and Stories
http://www.aypsite.org/forum/topic.asp?TOPIC_ID=289
Poetry and Quotations

It has been said that poetry is the language of divine experience and enlightenment. Somehow the divine can be more easily captured in concise verses than in long essays. The more concise the verses the more we can find between the lines. It is a paradox, really. Where there is paradox, God is always at work.

So, if you are one who writes poetry in your reverie, or if the poetry itself is your reverie, please share some with us. We will be very happy to savor it.

If someone else's writing has inspired you to greater spiritual heights, please share that also, so that we may be inspired too.

Here are two:

Keep walking, though there's no place to get to.
Don't try to see through the distances.
That's not for human beings. Move within,
But don't move the way fear makes you move.

~ Rumi

Why be vexed by the world?
It is the play of light and dark
It is being transformed
The world is you

~ Yogani

The guru is in you.

2005/08/04 17:02:28
Illuminated Poetry, Quotations and Stories
http://www.aypsite.org/forum/topic.asp?TOPIC_ID=381
The Parents of Invention

If necessity is the mother of invention, then stillness is certainly its father.

2005/08/05 13:07:34
Illuminated Poetry, Quotations and Stories
http://www.aypsite.org/forum/topic.asp?TOPIC_ID=386
What Is

It is not about what I want. It is about what is.

2005/08/07 13:03:43
Illuminated Poetry, Quotations and Stories
http://www.aypsite.org/forum/topic.asp?TOPIC_ID=393
The Greatest Teacher

Student: Who was your greatest teacher?

Teacher: They were all the greatest. When they were right, I grew. And when they were wrong, I grew even more.

2005/08/25 17:10:12
Illuminated Poetry, Quotations and Stories
http://www.aypsite.org/forum/topic.asp?TOPIC_ID=434
Unity

By definition, Unity will leave no one behind.

2005/08/28 11:50:36
Illuminated Poetry, Quotations and Stories
http://www.aypsite.org/forum/topic.asp?TOPIC_ID=438
Seeing

I see a world full with enlightened people.
"But where are they?" you ask.
They are everywhere, all around us.
It is all in our seeing.

2005/09/07 14:03:10
Illuminated Poetry, Quotations and Stories

http://www.aypsite.org/forum/topic.asp?TOPIC_ID=466
The Four Agreements

1. BE IMPECCABLE WITH YOUR WORD - Speak with integrity. Say what you mean. Avoid using the word to speak against yourself or to gossip about others. Use the power of your word in the direction of truth and love.

2. DON'T TAKE ANYTHING PERSONALLY - Nothing others do is because of you. What others say and do is a projection of their own reality, their own dream. When you are immune to the opinions and actions of others, you won't be the victim of needless suffering.

3. DON'T MAKE ASSUMPTIONS - Find the courage to ask questions and to express what you really want. Communicate with others as clearly as you can to avoid misunderstandings, sadness, and drama. With just this one agreement, you can completely transform your life.

4. ALWAYS DO YOUR BEST - Your best is going to change from moment to moment; it will be different when you are healthy as opposed to sick. Under any circumstance, simply do your best, and you will avoid self-judgement, self-abuse, and regret.

From "THE FOUR AGREEMENTS" by Don Miguel Ruiz
"A Toltec Wisdom Book and Practical Guide to Personal Freedom"

2005/09/09 17:57:06
Illuminated Poetry, Quotations and Stories
http://www.aypsite.org/forum/topic.asp?TOPIC_ID=466&REPLY_ID=622&whichpage=-1
The Four Agreements

Hi A & M:

The Four Agreements is an excellent little book that I highly recommend to anyone who is looking for yama/niyama (spiritual conduct) suggestions. With some inner silence added via daily deep meditation, it can be very effective.

As for making this topic sticky (perpetually on top), I don't want to be one-upping anyone here more than I have already, so I am shy to do that. So many have equally good quotes and poems to post here, I'm sure. If enough people add replies here, we can consider making it sticky -- by popular demand. A full-fledged discussion on The Four Agreements in "Books" or "Yamas & Niyamas" would be be a good way to go also.

It is up to you all.

The guru is in you.

2005/10/19 16:28:21
Illuminated Poetry, Quotations and Stories
http://www.aypsite.org/forum/topic.asp?TOPIC_ID=534&REPLY_ID=1042&whichpage=-1
Lit

So beautiful...

That's right up there with St. Theresa of Avila, St. John of the Cross and Rumi.

They also felt it to be a feeble expression while writing their stuff. Yet, we are still reading it hundreds of years later, and new divine odes like yours too. Thank you...

The guru is in you.

2005/11/25 11:22:33
Illuminated Poetry, Quotations and Stories
http://www.aypsite.org/forum/topic.asp?TOPIC_ID=606
Knocking

"I have lived on the lip of insanity,
wanting to know reasons,
knocking on a door.
It opens.
I've been knocking from the inside!"

~Rumi

2006/01/19 13:36:16
Illuminated Poetry, Quotations and Stories
http://www.aypsite.org/forum/topic.asp?TOPIC_ID=745&REPLY_ID=2647&whichpage=-1
We are the ones we have been waiting for

I once meditated in the middle of the Hopi lands in Arizona. A great depth of profound inner silence there. We are the ones they have been waiting for...

John C. Kimbrough
2006/09/29 10:03:33
Illuminated Poetry, Quotations and Stories
http://www.aypsite.org/forum/topic.asp?TOPIC_ID=934&REPLY_ID=11695&whichpage=-1
John Kimbrough on Teaching Yoga in Southeast Asia

quote:
_____
Originally posted by John C. Kimbrough

Freedom From Prison, Freedom From Drugs, Freedom From Defilements and Hindrances

We sometimes have a great interest in, and can even find a degree of enlightenment and insight when we see a movie that in some manner reflects our own life experiences...
_____

Hi John:

That is a moving story. I'm so glad we figured out a way for you to share your essays here without overrunning us. :-)
Here's to redemption...

The guru is in you.

2006/03/22 13:41:09
Illuminated Poetry, Quotations and Stories
http://www.aypsite.org/forum/topic.asp?TOPIC_ID=954&REPLY_ID=4885&whichpage=-1
I am

Beautiful, Sparkle.

Shanti, wasn't it you who were wondering about those living empty spaces? Well, you are doing it. No need to label them...
2006/03/28 12:03:55
Illuminated Poetry, Quotations and Stories
http://www.aypsite.org/forum/topic.asp?TOPIC_ID=984&REPLY_ID=5279&whichpage=-1
the Comforter

Oh yes. Thanks for sharing that, Alan.

In AYP, a parallel is drawn between kundalini and the holy ghost. Though purification is not always comfortable, it inevitably leads to infinite comfort. And "s/he" definitely does teach us all things. :-)

If you have read the Secrets of Wilder, you know I have a strong interest in seeing solid spiritual practices become available to Christians. And, of course, the great truths within Christianity have much to offer in the process of human spiritual transformation, as well. It is so in every religion.

The guru is in you.

2009/05/04 15:46:32
Illuminated Poetry, Quotations and Stories
http://www.aypsite.org/forum/topic.asp?TOPIC_ID=1591&REPLY_ID=49987&whichpage=-1
It is not you who suffers

quote:
_____
Originally posted by emc

A one hour video on Da Man! Go to "free audio/video" and "Awaken to the eternal"
http://www.theeternalstate.org/

"Wisdom is knowing I am nothing
Love is knowing I am everything
and between the two my life moves"
_____

Hi emc and All:

This video on the life and teachings of Nisargadatta Maharaj is excellent, and I highly recommend it. It ties in with many things we have been discussing in AYP over the years, and is very compatible.

Thanks so much for sharing it. :-)

The guru is in you.

2007/08/12 11:02:47
Illuminated Poetry, Quotations and Stories
http://www.aypsite.org/forum/topic.asp?TOPIC_ID=2839
Leonard Cohen

"They called me a poet, and I guess I used to be one."

"They called me a singer, though I could barely carry a tune."

"They called me a ladies man, which was a joke. I spent 10,000 nights alone."

"Nothing is perfect. The cracks let the light in."

From interview and songs on the DVD: "Leonard Cohen - I'm Your Man"

2007/12/20 17:11:46
Illuminated Poetry, Quotations and Stories
http://www.aypsite.org/forum/topic.asp?TOPIC_ID=3291
The Magnificat

--------The Magnificat--------

My soul sings in gratitude.
I'm dancing in the mystery of God.
The light of the Holy One is within me
and I am blessed, so truly blessed.

This goes deeper than human thinking.
I am filled with awe
at Love whose only condition
is to be received.

The gift is not for the proud,
for they have no room for it.
The strong and self-sufficient ones
don't have this awareness.

But those who know their emptiness
can rejoice in Love's fullness.

It's the Love that we are made for,
the reason for our being.

It fills our inmost heart space
and brings to birth in us, the Holy One.

An interpretation of Mary's Song -- Luke 1:46-55
by Joy Cowley, Auckland, New Zealand
http://www.joycowley.com

2008/01/21 08:46:49
Illuminated Poetry, Quotations and Stories
http://www.aypsite.org/forum/topic.asp?TOPIC_ID=3391&REPLY_ID=29121&whichpage=-1
Sylvan of the Heart

Hi Scott:

Thank you. Beautiful sharings. Do continue writing and publishing. We all become wiser by it.

The guru is in you.

2008/05/21 08:22:25
Illuminated Poetry, Quotations and Stories
http://www.aypsite.org/forum/topic.asp?TOPIC_ID=3938
Don't Sweat the Small Stuff...

Hi All:

A modern Buddhist quotation:

"Don't sweat the small stuff. It's all small stuff."

If we translate that into AYP terms, it comes out something like this:

"Don't sweat the scenery. It's all scenery."

:-)

The guru is in you.

Who, what, when and where...
http://www.aypsite.org/forum/forum.asp?FORUM_ID=41

2005/07/13 13:27:00
Member Announcements - Events, Classes & Retreats
http://www.aypsite.org/forum/topic.asp?TOPIC_ID=290
Announcements - Events, Classes & Retreats

Is your guru coming to town? Or have you heard of any enlightening events, classes or retreats?

This is the place for all those important announcements. Make sure to include who, what, when and where, so we can all find it.

See also the AYP Directory Links Section for yoga teachers, classes, retreats, organizations, etc. -- http://www.aypsite.org/LinksDirectories.html

The guru is in you.

2005/12/04 10:24:15
Member Announcements - Events, Classes & Retreats
http://www.aypsite.org/forum/topic.asp?TOPIC_ID=618&REPLY_ID=1761&whichpage=-1
AYP Group Forming in San Francisco

Thank you, Ramon!

Yes, this is very exciting. The next step in AYP is to "take it to the people." That is, the people around us in everyday life. It can be in informal settings like person-to-person anywhere or in casual gatherings, discussion groups, etc. It can also be in more structured seminars and classes. Any medium will do.

Up until now there has been a gap between the "whole enchilada" writings on practices contained in the AYP lessons and the Secrets of Wilder novel. These contain a multitude of practices and their interrelationships. I wanted to do these first because, as a practitioner, I knew from the beginning all those years ago that it has been largely missing in the spiritual literature. Well, now we have it and can build on it here in the AYP community. That is happening, and it is a joy to see.

But, let's face it, the AYP lessons and novel are a bit much to hand to beginners and expect them to grasp it all. What has been needed is easier doorways into the knowledge that can be practically applied by anyone from day one. Enter the new book, *Deep Meditation - Pathway to Personal Freedom*, with more "*AYP Enlightenment Series*" entry-level books on other practices to follow soon. These can be used to introduce the knowledge to the general public. That is what they are for.

So, Ramon, when you stepped up with this opportunity to try it out, naturally I was very interested.

Over the past couple of years, others have expressed interest in forming local groups to help transmit the AYP knowledge and for support to those who are doing the practices. I encourage anyone interested in doing that to move ahead. It can add another layer of growth to your path. Feel free to contact me for suggestions. I will provide whatever support I can, including some free copies of *Deep Meditation* to help get things started.

The **AYP Forums** are an ideal place to network for this. We can share ideas and field questions on practices here that are not already covered in the AYP writings. In time, we can develop a flexible AYP teaching guideline that anyone can use to start up a discussion group, seminar or class. So there are a lot of possibilities to expand the "horizontal teaching model," which is person-to-person transmission of the "open source" practices of AYP.

For those who are not inclined to participate in groups or seminars, there are always the AYP books to hand out. The new one, *Deep Meditation*, is very inexpensive and self-explanatory to anyone who picks it up. So handing them out is also a good way to spread the knowledge. See the AYP Helpers forum for more on ways to obtain AYP books for giving away.

The new book should be showing up on Amazon and in other retail distribution channels this month.

The guru is in you.

2005/12/06 07:52:56
Member Announcements - Events, Classes & Retreats
http://www.aypsite.org/forum/topic.asp?TOPIC_ID=618&REPLY_ID=1801&whichpage=-1
AYP Group Forming in San Francisco

Hi Sean:

Sounds great. See the free offer for *Deep Meditation* books to hand out over here. It is the least I can do to help out.

To others, you don't have to start an AYP group to be eligible for these free books. We just want to hand them out everywhere. The book itself will do the rest. So step right up! :-)

I hope someone in San Francisco will be able to get **Yoga Journal's** attention on AYP at some point (circulation over 300,000). I have been trying for over a year, without much luck. Even spent over $1,000 for an ad in there last summer, which did not produce much. They have offices in Berkeley with headquarters (and editorial bosses) now in San Francisco. Any ideas how to entice them to do an AYP book review? A Los Angeles yoga magazine is interested in doing one, but nothing has been published on AYP yet. We really need published book reviews to help get the word out.

The AYP books will be in the two major new age trade shows in the USA next year (INATS), which should help visibility.

Well, all of that is above and beyond nice cozy meditation get-togethers in your loft, Sean. John Wilder and friends were into that as well. I started out that way too. And look what is happening now. Gatherings, especially on practices, are one of the best ways to promote expanding world consciousness, whether they be in the living room, the classroom, or here in cyberspace.

The guru is in you.

2005/12/10 08:43:30
Member Announcements - Events, Classes & Retreats
http://www.aypsite.org/forum/topic.asp?TOPIC_ID=618&REPLY_ID=1868&whichpage=-1
AYP Group Forming in San Francisco

Hi Ute:

I hope that serious open source writings on yoga like AYP can help bring yoga back to its roots of inner silence and ecstasy, and bring the mainstream along with it. That is the goal here. It's a tall order, but we are up to the task, yes?

The tank tops are okay if the practice is for real. Just part of the scenery, you know. :-)

The guru is in you.

2006/01/07 15:44:49
Member Announcements - Events, Classes & Retreats
http://www.aypsite.org/forum/topic.asp?TOPIC_ID=703
Iyengar on PBS
Received in my email today:

Go to: http://www.pbs.org/wnet/religionandethics/week919/profile.html
and watch the segment with BKS Iyengar if you missed it.

Religion & Ethics Newsweekly
Friday, January 6, 7:30pm
CHANNEL 20 (WFYI TV 20)

A report on relief efforts in Kashmir following the October earthquake that claimed thousands of lives and left millions homeless. Also: Indian yoga master B.K.S. Iyengar; and a Carnegie Hall performance by cantor Rebecca Garfein.

Appears to repeat Sunday morn at 11:30 a.m.

Check your own area tv listings. Jyoti

Tune In For A Profile of B.K.S. Iyengar

Dear Jyoti,

Don't miss the opportunity to see Guruji on television this weekend.

RELIGION & ETHICS NEWSWEEKLY, WNET CHANNEL 13
Airing:
Saturday, January 7, 10:30 AM
Sunday, January 8, 6:30 PM
(Check local listings for other times)

Kim Lawton talks with Indian yoga master B.K.S. Iyengar about his revolutionary approach and impact on yoga in the U.S. and how his teachings encourage people of faith to use the practice as a way to enhance their own spiritual beliefs.

Namaste

Iyengar Yoga Association of Greater New York
info@iyengarnyc.org
(212)691-9642
http://www.iyengarnyc.org/

2006/06/13 14:41:43
Member Announcements - Events, Classes & Retreats
http://www.aypsite.org/forum/topic.asp?TOPIC_ID=1215
MapQuest Style Yoga Studio Locator

Hi All:

A map locator covering nearly 5,000 yoga studios in the USA:

http://find.mapmuse.com/re1/interest.php?brandID=YOGA_STUDIOS

Pretty amazing site. Have fun with it! :-)

The guru is in you.

2006/06/30 11:36:25
Member Announcements - Events, Classes & Retreats

AYP Long Distance Meditation Group?

Hi Shanti and All:

It is a wonderful idea and I wish you all the best in your group meditation(s). It will be best if I stay on the sidelines and bathe in your waves of bliss. Thank you for that! :-)

You are illuminating the world with the light of your inner silence -- the natural outcome of your individual and collective practice. Everyone on the planet will benefit.

The guru is in you ... Enjoy!

2006/06/30 16:15:00
Member Announcements - Events, Classes & Retreats
AYP Long Distance Meditation Group?

Hi All:

Not to butt in, but while routines can be kept according individual schedule, the group effect can be optimized by all beginning the meditation part of the routine at the same time. It's not mandatory, of course. Just some input for those who are interested in optimizing the group effect.

All the best!

The guru is in you.

2010/01/10 09:45:59
Member Announcements - Events, Classes & Retreats
AYP Long Distance Meditation Group?

quote:
_____
Originally posted by avinod

Note: Im re-sending this mail as I corrected the email-id in my profile.Thanks again.
_____

Hi Avinod and welcome.

I'm sure Shanti will address your request (ah, done!). I wanted to let you know that the email you registered with yesterday is not receiving mail from the forum, and you may want to update it. You can do so by clicking on the "profile" link at the top of this page, logging in, and making any corrections that you feel are necessary. The AYP forums have strong spam protection features, and you can elect not to receive mail from other members. A valid email is still needed for forum moderation notifications, periodic healing samyama list confirmations, etc.

All the best!

The guru is in you.

2010/11/13 11:40:51
Member Announcements - Events, Classes & Retreats
AYP Long Distance Meditation Group?

quote:
_____
Originally posted by singram61

I can be the host. I live 5 minutes from 95 right at exit 1--PA/DE border. I love AYP. It has helped me immensely.

You wrote:
Also, if you'd be interested in starting a group of you own or meet up with other AYP practitioners let me know, I know of someone else who is interested in joining a group. He lives in the King Of Prussia area.
_____

Hi singram61:

If you are interested, I will be happy to add you as a "planning contact" on the AYP website local contacts page. If so, let me know your town/city and name/handle you'd like to use on the list.

Thanks!

The guru is in you.

2006/07/10 10:36:13

quote:
_____

Originally posted by Shanti

In lesson#37 Yogani says..
[quote]Group meditations are not a substitute for your regular twice-daily meditations. Your individual practice is your primary practice, and should always be. This keeps your spiritual destiny in your hands, in your daily practice, regardless of other circumstances. Groups come and go. Group meditations can be a wonderful boost, but they will come and go too. Don't rely on them as core practice. Think of them as bonuses. Life is always changing on the outside. Be sure that your daily practice is ingrained as an inside aspect of your life, not subject to being waylaid by outer events.

_____

Hi All:

The intent in the above lesson was to discourage folks from relying on group meditations as a primary source of practice, which some of us might tend to do. Much more important is to have our home routine well-established and be self-sufficient in that. Then whatever else comes along in the way of group meditations, etc., we can regard as a bonus.

When preparing the lesson, I was not thinking of worldwide long-distance meditations, or their potential power for wide-scale purification and opening. In this case (or any powerful group meditation situation), it is incumbent on all of us to keep self-pacing in mind, as needed, whether the group meditation happens to be during our regular routine of practice, or in addition to it. It can be done either way. Each should weigh the results and make adjustments accordingly, as I see many of you are doing already.

Smart self-pacers, you are. :-)

The world meditations are a wonderful new program, with very promising long term potential. Thank you, Shanti!

Gee, how many thousands can join in, and what will be the long term effect on world consciousness? Let's find out...

The guru is in you.

2010/01/13 14:04:37

quote:
_____

Hi friends!

This evening i heard from a friend of another friend named Larry.
His doctors have told him he will soon have a leg amputated from below the knee. he has diabetes and fragmented bones in his foot, also drug complications (prescription) This has freaked me out completely, so i am calling to those who might help. If so, what info is needed to help it happen, or anything else?

With much Love (and squeaky tears)

Rael
_____

2006/07/24 18:25:54

Hi All:

Just to chime in here, Trip did a terrific job on his nine day solo retreat, mainly because he was able to stick with his pre-planned schedule. As in daily life, the activities on a retreat are as important as the practice routines in order to integrate purification that is occurring, and even more so while going deeper and deeper in retreat mode.

When we first started communicating on his retreat, Trip was planning on longer sessions, and on adding new practices, etc. Sort of a retreat free for all -- it would have been very tough to hold it together. I think he will tell you that he had more than enough to say grace over with 2+2 daily routines with his existing practices, only nuanced modestly for the retreat.

Several have asked me about AYP retreats over the past couple of years, and now maybe it is time to put a toe in the water. Trip's idea for online retreats is intriguing, and maybe it could work for those who have the discipline to stick with a schedule. Of course, actual group retreats would be better, and there is no reason why they could not evolve in time, perhaps even combined with the online ones -- simultaneous retreats spread around the planet, all connected via the internet. Interesting possibilities there ... but first things first.

It is true, Near, that the AYP practices are very powerful, and must be managed very precisely when in retreat mode. It is all about the schedule. If this is done, a retreat can produce a big step forward with relative safety. The key to online retreats will be good communications with the coordinator, and making any adjustments that are necessary during the retreat. As with regular practices, everyone reacts a little differently to multiple routines.

Trip has volunteered to be the first retreat coordinator. I told him that we could create one or more private forums here as needed for communications during online retreats. Not sure if chatrooms would be a help or a hinderance -- it is an open question. Perhaps for some light group interaction at predetermined times of the day.

Starting out with a weekend would be best, and not in a house full of busy activities. It would be good if meals could be taken care of, but not with a lot of interaction with family or friends who are not in retreat mode. That is why they call it a retreat. :-)

It is up to the interested parties to get it together. My role would as part time advisor only. I have plenty of experience in this area, so can provide useful guidelines. But I'm not available for ongoing interactions during retreats. The coordinator (in this case, Trip) would advise me of any special input needed from here. The retreat schedule would be set up in advance, so variations should be the exception rather than the rule.

Well, it is a start. Let's see what happens.

The guru is in you.

2006/07/30 13:41:34
Member Announcements - Events, Classes & Retreats
http://www.aypsite.org/forum/topic.asp?TOPIC_ID=1357&REPLY_ID=10055&whichpage=-1
AYP Group Retreats

quote:
───────
Originally posted by trip1

I'm not sure how effective a half-day retreat would be, but I think that so long as physical activity is utilized (as per the schedule), the extra morning practice shouldn't be a problem. Maybe Yogani can chime in with a bit more information on that, as this is only my guess.

─────────

Two plus one routines in a single day could be tried if there are no responsibilities or decisions to be dealing with on that day, going to light physical activity, study and rest instead, along the lines of Trip's schedule. Extra routines (beyond two per day) are not recommended when engaging in normal daily activities.

The smoothness (or lack) in the result of one day doing 2+1 will depend on the person. Obviously, it is not a big leap, so could not really be called a "retreat."

The real benefit of multiple routines in retreat mode is over several days or weeks. Like everything else in yoga, the benefits come with steady practice over time. In the case of retreats (short or long), they can be added periodically into regular life (several times per year) to bring an added dimension of growth which, over the long term, will make a significant difference in over all progress. And, as Trip will tell you, the results are quite noticable after one retreat. Imagine a few dozen of these spread out over years. It all adds up. :-)

The guru is in you.

2007/10/03 10:48:02
Member Announcements - Events, Classes & Retreats
http://www.aypsite.org/forum/topic.asp?TOPIC_ID=1416&REPLY_ID=25844&whichpage=-1
Weekend Solo Retreats - Schedule & Information

quote:
───────
Originally posted by bewell

Hi,

All the retreat directions make sense to me but this one in the study suggestions:

"Reading and/or posting in the private forum"

What is "the private forum?"

Thanks in advance to anyone who can clarify this one for me.

─────────

Hi Bewell:

The idea is that we would have a private forum available for AYP retreat participants for questions and communications between locations engaged in simultaneous practice, and with administrators who could answer questions.

So far, there have not been enough AYP retreat activities going on (individuals only to date) to warrant activating this feature. When the need is there for a group venue, we will create one.

Of course, internet will not always be available at retreat locations, so forum interaction would an optional feature, and not essential.

The emphasis is on working toward providing everything locally to support successful retreats, including on-site support in the case of groups.

678 – Advanced Yoga Practices

The realization of organized AYP retreats is in the embryonic stage, and is tied to the formation of meditation groups around the world, which could form the basis for periodic retreat gatherings. Establishing a meditation group is a first step toward organizing group retreats. It takes time...

Wanted: Meditation group leaders and retreat administrators. Apply within. :-)

The guru is in you.

2006/09/21 09:18:53
Member Announcements - Events, Classes & Retreats
http://www.aypsite.org/forum/topic.asp?TOPIC_ID=1524&REPLY_ID=11426&whichpage=-1
Free Books

Hi Hunter:

What a kind offer. I have sent this to these folks who are building a spiritual library in Romania:

http://www.aypsite.org/forum/topic.asp?TOPIC_ID=1247

Maybe you will hear from them. Of course, I'm sure there are plenty of folks closer by that may contact you too.

The guru is in you.

2006/11/08 11:17:02
Member Announcements - Events, Classes & Retreats
http://www.aypsite.org/forum/topic.asp?TOPIC_ID=1692
Yogani Radio Interview - Live Webcast - Nov 12th

Hi All:

I am scheduled to be interviewed on a one hour radio show -- Sunday, November 12th, at 7 pm eastern time, USA. The interview will be webcast live from this link:
http://1360wsai.com/pages/streaming.html

The radio station is 1360AM WSAI in Cincinnati, Ohio.

The show is called: "Yoga -- The Other Ninety-Eight Percent."
Sounds fitting for an AYP discussion, doesn't it? :-)

For those in other time zones, see this link showing times around the world matching Sunday, 8 pm eastern time, USA.

Note: See my next post below for a just discovered limitation on international access to the webcast.

If you have the ability to record live audio feed on your computer, feel free to do so and share it as you see fit. It is hoped that we can use a digital audio file to make the interview available for listening anytime on the AYP website. I am not familiar with how to record digitally or set it up for website listening, so anyone that can help with this, please let me know.

Looking forward to exploring this new level of communication for AYP on Sunday!

The guru is in you.

2006/11/08 13:57:01
Member Announcements - Events, Classes & Retreats
http://www.aypsite.org/forum/topic.asp?TOPIC_ID=1692&REPLY_ID=13056&whichpage=-1
Yogani Radio Interview - Live Webcast - Nov 12th

Hi All:

I just received the following note from someone outside the USA (Ireland). Apparently there is a restriction on the live audio stream outside the USA, which I was not aware of. All the more reason to record the interview and have it available on the AYP website, hopefully within a couple of weeks.

Apologies to all outside the USA for the limitation. I am checking to see if there is a way around it.

Thanks, Weaver, for the kind offer. Let me know via email if it is do-able for you. Anyone else with capability please record the interview also. Better we have several copies than none!

The guru is in you.

Hi Yogani,

I tried to access the link you provided to the streaming website and received the following message;

We are sorry but due to licensing restrictions we are not able to allow access to the content you are requesting outside of the United States. If you are US Military serving overseas please Click Here ... All others can send comments using the form below...

I am sure many people outside the US would love to hear this interview.

Can you contact them to make it easier for people outsde to listen in?

If they receive this message, that might be as far as they go.

I am going to fill in the form, and see what reply I get.

Good luck with your interview and keep up the good work...

2006/11/08 16:07:14
Member Announcements - Events, Classes & Retreats
http://www.aypsite.org/forum/topic.asp?TOPIC_ID=1692&REPLY_ID=13061&whichpage=-1
Yogani Radio Interview - Live Webcast - Nov 12th

quote:
_____
Originally posted by azaz932001

Got it now a few minor adjustments done the trick :-) so i should be recording the programme ok :-)

Richard
_____

Hi Richard:

That's great. You can listen in the UK? So there is hope for tapping in outside the USA.

If anyone has trouble accessing the live feed, kindly report it here.

The guru is in you.

2006/11/10 10:03:34
Member Announcements - Events, Classes & Retreats
http://www.aypsite.org/forum/topic.asp?TOPIC_ID=1692&REPLY_ID=13113&whichpage=-1
Yogani Radio Interview - Live Webcast - Nov 12th

Hi All·

The more recordings the better, so we will have plenty of backup copies, just in case. So record away! :-)

As things stand now, Trip will lead the effort to get the interview file in the best size and format for AYP website listening. He has professional experience in this area. There are several ways to do it, and we'd like to do it in a way that allows for both easy streaming audio on the website without the need for a separate player download, and optional download of an MP3, if desired.

Many thanks, and all the best!

The guru is in you.

2006/11/12 11:15:57
Member Announcements - Events, Classes & Retreats
http://www.aypsite.org/forum/topic.asp?TOPIC_ID=1692&REPLY_ID=13181&whichpage=-1
Yogani Radio Interview - Live Webcast - Nov 12th

Hi All:

Thanks much for your kind wishes. I am looking forward to "seeing" you tonight, radio gods willing.

As for a picture of me, it is not the way to go. Much better to take a good look in the mirror.

The guru is in you! :-)
2006/11/12 16:43:32
Member Announcements - Events, Classes & Retreats
http://www.aypsite.org/forum/topic.asp?TOPIC_ID=1692&REPLY_ID=13195&whichpage=-1
Yogani Radio Interview - Live Webcast - Nov 12th

Hi All:

I just spoke with the radio interviewer (4:30 pm here) and he informed me that <u>the **radio show will be at 7 pm**, not 8 pm tonight</u>. It will still be a one hour show. He was very apologetic.

So we will proceed accordingly.

Those who are recording, please adjust your times to be an hour sooner, so we can be sure to have something for the many who will likely tune in an hour late.

The guru is in you.

680 –   Advanced Yoga Practices

2006/11/13 08:57:57
Member Announcements - Events, Classes & Retreats
http://www.aypsite.org/forum/topic.asp?TOPIC_ID=1692&REPLY_ID=13241&whichpage=-1
Yogani Radio Interview - Live Webcast - Nov 12th

Hi All:

Thanks much for your support and feedback. That was fun last night! :-)

For those who missed the interview, a test version is up already here:
http://www.aypsite.org/forum/topic.asp?TOPIC_ID=1706

Thanks Trip!

If all goes well, it should be accessible on the AYP homepage soon.

The guru is in you.

2006/11/14 08:51:43
Member Announcements - Events, Classes & Retreats
http://www.aypsite.org/forum/topic.asp?TOPIC_ID=1692&REPLY_ID=13267&whichpage=-1
Yogani Radio Interview - Live Webcast - Nov 12th

quote:
_____
Originally posted by Sparkle

If you get time in your busy schedule would you consider making CD's of maybe lessons or Q and A sessions ?. I think, with that nice voice of yours they would go down a treat. Louis
_____

Hi Louis and All:

Thanks much for the vote of confidence on doing more audio.

The plan is to eventually do all of the AYP Enlightenment Series books (9 of them) in audio. If anyone knows audiobook publishers who might be interested, let me know. I think that will be much more useful audio than the interviews -- preplanned instructional material, which is many steps beyond the interview yak yak. We will likely hear more of the yak yak too. :-)

All the best!

The guru is in you.

2006/11/15 08:15:13
Member Announcements - Events, Classes & Retreats
http://www.aypsite.org/forum/topic.asp?TOPIC_ID=1692&REPLY_ID=13295&whichpage=-1
Yogani Radio Interview - Live Webcast - Nov 12th

quote:
_____
Originally posted by Yoda

[i]Awesome news! I was hoping so!! Sean at taobums said he could help you set up downloads for your site probono. He's busy at the moment, but he said he'd love to help.
_____

Hi Yoda:

Trip has done a fine job of enabling AYP for audio downloading already (see here). It is good to know that Sean can help also if needed. In fact, he has helped tremendously already through the Tao Bums website, as have many of you over there. Many thanks!

Regarding the Enlightenment Series audiobooks, those will be available through Amazon and others whenever they get done. I have to write the rest of the books first. We only have 4 of 9 done so far, with another one on the way. The plan is to have them done by the end of 2007, assuming I am not spending too much time yak yaking between now and then. :-)

The audiobooks would be done after that, unless an interested audiobook publisher steps forward to take the lead on it before then.

The guru is in you.

2006/11/12 16:46:44
Member Announcements - Events, Classes & Retreats
http://www.aypsite.org/forum/topic.asp?TOPIC_ID=1704
Yogani Radio Interview moved up an hour!

Hi All:

I just spoke with the radio interviewer (4:30 pm here) and he informed me that **the radio show will be at 7 pm, not 8 pm tonight** (eastern time, USA). It will still be a one hour show. He was very apologetic.

So we will proceed accordingly. The webcast link is http://1360wsai.com/pages/streaming.html

Those who are recording, please adjust your times to be an hour sooner, so we can be sure to have something for the many who will likely tune in an hour late.

The guru is in you.

2006/11/13 09:05:53
Member Announcements - Events, Classes & Retreats
http://www.aypsite.org/forum/topic.asp?TOPIC_ID=1704&REPLY_ID=13242&whichpage=-1
Yogani Radio Interview moved up an hour!

Thanks much, Andrew. :-)
2006/11/29 16:19:08
Member Announcements - Events, Classes & Retreats
http://www.aypsite.org/forum/topic.asp?TOPIC_ID=1767&REPLY_ID=13881&whichpage=-1
New AYP group meditation started
Congratulations, Louis!

I'm sure Shanti and Sadhak can give you a few tips, having been at it for a while.

With best wishes to all in your new meditation group, and in meditation groups everywhere. The more the merrier!

The guru is in all of you. :-)
2006/12/13 14:34:26
Member Announcements - Events, Classes & Retreats
http://www.aypsite.org/forum/topic.asp?TOPIC_ID=1767&REPLY_ID=14468&whichpage=-1
New AYP group meditation started

quote:
_____
Originally posted by Sparkle

A question for Yogani:
Some of my group have been doing meditations through the crown for years. I wonder about the effects of AYP practice if they continue with these crown practices. My advice to them would be to stop, but old habits die hard.
How big is the inherent danger here if the kundalini starts rising and they are continuing with their crown practices?
I know this is a very general question and probably varies from individual to individual, but what I need to ask myself is: Should I be teaching AYP practices to people whilst knowing they are also doing crown opening meditations?

Louis

_____

Hi Louis:

I don't think AYP is going to exacerbate problems related to crown practices that others have been doing. If anything, doing deep meditation, spinal breathing and other AYP practices will help bring things to a head and provide the motivation for folks to find more balance in their practices. To hold off from deep meditation in such cases will only delay the inevitable. Don't forget, in addition to its stimulative effects, AYP has many cushions built in that offset the risks.

There are many who have come to AYP with a history of crown practices and the associated difficulties, and found understanding, relief and much better balance going forward. I think it is safe to assume that anyone who is doing crown practices who hasn't blown it out the top yet is going to find the same with AYP. Yes, their path will be accelerated, most likely with less severe dislocations than they would have experienced otherwise.

Regarding crown practices and related openings, we should not regard these things as the boogy man. Maybe that is my fault for offering so many cautions, to beginners especially (there have been so many unnecessary disasters). Still, the crown will open with the practices we have in AYP, and there are pointers in the lessons for exploring and expanding on that with relative safety. In the new book on Samyama, we are going to do some more with the crown, and go far beyond. :-)

The AYP suggestion is not to avoid the crown under all circumstances. It is to undertake purification and opening in an order and a way that will provide for maximum progress with good comfort and safety. I think everyone is looking for that.

So I don't think anyone should be shielded from the AYP knowledge. It may be just what they need. With it, each person will be in a better position to determine how to proceed based on their own experiences. The rest is up to them.

The guru is in you.

2007/04/10 12:53:17
Member Announcements - Events, Classes & Retreats
http://www.aypsite.org/forum/topic.asp?TOPIC_ID=1767&REPLY_ID=20121&whichpage=-1

New AYP group meditation started

Hi Louis:

Sounds like terrific happenings there. Plowing new ground!

While it is only a matter of perspective, the "main" meditation group could be seen as the one open to the public, where anyone could walk in and sit and meditate with the group. That group would be only for meditation, discussion/satsang and snacks. That kind of "introductory group" can grow pretty large, providing a "wide gate" for the community. It is a great idea. The introductory group can serve for both public relations and meditation training, plus reviewing the broad system of practices, but not practicing beyond deep meditation in that group. Of course, the larger the group gets, the trickier it will be to manage.

Many years ago we used to run a similar group here, and once it got over 20 people, the dynamic changed -- there was much more spiritual power generated, and also a few flies started showing up in the ointment -- people who were there for the wrong reasons. Then more structure became necessary to keep the thing from spinning off on tangents. It takes some leadership and structure, which is somewhat opposed to the free-flowing nature of such gatherings. If left to their own devices, such gatherings tend to become unstable and fly apart, so some sort of structure has to be implemented.

The other group you mentioned (your current "main group") could continue to be for the fuller practice routine, open to those who have progressed and are interested in that. But it should not be considered to be a replacement for daily pracice, as you mention. For those who have gotten the daily practice part of it in place, the practice group could eventually lead into weekend retreats, and beyond. That is an area where we have information resources in place already -- see the first two topics in this forum.

Do keep us posted on how things develop. I'm sure many will benefit from your experiences as they consider starting and expanding their own groups.

The guru is in you.

2006/12/29 13:03:37
Member Announcements - Events, Classes & Retreats
http://www.aypsite.org/forum/topic.asp?TOPIC_ID=1865
New Yogani Live Radio Interviews in Dec & Jan
Note (added Jan 2): Radio interviews are scheduled for every Sunday evening in January. Details can be found on the AYP Audio Page.

Hi All:

Have just received word that I am scheduled to be interviewed live on the radio again, Sunday, Dec 31, at 7 pm eastern time (one hour show), USA.

That's this Sunday, New Year's Eve!

The radio station is 1360AM WSAI in Cincinnati, Ohio.
The interview will be webcast live from this link:
http://1360wsai.com/pages/streaming.html

For those in other time zones, see this link showing times around the world matching Sunday, 7 pm eastern time, USA.

Many locations outside the USA will not be able to listen live. We have plans to record the show and put it on the AYP website like we did the November interview.

If you have the ability to record live audio feed on your computer, please do so. It is always good to have backup recordings in case our recording efforts here don't work.

Here we go again! :-)

The guru is in you.

2006/12/29 23:04:41
Member Announcements - Events, Classes & Retreats
http://www.aypsite.org/forum/topic.asp?TOPIC_ID=1865&REPLY_ID=15070&whichpage=-1
New Yogani Live Radio Interviews in Dec & Jan

Hi Andrew:

Call-ins would be great, and it is pretty much wide open, since this has happened so fast that there is no planned subject for the show yet. Just keep in mind that there may be a lot of folks new to yoga listening. So I would not expect to be giving a detailed dissertation on kechari mudra. :-)

Hi Weaver:

Yes, Brett is on it. A few backup recordings would not hurt, just in case.

Hi Vil:

Rumi is one of my favorites.
"Keep walking, though there is no place to get to ... Move, but not the way fear makes you move..."

The guru is in you.

2006/12/30 09:26:33
Member Announcements - Events, Classes & Retreats
http://www.aypsite.org/forum/topic.asp?TOPIC_ID=1865&REPLY_ID=15100&whichpage=-1
New Yogani Live Radio Interviews in Dec & Jan

Hi All:

It might be good to focus this interview more on deep meditation, including some basic instructions. Call-ins can be on that, or anything -- the more the merrier. We can always bring the discussion back to deep meditation. Everything always gets back to that -- inner silence. :-)

I will see what Scott (the host) thinks about this approach.

Also, it should be mentioned that the show has had some financial shortfalls, and donations to the the non-profit charity announced on the show can be earmarked for the radio show. The future of the show is somewhat in question for financial reasons, so they can use any support folks can offer. The cost per show is $300, I believe.

Originally, I was scheduled to be on every weekend in January to fill in for the sponser, Will, who just left for a month in India. Not sure where that stands with the financial shortfall. Donations could make the difference. I am willing to do the interviews in January if the show stays on the air.

The guru is in you.

2006/12/30 14:58:29
Member Announcements - Events, Classes & Retreats
http://www.aypsite.org/forum/topic.asp?TOPIC_ID=1865&REPLY_ID=15137&whichpage=-1
New Yogani Live Radio Interviews in Dec & Jan

Hi Andrew:

I plan on doing that later today or early tomorrow. Have been backed up here with family matters.

Hunter, have you got MySpace covered?

Thanks.

TGIIY

2007/01/01 12:11:42
Member Announcements - Events, Classes & Retreats
http://www.aypsite.org/forum/topic.asp?TOPIC_ID=1865&REPLY_ID=15246&whichpage=-1
New Yogani Live Radio Interviews in Dec & Jan

Hi All:

Compliments of Brett -- the interview recording (great job!):

Play now -- http://www.aypsite.com/audio/interview1206.html

MP3 Download -- http://www.aypsite.com/audio/downloads/Yogani_Interview-12-31-2006.mp3

The AYP Audio Page on the website is being updated with the recording and other new information, and will be up today. (PS: It is up now.)

All the best for 2007!

The guru is in you.

2007/01/01 22:13:31
Member Announcements - Events, Classes & Retreats
http://www.aypsite.org/forum/topic.asp?TOPIC_ID=1865&REPLY_ID=15267&whichpage=-1
New Yogani Live Radio Interviews in Dec & Jan

Thanks, Andrew. It was fun. :-)

Next week we will do Spinal Breathing Pranayama -- same time, same place. The particulars are on the AYP Audio Page now.

I'm pretty sure both phone numbers were given on the show, but just in case, they are:

Toll free: 877-345-3779
Local number (toll call outside Cincinnati): 513-749-1360

If I am going to be on every Sunday in January, I'm going to see if it will be okay to go through the topics of the E-Series books in order. That would be:

Dec 31 -- Deep Meditation (done!)
Jan 7 -- Spinal Breathing Pranayama

Jan 14 -- Tantra (tiptoeing through on live radio)
Jan 21 -- Asanas, Mudras and Bandhas (good for Will's Cincinnati Yoga School)
Jan 28 -- Samyama (the book will available by then)

That is tentative beyond Jan 7. Not sure how many weeks we have to work with yet. We'll see what Will and Scott think. It is their show.

All the best!

The guru is in you.

2007/01/02 10:21:08
Member Announcements - Events, Classes & Retreats
http://www.aypsite.org/forum/topic.asp?TOPIC_ID=1865&REPLY_ID=15284&whichpage=-1
New Yogani Live Radio Interviews in Dec & Jan

Hi Sadhak:

Can you listen online?

The guru is in you.

PS: It could be traffic. There have been hundreds of downloads since yesterday. We have plenty of bandwidth, but not sure how many can be downloaded simultaneously. Maybe there are some limits internationally.
2007/01/03 08:12:10
Member Announcements - Events, Classes & Retreats
http://www.aypsite.org/forum/topic.asp?TOPIC_ID=1865&REPLY_ID=15321&whichpage=-1
New Yogani Live Radio Interviews in Dec & Jan

Hi Sadhak:

If you are on dialup, that may be a sticking point. It is 20 MB.

Maybe someone can email you the mp3 file.

Shanti, can you help with that?
That may or may not work for download through your email.

We'll get it to you somehow, and you can pass it on accordingly. :-)

The guru is in you.

2007/01/03 13:57:47
Member Announcements - Events, Classes & Retreats
http://www.aypsite.org/forum/topic.asp?TOPIC_ID=1865&REPLY_ID=15343&whichpage=-1
New Yogani Live Radio Interviews in Dec & Jan

Hi All:

We got the go-ahead for the interview topic schedule for the rest of January.

The AYP Audio Page has been updated. So now we are scheduled to introduce topics from the first five AYP Enlightenment Series books:

Deep Meditation
Spinal Breathing Pranayama
Tantra
Asanas, Mudras & Bandhas
Samyama

With a little luck, we will be able to get it all on the air, and recorded. Keep your fingers crossed.

I also added the call-in numbers (at bottom of audio page) for those who would like to plan ahead. Would love to hear from you live on the radio.
:-)

All the best!

The guru is in you.

2007/01/03 17:53:12
Member Announcements - Events, Classes & Retreats
http://www.aypsite.org/forum/topic.asp?TOPIC_ID=1865&REPLY_ID=15352&whichpage=-1
New Yogani Live Radio Interviews in Dec & Jan

Hi All:

This is a tip for online listening...

For those with dial-up or other slow internet, you can pause the online player and wait for the segment of the show you are on to download a bit, and then play it. As long as the moving track button does not catch up with the wiggly download progress bar, you will be okay. If it does, just pause the player and give the wiggly download bar a chance to get ahead again. That should make it possible for anyone to listen online.

Downloading the entire MP3 (20 MB) is another matter.

The guru is in you.

2007/01/09 23:57:02
Member Announcements - Events, Classes & Retreats
http://www.aypsite.org/forum/topic.asp?TOPIC_ID=1865&REPLY_ID=15713&whichpage=-1
New Yogani Live Radio Interviews in Dec & Jan

Hi All:

Due to more basketball games on WSAI, the AYP interviews will be starting at about 7:30 pm for the next two Sundays (instead of 7 pm), and running until 9:00 -- that is up to 1 1/2 hours on the air instead of 1 hour. I said thank you very much. :-)

The audio page has been updated accordingly: http://www.aypsite.com/audio.html
That is the place to look for the latest scheduling information.

The guru is in you.

2007/01/15 00:02:22
Member Announcements - Events, Classes & Retreats
http://www.aypsite.org/forum/topic.asp?TOPIC_ID=1865&REPLY_ID=16103&whichpage=-1
New Yogani Live Radio Interviews in Dec & Jan

Hi All:

The January 14th radio interview recording on Tantra is available for listening and download here: http://www.aypsite.com/audio.html

Many thanks to Brett for capturing it and making it available for everyone to listen to.

Wishing you all the best on your path. Enjoy!

The guru is in you.

2007/01/20 09:39:22
Member Announcements - Events, Classes & Retreats
http://www.aypsite.org/forum/topic.asp?TOPIC_ID=1865&REPLY_ID=16305&whichpage=-1
New Yogani Live Radio Interviews in Dec & Jan

Hi All:

Got the word from Scott Fitzgerald that we are on 7-8 pm this week (Jan 21st), instead of 7:30-9:00 pm. No basketball game, apparently.

I modified the audio page to suit.

This week we are covering Asanas, Mudras, Bandhas and Kundalini.
Looking forward to "seeing" you on the air. :-)

The guru is in you.

2007/02/24 10:54:21
Member Announcements - Events, Classes & Retreats
http://www.aypsite.org/forum/topic.asp?TOPIC_ID=2110&REPLY_ID=18032&whichpage=-1
AYP & Outside Retreats

Hi Brett:

I was recently asked the same question about an Adyashanti retreat, and here is what I wrote, which can apply to any retreat involving another teaching and/or practice routine:

Hi:

Depending on how intensive the specific practice routine at the retreat is, you might consider cutting back to short (maybe very short) deep meditations only -- to "honor the habit." That way it will not be a strain either during the retreat or getting started again with AYP practices afterward. In other words, self-pace it.

You can also ask Adyashanti what he suggests, as I am sure others will be there with practice routines from other traditions. Being the advaita (non-dual) guy that he is, he might say, "Forget practices," though he did a lot of them himself to get the to the "no-practice" mode. It is one of those Buddhist koans -- you don't need practices, except to get there, though there is no place to get to. :-)

Looking forward to doing the Self-Inquiry book this spring, where the advaita versus yoga practices (non-dual versus dual) stuff will be addressed from an AYP point of view (for a taste, see here).

I will be very interested in new perspectives you find on the retreat. Do let me know. (Feedback is welcome here in the forum, of course.)

Have a great retreat!

The guru is in you.

2007/03/08 10:23:48
Member Announcements - Events, Classes & Retreats
http://www.aypsite.org/forum/topic.asp?TOPIC_ID=2202&REPLY_ID=18503&whichpage=-1
Non-Dual vs. Dual - and AYP meets Zen on a Retreat

Hi Kirtanman:

Glad to hear you have landed.

Great info. Thank you!

Here are two topics that tie in where some "advaita/dvaita" friction has emerged:
http://www.aypsite.org/forum/topic.asp?TOPIC_ID=2096 (it started here)
http://www.aypsite.org/forum/topic.asp?TOPIC_ID=2195 (spin off)

These are good discussions, with deeper perspectives evolving about the relationship of practices and experiential non-dualism (advaita).

Also, there is an offline situation we are dealing with where an AYP person was blown to pieces at a recent Adyashanti Zen retreat. Too much of a good thing, resulting in a very sick aspirant. Total lack of "self-pacing" support at the retreat. So we have work to do in sorting out the relationship between AYP and Adya's approach -- which is, indeed, a powerful combination. He should be apprised also.

Aside from advaita/dvaita issues, this comes under the occasionally asked "non-AYP retreat" question. Maybe we need our own retreats? And certainly a better understanding about the potential benefits and risks for AYP practitioners participating in various other kinds of retreats.

This is all very exciting stuff, because we are going to bridge the gap between non-dual and dual one way or another. It is cropping up in multiple places these days, which means we are putting a face on it experientially. No more philosophical arguments about it are necessary. We are nailing "the thing itself." We are not talking about a few people having unity experiences. We are talking about consolidating practical means for everyone to cross over, and gracefully too. Much needed, yes?

Thanks for helping bridge the gap. :-)

The guru is in you.

2007/03/08 23:37:33
Member Announcements - Events, Classes & Retreats
http://www.aypsite.org/forum/topic.asp?TOPIC_ID=2202&REPLY_ID=18548&whichpage=-1
Non-Dual vs. Dual - and AYP meets Zen on a Retreat

Hi Kirtanman:

Thanks for the perspectives. Yes, I think it was overdoing in sittings in the first full day on the 5 day retreat. No other extenuating issues were brought in that I am aware of, except a couple of years of AYP "pre-cultivation." The reported experience actually started out quite good (very advaita-like), but then went into an extreme energy overload with practically no sleep for days, leading to illness. The person is doing better now.

Bottom line: AYP deep meditation and Zen meditation are not the same, and someone with an established deep meditation background is going to go deep in a Zen-style sitting (zazen or vipassana), even without consciously using the mantra. With deep meditation, we gradually develop the habit of going deep simply by closing our eyes. Do that 4-5 times in long sittings on the first day of a Zen retreat, with lots of group satsang added, plus someone like Adyashanti around, and what have you got? Overload!

So, watch out for those multiple long sittings on a Zen (or any other kind of) retreat if you are established in AYP deep meditation practice.

Weekend and extended AYP retreat schedules were worked up some months back. They are very structured and measured on the number and duration of meditation sessions. We know that these schedules deliver more than enough purification and opening. To attempt to do more than this is risky:

Weekend Schedule: http://www.aypsite.org/forum/topic.asp?TOPIC_ID=1416
Extended Schedule: http://www.aypsite.org/forum/topic.asp?TOPIC_ID=1428

These schedules are for solo retreats, but can be applied for groups also, with an experienced practitioner appointed as leader for schedule management and monitoring of participants. Guidance in self-pacing should be an integral part of any retreat, certainly any time that AYP practices (or practitioners!) are involved.

The guru is in you.

2007/03/09 14:07:17
Member Announcements - Events, Classes & Retreats
http://www.aypsite.org/forum/topic.asp?TOPIC_ID=2202&REPLY_ID=18574&whichpage=-1
Non-Dual vs. Dual - and AYP meets Zen on a Retreat

Hi Kirtanman:

Did not intend to depart from the advaita/dvaita discussion you so eloquently embarked on in the first post here. The retreat situation was a pressing matter, and it turns out, we think, it had less to do with advaita than with overdoing in practices (with an inner AYP tendency) in an already highly stimulative environment.

Regarding advaita (non-duality) vs. dvaita (duality), my two cents are in a short post over here:
http://www.aypsite.org/forum/topic.asp?TOPIC_ID=2195#18510

Sort of a koan, really: "Stillness in action," the paradox of upholding both non-dual and dual via the ongoing experience of "the thing itself." It puts a twist on the philosophical/logical approach (which can't go there), and makes for interesting self inquiry too.

It is also in full support of "practices," which I don't think anyone can argue against effectively anymore. Seeking non-duality through non-doing is a doing. Those who insist on an attitude of non-doing may be expressing their own need to sustain a polarity that is intellectually unsustainable, though definitely experientially sustainable if we let inner silence move. Paradox! Non-doing comes only when we allow inner silence to do -- to flow out as divine love.

This world is stillness in action, and so are we. When we have come to that via practices, all is experienced as the eternal unmoving omnipresent silent One in perpetual radiant motion.

Do we stop "practice" then? No, we continue on for the benefit of everyone, who are an expression our self. Does the pure advaitist practice? Yes, in telling us what is the truth, he or she is practicing, though they may deny it. That denial is practice. Or they may go completely silent. That too is practice. :-)

The guru is in you.

2007/03/09 15:52:07
Member Announcements - Events, Classes & Retreats
http://www.aypsite.org/forum/topic.asp?TOPIC_ID=2202&REPLY_ID=18585&whichpage=-1
Non-Dual vs. Dual - and AYP meets Zen on a Retreat

Hi Jill:

Asanas are normally part of our practice routine -- asanas, pranayama, meditation, etc., in order like that. As you can see from the AYP retreat schedules (links above), it is the number of practice routines we are managing in relation to time on the retreat, physical activity, mental activity, meals, sleep, etc. Each person's practice routine may be a bit different, depending on where they are with building their routine, but the over all retreat schedule stays the same. It is designed to accommodate varying individual practice routines.

The activity during a retreat is for grounding in-between our practice sessions. Asanas can bring some grounding, but can also stimulate energy flow, so we keep them pretty measured in the retreat schedule as part of the practice session, along with spinal breathing pranayama and deep meditation. If we have not been doing asanas before a retreat, it is okay to begin a light set on the front end of the practice routine during the retreat. But we do not add on other practices during the retreat, like increasing practice times, mantra enhancements, mudras, bandhas, or whatever. -- that is a formula for potential energy overloads. Better to do additions other than asanas outside the retreat, and have them well-stabilized before we go on retreat.

If you are interested in doing a retreat, either solo or pulling a group together, I'm sure Trip/Brett (author of the AYP retreat schedules) will be happy to answer any questions you have.

An ideal way to get a group retreat together is to first form a weekly meditation group at home, and then, later on, move to doing occasional local retreats. Who knows where it might go from there? Maybe all the way to non-dual duality! :-)

The guru is in you.

2007/03/09 22:10:15
Member Announcements - Events, Classes & Retreats
http://www.aypsite.org/forum/topic.asp?TOPIC_ID=2202&REPLY_ID=18601&whichpage=-1
Non-Dual vs. Dual - and AYP meets Zen on a Retreat

Hi Brett:

Thanks for chiming in on the advaita/retreat discussion. I am looking forward to receiving more feedback on our Adyashanti retreat participant. Obviously, the ongoing experience there over time will determine what the result of this event has been, not what anyone might think it is, including me.

My main concern is that we don't have AYP folks going off and getting blown to pieces on retreats. Or, if they choose that, at least it can be done with eyes open. And maybe sometimes it will be unavoidable (like in this case?) -- when the divine call comes, that's it, we have to go, regardless of the consequences. I'm sure there are more than a few AYP practitioners out there who would choose to go through the "week of hell" if it really would produce realization. Of course, no one will be exactly the same as the participant who had the recent experience, so nothing is guaranteed, except maybe the week of hell for those who either seek it or stumble into it.

In retrospect, my original advice on this matter was inadequate, and we have to look deeper so we can better advise on the potential rewards and risks of non-AYP retreats. Since we do not have a full scope AYP retreat program in place yet, I suspect we will be in this mode of looking at AYP practitioners meeting other systems of practice (or "non-practice") in retreat mode for some time. Perhaps there will be some good fits, and effective crossovers will go on indefinitely.

From the AYP point of view, it is a practical matter of optimizing progress with safety. With thorough information, each can choose for themselves. If we do what has to be done information-wise, no one will have to be flying completely blind, and the knowledge-base can keep building indefinitely on top of that. Who knows, maybe someday the enlightenment journey will be as smooth and reliable as air travel. Then everyone can go. Wouldn't that be nice?

On this journey, we'd like to lose all our baggage. :-)

All the best!

The guru is in you.

2007/06/02 14:53:41
Member Announcements - Events, Classes & Retreats
http://www.aypsite.org/forum/topic.asp?TOPIC_ID=2633
Yogacharya Festival in California July 2007

Hi All:

Just when it was beginning to look like there is no such thing as a "yoga convention" in the USA, I heard about this July 12-15 festival in Santa Clara, California, which looks to be a good-sized gathering (~1500) with some of the big names in yoga involved. This

The Yogacharya Festival is dedicated to BKS Iyengar and his teachings.
http://yogacharya.org

While unable to attend, I hope we can make AYP and the AYP books visible there in some ways. East-West books has already been contacted -- they will have a bookstore in the convention lobby, and we are hoping to have the books in there.

Would anyone in the area where the convention will held be interested in seeking an exibitor who might be willing to display the AYP books (for a modest cost), and find other ways to increase our visibility at the convention?

Many thanks!

The guru is in you.

2007/06/04 16:56:29
Member Announcements - Events, Classes & Retreats
http://www.aypsite.org/forum/topic.asp?TOPIC_ID=2633&REPLY_ID=22767&whichpage=-1
Yogacharya Festival in California July 2007
Note: See these two related posts:

http://www.aypsite.org/forum/topic.asp?TOPIC_ID=2621#22748
http://www.aypsite.org/forum/topic.asp?TOPIC_ID=2621#22766

The AYP books will be there!

The guru is in you.

2007/06/10 09:12:40
Member Announcements - Events, Classes & Retreats
http://www.aypsite.org/forum/topic.asp?TOPIC_ID=2657&REPLY_ID=22979&whichpage=-1
retreat schedule clarification - asanas, breakfast

Hi Tadeas:

An alternative would be to have a very light snack upon rising, before the morning sessions, and then not eat until lunch.

I'd also suggest you be careful about doing 90 minutes of asanas in addition to morning and evening sessions, which already include asanas prior to sitting practices. In retreat mode, all of our practices become much more powerful, including asanas, so you may find yourself overdoing with all those asanas. Careful self-pacing is in order for any variations in the basic retreat routine. Also keep in mind the delayed effects that can happen with practices. This is especially true on retreats. Everything can be going along fine, and all of a sudden we can find ourselves in an overload. Much better to learn to walk before we run. Easy does it ... you will find your balance that way for maximum progress with the fewest upheavals... :-)

All the best!

The guru is in you.

2007/06/10 20:12:01
Member Announcements - Events, Classes & Retreats
http://www.aypsite.org/forum/topic.asp?TOPIC_ID=2657&REPLY_ID=22999&whichpage=-1
retreat schedule clarification - asanas, breakfast

quote:
_____
Originally posted by tadeas

Thanks for the advice, Yogani. I'll certainly self-pace if necessary.

My idea was to leave out the morning and evening (ayp) asanas and only do my one daily ashtanga vinyasa series in the morning (approx. 90 minutes). Because it would be too much to also include the ayp asanas (which I don't practice anyway).
What do you think about that?
_____

Hi Tadeas:

Actually the asanas are the first part of the process of going in with spinal breathing pranayama, deep meditation, etc., cycling progressively deeper with each session on retreat.

Not sure how it would play without asanas before each of the sitting sessions and doing a long session of asanas separately during the day. Maybe it would be fine. If you go that route, let us know how it works out. I suggest you begin with a short retreat rather than a long one, so you can test the waters.

All the best!

The guru is in you.

2007/07/13 09:39:36
Member Announcements - Events, Classes & Retreats
http://www.aypsite.org/forum/topic.asp?TOPIC_ID=2769
Yoga Evolution Conference - New York: Aug 7-9
For those in the NYC area:

http://www.fityoga.com/html/conferences.htm

Anything that can be done to help make AYP visible at this August 7-9 yoga conference will be much appreciated.

The AYP books are being displayed in the conference bookshop (run by East West Bookstore) at the Yogacharya (Iyengar) Festival this weekend in California.

Something like that in New York next month would be great -- contact me for display copies. Or even just handing out a few AYP website cards or book flyers. Or even the AYP flying yogini! :-)

All the best!

The guru is in you.

2009/06/10 10:08:33
Member Announcements - Events, Classes & Retreats
http://www.aypsite.org/forum/topic.asp?TOPIC_ID=3033&REPLY_ID=52207&whichpage=-1
AYP Global Meditation Group-East...

Hi Shanti:

Reactivating the Global Group Meditation - East is a great idea. I assume you will include this in the main Global Group Meditation and Healing Samyama announcements also, so many will see it.

All the better to illuminate the planet with pure bliss consciousness. :-)

The guru is in you.

2008/01/04 17:12:16
Member Announcements - Events, Classes & Retreats
http://www.aypsite.org/forum/topic.asp?TOPIC_ID=3330
Ayurveda/Yoga Conference in Rishikesh -- Feb 21-25

Hi All:

FYI -- received here today...

The guru is in you

An Indian Knowledge Systems Conference

"AYURVEDA AND YOGA: WHERE SCIENCE MEETS CONSCIOUSNESS"

RISHIKESH - In the Himalayas... ' Where It All Began!'

FEBRUARY 21-25, 2008

Dear Friend

Namaskar! Here is conveying you Season's Greetings from Punarnava Ayurveda!

We thank you for your trust in Punarnava Ayurveda & let us welcome you yet again to be part of our journey towards the Vision of universal well-being! Our International Conference Ayurveda and Yoga: Where Science Meets Consciousness will be hosted at Parmarth Niketan Ashram in Rishikesh - India from February 21-25, 2008 .

Do register yourself for the Conference before January 15, 2008 , & avail the opportunity to register at a discounted Registration fees ! For all details & to register, please go to http://www.AyurvedaConference.com and we are at conference@punarnava.com to help you be there.

As the world-renowned speakers share their wisdom on Ayurveda and Yoga, a special learning & spiritual experience will get created at this Conference, just for you!

You may please support the cause of the Conference, by spreading the word about the Conference and thus let more people benefit from this experience in the Himalayas ! We would really look forward to welcoming you in Rishikesh! Thank you.

Warm regards,

Aparna

Event Co-ordinator

Conference Organised By

Punarnava Ayurveda Trust

A-21, Parsn Galaxy,

Nanjundapuram Road

Coimbatore 641 036 INDIA

Phone - +91 422 2311521

Fax - +91 422 4308081

Mobile - +91 93603 15495

Email - conference@punarnava.com

Web - http://www.punarnava-ayurveda.com , http://www.ayurvedaconference.com

2008/03/28 10:42:05
Member Announcements - Events, Classes & Retreats
http://www.aypsite.org/forum/topic.asp?TOPIC_ID=3676&REPLY_ID=31864&whichpage=-1
Interview with an AYP'er on the radio/net

Thanks much, Scott and Guy.

Here is an MP3 link for the talk (12min, 5.8MB): http://www.aypsite.com/audio/downloads/Scott-and-Guy-03-28-2008.mp3

I loved it! :-)

The guru is in you.

2008/03/31 13:35:48
Member Announcements - Events, Classes & Retreats
http://www.aypsite.org/forum/topic.asp?TOPIC_ID=3677&REPLY_ID=31993&whichpage=-1
SW Florida Group -- Anybody Know or Interested?

Hi Nancy:

None that I know of.

You may want to check with these folks, though they are on the other coast of Florida -- Boca Raton/Miami area.
http://www.aypsite.org/forum/topic.asp?TOPIC_ID=2244

I know there are folks doing AYP in Tampa/St Pete, but few down Ft Myers way. It may be best to start a local group and teach them deep meditation yourself. That is what others have been doing. If you can't find local AYP practitioners, then help create them. Where there is the will, there is a way... :-)

The guru is in you.

2008/08/20 09:06:03
Member Announcements - Events, Classes & Retreats
http://www.aypsite.org/forum/topic.asp?TOPIC_ID=3677&REPLY_ID=36579&whichpage=-1
SW Florida Group -- Anybody Know or Interested?

Hi Nancy:

Yes, it is best to start small with a few friends who have interest, meeting in someone's home once a week. Meditate, talk a while, have a snack. Making it a regular weekly thing is good, so everyone will know it is coming up and be looking forward to it.

Plowing through the lessons (the big book) may be too much for some. If that's the case, the little Deep Meditation book is also a good starting point. The Enlightenment Series books can be used for spoon-feeding like that, a series of courses on the practices. Whatever works. :-)

All the best!

The guru is in you.

2008/08/05 11:04:45
Member Announcements - Events, Classes & Retreats
http://www.aypsite.org/forum/topic.asp?TOPIC_ID=3805&REPLY_ID=36054&whichpage=-1

quote:
_____

Originally posted by Sparkle

Hi
Just to say the retreat was a major success.
Personally I am still reeling after it and will not say much.

What I can say is that if I did that amount of practice and experienced that much silence on my own I would be blown out of it. The group energy, opportunities to express ourselves honestly and lots of beautiful walks in the country seemed to balance us all out.

Love to all
Louis
_____

Hi Louis:

Bravo! Have been very interested to hear when someone came up for air. :-)

I hope more of these will be occurring around the world. From your few words, it sounds like you have the essence of it. Well run balanced retreats are not only good for the participants -- they are good for everyone everywhere. The more who attend a retreat, the more penetrating the effects. It is the awesome power of human spiritual transformation in your hands.

The guru is in you.

2008/09/10 09:49:47
Member Announcements - Events, Classes & Retreats
http://www.aypsite.org/forum/topic.asp?TOPIC_ID=4399&REPLY_ID=37500&whichpage=-1
Boston or Massachusets group

Hi Near:

It is good to announce your intention to form a meditation group here, but in reality the members will come mainly from outside the internet in your local community and network of friends and acquaintances. You can also advertise by putting a flyer up in local yoga studios, new age stores, etc. But starting small in the home is usually best -- one step at a time. This is how AYP will overflow from the internet into the broad society, and I am all for it as you know.

It is a great thing to do for your community. Outpouring divine love...

Thank you!

The guru is in you.

2008/10/17 16:12:02
Member Announcements - Events, Classes & Retreats
http://www.aypsite.org/forum/topic.asp?TOPIC_ID=4579&REPLY_ID=39078&whichpage=-1
Weekend Retreat Questions

Hi Carson:

A retreat is doing less, except for possibly a pre-planned extra practice routine each morning, and staying put more or less. The more stuff you add, the more likely the chance for an imbalance and/or overload.

If you want to do a food fast and get in the car to go do Bikram, then perhaps better to do regular practices like always and do those other things. That could be overdoing too, so be prepared to self-pace sooner rather than later. :-)

The key elements of a retreat are a highly structured schedule, no responsibilities (except for keeping the schedule), and no major decision making. Satsang (spiritual company) is also important on a retreat, especially for beginners, so maybe better not to do a first retreat by yourself.

Just some food for thought.

All the best!

The guru is in you.

2008/11/13 09:50:14
Member Announcements - Events, Classes & Retreats
http://www.aypsite.org/forum/topic.asp?TOPIC_ID=4694&REPLY_ID=40437&whichpage=-1
Shaktipat Offered

quote:
_____

Originally posted by krcqimpro1

I have also just 'enrolled' for it . Early feb.2009 is the scheduled date. I also spoke to Jayant, who posted the idea. It was amazing talking to him. Just 27 yrs.old and what he seems to have recd. is mind boggling ! He says, after shaktipath in 1999, without even willing it, he just

692 – Advanced Yoga Practices

'automatically' starts doing the asanas, mudras and pranayam need every day to keep the Kundalini rising. I wonder what Yogani has to say on this.

_____

Hi krcqimpro1:

Here is an AYP lesson on shaktipat: http://www.aypsite.org/146.html

All the best!

The guru is in you.

2009/01/04 11:19:58
Member Announcements - Events, Classes & Retreats
http://www.aypsite.org/forum/topic.asp?TOPIC_ID=4979
Yogani on the Radio - 2009 - KKCR Hawaii

Hi All:

I will be interviewed today (Jan 4th) on http://www.kkcr.org radio Hawaii at 12:15pm Hawaii time, which is 5:15pm eastern time USA. The interview can be listened to via live webcast.

The interview will be hosted by Dr. Ann West: http://kkcr.org/djs/annwest.htm
Her program is called "Truth From the Source," and is broadcast 12:00-1:00pm Hawaii time the first Sunday of each month.

The plan is to have the interview recorded and available for listening within a few days on the the AYP website at: http://www.aypsite.org/audio.html

All the best!

The guru is in you.

2009/01/05 09:56:23
Member Announcements - Events, Classes & Retreats
http://www.aypsite.org/forum/topic.asp?TOPIC_ID=4979&REPLY_ID=43051&whichpage=-1
Yogani on the Radio - 2009 - KKCR Hawaii

Hi All:

The Jan 4th interview with Dr. Ann West is now up on the audio page, here: http://www.aypsite.org/audio.html

Enjoy! :-)

The guru is in you.

2009/01/05 16:46:43
Member Announcements - Events, Classes & Retreats
http://www.aypsite.org/forum/topic.asp?TOPIC_ID=4979&REPLY_ID=43065&whichpage=-1
Yogani on the Radio - 2009 - KKCR Hawaii

Hi Carson:

There was a problem with the online streaming audio player yesterday, but that was fixed before the new interview was added. Try clearing your browser cache. That might fix it.

You also have the option to click left on the "Download MP3" link, and you may get a default player to open on your computer. Or you can click right on that link and download the MP3 file to your computer and play it on any MP3 player. So there are several options.

We will also be adding the interview to the AYP Youtube page, probably in a week or so.

Thanks, All. It was fun. Dr. Ann did a wonderful job hosting. Looking forward to doing more of these. :-)

The guru is in you.

2009/01/28 11:48:02
Member Announcements - Events, Classes & Retreats
http://www.aypsite.org/forum/topic.asp?TOPIC_ID=4979&REPLY_ID=44367&whichpage=-1
Yogani on the Radio - 2009 - KKCR Hawaii

Hi All:

We have another one-hour radio interview with Dr. Ann West coming up on Sunday, Feb 1, at 12 noon Hawaii time (5pm Eastern USA) on http://www.KKCR.org. You can listen to it there via live streaming audio.

The topic is Deep Meditation, with basic instructions, and a discussion of experiences with Dr. Ann, who has been doing AYP Deep Meditation since our last interview on Jan 4. That should be very interesting. :-)

The new interview will be available soon after broadcast for listening anytime on the AYP website audio page and on Youtube.

Enjoy!

The guru is in you.

2009/01/29 10:53:00
Member Announcements - Events, Classes & Retreats
http://www.aypsite.org/forum/topic.asp?TOPIC_ID=4979&REPLY_ID=44414&whichpage=-1
Yogani on the Radio - 2009 - KKCR Hawaii

quote:
_____
Originally posted by Ananda

Hi yogani,

what i'm going to ask might be too much but in case you have the time well...

while you're at it, can you speak during the interview a bit concerning samad
Hi and why is it that she overtakes us in such force while we are off guard during deep meditation and it's increase in power over time.

what i mean is i would like to hear more about the state of samad
Hi in relation to deep meditation (a bit of the stuff under the hood!)

and if it's possible, would you expand a little on the mechanics involved in lesson mantra design 101 and about the mechanics of the removal of obstructions.

i am just asking this to spice things up if possible, bcz i don't know if anyone feels the same as i do but it sounds like these talks are headed toward being a lot the same like the old ones...

kindest regards,

Ananda
_____

Hi Ananda:

I'd love to, but the interview is already done and will be broadcast on Sunday. It is the first time I have been involved in a prerecorded interview, a new experience. Some of what you are asking is in there, and some is not. Whatever is not, feel free to come back and ask here afterward.

There are also a few omissions and fumbles in the interview. Anyone who spots them can bring them up here. That is what happens in casual conversations versus writings. I plan to address these things in the next interview, which will be on spinal breathing pranayama.

There is some great stuff in the interview related to Dr. Ann's experiences as a new AYP deep meditation practitioner. She has long experience with spiritual traditions and practices, so she has had a very interesting start, to say the least. :-)

The guru is in you.

2009/02/11 14:02:17
Member Announcements - Events, Classes & Retreats
http://www.aypsite.org/forum/topic.asp?TOPIC_ID=4979&REPLY_ID=45079&whichpage=-1
Yogani on the Radio - 2009 - KKCR Hawaii

Hi All:

A short interview occurred yesterday with Scott Fitzgerald on WPTF Radio, North Carolina. It is called "Why Real Men Do Yoga." :-)
See the top one here: http://www.aypsite.org/audio.html

Also, along with the new interviews, we have been adding new AYP audiobook previews with video to the AYP Youtube page. One on Tantra was added a day ago that is receiving a lot of views. For that, see the lower right section of the page here: http://www.youtube.com/user/yogani99

Enjoy!

The guru is in you.

2009/02/25 17:41:02
Member Announcements - Events, Classes & Retreats
http://www.aypsite.org/forum/topic.asp?TOPIC_ID=4979&REPLY_ID=45984&whichpage=-1
Yogani on the Radio - 2009 - KKCR Hawaii

Hi All:

We have another one-hour radio interview with Dr. Ann West coming up on Sunday, Mar 1, at 12 noon Hawaii time (5pm Eastern USA) on http://www.KKCR.org. You can listen to it there via live streaming audio.

The topic is Spinal Breathing Pranayama, with basic instructions, and a discussion of experiences with Dr. Ann, who has added spinal breathing before her deep meditation sessions since our last interview on Feb 1.

The new interview will be available soon after broadcast for listening anytime on the AYP website audio page and on Youtube.

Enjoy!

The guru is in you.

2009/02/28 16:13:59
Member Announcements - Events, Classes & Retreats
http://www.aypsite.org/forum/topic.asp?TOPIC_ID=4979&REPLY_ID=46230&whichpage=-1
Yogani on the Radio - 2009 - KKCR Hawaii

quote:
_____
Originally posted by Guy_51

Hi Yogani:

Is this broadcast live, and if yes will Dr. West take calls from listeners?
Mahalo,

Guy
_____

Hi Guy:

This one is prerecorded like the last one, so no phone-in is possible. Sorry.

Many of Dr. Ann's programs are prerecorded, because she travels regularly. She is in Europe now. The first one we did in early January was "Aloha live." :-)

The guru is in you.

Yogani

2009/04/05 11:17:03
Member Announcements - Events, Classes & Retreats
http://www.aypsite.org/forum/topic.asp?TOPIC_ID=4979&REPLY_ID=48378&whichpage=-1
Yogani on the Radio - 2009 - KKCR Hawaii

Hi All:

We have another one-hour radio interview with Dr. Ann West coming up today Sunday, April 5th, at 12 noon Hawaii time (6pm Eastern USA) on http://www.KKCR.org. You can listen to it there via live streaming audio.

The topic is **Tantra**.

The new interview will be available soon after broadcast for listening anytime on the AYP website audio page and on Youtube.

Enjoy!

The guru is in you.

2009/04/05 19:07:21
Member Announcements - Events, Classes & Retreats
http://www.aypsite.org/forum/topic.asp?TOPIC_ID=4979&REPLY_ID=48393&whichpage=-1
Yogani on the Radio - 2009 - KKCR Hawaii

Hi All:

Those who tuned in today will have found that the AYP interview on Tantra was not on. Not sure what happened, and I have inquired. The interview was pre-recorded earlier this week, so it does exist, and has in fact been set up for the AYP website in preparation for public posting later today.

Until this is cleared up, the interview recording will not be added to the public audio page on the website. However, those who have been reading here and expecting to hear the interview can find it on a hidden (unlinked) website page here: http://www.aypsite.org/audio.html

The guru is in you.

2009/04/06 10:55:25
Member Announcements - Events, Classes & Retreats
http://www.aypsite.org/forum/topic.asp?TOPIC_ID=4979&REPLY_ID=48417&whichpage=-1
Yogani on the Radio - 2009 - KKCR Hawaii

Hi again All:

I heard back from Dr Ann. She is not sure what happened with the broadcast, but told me the Tantra interview would air at some point. In the meantime, she said to put the recording up for public listening as we normally do, and we will do that shortly.

Enjoy! :-)

The guru is in you.

2009/05/12 18:33:02
Member Announcements - Events, Classes & Retreats
http://www.aypsite.org/forum/topic.asp?TOPIC_ID=4979&REPLY_ID=50629&whichpage=-1
Yogani on the Radio - 2009 - KKCR Hawaii

Hi All:

Here is an update on the KKCR interviews via email correspondence today:

Q: ...just a quick note to inquire about the much anticipated May radio interview with you by Dr Ann West. Did it occur? Will it be posted soon? I very much appreciate all you've done and are doing. Thank you so very much.

A: Thank you for your kind note.

The interview for May 2nd did not happen for two reasons: First, the station was doing fund-raising and Dr Ann's program was preempted. Second, Dr Ann just moved to a new house and did not have web conferencing capability yet, so we postponed recording of the "Asanas, Mudras and Bandhas" interview until later this month. She is in Europe now, so the programs are being prerecorded (over web conference) and sent to KKCR in Hawaii.

There is another wrinkle in this, in that the Tantra interview did not air in early April as planned (we don't know why), and Dr Ann may have that broadcast first, perhaps on June 7th. We'll see. She did give permission for the Tantra interview to be posted by us last month, so it can be found on the AYP audio page and on Youtube.

I will post this in the forum announcement topic, so others with interest will know what is happening. Further updates will be posted there as we have them.

All the best!

The guru is in you.

2009/05/14 14:11:10
Member Announcements - Events, Classes & Retreats
http://www.aypsite.org/forum/topic.asp?TOPIC_ID=4979&REPLY_ID=50755&whichpage=-1
Yogani on the Radio - 2009 - KKCR Hawaii

Hi All:

Update: It turns out the Tantra interview did broadcast from KKCR Hawaii on May 3rd at 1pm, an hour later than originally scheduled due to an on-air fund-raising drive occurring that day.

The Asanas, Mudras and Bandhas (AMB) interview with Dr. Ann West will be prerecorded soon, and is scheduled to be broadcast on Sunday, June 7th at 12 noon Hawaii time here: http://www.kkcr.org
That's 6pm eastern time USA.

The AMB interview recording will be available on the AYP website and AYP Youtube channel shortly after broadcast.

An "Interviews" link has been added to the top menu of the AYP main website, making it easier to find all the interview recordings.

The guru is in you.

2009/05/28 12:04:51
Member Announcements - Events, Classes & Retreats
http://www.aypsite.org/forum/topic.asp?TOPIC_ID=4979&REPLY_ID=51585&whichpage=-1
Yogani on the Radio - 2009 - KKCR Hawaii

Hi All:

The next one hour interview with Dr. Ann West on "Asanas, Mudras and Bandhas" was prerecorded yesterday, and is scheduled to air (and webcast) on Sunday, June 7th at 12 noon Hawaii time (6 pm eastern time USA) on http://www.kkcr.org

Soon after, the recording should be available on the AYP interviews page.

The interview provides perspective on yoga postures and subtle inner physical maneuvers in relation to the broad scope of the eight limbs of yoga, ecstatic kundalini awakening, and the emergence of higher states of consciousness on an individual and global scale.

We managed to discuss the weekly AYP global group meditation and samyama healing sessions too. :-)

The guru is in you.

2009/05/28 16:50:35
Member Announcements - Events, Classes & Retreats
http://www.aypsite.org/forum/topic.asp?TOPIC_ID=4979&REPLY_ID=51603&whichpage=-1
Yogani on the Radio - 2009 - KKCR Hawaii
Correction:

The KKCR broadcast will be Sunday June 7th, the first Sunday of the month -- same time, same place.

Dr. Ann and I got a week ahead of ourselves.

I am correcting the above announcement also...

The guru is in you.

PS: Shanti, The global group meditations are one the best things coming out of AYP. Thanks so much for creating and nurturing them. :-)

2009/07/03 10:42:59
Member Announcements - Events, Classes & Retreats
http://www.aypsite.org/forum/topic.asp?TOPIC_ID=4979&REPLY_ID=53163&whichpage=-1
Yogani on the Radio - 2009 - KKCR Hawaii

Hi All:

The next one hour interview with Dr. Ann West on **Samyama** was prerecorded a few days ago, and is scheduled to air (and webcast) on Sunday, July 5th at 12 noon Hawaii time (6 pm eastern time USA) on http://www.kkcr.org

Soon after, the recording should be available on the AYP interviews page and Youtube channel.

The interview provides an introduction to the AYP Samyama book, with an overview of essential principles, techniques, and implications for individual practitioners and the world. Cultivating stillness in action, siddhis and miracles! :-)

The guru is in you.

2009/07/31 17:45:18
Member Announcements - Events, Classes & Retreats
http://www.aypsite.org/forum/topic.asp?TOPIC_ID=4979&REPLY_ID=54414&whichpage=-1
Yogani on the Radio - 2009 - KKCR Hawaii

Hi All:

We are back for another one. :-)

The next one hour interview with Dr. Ann West on **Diet, Shatkarmas and Amaroli** was prerecorded today, and is scheduled to air (and webcast) on Sunday, August 2nd at 12 noon Hawaii time (6 pm eastern time USA) on http://www.kkcr.org

Soon after, the recording should be available on the AYP interviews page and Youtube channel.

The interview provides an introduction to the AYP Diet, Shatkarmas and Amaroli book, with an overview of key principles and techniques, how these tie in with the broad scope of yoga practices, and the rise of ecstatic conductivity via the nectar cycle in the human neurobiology.

Next, we are planning to do **Self-Inquiry**. Looking forward to that here, and letting it go in stillness. :-)

The guru is in you.

2009/10/03 12:50:17
Member Announcements - Events, Classes & Retreats
http://www.aypsite.org/forum/topic.asp?TOPIC_ID=4979&REPLY_ID=57994&whichpage=-1
Yogani on the Radio - 2009 - KKCR Hawaii

Hi All:

The next one hour interview with Dr. Ann West on **Self-Inquiry** was prerecorded, and is scheduled to air (and webcast) on KKCR Hawaii, Sunday, October 4th at 12 noon Hawaii time (6 pm eastern time USA) on http://www.kkcr.org

Soon after, the recording should be available on the AYP interviews page and Youtube channel.

The interview provides an introduction to the AYP Self-Inquiry book. It also covers more recent developments highlighted in AYP Lesson 350 and Lesson 351. The interview also reviews the strengths and weaknesses of non-duality (jnana/advaita) approaches, ancient and modern, in relation to the presence of abiding inner silence (the witness) in the aspirant.

Next month, we are planning to do **Bhakti and Karma Yoga**.

All the best!

The guru is in you.

2009/10/30 12:40:26
Member Announcements - Events, Classes & Retreats
http://www.aypsite.org/forum/topic.asp?TOPIC_ID=4979&REPLY_ID=59168&whichpage=-1
Yogani on the Radio - 2009 - KKCR Hawaii

Hi All:

The next one hour interview with Dr. Ann West on **Bhakti and Karma Yoga** was prerecorded a few days ago, and is scheduled to air (and webcast) on KKCR Hawaii, Sunday, November 1st at 12 noon Hawaii time (5 pm eastern time USA) at http://www.kkcr.org

Soon after, the recording should be available on the AYP interviews page and Youtube channel.

The interview provides an introduction to the AYP Bhakti and Karma Yoga book, discussing the relationship of desire, our chosen ideal, and action for advancement on the spiritual path, and for transforming the consequences of our karma.

Next month, we are planning to do **Eight Limbs of Yoga**, covering the overall structure and pacing of self-directed spiritual practice. That is currently the last book in the Enlightenment Series, and will complete the 2009 series of 10 interviews on KKCR Hawaii.

Dr. Ann has been a terrific host throughout, and I am very grateful to her for making this series of talks possible.

The guru is in you.

2009/11/01 18:09:56
Member Announcements - Events, Classes & Retreats
http://www.aypsite.org/forum/topic.asp?TOPIC_ID=4979&REPLY_ID=59235&whichpage=-1
Yogani on the Radio - 2009 - KKCR Hawaii

Hi All:

As those who tuned in today surely noticed, the Self-Inquiry interview was broadcast again on KKCR, instead of the new Bhakti and Karma Yoga interview.

Not sure what happened, but our next broadcast opportunity will be December 6th. Will confirm the schedule here before then.

The guru is in you.

2009/11/02 11:25:05
Member Announcements - Events, Classes & Retreats
http://www.aypsite.org/forum/topic.asp?TOPIC_ID=4979&REPLY_ID=59257&whichpage=-1
Yogani on the Radio - 2009 - KKCR Hawaii

quote:

Originally posted by yogani

Hi All:

As those who tuned in today surely noticed, the Self-Inquiry interview was broadcast again on KKCR, instead of the new Bhakti and Karma Yoga interview.

Not sure what happened, but our next broadcast opportunity will be December 6th. Will confirm the schedule here before then.

The guru is in you.

Update: There was a mix-up and the wrong recording was put on for the broadcast yesterday. The Bhakti and Karma Yoga interview has been rescheduled for Dr. Ann's next program on December 6th.

The good news is that Dr. Ann has given permission to put the Bhakti and Karma Yoga interview up on the AYP website and Youtube now, so look for those soon -- on the website today sometime, and on Youtube in a couple of days.

Enjoy!

The guru is in you.

2009/12/30 18:35:59
Member Announcements - Events, Classes & Retreats
http://www.aypsite.org/forum/topic.asp?TOPIC_ID=4979&REPLY_ID=61951&whichpage=-1
Yogani on the Radio - 2009 - KKCR Hawaii

Hi All:

Update: The **Bhakti and Karma Yoga** interview (#9) did broadcast from KKCR Hawaii on December 6th. As you may recall, the November broadcast was delayed. The interview recording has been on the AYP interviews page since early November, along with all the others we have done.

New Interview: The next one hour interview (#10) with Dr. Ann West on **Eight Limbs of Yoga** has been prerecorded, and is scheduled to air (and webcast) on KKCR Hawaii, Sunday, January 3rd at 12 noon Hawaii time (5 pm eastern time USA) at http://www.kkcr.org

Soon after the broadcast, the recording should be available on the AYP interviews page and Youtube channel.

The interview provides an introduction to the AYP Eight Limbs of Yoga book, discussing the compilation of these categories of practice in the Yoga Sutras of Patanjali centuries ago, and how we have adapted them in the AYP system for practical utilization in modern times.

That will complete the series of 10 interviews we started a year ago. Many thanks to Dr. Ann West!

The guru is in you.

2009/10/11 11:21:15
Member Announcements - Events, Classes & Retreats
http://www.aypsite.org/forum/topic.asp?TOPIC_ID=5752&REPLY_ID=58281&whichpage=-1
Byron Katie in Toronto, October 2 to 4, 2009
Bravo! :-)

2010/10/23 13:55:08
Member Announcements - Events, Classes & Retreats
http://www.aypsite.org/forum/topic.asp?TOPIC_ID=8292&REPLY_ID=74117&whichpage=-1
Register Now-AYP retreat: Northeast USA, Oct 22-24

quote:
_____
Originally posted by Emil

Hi all,
As I'm writing this, you guys are experiencing pure bliss consciousness. which is fair :) I just wanted to say, isn't one weekend a bit too short? I mean If I was going to attend this I would have to spend $3000 on air fare and fly for 20 hours and back which would be just too much for one weekend. However for a week long retreat I wouldn't mind making that sort of investment. Just as a suggestion.

Please update us with your experiences from the retreat.

Cheers,
Emil
_____

Hi Emil:

The answer is to organize a retreat in Australia, assuming that is where you are. Plenty of AYP practitioners there. There are also possibilities for retreats in Asia. In time, we hope to have them going on everywhere. It is largely a function of those who are willing to make local arrangements (support for this can be made available by contacting me).

We are gradually having more experienced leaders available to come and run AYP retreats anywhere in the world, while training interested local practitioners/leaders to do the same. Lot's of opportunities...

All the best!

The guru is in you.

PS: Arrangements are currently in progress for a 5 day AYP retreat to be held March 20-25, 2011 at Kripalu Yoga Center in Massachusetts, USA. That is still a long way to come from Australia though.

2010/10/23 14:26:38
Member Announcements - Events, Classes & Retreats
http://www.aypsite.org/forum/topic.asp?TOPIC_ID=8292&REPLY_ID=74118&whichpage=-1
Register Now-AYP retreat: Northeast USA, Oct 22-24
PPS: Local contacts for planning AYP meditation groups, training and retreats around the world (including Australia) can be found here: http://www.aypsite.org/events.html That is a good place to start local/regional discussion for doing something.

For All: No matter where you are, if you would like to become a "planning contact" for local/regional AYP networking, let me know. It is not the kind of thing that produces a flood of email -- more of a long term networking thing to help get people with similar interests in touch.

2010/10/15 10:15:34
Member Announcements - Events, Classes & Retreats
http://www.aypsite.org/forum/topic.asp?TOPIC_ID=8577&REPLY_ID=73841&whichpage=-1
Czech AYP retreat 2010 - a short report
Bravo! :-)

2010/11/16 16:10:54
Member Announcements - Events, Classes & Retreats
http://www.aypsite.org/forum/topic.asp?TOPIC_ID=8747

AYP Retreat - Kripalu, USA, Mar 20-25, 2011

Hi All:

An AYP retreat will be occurring at the Kripalu Center for Yoga and Health - March 20-25, 2011 at Stockbridge, Massachusetts, USA.

A retreat is an opportunity to step away from our normal daily activities for enhanced cultivation of deep abiding inner silence in a comfortable structured program designed to enhance our quality of life when we come back home. See Lesson 387 for a discussion on retreats and the AYP baseline retreat structure.

The Kripalu retreat will be run by Katrine and Carson, will be open to AYP practitioners at all levels of experience ("from beginners to advanced"), and will be the longest AYP retreat yet (5 days). We are hoping it will be the biggest too, with plenty of room at this well-known international facility. The more who show up, the more powerful the retreat will be.

For newcomers to AYP, training in deep meditation will be provided at the retreat. All are welcome.

Given the impressive results from the October 22-24 Mensch Mill/Allentown, Pennsylvania retreat, having one twice as long at Kripalu should be a major inner silence awakener and stabilizer for those who attend. There is plenty of time to plan ahead, so do make it there if you can. I don't think you will regret it.

Sign-up for the retreat is through Kripalu at the link provided, or it can be done by calling 800-741-7353.

There is also a Kripalu PDF flyer for the retreat, which can be viewed and downloaded here. You can print and pass this flyer around, post it in your local yoga studio, new age shop, or anywhere. The more people who hear about the retreat, the better.

If you have any questions relating to this event, feel free to post them here, or you can email Katrine, Carson or me by clicking on our forum name links (forum sign-in required to post or email).

Wishing you all the best on your continuing path. Enjoy!

The guru is in you.

2010/12/31 13:26:24
Member Announcements - Events, Classes & Retreats
http://www.aypsite.org/forum/topic.asp?TOPIC_ID=8747&REPLY_ID=77699&whichpage=-1
AYP Retreat - Kripalu, USA, Mar 20-25, 2011

Hi All:

Kripalu's Spring 2011 catalog has been received here, in a glossy magazine format.

I have scanned a few of the pages to give an overall idea of the breadth of programs they having going on (hundreds), and the specific pages where AYP is covered (marked with asterisks), including a description of the March 20-25, 2011 AYP retreat. See here:
http://www.aypsite.org/images/Kripalu-Spring-2011.pdf

More information on the Kripalu AYP retreat can be found in the first post of this topic.

Wishing you all the best on your retreats in 2011!

The guru is in you.

Forum 22 – AYP Helpers

A place for discussing ways to help out with the AYP work.
http://www.aypsite.org/forum/forum.asp?FORUM_ID=34

2005/07/13 13:42:21
AYP Helpers
http://www.aypsite.org/forum/topic.asp?TOPIC_ID=291
Paying It Forward - AYP Helpers

If you have found AYP to be a useful resource, please pass the word to as many as you can so others might benefit also.

In AYP Lesson #166, the concept of "Pay It Forward" is discussed. It is doing for others what others have done for us in making AYP visible in some way. That way the word can keep getting around to those who may have interest. See http://www.aypsite.org/166.html

This forum is for those who would like to be AYP helpers, for networking and sharing ideas on how to spread the word. Even just mentioning AYP in another forum with a direct link included can make a huge difference. There are hundreds of ways both on the Internet and off it that this work can be made more visible. Anything that is done along those lines will be a blessing.

But no spam in the name of AYP, please, especially not the offensive automated kind that turns people off. Let's keep it respectable and on the highest level of integrity. There are many ways to do that.

AYP is a horizontal teaching, meaning everyone can bring the knowledge to everyone else, and that is how these writings will naturally grow in their influence.

"Candles lighting candles until all candles are lit."

Many thanks to all who have helped in this labor of love...

The guru is in you.

2005/08/28 16:25:59
AYP Helpers
http://www.aypsite.org/forum/topic.asp?TOPIC_ID=440
International Translations of the AYP Lessons
Since 2004 there have been a number of international translations of the AYP lessons undertaken. They are:

Arabic -- http://groups.yahoo.com/group/theguruisinyou (added 3/7/08)
..........or http://www.ayparabia.com (added 7/18/10)

Bulgarian -- http://www.bg-ayp.dir.bg/index.html (added 2004)

Chinese -- http://blog.sina.com.cn/aypchinese (added 8/27/10)

Czech -- http://ayp.cz/ (added 9/24/07)

Dutch -- http://sites.google.com/site/aypnederlands (added 11/9/10)
..........or http://www.odysseyofthesoul.de/AYP (added 10/13/06)

Farsi/Persian -- http://aypfarsi.blogspot.com (added 12/30/10)

French -- http://fr.groups.yahoo.com/group/Pratiquesavanceesdeyoga (added 2004)
..........or http://www.aypsite.ch (added 8/16/10)

German -- http://www.fyü.de (added 4/23/10, revised 8/12/10)
..........or http://aypsite.at (added 6/1/10)
..........or http://groups.yahoo.com/group/AYPdeutsch (added 9/27/05)

Hebrew -- http://sites.google.com/site/ayphebrewsite (added 5/9/09)

Hindi -- http://groups.yahoo.com/group/AdvancedYogaPractices_Hindi (added 2004)

Norwegian -- http://www.satsangwithkatrine.com/AYPLeksjonerpNorsk.html (added 5/5/10)

Portuguese -- http://ayppt.wordpress.com (added 6/20/08)

Spanish -- http://sites.google.com/site/aypcas (added 5/26/09)
..........or http://es.groups.yahoo.com/group/aypcastellano (added 5/9/09)
..........or http://www.namaste.com.mx/practicas (added 2004)

The International Translations are also listed on the main website here.

Note: On 12/3/08, a Google Automated Translation Tool covering about 60 languages was added at the bottom of all website and forum pages. 35 languages appear in the translator icon pull-down menu, and nearly 60 languages in another pull-down menu once the translator is launched with any language. The Google automated translations are gradually improving over time, and can be helpful with AYP lessons and forum discussions that are not covered in the human (manual) translations above.

The people who have been doing the international translations are the unsung heroes of AYP, and have my deepest gratitude. Because of them, many around the world have been able to read the lessons who would not have access to them otherwise.

If you are interested in translating part or all of the AYP lessons to another language, or assisting on an existing translation effort, please contact me directly. It is a wonderful way to help others, while at the same time deepen your experience of yoga. Here is what one translator had to say about his experience:

"I did a translation of the AYP site into Bulgarian, my native language. While doing this I have had experiences very similar to the shaktipat..."
http://www.aypsite.org/forum/topic.asp?whichpage=0.52&TOPIC_ID=350#336

The other translators have had similar experiences. In fact, I too consider myself to be a translator of the lessons -- into English from the original Inner Silence - Pure Bliss Consciousness -- and the experience of being filled with divine light by the work has been the same for me.

So, there is much to be gained from doing a translation of the AYP lessons. In the giving, we receive a thousand times over.

Any questions or comments you may have on international translations are welcome here.

The guru is in you.

2005/09/27 09:03:57
AYP Helpers
http://www.aypsite.org/forum/topic.asp?TOPIC_ID=440&REPLY_ID=774&whichpage=-1
International Translations of the AYP Lessons
A German translation of the AYP lessons has been started at http://groups.yahoo.com/group/AYPdeutsch/

Thank you!

The guru is in you.

2006/09/22 17:56:05
AYP Helpers
http://www.aypsite.org/forum/topic.asp?TOPIC_ID=440&REPLY_ID=11482&whichpage=-1
International Translations of the AYP Lessons

Hi Yogini:

Yes, by all means, do it. The internet medium (website, blog, etc.) and URL are your choice. Whatever works best for you and your readers. Sorry, I can't accommodate it on the AYP site.

The AYP website materials are fair game for translation and public viewing on the web. That is what they are for. Just provide one or more links back to http://www.aypsite.org for reference.

Beyond the online lessons are the AYP books, which are not available for free web viewing. If you want to translate the books, then we are talking about publishing books in Dutch, which would be wonderful. We can work with whatever your inclinations are.

Regarding open source practices, freedom and responsibility, you can bet I was holding my breath when AYP first went out for public viewing -- there have been so many dire predictions about how people will hurt themselves with open access to powerful spiritual practices. Well, it is not true. Everyone has been very responsible and actually brilliant in applying the practices with self-pacing. The level of responsibility displayed by everyone has been so impressive that there is even a short lesson on the subject here: http://www.aypsite.org/217.html

It is exactly the opposite of the dire predictions -- more information leads to more responsibility, while less information leads to more desperate measures and more danger. So much for the dire consequences of open source spiritual practices.

Once you have a URL let me know and we can post it.

My Dutch genes say, thank you. Oops, the secret is out. Yogani wears wooden shoes and lives in a windmill in Florida! :-)

The guru is in you.

2006/10/04 11:32:53
AYP Helpers
http://www.aypsite.org/forum/topic.asp?TOPIC_ID=440&REPLY_ID=11896&whichpage=-1
International Translations of the AYP Lessons

Thanks very much, Yogini and Wolfgang.

Looks great, even if I can't read it. :-)

Just a reminder to translate the "I AM" (AYAM) mantra phonetically for sound, and not for meaning.

I will add the Dutch link to the AYP translations list once a few more lessons are done. Same goes for your German effort, Wolfgang. Post the link here whenever you are ready.

Carry on!

The guru is in you.

2006/10/06 10:23:15
AYP Helpers
http://www.aypsite.org/forum/topic.asp?TOPIC_ID=440&REPLY_ID=11971&whichpage=-1

International Translations of the AYP Lessons

Hi Yogini and Wolfgang:

There have been long discussions on the pronunciation of the "I AM" (AYAM) mantra here in the forums. There is no perfect version of it, and neither is it crucial. But we do need a reasonable starting point.

The pronunciation I intend in the lessons is "I AM" as they say it on the American or British evening news -- minus the meaning, of course.

Deep meditation is an inner picking up of the sound vibration in thought, soon fading to fuzziness where the pronunciation becomes indistinct. It is only a faint feeling at those very silent levels of the mind, with corresponding slow-down in body-wide neurobiological activity. In following the procedure of deep meditation, we may come back to the mantra faintly and indistinctly also, depending on the course of purification occurring in the nervous system, which determines the level of our mental activity. We gently favor less, letting the mantra refine naturally.

So, in the translations, we are giving a starting point for deep meditation. The "I AM" sound vibration is what we use in AYP. The same goes when we are adding mantra enhancements, which come later in the lessons. The mantra enhancements provide a broader starting point in thought and, upon refinement in deep meditation, give us a bigger footprint in inner silence.

The guru is in you.

2006/10/18 13:37:17
AYP Helpers
http://www.aypsite.org/forum/topic.asp?TOPIC_ID=440&REPLY_ID=12407&whichpage=-1
International Translations of the AYP Lessons

Hi Yogini and Wolfgang:

The Dutch translation site has been added today to the links sections of the three AYP websites and main AYP Yahoo group. The list has also been updated at the beginning of this topic. The German translation site (a joint effort) has already been posted in all these places for some time.

So, currently, we have six translation sites in all. Thank you translators!

The guru is in you.

2007/09/24 10:31:18
AYP Helpers
http://www.aypsite.org/forum/topic.asp?TOPIC_ID=440&REPLY_ID=25647&whichpage=-1
International Translations of the AYP Lessons

Hi All:

A **Czech translation** of the AYP online lessons has begun here -- http://ayp.cz/
There are plans to include a forum as well.

Also, several have asked about **translating the AYP books** into other languages. While this can be a challenge with all the hurdles associated with publishing physical books, it can be very easily done in eBook form. PDF eBooks in any language can be downloaded directly from the AYP website for a small cost, like is presently being done for the special edition English versions with audio introductions. An eBook can be printed, so it can go into physical form that way. To publish a translated AYP book, all that is needed here is a formatted MS Word document in the translated language, and it can be converted into PDF eBook form for download through the AYP website.

Many thanks to all who are translating!

The guru is in you.

2008/03/08 09:48:46
AYP Helpers
http://www.aypsite.org/forum/topic.asp?TOPIC_ID=440&REPLY_ID=31018&whichpage=-1
International Translations of the AYP Lessons

Hi All:

A translation of the AYP online lessons to **Arabic** has begun here: http://www.bafree.net/forums/showthread.php?t=75280
or --- http://www.ebnalnil.com/vb/showthread.php?t=34423
(This site has certain posting requirements to gain access -- see instructions there.)

A hearty welcome to Arabic readers everywhere!

The guru is in you.

2008/06/20 13:54:05
AYP Helpers
http://www.aypsite.org/forum/topic.asp?TOPIC_ID=440&REPLY_ID=34710&whichpage=-1
International Translations of the AYP Lessons

Hi All:

A translation of the AYP online lessons to **Portuguese** has begun here: http://ayppt.wordpress.com

A hearty welcome to Portuguese readers everywhere!

The guru is in you.

2008/12/03 14:08:26
AYP Helpers
http://www.aypsite.org/forum/topic.asp?TOPIC_ID=440&REPLY_ID=41820&whichpage=-1
International Translations of the AYP Lessons

Hi All:

A "**Google Translator**" tool has been added on a test basis at the bottom of every AYP website and forum page, providing automated translations from English to about 35 other languages.

I don't know if the translator tool is very accurate, and would appreciate feedback here from anyone knowledgeable in any of these languages.

Many thanks!

The guru is in you.

2008/12/03 14:51:36
AYP Helpers
http://www.aypsite.org/forum/topic.asp?TOPIC_ID=440&REPLY_ID=41832&whichpage=-1
International Translations of the AYP Lessons

Hi Yogaislife and Shanti:

Thanks for the feedback. I figured accuracy would be mixed. The question is whether it will be a help or a hindrance to keep the translation tool on the website.

The AYP lessons are the main reason I installed it, and was not even sure if it would work at all in the forums due to the technology differences. It is nice that it does work in the forums. It's a good thing people cannot sign in when in other language modes. We don't want to encourage posting here in Portuguese, Hindi, Chinese, etc. :-)

The guru is in you.

2008/12/03 15:59:56
AYP Helpers
http://www.aypslte.org/forum/topic.asp?TOPIC_ID=440&REPLY_ID=41836&whichpage=-1
International Translations of the AYP Lessons
PS: It is not expected that the Google translator tool can replace the fine translation work occurring on the dedicated translation sites listed at the beginning of this topic.

The tool might help with AYP lessons not yet translated by knowledgeable practitioners, or for languages that are not being covered so far.

2008/12/04 09:42:36
AYP Helpers
http://www.aypsite.org/forum/topic.asp?TOPIC_ID=440&REPLY_ID=41872&whichpage=-1
International Translations of the AYP Lessons

Hi Ananda:

Thanks much for the feedback and suggested alternative for Arabic.

Yes, we are a long way from accurate automated translating, so don't give up your great translating effort for putting the AYP lessons into Arabic! :-)

The good news is that automated translating will keep improving over time, and Google will surely be a leader in this due to their global reach and vested interest in world languages. So hopefully the Google translator gadget will get smarter in a few years.

More feedback from everyone on the Google (or any other) translator is welcome here. The more input we have, the more new ideas and solutions will be stimulated.

All the best!

The guru is in you.

2008/12/05 18:11:12
AYP Helpers
http://www.aypsite.org/forum/topic.asp?TOPIC_ID=440&REPLY_ID=41928&whichpage=-1
International Translations of the AYP Lessons

quote:
_____
Originally posted by Ananda

hello yogani and thk you.

and since it's out in the open that i am the arabic translator, i would just like to attest to the credibility of this part in the intro on this post:

quote:

Originally posted by yogani

"I did a translation of the AYP site into Bulgarian, my native language. While doing this I have had experiences very similar to the shaktipat..."
http://www.aypsite.org/forum/topic.asp?whichpage=0.52&TOPIC_ID=350#336

—————

plus i think that the fast success i'm having with the practices has a lot to do with the translation i've done till now.

and it's an honor to be part of smthg this great and it's a good way to help others plus leave a good trace behind (karma yoga).

namaste my brothers and sisters,

Ananda

—————

Bravo! :-)

2008/12/06 11:22:03
AYP Helpers
http://www.aypsite.org/forum/topic.asp?TOPIC_ID=440&REPLY_ID=41952&whichpage=-1
International Translations of the AYP Lessons

quote:

Originally posted by mimirom

Hi all,

could anyone provide me contact info to the Czech translation group please? I believe I could help there. I've been to the http://ayp.cz/ site, but there doesn't seem to be any contact section.

mettá,

Roman

—————

Hi Roman:

Here is a contact: http://www.aypsite.org/forum/pop_profile.asp?mode=display&id=1611

Many thanks for your interest in helping out!

The guru is in you.

2009/01/14 12:41:02
AYP Helpers
http://www.aypsite.org/forum/topic.asp?TOPIC_ID=440&REPLY_ID=43470&whichpage=-1
International Translations of the AYP Lessons

quote:

Originally posted by Ananda

may i suggest this free tool as well for help in the translation work:
http://www.appliedlanguage.com/free_translation.shtml

—————

Hi Ananda:

Thank you for the additional translation tool. If this offers a better translation for any languages than the Google tool we are currently using at the bottom of every AYP web page, do let me know. If so, we will see about trying it out. It does not seem to be a clean install, and there are commercial hooks in it, so it would have to offer significant advantages over the free Google translator tool to be considered.

All the best!

The guru is in you.

2009/01/15 10:09:12
AYP Helpers
http://www.aypsite.org/forum/topic.asp?TOPIC_ID=440&REPLY_ID=43519&whichpage=-1
International Translations of the AYP Lessons

quote:
_____
Originally posted by Ananda

i didn't compare between the two sorry about that, and speaking for myself i don't use the google gadgets i found it to be not such a good tool in the arabic translation.

i just posted this free program as a replacement for babylon whom i think to be as the best tool among translators.

this translator does a good work on french to english and english to french plus arabic to english and english to arabic as far concerning the languages i know of.

and sorry about the commercial hooks i didn't give too much thought for that when i posted the subject.

kindest regards,

Ananda
_____

Hi Ananda:

If there is a way to put a Babylon automated translation tool on the AYP website without breaking the bank, I would be interested.

If they do not have such a tool now, perhaps in the future. Do keep us posted.

Thanks!

The guru is in you.

2009/05/09 14:45:21
AYP Helpers
http://www.aypsite.org/forum/topic.asp?TOPIC_ID=440&REPLY_ID=50392&whichpage=-1
International Translations of the AYP Lessons

Thank you, Yonatan. :-)

The Hebrew translation site link has been added to the listing in the first post of this topic, which is linked from the left border of every page of the AYP website and forums.

Also, Miguel has started a new Spanish translation site, continuing to translate beyond lessons #41, which is as far as the prior translation went as of 2006. The new Spanish site link has also been added to the list in the first post of this topic. The link is:
http://es.groups.yahoo.com/group/aypcastellano

Both the Hebrew and Spanish translation links will also soon be added to the listing of translations in the Links Section of the AYP website.

Much appreciation to you both, and happy translating. Many will benefit, not least of all the translators. :-)

The guru is in you.

2009/05/14 13:14:49
AYP Helpers
http://www.aypsite.org/forum/topic.asp?TOPIC_ID=440&REPLY_ID=50750&whichpage=-1
International Translations of the AYP Lessons

quote:
_____
Originally posted by Haksun

Hello,

I find the AYP site very informative and, if allowed to do so, would like to translate the lessons on the AYP site into Korean, which would then be published on an internet forum (to be created for AYP) open to the public free of charge. Would this be fine?

I look forward to your reply. Thank you. haksun
_____

Welcome Haksun!

A translation of the AYP online lessons to Korean for free viewing would be wonderful. Thanks so much for volunteering.

The choice of type of online forum or website is up to you. You can get some ideas by checking the translations listed in the first post of this topic: http://www.aypsite.org/forum/topic.asp?TOPIC_ID=440

The only requirement on this end is to provide a link back to the main AYP website (http://www.aypsite.org), so readers will know where all this is coming from, and can find us.

Translations of the AYP books are possible also, but those cannot be posted for free on the internet, since the books are the primary source of financial support for AYP. Anyone interested in doing AYP book translations can contact me via email.

Let me know when you have a Korean site up and running with the first lessons translated, and we can add the link on the AYP website listings.

All the best!

The guru is in you.

PS: A few days ago, a "Languages" link was added to the top menu on the main website, so it will be easier for new visitors to find the international translations (the link in the left border is still there too). This suggestion came from Miguel, and it is a great idea. Thanks Miguel! :-)

2009/05/27 11:10:28
AYP Helpers
http://www.aypsite.org/forum/topic.asp?TOPIC_ID=440&REPLY_ID=51524&whichpage=-1
International Translations of the AYP Lessons

Hi All:

Miguel has the Spanish translation website up and running. That is in addition to the Yahoo group that was recently added. Both are included in the AYP translation listings.

Thanks Miguel! :-)

The guru is in you.

2009/05/28 11:37:10
AYP Helpers
http://www.aypsite.org/forum/topic.asp?TOPIC_ID=440&REPLY_ID=51582&whichpage=-1
International Translations of the AYP Lessons

quote:
_____
Originally posted by Akasha

Impressive, Miguel.

As is that page of links, Yogani (never seen so many yoga links,interesting ones too, on one page)

Much Respect,:-)

_____

Hi Akasha:

Beyond the international translation links, which are kept up to date, the links page is in need of updating, with many new links to be added, and some dead ones to be removed. The same goes for the extended booklist and testimonials. So much has happened in the past few years, with the experiences of many practitioners advancing by leaps and bounds. The website sections mentioned will be brought up to date with the community of practitioners eventually. In the meantime, posting of new lessons will continue to be the first priority here. :-)

Carry on!

The guru is in you.

2009/05/28 13:37:58
AYP Helpers
http://www.aypsite.org/forum/topic.asp?TOPIC_ID=440&REPLY_ID=51593&whichpage=-1
International Translations of the AYP Lessons

quote:
_____
Originally posted by miguel

Wow,i didnt know about the extended booklist section.
My sincere and humble congratulations yogani,you are creating and incredible huge source of knowledge with ayp.And in the best place for reaching maximum spiritual searchers:the world wide web.
Im really overwhelmed.:-)
_____

Hi Miguel:

The tool box keeps growing. More importantly, those who are using the tools keep growing by their own effort. :-)

Bravo!

The guru is in you.

2010/02/18 11:00:57
AYP Helpers
http://www.aypsite.org/forum/topic.asp?TOPIC_ID=440&REPLY_ID=65031&whichpage=-1
International Translations of the AYP Lessons

quote:
_____
Originally posted by kashiraja

As far as I can see the translation into german has only reached lesson 36. Is that true?

Maybe I could go on translating other lessons.
_____

Hi kashiraja:

That would be wonderful. I will email the person administering the German translation site, Wolfgang, with copy to you, and hopefully the German translation can be carried forward.

It is also possible to copy from the existing translation and then carry it forward on your own site, with the link added to the AYP website where many can find it. This has happened with the Spanish translation, and it is fine. Whatever can get the job done. :-)

Many thanks, and all the best!

The guru is in you.

2010/04/23 15:29:25
AYP Helpers
http://www.aypsite.org/forum/topic.asp?TOPIC_ID=440&REPLY_ID=67699&whichpage=-1
International Translations of the AYP Lessons

Hi All:

A new translation link for German has been added to the listings in the first post of this topic and on the links page of the main website.

This translation is carrying on with new lessons, beyond the work that was done years ago, and is being provided by Bernd. Thank you Bernd! :-)

The guru is in you.

2010/05/07 11:00:11
AYP Helpers
http://www.aypsite.org/forum/topic.asp?TOPIC_ID=440&REPLY_ID=68373&whichpage=-1
International Translations of the AYP Lessons

Hi All:

A new AYP lessons translation link for Norwegian has been added to the listings in the first post of this topic and on the links page of the main website.

Katrine has recently started this one, among her many other projects to help spiritual practitioners in Norway and Ireland. Thank you Katrine! :-)

The guru is in you.

2010/05/07 11:22:59
AYP Helpers
http://www.aypsite.org/forum/topic.asp?TOPIC_ID=440&REPLY_ID=68374&whichpage=-1
International Translations of the AYP Lessons

quote:
_____
Originally posted by ConsciousEvolution

I can help with translating more lessons in Hebrew if needed and my friend said she could help with Spanish.
Let me know.

Peace
_____

Hi ConsciousEvolution:

That's wonderful! :-)

There are two possible paths. First is to contact the active translator, if any, and see if a combined effort can work. I say "if any" because several of the translations are not being actively worked on. In some cases, the former translator may not be reachable anymore.

If there can be a collaboration, great. Try for that first, as the translation work can go faster that way.

If a collaboration is not feasible, for whatever reason, then you are free to use what has been done (copy it), start your own site, and continue on translating new lessons. It may seem to be a sloppy approach, with multiple translations out there at various levels of completion, but this is the best way I have found to keep the translations going. It is challenging work, and no one is to be faulted for stopping after while. The main thing is for others who are inspired to be able to pick up what has been done and run further with it. That way, eventually all the translations will be done. :-)

I will be happy to list any new translation links on the AYP website and forums.

Maybe Miguel can use some help. The Spanish translation is up to Main Lesson 90 and Tantra Lesson 4.

The Hebrew translator is Yonatan. You can find an email link for him by clicking on his ID in the member list or anywhere in the forums. (There is an email link on the Hebrew website too.) The Hebrew translation is up to Main Lesson 17. If you can help it go further, that would be terrific.

Many thanks!

The guru is in you.

2010/05/13 10:54:02
AYP Helpers
http://www.aypsite.org/forum/topic.asp?TOPIC_ID=440&REPLY_ID=68704&whichpage=-1
International Translations of the AYP Lessons

quote:
_____
Originally posted by Panthau

Hey,

Do i see it right, that there are two german translations which end up early in the pranayama part?

If so, and im willing to translate, can i use these resource and start a new site? How free am i in design questions? Its just that it would be a lot more fun, not only to translate but also to place it in a whole new environment... because these german resources are rather... not so... beautiful as they could be :)

Thanks
Pan
_____

Hi Pan:

You can do whatever you like with presentation, as long as you are not altering the content of the lessons (including mixing with other content like reader discussions on the same page), and link back to the main English website so readers can find us.

FYI, the German translation listed first is active (the second is inactive). The translator is kashiraja. You may want to drop him a line to see if a joint effort makes sense. Or do your own thing, as described in my post above. If you develop a site, let me know the link so we can add it to the list. The one with the most lessons completed goes on top. :-)

Many thanks, and all the best!

The guru is in you.

2010/05/13 11:39:22
AYP Helpers
http://www.aypsite.org/forum/topic.asp?TOPIC_ID=440&REPLY_ID=68711&whichpage=-1
International Translations of the AYP Lessons

quote:
_____
Originally posted by Panthau

I just wondered about the translation of "i am" which kashiraja translated as "AYAM" (which sounds different to me).
_____

It is the same sound as the English words "I AM," however that may be spelled in German. In English "AYAM" is pronounced the same. AYAM can be viewed as a Sanskrit derivation, which would be pronounced the same everywhere. This additional spelling was provided in the lessons to make it clear that the mantra is a sound without meaning used in deep meditation. The important thing is to convey the sound, not any meaning.

The guru is in you.

2010/05/14 13:59:00
AYP Helpers
http://www.aypsite.org/forum/topic.asp?TOPIC_ID=440&REPLY_ID=68786&whichpage=-1
International Translations of the AYP Lessons

Hi Pan:

When you have some lessons up there (say at least 5-10), let me know and we can post the link then.

Many thanks!

The guru is in you.

2010/05/16 10:30:35
AYP Helpers
http://www.aypsite.org/forum/topic.asp?TOPIC_ID=440&REPLY_ID=68847&whichpage=-1
International Translations of the AYP Lessons

quote:
_____
Originally posted by ConsciousEvolution

A question for Yogani:

I'm translating from English to Hebrew right now, at a pretty good pace.
Reading through my translations, they look alright. They seem professional and the vocabulary used is quite good.
The original meaning is conveyed.
The thing is, that they feel mechanical to some extent. There's something a bit lifeless about them.
Remember, Hebrew does not come from Latin so it's quite a different language.
I've been trying to be very loyal to the original text but the problem is that that somehow renders my translations a bit cold, with not enough soul.
On the other hand, I might have to wander off quite a bit from the original in order to render them friendlier and more soulful, and then they might not be as accurate and loyal to the original text as they are now.

Anyway, you get my drift...

So? What's your advice? What are the guidelines, what's the preference?
In short, may I take the liberty to simplify it and make it more user-friendly in Hebrew, a different language, or do I stay loyal to source as literally as I can?

Thank you Kindly,

CE
_____

Hi CE:

The purpose of the translation is to convey the content. If it can be done with some "flair" in the language being used, so much the better. Then it is coming alive in stillness.

You have good input from several here with experience translating the lessons, and I concur with their sharings.

My own "translation" went from inner silence to English, and whatever flair is in there just happened. I am sure as you get into it, you will find the same.

Many thanks, and enjoy!

The guru is in you.

2010/05/16 10:33:51
AYP Helpers
http://www.aypsite.org/forum/topic.asp?TOPIC_ID=440&REPLY_ID=68848&whichpage=-1
International Translations of the AYP Lessons

quote:
_____
Originally posted by Panthau

Hi again,

I just realized that my intension to make this translation, was born after a phase of stillness, as my mind desperately tried to grab something to hold on to.

As Papaji said, the concept of every exhausting spiritual practices which gets you to your desired goal, is a new entanglement in the game of light without substance.

All that is needed, is stillness, to get back and experience what we are.

So if anyone wants to use the stuff i created so far, is welcome. If needed, i can finish the structure of the site.

Atb,
Pan

———————

Hi Pan:

Whatever you need to be doing in the present will be best. It was a good start. Maybe you will come back to it later. Tuck it away safely until then.

Many thanks!

The guru is in you.

2010/05/31 10:46:25
AYP Helpers
http://www.aypsite.org/forum/topic.asp?TOPIC_ID=440&REPLY_ID=69396&whichpage=-1
International Translations of the AYP Lessons

quote:
———————
Originally posted by kashiraja

Hi Yogani,
Lesson 46, A. first paragraph
"This will manifest as an emptying of the lungs and then a drawing up from near the bottom of the spine".
What is drawn up. Do you mean just a drawing up of muscles or Prana and can I express that in my translation for clarification.
———————

Hi kashiraja:

It is both physical and energetic (pranic). In time, it is less physical and more energetic, which is the whole body mudra effect. But that is jumping ahead. :-)

Hope that helps.

The guru is in you.

2010/06/01 11:14:54
AYP Helpers
http://www.aypsite.org/forum/topic.asp?TOPIC_ID=440&REPLY_ID=69431&whichpage=-1
International Translations of the AYP Lessons

quote:
———————
Originally posted by Panthau

It seems like AYP is helping me to let go. This again, helps me to translate :)

I hope it isnt a problem, that ive chosen the same domain name. I thought thats also a good way to find it through google.

http://aypsite.at

Done so far:
Lesson 10-15
FAQ 1-28

Todo:
Rest of Mainlessons
Rest of FAQ
Tantra Lessons
Topic-Index
Ayurveda Diet
Forum

Still a lot to go, but i thought its time to publish it, so maybe people can benefit from the first FAQ translations.

Thanks!
Pan

———————

Hi Pan:

Thanks for taking the initiative. The site looks great.

While I do not read German, it appears you are using Wikipedia links to describe terms like meditation, mantra, pranayama, samyama, etc, in the AYP introduction. This can be confusing for those reading the translation, because those links many not provide a view on these terms consistent with the AYP writings. This is not to say that one is right and the other is wrong, only that they are not going to be consistent. It would be fine to use such links in a general discussion about spiritual practices, but not in an introduction that is specific to the AYP system. The Yogani Wikipedia link is fine, but it is requested to move the others out of the AYP introduction. Then I will be happy to add your translation link to the list.

The same goes for any definitions, commentary or forum discussions by others. They should be kept separate from the AYP lessons to minimize confusion about what is AYP writing and what is coming from other sources.

Regarding translating the Forum FAQs, that may not be an easy task. These will be changing over time, and they usually link to multiple other forum topics. It may be best to leave translation of the forum FAQs, and the forums in general, to the automated **Google Translator Tool** found at the bottom of every website page. That tool is far from perfect, but does address what is current. There is no way anyone can manually translate the thousands of topics in the forums, at least not in this lifetime. :-)

Many thanks!

The guru is in you.

2010/06/01 20:38:23
AYP Helpers
http://www.aypsite.org/forum/topic.asp?TOPIC_ID=440&REPLY_ID=69448&whichpage=-1
International Translations of the AYP Lessons

quote:
_____
Originally posted by Panthau

Done :-)

(I may be sometimes a bit over the top, but not enough to ever translate a whole forum :P)

Thanks
Pan

I wonder, why am i not moderated?
_____

Thanks much, Pan.

Have added your German translation link to the list.

The guru is in you.

2010/06/04 11:10:48
AYP Helpers
http://www.aypsite.org/forum/topic.asp?TOPIC_ID=440&REPLY_ID=69527&whichpage=-1
International Translations of the AYP Lessons

quote:
_____
Originally posted by kashiraja

Hi Yogani,

Lesson 47, A. 6th paragraph.

"So, the effect of meditation on chakras is to calm them, to still them."

It is clear to me what I have to translate.

But, to my understanding the calming concerns only the lower three chakras. The upper three chakras are stimulated.
_____

Hi kashiraja:

I'll stick by what is said in the lesson. Deep meditation cultivates inner silence throughout the nervous system, and beyond. Experiences may vary from time to time. Such is the process of purification and opening in each of us, and the unfathomable karma behind it. It is all stillness in action. :-)

Many thanks!

The guru is in you.

2010/07/12 19:21:30

quote:

_____
Originally posted by kashiraja

Therefore my suggestion: Isn't it possible to integrate into each of your sits a flag with the link(s) of the language where a translation is available as it has become standard for websites.

Everyone interested in a translation will first look out for such a flag indicating his own language.

_____

Hi kashiraja:

Flags would be great, but so far I have not figured out how we could do that with multiple translations at different levels of completion. That is why we have kept using a list.

The list is actually in two places, at the beginning of this topic, and in the AYP website links section. On the main website, direct links to the list are given in three places on every page (top menu, left side menu, and bottom link along with the Google translator tool), and in the forums in two places on every page (left side menu and bottom link along with the Google translator tool). Admittedly, the reader has to be able to recognize the words "languages" or "international translations" to find these.

It would certainly be a plus to use a masthead of flags somewhere and link that to the translations list in the links section. Will put it on the "to do" list.

Thanks for the suggestion, and for the German translation work. I am sure the traffic will grow over time. We'll do what we can on this end to help.

The guru is in you.

PS: I was informed recently that the Arabic AYP translation has over 100 readers now. That is pretty exciting. It is not so much about absolute numbers as it is about how we are doing this year compared to last year. It is all growing... :-)

2010/07/13 14:26:33
AYP Helpers
http://www.aypsite.org/forum/topic.asp?TOPIC_ID=440&REPLY_ID=70910&whichpage=-1
International Translations of the AYP Lessons

Hi kashiraja and All:

A "flags icon" has been added on top of the left side border on all AYP website and forum pages. It links to a new translations page that replaces the translation links that were on the links page.

It was not practical to provide individual flag links to translations in the various languages, because we have more than ten human (manual) translations (more than one for some languages), plus the Google Automated Translation Tool covering about 35 languages. So we are linking to one page that has everything on it, and hopefully easier to find now with the "flags icon" on the top-left of every page.

Thanks for the suggestion. May many more people easily find the AYP writings in their own language. :-)

The guru is in you.

2010/07/13 18:45:13
AYP Helpers
http://www.aypsite.org/forum/topic.asp?TOPIC_ID=440&REPLY_ID=70920&whichpage=-1
International Translations of the AYP Lessons

quote:

_____
Originally posted by kashiraja

Thanks Yogani,

great, I think that's a pritty good solution you found.

_____

Hi kashiraja:

Just added individual flags for the various languages shown on the new translations page. :-)

The guru is in you.

2010/07/14 08:38:51
AYP Helpers
http://www.aypsite.org/forum/topic.asp?TOPIC_ID=440&REPLY_ID=70941&whichpage=-1

International Translations of the AYP Lessons

quote:
_____
Originally posted by yogani

Just added individual flags for the various languages shown on the new translations page. :-)

The guru is in you.

_____

Hi All:

There could be some complaints about using the Arab League flag for Arabic and the Spanish flag for Spanish, since both languages are used elsewhere. The idea was to designate each language with a small graphic that would be easily recognizable by those who would not recognize their language spelled in English. Using the flag for the source country/region seemed reasonable, and unmistakable.

An alternative would be to spell the language out in its corresponding script, like is done in the Google Translator, which would be more difficult.

Hopefully what has been done is reasonable and will not offend anyone. There is much else to be working on here.

The guru is in you.

2010/07/14 10:54:00
AYP Helpers
http://www.aypsite.org/forum/topic.asp?TOPIC_ID=440&REPLY_ID=70946&whichpage=-1
International Translations of the AYP Lessons

Hi Miguel:

Well, the Spanish flag is the accepted icon for Spanish in translator devices and services, as is the Arab League flag for Arabic. Both are also found in the multi-flag icon added on the top-left of the website and forum pages, which is a standard layout used for language translators. In this case, the flag icons are not country designations. They are easy-to-recognize language designations. No politics in that.

The guru is in you.

PS: Brazil could complain about the Portuguese flag, and the USA could complain about the UK flag (if we used it). It could go on and on. From a practical standpoint, the places where the languages originated are the most logical icons to use -- easily recognized.

2010/07/21 11:12:55
AYP Helpers
http://www.aypsite.org/forum/topic.asp?TOPIC_ID=440&REPLY_ID=71132&whichpage=-1
International Translations of the AYP Lessons

quote:
_____
Originally posted by Panthau

Has lesson 63 been written before 62 or is there a mistake?

Lesson 62:
"Date: Wed Dec 31, 2003 1:17pm"

Lesson 63:
"Date: Wed Dec 31, 2003 0:49pm"

Thanks!
Pan
_____

Hi Pan:

They were written in the order shown. The time stamps were copied from Yahoo Groups, and there must have been a discrepancy. Lessons 62 and 63 are shown as 1:23 pm and 1:24 pm on Yahoo now, both on Dec 31, 2003.

We have not used time stamps on website lessons for some time, and you are not required to use them. The date is good enough.

Many thanks for your translating work!

The guru is in you.

714 – Advanced Yoga Practices

2010/08/04 10:11:09
AYP Helpers
http://www.aypsite.org/forum/topic.asp?TOPIC_ID=440&REPLY_ID=71577&whichpage=-1
International Translations of the AYP Lessons

quote:
_____
Originally posted by kashiraja

Hi Yogani,

a technical question.

Did you organize your website in a way that you had only to change one or two pages or files in order to integrate the flag icons or had you to go through all pages and change them.

If the first case, how did you do that?

Best regards and thanks.
_____

Hi kashiraja:

The AYP website is managed with MS Frontpage, with optional top, bottom, left and right borders. The borders can be applied to all pages with one action. So a change or addition in a border is reflected on all pages that are turned on for borders. Other website software packages have similar (and more advanced) capabilities. It is very common for menu maintenance and other site-wide display information. Frontpage is a bit out-of-date, but it works for us.

In the early days, we did not have border capability, and it made website maintenance much more labor-intensive, with severe limitations on what additional information (and menu modifications) we could display on the hundreds of pages on the website. Thank goodness we got beyond that, because now we have twice as many pages. :-)

The guru is in you.

PS: The AYP Support Forums software has border capability also (not part of MS Frontpage), and that is how the same border information and features (like the Google Translator on bottom of page) are shown on the thousands of pages in the forums.

2010/08/12 22:46:33
AYP Helpers
http://www.aypsite.org/forum/topic.asp?TOPIC_ID=440&REPLY_ID=71878&whichpage=-1
International Translations of the AYP Lessons

Hi kashiraja:

Nice start with Frontpage. :-)

Which link do you want to use for your German translation?

Yes, the "ü" might create some difficulties. It already has in your post above, where the forum cannot automatically create the link. Perhaps it can be manually inserted. Not sure about displaying it with a working link on the AYP website. Will have to see.

Regarding getting the forums together with the lessons, we have the English AYP lessons and support forums hosted together on the same server under the same domain -- http://www.aypsite.org. This was possible because the forum software we are using can be installed under any domain on a server with suitable database capability. You may or may not have that flexibility with your forum software. There is an advantage having both the AYP lessons and forums under the same domain name, and kept public. It greatly increases search engine exposure for both. This has made AYP easy to find (on purpose or accidentally) on the web.

The guru is in you.

2010/08/13 11:04:46
AYP Helpers
http://www.aypsite.org/forum/topic.asp?TOPIC_ID=440&REPLY_ID=71896&whichpage=-1
International Translations of the AYP Lessons

Hi kashiraja:

I was able to instal the www.fyü.de link both in the first post of this topic and on the translations page of the main website. The link is made active (including in this post) with manual coding of the URL.

FYI, the link is hijacking the browser address window (in Firefox) with itself for all pages opened from your website. This may have to do with the forwarding function.

Many thanks to both you and Panthau for all your efforts in German translation.

Onward!

The guru is in you.

2010/08/16 15:25:32
AYP Helpers
http://www.aypsite.org/forum/topic.asp?TOPIC_ID=440&REPLY_ID=71973&whichpage=-1
International Translations of the AYP Lessons

quote:
_____
Originally posted by Buffle37

Hi all,
I am happy to annonce that to day the new site for the french translations is on the web at:

http://www.aypsite.ch/

with 60 main lessons and 2 tantra lessons
_____

Bravo! :-)

The translation lists have been updated.

The guru is in you.

2010/08/19 12:23:25
AYP Helpers
http://www.aypsite.org/forum/topic.asp?TOPIC_ID=440&REPLY_ID=72098&whichpage=-1
International Translations of the AYP Lessons

Hi Kashiraja and Pan:

Kashiraja, I see the individual URLs are now coming up when going from fyü.de, and these are on fyue.de. Do you want to leave the translation link as fyü.de, or change it to fyue.de? It seems to be working okay now. If it isn't broken, maybe we don't have to fix it.

Regarding the forum, nothing wrong with leaving it where it is and linking back and forth between the lessons and forum. This too has advantages -- not all the eggs in one domain/server basket. To get it under the AYP lessons domain would require either resident software on your hosting service (which could not be moved), or an installable (and movable) software. The one being used here (Snitz) is installed in a folder ("forum") on the aypsite.org server and can be moved if needed. Yes, the Snitz software has a border feature similar to MS Frontpage, so the borders look the same, even though they are coming from two different sources. You may or may not be able to do something similar on resident forum software, or on a separate forum/blog site like you have.

While I prefer that you and Pan work it out on how to proceed with lessons and forum(s), I do agree with Pan that one German AYP forum community would be better than two. Building an online community is a long and tedious process, and is best undertaken as a group effort in one place. Not so with lesson translations, which can be put up on the web by anyone who is translating. Translation collaborations are fine, but not essential. I'd say a collaboration to build an online forum community is essential. There have been many involved in building the AYP community here, and I am very grateful to everyone who has pitched in.

My interest is in seeing the AYP lessons out there, and however that gets done is fine here. The reason we got into multiple translations in the same languages is because it is a big effort and there is a fatigue factor that sometimes comes, and any translation effort may stop at some point. This is perfectly understandable. New translators who come along can rarely gain access to existing translation websites to continue them, so we came up with the "copy and continue" scheme, which has worked pretty well. It is sort of like a relay race -- one person carries the baton, and then another person carries it. It was not originally intended to be a competition between two active translations, but if the two of you are enjoying it, that's fine too. Whatever works. :-)

It is up to the two of you to work it out, or continue separately -- your choice. Btw, someone in Berlin emailed me recently, asking if they could assist in German translation of the lessons. I suggested he contact either or both of you and offer services. Or if that did not work, he could continue the relay with yet another German translation! We don't want to hold anyone back who wants to translate. Don't know if you will hear from this person, but thought to mention it. It is wonderful that interest for AYP in Germany is on the rise.

Pan, I was looking at your site to see where you are in translating the lessons. With all the lesson titles translated in the directory, it was difficult to see how far the actual translated lessons go. Most lesson titles in the directory give a "nothing here" message when clicked on. Maybe I missed something, not being a German reader. How does one find out how far the translated lessons go without having to click on a bunch of the titles?

Many thanks to both of you, and onward with German AYP! :-)

The guru is in you.

2010/08/23 18:56:10
AYP Helpers
http://www.aypsite.org/forum/topic.asp?TOPIC_ID=440&REPLY_ID=72298&whichpage=-1
International Translations of the AYP Lessons

Hi kashiraja:

Sounds like a good plan. :-)

If you save this file to your hard drive and put it in the same folder with your website HTML files, the icon should show up in the browser tabs and elsewhere:

http://www.aypsite.org/favicon.ico

The guru is in you.

2010/08/25 13:23:01
AYP Helpers
http://www.aypsite.org/forum/topic.asp?TOPIC_ID=440&REPLY_ID=72361&whichpage=-1
International Translations of the AYP Lessons

quote:
_____
Originally posted by Buffle37

mains lessons 61 to 90 have been added to day on french web site:

http://www.aypsite.ch/index.php

_____

:-)
2010/10/14 10:42:55
AYP Helpers
http://www.aypsite.org/forum/topic.asp?TOPIC_ID=440&REPLY_ID=73793&whichpage=-1
International Translations of the AYP Lessons

quote:
_____
Originally posted by kashiraja

Hi Yogani,

I have some difficulty understanding and translating this sentence:

"Everything we have done so far as been from the root on up, above siddhasana, which is systematic stimulation at the perineum." Tantra 1 penultimum Paragraph first sentence.

Can I read this sentence as: "Everything we have done so far [h]as been from the root on up, above [all] siddhasana, which is systematic stimulation at the perineum."
_____

Hi kashiraja:

Yes, that is a typo, and should read, "Everything we have done so far <u>has</u> been from the root on up..."

That typo has been hiding there for for nearly 7 years, and you are the first to mention it! It has been corrected (in the last paragraph) here: http://www.aypsite.org/T1.html

Not sure what you mean adding the word [all]. The reference is meant to be physical and energetic, meaning that in sitting practices we work mainly from the perenium upward. When working with sexual energy in tantric mode, a much wider range of energy flow is accepted. As we know, sexual energy can go either way. This is why success with tantric sex depends largely on our sitting practices, because the upward bias for sexual energy comes from abiding inner silence. The techniques of tantric sex do not work very well without that necessary prerequisite, as many have found. The good news is that tantric sexual techniques work very well when abiding inner silence is present.

Many thanks!

The guru is in you.

2010/10/14 11:52:51
AYP Helpers
http://www.aypsite.org/forum/topic.asp?TOPIC_ID=440&REPLY_ID=73797&whichpage=-1
International Translations of the AYP Lessons

quote:
_____
Originally posted by kashiraja

Hi Yogani,

I wondered whether "above siddhasa" is meant to stress Siddhasana es technique so I thought it should read "above all"

So "above" is meant locally. But with this you are excluding all those who don't or can't practice siddhasana for any reason. But of course one can use a prosthetic.

Thanks.

P.S.: In your AYP book "Easy lesssons for an ecstatic living" I find typos now and then. Should I make a list or do you have enough feedback already.

_____

Hi kashiraja:

No, siddhasana is not being emphasized as essential. It is only mentioned as an example to point out where sitting practices have their "floor." Of course, it is not that precise, because the rise of ecstatic conductivity, with or without tantric sexual methods in the picture, is a "whole body" experience. The point of the lesson is to say that we can look beyond (or below) the sushumna (spinal nerve) to illuminate the sushumna, which is the role that tantric sex plays in the overall scheme of things. That simple idea overrides many stigmas about sex, and sets the stage for introducing the practical methods in the tantra lessons.

Keep in mind that each lesson was written at a point in time, with a particular frame of reference related to the structure of practices that had been introduced at that time. It would be accurate to say that the lessons have evolved quite a lot over time to take an increasingly broader view corresponding with the evolution of the community of practitioners. In doing so, we have been continually building understanding and refined application of the core practices that were introduced in that first year. So, ultimately, the best way to regard any particular lesson is from the perspective of the whole of AYP we see today, and what people are experiencing in using the baseline system of practices. It continues to evolve, and with pretty good results, I think.

Of course, each lesson should be translated "as is" to reflect what it delivered when written, minus the typos. :-)

Any typos found in the AYP books can be emailed to me. Records of these are being kept, and someday they can be incorporated in future editions.

Thanks!

The guru is in you.

2010/10/25 15:49:52
AYP Helpers
http://www.aypsite.org/forum/topic.asp?TOPIC_ID=440&REPLY_ID=74203&whichpage=-1
International Translations of the AYP Lessons

quote:
_____
Originally posted by Philaboston

Hi Yogani and fellow translators,

I write to you for advice on launching a sister (2nd) Chinese translation site. As you know, there are two sets of Chinese characters: the simplified used in mainland China and the unsimplified in Taiwan and Hong Kong. It's not very difficult to learn to recognize the simplified if one already knows the unsimplified. But there still be some difficulties that I worry might become an obstacle for readers from Taiwan and Kong Kong (It's more complicated for Hong Kong people, because their writing often reflect Cantonese in stead of Mandarin.) I'm thinking of launching a parallel blog in unsimplified Chinese. Will this cause confusion or possible communication complex between the two groups of aypers?

Phil

_____

Hi Phil:

No problem with that. When you have the second link, just let me know. We can list both, each with a clear designation of what it is.

Many thanks!

The guru is in you.

2010/10/30 09:57:00
AYP Helpers
http://www.aypsite.org/forum/topic.asp?TOPIC_ID=440&REPLY_ID=74450&whichpage=-1
International Translations of the AYP Lessons

quote:
_____
Originally posted by Medea

I have a question on the Dutch translations. It seems that the process of translating has been stopped for a while, and I would like to offer my assistance. Maybe the Dutch translator can contact me to share his/her ideas on this?

I also had an idea about the international translations page. All the different languages are named in English. There are of course also the flags, but maybe the accessibility for non English speakers would be improved if their language was also named in their native tongue. For example: the word 'Dutch' in the Dutch language is very different from English, namely *Nederlands*. It could be confusing for some. Just an idea :)

_____

Hi Medea:

The Dutch translator is no longer available. It is a long time since anything has been done with it. If you would like to pick it up, you can copy what has been done, edit it as needed, and use your own website to share it. The current Dutch site is not accessible for editing or additions, so it would be very good to launch a new site for active translation work. I will be happy to add the link to the list of translations. There are plenty of tips on getting started in this topic. Check my previous posts here.

Regarding the naming of languages in their own language, it had occurred here, but I was not sure we could handle the fonts in all cases. It is one of those things on the list of things to do. Thanks for pointing out the benefits of doing it sooner rather than later. :-)

Btw, if you would like to be listed as a "planning contact" on the AYP contacts page for the Netherlands, email me with preferred name, location (city/region) and email to use. We can also put your website link there, if and whenever you have one.

Many thanks!

The guru is in you.

2010/11/09 10:10:11
AYP Helpers
http://www.aypsite.org/forum/topic.asp?TOPIC_ID=440&REPLY_ID=74976&whichpage=-1
International Translations of the AYP Lessons

quote:
_____
Originally posted by Medea

Hi all,

So, I built a website and started editing lessons. The site is open for all now and can be found at http://sites.google.com/site/aypnederlands/ Feedback is welcome of course!

Love, Marleen
_____

Hi Medea:

Looks very good. Will add it to the lists today.

Many thanks!

The guru is in you.

2005/09/24 16:27:00
AYP Helpers
http://www.aypsite.org/forum/topic.asp?TOPIC_ID=493&REPLY_ID=751&whichpage=-1
website volume

Hi Andrew:

Great question -- very relevant to where we are all going with this. Here are a few perspectives, and where I'd like to head with it over the next few years.

I may have corresponded with 500 people over the last two years (maybe more - haven't counted), but never all in one day! There is always a rotation going on with who is writing, which determines who I am corresponding with. These days I usually have only a few correspondences going on at any one time, occasionally spiking to half a dozen or so. Last year, before the lessons reached critical mass, it was more like a dozen rotating correspondences going on all the time, and spiking to 20 or so every now and then. Pretty crazy back then.

As the lessons have become more complete the emails have become much less, even as the lesson readership and website volumes have gone way up. That is what I have been hoping for -- a body of written knowledge that can eventually stand on its own. With the forums coming up now and beginning to fill in many of the questions that used to come to me (thank you!), there is the opportunity for AYP to evolve into a self-propelled worldwide community of practitioners using an open source integrated system, according to each person's needs. That is my wish for what AYP will become, and we are making progress.

Before aypsite.org was launched in June 2005, the Geocities site was running 10,000 page visits per month -- about 300/day. aypsite.org (including the forums launched in July) went almost straight to 50,000+ page visits per month -- averaging about 2,000/day now, with about 2/3 of that in the forums, so you are getting a lot of unregistered readers over here for sure. The Geocities site has dropped about in half since aypsite.org came out. Also, there are still folks who prefer the Yahoo groups for reading the lessons, but I have no way to measure that activity.

Here is an amazing statisitic: Since opening in June, aypsite.org has seen 18,000 visitors (individual readers) from 90 countries. The breakdown on readers is:

USA - 73%
Canada - 6%
UK - 4%
India - 4%
Australia - 2%

Germany - 1%
...with the remaining 10% spread out among 85 other countries.

The numbers indicate that the West will be carrying the ball on the expansion of applied spiritual practices in the years to come, though these are AYP numbers only and do not necessarily represent what is happening in all systems of spiritual practice. An interesting data point though, isn't it?

As for what I will be doing from here on, I am beginning what will likely be a fairly long list of small books, each on a single practice, or same-in-class group of practices. There could be a dozen or more of these small books coming out over the next couple of years, starting with the first few in late 2005 or early 2006. They will be "entry level" and aimed at the average person who may have a glimmer of an interest in any practice like deep meditation, pranayama, tantra, mudras/bandhas, asanas, etc. The idea will be to create multiple entry points into AYP in the book market for many people with diverse interests.

I'd also like to continue filling in the remaining knowledge gaps in the AYP online lessons, as was mentioned in the last lesson #275. In the end, the additional lessons since the first book, along with a lot of unpublished Q&As piling up here, can be put together into a "Volume 2" AYP Easy Lessons book.

If I can get all that done, then maybe take a break for a while? :-)

The guru is in you.

Yogani

2005/09/26 11:17:09
AYP Helpers
http://www.aypsite.org/forum/topic.asp?TOPIC_ID=493&REPLY_ID=767&whichpage=-1
website volume

Hi Andrew:

I believe self-pacing never had much opportunity to evolve before now because the practices were so little available, and fragmented among multiple traditions besides -- not much to self-pace with. The methods of dissemination precluded the need for pacing, except by the personal supervision of the guru, of course. And that was the way it had to be when the means for communicating with aspirants was so limited. The solution was to collect people together into ashrams and communities where the guidance was available. That was limited access for the public, of course, and also inevitably led to the social and political complications within the communities, and all that cult nonsense.

With the Internet, maybe we have found a good compromise -- maximum information flow to everyone, with minimum distractions. Well, it's not the same as being in a physical community, but the fact that self-pacing is evolving naturally out of it means something new and exciting is happening. Could self-directed practitioners travel this fast in significant numbers before? It will be interesting to see how it pans out.

As for Babaji, Jesus, Buddha, Krishna and the like, I hope this will meet with their approval. I have heard no complaints, so far. We're all on the same team...

Thanks all for being part of it ... this illuminating experiment in applied yoga science.

The guru is in you.

Yogani

2005/09/26 15:17:30
AYP Helpers
http://www.aypsite.org/forum/topic.asp?TOPIC_ID=493&REPLY_ID=769&whichpage=-1
website volume

Hi again Andrew:

Would you mind if we move this topic to "AYP Helpers?" It says a lot about the nuts and bolts of the human side of the AYP work, and where we can all take this together.

This ties in with David's "infallibility" discussion too -- the wisdom of taking what works from a teacher and leaving the rest behind. Getting past the "perfect or nothing" syndrome -- neither is reality. That goes for students and teachers, both...

Bottom line: I'm a person who can organize the practical aspects of yoga, write it down, and offer advice based on my own long-time journey. The rest is in everyone's own hands. It is cause and effect -- not a mystical deliverance beyond our own making. Is that a disappointment, or a revelation? It depends on who is reading, who is practicing, and what the experiences are, yes?

Whatever the case may be, whittling the pedestal(s) down to horizontal is in everyone's best interest. Eventually, it will spread the work out too. Hence, the move to AYP Helpers ... :-)

The guru is in you.

Yogani

2005/09/26 22:32:12
AYP Helpers
http://www.aypsite.org/forum/topic.asp?TOPIC_ID=493&REPLY_ID=773&whichpage=-1
website volume

Thanks Andrew.

For those who are interested, this topic provides an overview of where we are with AYP readership numbers, and where we can go. With many pitching in, I know we can create that worldwide open source community for spiritual practices. It is within our reach. All we have to do is keep moving ahead. Each person's individual progress is everyone's progress, and vise versa!

The guru is in you.

2005/10/04 17:40:05
AYP Helpers
http://www.aypsite.org/forum/topic.asp?TOPIC_ID=504
Forum connection problems, tech help & money
This is an email exchange with Paul regarding hitting the database connection limit:

Q: I was unable to access the AYP forum site.
This is the error message that I got. Maybe it is at my end but I thought that I would give you a heads up!
Paul

"The page cannot be displayed
There is a problem with the page you are trying to reach and it cannot be displayed..."

A: Hello Paul:

I experienced the same access problem to the forums last Friday night, and investigated it with our hosting service, GoDaddy.com. It turns out that while we have plenty of bandwidth and data storage capacity, the ASP language MySQL database configuration used by the forum has a limit of 50 simultaneous connections, and this is what we are bumping up against. You should not have this problem with the online lessons. If you do, let me know.

Obviously, this database connection limit (which is buried in the hosting service documentation) will not serve us for the long term, or even the short term considering how fast the AYP readership is growing. The only way to fix it with GoDaddy is to go to a dedicated server setup, which requires setup skills I do not have (yet), and it costs significantly more too. There are other hosting services, but I have not been able to locate one with preconfigured large connection capacity to MySQL database hosting.

Another solution (a stop gap) would be to allow access to forum members only. This would take the forums out of the search engines (ouch) and greatly reduce the readership. That would reduce the AYP forum's database connection load. If access problems become chronic, we may have to close the forums to non-members until we can find a long term solution.

If anyone else has been hitting this limit, let me know. I'm not sure how quickly it can be addressed with a long term fix, given the technical hurdles.

We were starting to have capacity problems on the Geocities site before aypsite.org was launched in June. Here we are four months later, bumping the ceiling again.

Suggestions?

The guru is in you.

Yogani

2005/10/05 12:35:14
AYP Helpers
http://www.aypsite.org/forum/topic.asp?TOPIC_ID=504&REPLY_ID=837&whichpage=-1
Forum connection problems, tech help & money

Hi Andrew:

The solution will probably be to set up in dedicated server mode, which will take some time. That will give us control of all the parameters. We may have to turn off non-member viewing here for a while until we can get upgraded. That would remove the forums from the search engines, reduce traffic, and increase forum sign-ups at the same time.

I'll put a note in the announcements and AYP helpers forums soon to address this. Will also ask for help in the Snitz forums (link at bottom of this page).

The AYP forums are slow here this morning, but not locked out on connections so far. These are tech issues that will be resolved in time. Please note further access or speed problems here so we will have more data points.

The postings in the forums continue to be terrific. Very useful explorations of applied yoga science -- a gold mine for independent practitioners! We will do what is necessary to keep it available for everyone.

The guru is in you.

Yogani
2005/10/06 00:07:11
AYP Helpers
http://www.aypsite.org/forum/topic.asp?TOPIC_ID=504&REPLY_ID=846&whichpage=-1
Forum connection problems, tech help & money

Hi Andrew:

A couple of other hosting options have come up from the Snitz community forum that I am investigating, though it still may go to a dedicated server on GoDaddy. Once it becomes clear where we are going with the forum, I will let everyone know. The cost of a virtual dedicated server on GoDaddy is $30-35/month, depending on the length of commitment -- not cheap.

On donations, there was a donation page on the AYP Geocities site for about six months last year. It netted $13 from one kind person and some negative PR from others who were not so kind. Everyone else ignored it, so I ended the donation page when the first AYP book came out. Since then, one person has stepped forward with a generous unsolicited donation, for which I am very grateful. I will also be grateful if others are inclined to do the same, but I am not comfortable advertising publicly for it anymore.

Any other donations that do come, if ever, I request be for value perceived to have been received already, not for anything expected to happen in the future. That way, there cannot be any misunderstandings about it. What would be ideal would be if the word got around without me having to solicit. I still have a http://www.paypal.com account using the yogani99@yahoo.com email address. Haven't checked it for some time. Gee, maybe there is a fortune in it! Not likely. :-)

Thanks for your concern on money matters. It is a concern here too. So I keep writing...

The guru is in you.

Yogani

PS -- I would not be opposed to seeing this topic moved to AYP helpers at some point. If so inclined, one of you can move it with an appropriate message at the end, posted after the move. As long as it is not me asking for money. Somehow that does not fit into the equation for this work anymore. I feel that balancing of the financial equation has to come freely from the other side, or not at all. It is an energy thing related to receiving and giving. It should come naturally from within, like everything else we do here.

2005/10/10 12:53:05
AYP Helpers
http://www.aypsite.org/forum/topic.asp?TOPIC_ID=504&REPLY_ID=915&whichpage=-1
Forum connection problems, tech help & money

Hi All:

To follow up on this discussion, the AYP forums have been moved to a new server host as of 10/9/05. This hosting service includes technical support for the Snitz forum software we are using here, and is designed for growth. Thank goodness for that!

Make sure you bookmark the new forum address, which is http://www.aypsite.org/forum There is currently automatic forwarding from the old address, but maybe not forever.

For more information on the move and the new ".org" website, see http://www.aypsite.org/forum/topic.asp?TOPIC_ID=512

The guru is in you.

2005/10/10 15:53:51
AYP Helpers
http://www.aypsite.org/forum/topic.asp?TOPIC_ID=511&REPLY_ID=920&whichpage=-1
Giving & Receiving

Hi Andrew:

A very interesting inquiry. What is giving? What is receiving?

This raises related questions: What is expecting? What is taking? What is resisting giving or receiving?

Can we be giving if we are expecting? Can we be receiving if we are taking? What does it mean if we do not want to give or receive?

And how does spiritual progress enter into all these considerations?

I don't think we can answer all this on the level of mind (the intellect) other than to observe and recognize known causes and effects. Beyond that, it is a matter of our heart and our conduct. With yoga practices in the picture, the role of spirit in these processes is increased greatly. I think that is the key. It is in this context that I said, "It (giving) should come naturally from within."

We all know people who give and give. We also know people who take and take. And we know people who find it difficult to give or receive. It seems we are born with certain inclinations. Wherever we start out, the anvil of life seeks to lead us to more. Perhaps that is the clue. There is a force of evolution involved, and we know that our practices are part of that.

Our choices about interacting are part of the process of evolution also. As we open from within, we have more options. Inner silence eventually lays it all out for us. We see things more and more as they really are -- a play of divine energy everywhere, forever flowing and growing on the blissful screen of our inner stillness.

I think the secret of giving and receiving is in that – developing our ability to be a conscious part of the never-ending flow of life toward more. Without giving and receiving, nature is thwarted -- constipated. Our own inner silence is the best stimulator of the natural processes of nature.

When we become an intimate part of the divine process by cultivating inner silence, we find that giving involves no bargaining. It is the opposite of much we have been taught about the "business" of life. Yet, giving depends on receivers, just as you point out. A receiver is part of the process. And like a true giver, a true receiver has no expectations.

In Rig Veda it says, "The physician longs for the sick." Just so, a giver longs for receivers. Not takers. There is a difference. The first is divine process. The second is dysfunction. But you know, a true giver will settle for a taker too. Because it does not matter. Every taker today will be a

722 –   Advanced Yoga Practices

receiver tomorrow, and a giver the day after. That is how it works. Giving is contagious. Everyone should catch this divine bug.

With yoga practices, you will catch the bug. It will happen. That's because inner silence and ecstatic bliss are the source of it. The source of all giving and receiving. Giving is the outpouring of divine love. Receiving is the in-pouring of divine love. Outpouring becomes in-pouring and in-pouring becomes outpouring. Through our practices we gradually open to this. It is the natural flow of things.

"Expecting" is a blockage of divine energy within us. So is "taking." These are from a limited view of life -- a blocked view. Not feeling free to give or receive is another form of blockage. It all dissolves with our spiritual growth. And then the increasing flow of giving and receiving enhances our spiritual growth even more.

But it has to be spontaneous, you know. If I tell you, "Give!" it can make a lot of discomfort, because the energy isn't ready to flow. If I say, "Receive!" it is just the same. It has to come from within each of us. And it will if we have some bhakti (really want to grow) and are doing daily practices.

Giving and receiving are yoga practices, and they cannot be instantly manifested in the advanced stage from out of nowhere. As with all of AYP, we only can do what we are ready to do. If I tell you, "Do kechari!" what help is that if you are not ready? Not much. It can even be harmful. But we can talk about kechari -- the particulars to know for whenever they may come in handy, according to your own development and need.

We can talk about the particulars of giving and receiving like that too. Maybe it will provide a little inspiration.

I especially like the "Pay It Forward" model http://www.aypsite.org/166.html
It encourages us to become givers, inspired by what we have received, and request others to do the same with what they receive from us. It is a self-perpetuating and exponential process. It is just the kind of spiritual dynamic I hope we can create with the open resource knowledge in AYP. "Pay It Forward" is also in line with the "horizontal teaching model" we are creating in the AYP forums and in other ways around the world – "Candles lighting candles until all candles are lit."

As for the part of your question about creating debts between people, I don't believe in that. Can we create or dissolve blockages in the divine flow with our conduct? Absolutely. But who is to say how those will be worked out? Since everything is connected, what we do here will have an effect everywhere else. It is not limited to this or that person. It is very liberating to let go of the "I owe you, you owe me" thing. If we give of ourselves freely, the entire universe will be enlivened. And if we can't, the entire universe will be that little bit more constipated. It should be obvious which is best for us, and for the universe.

It is impossible to express how transforming it has been for me these past few years doing the AYP work. Having all of you to write to has been the greatest blessing. So, while you may think I am the one to be thanked, it is to you I say, thank you.

I hope others will put in their two cents on this topic. It is an important one. C'mon, give a little. :-)

We can't have enlightenment until we learn to give it away.
See http://www.aypsite.org/120.html

The guru is in you.

2005/10/10 13:08:47
AYP Helpers
http://www.aypsite.org/forum/topic.asp?TOPIC_ID=513
Is anyone experiencing forum load time delays?

Hi All:

I have seen some intermittent load time delays on the new hosting service since it started up Sunday, 10/9/05.

Have you experienced any delays when you call up the AYP forums since the new host came online? If you have, please report it here.

A delay would be a load time of more than a couple of seconds on fast internet, and whatever you consider to be abnormal if you are on dial-in. The timer feature for the forum has been turned on (see bottom of page), so you can measure load times.

Thanks for helping out. The tech folks would like to know how widespread such delays might be. It will help them pinpoint and resolve any problems.

And if the load times you are experiencing are terrific, we'd like to hear from you too. :-)

The guru is in you
2005/10/12 12:17:58
AYP Helpers
http://www.aypsite.org/forum/topic.asp?TOPIC_ID=513&REPLY_ID=954&whichpage=-1
Is anyone experiencing forum load time delays?
That's a good load time, Richard. May we all do that well.

I am still getting occasional load times of 10-15 seconds here, and sometimes a complete time out with an ASP script error.

Since no one else has mentioned delays here yet, perhaps I am the only one. That would be good!

Anyone having delays, please do report it.

The guru is in you.

2005/10/13 08:02:24
AYP Helpers
http://www.aypsite.org/forum/topic.asp?TOPIC_ID=513&REPLY_ID=965&whichpage=-1

Is anyone experiencing forum load time delays?

Thanks much.

These inputs will lead to more digging for a solution.

Anyone else?

The guru is in you.

2005/10/13 23:36:37
AYP Helpers
http://www.aypsite.org/forum/topic.asp?TOPIC_ID=513&REPLY_ID=973&whichpage=-1
Is anyone experiencing forum load time delays?

Hi All:

Thanks much for those additional inputs.

Other load time experiences anyone is having are welcome here also.

The problem is being worked on as we speak -- the tech folks are trying to track down the source of it. It is one of those mysterious gremlin things...

The guru is in you.

2005/10/15 10:07:51
AYP Helpers
http://www.aypsite.org/forum/topic.asp?TOPIC_ID=513&REPLY_ID=982&whichpage=-1
Is anyone experiencing forum load time delays?

Hi again all:

Some tech things were done over the past couple of days, and the load times (here anyway) have improved quite a bit.

If anyone is still experiencing forum load time delays, please let us know.

The guru is in you.

2005/11/03 16:58:28
AYP Helpers
http://www.aypsite.org/forum/topic.asp?TOPIC_ID=513&REPLY_ID=1367&whichpage=-1
Is anyone experiencing forum load time delays?

Hi All:

Has anyone been experiencing load time delays for the AYP forums lately?

If so, please advise on how often and how long the delays have been. There is a load time given at the bottom of every page.

If you have had any timeouts with an error message, please advise also.

Thanks.

The guru is in you.

2005/10/29 16:43:15
AYP Helpers
http://www.aypsite.org/forum/topic.asp?TOPIC_ID=558
Quantity "Deep Discount" on AYP Books

Hi All:

Over the months, several have asked about obtaining "quantity discounts" on the purchase of the AYP books for gift-giving and sharing with others. I have hesitated to do that so as not to undercut the booksellers, but I now recognize that if many AYP books are being handed out, that will be a big benefit to everyone, including the booksellers.

So, now I am offering a "deep discount" from the suggested retail prices of the AYP books to those who are interested in buying at least five copies. If you would be interested in exploring this further, please write to me for the specifics -- yogani99@yahoo.com

Note: Due to shipping costs for "drop shipments" from the printer in Nashville, Tennessee, this offering is only economically feasible for the continental USA. Outside the continental USA, it will likely be less expensive to order the books from the Amazon site nearest you, where price discounts and free shipping are often available.

Post Note: Arrangements have been made, and now we can ship direct from the printer in London, UK also.

Thank you very much to Anthem who has been so kind to put up the "AYP needs your help" posting. To all who have responded with donations, I am extremely grateful. It is a relief to have some help with the operational and promotional costs associated with making the AYP knowledge available to as many people as possible around the world.

It is requested that any donations be based on the perception of value already received from AYP. That is what I am most comfortable with in a donation situation.

Wishing you all the best on your path. Practice wisely, and enjoy!

The guru is in you.

2005/10/30 10:34:11
AYP Helpers
http://www.aypsite.org/forum/topic.asp?TOPIC_ID=558&REPLY_ID=1260&whichpage=-1
Quantity "Deep Discount" on AYP Books

Hi Richard:

Thank you for your valuable feedback. Yes, I don't think the pricing situation in the UK is very good either. There are several reasons for it:

1. Historical versus current exchange rates - The American books I checked are priced at 1.4-1.5 $/BP instead of the current rate of 1.78, which is favoring historical rates over current rates. That means higher prices in the UK compared to USA right off the bat. When setting this up last year, I used about 1.4 $/BP, which yields the AYP book UK price of 29BP, or about $52 (29 x 1.78), not the $76 you mentioned. With the printing costs over there, this would produce the same royalty here, or so I thought.

2. Currency conversion costs. I did not know about this when starting out. In my case, it is 10% right off the top to the bank here. This might explain part of why cross border prices are higher in general.

3. Amazon UK refuses to discount the AYP books. This has nothing to do with the suggested retail price, but was unexpected. In the USA Amazon discounts the AYP book 34%. In Canada, 30%. In France, 15%. In Germany, none. In Japan, none. Amazon Germany and Japan also use exchange rates favorable to themselves in setting their retail prices, besides not discounting them.

All of this cross-border finagling helps explain why European cars are more expensive in America, and vise versa.

The only prices set by me are USA and UK. All the rest are translations by others. **I am going to make an adjustment in the UK price for both the AYP book and Secrets of Wilder to try and improve the situation.** But I hope you can see that the price differential is also in the hands of others, built into the system, so to speak. I'll do the best I can on this end.

Also, price changes are not instant. It might take a few months to come through the distribution chain.

Finally, besides in Nashville Tennessee, the AYP books are also printed in London, UK. One might ask, why can't drop shipments for quantity purchases be sent from London? That option does not exist in the web-automated ordering system at the printer, and I am investigating to see if drop shipments can be ordered from London by other means. If it can be done, I will let you know here. That would enable us to do the deep discount for quantity purchases in Europe as well, hopefully with shipping costs that are feasible.

I apologize for any missteps made on this end. All of this international stuff is new to me, and I am learning. Please do correct me if anything has been missed in the figuring here. I'd like for the AYP books to be available everywhere as equitably as possible.

The guru is in you.

2005/10/30 11:46:09
AYP Helpers
http://www.aypsite.org/forum/topic.asp?TOPIC_ID=558&REPLY_ID=1262&whichpage=-1
Quantity "Deep Discount" on AYP Books

Hi Richard:

Agreed. I'll see what can be done. UK prices will come down.

The guru is in you.

2005/10/30 13:46:16
AYP Helpers
http://www.aypsite.org/forum/topic.asp?TOPIC_ID=558&REPLY_ID=1264&whichpage=-1
Quantity "Deep Discount" on AYP Books

Hi Richard:

The Secrets of Wilder novel and the AYP easy lessons book will be in both of the 2006 International New Age Trade Shows (INATS) -- Orlando in February and Denver in June. These are the biggest shows, I am told. The books will be in the booth of New Leaf Distributing, the largest new age book distributor in the USA. These are wholesaler shows, not open to the general public. There will be store and chain buyers there from the USA, Europe and many other places. "Yogani" has no plans to be at either of these shows...

There will also be new "entry-level" AYP books included in these shows: One for February - "Deep Meditation," and two more added for June - "Spinal Breathing Pranayama" and "Tantra." So there will be a total of three AYP books in the Feb show, and five in the June show. The new books are designed for mass market readership, much more so than the current AYP books. They will include concise instructions on specific practices with no mumbo-jumbo, and will be inexpensive.

In addition to the shows, flyers are being sent to all the New Age bookstore outlets in the USA. There have been AYP press releases going out regularly to the entire American media, print advertising has been bought, and other promotions have been done also. All of this has been USA only. The funding available is limited, so I am picking promotions very carefully, and not able to do many of the things I would like. Considering that over 70% of the AYP website readership is the USA, that is where I am focusing.

The AYP books are "self-published." That limits the reach of promotional activities, which are very expensive. While book production and distribution are no longer major issues in self-publishing due to the great new technologies, the "mass marketing," as you call it, continues to be a big challenge.

Attracting a publisher to do all of this for AYP was not possible in the beginning, but maybe there will be more interest moving forward. That would be a big help for the Secrets of Wilder, especially, because it can reach far beyond the "yoga circuit."

For the reasons you have mentioned, during this development period, I think the Secrets of Wilder will continue to be a "sleeper," with its potentially huge public appeal. It was written for that purpose -- to put a human "everyman" face on what we could not even be talking about a couple of years ago -- an integrated self-directed program of practices for cultivating human spiritual transformation, plus sharing in the complete journey with modern practitioners in a western cultural setting.

From the standpoint of practical spiritual knowledge, the Secrets of Wilder is like Jonathan Livingston Seagull with big teeth. :-)

So I do agree with you about the Secrets of Wilder. It may be a few years ahead of its time, but its time is surely coming. Lacking the advantage of a big marketing budget, it will most likely happen mainly by word-of-mouth.

Any help with promotions is much appreciated -- financial or time and effort anyone can spare for helping increase AYP visibility. I will continue to do all I can here.

The guru is in you.

2005/10/31 10:56:46
AYP Helpers
http://www.aypsite.org/forum/topic.asp?TOPIC_ID=558&REPLY_ID=1278&whichpage=-1
Quantity "Deep Discount" on AYP Books

Hi Lili:

The Secrets of Wilder is available for any channel that can help it find the broad audience it was written for. It is available for reissue with a large book publisher, and for being turned into a screenplay. No one has come knocking on either of these yet.

The novel is a sleeper that will "wake up" sometime in the future. It is a metaphor for all of humanity.

If we look at it that way, the prospects are pretty exciting for everyone!

Thanks for chiming in. It is a great suggestion.

The guru is in you.

2005/11/04 14:04:01
AYP Helpers
http://www.aypsite.org/forum/topic.asp?TOPIC_ID=558&REPLY_ID=1379&whichpage=-1
Quantity "Deep Discount" on AYP Books

Hi Yoda:

Yes, the Secrets of Wilder is very hands-on with practices, and on what it is like to live through the process of human spiritual transformation. I wanted the story to have that level of realism, while at the same time have the universal elements of the Campbell mythological structure, so it might both inspire and instruct like no spiritual novel has before. That was the goal -- a tall order. We'll see what the verdict is as awareness of it in the marketplace increases. Pretty good reviews on Amazon so far.

The growth scenario you describe sounds good to me. May your words be prophesy. :-)

It's that first 0.1% that takes the most time, work and money for sure.

It is interesting to note that the most popular "new" spiritual books today, like "The Power of Now" and "The Four Agreements," were written back in the 1990s. They have followed the scenario you describe, with most of the growth in awareness of these writings happening in recent years.

The guru is in you.

2005/11/07 13:01:49
AYP Helpers
http://www.aypsite.org/forum/topic.asp?TOPIC_ID=558&REPLY_ID=1444&whichpage=-1
Quantity "Deep Discount" on AYP Books

Post Note: Arrangements have been made, and now we can ship direct from the printer in London, UK also.

2005/12/01 19:42:52
AYP Helpers
http://www.aypsite.org/forum/topic.asp?TOPIC_ID=558&REPLY_ID=1740&whichpage=-1
Quantity "Deep Discount" on AYP Books

Hi All:

As promised in my postings of October 30th above, the UK prices for the *AYP Easy Lessons* book and the *Secrets of Wilder* have been substantially reduced. You can check by going to the appropriate Amazon UK links here.

Also, the new book **"Deep Meditation - Pathway to Personal Freedom"** will be showing up in all the distribution channels soon! It is available for the quantity deep discount also from both the USA and UK. It is an inexpensive little book that enables anyone to easily learn deep meditation and manage the practice long term, including handling the many experiences that can come up as purification progresses in the nervous system and full potential unfolds.

If you are interested in handing out any of the AYP books to help spread the word, please write me for details.

Btw, all of the AYP books are also available in eBook format worldwide, for much lower cost than the physical books. Those links are on the AYP books page as well.

The guru is in you.

2006/01/29 14:23:30
AYP Helpers
http://www.aypsite.org/forum/topic.asp?TOPIC_ID=558&REPLY_ID=2852&whichpage=-1
Quantity "Deep Discount" on AYP Books

Hi Cosmic:

Somehow missed your note here until now.

All of the AYP books were sent to Oprah's book club (and to other well-known people) shortly after they were published. No responses received so far. So the writing continues...

The theory is that the bigger the spiritual wave gets the less it can be ignored. Thank you to all you spiritual wave makers. :-)

When you get around to it, I hope you enjoy the Secrets of Wilder. It is a blend of many things. Most of all, it is a tale about how one person's journey (using real practices) leads to the rise of worldwide spiritual science. It begins with one very determined teenager on a pregnant windswept Florida beach... Whewee!

It could be any of us taking the bull by the horns in this way. It could be all of us!

Imagine it...

The guru is in you.

2006/06/09 17:44:47
AYP Helpers
http://www.aypsite.org/forum/topic.asp?TOPIC_ID=558&REPLY_ID=7905&whichpage=-1
Quantity "Deep Discount" on AYP Books

Hi All:

With the new Tantra book out, just a reminder that the **quantity deep discount** is still active. That is **55% off suggested retail plus shipping** for as many books as you want.

Due to shipping costs from the printer (USA or UK), it only works economically for 5-10 books or more (combining titles if you want). For fewer than 5-10 books, it is usually less expensive to buy them with discounts from a large retailer like Amazon.

If interested in the quantity discount, let me know. It is easy to do, and is a big help to AYP.

Would anyone like to stand on the street corner handing out Tantra books? :-) Well, maybe handing out Deep Meditation or Spinal Breathing books would be safer. They all lead to the same place. It is only a matter of which door one wants to walk through first ... all doors lead inward...

The guru is in you.

PS -- Retail prices can be found individually using the Amazon links on the books page, or you can find book info and USA suggested retail prices for all the AYP books on the flyer here -- http://www.aypsite.com/11-AYP-Flyer-5-2-06.pdf (big PDF file - it takes a while to load the first time - also accessible via link on the bottom of the books page)

2005/11/07 12:58:02
AYP Helpers
http://www.aypsite.org/forum/topic.asp?TOPIC_ID=578&REPLY_ID=1443&whichpage=-1
Ideas for making AYP money

Thank you for your thoughtful suggestions, Etherfish.

Donations are appreciated, as long as they are on the basis of the perception of value received already. Anthem has been kind enough to cover that here - http://www.aypsite.org/forum/topic.asp?TOPIC_ID=556 including the appropriate Paypal link.

I am not inclined to make a structured program out of donations, having trust in the opening hearts that are out there.

Several website advertising approaches have been reviewed, and for now I am going to use the space for the AYP books. It is hoped that the addition of several new books in the coming months, along with promotions, will be enough to provide sufficient financial support. If the books do not do that, then by sometime next year, outside advertising would be seriously considered. The hope is to keep the websites all AYP.

In addition, I am offering a quantity deep discount on the AYP books for those who would like to hand them out. The more of them that are out there, the better.

See http://www.aypsite.org/forum/topic.asp?TOPIC_ID=558

(Note: This discount is available with shipping from both the USA and UK now)

Suggestions are always welcome on how we can reach more people with the AYP writings. And direct action in whatever way one may be inclined to help is even better.

The guru is in you.

2005/11/08 08:28:13
AYP Helpers
http://www.aypsite.org/forum/topic.asp?TOPIC_ID=578&REPLY_ID=1451&whichpage=-1
Ideas for making AYP money

Hi Etherfish:

The AYP booklist with over 400 titles is set up this way through Amazon Associates. It is a 5-8% commission from Amazon, depending on volume, for books purchased through those links.

Keep in mind that at the current traffic level of AYP, we are talking about very small amounts of money for both book link commissions and the sale of website advertising space.

More importantly, anyone with a website can use Amazon Associates to display the AYP books and receive the 5-8% commission for AYP book sales. I like that best, because it helps get the AYP books out there.

The more AYP books out there, the better.

The guru is in you.

2005/11/18 11:43:31
AYP Helpers
http://www.aypsite.org/forum/topic.asp?TOPIC_ID=591&REPLY_ID=1548&whichpage=-1
Amazon

Hi Yoda:

I wanted to say thank you for your wonderful Amazon reviews of the AYP books, and for encouraging others to do reviews also.

There is a new AYP book coming out in a few weeks called "*Deep Meditation - Pathway to Personal Freedom*," which is aimed much more at a mass audience than the first two books. There will be a series of concise primer books on individual practices like this to provide more doorways for the general public into the broad body of AYP knowledge. I hope to have four more of these instruction books out in 2006. And a few more in 2007.

You know, like you, I was a voracious reader when I first stumbled onto the spiritual path over 30 years ago. It did not take long to see that there was an acute shortage of written instructions on spiritual practices. As time went on, I also realized that the traditions, while each being strong in their area, were not offering a full range of practices covering every aspect of human spiritual transformation. So, besides there being a need for documenting practices, it became obvious that an integration of practices across the board was needed. Well, I first had to do the integration for myself, which took over 20 years of crossing boundaries and doing personal research – being my own guina pig. It worked. (*The Secrets of Wilder* is a record of the sequence of discoveries, though much compressed in time, recast in events, and raised to the level of an epic "hero's journey," in the spirit of Joseph Campbell's work.)

A few years ago, I realized it would be a shame if all the research went into the well with me, and that it was time to write it down. So AYP was born. It has turned out to be a wonderful expansion on my own path — an outpouring of divine love in service to others -- and I have been very happy to see many finding benefits in the writings.

As you know, I do not consider AYP to be the last word on yoga. I strongly encourage others to carry the exploration further in an open source way, so we can see yoga evolve into a real applied science in the mainstream of society. It is much needed. Then we will have done the right thing for present and future generations.

Wishing you all the best as you continue on your path. The next two decades ought to be at least as interesting for you as the first two. :-)

The guru is in you.

2005/11/18 12:44:56
AYP Helpers
http://www.aypsite.org/forum/topic.asp?TOPIC_ID=591&REPLY_ID=1554&whichpage=-1
Amazon

Hi Near:

Yes, I agree about a tantra book ... From the last page of "Deep Meditation," which includes the schedule for 2006:

"...In the order published, his books include:

Advanced Yoga Practices – Easy Lessons for Ecstatic Living
A large user-friendly textbook providing 240 detailed lessons on the AYP integrated system of advanced yoga practices.

The Secrets of Wilder – A Novel
The story of young Americans discovering and utilizing actual secret practices leading to human spiritual transformation.

The AYP Enlightenment Series
Easy-to-read instruction books on yoga practices, including:

--**Deep Meditation – Pathway to Personal Freedom**

--**Spinal Breathing Pranayama – Journey to Inner Space**
(Due out spring 2006)

--**Tantra – Discovering the Power of Pre-Orgasmic Sex**
(Due out spring 2006)

--**Asanas, Mudras and Bandhas – Secrets of Inner Ecstasy**
(Due out second half 2006)

--**Samyama – Manifesting the Power of Inner Silence**
(Due out second half 2006)

Additional AYP Enlightenment Series books are planned..."

It will continue to be busy here!

The guru is in you.

2005/11/20 22:24:23
AYP Helpers
http://www.aypsite.org/forum/topic.asp?TOPIC_ID=591&REPLY_ID=1587&whichpage=-1
Amazon

Hi Roberto:

Sorry to hear that. Let me know if you do not receive an immediate exchange on that from Amazon at no cost to you. If you don't, I will make sure you are sent the right book. It was obviously a printing error. Hopefully not a whole batch. I will alert the printer...

Thanks for reporting it.

The guru is in you.

2005/11/21 11:46:33
AYP Helpers
http://www.aypsite.org/forum/topic.asp?TOPIC_ID=591&REPLY_ID=1593&whichpage=-1
Amazon

Hi Roberto:

I don't imagine there is much similarity between the ancient secrets of Wales and the ancient secrets of yoga, or, for that matter, the Secrets of Wilder. But who knows?

Anyway, they ought to go find their own cover. :-)

The printer has been notified. Do let me know if there is any problem straightening this out on your end. I want it to be right for you, in every respect...

The guru is in you.

2005/11/24 14:19:32
AYP Helpers
http://www.aypsite.org/forum/topic.asp?TOPIC_ID=605&REPLY_ID=1638&whichpage=-1
Long load times

Thanks for posting this, Paul.

Indeed, long load times have been an issue for some from time to time, and it is important for such incidents to be reported so we can track down the gremlin that is responsible.

The guru is in you.

2005/12/09 17:32:34
AYP Helpers
http://www.aypsite.org/forum/topic.asp?TOPIC_ID=605&REPLY_ID=1859&whichpage=-1
Long load times

Thanks Anthem:

It happens here on my end quite often. I was hoping I was the only one.

If it continues, and others are reporting load time and timeout problems, we will probably move the forum to a new host. It should not affect operations at all, except for a short shutdown. This has been discussed with our Snitz expert, Ruirib, and he is willing to continue with us in that mode, which is very good. Tech support like he has been providing so well is essential to run the forum. As far as we can tell, it is the hosting service, and affecting only the AYP forum, not the other forums he is handling.

Karma?

That's okay, we have the inner silence and we will just keep on trucking. That is stillness in action.

The guru is in you.

2006/01/30 16:33:08
AYP Helpers
http://www.aypsite.org/forum/topic.asp?TOPIC_ID=605&REPLY_ID=2890&whichpage=-1
Long load times

Hi All:

The forum was not moved to a new host last month (discussed in last post) because the load time delays we were experiencing became less for a while. Now they seem to be back, with several commenting about it offline.

Is anyone else experiencing load time delays and timeouts with the AYP forums?

The guru is in you.

2006/02/01 17:29:29
AYP Helpers
http://www.aypsite.org/forum/topic.asp?TOPIC_ID=605&REPLY_ID=2956&whichpage=-1
Long load times

Thanks Guy:

Apparently not many are having load delay problems. Thank goodness for that. For the few who have this probem, it can deteriorate steadily and become severe.

I am running old technology here (Win98 -- can't bring myself to upgrade and start over reloading the huge amount of software running pretty well here), and have tried several things to improve performance on a couple of applications. Both are browser-based. The AYP forum is one of them. Yahoo mail is the other.

One thing that seems to help, is purging the browser cache -- temporary files. This can be done in the browser tools menu (delete temp files), or using a cleanup utility like Windows disk cleanup or Norton clean sweep. I use the latter.

This improves both the forum load times and Yahoo mail performace. These seem to bog down over time in unison. Then I purge the temp files and they run okay again. Anyone know why?

The guru is in you.

2006/02/01 23:04:45
AYP Helpers
http://www.aypsite.org/forum/topic.asp?TOPIC_ID=605&REPLY_ID=2965&whichpage=-1
Long load times

Hi Weaver:

Thanks for the tech info.

I am still on 256 MB RAM, which has not been a problem until the past six months or so, since we started with the Snitz forum SW. Perhaps the temp file backlog has gotten much bigger with the forum SW, and more memory is needed to go through it all with each click. Within a week or so, 500 MB or more in temp files can build up here (thousands of small files), and by then the AYP forums and Yahoo mail will be choking. I think we are finally getting a handle on managing it (purge the temp file regularly), though this does not explain clocked long load times (bottom of this page) or timeouts on the database server, unless the big temp file backlog is causing corrupted scripts to be sent to the database which it can't read properly. It could be a particular type of temp file being produced by the database or forum SW that is causing the problem. Comments on that, anyone?

The guru is in you.

2006/02/02 15:04:13
AYP Helpers
http://www.aypsite.org/forum/topic.asp?TOPIC_ID=605&REPLY_ID=2991&whichpage=-1
Long load times

Hi Weaver:

I have 700 MHz, 256 MB RAM and IE 6.0. This is not the host server, user only, but as administrator, which may or may not have extra tech baggage attached. For some reason, the temp file limit was set at 1 GB. I just reduced it to 100 MB. Hopefully that will not limit performance.

Here is an interesting wrinkle. As soon as I go into the forum, the temp files go up several MB and up 5-10 MB after a few rounds of surfing the forum.

In additon, if I go to the MS Disk Cleanup utility and view the internet temp files, there are 33 Snitz folders plus a 16 MB "index.dat" file there. The folders all have a few thousand Snitz files in them (each!), about 100 MB per folder. A lot of stuff. What is even stranger is that after I do the cleanup, the value on the cleanup utility goes to zero, but all the files just mentioned are still there. What is all this? I have no idea. Finally, the temp file is called C:\WINDOWS\Local Settings\Temporary Internet Files\Content.**IE5**, and I am on **IE6**. There is no IE6 temp file, so this folder maybe is a holdover from a previous version of IE? It is the one the cleanup utility pulls up, and there are no others at this location in Windows.

I am tempted to delete all of this Snitz stuff manually, as the utility shows nothing there and can't seem to touch it, but better see what the Snitz expert has to say first.
Rui! :-)

I have not checked or done anything with the temp files for Firefox, but have experienced similar delays there the few times I tried it. Maybe it uses the same temp files as IE?

Am I putting anyone to sleep yet? Back to yoga...

The guru is in you.

2006/02/02 19:48:52
AYP Helpers
http://www.aypsite.org/forum/topic.asp?TOPIC_ID=605&REPLY_ID=3004&whichpage=-1
Long load times

Hi Rui:

I deleted the 3 GB of Snitz files manually, but the 16 MB "index.dat" file could not be deleted or moved -- "access denied." Is that a Snitz file? The first time I went back into the forum, 18 new Snitz folders showed up in the temp file. None of this is visible in the cleanup utilities, so you may have it too, invisible stuff piling up in there. On top of that there is the rapid pile-up of visible temp files here which can (and must) be deleted with utilities regularly or the whole thing jams up.

Is there a history of Win98 having difficulties with Snitz? What is happening here does not seem normal based on everything you and others are telling me.

Weaver, the 100 MB temp file limit did not work. It jammed up quickly. So I set it to 5 GB to account for the 3 GB of invisible files (now deleted but coming back) plus the ongoing pile-up of visible files. Fortunately I have a big hard drive. It is running better!

Thanks.

The guru is in you.

2006/02/02 23:51:54
AYP Helpers
http://www.aypsite.org/forum/topic.asp?TOPIC_ID=605&REPLY_ID=3014&whichpage=-1
Long load times

Thanks much, Weaver.

I will continue to tinker with it as necessary to keep the forum reasonably accessible here. Can't afford to make it much more of a project than that at this stage. Too much other AYP stuff to get done. Hence, no upgrades likely either for a while.

I am very happy that nearly everyone has pretty good access. That is what counts. Hmmm ... that is a metaphor for what I hope AYP will become -- a resource that many can share in and use effectively without needing so much support from the guy who happened to write the information down.

The guru is in you.

2005/12/04 10:13:39
AYP Helpers
http://www.aypsite.org/forum/topic.asp?TOPIC_ID=620
Donations to AYP

Hello All:

Donations for helping make the AYP writings available to everyone around the world are accepted, and may be made to AYP on Paypal.com.

Paypal membership is not required. Just enter an amount and go to the bottom of the page to use the credit/debit card option.

It is preferred that any donations be for value that you feel has already been received, rather than for expectations about the future. In this way, the benefits that you have received can be translated into opportunities for others to receive similar benefits.

Also see the AYP Book Quantity Discount Program for obtaining copies of the AYP books for handing out or reselling. If you would like to participate directly in promoting, translating, publishing, or selling the AYP books, please write to Yogani at yogani99@yahoo.com. All assistance is greatly appreciated.

If you would like to start or participate in a local AYP meditation group or retreat, see related topics in the AYP Helpers forum category, or start a topic there for your own area.

The guru is in you.

Note: AYP is not a non-profit, tax exempt entity, and donations are not deductible for tax purposes.

2009/03/05 18:57:52
AYP Helpers
http://www.aypsite.org/forum/topic.asp?TOPIC_ID=620&REPLY_ID=46535&whichpage=-1
Donations to AYP

quote:
_____
Originally posted by SeekingShiva

Yogani-

Before donating I have a quick question:

The email address is yogani99@yahoo.com but I read somewhere that this is not your address. I just wanted to confirm before hitting the donation button.

Thanks

_____

Hi SeekingShiva:

Yes, that is the correct email address.

Thanks much for your support!

The guru is in you.

2009/03/05 20:52:43
AYP Helpers
http://www.aypsite.org/forum/topic.asp?TOPIC_ID=620&REPLY_ID=46544&whichpage=-1
Donations to AYP

quote:
_____
Originally posted by anthony574

Is that PayPal link still valid? How do you donate?
_____

Hi Anthony:

Yes, the "AYP on Paypal" link in the first post of this topic is still good. Or the aforementioned yogani99 email address can be used on Paypal as well.

Thanks!

The guru is in you.

2010/01/03 08:28:15
AYP Helpers
http://www.aypsite.org/forum/topic.asp?TOPIC_ID=620&REPLY_ID=62054&whichpage=-1
Donations to AYP

Hi Anil:

Your interest is supporting AYP is much appreciated. But please don't create a burden for yourself with it.

There are many ways to help, and each will do what they can according to the heart.

From my side, the preference is for any donations to be for the perception of benefits received already, not for anything in the future. No expectations. :-)

Wishing you all the best on your path. Practice wisely, and enjoy! I have that wish for everyone, released in the stillness we all share...

The guru is in you.

2005/12/19 10:14:19
AYP Helpers

http://www.aypsite.org/forum/topic.asp?TOPIC_ID=657
Deep Meditation for Barnes and Noble Bookstores

Hi All:

Nearly 1000 free copies of **Deep Meditation** have been sent out to over 100 people by now, with good reports coming back, so the book is beginning to circulate.

The following is from my email today, raising the question about Barnes and Noble in the USA (largest bookstore chain). Approaching individual stores (Barnes and Noble or any other) with a copy or two would be good. There is also a central purchasing office where I am applying, but that is difficult without demonstrated demand in the field, so any promoting you can do with local stores will be very helpful.

Also, please don't forget those Amazon reviews. Very important, and much appreciated.

Q:
I read your book on **Deep Meditation** this afternoon it is a wonderful book and I'm looking forward to the following books you promised in spring 2006.

I decided to send a book to my friend in Holland and another to my friend in Seattle. With your permission, I would like to introduce all 3 of your books to my local Barnes and Noble bookstore to carry locally.

Keep up the Great Work.

A:
I'm very glad you liked it. :-)

Yes, Barnes and Noble sounds great. See what they say. They can order direct from the printer using the ISBN numbers. **Deep Meditation** is already listed on their web site along with the other AYP books here, but I don't think that means much to the physical stores. Wouldn't hurt to mention it though. The ordering info for bookstores is also on the AYP books page.

All the best!

The guru is in you.

2005/12/23 14:16:18
AYP Helpers
http://www.aypsite.org/forum/topic.asp?TOPIC_ID=657&REPLY_ID=2117&whichpage=-1
Deep Meditation for Barnes and Noble Bookstores

Hi All:

It can be done at Barnes and Noble with a walk-in. See this from my email today. And do the same if you like... :-)

The guru is in you.

"Dear Yogani: I went to my local Barnes and Noble book store yesterday and handed the manager a sheet I printed from the Amazon website on the review of your books. After he read the reviews he said, "Why am I not carrying these books?" I said, "I don't know," and handed him all three books (AYP, Wilder and Deep Med). He walked to the computer and ordered 5 of each. So Twin Falls, Idaho Barnes and Noble is now carrying your books!"

PS -- This story also highlights the importance of those Amazon reviews -- doing them, and also using copies of them as this person did for the bookstore walk-in. It worked!
2006/01/13 15:19:08
AYP Helpers
http://www.aypsite.org/forum/topic.asp?TOPIC_ID=729
AYP Books - Marketing Plans for 2006

Hi All:

For the many of you who in your own way have been (or would like to be) helping spread the word on AYP, I thought to give a summary of the evolving 2006 marketing plans for the AYP books. Perhaps this information will be useful to you in your travels. Maybe you will encounter people who will have interest in some of what follows below.

As always, all suggestions and help for increasing AYP exposure are much appreciated.

I am most grateful to everyone who has put "an oar in the water" for helping spread the word on AYP, whether is has been financial or in speaking to others about the AYP lessons and books. Thank you!

As some of you know and have told me, breaking into the "book trade" is tough to do. With what has been done so far (a lot I thought), the AYP books have achieved miniscule sales -- about 700 total books sold in 2005. So the marketing program is being beefed up substantially in 2006. Here is a summary:

1. Press Releases -- Four have been issued to 3,000 US newspapers, radio stations, and college newspapers since last summer. See here for links. The most recent one was on the new **Deep Meditation** book -- 1/03/06. We are covered for one more press release to be issued in the spring when the **Spinal Breathing Pranayama** and **Tantra** books come out. All of these press releases have been paid for with a kind donation that was received last spring.

2. Press reviews -- Review copies of the **Deep Meditation** book have been sent to the book review editors of 75 large US newspapers, yoga/spiritual magazines and independent book review publications. This was also done with the other two AYP books last year. Believe it or not, the AYP books are yet to receive one press review, though there have been a few nibbles. It is very tough to break into the established literary review system that tends feed on itself and shun anything new and original, unless of course it is something achieving popularity on its own -- then everyone wants to jump on the bandwagon. We're not there yet, but heading in the right direction...

3. Book Handouts -- Over 1,000 copies of **Deep Meditation** are in the process of being shipped to and handed out by over 100 people. Most of these are in the USA, with copies also distributed in Canada, South America, the UK and Europe, India, Australia, the Middle East and Africa. This activity has been covered in part by donations and is being wound down now due to lack of additional funding to support it in lieu of other things going on (see below). I hope the books find their way into the hands of lots of people who will be inclined to spread the word. Many thanks to all who are handing them out!
Note: The deep discount program is still available for obtaining AYP books for handing out -- write me for details.

4. Approaching bookstores, libraries and educational institutions -- This has been happening on a limited basis via a few volunteers (see this bookstore "walk-in" success story). It is a huge mountain to climb -- the single greatest challenge the AYP books are facing -- penetrating the above mentioned channels. If anyone is inclined to participate in introducing the AYP books to any of the mentioned channels (like your local Barnes and Noble), please contact me. Sample AYP books, fliers and other handout materials are available to aid in "walk-ins." Obviously, this is not for everyone. If you are inclined to do walk-ins to help place the AYP books in your local bookstores, do write me. It is really important.

5. Submittal to book chains -- Recently, the three AYP books have been submitted with applications to the small press buyers at the Barnes and Noble and the Borders book chains in the USA. No word yet. This is in addition to approaching local stores. It's a dual strategy -- top down and bottom up.

6. Trade shows -- The AYP books are signed up for exhibition in four trade shows in 2006 so far: Two International New Age Trade Shows ("INATS" - Orlando/Feb and Denver/June - New Leaf Distributors booth), the Public Library Association Trade Show (Boston/Mar), and Book Expo America (Wash DC/May - largest book trade show in the USA). The last two were just added to increase national exposure and the AYP books will be in the Publishers Marketing Association (PMA) booth at both shows. All of these events are for the book trade only (publishers, wholesalers and retailers) - not open to the public. If you know anyone in the book trade, you can let them know the AYP books will be exhibited at these shows.

7. Getting a real distributor -- Currently the AYP books are distributed through "passive" channels that include no active marketing to the book trade. As a result, very little is happening, except what you are reading here, which is a drop in the bucket compared to what must be done to achieve visibility and acceptance in the book trade -- every little bit helps, bringing us one step closer. Achieving book trade presence will be a big step toward achieving public acceptance of open source spiritual practices. A strategy is being pursued to achieve placement with a major distributor who will actively market the AYP books through a large professional sales network in the USA and abroad. If we can get in with a large distributor with a marketing organization, it will be a huge step forward.

8. Continuing to build the AYP websites and forum community -- As you know, AYP started on the web, and I see the AYP web presence continuing to be in the central role. So the focus on expanding the usefulness of the free online lessons and forums will continue. All of you who are participating in this community are playing an important role in lifting world consciousness. I am convinced that self-directed spiritual practice utilizing open source systems like AYP is the wave of the future. It is how everyone will be able find equal access to the divine within.

9. Financial contributions are still welcome -- As you can imagine, all of this costs money. Whatever comes in here is going right back out the door (and then some) to support all of these activities. So if you would like to help out financially, you may do so at AYP on Paypal.com. All I ask is that any financial giving be in line with what you feel you have gained from AYP already. All contributions are used to help make the AYP knowledge available to everyone around the world.

Wishing you the best on your chosen path. Practice wisely, and enjoy!

The guru is in you.

2006/01/22 23:29:21
AYP Helpers
http://www.aypsite.org/forum/topic.asp?TOPIC_ID=729&REPLY_ID=2735&whichpage=-1
AYP Books - Marketing Plans for 2006

Hi Cosmic:

Thanks for the feedback. iUniverse (partially owned by Barnes and Noble) is one of several print-on-demand publishers that were considered when the first AYP book was in preparation in 2004. Most of the print-on-demand publishers use http://www.lightningsource.com for their printing and central distribution point. In the end it was decided to go direct with LightningSource as a new independent publisher (AYP Publishing) for a number of reasons, including complete control of the books themselves and the automatic listing with the major US and European distributors, plus Amazon and Barnes and Noble, with no middlemen or biased parties involved.

Beyond the listings (which enable orders to come in from almost any market segment, be filled print-on-demand and shipped within 48 hours), getting all of those channels to actually stock the books in their warehouses and on their shelves is another matter having more to do with generating public demand than pushing the books through the distribution channels from the inside. Of course, we'd like to be doing both, without giving up our autonomy.

We have made good progress with Amazon, who now stocks the AYP books and ships them within 24 hours in the USA. That took many months to build. We are now going through a similar process with the rest of the wholesale and retail distribution channels -- slowly building public market demand as they slowly build confidence to stock the AYP books in their warehouses and on the shelves for immediate availability. Barnes and Noble central purchasing is reviewing the AYP books for stocking as we write, and the store walk-ins that are being done by AYP volunteers are definitely helping. The Amazon reviews are helping a lot too in many venues where the books are being presented, so please keep them coming.

It all takes time. We have some time. The AYP books are not going out of style any time soon. I suspect they will ripen with age. And the more time that goes by, the more AYP books there will be, typing fingers willing. So we will just keep pecking away at it, continuing to make the lessons and books as visible to the public as possible with whatever resources we have available to do that with, and at the same time continue to build the free online resources and community here on the web...

I am very grateful to all of you who are inclined to pass the word and help out in any way you can. Thank you!

The guru is in you.

2006/05/23 23:34:22
AYP Helpers
http://www.aypsite.org/forum/topic.asp?TOPIC_ID=729&REPLY_ID=7284&whichpage=-1
AYP Books - Marketing Plans for 2006

Hi Sadhak:

The Wilder movie topic you mentioned is here, along with my reply to your posting there. As mentioned there, the AYP paperback books are not available in India, but the ebook versions are. See http://www.aypsite.org/books.html

I did not see your note on publishers anywhere. The names of the publishers and distributor you know would be appreciated either here or via email. I am aware of MLBD and B. Jain, and plan to submit to them later in the year after the next AYP Enlightenment Series books comes out. "Tantra" is coming out in a few weeks. Then "Asanas, Mudras & Bandhas" in the autumn, "Samyama" later in the year, and "Shatkarmas & Amaroli" by early 2007. That will leave about three more to finish off the series by the end of 2007 -- Planned: "Self-Inquiry," "Bhakti and Karma Yoga" and "Eight Limbs of Yoga (with heavy focus on self-pacing and related matters)." Whew! :-)

At some point I'd like to submit all the books to as many qualified publishers in India as possible. Then the books will have a good chance to become available at reasonable cost locally over there -- very important. Until then, the ebooks are the main way to read the AYP books in India. Hopefully we can fix that in the not-to-distant future.

Thanks for any suggestions you may have!

The guru is in you.

2006/05/25 22:47:04
AYP Helpers
http://www.aypsite.org/forum/topic.asp?TOPIC_ID=729&REPLY_ID=7334&whichpage=-1
AYP Books - Marketing Plans for 2006

Hi Sadhak:

Oh, that is wonderful about the publishers. Full Circle is a one I was not aware of. I look forward to the others you are researching. The more good ones we can approach the better. If we contact 10, maybe one will have a serious interest in publishing and distributing the AYP books in India.

Thanks much!

The guru is in you.

2006/05/26 10:11:20
AYP Helpers
http://www.aypsite.org/forum/topic.asp?TOPIC_ID=729&REPLY_ID=7348&whichpage=-1
AYP Books - Marketing Plans for 2006

Hi Hunter:

Great suggestion. Is there anyone conveniently located in California who would like to make contact with East West on behalf of AYP?

The same goes for similar publications in other states across the USA, and in countries around the world.

Many thanks!

The guru is in you.

PS -- The AYP books are carried by New Leaf, Ingram and Baker Taylor in the USA and by major UK based European distributors too. For more on distribution, see the first paragraph here: http://www.aypsite.org/books.html

2006/05/28 13:44:29
AYP Helpers
http://www.aypsite.org/forum/topic.asp?TOPIC_ID=729&REPLY_ID=7443&whichpage=-1
AYP Books - Marketing Plans for 2006

Hi Sadhak:

Thanks very much for those. You can be sure they will be fully explored. And feel free to add further perspectives and publishers as they come to you.

It is about time we got AYP going in India. For heaven's sake, all this came from there, and we are only trying to send it back in a refined and highly useable form. You know, like the Japanese did with cars in America. :-)

I wonder if Bharatiya Vidya Prakashan (K C Jain) is part of B. Jain Books. Do you know? If so, we have them covered. In fact, just today, we got a tiny nibble from B. Jain. Time will tell on that...

New Age Books is part of MLBD (the biggest in spiritual books in India), which we also have covered -- with no interest so far.

All the rest are new territory and of great value in the over all effort to get AYP going in India. Terrific inputs!

The guru is in you.

2006/05/29 10:39:33
AYP Helpers
http://www.aypsite.org/forum/topic.asp?TOPIC_ID=729&REPLY_ID=7476&whichpage=-1
AYP Books - Marketing Plans for 2006

Hi Sadhak:

Thank you. As I understand, some (or many?) publishers in India are connected with spiritual organizations and only publish material related to that organization's teachings. This is fine, of course, but not the kind of publisher we are looking for -- we'd like to be with one that is non-sectarian ... and having a website store (essential) and with good physical distribution throughout India.

Also, and this might be tricky and not immediately achievable, we'd like to find a publisher that is willing to take on the entire (and growing) list of AYP books -- it's especially important for the Enlightenment Series books, which are interconnected -- a series. I realize a multi-book arrangement may not be easy to achieve on the front end, so we will have to see what they say, and remain flexible.

Time is on our side because the readership will likely continue to grow along with the list of AYP books, so the publishing opportunity will hopefuly become more attractive as time goes on. Maybe at some point it will become a "no-brainer" for the the Indian publishing houses, though I think it is a no-brainer already. A slight bias here, of course... :-)

The guru is in you.

2006/05/30 08:51:31
AYP Helpers
http://www.aypsite.org/forum/topic.asp?TOPIC_ID=729&REPLY_ID=7510&whichpage=-1
AYP Books - Marketing Plans for 2006

Hi Sadhak:

It should be mentioned that the route taken in the USA and UK has been to "self-publish" through a large "print-on-demand" company -- http://www.lightningsource.com. It was by necessity, due to the similar challenge of finding a traditional western publishing company that would be interested in the AYP writings.

It has turned out to be a very good way to go, because this approach enables us to cut through all the red tape and put the books out in rapid succession, including timely delivery into the distribution channels with no investment in inventory required. Plus, the concern about getting and keeping all the AYP books in print is taken care of with this approach. They are all there in secure digital files at the printer, available indefinitely for print-on-demand as needed, and shipped within 48 hours. It is working very well as the books move slowly but surely out into more and more distribution channels.

Last year, I looked for self-publishing print-on-demand companies in India, but could not find any that were viable. If you run across any, do let me know. The next best thing (maybe) would be a reputable self-publishing firm with distribution capability. In that case, we would probably have to pay for pre-printed inventory and warehousing, which would be a problem with a big list of books. For distribution, a web store covering India could do it for us starting out. What we need right now is a place to send readers to buy the books in India at local prices, and a web store would suffice until broader distribution could be achieved.

There are all sorts of ways to publish the AYP books in India. It is just a question of finding a reliable way that will not run us into costs we cannot afford. That is why the focus remains on the traditional publishers who can do it all, but with the associated big loss in speed and efficiency. You can be sure if we could find a company like Lightning Source operating in India, we'd have all the AYP books up and running there in no time. So it is worth keeping an eye open for that.

And, yes, the AYP books are head and shoulders above the online lessons -- the next generation of AYP writing.

Thanks for looking into all this...

Btw, I updated the books page over the weekend, so now it has the full list of AYP Enlightenment Series books on it (nine in all), scheduled out through 2007, plus the **website cards** (thank you Trip!) and the current **AYP books flyer** printable from links at the bottom of the page.

The guru is in you.

2006/06/07 13:18:58
AYP Helpers
http://www.aypsite.org/forum/topic.asp?TOPIC_ID=729&REPLY_ID=7814&whichpage=-1
AYP Books - Marketing Plans for 2006

Thank you, Sadhak.

There is a letter here used in the last "India campaign" well over a year ago, which can be updated for Macmillan/India and others. There is also an "AYP publisher's page" made up with all that you mentioned and more: http://www.geocities.com/advancedyogapractices/publish
That was for the first book nearly 18 months ago, before the Secrets of Wilder and the Enlightenment Series books, and also before the current ad-free websites, so it needs updating and migration to an ad-free domain. But there it is...

The track we are on now is to get the next book is out in September ("Asanas, Mudras & Bandhas - Awakening Ecstatic Kundalini") and then submit to as many publishers in India as we can. That is how the above list of publishers will most likely be used. Right now I am in the thros of writing and a few other things, and am not ready to drop everything to embark on a new India publisher campaign. But we will this year!

In the meantime, if any serious interest can be generated among publishers in India, that will be very much welcome. Feel free to pass on any and all information you have on AYP. The books flyer has been recently updated and tells the story for existing books, and details Enlightenment Series books coming out over the next 18 months (see link at bottom of the books page). Add to those books a big AYP Easy Lessons Volume 2 and the Secrets of Wilder screenplay, and that is the entire schedule at this point. The last two items are beginning to take shape here as well, so it will be busy here for some time to come.

The strategy is to remain focused first and foremost on the writing, with the assumption that many who are interested in the field of yoga will notice, and tell others until eventually everyone knows, even the publishers in India! We're all doing what we can... :-)

As for rights, yes, I think it would be beneficial for the Indian publisher to cover all of South Asia, and perhaps beyond.

The guru is in you.

2006/06/08 10:54:02
AYP Helpers
http://www.aypsite.org/forum/topic.asp?TOPIC_ID=729&REPLY_ID=7834&whichpage=-1
AYP Books - Marketing Plans for 2006

Hi Sadhak:

Yes. Do it. It is time when you think it is -- it is time when each person thinks it is. I think it is time, but can only do so much ... so others must decide and do also.

As they say in China: "Many hands make light work."
Do they really say that, Alvin? :-)

But you get the idea. The more AYP buzz that can be created, the sooner the Indian publishers will say, "Hmmm, there is something going on here." It is the same everywhere, and everyone has my okay to buzz away. I wish everyone would...

There are only two hands here, and a big world to transform. So, having to choose, I choose the writing. The rest can follow from that, sooner or later. The sooner the better!

Put another way, better to have good writing and half-baked promotion than half-baked writing and good promotion, though I know that flies in the face of the way things are often done. If AYP promotion is going to be better than half-baked, others will have to make it so. It is as simple as that. It is about the people ... about what each person chooses for their own life, and for the life of the world...

Many thanks!

The guru is in you.

2006/06/09 12:21:51
AYP Helpers
http://www.aypsite.org/forum/topic.asp?TOPIC_ID=729&REPLY_ID=7888&whichpage=-1
AYP Books - Marketing Plans for 2006

Hi Alvin:

The ideal cover for the AYP Easy Lessons book would have been a mirror ... but the printer could not do it, so I dedicated the book to "you who seek the truth within" instead. It was the best these two hands could do at the time... :-)

Perhaps in the future there will be more time and money to upgrade the cover. Of course, by then it may be "branded" (widely recognized - let's hope so), so we may be stuck with it.

The real task at hand is taking AYP as it is and reaching more people. The best way to do that is to get it in the public media in the form of book reviews and possible author interviews (did I say that?). With growing public demand, distribution will follow.

Hi Sadhak: That's the spirit!

The guru is in you both, and in everyone!

PS -- see the printable **website cards** and updated **four page flyer** providing essential details on all the AYP books (current and scheduled) at the bottom of the books page -- http://www.aypsite.org/books.html

2006/02/11 15:13:36
AYP Helpers
http://www.aypsite.org/forum/topic.asp?TOPIC_ID=817&REPLY_ID=3261&whichpage=-1
AYP Website Cards to Hand Out (print them here)

Hi Trip:

That is a great idea. Something simple -- an AYP site card with a couple of lines of information and the website address. A webpage template that anyone can print on standard business card paper is a good way to pass it on. Even printed on regular paper it could work if one does not mind doing some cutting.

Let me mull over what could be on it and I will be in touch. Or contact me if you have something already.

The guru is in you.

2006/02/13 12:29:03
AYP Helpers
http://www.aypsite.org/forum/topic.asp?TOPIC_ID=817&REPLY_ID=3315&whichpage=-1
AYP Website Cards to Hand Out (print them here)

Hi All:

Trip did a great job designing an AYP card that can be used to hand to people you would like to pass the website address to.

They are laid out 10 on a page in Adobe PDF format, here:

http://www.aypsite.org/aypcards.pdf

They can be printed in either black and white or color (logo is in color).

They are set up for standard scored 10 card business card stock for easy separating, and the corners are marked for cutting too. I have not tried the scored card stock yet, but have printed some on plain white paper and they look good. Have a few in the wallet already.

Feel free to print these out in mass so everyone on the planet can have one. :-)

Thanks much, Trip!

The guru is in you.

2006/03/04 16:05:51
AYP Helpers
http://www.aypsite.org/forum/topic.asp?TOPIC_ID=817&REPLY_ID=4104&whichpage=-1
AYP Website Cards to Hand Out (print them here)

Hi All:

Here is the single high resolution card image Trip made for professional level printing:

http://www.aypsite.org/aypcard300dpi.jpg

Here are his comments that go with it:

"I've attached the single business card in JPG format to this email. The reason it looks bigger than usual on your screen is because it is 300DPI as opposed to standard screen 72DPI. I've printed many cards/flyers in the past through professional printers, and this is the way they request the files be sent. I substituted the high-res AYP logo into the card so when printed it should turn out beautiful."

Thanks much Trip!

The guru is in you.

2006/02/15 18:54:40
AYP Helpers
http://www.aypsite.org/forum/topic.asp?TOPIC_ID=827&REPLY_ID=3385&whichpage=-1
taking responsibility for AYP

Hi Guy and Weaver:

You got me thinking...

I wonder if we have a franchising expert in our midst. The thought occurred that if we could muster the expertise, a chain of AYP Schools could happen someday. Of course, it would depend on the presence of skilled practitioners interested in moving into teaching. I see people with those skills rising quickly among us already. As our numbers grow, the skills will be there.

It would be the perfect venue for the AYP writings to be applied in the teaching environment on the local level.

We would obviously need professional educators, as well, to develop and administer the curriculum.

It could all be set up centrally and reproduced thousands of times in franchised AYP Schools all over the world. It could be set up as a real business, so those involved could make a living and provide for their families -- a small detail that all yogis and yoginis must attend to.

The interview question to the franchising expert might be, "What would you rather be doing with your life, selling hamburgers or worldwide enlightenment?"

And to the educator: "Would you rather be churning out diplomas or seers?"

:-)

The guru is in you.

PS -- If it evolved to become a successful corporation, that would also go a long way toward addressing the challenge of preserving the teachings long term, beyond all of our lifetimes.

2006/02/16 09:48:03
AYP Helpers
http://www.aypsite.org/forum/topic.asp?TOPIC_ID=827&REPLY_ID=3404&whichpage=-1
taking responsibility for AYP

Hi Etherfish:

I both agree and disagree -- for present and future. It would certainly be difficult to successfully launch such a chain of schools now. But with more reputation (franchise recognition), more awakening in society, an organized curriculum that works and a solid business plan, it can fly. I think it must. Where else can humanity go with all this knowledge? We will never be the same.

Just to emphasize the importance of pressing ever-forward, here is a quote from JFK:
"If not us, then who? If not now, then when?"

We all have much more power to make a better world than we realize. It can only be revealed in our doing.

The guru is in you.

2006/02/18 00:07:32
AYP Helpers
http://www.aypsite.org/forum/topic.asp?TOPIC_ID=827&REPLY_ID=3514&whichpage=-1
taking responsibility for AYP

Hi All:

I've been reading along here, and wow what a lot of great insights and suggestions.

We all know that there will be a market for self-directed integrated practices for a long time to come. What we don't know is how fast it will grow or how big it will get. I think assuming it will continue to be a growth market (and possibly big) is a safe bet. We also know that no one is servicing it very well right now -- speaking of everything else besides asanas, as Jim points out.

Maybe this market has not even been defined until we came along with self-directed integrated practices, and it, like AYP, is still forming. It has been in 1000 tiny pieces until now. Are we the market here in AYP, and determining its growth? If so, we may be sitting on something far bigger than we can imagine, particularly if society is in the process of making a major shift in this direction. How to play it?

I think it is a matter of timing our actions so as not to get too far ahead of ourselves, while at the same time having a blueprint for addressing demand as it emerges. Setting up $50,000 AYP franchises willy-nilly now, or any time soon, would be sure to fail. But five years from now, who knows? Maybe even renting space for gatherings right now is premature. Living rooms are the best place for the grassroots to take root, I think, and then see where it goes from there. It is a lot easier to expand to meet growing demand than to retreat from insufficient demand. Much easier on the pocket book too.

Getting the yoga teachers involved is a great idea. I guess there are several ways to do that. Maybe they can be our guinea pigs, since they already have studios and students. They can find out in a hurry how many of those folks on the mats are looking for more. Would we lose control by going that route? I don't think so. AYP owns the books.

For me it is all about the books right now -- both writing them to address the mainstream, and selling them. It is also about completing the material for advanced practitioners. Books -- maybe 10 more over the next few of years. After that, we'll see what is happening.

Groups can use the books. Yoga teachers can use the books. Word of mouth can use them. Everyone that is involved in the expansion of AYP will need the books. And that is good for both the practitioners and funding the growth of AYP from here. At this early stage, donations are still accepted too. It is all still on a shoestring here.

Obviously, for expanding the knowledge horizontally, it isn't only about distributing the AYP books. It is about teachers gaining the necessary experience to teach the AYP knowledge. I'm not sure how to do that. Certifications? Not sure. That part I know little about, so someone with experience in that would be needed. I'm willing. I just don't know anything about running training and certification programs.

As the market begins to take shape, and I expect it will in the coming years (we seem to be creating it as we go), then it will become clearer how far we can go with this. If it looks like a huge growth market coming up, then we should have a plan for expanding to meet the demand as far as it can go. This isn't really about me. It is about creating something that will have international reach and be able to carry the knowledge of self-directed integrated practices forward and far into the future. It is also about creating something that meets the demand in an attractive economic way, and provides a living and long term economic security for those who are doing the work. We should not repeat the mistakes made by others in the past.

A normal business model has not been a good match-up for spiritual teachers in the past (good economic supply to the market with reasonable compensation for providers), but do we know that it cannot be achieved in the future? We do not know. Just because others have failed in the past, this does not mean it cannot be done. This is spiritual, but it is also business. And we may be sitting on top of one of the biggest business opportunities of the 21st century. If we do not address it, you can be sure others eventually will. Right now, who is in a better position to do it than us?

I know nothing about non-profit organizations, but do know something about business, having spent 30 years in it and having the degrees as well. I'm certified in business, but not in yoga! :-)

I'm sure much can be done with a non-profit structure. But I have no experience with that. If we go that route, experts will be needed. I do know that a lot can be done with a for-profit business structure also -- the possibility for shared ownership among the participants and long term continuity being a couple of the most important things from my point of view.

Whichever way it goes, there will be the need for business plans, curriculums, finance, facilities, marketing, administration, all that stuff. I am not the world's greatest manager of people, so we would need to find expert managers too.

But not all for today…

I am only projecting some general ideas, just in case we are sitting on the equivalent of what the PC revolution was in 1980. At that time, a man with a vision came along and said, "There will be a PC on every desk." And 25 years later we all know that he was right.

Well, there is a man here with a vision too -- "There will be self-directed integrated practices in every home." It is a shared vision among many of us. Will we be right 25 years from now? Time will tell.

I hope the brain-storming will continue, and that it will translate into action.

It is an honor to be here among so many wise souls...

The guru is in you.

2006/02/18 10:20:22
AYP Helpers
http://www.aypsite.org/forum/topic.asp?TOPIC_ID=827&REPLY_ID=3523&whichpage=-1
taking responsibility for AYP

Hi again All:

There is also the simpler leveraged "software only" approach which is the early growth model of Gates/Mircosoft. They got the contract to provide the operating system for IBM's new PC in the early 1980s, and the rest is history. Before that, they were just another struggling little software company.

So the question is, who is the IBM of the yoga business, the one who has the ability to quickly take it to the next level? It is Iyengar, isn't it?

How difficult would it be to obtain "the contract" for taking Iyengar yoga decisively beyond asanas? It seems the places where he has gotten stuck (deep meditation, spinal breathing, kundalini, etc.) are the same places where we have broken through. Is there a way for AYP to get together with Iyengar? They have the reputation, teachers, facilities, etc. We have the software. A good marriage?

Barring a big break like that, we will no doubt keep plugging along as per my note above, developing this market by ourselves if we have too. But it sure would be nice if we could find a big springboard to take everyone to the next level overnight.

See what you started with your Gates quote, Guy? Not bad... :-)

The guru is in you.

2006/02/19 14:11:52
AYP Helpers
http://www.aypsite.org/forum/topic.asp?TOPIC_ID=827&REPLY_ID=3588&whichpage=-1
taking responsibility for AYP

Hello Star, and welcome!

That is a very kind suggestion on tithing. For those who do not know, donations are accepted at AYP on Paypal.com.

My suggestion is that donations be primarily for what you feel AYP has given to you, rather than for what you think AYP needs. That way there will always be a measure of fairness in it. All funds are used to make the knowledge available to as many people as possible around the world. So, like any other kind of helping that is done, donations are part of the horizontal transmission of AYP.

All forms of assistance are much appreciated.

And, yes, it would be very nice to be doing this work without having the bills pile up. Someday it will be like that, I hope. :-)

The guru is in you.

2006/02/19 15:02:06
AYP Helpers
http://www.aypsite.org/forum/topic.asp?TOPIC_ID=827&REPLY_ID=3590&whichpage=-1
taking responsibility for AYP

Hi Victor:

Thanks for your insights on the Iyengar situation.

Certainly almost anyone of good reputation endorsing the AYP work would be a huge plus. I thought of Iyengar because of the large influence and reach he and his organization have, and the apparent matchup between what they teach and what AYP offers.

While it is true they can move to make the necessary additions themselves, they have not so far. It is something of a mystery. In fact, this same mystery is found in all the major traditions. They seem to have difficulty innovating beyond the original yoga tool set that has been developed or inherited. Of course, the tendency to avoid integrative innovation within the ranks also makes it difficult to accept innovation from the outside.

Nevertheless, if Iyengar yoga teachers (or any others) have the flexibility to bring in what you call "internal" methods (deep meditation, spinal breathing, etc.), then that would be good for everyone.

So we are talking about two things here:

1. Obtaining public endorsements of AYP by reputable people in the field of yoga.

2. Direct utilization of AYP by yoga teachers at all levels who have the independence to do so. There are currently no requirements or restrictions from this end on how this might be done.

To address Guy's earlier comment, what we are not talking about here is getting into bed with a big brother and selling out the AYP mission to someone else. It is about finding synergies in the marketplace and leveraging them to everyone's advantage. It is the students who will benefit the most, and that is what it is about, after all.

So, Victor, Jim, and everyone who has contacts with yoga teachers, famous or not, I'd appreciate anything you can do to make the connections that can help take AYP, and all of yoga, to the next level.

We are having a taste of the possibilities of self-directed integrated practices with the AYP approach. There is no reason why everyone can't have the experience, without upsetting the existing apple carts. It is simply a matter of communications and moving toward integration of the most effective methods. That is the thrust of all good science, including good yoga science.

The guru is in you.

2006/02/19 22:39:27
AYP Helpers
http://www.aypsite.org/forum/topic.asp?TOPIC_ID=827&REPLY_ID=3610&whichpage=-1
taking responsibility for AYP

Hi Shanti & Etherfish:

Well, it is not intended as a requirement. Only a way of avoiding future expectations on the AYP work, which I am a bit sensitive about.

In any case, I am very happy that you feel you are benefiting. There are lots of ways to help out, and I know you are in your own way. It is all balanced in the long run. We are all giving to someone -- paying it forward. It is the nature of what we are cultivating within ourselves.

The guru is in you.

2006/02/20 10:18:49
AYP Helpers
http://www.aypsite.org/forum/topic.asp?TOPIC_ID=827&REPLY_ID=3618&whichpage=-1
taking responsibility for AYP

Hi All:

To follow up on the yoga teachers discussion, where do yoga teachers and suppliers of yoga supplies and books gather to share? Are there yoga trade shows and conventions? I have not found any so far. Do Iyengar, International Yoga Federation or other large yoga organizations sponsor any? Do Yoga Journal or other large yoga publications sponsor any?

I think we have not found AYP's main audience yet. We have been relying on the audience finding AYP, which has been happening here on the websites. But it is only the tip of the iceberg.

The AYP books were exhibited heavily at a recent new age trade show. It has hardly made a ripple in book sales. I realize now that, for the most part, new agers are not AYP's main audience. We will dutifully exhibit in another new age trade show in June, a large librarian's trade show in March, and the world's largest book trade show (Book Expo America) in May. But I think all of these will miss our primary audience, which is serious practitioners -- yoga teachers and avid yogis and yoginis. Where do these rare birds gather in groups? Birds of a feather, you know. That is where we should be exhibiting the AYP books.

Any ideas?

The guru is in you.

2006/02/20 12:29:06
AYP Helpers
http://www.aypsite.org/forum/topic.asp?TOPIC_ID=827&REPLY_ID=3624&whichpage=-1
taking responsibility for AYP

Hi Jim:

I agree with you. If the thing is truly an innovation, a sea change, it will almost certainly be discovered eventually. But it must be seen by someone somewhere for this process to begin and progress. There is little doubt that if it is seen by many someones in many places the dissemination will happen faster.

It is a question of preference for velocity. Can we walk to Los Angeles from New York? Sure. Very few will want to go that way. Some may prefer to drive. Most will fly. All options are available, and we know what our choices are. The key is in knowing the choices -- having them visible, and being free to choose.

Exhibiting the AYP books (having them visible to the right audiences) is a pretty benign process. So is word of mouth. Yes, it surely is a hybrid. Everyone has their own approach to passing information, and that is honored and appreciated here.

I remind you that this community would not be here now if AYP had not been very heavily promoted in the early Yahoo days, and again when the several websites were launched. Would a slower path have been okay? Sure, but maybe you would not have run across it by now either. Well, I am very glad you did... :-)

The guru is in you.

2006/02/21 10:52:29
AYP Helpers
http://www.aypsite.org/forum/topic.asp?TOPIC_ID=827&REPLY_ID=3655&whichpage=-1
taking responsibility for AYP

Hi All:

I'm afraid I have to take issue. The reason good products and services are not well known is almost always because they have not been effectively promoted/marketed. And the reverse is true also. Chopra's and Tolle's fine works are well known not because they are better than other works, but because they have been effectively marketed.

"Marketing" is a sort of dirty word among purists. I think that is naive. It is easy to take the purist position when we think we already have the thing. But do we?

Consider this. Our spiritual progress depends as much on the other person finding their path as on the perception that we have found ours. It is a fact. So there is an urgency involved.

This is what drives all genuine spiritual teachers. It is a maturing of bhakti -- spiritual desire extending beyond our personal self to everyone else. We will know we have it when we become just as concerned about the spiritual progress of others as we are about our own, writing no one off as unworthy or unready -- no one. It is not for us to decide. It is for them to decide, and they cannot do that without adequate information.

Personal and global spiritual progress cannot be separated. When they are, the path is incomplete.

The guru is in you.

2006/02/21 13:11:11
AYP Helpers
http://www.aypsite.org/forum/topic.asp?TOPIC_ID=827&REPLY_ID=3661&whichpage=-1
taking responsibility for AYP

Hi All:

I promise not to insist that we shave our heads and hand out copies of Deep Meditation in airports. For those who are too young to know about that, consider yourselves lucky. :-)

But seriously, I understand you, Jim, but I do not think you have been accurately interpreted. It is not necessarily "better" to go slow -- or even fast. What is "better" is for each person to follow their heart on this, and not subscribe to any particular point of view or dogma about it.

Do what makes your heart sing. That is the real bhakti in us. The rest is all a bunch of ideas, not to be imposed on anyone.

At the same time, there are certain facts of business that we should all be aware of. Contrary to popular belief, good things do not fall from the sky like manna from heaven. If you have heard about something good, you can be sure that someone (more likely many someones) has put in a lot of work to provide the visibility of that good thing for your benefit.

But listen, inside we all know what is the right thing to do. I'll take that over a dogmatic approach any day. But at the same time let us be realistic about causes and effects. We do that with our practices too, yes?

And if anyone feels like handing out AYP books at the airport, be my guest. :-)

The guru is in you.

2006/02/21 16:29:18
AYP Helpers
http://www.aypsite.org/forum/topic.asp?TOPIC_ID=827&REPLY_ID=3668&whichpage=-1
taking responsibility for AYP

quote:
─────────
Melissa wrote: What does everyone think of say a five day AYP retreat?
─────────

Hi Melissa:

Sounds nice. Wish I could. Maybe when all the books are done. Or maybe by then that long walk in the woods alone that Jim mentioned will be the best thing. If you all want to gather, go ahead. Don't let me hold you back.

The story you told me about your mother running off with your copy of Deep Meditation is a perfect example of it being impossible to know who will be interested. That is why everyone is a reasonable suspect. There is just no telling, especially with the small AYP E-Series books, which are designed for digestion by everyone.

On the other hand, we have to do some targeting or we will scatter our resources too thin. I think anyone involved in (or considering) yoga is fair game, especially teachers. I'll ask the question again -- Where do teachers gather in numbers? And, relating to Guy's question, what trade magazines do they read?

Yes, there are rigid types in yoga. But also plenty of people who have seen the value of daily practice who know there must be more than what they have experienced so far.

Welcome to the AYP smorgasbord, complete with instructions on how to eat it all without exploding! :-)

742 –   Advanced Yoga Practices

The guru is in you.

2006/02/21 19:07:35
AYP Helpers
http://www.aypsite.org/forum/topic.asp?TOPIC_ID=827&REPLY_ID=3672&whichpage=-1
taking responsibility for AYP

Hi All:

Okay, so it is unanimous (almost). We all should drop in on our local yoga teachers and hand them the AYP website card as a minimum. Better yet, leave a healthy stack of them. Handing over an AYP book or two besides is best of all.

Picking up on Etherfish's suggestion to "mainstream-ize" the AYP message (you didn't think I was reading, did you, Etherfish?), how about these snippets for the first five AYP E-Series books? Keep in mind these concepts are for public consumption leading to exploration of the practices and finding the reality of what they bring, which may not be exactly what new practitioners are looking for to begin with -- much more, in fact!

The list is only embryonic (maybe idiotic), so please add on, with special emphasis on **who** could be approached in each category. Keep in mind that those AYP website cards are cheap and can be sprinkled just about everywhere. Many of the "who's" here deserve a stack, at least.

#1 Deep Meditation -- less stress, more creativity, better productivity, more intelligence, inner peace and bliss
Who? Doctors, psychologists, educators, therapists, capitalists, workaholics, artistic types, college students

#2 Spinal Breathing -- relaxation, better health, more energy, ecstasy
Who? Healthcare professionals, patients, athletes, people who want to learn how to breathe

#3 Tantra -- better sex, spiritual sex, sexual power
Who? Tantra teachers and groups, sex therapists, romantics, and everyone gathering in all those places where people go to find each other

#4 Asanas, Mudras & Bandhas -- relaxation, flexibility, energy, ecstasy
Who? Those looking for a simple way into postures, a compact physical exercise routine, plus powerful supplements (Ms&Bs) to meditation and pranayama. People who have interest but don't necessarily want to become asana experts -- little do they know what they are getting into here!

#5 Samyama -- desire fulfillment, personal power, road to riches
Who? Power types, magicians, wiccans, capitalists, astral travelers, miracle mongers

A little tongue in cheek there, but if you saw my emails over the last couple of years, you would know all of these have been represented, and some of the least likely have stuck with AYP...

So, who else? And how many of these are on your normal travel route? You don't have to admit to anything -- just hand out the cards! :-)

The guru is in you.

2006/02/21 23:01:21
AYP Helpers
http://www.aypsite.org/forum/topic.asp?TOPIC_ID=827&REPLY_ID=3685&whichpage=-1
taking responsibility for AYP

Hi Etherfish:

Lots of great ideas, and lots and lots and lots of work. Who is going got do all that work?

We can represent the product in different ways, within limits, but redesigning and redoing it (the books) over and over for every application will not work, not this year anyway, or next, and probably the year after. There is not enough of me here for that.

It would be like redesigning and rebuilding this whole forum to make it more appealing to some people -- months of work -- I can tell you from experience. Rewriting books takes much longer. Not feasible in real time. We have to get real about this. See? :-)

But there is a lot we can do with what we do have, and what we will have soon (more small AYP books as listed above). If we cannot redesign the product, we can certainly redesign the presentation in different ways to accommodate each kind of audience in our talking, sharing, and even alter marketing materials like cards, fliers, posters, etc., which also takes work, but not nearly as much as republishing books willy-nilly at the drop of a hat.

The AYP books themselves will not be changed any time soon. There are only so many babies I can give birth to per year and the maternity ward is full already. (And a new web site? Not by me!)

So, I suggest we focus on the presentation, rather than the product.

By the way, that reminds me of the classic "Four P's of Marketing." Here they are:

Product -- Set for this year, with plans crystallizing for next year and the year after (no rewriting of current books planned).

Price -- These are fairly set also. A few small changes are in the works.

Point of Sale -- Internet retail availablity is good, and improving. Placement in physical retail stores is poor -- anyone done any walk-ins lately? With more reader demand, store placement will get easier. In fact, with strong reader demand, store placement will take care of itself. The present wholesale distribution channels we have in place are good and can handle industrial strength demand.

Promotion -- Well, that is what we talking about here. Promotion is not redesigning the product. It is selling the product we have, and includes PR, advertising, networking and direct sales. Maybe a little packaging too, but don't put too much strain on the factory.

So, the bottom line is, what can we do now with what we have? Operative word -- now. And what can we add in a timely fashion to do more? AYP E-Series books #2 and #3 are coming in a few months, and #4 and #5 in the second half of the year. What can we do with these in the near term once they are out? And so on... The same audiences will be there. It is only a matter of approaching them in the best way with what we have.

The concept you have of addressing different interest groups is good. AYP has all kinds of potential with these, and can be presented in many different ways. However, the implementation needs to be in line with real products available now and in the near term. Then we can be connecting with the market segments that are there as best we can, instead of making dream schemes that cannot be implemented in real time.

Most important is these things we are talking about being done without my labor much involved. There just is not any more of me available beyond what you see here. In other words, it is not about what more I can do. It is about what everyone else can do. That makes sense, doesn't it?

The guru is in you.

2006/02/22 09:49:48
AYP Helpers
http://www.aypsite.org/forum/topic.asp?TOPIC_ID=827&REPLY_ID=3706&whichpage=-1
taking responsibility for AYP

quote:
_____
Originally posted by Etherfish

A lot of marketing has to do with packaging and presentation (image).
_____

Hi Etherfish:

Yes, that has been taken into account as much as possible already for the AYP Enlightenment Series books. They are being written for the mainstream and for longevity. We will not be turning the AYP writings into cheesy stuff, though. We won't go that far. We are willing to meet everyone half-way.

Present it however you like, but please do present it. Thanks much! :-)

The guru is in you.

2006/02/26 11:20:23
AYP Helpers
http://www.aypsite.org/forum/topic.asp?TOPIC_ID=827&REPLY_ID=3876&whichpage=-1
taking responsibility for AYP

Hi Etherfish:

It sounds good. I prefer we use the http://www.aypsite.com link for public display instead of .org. That is the current approach in all AYP PR and advertising. The two sites are mirrors.

www.advancedyogapractices.com is also used for public display. It is routable and is currently routed to the .com AYP books page. It is a bit long, so I generally only use it in the AYP books where a rerouting may be necessary in the future.

www.secretsofwilder.com is another link that can be used, as appropriate. It is also routed to the .com AYP books page.

The guru is in you.

2006/03/20 12:53:36
AYP Helpers
http://www.aypsite.org/forum/topic.asp?TOPIC_ID=945
AYP Around the World

Hi All:

Over the past three months, AYP has had visitors from about 100 countries around the world. The data below is for http://www.aypsite.com (Dec 20, 2005 - Mar 19, 2006) showing the country, number of visitors and percentage of the total. Of course, http://www.aypsite.org is also very active due to this forum, but a country breakdown is not available for .org. The Geocities site and Yahoo groups also continue to receive healthy traffic. So the stats below are a partial snapshot of the whole picture.

.Org has had 16,000 visitors of its own so far this year -- not included below. The total traffic on all AYP sites is running at 10-15,000 hits per day now, more than 10 times what it was a year ago.

The dominance of the USA in the stats is surprising. What does this mean?

Still waiting for more of this to show up in AYP book sales, so we can expand even more proactively. Still waiting, and writing... :-)

The guru is in you.

UNITED STATES 16,842 visitors 78.2%
INDIA 680 3.16

744 – Advanced Yoga Practices

CANADA 618 2.87
UNITED KINGDOM 523 2.43
GERMANY 323 1.5
AUSTRALIA 215 1
CHINA 208 0.97
BULGARIA 189 0.88
FRANCE 181 0.84
UNKNOWN 123 0.57
NETHERLANDS 122 0.57
JAPAN 92 0.43
SAUDI ARABIA 82 0.38
ISRAEL 82 0.38
SWEDEN 80 0.37
SWITZERLAND 68 0.32
BELGIUM 65 0.3
SPAIN 60 0.28
MALAYSIA 57 0.26
MEXICO 57 0.26
NORWAY 55 0.26
FINLAND 51 0.24
PORTUGAL 45 0.21
BRAZIL 39 0.18
UNITED ARAB EMIRATES 38 0.18
PHILIPPINES 33 0.15
ITALY 31 0.14
SINGAPORE 29 0.13
IRELAND 28 0.13
HONG KONG 28 0.13
MALAWI 27 0.13
AUSTRIA 26 0.12
SOUTH AFRICA 25 0.12
RUSSIAN FEDERATION 25 0.12
THAILAND 24 0.11
CZECH REPUBLIC 22 0.1
POLAND 21 0.1
PAKISTAN 20 0.09
SLOVENIA 19 0.09
TURKEY 18 0.08
COLOMBIA 18 0.08
INDONESIA 16 0.07
EGYPT 16 0.07
ROMANIA 16 0.07
GREECE 13 0.06
NEW ZEALAND 13 0.06
MALTA 10 0.05
DENMARK 10 0.05
HUNGARY 9 0.04
SERBIA AND MONTENEGRO 9 0.04
ARGENTINA 9 0.04
CHILE 7 0.03
KUWAIT 7 0.03
CROATIA 7 0.03
ESTONIA 7 0.03
VENEZUELA 6 0.03
ICELAND 5 0.02
BAHRAIN 5 0.02
ECUADOR 5 0.02
VIET NAM 5 0.02
PUERTO RICO 4 0.02
MAURITIUS 4 0.02
ALGERIA 4 0.02
PERU 3 0.01
LITHUANIA 3 0.01
SRI LANKA 3 0.01
BOSNIA AND HERZEGOVINA 3 0.01
TAIWAN 3 0.01
URUGUAY 3 0.01
TRINIDAD AND TOBAGO 3 0.01
BARBADOS 3 0.01
SYRIAN ARAB REPUBLIC 2 0.01
PANAMA 2 0.01
COSTA RICA 2 0.01
LEBANON 2 0.01
NIGERIA 2 0.01
MOROCCO 2 0.01
GUYANA 2 0.01
ANGOLA 2 0.01
LATVIA 2 0.01
GAMBIA 1 0
LUXEMBOURG 1 0
MACAO 1 0
UZBEKISTAN 1 0

SENEGAL 1 0
PARAGUAY 1 0
TUNISIA 1 0
MYANMAR 1 0
BANGLADESH 1 0
SLOVAKIA 1 0
CYPRUS 1 0
BOTSWANA 1 0
RWANDA 1 0
SERBIA AND MONTENEGRO 1 0
QATAR 1 0
CAYMAN ISLANDS 1 0
NEPAL 1 0
DOMINICAN REPUBLIC 1 0

2006/03/20 13:57:01
AYP Helpers
http://www.aypsite.org/forum/topic.asp?TOPIC_ID=945&REPLY_ID=4756&whichpage=-1
AYP Around the World

Hi Melissa:

"Hits" include all page requests, including multiple requests from individual visitors.

There are several translations of the AYP lessons being done on the web by volunteers. Some are further along than others. They are listed here: http://www.aypsite.org/forum/topic.asp?TOPIC_ID=440 ...and also listed in the AYP links section.

Someday the international translations will become a more organized project, with books being published. That too is a function of how the English language AYP books do. It all takes time...

The guru is in you.

2006/03/20 14:39:46
AYP Helpers
http://www.aypsite.org/forum/topic.asp?TOPIC_ID=945&REPLY_ID=4763&whichpage=-1
AYP Around the World

Hi Weaver:

Yes, the web is strong here. The skewing toward USA is probably language related too   English.

What I am really wondering is if the USA is leading the charge in yoga worldwide. It seems so. It is a huge responsibility, given our youth in the field as compared to India -- there is no comparison! Well, maybe that is an advantage. We have fewer laurels to rest on, and so have to dig out the truth of human spiritual transformation and rely on actual results instead of long history, legends and lore. It is like so many things in America. It is the practical results and forward progress that count the most. It works in yoga like it does in most things...

But let's face it, we would not be here doing all this were it not for the greatness of India. I bow to Mother India. May we take what she has so generously shared and make the very best of it.

The guru is in you.

2006/03/20 17:26:55
AYP Helpers
http://www.aypsite.org/forum/topic.asp?TOPIC_ID=945&REPLY_ID=4782&whichpage=-1
AYP Around the World

Hi David:

Thank you for the overall internet stats.

Since the USA AYP traffic in relation to India and Canada is on the order of 25 times more, where the ratios in the figures you gave for overall internet usage are much smaller, this may point to something unique relating to yoga going on in the USA. The AYP ratios for the USA versus the UK and Australia are even further apart.

Could we say that the wide differences in the ratios between AYP and general internet usage are due to involvement in yoga? If so, then it indeed does point to the USA being the source of a worldwide renaissance in yoga -- especially self-directed practices, which is what AYP is about.

On Melissa's comments on Jesus and yoga, the "Aquarian Gospel of Jesus the Christ" by Levi (said to be transcribed from the "akashic records") is another good one, covering the years Jesus spent in India and elsewhere between the time when he left Palestine as a youth and finally returned near the age of thirty. This long period is known as the lost (or missing) years of Jesus. It can be found on the AYP book list here: http://www.aypsite.org/booklist5.html There are other accounts of Jesus in India, including some local lore within India itself. Where I read about it slips my mind right now. Maybe someone knows. Or look it up in the Aquarian Gospel, which has an amazing amount of detail in it. Levi was either reading the akashic records or had a terrific imagination. :-)

Anyhow, none of this changes the fact that something profoundly good is happening when we do our daily practices. Results! Now it is up to us to get the word out.

The guru is in you.

2006/03/21 09:52:45
AYP Helpers
http://www.aypsite.org/forum/topic.asp?TOPIC_ID=945&REPLY_ID=4819&whichpage=-1
AYP Around the World

Hi Richard:

Where would we be in the USA without the high British standards of democracy, industry and culture? These are the mainstays of American society. The difference between the two nations has been environment and age.

One thing I have noticed in dealing with the UK on practical matters is a bit of slowness to act if it is something new. The same with India. Both countries seem somewhat set in their ways due to long history in the ways of doing things. The urgency for change is not there as much as in the USA. Someday the USA will get old and more set in its ways too. But for now we still seem to have enough energy and flexibility to pave new roads.

None of this means that the British are not interested in enlightenment, or anyone else anywhere in the world. People everywhere are interested in enlightenment. It is wired into all of us. AYP has seen visitors from 100 countries in the past three months! It is always a matter of personal choice, yes? But the national personality can make a difference also. There can be some inertia in a society (including in the USA) ... but I think it can be overcome. When the benefits of an efficiently applied technology become obvious, nearly everyone will take advantage.

In any case, if the British had not been in India 150 years ago, we would not have seen yoga in the west as soon as we did, and maybe barely at all by now. For some history on how yoga found its way westward, and the pivotal role of the British, see lesson 253 --
http://www.aypsite.org/253.html

As for the Maharishi, he has had his own agenda, and unfortunately the spiritual aspirations of people everywhere have gradually slipped into a distant second place from his point of view. It is no reflection on the UK or any other nation that has seen the teaching of Transcendental Meditation whither away. It has happened in the USA too, and I think we have been similarly blasted. When someone blames others for their own problems, it is pretty much over, isn't it?

The unstoppable force of spiritual evolution goes on at an ever-increasing rate. Interestingly, and very much to his credit, the Maharis Hi played an important role in fostering the shift of human consciousness during the 20th century. But now we are in the 21st century and the rules of the game are changing fast. We are moving into powerful integrated systems of self-directed practice. The age of wide open yoga science is dawning!

We owe much to the people and nations, warts and all, who have played a role in getting us to this point. Hopefully we, warts and all, can do as good a job as they did in passing something useful on to our successors.

The guru is in you.

2006/03/22 10:51:50
AYP Helpers
http://www.aypsite.org/forum/topic.asp?TOPIC_ID=945&REPLY_ID=4878&whichpage=-1
AYP Around the World

Hi Melissa:

100th monkey? I had to look that one up. Fascinating -- "Sudden shift." "Leap of consciousness." "Sea change." "Phase transition." "Critical mass." The rising of the coquinas in the Secrets of Wilder!

Could we be the 100th monkey? Or maybe the 99th? The 100th couldn't be far off. :-)

http://skepdic.com/monkey.html

"The hundredth monkey phenomenon refers to a sudden spontaneous and mysterious leap of consciousness achieved when an allegedly 'critical mass' point is reached. The idea of the hundredth monkey phenomenon comes from Dr. Lyall Watson in his book Lifetide (1979)."

Very interesting ... let's keep going!

The guru is in you.

2006/03/26 15:53:10
AYP Helpers
http://www.aypsite.org/forum/topic.asp?TOPIC_ID=980&REPLY_ID=5172&whichpage=-1
Yoga class

Hi Guy:

Wow! That is terrific. If we could repeat that scenario a few thousand times around the world, I think we'd break through.

I agree, the "yoga industry" is where we need to be. It is a vast field of opportunity for folks to find benefits from AYP.

I still have not found a wholesale distributor that focuses solely on the yoga industry. If anyone knows of one, please do let me know.

Thanks much!

The guru is in you.

2006/04/04 07:48:57
AYP Helpers

http://www.aypsite.org/forum/topic.asp?TOPIC_ID=1010&REPLY_ID=5593&whichpage=-1
Helping AYP

Hi Guy and All:

Thanks for this topic. I am very appreciative of anything anyone is inclined to do to help spread the word on AYP.

On the practical financial side, the donations and quantity discount purchases of books to hand out have been especially helpful for both getting the books out there and providing necessary support for expenses here.

Along those lines, I have some leftover books from the last trade show that I would like to clear out of here. I wish I could give them away, but can't afford it at this stage. We could do about 65% off suggested retail, including mainland USA shipping, for combined lots of 20 or more. Here is what is available:

Deep Meditation -- 100 (at $4 each)
AYP Easy Lessons -- 10 (at $14 each)
Secrets of Wilder -- 5 (at $7 each)

Please write if you'd like to help clean out the office here. :-)

Many thanks...

The guru is in you.

2006/04/06 12:56:08
AYP Helpers
http://www.aypsite.org/forum/topic.asp?TOPIC_ID=1020
"Spinal Breathing" Available for Quantity Discount

Hi All:

It will be a week or two before the new Spinal Breathing book is available in the retail distribution channels. Maybe sooner for the eBook. When it happens, it will be announced here in the forum and on the home page and books page on the website.

In the meantime, the Spinal Breathing book is available now for direct ordering though me via the quantity discount program, which is 55% off, plus shipping, for ten or more books. These are shipped direct from the printer within 48 hours. The retail price on this book is $11.95, so the quantity discount price is $5.38. To order, write me.

While not many have seen the new book so far, those who have say it is up to the AYP standard, and goes beyond in some ways. It is a practical distillation on spinal breathing that has not been available in print before. I think it is a good one to hand to yoga teachers everywhere. And the Deep Meditation book also, of course.

Speaking of the Deep Meditation book, and the other AYP books, there are still some left in the office here at the 65% discount offer posted the other day. See my post of April 4th here. Please do take advantage. When the office copies are gone, it will revert to the 55% quantity discount offer for all of the books.

With the growing number of strong practitioners here, I hope many of you will take to buying and handing out the books. That is good for everyone, and helps tremendously to ensure the growth and longevity of AYP.

Many thanks for helping out.

The guru is in you.

2006/04/06 16:42:55
AYP Helpers
http://www.aypsite.org/forum/topic.asp?TOPIC_ID=1020&REPLY_ID=5712&whichpage=-1
"Spinal Breathing" Available for Quantity Discount
PS: For those who are in Europe, the 55% quantity discount mentioned above is available for shipping direct from the printer in London also.
2006/04/08 22:55:42
AYP Helpers
http://www.aypsite.org/forum/topic.asp?TOPIC_ID=1020&REPLY_ID=5780&whichpage=-1
"Spinal Breathing" Available for Quantity Discount

Hi All:

The Spinal Breathing Pranayama eBook showed up on Diesel today -- http://www.diesel-ebooks.com/cgi-bin/item/0976465574
Contrary to what it says there, read aloud and printing are enabled (for all the AYP ebooks).

It won't be long before the new book is in all the channels.

The guru is in you.

2006/04/10 23:52:09
AYP Helpers
http://www.aypsite.org/forum/topic.asp?TOPIC_ID=1020&REPLY_ID=5841&whichpage=-1
"Spinal Breathing" Available for Quantity Discount

quote:

Will you be putting up a picture link from the main AYP sites as well?

————————

Hi Anthem:

Oh yes, as soon as the paperback is on Amazon, the Spinal Breathing cover link will be added to the others going down the right side of every web page. An announcement will go on the homepages and the books pages will be updated.

The guru is in you.

————————

2006/04/11 11:06:52
AYP Helpers
http://www.aypsite.org/forum/topic.asp?TOPIC_ID=1020&REPLY_ID=5853&whichpage=-1
"Spinal Breathing" Available for Quantity Discount

Hi Near and Anthem:

Thank you! Hope you enjoy it. All feedback and discussion welcome, as are Amazon reviews.

The guru is in you.

————————

2006/04/13 00:24:16
AYP Helpers
http://www.aypsite.org/forum/topic.asp?TOPIC_ID=1020&REPLY_ID=5915&whichpage=-1
"Spinal Breathing" Available for Quantity Discount

Hi All:

Both the paperback and ebook for "Spinal Breathing Pranayama" showed up on Amazon USA today, and the paperback on Amazon UK. If it is not on Amazon Canada, France, Germany and Japan already, it will be soon.

For now, check the bottom of the list on Amazon USA here, and also on Amazon UK here.

I'll get the Amazon cover image, book description and AYP website updates (including links on the AYP books pages) done in the next few days. In the meantime, the book is available for ordering now.

The guru is in you.

————————

2006/04/13 15:26:23
AYP Helpers
http://www.aypsite.org/forum/topic.asp?TOPIC_ID=1020&REPLY_ID=5930&whichpage=-1
"Spinal Breathing" Available for Quantity Discount

Hi All:

Okay, "Spinal Breathing Pranayama" is up on all the Amazon sites now (cover image and description coming soon), and the AYP home page and AYP books page have been updated, including live links to Amazon USA, UK, Canada, France, Germany and Japan. The cover image (linked to Amazon USA) has also been added to the right border of all the website pages.

The guru is in you.

————————

2006/04/14 12:30:34
AYP Helpers
http://www.aypsite.org/forum/topic.asp?TOPIC_ID=1020&REPLY_ID=5957&whichpage=-1
"Spinal Breathing" Available for Quantity Discount

Hi Anthem:

Still a negative cash flow here, and a factor of times 10 needed on the current level of book sales to begin to break even.

It is not as bad as it sounds. Books are moving at least twice as fast now as a year ago, and a few more "doublings" like that will have us there -- 2 x 2 x 2 x 2 = 16. It is not impossible to achieve this in a year or two when the numbers are small.

To put it into the actual numbers, AYP sold 765 books in 2005, has sold about 500 to date this year, and will likely do well over 1,500 in 2006 at the present rate. If the rate increases as we move along here, then 2006 could be much more... The break-even is around 15,000/year, and solid self-financed growth (like a snowball rolling downhill) will be when we get into the 20-30,000 range. Those numbers sound big, but there are a lot of things happening now that can help make it happen.

Many are helping in their own way, and I am very grateful to all for that. Thank you.

One of the biggest contributors right now is the quantity discount program (the 55% off retail offer) which is helping both the book sales and spreading the books to more and more people. Thank you to all who are helping in this way. The quantity discount program is win-win all the way around. Those interested in participating in this, please write me directly.

A few are actively marketing in their sphere of travel and/or in certain market segments, and that too is a big help. Of particular importance is finding more in-roads into the "yoga industry," which is AYP's single greatest opportunity. Very little has been done there so far. We do not yet have a distributor focused entirely on the yoga industry, and do not have an organized program to approach yoga teachers, studios and suppliers. There is a lot to do in the yoga industry, so any help we can get with that will be great. Even just dropping off a few AYP books with local yoga teachers and studios would be a huge help.

Another big contributor to growth will be adding more "Enlightenment Series" books to the mix, so there will be more entry points into AYP for those coming with different kinds of backgrounds and interests. So, I keep writing!

Over all, I am more optimistic about AYP finances now than at any time in the past, even though we have a long way to go to be solvent. There is a glimmer of light at the end of the tunnel. It is my hope that book sales alone will eventually be enough to support the free online lessons and community, and the ongoing writing effort here.

To have this growing open resource freely available long-term for everyone around the world would be fantastic. That is my dream. Along the way, all support is greatly appreciated, including direct donations, which were a major factor in helping keep the boat afloat last year. Many thanks to all who have and continue to help in that way.

Oh, and don't forget to print those AYP website cards and leave them in suitable locations. It can be done anonymously in charming ways. I am in the habit of sticking them on benches and in other places where people might go to reflect on their lives. When I have gone back they have always been gone... Serendipity... :-)

The guru is in you.

2006/04/22 17:36:05
AYP Helpers
http://www.aypsite.org/forum/topic.asp?TOPIC_ID=1067&REPLY_ID=6258&whichpage=-1
Group Meditation

Hi Meg:

A good way to talk about AYP is to put it in terms of what the other person might be looking for. No two people are the same, of course, but generally, most are seeking less hassle in life, better health, prosperity, good relationships and happiness in general.

Ecstatic bliss and enlightenment are further up the needs scale for most people, but it is surprising how quickly they will ascend once they see the positive effects of practices on their basic needs and begin to comtemplate their greater possibilities.

If you use deep meditation as an opener, the following, borrowed from the back of the Deep Meditation book, might be helpful:

"Deep Meditation" is a concise step-by-step instruction book for a simple yet powerful method of daily meditation that will systematically unfold inner peace, creativity and energy in daily life. Whether you are seeking an effective tool for reducing stress, improving your relationships, achieving more success in your career, or for revealing the ultimate truth of life within yourself, "Deep Meditation" can be a vital resource for cultivating your personal freedom and enlightenment.

If you want to take the discussion further up the scale, consider this, borrowed from the back of the AYP Easy Lessons book:

The premise of Yoga is simple. There is an outer reality and an inner one, and our nervous system is the doorway between them. Effective Yoga practices stimulate and open that doorway. The result? Peace, creativity, happiness, and a steady rise of ecstatic bliss radiating from within us... Advanced Yoga Practices (AYP) brings together the most effective methods of Yoga in a flexible integrated system that anyone can use. Instructions are given in plain English for deep meditation, spinal breathing pranayama, bodily manipulations (asanas, mudras and bandhas), tantric sexual practices, and other methods that are systematically applied to swing open the door of our nervous system to permanent higher experience. This is a non-sectarian approach that is compatible with any belief system or religious background.

Now that is moving up the scale, and it generally only works for those who are contemplating these things already. So proceed accordingly.

The trick is to discuss it from the perspective of the person who we are talking to, which means first finding out where their head and heart are at, and then gearing the discussion to that.

All the best!

The guru is in you.

2006/04/22 19:21:21
AYP Helpers
http://www.aypsite.org/forum/topic.asp?TOPIC_ID=1067&REPLY_ID=6261&whichpage=-1
Group Meditation

Hi Shanti:

What a nice way to share AYP with your friends and acquaintances. There is nothing like a group meditation to convince people in a hurry that something profound is going on in deep meditation.

There is that line from the Bible:
"Where two or three are gathered in my name, there I am in their midst."

It is really true, and is quite noticeable. With six or more the effect goes up exponentially.

The wonderful thing about this kind of sharing is that we don't have to do anything beyond the mechanical part. The real content of the work comes through us and through everyone who is involved. This is divine life -- stillness in action!

I hope others here will be inspired by your experience and consider doing the same in their area. It does not require anything special in the way of facilities -- just a place for everyone to sit comfortably. Keep us posted on how it goes!

The guru is in you.

2006/04/24 13:53:26
AYP Helpers
http://www.aypsite.org/forum/topic.asp?TOPIC_ID=1067&REPLY_ID=6309&whichpage=-1
Group Meditation

quote:
_____
David said: Teaching for a fee and including the book as part of the deal is a great win-win situation for everyone.
_____

Hi All:

Sounds very good, with or without the fee -- casual or structured gatherings. Whatever works for those involved...

Would anyone like to volunteer to help others get started on the hosting/teaching side? If we have a general scenario to follow for hosts/teachers, with support as needed, it might be easier to invite friends and acquaintances into the home for sharing, assistance and tasting inner silence deeply via group meditations. It is also an excellent way to give and receive ongoing support.

The AYP books are intended for both individual and group instruction and follow-up. It is yet to be seen exactly how the group aspect of it will develop. All in good time.

I'm moving this topic over the the AYP Helpers forum, as that seems to be a better fit with the way the discussion has evolved here. Thanks much!

The guru is in you.

2006/04/24 16:10:53
AYP Helpers
http://www.aypsite.org/forum/topic.asp?TOPIC_ID=1067&REPLY_ID=6313&whichpage=-1
Group Meditation

Hi Shanti:

What I have in mind is someone (or several someones) who can give folks a nudge on setting up group meditations, and offer encouragement and support on how to do it. You know that having a group meditation is pretty easy to do, because you are doing it now. But for some it might seem complicated. It isn't really. It is just a matter of asking a few folks if they are interested, getting a hold of some Deep Meditation books, and opening the door on a day of the week that suits everyone.

I recommend meditating first. One person can keep the time, so the others don't have to think about it. Then, after coming out slowly, some discussion can take place as the group would like. If there are no sharings or questions, a few sentences or paragraphs from an AYP book, or other relevant writings, can be read to stimulate the group. That almost never fails to open up an interesting discussion. Most people experiencing this simple format are amazed at how easily it flows. Something deep inside us becomes free to express in that kind of group environment, perhaps for the first time in our lives. Egos are checked at the door, just like here in the forum, so it is often a special experience and everyone walks away with something valuable -- some nice inner silence, clarity and new understandings about their path and life.

It can also be done the other way -- discussion first and then meditation at the end -- but that is usually not as relaxed as the former approach, especially for beginners who are likely to have experiences to share right after their first meditations. Even we "old pros" might be more in-the-groove on discussing practices and experiences after meditation than before.

Also, with beginners in the group, it might be best to limit the group meditation to 10-15 minutes until sure that everyone will be all right. Group self-pacing, you know.

Of course, group meditations are not a replacement for our daily practice at home, or wherever we happen to be at the appointed time.

A lesson on group meditations can be found here: http://www.aypsite.org/37.html

And, as someone mentioned recently, group meditations are covered in the Secrets of Wilder novel also. Boy, are they!

So, if you are encouraging group meditations there, it is only one small step to be encouraging them everywhere. This AYP cheerleader can use all the help he can get. :-)

The guru is in you.

2006/06/01 23:21:59
AYP Helpers
http://www.aypsite.org/forum/topic.asp?TOPIC_ID=1067&REPLY_ID=7669&whichpage=-1
Group Meditation
Sadhak wrote: "But perhaps Yogani will address my concern about mixing old and new practitioners in group sessions, and why there are adverse effects on some."

Hi Sadhak:

If we are are going to provide everyone on the planet with the same opportunity, then all the doors must be flung wide open and everyone should have the option to come in -- it is their choice. The arbitrary "slicing and dicing" must end -- that is another phrase for "sectarian hierarchy."

My opinion is that the benefits of inviting everyone to come together in spiritual practices in an open way far outweigh the minor disruptions that may be encountered in something like a group meditation. It is increased purification and opening. That's all. And we have ways to deal with it.

This forum, and AYP in general, is a good example of blending old timers with newcomers, and many different spiritual backgrounds as well. The synergies are amazing, and it works. Yes, the gears do grind occasionally, and we work through it. The USA is another example of this kind of synergistic phenomenon -- a melting pot of many cultures and peoples, each retaining their roots. They said it couldn't be done. The fact is it can be done, and the whole is far greater than the sum of the parts.

It can happen in yoga too -- a worldwide democratization of the tools and knowledge. That is worth far more than preventing a few grinding gears here and there. Chances are they will grind anyway, and why not have it be among friends? :-)

Reminder: Self-pacing works in groups too, as needed ... there are ways to deal with excess energy flow in just about any setting ... that is really what we are talking about here. Who are we to decide who is ready for a spiritual energy surge and who is not? That is what happens in group meditations. If people are feeling it in the room, they will be feeling it down the block, on the other side of town, and on the other side of the world. That is the purpose of group meditations -- to soak the world with inner silence. So it is for everyone, both in the room and everywhere ... better to be in the room if it is not too much, and each can decide that for themselves -- self-pacing.

Some beginners can conduct more energy than old timers, which means they are old souls disguised as beginners. Let them all in!

The guru is in you.

2006/07/04 13:04:14
AYP Helpers
http://www.aypsite.org/forum/topic.asp?TOPIC_ID=1067&REPLY_ID=8903&whichpage=-1
Group Meditation

Hi Jim:

AYP groups and gatherings are inevitable. They will happen even if they are not mentioned. And there are real benefits, as many are noticing. Indeed, group practice is a powerful tool to help accelerate the rise of world consciousness.

We really haven't scratched the surface yet in AYP on groups, retreats, and organized educational programs. There are endless possibilities -- all of them good for raising individual and world consciousness.

All of these things need some structure, and we are in the very early stages of filling it in. Several have gone on retreats and have asked for routines to do there, and suggestions have been offered to optimize progress and avoid overloads in an intensive practice situation. I can see large AYP group retreats someday. There is so much to do! Eventually it will be done, definitely not all by me.

As for the open discussions on experiences, it's sort of like democracy, you know ... sometimes messy, but much better than the alternative. Some of us old timers have seen the alternative, living under hierarchies that prohibit discussions on experiences, and it does not work.

As long as we are clear about real spiritual progress being beyond the multitude of our experiences, no matter how long it takes us to catch on, eventually we will. It was mentioned way early in the original AYP lessons -- experiences will be there and we will favor the practice. The way I see it, we can't hide from our own evolutionary process. The more we know about it the better. If we try and sweep it under the rug, what good will it do? The rug is an experience too!

It is the same with the guru. No matter what we say, many will stay focused on the external guru. That's okay. But where is the guru really? Inside, beyond our external experiences of guru. It is the same thing. In time, we grow and understand what is real and what is a reflection of our inner condition and bhakti. In stillness we know.

In the meantime, we can talk about it. It is good for our motivation to see the signposts along the highway, ours or someone else's, as long as we don't get stuck staring at them. Better to be practicing than gawking at the scenery. :-)

The guru is in you.

2006/05/11 22:10:42
AYP Helpers
http://www.aypsite.org/forum/topic.asp?TOPIC_ID=1154
Secrets of Wilder -- The Movie!

quote:
_____
Originally posted by yogani
I even have a crazy idea to write a screenplay for the Secrets of Wilder, and have been studying up a bit for that. Maybe in a year or two, as time permits. Doing a reasonable first pass on a screenplay is the way to help get that ball rolling. A movie could take a very long time to happen -- years and years. The process has to start somewhere, like here on this old computer. Any movie industry people out there? :-)

Originally posted by Sean
My brother and I are amateur film makers, he's currently editing a documentary down in LA that will come out soon. He owns a high end prosumer camera, an Apple G5 and Final Cut editing software which is about all you need to make a decent indie flick on a low budget these days. And I can even simulate explosions and aliens using 3D software if need be and then we can get Tom Cruise to star in it, etc. Seriously though, I'd love to work on this film.

Sean

http://www.thetaobums.com/forum
_____

752 – Advanced Yoga Practices

Hi Sean:

That's great news. I will keep you in the loop. It will be a long term project. No screenplay here for a year or two (more AYP books first), and then a rough first effort when it does happen -- no doubt needing many improvements. I'm reading up on screenwriting and cinematic story-telling now. Lots of possibilities...

So, do you think the Secrets of Wilder story would make a decent movie? I heard recently that the Celestine Prophesy is being made into a movie. I like the Wilder story better.
Of course, I am biased. :-) (those are my Hollywood sunglasses)

The guru is in you.

2006/05/15 15:10:33
AYP Helpers
http://www.aypsite.org/forum/topic.asp?TOPIC_ID=1154&REPLY_ID=7017&whichpage=-1
Secrets of Wilder -- The Movie!

Hi Sean:

Thanks for the vote of confidence on the story. It sure would be fun to make a Secrets of Wilder movie, wouldn't it?

Have not seen Magnolia. Will take a look. I happened to see AeonFlux (the movie) recently and it has some impressive "neurobiological" internal animation in it, not related to anything spiritual, but an interesting effect.

Yes, the cinematic "internals" (animation) and external special effects covering the wide range of spiritual experiences in the story would be important in a Wilder movie. One way to get the movie to stand out and attract a following would be to take those aspects to a new level well beyond what has been done before -- making it one of those "gotta-see" movies. Not sure exactly what that means in terms of effects, but innovation does attract an audience, and that is what AYP is about in the first place.

Innovation in the artform is, in large part, what created the Star Wars legacy -- special effects that no one had ever seen before, way back in 1977. It paved the way for a whole new era of Sci-Fi movies using such effects. It would be very beneficial if a Wilder movie could make a quantum leap in portraying spiritual experiences, not to mention be top notch in terms of the story adapted for the screen, quality of acting, traditonal film craft, etc. In other words, a captivating portrayal of the enlightenment process occurring in modern times, taken to a level of expression not seen before. We certainly have the raw material to work with -- the novel. Doing it right will be a big project and will take time and money. I'd rather do that than rush through and come up short with the end result.

The goal here will be to aim high and try and attract a major film maker with strong resources, financing and distribution to do this sort of project. If no one steps up, it may well end up as a small independent production, if it happens at all, but shouldn't we try with the majors first?

As mentioned, it will be a year or two and a few more AYP books before I can focus on a screenplay. In the meantime, I will continue studying the craft on the side. If a top-notch professional screenwritier comes along before I can take a serious stab at it, then that could work too. All options are open right now.

Any other ideas on this are welcome!

The guru is in you.

2006/05/16 14:00:22
AYP Helpers
http://www.aypsite.org/forum/topic.asp?TOPIC_ID=1154&REPLY_ID=7062&whichpage=-1
Secrets of Wilder -- The Movie!

Hi Sean:

Is it common now-a-days to do a few scenes in an independent (or amateur) film mode to present to major film makers along with the screenplay?

It would basically be a low-tech preview of the movie on DVD included with the screenplay and other pre-production information that would help make the reviewers' job easier ... in our favor, of course. :-)

The guru is in you.

2006/05/17 10:38:24
AYP Helpers
http://www.aypsite.org/forum/topic.asp?TOPIC_ID=1154&REPLY_ID=7096&whichpage=-1
Secrets of Wilder -- The Movie!
Thank you, Bill.

Robert McKee is recommended in one of the screenwriting books I have read: "Save the Cat!" by Blake Snyder, a fun book that covers the essentials very well.

Snyder also recommends books by Syd Field, the "master of the craft," and Viki King. And, of course, Joseph Campbell's "Hero With a Thousand Faces," which was an important part of the groundwork for the Secrets of Wilder novel also. Fortunately, we have our story already. It is only a matter of moving it from the book to the screen -- no small task.

I am looking at resources on movie-making as well, in an attempt to minimize the gap that often occurs between screenwriting and cinematography.

The guru is in you.

2006/05/19 11:53:14
AYP Helpers
http://www.aypsite.org/forum/topic.asp?TOPIC_ID=1154&REPLY_ID=7146&whichpage=-1
Secrets of Wilder -- The Movie!

Hi Sean:

Thanks much. A serious effort is lurking in the background here, though it is not like what someone wrote to me recently: "I'm so happy to hear you have a movie deal for the Secrets of Wilder!"
We wish... :-)

Well, we will need a screenplay first. Between now and then there are lots of possibilities to consider, and a lot more to learn from the many professionals who have so generously recorded their experiences in the trade.

The initial strategy here is to try and get a major player involved in making the movie. If none will, then, at the same time, we can be moving to do it ourselves -- either in part to further attract the industry, or the whole thing -- we'll just keep working on it, favoring the path of least resistance to get it done. That has been the approach taken with all the AYP material so far, and it is working okay, thanks to the wonderful technologies we have available today that can empower anyone who wants to make a contribution and is willing to do the work. Perhaps it will be similar in approaching the movies?

One of the most important things I am learning about script writing, besides the artistic craft side of it, is to tailor the presentation of the story in a way so it can be filmed in one geographical area. That could be Florida or California, depending on how the chips fall, with distant story locations like DC, Blue Ridge Mountains, etc. put in visually for effect, as needed, with the actual scenes shot locally. A good example of this approach is the globe-trotting "Alias" spy TV series, which convincingly goes to many countries around the world, yet, was filmed almost entirely in Southern California. Keeping the shooting locations in one area is about containing costs, of course, and saving time too.

The spiritual experience special effects side of it is another area to be investigated. That will be an important part of the movie, and we'd like for it to be a standout, as mentioned previously. Again, the screenplay will be be tailored to try and make the best economic use of special effects.

The guru is in you.

2006/05/22 11:18:39
AYP Helpers
http://www.aypsite.org/forum/topic.asp?TOPIC_ID=1154&REPLY_ID=7255&whichpage=-1
Secrets of Wilder -- The Movie!

Hi Sadak, and welcome!

The Secrets of Wilder novel presents the discovery, application and resulting experiences of real spiritual practices (AYP style) in an American adventure/romance story. No Sanskrit terms are used. The purpose is to approach a modern western Christian audience with the integrated non-sectarian practices in a familiar setting. Even so, the story reaches far beyond what most westerners might expect. Maybe beyond what most Indians might expect too, because the "Secrets of Wilder" do not stay secret for very long. And neither do the practices or their progressive effects stay secret in AYP. The doors are flung wide open...

In addition to paperback, all of the AYP books are available worldwide in ebook format, so you should be able to download the novel there. For links, see: http://www.aypsite.org/books.html

AYP has at least a few thousand internet readers in India. We have been inquiring for over a year to find a publisher for the AYP books there so they can be readily available at local cost -- no success in getting published in India so far. If you have any suggestions on this, let me know.

As things evolve here with the screenplay and related movie-making matters, I'd be happy to keep you in the loop. Keep in mind that this is a long term project -- the screenplay is not expected for at least a year. By then, there will be several more AYP instruction books on practices out, and increasing visibility to the public. In that sense, time is on our side...

Who knows? Maybe the Secrets of Wilder will play well in India. Check out the novel and let us know what you think.

Bollywood, here we come?! :-)

The guru is in you.

2008/10/15 13:20:58
AYP Helpers
http://www.aypsite.org/forum/topic.asp?TOPIC_ID=1154&REPLY_ID=38937&whichpage=-1
Secrets of Wilder -- The Movie!

Hi Markern:

Many thanks for all the new ideas. Of course the only way any of this can get done is if you and others of like mind go out and make it happen. Go for it!

But maybe better read the Secrets of Wilder novel first. Most like it, but some do not. As they say, "There's no accounting for taste." :-)

To add an update to my posts above from 2006 on a Secrets of Wilder movie, the strategy here has shifted to more of a wait and see mode on that. This is due to learning about the industry, and what is involved in any movie getting made. It is generally a long and serendipity journey, having to do more with who in the industry wants to adapt a book to the screen than whether or not an author has written a screenplay.

The Secrets of Wilder has been read by at least one movie mogul who liked it, but this is no guarantee that anything will happen with it within a decade!

So, circulating the book to studios, producers, directors, agents and stars is the way to go, knowing that in time the odds will tilt toward someone wanting to do something. Then the adaption process can start, which is taking 15 hours of reading and converting it into 2 hours of movie screenplay -- no small task, probably best left to the professionals, and even that will likely get rewritten two or three times at least before (and sometimes during) shooting. That is how it goes in the movie business.

The main thing on our end is to see that as many key players as possible see and/or hear about the book, and when someone does come forward with some interest, to be sure they have the intention to be as true to the story as possible in adapting it to the screen. Once the movie rights are obtained, it is in the hands of the movie makers, to make or not to make, and how it will be made. So a meeting of minds on the front end is very important.

What the Secrets of Wilder has going for it as a potential movie is that it deals with the universal theme of human enlightenment in a Joseph Campbell-esque way, and can be presented as a pretty exciting adventure as well. Not sure the spiritual practices in the book would translate well to the screen, but the experiences certainly could with state-of-the-art special effects. From there, the viewer may be inspired to dig deeper into the practices themselves. That is the reason the novel was written in the first place -- not only to instruct, but to inspire further study leading to daily practice. All the rest of the AYP writings are in place for that.

So, if you like the novel, any help along these lines will be much appreciated. The same goes for any other passing of the word you may choose to undertake (as you mentioned here and elsewhere).

Thanks, and all the best!

The guru is in you.

2008/10/15 14:17:57
AYP Helpers
http://www.aypsite.org/forum/topic.asp?TOPIC_ID=1154&REPLY_ID=38942&whichpage=-1
Secrets of Wilder -- The Movie!

Hi Carson:

No disagreement on your thoughts, and that is why the strategy has shifted to simply making as many people in the industry as possible aware of the Wilder story, and sitting back and waiting (samyama is definitely going on in that :-)) . If nothing else, readers in the industry may be spurred along on their own spiritual path.

I believe as the shift in global consciousness continues, the demand for Wilder-style stories will increase, including more commercial viability.

A couple of years ago, both the Celestine Prophesy and the Peaceful Warrior came out -- the first as a do-it-yourself independent production, and the second as a Hollywood production. The latter is far better made than the first, so there is something to be said for waiting for professionals to develop a sincere interest in doing such a project, which I do favor now. I don't know if either of those movies was a commercial success (I suspect Peaceful Warrior did better), but the fact that both were made is noteworthy.

So, we'll see how it goes. The trade-off is that if a Wilder movie eventually gets made, and it is reasonably well-done (that front-end meeting of the minds), it can greatly expand the number of spiritual practitioners around the world. That is worth aiming for.

So please continue to pass the novel on, and we'll continue to do samyama on it too. :-)

The guru is in you.

2008/10/15 15:09:21
AYP Helpers
http://www.aypsite.org/forum/topic.asp?TOPIC_ID=1154&REPLY_ID=38946&whichpage=-1
Secrets of Wilder -- The Movie!

Hi Carson:

Yes, if Wilder can eventually do as well as Peaceful Warrior did in the translation to screen (even though quite piecemeal), it will be worthwhile. I am open to it, and recognize that it could be many years before someone able to do a decent piecemeal job comes along. As Millman points out, it is a net plus -- an audience widener. So why not, if and when the opportunity presents itself?

On the opposite end, the adaption to the screen of the Da Vinci Code was so true to the myriad details in the book that it tended to drag on the screen, getting bogged down in itself. It is just not possible to get a whole book onto the screen gracefully, so it is all in the adaption, which means leaving a lot out. Of course, the Da Vinci Code was guaranteed a degree of commercial success due to the popularity of the book and the Hollywood horsepower that was poured into it.

I don't think Wilder has to worry about being over-articulated in movie form the way the Da Vinci Code was. It is pretty expensive. We'd love to have that problem though.

I also remember that Carl Sagan was furious with what Hollywood was doing with his novel, Contact, and that there was even legal action about it. It is ironic, because Contact turned out to be a great movie, and a wonderful tribute to Carl Sagan and his work. Unfortunately, he passed away before he could see it.

Well, just to point out a few of the many contradictions and cross-currents that can be found in the movie business. So let's not take it too seriously, while keeping the door open at the same time. I think we are on the same page with that. Keep passing out those copies of Wilder! :-)

The guru is in you.

2010/10/15 23:59:22
AYP Helpers

Secrets of Wilder -- The Movie!

Hi Kavelian, and welcome. :-)

Thanks much for the overview from your perspective inside the industry.

I agree that the screenplay is the key. It is a matter of coming up with a good one. That is what drives the whole process. Can't blame production companies for being picky -- many millions are spent to put a story on the screen based on those 100 or so double-spaced pages. The screenplay had better be good -- very good.

As you will "see" when you read it, the Secrets of Wilder is largely a visual story, because that is the way it came to me. The spiritual journey of John Wilder is conveyed with elements of adventure, drama, romance/sexual tension, and comedy. Of course, important parts of the imagery are "internal." Some of that can be expressed beautifully with digital effects, to a degree that supports the overall flow of the story (not to overdo it).

It is a given that we will not be able to put all of the Wilder story into a screen adaption. As you point out, it will have to be distilled into a much shorter visual experience that illuminates the essence, while making it an even more captivating story at the same time. That is the creative challenge.

The Wilder movie project has been on the back burner since my last post above two years ago. There have been a series of other projects demanding full attention here since then. Perhaps at some point circumstances will permit work to begin in earnest on a screenplay. I have mixed feelings about tackling it by myself. A talented screenwriter assisting would be much preferred. Whenever the time comes to address it, we will do the best we can with what we have.

Thanks again for your sage advice, and all the best on your continuing path in practices!

The guru is in you.

2010/11/12 20:25:09
AYP Helpers
Secrets of Wilder -- The Movie!

quote:
_____
Originally posted by faileforever

Hope this will one day be on the big screen and reaching out to millions.
_____

Me too. :-)

2006/06/09 13:12:34
AYP Helpers
an inexpensive and effective way to promote AYP

Hi Alvin:

Excellent idea to write reviews for yoga and self-help books on Amazon, referring to the AYP book(s). Of course, such reviews should be sincere, knowledgeable and informative. In most cases, AYP can be presented as a complement to a good book or teaching. Being seen as a useful addition rather than a replacement is a good way to win hearts.

Amazon searches on any of the terms you mentioned above will turn up books, which can then be ranked from best selling on down. Best selling is where the viewers are, so that is where the reviews mentioning AYP will do the most good.

For example, Iyengar's "**Light on Yoga**" has been the best selling yoga book on Amazon for as long as I have been looking. It so happens that AYP can be an excellent complement to Iyengar training. Jim, Victor and others can verify that. AYP can be a real benefit there, and we should not be shy to communicate it to all people in Iyengar, or considering Iyengar -- it is at the heart of the yoga market, which is where we need to be. The same goes for other popular teachings, as you mentioned.

Can anyone list the most popular yoga and self help books? You are off to a good start, Alvin, but how about we take aim at best sellers? There are many nipping at Iyengar's heels. We'd like to put AYP square in the middle of that pack as a co-training tool -- an open resource to all.

Another approach is, if anyone has read a good book, regardless of popularity/sales rank, and want's to review it on Amazon, then do so, pointing out the relationship it might have to the role of the AYP books in your life. The more places AYP can be mentioned the better.

Also, keep in mind that probably 75% of the Amazon yoga traffic flows through the Amazon USA site (AYP website traffic mirrors this too) with the rest of the Amazon yoga traffic through Canada, UK, France, Germany/Austria and Japan. Not that I would not like to see AYP mentioned in reviews on all the Amazon sites. But if it is numbers we are seeking, Amazon USA is the place to start.

Now, great suggestions like this for promoting AYP are wonderful, but who is actually going to go out and do something? As we say in America, it is in the doing where the rubber meets the road ... or did that one come from China too?

So far about half of the suggestions to promote AYP have been for me to do something (thanks, I needed something else to do), and the other half have been great ideas that very few have acted on. The ones who have stepped up are making a difference (thank you!), but we are still way short on having the many hands that make light work...

The guru is in you.

756 –   Advanced Yoga Practices

2006/06/10 18:39:50
AYP Helpers
http://www.aypsite.org/forum/topic.asp?TOPIC_ID=1202&REPLY_ID=7928&whichpage=-1
an inexpensive and effective way to promote AYP

Hi Alvin:

Thanks for those, and for your reviews of the AYP books on Amazon too. They make a big difference.

Here is a search for "**Yoga**" on Amazon USA, ranked for best-selling: click here (4,300 books)

Try a few searches of your own. Check the book rankings on Amazon to see how each category fares in relation to the over all universe of books. For example, Iyengar's best-selling "**Light on Yoga**" is usually ranked somewhere between 500-1000. Waynes Dyer's book on meditation is in that range too. That is about as good as it gets for yoga books. Maybe there are some self-improvement books that do better where aspects of AYP might be appreciated? Look and see.

Here are a few others:

Meditation -- click here (9,300 books!)

Pranayama -- click here (42 books) AYP Spinal Breathing Pranayama comes up #5 on this list, which isn't saying much -- sales are very small (rank over 100,000). The best selling book on this list "Light on Pranayama" by Iyengar ranked 5,000-10,000, so pranayama books are not nearly as lively as yoga and meditation books.

Breathing -- click here (1,100 books) Similar to pranayama, with many added.

Kriya -- click here (77 books) Best seller here is Satyananda's "Systematic Course in the Ancient Tantric Techniques of Yoga and Kriya" - rank over 100,000, not an active book category. "Yoga" and "Meditation" seem to be where the action is.

Oh, and of course, let's not forget...

Tantra -- click here (490 books) The rankings fall off fast here. We'll see how AYP Tantra does. Anyone feel like planting a few seeds in the reviews for top seller "Sex and the Perfect Lover - Tao, Tantra and Kama Sutra" by Mabel Iam (what a name! :-)), ranked 600.

There is no doubt that if readers of best-selling yoga and self-improvement books hear about AYP, it will make a big difference. Help with that will be much appreciated.

The guru is in you.

2006/06/11 12:00:41
AYP Helpers
http://www.aypsite.org/forum/topic.asp?TOPIC_ID=1202&REPLY_ID=7944&whichpage=-1
an inexpensive and effective way to promote AYP
Further thoughts:

The **Secrets of Wilder** is relevant to mention in reviews for the **Da Vinci Code**, the hottest book (and movie) on the planet at the moment.

Wilder shares the defiance of religious hierarchy theme with the Da Vinci code, and the implication that spirituality is to be found in the human being, not in the church.

As you know, Wilder then takes a different direction, focusing on the actual methods of human spiritual transformation, their transmission to many, and the far-reaching consequences of that. And, interestingly, the Wilder secrets, at times, come from within Christendom itself, validating the teachings of Jesus, while at the same time refuting the distortions of organized religion.

Other books where the Secrets of Wilder can be mentioned usefully in reviews are:

The Celestine Prophesy -- Redfield (new movie, not well-received, self-produced - lessons on how **not** to do it)

Way of the Peaceful Warrior -- Millman (also a new movie out, doing better than Celestine, thanks to a professional Hollywood production.)

Jonathan Livingston Seagull and **Illusions** -- Bach

Converstations With God -- Walsch (not a novel, but comparable)

Maybe you know of others? Give it a whirl. John Wilder can use all the help he can get. :-)

The guru is in you.

2006/06/12 12:56:55
AYP Helpers
http://www.aypsite.org/forum/topic.asp?TOPIC_ID=1202&REPLY_ID=7970&whichpage=-1
an inexpensive and effective way to promote AYP

Hi Will:

The AYP Geocities site (http://www.geocities.com/advancedyogapractices) does not display the books on every page (Yahoo ads instead), but it has limited bandwidth.

Thanks much for helping out. Yes, lots of AYP links in all the places where there is relevant traffic certainly do help.

The guru is in you.

2006/08/11 15:56:46
AYP Helpers
http://www.aypsite.org/forum/topic.asp?TOPIC_ID=1202&REPLY_ID=10407&whichpage=-1
an inexpensive and effective way to promote AYP

quote:
_____
Originally posted by Alvin Chan

I've tried posting two reviews on amazon, but they never show up. May be they've banned any reference to any products on the reviews?
_____

Hi Alvin:

Sorry to hear that.

Amazon frowns on links (or products?) leading away from their site. There has not been a problem with mentioning other books, assuming it is done as part of a legitimate full scope review. All the better for Amazon...

Thank you for trying. I hope you will try again. Amazon USA is the place to do it -- the most traffic there by far.

As you know, Amazon reviews are one the easiest and best ways to lend AYP a helping hand. They end up in the search engines too!

The guru is in you.

2006/08/12 10:55:46
AYP Helpers
http://www.aypsite.org/forum/topic.asp?TOPIC_ID=1202&REPLY_ID=10424&whichpage=-1
an inexpensive and effective way to promote AYP

quote:
_____
Originally posted by Alvin Chan

I see. One year ago, I wrote a review on a good piano book and link to the website of the author, it did work and is still there. May be they change the rule now.

OKOK, I know what Amazon wants now. Let me try link back to its own page of AYP book this time!!
_____

Hi Alvin:

I suggest putting no links in book reviews, Amazon's or others. The name of the book and author is enough, and should not set off alarms.

TGIIY
2006/08/12 14:45:31
AYP Helpers
http://www.aypsite.org/forum/topic.asp?TOPIC_ID=1202&REPLY_ID=10433&whichpage=-1
an inexpensive and effective way to promote AYP

quote:
_____
Originally posted by Alvin Chan

It works!

http://www.amazon.com/gp/product/0007107005/ref=cm_aya_asin.title/102-3678896-2477765?%5Fencoding=UTF8&v=glance&n=283155

And I've picked the edition of Iyengar's classics with the fewest reviews (just 3 counting mine) so as to attract more attention.

Anyone can give me some comments on my review. I will be happy to edit it for improvement. I'm brain-storming and you know, I am not a native English speaker. So advice on grammer, use of words, style, etc are particularly welcomed.

_____

Good job, Alvin. Thanks!

Keep in mind that Amazon page readership is indicated by the sales ranking -- about 175,000 on this 2001 edition of Iyengar's Light on Yoga -- pretty high. Whereas the 1995 edition is usually ranked under 1000 -- the best selling (highest volume) book on yoga on all of Amazon. You could probably get away with putting the same review there, since it is the same book.
http://www.amazon.com/gp/product/0805210318/sr=1-1/qid=1155407726/ref=sr_1_1/103-4923313-7675054?ie=UTF8&s=books

758 – Advanced Yoga Practices

Check this list for bestselling books on yoga:
http://www.amazon.com/s/ref=sr_st/103-4923313-7675054?keywords=yoga&page=1&rh=n%3A1000%2Ck%3Ayoga&sort=salesrank&x=8&y=5

Editing Amazon reviews is hit or miss at best -- sometimes they disappear forever. If you get one up there, it is usually best to leave it alone. You know the old saying, "Let sleeping dogs lie." :-)

The guru is in you.

2006/06/25 09:15:25
AYP Helpers
http://www.aypsite.org/forum/topic.asp?TOPIC_ID=1248
Take Advantage of Quantity Discount for AYP Books

Hello All:

Just a reminder that we have an ongoing program offering a deep discount on any combination AYP books bought in quantity. It is 55% off the suggested retail prices plus shipping within a couple of days direct from the printer in either Tennessee, USA or London, England. The suggested retail prices can be found through links or the downloadable books flyer on the AYP books page.

There is no minimum quantity requirement to order. The economics of it are determined by shipping cost. In most cases, less than 5 books will be less expensive to order from Amazon or other discount retailer.

If you are interested in obtaining more than 5 books (any combination of AYP titles), using the deep discount will usually be a good deal. The more books ordered, the better the deal, as shipping cost becomes less of a factor.

If you would like to help spread the word on AYP, handing out books to others who you feel can benefit (and who can also spread the word) is an excellent way to do it. Books you obtain through this discount program may also be resold.

For quotes on delivery of AYP books to your area, write me at yogani99@yahoo.com.

If you would rather make a donation to help spread the word on AYP, see this forum topic.

Wishing you all the best on your path. Practice wisely, and enjoy!

The guru is in you.

Note: We can now also do quantity discount orders from New Del
Hi with the India editions, covering India, Asia, Indonesia, Australia and Africa.

2008/09/28 00:24:46
AYP Helpers
http://www.aypsite.org/forum/topic.asp?TOPIC_ID=1248&REPLY_ID=38201&whichpage=-1
Take Advantage of Quantity Discount for AYP Books

Hi Machart:

eBooks are not intended to be shared outside a household. If they are shared beyond that, this would begin to undermine the primary source of financial support for AYP -- the books.

It is preferred to keep the online lessons free to all, and the books available for a modest cost. The free online lessons are available because the books provide some financial support. That support is yet to reach break-even here. In other words, the personal bank account is still subsidizing it to a degree, though not as much as in the past. I am hopeful that AYP will be fully self-supporting in the not-too-distant future. As it is, our ability to invest in promotion remains very limited. AYP continues to be a global knowledge transmission strategy being run on a shoestring.

It is an interesting idea you raise about gifting AYP ebooks. It can apply to the AYP audiobooks too. This could be done through donations with email addresses provided to me on where to send the gifted ebook(s). While I'd like to offer a discount for ebook/audiobook gifting orders, it is not the same scenario as for the paperbacks, which are physical products that can be ordered in quantity, given away or resold (for a profit if desired). eBooks and audiobooks do not lend themselves to that kind of distribution structure. Plus, the ebooks are inexpensive to begin with -- 1/2 the paperback retail cost, or less, depending on the book. To go lower for a small quantity of ebooks (for the e-series especially) would see a large percentage eaten up in Paypal transaction costs.

So, bottom line, ebooks or audiobooks can be gifted by contacting me and doing the transaction at the direct download cost (see here for those).

Does this sound interesting?

Thanks for the suggestion.

The guru is in you.

PS: Your reply got in front of this post because I removed it and edited to include audiobooks and a few other points. Glad you like it. :-)
2006/07/04 12:23:03
AYP Helpers
http://www.aypsite.org/forum/topic.asp?TOPIC_ID=1278&REPLY_ID=8900&whichpage=-1
Wikipedia

Hi Shanti, Jim and All:

Guy followed up on the Hunter/East-West, Calif lead. Not sure where that one is right now. Keep in mind that most areas have a local new age and/or yoga publication, and one way or other they can hear about AYP -- hint, hint... :-)

Someone put AYP on Wikipedia a month or two ago and it got shot down, supposedly because it was too commercial with books on it. What??? Tolle and others have books on their sites. AYP does not sell anything directly on the site, not to mention the more than 300 free lessons on practices there, plus this terrific forum.

So, the question is, who is opposed to AYP on Wikipedia? Could it be the sectarians?

A multi-person effort on Wikipedia, as suggested by Jim, would be wonderful.

Note: For a few ideas, see Trip's fine work on **Zaadz** at: http://ayp.zaadz.com

Thanks for bringing Wikipedia up, Cosmic. It is an important one.

The guru is in you.

2006/07/04 19:01:43
AYP Helpers
http://www.aypsite.org/forum/topic.asp?TOPIC_ID=1278&REPLY_ID=8927&whichpage=-1
Wikipedia

Hi All:

Here was the previous attempt with AYP on Wikipedia -- see will.iam's June 12th post at
http://www.aypsite.org/forum/topic.asp?TOPIC_ID=1202&SearchTerms=wikipedia

It seems what AYP is, how it works, and how people can use it would be of interest to many, without mention of the books. Whoever had a problem with the book links on the website obviously didn't look far enough to find that there is a huge amount of free instructional material there. Isn't it odd? It used to be that most people had a hard time seeing the books because of the free lessons. Now they can't see the free lessons because of the books! :-)

As for my background, the most that is available on this is in the first press release last year -- http://www.aypsite.org/pressrelease1.html

You are welcome to use content from there.

All the best!

The guru is in you.

PS -- Ah, there you are will.iam! Thanks for chiming in.

2006/07/05 11:09:17
AYP Helpers
http://www.aypsite.org/forum/topic.asp?TOPIC_ID=1278&REPLY_ID=8976&whichpage=-1
Wikipedia

quote:
_____
Originally posted by Etherfish

how about this: Put up information about Yogani and AYP being non profit, mention free lessons and don't put any information whatsover about things that can be purchased.
Then later on add that information. Wiki is always up for additional information.
_____

Hi Ether:

Just to be clear, AYP is <u>not</u> a non-profit organization. It isn't an organization at all. It is just an old guy writing like crazy :-) ... and all of you wonderful practitioners ...

Even so, there is no profit -- not even close. Maybe in a few more years book sales will pay the bills. The crazy writer certainly hopes so. There will be no regrets about profit if and when there is any. And I expect the writing will go on as long as the brain and fingers are working ... though a vacation certainly wouldn't hurt.

For whatever it is worth...

The guru is in you.

2006/07/19 13:48:51
AYP Helpers
http://www.aypsite.org/forum/topic.asp?TOPIC_ID=1278&REPLY_ID=9675&whichpage=-1
Wikipedia

Hi All:

Off-forum efforts have led to one AYP article being successfully launched on Wikipedia, and a second one that is being worked on in communication with the Wiki editors and may or may not make it (the first "learning curve" effort -- deemed too promotional in present form).

Launched: http://en.wikipedia.org/wiki/Yogani

Questionable: http://en.wikipedia.org/wiki/Advanced_Yoga_Practices_%28AYP%29

Many thanks to all who have been contributing ideas and effort!

The guru is in you.

2006/07/19 16:58:41
AYP Helpers
http://www.aypsite.org/forum/topic.asp?TOPIC_ID=1278&REPLY_ID=9679&whichpage=-1
Wikipedia

Hi All:

Okay, an attempt has been made to clean up our questionable Wiki article. Let's see what the Wiki people say.

http://en.wikipedia.org/wiki/Advanced_Yoga_Practices_%28AYP%29

The guru is in you.

2006/07/20 11:16:24
AYP Helpers
http://www.aypsite.org/forum/topic.asp?TOPIC_ID=1278&REPLY_ID=9717&whichpage=-1
Wikipedia

Hi Alvin:

There is some support for the questionable AYP article among the Wiki editors. In fact, it has been edited by them to bring it closer to their standard. The current issue is that, early on, a few spoke up against the article on the issues of "notability" and "promotional advertisement," and lately the tide is shifting. Not sure how long or if the edits by us and Wiki editors will lead to an approval. If not, the article (possibly further edited) will be resubmitted under the name "Advanced Yoga Practices" (no acronym). That would likely pass, because the tide is already turning on this matter. The "notability" of AYP (their term) has now been recognized among Wiki editiors, though it was not in the beginning. In the meantime, the article has been cleaned up quite a bit and no longer looks like a promotion.

Meanwhile, the "yogani" article flew right through with no complaints so far. Once the other one is approved in some form, the two will be linked together, which will help fill in from both directions on your question about the generic sounding name of AYP. But preferably no cross linking before the pending article is approved. It is about "brand recognition" really. Any combination of words can be meaningless, or have a lot of meaning, depending on the degree of recognition in society -- what the Wiki folks call "notability." Slowly but surely, we are getting there. :-)

Once the AYP article is approved in some form, the door will be open to do many more articles on the practices listed -- most which do not exist on Wiki at present. There is some interest from Wiki on this, because dead end (article invitation) links have been placed on all the practices in the AYP article by a Wiki editor. So there is a great opportunity for both Wiki and us here. I will be happy to do the work if they are willing to open the door.

Thanks for your input.

The guru is in you.

2006/07/20 16:27:25
AYP Helpers
http://www.aypsite.org/forum/topic.asp?TOPIC_ID=1278&REPLY_ID=9725&whichpage=-1
Wikipedia

Hi Alvin:

Great idea. Yes, we can gain a lot of exposure with linking to AYP related pages from articles that cover common ground, done according to Wiki rules, of course.

But I suggest waiting until we sort the matter out on the AYP article in question. According to Wiki rules, there is a five day discussion period on an article proposed for deletion, and then the article will be either deleted or approved -- that would happen around July 22 in this case. If it is deleted, we are permitted to resubmit it with improvements, which we surely would do, as mentioned above.

Regarding linking back from other articles, including ones we may write ourselves on practices, we can do that as long as we are balanced in the presentation, including citing relevant scriptures, traditions and/or teachers as appropriate. It can be done with internal links to other Wiki articles, and/or with "External Links" which go at the end of the article.

Check this article on kechari mudra for one that I edited the other day (not my article) adding text and internal Wiki links to "Hatha Yoga Pradipika" and "Yogani." I also added two other teachers who are noted for kechari (no Wiki articles available for them), so the AYP addition is low-key and relevant. I'm pretty sure that external links could also be added at the end of that article for Paulsen, Shailendra and Yogani's kechari lesson #108 without complaints. I just haven't gotten around to it yet. You can see what external links look like by clicking back to the Yogani page. The links are supposed to be embedded, but I didn't get around to that yet either. Code for adding an external linking section at the end of an article and the method for embedding links can be copied from the edit page of any Wiki article that has external links.

From what I gather, it is taboo to put external links within a Wiki article -- only in the external links section at the end. So there are two ways to link:

1) Internal within Wiki direct from the article.
2) External after the article.

The guru is in you.

2006/07/23 12:20:00
AYP Helpers
http://www.aypsite.org/forum/topic.asp?TOPIC_ID=1278&REPLY_ID=9789&whichpage=-1
Wikipedia

Hi All:

Well, both of the AYP Wiki articles are up for deletion now, and it is pretty much out of my hands, since both have been labeled "vanity articles." Only input from others can change it. Here are the articles, which include links to talk pages for discussion and debate on the deletions:

http://en.wikipedia.org/wiki/Advanced_Yoga_Practices_%28AYP%29

http://en.wikipedia.org/wiki/Yogani

Wiki also has rules about supporters of an article getting organized and piling in to defend it, though they admit it happens all the time, and it does make a difference. Credible sources will make the biggest difference. It would be logical to assume that personal experience constitutes credibility, but it is not so simple in the Wiki world. Wiki rules encourage maintenance of the status quo, which we are certainly not for in AYP when it comes to teachings on spiritual practices. We can look forward to the day when open, easy-to-use systems of practice become the status quo. Until then, we will be viewed as promoters. So be it ... there are far worse things to be in favor of... :-)

Suggestion: If you have an idea to help AYP and bring it here, please consider following through on it. Good ideas are ten for a penny, while even a small amount of implementation is priceless.

Wiki is a case-in-point. AYP will only fly on Wiki when sufficient numbers of people believe it belongs there and are willing to weigh in to make it happen. It is in your hands.

The guru is in you.

2006/07/23 17:25:42
AYP Helpers
http://www.aypsite.org/forum/topic.asp?TOPIC_ID=1278&REPLY_ID=9797&whichpage=-1
Wikipedia

Hi Anthem:

Yes, all Wiki stuff is done through postings by anyone who is there. It tells you where to go for the deletion discussions in the notes on the above page links.

Posting is a bit odd, particularly on behind the scenes talk pages, as opposed to articles. Both are formatted and updated the same way. In either case, you go in and edit the page -- in the case of a talk page, adding your comments at the bottom. The best way to learn is to go into edit pages and see how others are doing it. To sign a talk page entry, Wiki sign-up is necessary, and then signing a talk page note is done by adding four squiggles like this: ~~~~ You can also post without Wiki signup, but maybe no one will pay attention. Not sure.

It is a pretty strange system, but there are detailed instructions for everything, and the learning curve is short.

Getting through the morass of "shoot from the hip" Wiki elves is something else. As far as I can tell, it is a dream world, with limited connection to reality, and certainly not toward innovations that are occurring in the field of yoga. But, oh, what great search engine exposure! Of course, there are a lot of ways to get that. :-)

The guru is in you.

2006/07/24 07:05:00
AYP Helpers
http://www.aypsite.org/forum/topic.asp?TOPIC_ID=1278&REPLY_ID=9813&whichpage=-1
Wikipedia

Hi All:

The AYP article is now gone -- the 5 day discussion window passed. The article can be reposted, but not by me. Anyone interested can do it -- I have the code saved here.

The second "Yogani" article is slated for deletion also. I put a note on the deletion talk page this morning (at the bottom) for the 10 Wiki elves who nominated the article for deletion:

http://en.wikipedia.org/wiki/Wikipedia:Articles_for_deletion/Yogani

It speaks to a fundamental flaw in the Wiki service that has become quickly apparent -- an inability to incorporate new innovations in knowledge. Perhaps that is the nature of an encyclopedia -- it is yesterday's news. But we expect better from the internet, don't we?

The guru is in you.

2006/07/24 11:17:23

AYP Helpers
http://www.aypsite.org/forum/topic.asp?TOPIC_ID=1278&REPLY_ID=9822&whichpage=-1
Wikipedia

Hi Alvin:

Yes, encyclopedias were invented as a proxy for the library we could not fit in the house. Does the internet (thousands of libraries on our desk) need a proxy?

If you are saying that Wiki is a viable proxy because what it has on yoga practices is well tested, I must disagree. What is there is a tangled rehash of media coverage and other information which can be found elsewhere on the web. Wiki is not about truth. It is about prominence -- truth and prominence are rarely the same thing in the field of yoga these days, certainly not in the sense of revealing a practical path.

If you do not have fame, Wiki has no interest, whether what you have is truth or not. The Wiki rules exclude new ideas and approaches to knowledge, wholesale -- no questions asked. Not just AYP, but many spiritual efforts going on around the world are excluded. When something reaches national and international prominence, for reasons relevant to truth or not, then Wiki is happy to jump on the bandwagon. On today's modern internet, that is both redundant and incomplete. And, in the case of yoga, it is misleading and confusing also...

Google is much better because it leaves nothing out.

Due to its narrow inclusion policy, Wiki is very limited as a research tool on spiritual matters. These days in the spiritual field, there is much more going on under the radar than on top of it. It is, in fact, where the action is. Wiki by its own policies does not show you any of that. So, when doing serious spiritual research, better use Google and the other search engines. Unless you are only looking for famous public domain stuff. Then use Wiki. And good luck with finding the truth in there.

Come to think of it, AYP is a sort of Wiki for yoga practices, having cut things away left and right. What we keep is not based on prominence, but on what works. That's the fundamental difference between AYP and Wiki. Will the two ever meet? :-)

As for what works in yoga practices, in the case of AYP, what is happening at home for each of us is obviously most important. But if it isn't happening at home, let's not ignore the growing list of recorded experiences under the bell curve.

The proof is in each of us, and in the statistical relevance of the experiences recorded by all of us. If the latter is true, the former should be true also, sooner or later.

Just some food for thought...

The guru is in you.

2006/07/24 11:47:24
AYP Helpers
http://www.aypsite.org/forum/topic.asp?TOPIC_ID=1278&REPLY_ID=9824&whichpage=-1
Wikipedia

quote:
_____
Originally posted by david_obsidian

The strategy that I would have liked to follow is to put up a very bare, unambitious article on AYP and have it accepted and let it lie low for a while before anything more ambitious is done. Maybe next time.
_____

Hi David:

It is not too late. But it can't be done quietly as you suggest, because if you are not linked within Wiki, you are flagged and there is no way to avoid the back room battle, at least at AYP's present level of "prominence." Still, with a half dozen or more people backing you up in the back rooms, it may be possible, most likely as an ongoing war.

But, honestly, if we are really on to what we think we are on to here, within a few years AYP will be on Wiki automatically. The national media will have to pick up on it first though. Wiki is pretty far behind the real world of yoga -- this one below the radar where the action is... :-)

The guru is in you.

2006/07/24 11:59:46
AYP Helpers
http://www.aypsite.org/forum/topic.asp?TOPIC_ID=1278&REPLY_ID=9827&whichpage=-1
Wikipedia

quote:
_____
Originally posted by Alvin Chan

One current suggestion is to write a detail and balanced article(with some history, quotes in the classics, etc) on kechari and include AYP as the external link. Include other books, of course, like the classics and Theos Bernard's books which teach the frenum snipping 40 years before yogani's (though not in that much detail). I'm sure this will do if the article is well-written.
_____

That's a good idea, Alvin. Would you like to try? See:

http://en.wikipedia.org/wiki/Kechari_mudra

If that one works, others could be tried, via external links to appropriate AYP lessons.

The guru is in you.

2006/07/24 16:34:51
AYP Helpers
http://www.aypsite.org/forum/topic.asp?TOPIC_ID=1278&REPLY_ID=9835&whichpage=-1
Wikipedia
Yes, great job, Alvin.

Other existing pages include kundalini, yoga sutras, tantra and asanas.

There are a lot of practices that are not covered in Wiki that are covered in AYP, and can be written up with historical background in scriptures, traditions and teachers. This was an idea I had in mind to do for linking back to an AYP page. They can also be done without an AYP page, like the kechari article was just done, assuming it sticks. Just go down the list on the AYP topic index and tie in the appropriate lessons to existing or new articles in a similar manner. Maybe start slow to make sure it will work. Don't want to have a lot of work deleted, like just happened.

There are no Wiki pages for Deep Meditation (only meditation), Spinal Breathing Pranayama (only pranayama), Siddhasana, Sambhavi, Mulabandha, Bastrika, Uddiyana, Nauli, Amaroli and most of the other practices we have here. This reveals how weak Wiki is on yoga -- what they have now is mostly sectarian fluff. We'd actually be doing them a favor by filling in on in-the-trenches practices. A nice project for a few someones, and educational too, because research would be necessary to pick up the additional sources to create non-biased articles, not to mention reviewing the corresponding AYP lessons. If one or two are done per week, it will add up over time.

Thanks, and good luck!

The guru is in you.

2006/07/24 16:53:21
AYP Helpers
http://www.aypsite.org/forum/topic.asp?TOPIC_ID=1278&REPLY_ID=9836&whichpage=-1
Wikipedia
Here is a reply to my note this AM. See Alvin, Wiki is not about "truth," but maybe something can still be done with it per above posts. Check the link below too for guidelines...

Response to Dear Wikians:

Yogani, your comment on the AfD shows you haven't really looked into precisely what Wikipedia is intended to be. An encyclopedia. Just like the dusty ones on the shelf. An encyclopedia summarizes published information. Its criteria is verifiability in published third-party sources, not truth. Also, writing an article about yourself is strongly discouraged. I see someone posted a welcome message for you, did you read any of the suggested material???

Of course, we welcome your verifiable contributions to articles on yoga, etc. but please take the time to read about what WP is supposed to be, what the criteria for inclusion are, and refrain from writing about yourself or your activities. And by the way, if you want to remain anonymous, an article on WP is the last thing you want. It would take only one person who knows who you are to add it to the article and then you could never remove it, as no one can own an article on WP, not even one about yourself. And if there is any verifiable or even unverifiable dirt or even nasty rumours about you, if you have even one enemy, you'll end up battling to keep that info out of the article and end up nominating the article for deletion yourself. It happens all the time when people post autobiographies... —Hanuman Das 13:07, 24 July 2006 (UTC)

Retrieved from http://en.wikipedia.org/wiki/User_talk:Yogani

2006/07/25 10:15:02
AYP Helpers
http://www.aypsite.org/forum/topic.asp?TOPIC_ID=1278&REPLY_ID=9849&whichpage=-1
Wikipedia
A note to Hanuman on his note above, and an encouraging reply:

Yogani to Hanuman:

Thank you, Hanuman Das. I am learning. Cannot help but notice a lack of articles on individual yoga practices in Wiki, let alone their integration into effective practice routines. Are verifiable articles on practices welcome? Also, can the Yogani article be placed on my user page with links intact? Can others edit that? Nothing to hide here ... no hidden agenda. In AYP, what you see is what you get. The guru is in you.
 Yogani 21:10, 24 July 2006 (UTC)

Hanuman to Yogani:

Yes, I think you have to ask an admin to move it, though. I think regular users can't move between namespaces, like from article space to user space. Put a note on the AfD (article for deletion) and the closing admin should be able to do it.
On article for individual yoga practices, postures, asanas, etc. I think that would be great. I wasn't even aware that so many were missing until getting involved in these AfDs... They are really needed and as long as references and citations are given, should be perfectly fine. If you have any problem with them let me know and I may be able to give you a hand with formatting or other details to make sure they are acceptable WP articles. —Hanuman Das 23:36, 24 July 2006 (UTC)
Retrieved from http://en.wikipedia.org/wiki/User_talk:Yogani

2006/07/28 15:51:59
AYP Helpers
http://www.aypsite.org/forum/topic.asp?TOPIC_ID=1278&REPLY_ID=9956&whichpage=-1
Wikipedia

Hi All:

Okay, the original AYP articles are both deleted now. Actually, the Yogani one has been moved to my user page, and I believe it is safe there for the time being. Hard to tell in the crazy Wiki world. :-)

http://en.wikipedia.org/wiki/User:Yogani
(previously edited by others -- article not entirely by me)

This user page gives some guidelines for anyone wishing to add articles on practices. All the red and brown links are missing articles on Wiki that we can do as and when we find time. Obviously, anything we write on practices should cite "notable" sources and have an AYP lesson link in the external links. Not sure if we can do more than that with AYP on Wiki, though we did manage to stay "notable" so far in the kechari mudra article. Time will tell...

Kindly place links here in this topic for any Wiki articles written, or for articles where AYP external links or other edits are added, like Trip and Alvin have done above. Those AYP external links on Wiki have stuck so far.

Many thanks!

The guru is in you.

2006/08/13 11:08:00
AYP Helpers
http://www.aypsite.org/forum/topic.asp?TOPIC_ID=1278&REPLY_ID=10449&whichpage=-1
Wikipedia

Very nice job, Trip. Thanks!

I will be amazed if it sticks, unless AYP/Yogani has become more "notable" in Wiki's eye over the past 30 days. Stranger things have happened in Wiki world. :-)

Failing to get an AYP article to stick on Wiki before, the strategy shifted to placing external links to relevant AYP lessons in articles on practices, and creating new articles on practices, using the Yogani user page (which seems to be a secure outpost) as a checklist for links to articles:

http://en.wikipedia.org/wiki/User:Yogani

As you can see by checking the practice links here, they don't have many articles on yoga practices on Wiki.

If your new article sticks, the links on practices could be duplicated in there over time also. We already have one good beachhead in the kechari article, and it links back to your article!

One thing is for sure. Anything I personally do on Wiki can raise red flags on "self promotion," so I have to be careful, sticking to new articles only on practices like the ones mentioned in the user profile linked above -- deep meditation, spinal breathing pranayama, etc. I have not had a chance to do any yet. Anyone who is so inclined, please feel free to take the lead...

The guru is in you.

2006/08/13 13:15:05
AYP Helpers
http://www.aypsite.org/forum/topic.asp?TOPIC_ID=1278&REPLY_ID=10455&whichpage=-1
Wikipedia

quote:
───────
Originally posted by Alvin Chan

When the name "yogani" is mentioned by someone else, it sounds much greater and more famous, isn't it? :-)
─────────

Maybe there are some advantages to mythologizing after all, though I'm sure David would disagree. :-)

The guru is in you.

2007/01/10 23:38:28
AYP Helpers
http://www.aypsite.org/forum/topic.asp?TOPIC_ID=1278&REPLY_ID=15771&whichpage=-1
Wikipedia

Hi All:

It should be mentioned that Brett never gave up on AYP's worthiness to be in Wikipedia, and after several go arounds since last summer, has convinced the powers that be that AYP belongs. As of today, the AYP page (enhanced) has been restored with deletion tags removed. Bravo!

http://en.wikipedia.org/wiki/Yogani

The guru is in you.

2007/01/11 00:08:29
AYP Helpers

http://www.aypsite.org/forum/topic.asp?TOPIC_ID=1278&REPLY_ID=15774&whichpage=-1
Wikipedia

quote:
_____
Originally posted by weaver

I say the same and thank you for your hard work Brett!

(The first external link should probably point to http://www.aypsite.org?)
_____

Hi Weaver:

Brett used the Geocities site because it does not have the AYP book covers on it. Wiki frowns on articles that point to "advertising." Nevermind that "notables" like Chopra and Tolle are selling stuff all over their websites. The difference between them and us is that they have been on Oprah -- we don't want to rush into that one. :-)

The guru is in you.

2007/01/16 11:37:21
AYP Helpers
http://www.aypsite.org/forum/topic.asp?TOPIC_ID=1278&REPLY_ID=16190&whichpage=-1
Wikipedia

quote:
_____
Originally posted by Etherfish

Why is it being considered for deletion? Is it because of lack of citations from relevent third party sources?
Are there articles about yogani or AYP? maybe the radio interviews would help?
_____

Hi Ether:

Yes, third party interviews and reports is the primary shortcoming we have with Wikipedia, particularly in magazines and newspapers. There is currently nothing suitable out there in the print media in the way of independent articles on AYP.

The radio interviews will help, but what we really need is independent articles in print that can be referenced.

If anyone here has a background in public relations, especially in setting up interviews for print publications, then we could sure use your help. I am willing if willing interviewers can be found.

The guru is in you.

2006/08/21 10:31:26
AYP Helpers
http://www.aypsite.org/forum/topic.asp?TOPIC_ID=1289&REPLY_ID=10760&whichpage=-1
Minimal donation list

Hi All:

The interest in supporting the AYP work is very much appreciated.

As you may know, AYP is already set up on Paypal here:
https://www.paypal.com/cgi-bin/webscr?cmd=_xclick&business=yogani99%40yahoo%2ecom&item_name=Donation%20to%20Advanced%20Yoga%20Practices&no_shipping=0&no_note=1&tax=0&cy_code=USD&bn=PP%2dDonationsBF&charset=UTF%2d8

There is no fee to the sender on Paypal, only to the recipient, which is $.30 + 2.9% of the amount. If a currency translation is involved, an additonal 2.5% is charged if on the recipient's end. All of that is a pretty big chunk out of a $2.00 donation, but still appreciated. I do not believe Paypal has the ability for periodic automatic payments.

Bank transfers are another matter, not familiar with exact charges there, but you can be sure there are some -- perhaps similar to Paypal. In any case, the bank account number here is not available except for special situations. Same for snail mail address to AYP Publishing. Where there is the will, there is a way.

Thank you, and all the best!

The guru is in you.

2006/07/28 16:29:00
AYP Helpers
http://www.aypsite.org/forum/topic.asp?TOPIC_ID=1366
MySpace, Zaadz and other Online Communities

766 –   Advanced Yoga Practices

Hi All:

Does anyone have experience on http://www.myspace.com?

Would this be a good place to establish a presence for AYP like Trip did on Zaadz?

http://ayp.zaadz.com (nice job, Trip!)

The reason I ask is because I read recently that the U.S. army is recruiting on MySpace. There must be a lot of young people there.

Better they join the yoga army, yes? :-)

The guru is in you.

2006/07/29 10:40:02
AYP Helpers
http://www.aypsite.org/forum/topic.asp?TOPIC_ID=1366&REPLY_ID=9983&whichpage=-1
MySpace, Zaadz and other Online Communities

Thank you for your feedback, Kathy and Scott.

You know, we all own the present, but the future belongs to the young. I'm not sure most of us realize that until we get old and think, "Oh, did we do that?" :-)

So I would be very happy to see many young people pick up the ball for the sake of the spiritual destiny of humanity. Who else can do it?

Thank you, Scott, for doing so. I'm sure we can find a way into the colleges too, and every other nook and cranny of human enterprise, because self-directed to-the-point spiritual development makes so much sense.

It has been said, "The best ideas are the ones that are implemented."

Go for it!

The title of this topic has been expanded to accommodate. There are no limits to what you can accomplish in this life...

The guru is in you.

2006/07/30 10:38:50
AYP Helpers
http://www.aypsite.org/forum/topic.asp?TOPIC_ID=1366&REPLY_ID=10030&whichpage=-1
MySpace, Zaadz and other Online Communities

Hi Scott:

I don't see an external link to the AYP site there. If it is permitted, the one to use is:

http://www.aypsite.com

Thanks for doing this.

Trip, are there liabilities in being on MySpace?

The guru is in you.

2006/10/05 10:33:57
AYP Helpers
http://www.aypsite.org/forum/topic.asp?TOPIC_ID=1568&REPLY_ID=11932&whichpage=-1
Myspace
Nice job, Hunter.

The diversity of links is especially good, offering readers multiple alternatives for finding their way in, according to their interest. We have lots of doors these days, and more coming. :-)

Thank you very much.

The guru is in you.

2006/12/20 13:32:27
AYP Helpers
http://www.aypsite.org/forum/topic.asp?TOPIC_ID=1568&REPLY_ID=14654&whichpage=-1
Myspace

quote:
_____
Originally posted by Hunter

Yogani,
Someone has posted a comment for you that I wanted you to read:

"yogani, in your teachings there is something rare and precious,
and at the same time, something universal, and intimate to all life. your websight is a tremendous resource, i can't thank you enough -
wahn luhv -agon"

Posted by: http://www.myspace.com/agonmizelle
_____

Thank you, Hunter.

That is a very kind note, and is much appreciated. You have been doing a great job over there on MySpace, helping folks find open resources here for paving their own way along the path.

The guru is in you.

2006/11/13 09:15:54
AYP Helpers
http://www.aypsite.org/forum/topic.asp?TOPIC_ID=1706&REPLY_ID=13243&whichpage=-1
Testers Needed! -- Yogani Interview Recording

Hi Trip:

Works great here too, on old Win98 technology -- tested on both MSIE and Firefox. The latter required a flash player plug-in download which took about 10 seconds.

Has anyone tried the Mac?

Good job. This is just what we need. So everyone will know, we are also looking into mp3 "Podcast" downloads as an additional option.

The guru is in you.

2006/12/03 17:09:58
AYP Helpers
http://www.aypsite.org/forum/topic.asp?TOPIC_ID=1782&REPLY_ID=14030&whichpage=-1
Updating websites?

Hi Christi:

Oh, how nice it would be to do that. However, each website is a little different for good reasons and requires unique attention when updating. Besides that, each site is stand alone, so if one goes down the others will still be there.

In addition to the websites, we do have some forwarded links. Try these: http://www.advancedyogapractices.com and http://www.secretsofwilder.com

All of that aside, the underlying reason why lesson posting has slowed down is because the focus here has shifted to book writing over the past year, and will stay there for another year or two. By then, I am hoping AYP will be self-supporting and we can do a lot more web stuff, typing fingers able. :-)

Thanks much for the suggestions. New ideas are always welcome!

The guru is in you.

2006/12/04 11:32:47
AYP Helpers
http://www.aypsite.org/forum/topic.asp?TOPIC_ID=1786&REPLY_ID=14068&whichpage=-1
AYP Forum 2.0? -- RSS

Hi Kirtanman and Wolfgang:

The Snitz forum software has many more features than we are currently using -- just about everything you mentioned. The options have been kept to a bare minimum in the current setup for simplicity's sake, to save on server storage and bandwidth, and to minimize hacker/spammer/virus invasions (they are always trying to break in, and we have a pretty good system in place now for preventing it).

Maybe other Snitz features will be turned on someday. If you want to see more of what Snitz can do, go to the link at the bottom of this page. It is open source freeware -- not counting hosting and upkeep.

Transforming what we have here to another forum software and database would be a large technical challenge, not to mention an administrative nightmare, so I don't think that is in the cards. Just increasing the options turned on here in Snitz would add considerable upkeep and administration -- not something I can entertain right now. In the digital world, things are seldom as simple as they seem, under the hood that is. :-)

Thanks for the suggestions. Keep the good ideas coming!

The guru is in you.

2006/12/06 12:01:29
AYP Helpers
http://www.aypsite.org/forum/topic.asp?TOPIC_ID=1786&REPLY_ID=14162&whichpage=-1

AYP Forum 2.0? -- RSS

Hi Kirtanman and All:

I am very interested in any sort of web "viral marketing" programs (RSS and others -- but not spam or unsolicited popups) that could be set up to increase AYP visibility -- preferably the online lessons before the forums, for clarity sake for newcomers.

But I have no time to implement such a thing myself. Any volunteers? :-)

Many thanks!

The guru is in you.

PS -- Having said that, the place to check about an RSS mod for Snitz is with the Snitz folks. It is probably available already. They have every other kind of mod. But remember what I said about AYP forum upgrades in the near term.

But tasteful (non-invasive) technology for spreading the word on AYP far and wide? Oh yes! :-)

2006/12/06 16:00:18
AYP Helpers
http://www.aypsite.org/forum/topic.asp?TOPIC_ID=1786&REPLY_ID=14172&whichpage=-1
AYP Forum 2.0? -- RSS

quote:
_____
Originally posted by Athma_Shakti

Dear Yogani

having vast experience in developing web based sys, i will be happy to offer volunteership to aypsite :-)
_____

Hi AthmaShakti:

That's great. Thank you. What do you recommend for "viral marketing" that will not eat the webmaster (little me) alive? :-)

The guru is in you.

2006/12/06 19:13:02
AYP Helpers
http://www.aypsite.org/forum/topic.asp?TOPIC_ID=1786&REPLY_ID=14182&whichpage=-1
AYP Forum 2.0? -- RSS
PS: Just a reminder that we have what some have called a pretty good "AYP ambassador" in the form of the radio interview -- 45 minutes long, 20MB downloadable MP3. http://www.aypsite.com/audio.html

The more file sharing that can be done with this the better.

The guru is in you.

2006/12/07 10:26:02
AYP Helpers
http://www.aypsite.org/forum/topic.asp?TOPIC_ID=1786&REPLY_ID=14195&whichpage=-1
AYP Forum 2.0? -- RSS

quote:
_____
Originally posted by Anthem11

Any news Yogani if you will be doing this again?
_____

Hi Andrew:

Tentatively, I am to be on the same show every Sunday evening in January. It will be announced when it is firm.

Or did I just announce it? :-)

The guru is in you.

2006/12/08 07:03:21
AYP Helpers
http://www.aypsite.org/forum/topic.asp?TOPIC_ID=1786&REPLY_ID=14235&whichpage=-1
AYP Forum 2.0? -- RSS

quote:
_____

viral marketing is a powerful technique to reach the media easily using email broadcasts, IM's, pop's etc..

this will increase number of hits/users also the traffic/load of the server.

and for webmasters and moderators maintaining the forums is the difficult think in the world haha.

Hi AthmaShakti:

Can you suggest specific programs you can implement yourself? If so, those would be much welcome.

Unsolicited email, IMs, popups or desktop icons are not appropriate -- these are spam.

AYP supporter produced "opt in" marketing programs are what we want, like networking sites (all of them), shared files (interview), links (but not "link exchange" spam), maybe RSS, etc.

Kirtanman, on RSS, I will look into it with Ruirib, our Snitz consultant, and see what can be done. The Taobums RSS only produces a page of code here, maybe because I am still on Win98. This old computer is a well-oiled publishing machine that only requires the writing itself to do it all. Would not want to reinvent that on a new machine until the books are done. Same with the forums and anything else that is working reasonably well on the existing AYP sites. It is a matter of maintaining maximum productivity and efficiency over the next 18 months or so -- a lot of writing still to do!

But spreading the word/marketing programs? Yes, we need much more of it. For that, many hands make light work. :-)

Many thanks to all!

The guru is in you.

2006/12/08 11:34:00
AYP Helpers
http://www.aypsite.org/forum/topic.asp?TOPIC_ID=1786&REPLY_ID=14241&whichpage=-1
AYP Forum 2.0? -- RSS

Hi Kirtanman:

With some checking, come to find that a reader download is needed for RSS for most computers, and neither Taobums nor Snitz RSS cue the user for that. What you end up with instead is a page full of code. Therefore, it would appear RSS is not ready for the teeming masses out there yet, which is the only reason I would be interested at this time. Maybe later when universality has been better-established.

Unless I am missing something?

The guru is in you.

2006/12/08 16:12:53
AYP Helpers
http://www.aypsite.org/forum/topic.asp?TOPIC_ID=1786&REPLY_ID=14249&whichpage=-1
AYP Forum 2.0? -- RSS

quote:

Originally posted by Wolfgang

quote:

Originally posted by yogani

Unless I am missing something?

May be an isssue of operating system (WIN98)
Or a browser issue ?
L&L
Wolfgang

Hi Wolfgang:

I was given to understand that a reader download is needed by many for RSS. I have both MSIE and Firefox here, neither is that far out of date (even though the operating system is old), and neither works with RSS.

Well, one way to settle it is to see who can see this and who can't:

http://www.aypsite.org/forum/rss1.asp

What does everyone say?

I just don't think we should be putting up a feature that will confuse lots of folks, and not be useful for spreading the word.

On another matter, your request for gender identification in the member profile did not go unnoticed. It was deliberately left out from the beginning so no one would feel pressured to reveal more about themselves than they wish. If it were active, the gender question would not be mandatory, but just having it there could send the wrong message, particularly in view of some of the subject matter we are covering here. Keep in mind that many experiences are being shared here that have rarely been revealed in public before, and with very good benefits so far. We do not wish to jade it in any way. Less on exactly who is doing the sharing can be more! Those who want to reveal their gender will find a way ... that has been the philosophy so far, and it seems to work. "If it ain't broke, don't fix it." :-)

The guru is in you.

2006/12/09 11:01:22
AYP Helpers
http://www.aypsite.org/forum/topic.asp?TOPIC_ID=1786&REPLY_ID=14286&whichpage=-1
AYP Forum 2.0? -- RSS

Hi All:

I'm afraid I don't have a clue what all this RSS talk is about. If we can't show a simple icon that <u>everyone</u> can point and click for the result, it will not be implemented here. It is as simple as that.

But feel free to use the beta link above.

If at some point it becomes a simple point and click feature for everyone, then let me know. Keep in mind that administrative time available here for setting up and operating this sort of program is zero. So if it is going to be done, someone else has to do it. Right now it looks like a can of worms.

Sorry, that's just how it is at this stage of AYP development. It is as much about the offline stuff as the online stuff, and there are only so many hours in the day.

The guru is in you.

2006/12/09 17:10:16
AYP Helpers
http://www.aypsite.org/forum/topic.asp?TOPIC_ID=1786&REPLY_ID=14307&whichpage=-1
AYP Forum 2.0? -- RSS

Hi All:

Our Snitz consultant must have removed it today. I have been away. Would anyone like it back?

The guru is in you.

2006/12/09 17:54:22
AYP Helpers
http://www.aypsite.org/forum/topic.asp?TOPIC_ID=1786&REPLY_ID=14314&whichpage=-1
AYP Forum 2.0? -- RSS

quote:

Originally posted by Athma_Shakti

Hi Yogani

yes it will be helpful to develop the reader.

AthmaShakti: Sorry about that. I'll see about having it put back.

Christi: That is very telling. Up-to-date XP/IE not seeing it either?

The guru is in you.

2006/12/10 10:40:12
AYP Helpers
http://www.aypsite.org/forum/topic.asp?TOPIC_ID=1786&REPLY_ID=14363&whichpage=-1
AYP Forum 2.0? -- RSS

Hi All:

I hope everyone is aware that there is an "active topics" link at the top of this page that pulls up all new posts (by topic) since the last visit. Any past time period can be selected as well. Using the pink folders on the main page is not a very reliable way of finding new postings. It does not always reflect reality.

As for RSS, I'll stand by the assertion that any link we place on public AYP pages must work in all browsers that can see the page, either as direct information, or a prompt to download a reader (like our recent addition of flash audio does). Keep in mind that AYP is being viewed on computers all over the world of every operating system and browser type, both new and old. The gig is global and not everyone has the latest whiz-bang browser, or has the ability to get it.

The guru is in you.

2006/12/11 11:20:52
AYP Helpers
http://www.aypsite.org/forum/topic.asp?TOPIC_ID=1786&REPLY_ID=14400&whichpage=-1
AYP Forum 2.0? -- RSS

Hi AthmaShakti:

It works!

Excuse me for asking, but isn't all of this RSS stuff redundant with the more robust forum "active topics" feature, which can be bookmarked by anyone?

On the HTML side, all new AYP lessons are transmitted via Yahoo group email. Anyone who wants them hot off the press can sign up for email delivery on Yahoo. New lessons are also announced on the website homepage, which links to a reverse chronological index of lessons for easy reference from the present going backwards. This is in addition to the chronological lesson indices on the website (links above). I am told setting up RSS for HTML can be a big job, something completely different from the forum RSS. How much additional navigation will be gained per hour of setup work?

Navigation has been a priority as AYP has grown, and that is why we have all that has been mentioned, plus topic index, site search, etc.

It is still not clear what practical addition this exciting and time consuming RSS discussion is leading to. Well, maybe the forum RSS holds some promise, though redundant, as mentioned, and a little tedious. :-)

The guru is in you.

2006/12/11 13:01:07
AYP Helpers
http://www.aypsite.org/forum/topic.asp?TOPIC_ID=1786&REPLY_ID=14404&whichpage=-1
AYP Forum 2.0? -- RSS

quote:
_____
Originally posted by Kirtanman

Hi Yogani,

"All will be revealed ...!"

:-)

Patiently continue your study (Googling technology terms), and your daily practices (spending time online), and before long, you will notice a new conductivity (aka enthusiasm) arising in your system ("Hey, this weird acronym-heavy Web technology is really kinda cool!") combined with a silent awareness of deeper technology truth ("Whoa ... I understand RSS! I really do! On to SaaS, SOA, AJAX, Etc. Etc. Etc.")

This awareness and energy is not to be found solely in people such as Athma Shakti, Ruirib and myself -- but is in you, as well.

And formal teachers of technology are no longer needed ("Google is our friend.") - you can chart your own course, and captain your own development - for in reality, the technology geek with the answers is not "out there" somewhere .....

The geek is in you.

PNW2*,

Kirtanman

*Peace, Namaste & Web 2.0 - I had to work a tech-ish acronym into the sign-off, somehow!

THIS POST HAS BEEN BROUGHT TO YOU BY THE "SORRY I HAD TO" DEPARTMENT OF KIRTANMAN'S MIND.

:-)
_____

I will have to give up yoga for this, and move into one of those tech caves where they slide a pizza under the door once a day. :-)

TGIIY

2006/12/11 13:08:45
AYP Helpers
http://www.aypsite.org/forum/topic.asp?TOPIC_ID=1786&REPLY_ID=14405&whichpage=-1
AYP Forum 2.0? -- RSS
PS: By all means, go out there and build lots of feeds to AYP! :-)

2006/12/12 13:42:20
AYP Helpers
http://www.aypsite.org/forum/topic.asp?TOPIC_ID=1786&REPLY_ID=14437&whichpage=-1
AYP Forum 2.0? -- RSS

quote:
_____
Originally posted by Athma_Shakti

Hi Yogani

Sure active topics can also be used.

yes various enhancements and navigation capabilities can be done in both sides(user/server).
----

it seems RSS may not be compatible here.

It was a good team work from all of us. I thanx for everyone in this thread, Yogani, RSS generators(is an intricate process), and Kirtanman who took the initiative.
_____

Hi AthmaShakti:

Thanks much for the work you have done on this. I hope you will leave the RSS reader up there on Geocities for anyone who would like to download it. Perhaps someday we will get into customized RSS to show things that are not easily accessible in the forums now. Obviously, a 10 post history is not going to cover everything that has gone on even in one day's time, but I'm sure there are things RSS can do that "active topics" cannot. Your work will not go to waste. Nothing ever does, especially in our yoga practices. :-)

All the best!

The guru is in you.

2006/12/12 14:27:15
AYP Helpers
http://www.aypsite.org/forum/topic.asp?TOPIC_ID=1786&REPLY_ID=14439&whichpage=-1
AYP Forum 2.0? -- RSS
PS -- Kirtanman, make my pizza veggie, and hold the onions. Juice is preferred over soda. How do they get the drink under the door? :-)
2008/03/15 18:18:31
AYP Helpers
http://www.aypsite.org/forum/topic.asp?TOPIC_ID=1786&REPLY_ID=31344&whichpage=-1
AYP Forum 2.0? -- RSS

Hi Jupiter:

Thanks for bringing this up. If RSS is something that can be useful to the readership, I'll be happy to add a link on all the website and forum pages, perhaps near the top of the right-hand border.

I am a few years behind most folks with technology here, hopefully making up for it in other ways.

What does the RSS link you found show? Is it one that would be useful to readers for keeping up with new forum postings? I don't recall who created it, and would not know how to edit it or make a better one, if needed. Do you know how?

Thanks!

The guru is in you.

2008/03/16 13:30:54
AYP Helpers
http://www.aypsite.org/forum/topic.asp?TOPIC_ID=1786&REPLY_ID=31374&whichpage=-1
AYP Forum 2.0? -- RSS
PS: The RSS Feed link has been added to the upper right corner of all website and forum pages. Thanks much for the heads up, Jupiter! :-)

2008/03/16 14:07:16
AYP Helpers
http://www.aypsite.org/forum/topic.asp?TOPIC_ID=1786&REPLY_ID=31377&whichpage=-1
AYP Forum 2.0? -- RSS

Hi Echo:

From what little I know, you need a late model browser (Firefox 2.0 can be downloaded for free), Google Reader (add the feed link as a new subscription there), or other live feed reader.

Firefox 2.0 works here and it updates new posts immediately. Google Reader works here too but has not been updating immediately.

I am sure others with experience can add useful pointers.

Good luck!

The guru is in you.

2008/03/16 19:19:54
AYP Helpers
http://www.aypsite.org/forum/topic.asp?TOPIC_ID=1786&REPLY_ID=31387&whichpage=-1
AYP Forum 2.0? -- RSS

Thanks much, Jupiter.

The Google Reader does not update the feed in real time here like Firefox does. Only every few hours.

We have had some intermittent delays with the RSS link. That is being looked at, so bear with us.

I will see about adding the icon.

How are live feeds shared in social networks, etc? Can you offer some advice on that to AYP forum readers? The more we can spread this around (ethically and legally), the better. :-)

All the best!

The guru is in you.

2008/03/17 13:53:11
AYP Helpers
http://www.aypsite.org/forum/topic.asp?TOPIC_ID=1786&REPLY_ID=31414&whichpage=-1
AYP Forum 2.0? -- RSS

Thanks Jupiter and Echo:

Great stuff!

I'll add a few updates to the RSS announcement page reflecting your comments, and add a "help link" under the RSS link leading to the announcement page.

All the best!

The guru is in you

2007/01/10 23:21:40
AYP Helpers
http://www.aypsite.org/forum/topic.asp?TOPIC_ID=1891&REPLY_ID=15770&whichpage=-1
Lesson 141 - AYP Articles - Hindustan Times, India

quote:
_____
Originally posted by Shanti

Hi Yogani,
I wonder if there is a way for you to post that article or make another lesson of it and point lesson 141 to this new lesson or change this lesson to show the article?... or would there be copyright issues?
_____

Hi Shanti:

I'm afraid that the Hindustan Times article on "Bhakti - Science of Devotion" has been lost. It was one of two that came and went on their server in 2004-5, and I do not have a backup for the Bhakti one. However, the article was an abridged version of lesson 67, so the the original content is still here. Lesson 67 is linked in lesson 141 already.

The other article was from lesson 132 -- "What is Sin?" I do have an image file of that one.

Now that we have AYP books available in India Editions, more articles can make a much bigger difference, and we are working on that.

The guru is in you.

2007/01/17 12:03:51
AYP Helpers
http://www.aypsite.org/forum/topic.asp?TOPIC_ID=1891&REPLY_ID=16234&whichpage=-1
Lesson 141 - AYP Articles - Hindustan Times, India
PS: A note has been added to lesson 141 regarding this issue: http://www.aypsite.org/141.html

2007/04/12 16:23:58
AYP Helpers
http://www.aypsite.org/forum/topic.asp?TOPIC_ID=1891&REPLY_ID=20269&whichpage=-1

Lesson 141 - AYP Articles - Hindustan Times, India

Thank you, David and Jim, and Gray for bringing this up originally.

I have placed both of the Hindustan Times articles on the AYP server, accessible at this link: http://www.aypsite.org/hindustan.html

Lesson 141 has also been updated.

The guru is in you.

2007/01/17 12:20:52
AYP Helpers
http://www.aypsite.org/forum/topic.asp?TOPIC_ID=1963
Public Relations Assistance Needed -- Print Media

Hi All:

The post below has been copied from the Wikipedia topic to highlight the need for assistance in setting up AYP print media interviews. All help is appreciated! :-)
----

quote:
_____
Originally posted by Etherfish

Why is it being considered for deletion? Is it because of lack of citations from relevent third party sources?
Are there articles about yogani or AYP? maybe the radio interviews would help?
_____

Hi Ether:

Yes, third party interviews and reports is the primary shortcoming we have with Wikipedia, particularly in magazines and newspapers. There is currently nothing suitable out there in the print media in the way of independent articles on AYP.

The radio interviews will help, but what we really need is independent articles in print that can be referenced.

If anyone here has a background in public relations, especially in setting up interviews for print publications, then we could sure use your help. I am willing if willing interviewers can be found.

The guru is in you.

2007/01/17 17:28:34
AYP Helpers
http://www.aypsite.org/forum/topic.asp?TOPIC_ID=1963&REPLY_ID=16242&whichpage=-1
Public Relations Assistance Needed -- Print Media

Hi Kirtanman:

Great suggestions, and I'm interested in all, as long as we can do it tastefully in relation to the AYP website and writings. Do not want to appear to be blatantly self-promoting. Frankly, it as about making AYP more visible, not me, and that is why I am willing to do the PR stuff, within reasonable limits.

So, we want to be available, but not throwing ourselves at the media in "red light district" fashion. It is a fine line to walk. Within that framework, I think we can do everything you have suggested, and more.

At this time I'd like to limit interviews to telephone or online text only. Also, there is little to no funding available here for this. The implementation of the worldwide AYP awareness strategy continues on a shoestring.

Contact me with specifics whenever you can. Perhaps you and Brett can work together to come up with something suitable for the AYP website, and for the appropriate direct channels to the print media.

Anyone else please feel free to chime in on this. Anybody from a national magazine or newspaper reading here? :-)

Many thanks!

The guru is in you.

2007/01/23 12:50:06
AYP Helpers
http://www.aypsite.org/forum/topic.asp?TOPIC_ID=1978&REPLY_ID=16406&whichpage=-1
paying it forward - amazon reviews

Hi Cosmic:

Thank you very much for those beautiful reviews.

Amazon reviews make a huge difference. It is one of the easiest and most effective ways to help out AYP. Write them from the stillness of heart, in truth.

Samyama anyone? :-)

The guru is in you.

2007/05/15 12:35:02
AYP Helpers
http://www.aypsite.org/forum/topic.asp?TOPIC_ID=2567
AYP Books Page Upgraded - Feedback?

Hi All:

After some offline suggestions and months of mulling, some upgrading on the AYP Books Page has been done. The idea is to give people more information on the books to help in the decision-making process.

To that end, the following has been added for each book:

1. A link to a separate page with description, table of contents and collected Amazon reviews (multi-site/country).

2. A "Read Sample Now" link to a PDF selection.

3. A "Hear Sample Now" link to an MP3 selection (Deep Meditation now, and the rest of the Enlightenment Series books as they come out in AudioBook format this year). The link is currently direct to to an MP3 file, but will be converted to flash audio soon (like the radio interviews) with no wait for loading.

All of these links open new windows, so the books page is not closed during the additional reading/listening.

The AYP Easy Lessons book and Secrets of Wilder short descriptions on the books page have also been fine tuned to be more engaging.

Any feedback on these upgrades plus suggestions for additional improvements are welcome.

Thanks!

The guru is in you.

2007/05/15 13:03:43
AYP Helpers
http://www.aypsite.org/forum/topic.asp?TOPIC_ID=2567&REPLY_ID=21920&whichpage=-1
AYP Books Page Upgraded - Feedback?

quote:
_____
Originally posted by Jim and His Karma

In my browser, the right hand margin of the text seems excessively to the left, making the text column unnecessarily narrow and wasting lots of empty space to the right (before the book cover column).
_____

Hi Jim:

What is your operating system and browser version? And which of the pages are doing that? The pages have been tested in Windows Internet Explorer 6.0 and FireFox 2.0, without having that issue.

We would like to fix it so these pages work properly in all the operating systems and browsers.

The guru is in you.

2007/05/15 14:58:31
AYP Helpers
http://www.aypsite.org/forum/topic.asp?TOPIC_ID=2567&REPLY_ID=21933&whichpage=-1
AYP Books Page Upgraded - Feedback?
Jim & Richard:

Does it do it on this page too? http://www.aypsite.org/books.html
That is the books page before the upgrade.

Thanks!

TGIIY
2007/05/15 15:23:00
AYP Helpers
http://www.aypsite.org/forum/topic.asp?TOPIC_ID=2567&REPLY_ID=21936&whichpage=-1
AYP Books Page Upgraded - Feedback?
Okay, so we don't have to go back to the old page to correct the issue. We will go forward with the new page and fix it! :-)

Will check back here once we think it is fixed.

Any more thoughts on books page strategy and content are welcome. Glad you liked the extra material, Richard.

The idea is to make the books page an interesting place to explore, beyond the online lessons and forums. Who knows, if people hang around there long enough, they might even order something. That would be okay. :-)

The guru is in you.

2007/05/15 15:52:41
AYP Helpers
http://www.aypsite.org/forum/topic.asp?TOPIC_ID=2567&REPLY_ID=21946&whichpage=-1
AYP Books Page Upgraded - Feedback?
Hi:

With some additional offline feedback, what I am hearing is that it is the difference between old screen and wide screen monitors. The AYP website is old screen format, and looks fine on old (narrow) screens. However, the book cover column on the right side (MS Frontpage border) will automatically (usually) go to the right hand edge of the monitor (any monitor), and the text margins will stay the same in narrow screen format. So the wider the screen the bigger the space between the book covers column and the text. All the pages on the website should have this configuration. Is that the case, Jim and Richard?

Meanwhile, anyone with an old screen monitor (narrow) should not see the big space in the middle between the text and book cover column.

Someday, we will convert the website to widescreen format, but not this week. It is nearly 400 pages of HTML! :-)

Most importantly, the text and associated links should be in the correct configuration on any computer, even if on the left side of a wide screen. If anyone has a problem matching up text and links to the corresponding books, or if things are out of alignment in a way that makes navigation difficult or is aesthetically unacceptable, let me know.

The guru is in you.

2007/05/30 16:32:35
AYP Helpers
http://www.aypsite.org/forum/topic.asp?TOPIC_ID=2567&REPLY_ID=22579&whichpage=-1
AYP Books Page Upgraded - Feedback?

Hi All:

The AYP book covers in the right hand border of every page on the web site now link directly to the corresponding books on the books page. From there you can go to individual book descriptions, tables of contents, reading and listening samples, and to book sellers around the world.

Also, Amazon USA has revamped the layout of reviews for all books to be much more favorable -- highlighting popular reviews, plus providing stats on all reviews. Feel free to add a review or two, if you have not done so already. Thanks! :-)

The guru is in you.

2007/05/30 16:21:54
AYP Helpers
http://www.aypsite.org/forum/topic.asp?TOPIC_ID=2621
AYP Artwork

Hi All:

Thought you might find this interesting -- promotional artwork used for ads in Canada:

http://www.aypsite.org/images/AYP-Canada-image.pdf
(click left to view, or click right to download)

Pretty modern, and much more attention-grabbing than the utilitarian AYP books flyer. :-)
http://www.aypsite.org/11-AYP-Flyer-5-2-06.pdf

Feel free to use either of these. There is some more promotional artwork (business cards and animated banner) at the bottom of the AYP books page.

Thoughts? Does anyone else have AYP artwork? If so, please point us to it. I believe there is more of it out there.

Anyone wanting to put together new AYP artwork let me know. We can make it available here also.

The guru is in you.

2007/06/02 15:56:25
AYP Helpers
http://www.aypsite.org/forum/topic.asp?TOPIC_ID=2621&REPLY_ID=22688&whichpage=-1
AYP Artwork

quote:
───────
Originally posted by Etherfish

Do you have any pictures of yourself with a cape in a flying position? ha ha just kidding.

The artwork is cool. Where does it come from? A member in Canada made it, or ???
Where is it used; in a magazine in Canada eh?
_____

Hi Ether:

No cape here :-), but I did add the "Flying Yogini" AYP Poster to the free download promotional materials on the bottom of the books page.

The artwork was done by someone in BC, Canada who is running print ads for AYP there, which is much appreciated. It looks like the same artwork may be used throughout India to help promote the new AYP India Editions there.

It never ceases to amaze how yoga begins in India, comes over here, and then goes back to India, flying yogini and all. Full circle...

Hey, whatever works to open the inner doorways worldwide to the divine flow. :-)

The guru is in you.

2007/06/03 13:28:15
AYP Helpers
http://www.aypsite.org/forum/topic.asp?TOPIC_ID=2621&REPLY_ID=22721&whichpage=-1
AYP Artwork

Thank you, All.

Yes, please feel free to print and send our yogini flying everywhere. :-)

Glad you like the new forum layout, Meg. The addition of the book cover border in the forums has been a long time coming. I did not want to do it until we could be sending folks to a much more interesting and informative books page, which we now have, and we will continue to build on it. Plus, I wanted to be sure we would not be crowding the forums space-wise on the page with a border. With most computers shifting to widescreen, the space situation is much better, so I feel okay adding the border now. And it is not too bad on my old 600x800 screen either. A couple of the smudged images will be cleaned up soon, and then I think we will have it in shape.

Comments and suggestions are always welcome.

All the best!

The guru is in you.

2007/06/04 10:24:19
AYP Helpers
http://www.aypsite.org/forum/topic.asp?TOPIC_ID=2621&REPLY_ID=22748&whichpage=-1
AYP Artwork

Hi All:

Would anyone be interested in handing out the AYP "flying yogini" at this yoga conference coming up in July:

Yogacharya Festival (honoring BKS Iyengar)
Santa Clara, California (near San Francisco)
July 9-15, 2007

Attendance is expected to be over 1,500. It is a great opportunity to introduce many hatha yoga practitioners to AYP.

Thanks!

The guru is in you.

2007/06/04 16:51:54
AYP Helpers
http://www.aypsite.org/forum/topic.asp?TOPIC_ID=2621&REPLY_ID=22766&whichpage=-1
AYP Artwork
PS: Just got the word that the AYP books will be displayed in the bookstore booth at the Yogacharya Festival.

The festival bookstore is being hosted by East West Bookstore of Mountainview, CA. Thank you, East West!

The guru is in you.

2008/10/09 15:57:41
AYP Helpers
http://www.aypsite.org/forum/topic.asp?TOPIC_ID=2621&REPLY_ID=38745&whichpage=-1
AYP Artwork

Hi All:

Just a note to let you know that the AYP Books Flyer has been updated to have more information, and is now on one PDF page instead of four pages, so it is much easier to view, print and download: http://www.aypsite.com/11-AYP-Flyer-5-2-06.pdf How is that for efficiency? :-)

A link for it can also be found near the bottom of the AYP Books Page, along with links for other promotional materials.

All the best!

The guru is in you.

PS: I am going to remove the ivory background shortly, so it can be printed more easily on white or colored paper.

2008/10/10 13:04:55
AYP Helpers
http://www.aypsite.org/forum/topic.asp?TOPIC_ID=2621&REPLY_ID=38766&whichpage=-1
AYP Artwork

quote:
_____
Originally posted by Christi
_____

Hi Yogani,

Nice new Canadian poster. She looks like she is levitating, or is that just some clever Photoshop thing? :-)

Christi
_____

Hi Christi:

I did not do the flying AYP yogini image. It came from someone who ran some ads with it in B.C., Canada. It is actually a couple of years old. It is a nice image, so it was added with the others at the bottom of the books page. If anyone out there has other AYP artwork that has been developed, let me know.

Btw, the new one page AYP books flyer now has a white background, so it can be easily printed on light colored paper. I usually use ivory (like the webpage background here), but everyone is encouraged to be creative and pass them out everywhere. :-)

All the best!

The guru is in you.

2007/09/05 15:37:50
AYP Helpers
http://www.aypsite.org/forum/topic.asp?TOPIC_ID=2898
Tips on Starting & Running an AYP Meditation Group

Hi All:

The following comes from email interchanges with Meg on starting and running an AYP meditation group in New York City. It is hoped other meditation group leaders around the world will chime in here with their feedback as well.

Comments from anyone interested in starting or joining a meditation group are welcome also.

The guru is in you.

. **Meg wrote:**

I'd like to get some advice on my meditation group. As you may know, I've started a med. group in my loft, but it's been pretty weak. A friend of mine who has a large penthouse office in midtown Manhattan is interested in learning to meditate, and has offered his space for free for me to start a group. It's a fantastic location, near the trains and buses, and I'm really excited to see what comes of it. I'm going to begin by advertising on Craig's List (which I didn't feel comfortable doing at my own place), and see where it goes.

We're going to start next week and I'm in the process of composing the ad. I could keep it generic ("Come meditate in a peaceful environment...discover inner silence...") The group would be more about building a spiritual community and less about the systematic cultivation of energy. It's a more predictable route to go, and for me, a beginner myself, probably the safer route. But I'm not so interested in predictability, and I feel pulled to move into the energy work. I'm not talking about diving in head first, but to follow the AYP book as a group, methodically building a platform of stillness through meditation, and adding to it very gradually. Slowly introducing new practices, cultivating energy, etc. This excites me...this is the route that I'd like to take. But I question my ability, since I consider myself to be only an advanced beginner. I also wonder what I'd do if someone had some serious energy overload issues. All I can do is stress the necessity of self-pacing, as Yogani does. But I've so much less experience than he that I do question if I'm out of my league, and should stick to a more solid and predictable platform of meditation and spinal breathing. Any thoughts on this?

Last question: since the location is so central, I'd like to let forum members know that we're there on Tuesday nights, in case anyone comes through the city and would like to drop in. How/where would I do this? Is it prudent for me to be so 'out there' with it? Craig's List and NYC are big pots, and I do think about some safety issues, but I'm more interested in meeting and meditating with interesting people than I am worried about attracting the deranged. There are always risks, right? Your thoughts appreciated.

I know that time will answer all the above questions, but I'd appreciate your wisdom while I'm in the planning stages. Thanks for your time! :)

Yogani wrote:

Go for it. :-)

You can put the word out to the AYP community in the "Member Announcements" forum, near the bottom of the list on the forums home page. Make sure to put an informative headline on it, Like "NYC Meditation Group Tuesday Nights," or similar.

Regarding your concerns about getting in over your head, there are all sorts of dynamics that occur in a meditation group, from kundalini cases walking in the door on day one, to folks overdoing with the AYP practices later on and having symptoms come up. Sooner or later, some issues will be there. But it is not your responsibility to solve everything for everyone. I can't do it. No one person can. But as a family of practitioners with a strong and growing written knowledge base, we can handle anything, regardless of our individual level of experience.

When issues come up, all you have to do is give your two cents and point people in the right direction for additional help. The AYP resources are becoming quite robust for handling just about anything that can come up. The forums are always there as a backstop for you (for group admin and practice issues) and for all practitioners. And I am there too.

One of the most important things about the AYP approach is that it is "self-directed." One of the fringe benefits of this is that no one (including me) has to stand up and pretend to be a know-it-all on practices and experiences. Anyone who learns how to refer people to the right resources will learn more themselves, while helping others. We are all working from the same core resources, and expanding on them as we go along. If you take that attitude in running a meditation group, you will do great and never be left holding anyone else's bag. It is an important point.

Of course, administration is needed, and someone has to take care of that. The knowledge on practices and the journey are something else, and we all share in that equally. If you are clear with everyone on that, the logical places people will go for help will be each other, the AYP writings, the AYP support forums, and to other sources of spiritual knowledge also. That is how it is designed to work, and it does work.

I suggest you contact Shweta, Louis and Sadhak, all who have experience running AYP meditation groups. Feel free to copy this email to them if you wish. I recommend it, since ideas on running AYP meditation groups are continuing to crystallize. It would also be appropriate to discuss it in the public forums, where more can contribute and benefit. I am not opposed to an epidemic of AYP meditation groups breaking out around the world. The more the merrier! :-)

The risk you are perceiving will be far outweighed by the rewards. A larger group will bring many benefits to you and everyone who attends. Just think admin -- the knowledge end of it is already taken care of.

Having this space come available in midtown Manhattan is a big break. Walk on through that door. There is a whole new world waiting for you.

As for the "energy cultivation," it will come naturally as everyone settles into inner silence, and that will be the right time for it. There is some admin associated with that too -- how to bring people at different levels of experience together fruitfully. There are various ways to handle it, but you don't have to worry about it now. Just go one step at a time. When the questions come up, the answers will be there. Inner silence will take care of it.

All the best!

Meg wrote:

I love your answer. :) I"m going to go for it. Will keep you posted - we're gearing up to start in a week.

On placing an ad:

I plagiarized your text book. Please consider this a first draft, and let me know if there are any corrections or suggestions. Thanks! I'm really excited - hope it floats.

New Meditation Group: Advanced Yoga Practices

The premise of yoga is simple. There is an outer reality and an inner one, and our nervous system is the doorway between them. Advanced Yoga Practices (AYP) stimulate and open that doorway. The result? Peace, creativity, happiness, and a steady rise of ecstatic bliss radiating from within.

AYP brings together the ancient methods of Yoga in a system that can easily be learned. Come join us on Tuesday nights and find the peace and joy that are your birthright. The teachings are non-sectarian: all belief systems are embraced and all methods of meditation are welcome. We'll build a solid platform of meditation, then gradually add the Advanced Yoga Practices. Classes are free. AYP books are available by donation.

Tuesday nights beginning September 11.
Instruction is from 7:00-7:30 p.m.
Pranayama and meditation are from 7:30 – 8:00.
Please bring your own pillow or mat.
(address and phone omitted in this post)

Yogani wrote:

Looks good. However, I would not start anyone in deep meditation without back support, unless they have experience and choose it. It will be a big obstacle for many people -- immediately cuts out most folks we'd like to invite to learn deep meditation. So I do not recommend advertising "bring floor mat or pillow."

The chair is a great invention, and most people know how to use one. :-)

I don't think seating should be mentioned in the ad. In fact, mentioning "comfortable seating available" would draw more people. Seating will work itself out over time. Some will go for the floor (or wall), and others will be happy in a chair. The instructional preference in the AYP lessons is for back support. Reason: No back support is a much bigger obstacle to beginning deep meditation than a help. To put any preference or peer pressure on no back support will surely reduce participation in the meditation group, and it isn't AYP.

Comfort, comfort, comfort.

I am copying the other meditation group leaders on this for a heads up. There have been occasional discussions in the forums on using no back support, and it is nearly always problematic for beginners. Nowhere in the AYP lessons is a preference for no back support expressed. There is good reason for it. 98% of the people on the planet will find it to be a major distraction, and that is the 98% we are interested in inspiring to take up daily practices. The other 2% can take care of themselves -- they tend to gobble up AYP in big bites, sometimes getting a little indigestion. :-)

You know, if these meditation group planning discussions were in the public forums, many may be inspired to chime in and start meditation groups. We ought to think about taking it public. Would you mind if I post our interchange in the forums?

The guru is in you.

Meg wrote:

Great points, Yogani. No, I don't mind - feel free to post whatever
you want on the forum. I'm not sure what kind of accommodations I'm
going to be getting - for sure there'll be walls, but I don't know
about any more than that. I'll check it out.

2007/09/05 23:51:36
AYP Helpers
http://www.aypsite.org/forum/topic.asp?TOPIC_ID=2898&REPLY_ID=25322&whichpage=-1
Tips on Starting & Running an AYP Meditation Group

quote:
_____
Originally posted by matangi

Yogani, given all of available resources, what is a practical amount of time with the practices before considering offering a class? I would see myself more as someone who is inviting a group of kindred spirits to join in the journey....learning together as we go...etc. I would serve as a resource point and certainly offer what I can....
_____

Hi Kathy:

That is good advice from Meg and Sadhak. It is not necessary to take it on in a "teaching" role. The "kindred spirit" approach you mention is a good one (pretty much how we do things around here), and only when you feel ready, as suggested. If you put in your two cents, it will be enough, and the rest of AYP is there to back you up. In time, your two cents will become a quarter, and finally a few dollars -- so much the better for everyone. It takes very little to get started -- only a desire ... and it grows from there.

Btw, there is no need to digest the entire AYP Easy Lessons book in one fell swoop. It represents decades of knowledge accumulation and application, and it will likely take years to absorb and apply it all. And there is a Volume 2 coming down the road too. :-) It will be good to read these a bit at a time as you are so inclined, but keep in mind that they are references for the long term.

A good way to introduce folks to the main practices in AYP is through the small Enlightenment Series books, and in some cases (especially for open-minded Christians), the Secrets of Wilder novel. These books are much easier to digest than the big book -- they are designed to be easy doorways leading inward toward integrated practices according to individual interests. For an AYP meditation group, pointing beginners to the little Deep Meditation book would be ideal. It can also be discussed in the group. Then, later on, the little Spinal Breathing Pranayama book, and so on.

Very happy to hear about your new openings. Keep in mind that there will be ups and downs along the way. That's why we favor the practice over the experience, enjoying ourselves along the way, of course. :-)

All the best!

The guru is in you.

2007/11/18 16:02:26
AYP Helpers
http://www.aypsite.org/forum/topic.asp?TOPIC_ID=3154
2007 Update and Plans for 2008 and Beyond

Hi All:

The below was posted in these AYP Yahoo Groups today:
AYP Yahoo Main Lessons
AYP Yahoo Tantra Lessons
AYP Forum on Yahoo (the original forum, now used only for occasional announcements)

All the best!

The guru is in you.

Hi All:

It has been a while since I have posted in the Yahoo groups. This is an update on what has been going on in Advanced Yoga Practices (AYP) this year, and on plans for the future. If you are a member of more than one AYP Yahoo group, you may receive more than one copy of this post. Apologies for that. I wanted to be sure to reach everyone who has an interest in AYP. Broadcast postings like this one are few and far between.

As many of you know, the purpose of AYP is to provide a fully integrated system of effective yoga practices as an "open resource" that is easily accessible for independent spiritual practitioners worldwide. The AYP routine is flexible and designed for implementation within a modern cultural setting, so no one has to leave their family and go off to the forest or change their lifestyle to engage in these practices with good results. We have been at it collectively for over four years now, and the community of practitioners has grown steadily.

More importantly, for those who have been taking advantage of the AYP practices over the past several years, the fruits are becoming quite apparent. There is more abiding inner silence, more ecstatic bliss, and more outpouring divine love. These are primary signatures of rising human enlightenment. Reports from many in the AYP Support Forums are confirming that we are indeed on to something. See for yourself by visiting the support forums here: http://www.aypsite.org/forum It is a dynamic community of nearly 2,000 practitioners, coming from just about every cultural and religious background around the world.

What we all have in common is our human nervous system, which is the doorway to the infinite and all divine experience. The practices are for opening our inner doorway, within whatever cultural or religious setting we happen to be in. Everyone has equal access to the natural process of human spiritual transformation. At least that is how it should be. NO MORE SECRETS.

We are doing everything possible to assure the long term availability of the AYP writings. The first priority has been to maintain ongoing free online access to the AYP lessons and support forums. Currently, more than 300 online lessons form the core. And thousands of postings by practitioners in the support forums form an ever-growing knowledge-base, documenting an ongoing refinement of the practices and experiences in the lives of many people around the world.

In addition to the online activities, a number of books are being written and published in paperback and ebook formats. The books so far include a large user-friendly textbook ("AYP Easy Lessons") expanding significantly on the online lessons, a spiritual novel ("Secrets of Wilder") -- a story about the evolution of practices in a modern cultural setting, and a series of smaller books ("AYP Enlightenment Series") covering individual aspects of practice in detail (six of these are complete to date).

Besides the paperback and ebook formats, the AYP Enlightenment Series books are also available in audiobook versions (read by me), in MP3 and CD formats.

For all of the AYP books, ebooks and audiobooks, visit the books page: http://www.aypsite.org/books.html There is a lot of information on the books available there, including content descriptions, reviews, and many free book text and audio previews.

AYP is a work in progress in many respects. Independent practitioners are steadily finding their wings, and the writing and communications go on… It will be interesting to see how it continues to unfold in the years to come.

In 2007, the following publishing activities occurred:

1. Two new Enlightenment Series books came out, #5 and #6 – "Samyama," and "Diet, Shatkarmas & Amaroli." And "Self-Inquiry" (#7) is due out by the end of the year.

2. MP3 audiobook downloads have been made available for all of the Enlightenment Series in 2007, plus, CD audiobook versions are becoming available now. The "Deep Meditation" CD version just came out, soon to be followed by "Spinal Breathing Pranayama" and additional titles. See here: http://www.aypsite.org/books.html#dm

3. All of the AYP books have been published in India in economical paperback editions covering India, Asia and Australia. This has been much needed. Now we have the paperback books available through many distribution channels worldwide from three publishing sources – America, England and India.

4. A series of six radio interviews were completed, covering my background and the core practices of AYP. These were recorded and are available for free listening on the website at: http://www.aypsite.org/audio.html

In 2008, it is hoped to complete the following writing and publishing activities:

1. Complete the remaining scheduled Enlightenment Series books – "Bhakti and Karma Yoga" and "Eight Limbs of Yoga" (on the important subject of "self-pacing" our practices).

2. Stay current with publishing audiobooks for new Enlightenment Series books, including MP3 downloads and catching up with the CD versions.

3. Begin, and maybe finish in late 2008, a second large textbook ("AYP Easy Lessons - Vol 2"), covering all that has been written online since the first volume, plus extensive new writings. This second large volume will "round out" the details of AYP as a full scope body of knowledge. Of course, the evolution of "applied knowledge" will continue indefinitely in the public arena. Volume two will be an attempt to bring a degree of closure, at least from this writer's perspective.

4. Continue participating in the AYP Support Forums, and resume posting new free online lessons in the Yahoo groups and on the AYP websites. New free lessons have been on hold while the intensive book writing has been going on. By the end of 2008, a shift back to more online writing is anticipated.

And beyond 2008:

There are several new Enlightenment Series book ideas bubbling up as possibilities for further writing (these are tentative) – "Yoga and Money," "Yoga, Death and Dying," "Yoga, Marriage and Family," and "Yoga, Politics and Religion." These might be useful add-ons. We'll see what happens…

While I continue to peck away at the keyboard, I hope all of you will continue to peck away with daily practices on your own path. And please feel free to bring your questions and comments to the AYP Support Forums, where there are many of like interest. I am there too. We'd love to hear how you are doing. There is strength in numbers.

Wishing you all the best on your chosen path. Practice wisely, and enjoy!

The guru is in you.

AYP Website: http://www.aypsite.org
AYP Support Forums: http://www.aypsite.org/forum

PS: There are many who have been helping the AYP work with generous sharing of their time and resources. You know who you are, and I thank you sincerely. It is our joy to be helping others to expand their inherent inner peace, creative energy, and happiness. It is worth doing.

2007/12/26 13:52:42
AYP Helpers
http://www.aypsite.org/forum/topic.asp?TOPIC_ID=3286&REPLY_ID=28263&whichpage=-1
Finally...

Hi All:

Great idea, and I hope many books are given away. As you know, I did a lot of that in the past myself, but it got to be too much.

Just so you will know, the income here is not eroded by using the AYP quantity discount program referred to by Shanti above. It is 55% off suggested retail, plus shipping. The 55% is what distributors and retailers make in the traditional channels, so giving that for a quantity discount order does not affect revenue here. When Amazon (or anyone) discounts the retail price, it comes out of the 55% and does not affect AYP financially either.

The 45% publisher share comes here no matter whether the books are sold to a distributor, large retailer, or to someone using the 55% off quantity discount. The 45% covers printing and overhead expenses to run AYP, or it is supposed to -- still not there yet volume-wise. In any case, how the books are obtained has no impact on that. The more volume the better by any channel, including quantity discount.

I greatly appreciate efforts along the lines being explored. The more books we can put out there by any means, the better. Thanks!

The guru is in you.

PS: Jim -- to clarify, the soon-to-be-completed Self-Inquiry book will be #7 of the 9 Enlightenment Series books currently scheduled. The last two (Bhaki/Karma Yoga and Eight Limbs) are planned to be done by next summer. Besides the E-Series, we have the big AYP Easy Lessons Vol 1 textbook and the Secrets of Wilder novel, so there are 9 books (nearly) available so far.

2007/12/26 16:17:27
AYP Helpers
http://www.aypsite.org/forum/topic.asp?TOPIC_ID=3286&REPLY_ID=28266&whichpage=-1
Finally...

Hi Jim:

Yes, any combination of titles or quantity of books can be ordered with the quantity discount:
http://www.aypsite.org/forum/topic.asp?TOPIC_ID=1248

The economics of the quantity discount are driven primarily by shipping cost from the printer in either Tennessee, USA, or London, UK, which can be quoted once a tentative order is generated. Anyone wanting to do that can just write me.

Thanks!

The guru is in you.

Note: We can now also do quantity discount orders from New Del
Hi with the India editions. Overseas shipping for that is not recommended.

2007/12/27 12:44:46
AYP Helpers
http://www.aypsite.org/forum/topic.asp?TOPIC_ID=3286&REPLY_ID=28293&whichpage=-1
Finally...

Hi Jim and All:

Sounds great!

Keep in mind that new members have to post in the forum several times before forum email is accessible (a spam defense), so publishing an email address (or emailing the person, which can then be responded to) may be appropriate.

The guru is in you.

2007/12/20 10:12:01
AYP Helpers
http://www.aypsite.org/forum/topic.asp?TOPIC_ID=3287&REPLY_ID=28075&whichpage=-1

New AYP book topics?!?!?!?!

Hi Cosmic Troll:

Thanks very much for your support. It goes both ways, of course. AYP can only be what independent practitioners make of it. I am very grateful to everyone who is making a go of it. We have a ways to go to get *human spiritual transformation* completely out of the closet. Some wonderful strides are occurring around here these days. Bravo!

On the writing and where it is going, this post covers writing plans here over the next couple of years: http://www.aypsite.org/forum/topic.asp?TOPIC_ID=3154 I can't make firm commitments beyond finishing the 9 Enlightenment Series books and AYP Easy Lessons Volume 2, all planned to be done by the end of 2008, or maybe into early 2009. Then I'll need a rest.

Beyond that, there are some tentative ideas for books like you are suggesting, on yoga applied in daily living. The ones that are on the *tentative* list so far include:

Yoga and Money - Keys to Financial Freedom
Yoga, Marriage and Family
Yoga, Death and Dying - A Practical Guide for the Living
Yoga, Politics and Religion - Role of the Individual in a Global Society

That last one is along the broad lines you are suggesting, and it is way simpler than one might expect. Become enlightened, and so will the world. All actions flowing out from that will be for the better -- the irresistible power of constant outpouring divine love, bringing unity to all.

The additional books would be done on a much looser schedule, if they are done at all. My hope is to have the essentials covered by the time AYP Easy Lessons Volume 2 is done. The view is that anything coming from here after that will be icing on the cake. Of course, all views are subject to change. :-)

If anyone has other topic suggestions, feel free to float them. No guarantees, of course.

I am not the only one who can write, and it is hoped that others will wield the keyboard in book-writing mode. Over the long term, the recorded word is far more influential than any living teacher. History has taught us that. What we record here and now has far-reaching consequences. So, by all means, let's do it.

The guru is in you.

2007/12/21 09:04:22
AYP Helpers
http://www.aypsite.org/forum/topic.asp?TOPIC_ID=3287&REPLY_ID=28117&whichpage=-1
New AYP book topics?!?!?!?!

quote:
_____
Originally posted by cosmic_troll

Okay, your *tentative* list covers what I'm talking about... I kind of take your response as a call to action... I do have some writing abilities... as many on these forums do as well.

Could books written by other people be published under the AYP banner?
_____

Hi CT:

Yes, writing by others is surely encouraged, here in the forums and in published articles and books. All is due course...

And, yes, AYP Publishing could be a vehicle for books. It is fairly easy to do direct download ebooks through the AYP website. Widely distributed paperbacks and Adobe secured ebooks are a bit more involved, but well within reach. When the time comes, the AYP books page could be expanded to cover books by others -- instant visibility to an ever-growing readership.

Of course, content will be the key. Anyone with a book project can contact me whenever it is coming together. Keep in mind that I am pretty tied up for the next year with the AYP writing projects. And after that, who knows? But where there is the will there is a way.

The guru is in you.

2008/01/09 14:55:30
AYP Helpers
http://www.aypsite.org/forum/topic.asp?TOPIC_ID=3348&REPLY_ID=28666&whichpage=-1
AYP on the farm

Hi Hunter:

It sounds very good. Feel free to copy any AYP instructions as you see fit. The Deep Meditation PDF eBook (direct download version) can be printed from as desired. Drop me an email and I'll send you one if you don't have it already. Of course, the physical Deep Meditation book is pretty compact, so that could also work very well to help people get started. Your choice.

Btw, the MySpace AYP page you started way back when is still going strong. We see new visitors coming from there regularly. Thanks much for that.

All the best!

The guru is in you.

2008/01/10 09:10:47
AYP Helpers
http://www.aypsite.org/forum/topic.asp?TOPIC_ID=3348&REPLY_ID=28700&whichpage=-1
AYP on the farm

Hi Hunter:

It should also be mentioned that for those who are established and stable in twice-daily deep meditation, retreat schedules are available here (see top of topic list) for engaging in more than two meditation sessions per day. It is not recommended to undertake more than two sittings per day except in retreat mode while following a structured schedule like the ones linked here.

Maybe some established meditators will want to come to the farm. There are plenty of them in California. :-)

All the best!

The guru is in you.

2008/01/10 19:02:28
AYP Helpers
http://www.aypsite.org/forum/topic.asp?TOPIC_ID=3348&REPLY_ID=28720&whichpage=-1
AYP on the farm

Hi Hunter:

If you are going to buy 5 or more books (mixing any titles), you can probably save money using the quantity discount:
http://www.aypsite.org/forum/topic.asp?TOPIC_ID=1248

All the best!

The guru is in you.

2008/02/03 14:32:18
AYP Helpers
http://www.aypsite.org/forum/topic.asp?TOPIC_ID=3426
Calling All INDIA Practitioners!

Hi All:

As you may know, after few years of effort, we managed to get all of the AYP books into print in **India Editions** about a year ago.

While the over all demand for the India editions was fair for the first year, it has waned during recent months and our distribution channels are losing interest in carrying the books. This has placed some hardship on our generous supporters in New Del
Hi who undertook this project out of their own pocket. We are looking for ways to keep the India editions in print and available over the long term.

If you are in India and are interested in seeing the AYP books continue to be available there, we need your help.

Things you can do to help are:

1. Buy the books online - they are listed on the AYP books page under each title, available though FirstandSecond.com (F&S), the largest online book store in India.

2. Ask your local book store to order the books for you. They can be obtained by stores from distributor Variety Book Depot at varietybookdepot@rediffmail.com, or direct from the publisher, Grasroutes at http://www.grasroutes.com/html/yoga.html. Both are in New Delhi. Or you can write me directly and I will make sure you are able to find the books.

3. Tell your yoga friends about the AYP India editions, and help them obtain them.

4. Order the AYP India editions via the Quantity Discount Program direct from the publisher at http://www.grasroutes.com/html/yoga.html, or from me at yogani99@yahoo.com. You can give the books away to anyone you feel would have interest, or resell them of you like.

5. Offer suggestions and/or direct help for securing long term and stable publishing and distribution for the AYP India editions. We have eight AYP titles in print in India (soon to be nine). This is a good start, far beyond the "idea" stage. We are open to any suggestions or solutions that can help carry the India editions forward. More needs to be done to assure the longevity of the books. It cannot be carried on the shoulders of one or two people. So please help.

There are many from India who visit the AYP website and support forums, which are free, as you know. It is hoped we can translate your interest into action to help make the AYP writings more available in India through the reasonably priced India editions.

The AYP books add new dimensions and clarity on integrated practices and experiences, reaching well beyond the free online writings. Plus, the AYP books can be kept near at hand for easy reference.

India is where the knowledge of yoga began. The desire is to send the efficient AYP approach back to Mother India as an offering of gratitude. It is the least we can do.

The demand for the AYP writings continues to grow steadily in the Americas and Europe. It is my hope that we can also inspire and support increasing interest in self-directed spiritual practice in India and throughout Asia.

All the best!

The guru is in you.

2008/03/20 12:10:09
AYP Helpers
http://www.aypsite.org/forum/topic.asp?TOPIC_ID=3426&REPLY_ID=31536&whichpage=-1
Calling All INDIA Practitioners!

Hi Ajna:

Many thanks. Yes, it would be wonderful to reach the many in India who are forward-looking in applied science. Yoga is science too, and there is great potential for improved applications.

A new era of self-directed spiritual practice is emerging worldwide and there is no reason why India cannot be a leader in it. You would think India has an advantage in this, but long-time traditions can present inertia that resists change for sure.

I believe that eventually many in India will press ahead into a renaissance of spiritual practice based on results rather than by-rote repeating of the cycles of the past. An optimized blend of old and new is needed -- sound applications of cause and effect in practices on the basis of individual experience. Then there will be a clear path to enlightenment for everyone.

Feel free to point others to this topic for further discussion. We are looking for a "core group" of spiritual innovators to emerge in India. I have great hope for it.

All the best!

The guru is in you.

2008/04/01 12:46:44
AYP Helpers
http://www.aypsite.org/forum/topic.asp?TOPIC_ID=3426&REPLY_ID=32030&whichpage=-1
Calling All INDIA Practitioners!

Hi Venkym and welcome!

Wishing you all the best in your efforts to inspire independent practitioners in India. May many take personal responsibility for their spiritual unfoldment. There is no one else who can do it for us. :-)

The guru is in you.

2008/10/16 15:25:11
AYP Helpers
http://www.aypsite.org/forum/topic.asp?TOPIC_ID=3426&REPLY_ID=39006&whichpage=-1
Calling All INDIA Practitioners!

Hi Markern, and All:

These two articles appeared in the Hindustan Times (one of the largest newspapers in India) in 2004 and 2005:
http://www.aypsite.org/hindustan.html

They are further discussed here: http://www.aypsite.org/forum/topic.asp?whichpage=1&TOPIC_ID=1891

The guru is in you.

2009/12/28 11:18:39
AYP Helpers
http://www.aypsite.org/forum/topic.asp?TOPIC_ID=3426&REPLY_ID=61862&whichpage=-1
Calling All INDIA Practitioners!

Hi Krish:

Many thanks. Very happy to hear this. We owe much to the rich spiritual heritage of India, and are fortunate to have an opportunity to return a practical distillation of knowledge that can be used by anyone in India to enrich everyday life.

The guru is in you.

2010/06/16 10:06:36
AYP Helpers
http://www.aypsite.org/forum/topic.asp?TOPIC_ID=3426&REPLY_ID=69933&whichpage=-1
Calling All INDIA Practitioners!

quote:

Originally posted by anillsinha

Yesterday I received the shipment for 6 books of AYP Enlightenment Series from First and Seconds. I wanted to get the 'Eight Limbs of Yoga' book also. But I find that the Indian Edition is not listed in the site of either First and Seconds or Grassroutes. Is it out of print?

———————

Hi anillsinha:

Sorry, the Eight Limbs of Yoga book is not out in paperback in India yet. Unlike in the Americas and Europe, economical "print-on-demand" publishing has not been available in India so far, so books have to be printed in quantity, stored and distributed, which is expensive and time-consuming. The sale of AYP books in India has not been enough to support the additional up-front costs for publishing Eight Limbs (or additional upcoming books) the old-fashioned way, so we are waiting for sales to catch up, or for economical print-on-demand to become available there. It is expected that print-on-demand will be available in India sooner or later. Technology marches on! :-)

In the meantime, all of the AYP books are available in non-DRM PDF ebook format worldwide. You can find the Eight Limbs of Yoga ebook available for direct download from AYP here: http://www.aypsite.org/books-xdirdownload.html

Note: The AYP books will become available in additional ebook formats (non-DRM ePub and Mobi) over the next 6-12 months to support all e-readers and tablet computers, including the Apple iPad. The AYP books are on the Amazon Kindle now, though needing a bit of format clean-up. Kindle books can also be obtained and read on the iPad.

If anyone here is familiar with the status of paperback print-on-demand publishing in India, feedback and suggestions are welcome. What we are looking for is something similar to the set-up we are using in the Americas and Europe, here: http://www.lightningsource.com
It works very well for on-demand printing and distribution through the major channels, with very little up-front cost or ongoing administration required.

All the best!

The guru is in you.

2010/06/17 11:09:59
AYP Helpers
http://www.aypsite.org/forum/topic.asp?TOPIC_ID=3426&REPLY_ID=69958&whichpage=-1
Calling All INDIA Practitioners!

Hi anillsinha:

Many thanks for the feedback. Looks like good progress for print-on-demand publishing has been occurring in India over the past few years. When we first started looking in 2005, there was none.

The piece that is still missing is direct connections and automatic fulfillment through major distribution channels -- print-on-demand ordered by and shipped direct to online booksellers and physical distributors, according to demand they see at the retail level. It is coming. This is how it works in the Americas and Europe. It is very efficient and cost-effective for all parties concerned.

We will be making a decision on this in 6-12 months, when the next two AYP books are coming out. When we address these in India, we will also begin shifting publishing of all the AYP books to print-on-demand there, preferably with automatic fulfillment through major distribution channels.

The Eight Limbs of Yoga book will go straight to print-on-demand publishing, along with the two new books (AYP Easy Lessons Vol 2 and Liberation).

The guru is in you.

2010/09/10 11:24:52
AYP Helpers
http://www.aypsite.org/forum/topic.asp?TOPIC_ID=3426&REPLY_ID=72786&whichpage=-1
Calling All INDIA Practitioners!

Hi njethwa, and welcome. :-)

Yes, the internet offers great opportunities for the recording and sharing of practical spiritual knowledge. It has been the lack of such communication tools that has kept knowledge limited and divided (sectarian) in the past. Those who came before certainly have done the best they could with the tools available, but all too often the result has been "personality cult" rather than open availability of applied knowledge. The cultures of the world are still doing it the old-fashioned way. But times are changing...

There are two shifts going on:

1. Increasing open availability of effective practices for cultivating the natural process of human spiritual transformation. AYP is only one symptom of this trend, which has been emerging and accelerating over the past 100+ years (see Lesson 253).

2. A growing recognition that the center of all spiritual development is found in each and every individual, not outside in a teacher or system of practices, no matter how capable. All spiritual knowledge is a reflection of what exists in each of us. The knowledge is only as good as its ability to enhance the natural process of purification and opening within us. Teachers and systems of practice are for serving the people in this endeavor, which every person is free to undertake according to their own inner spark of awakening (bhakti).

So here we are, with wonderful communications, powerful spiritual tools, and a growing awareness of the role of every human being on the planet being the doorway to the divine.

If you would like to use your technical skills to help make applied spiritual knowledge more visible to the the world-at-large, feel free to do so. Many hands make light work.

Let's do it! :-)

The guru is in you.

2010/09/10 14:21:54
AYP Helpers
http://www.aypsite.org/forum/topic.asp?TOPIC_ID=3426&REPLY_ID=72797&whichpage=-1
Calling All INDIA Practitioners!

Hi njethwa:

Actually, we are in pretty good shape with Google and the other search engines. Both the forums and the main website (lessons) are continuously site-mapped for Google, and about 50% of all traffic comes through the search engines. For traffic stats and history, see the "traffic" link on the top menu of the main website.

As far as blogging goes, these forums fill that need for many who wish to share and interact on spiritual practices and experiences. It has become a vast knowledge base here, above and beyond the AYP lessons and books, and growing all the time.

Some here have started their own blogs, which can be found under "AYP related" in the links section of the main website. There are also a dozen on-going translations of AYP into other languages, which have spawned spin-off activities on the web.

AYP also has a presence on Facebook (by others), Myspace, and Youtube (very active). Links for those can be found near the bottom of the left border on any page of the website and forums.

Then there is the real-world stuff -- meditation groups, hands-on training, retreats, research, etc., all on the upswing. See the contacts list on the main website, which is in very early stages of formation.

It goes on and on ... as it should.

Everything related to AYP has been evolving from rudimentary to gradually more sophistication. So it goes, with each step leading to the next. Obviously, there is a limit to what I can do here, but there is no limit to what everyone else can do. That is what I encourage, for everyone to reach out as so inclined through their own channels. And keep in touch here, as desired.

As you get your practices into long term stable daily mode, and with inner silence and ecstatic conductivity steadily coming up, doors will open pointing to what can happen next. Then just walk through. It is becoming like water flowing downhill. Stillness in action.... :-)

The guru is in you.

2010/09/10 14:30:30
AYP Helpers
http://www.aypsite.org/forum/topic.asp?TOPIC_ID=3426&REPLY_ID=72798&whichpage=-1
Calling All INDIA Practitioners!

quote:
_____
Originally posted by krcqimpro1

Yogani,

Is there a way of "sorting" the members list of AYPers to obtain just their co-ordinates?

Krish
_____

Hi Krish:

By clicking the column top labels on the member list, you can sort by any of them. You won't get more than country that way, and not everyone has country listed, but you can get an idea about who is in India, and contact them through the forum email service.

A good place to start would be to get in touch with those in India who have been active in the forums. Quite a few these days.

India is a big project, one with huge potential for self-directed spiritual practice on a mass scale. It is fitting that knowledge of the practical application of yoga should travel full circle, from east, to west, to east. It's the least we can do, to bring the precious knowledge we have learned to use back to mother. :-)

All the best!

The guru is in you.

2008/02/07 13:34:51
AYP Helpers
http://www.aypsite.org/forum/topic.asp?TOPIC_ID=3435&REPLY_ID=29788&whichpage=-1
Public Relations - Radio and Internet Radio

quote:
_____

Originally posted by Jim and His Karma

quote:
_____

Scott said: I don't think any attention should be given to Yogani, other than the "organizer" of this system.
_____

I agree that leading with a Fearless Leader angle may not send the truest message of what AYP is about. And Yogani has often stated that he doesn't want to be saddled with carrying the brand image long term, though he does do a great job (as we all know) answering questions and making the esoteric seem mildly attainable. But he's the only spokesman we've got (unless you want to help on that). Agreed, though, that it's truest for the practice, truest to Yogani's intentions, and most likely to attract press if we stress the practice rather than the individual who created it. We had some problems on Wikipedia last year when sight was lost on that, and the Wiki people concluded this was about self-promotion.
_____

Hi All:

This part is music to my ears, especially the part about other spokespersons.

My only interest in going on the air (or Wikipedia, or anywhere) is to broaden the visibility of AYP. I am very willing to do that, but hope to ride off into the sunset when others pick up that role as time goes on. I wonder if all this can be accomplished while staying anonymous, but that is my problem. It is a trade-off. Anonymity versus Oprah? -- A journey from from the sublime to the ridiculous, and hopefully back again. It is all the same really. :-)

All that aside, the intention is for AYP to become a self-perpetuating open resource that will have many spokespeople, a lot of public visibility, and play a role in promoting and supporting self-directed spiritual practice everywhere. That, plus help "Applied Spiritual Science" reach critical mass in the large research and educational institutions.

So I will duck out of here for now. Call me if you need me. :-)

Thanks much!

The guru is in you.

2008/02/07 23:06:24
AYP Helpers
http://www.aypsite.org/forum/topic.asp?TOPIC_ID=3435&REPLY_ID=29803&whichpage=-1
Public Relations - Radio and Internet Radio

quote:
_____
Originally posted by scottfitzgerald

Then what would be the approach? First non-linear, international, on-line open spiritual community? The first spiritual path that takes the Linux approach instead of the Microsoft approach?

Yogani? Intent?
_____

Hi Scott:

Thanks for chiming in on this. I'd say whatever will work in each venue. You know what people want to hear about. Just tell it like it is in a way that you know will draw interest. Every aspect of AYP leads to every other aspect, so the conversation can start anywhere, depending on audience interest.

AYP is not difficult to grasp by anyone who really wants to. And it's not difficult to produce lasting results. Way easier than considering all this back in the 1970s. Maybe that is the story. It is a new era of spiritual practice and experience... :-)

The guru is in you.

2009/03/26 17:01:09
AYP Helpers
http://www.aypsite.org/forum/topic.asp?TOPIC_ID=3456&REPLY_ID=48007&whichpage=-1
AYP is on Facebook

Hi All:

I finally got something started on Facebook, in addition to the other two AYP Facebook pages that we know of (they are linked above and on the new Facebook page). If you know of others, do connect up the network.

See "the wall" here for some initial entries, and feel free to add on: http://www.facebook.com/pages/Yogani/83306582904

The more the merrier. Thanks! :-)

The guru is in you.

2009/03/26 17:28:03
AYP Helpers
http://www.aypsite.org/forum/topic.asp?TOPIC_ID=3456&REPLY_ID=48008&whichpage=-1
AYP is on Facebook
PS: I don't see where people can become "members." Does that happen automatically when someone posts on the wall, or did I make the wrong kind of Facebook membership and page?

2009/03/26 20:04:32
AYP Helpers
http://www.aypsite.org/forum/topic.asp?TOPIC_ID=3456&REPLY_ID=48016&whichpage=-1
AYP is on Facebook

Thanks, Cosmic.

Do you think this will serve the purpose as it is currently set up? Anyone else have opinions about this? I am not very familiar with Facebook.

The guru is in you.

2009/03/26 22:54:27
AYP Helpers
http://www.aypsite.org/forum/topic.asp?TOPIC_ID=3456&REPLY_ID=48021&whichpage=-1
AYP is on Facebook

quote:
_____
Originally posted by CarsonZi

My opinion is that you should set up a group instead of a page.
_____

Hi Carson:

The other two AYP Facebook links mentioned above are groups. It isn't clear to me how to form a group, but I think an individual membership is needed first, which I do not have. I can't re-register with the same email address (preferred) without deleting the organizational membership and page just made today. Maybe I will play with it a bit before deciding whether or not to start over in another mode.

Here is the Facebook organizational page (same mode as the Yogani/AYP page made today), which shows members and many other features that might be useful for building into an AYP Facebook page over time:
http://www.facebook.com/facebook?ref=pf

We'd like to have their traffic. All in good time. :-)

The guru is in you.

2009/03/26 23:06:32
AYP Helpers
http://www.aypsite.org/forum/topic.asp?TOPIC_ID=3456&REPLY_ID=48022&whichpage=-1
AYP is on Facebook

Hi Cosmic:

We crossed posts. As mentioned, I'd like to mull it over a bit. Not opposed to having an AYP group on Facebook, but there are two there already by others. Of course, if/when I make one, it will be "official," and I can do much more with the content, like has been done on the restarted "official" AYP MySpace page, where lots of stuff has been added from the AYP website and Youtube: http://www.myspace.com/yogani

If a few of you add a couple of posts and memberships to the new AYP Facebook page, it will help us see what is going on with it.

Thanks!

The guru is in you.

2009/03/26 23:24:38
AYP Helpers
http://www.aypsite.org/forum/topic.asp?TOPIC_ID=3456&REPLY_ID=48023&whichpage=-1
AYP is on Facebook
PS: In terms of adding HTML code for inserts, Facebook looks pretty archaic compared to MySpace. Nevertheless, we'd like to have a good presence on both of these behemoth social networks. We have a good presence on Youtube already (another behemoth). In a few short months since we started there, we have risen to the top 1000 channels on Youtube for combined video views. That is way more than I was expecting. So, naturally, we are working to put AYP Youtube videos on MySpace, Facebook and anywhere else that makes sense from an online networking standpoint -- "viral videos."

Further networking suggestions are welcome. Better yet, post some of those AYP Youtube videos around yourself. It is not difficult. The most popular AYP videos are the ones on Tantra, naturally. :-)

Speaking of which, the next radio interview on KKCR Hawaii will be on Tantra, coming up on Sunday, April 5th. More on that will be posted in the forums next week.

The guru is in you.

2009/03/27 10:45:37
AYP Helpers
http://www.aypsite.org/forum/topic.asp?TOPIC_ID=3456&REPLY_ID=48037&whichpage=-1
AYP is on Facebook

Hi Cosmic:

Thanks (all) for putting some info on the Facebook page so I can see a bit of how things work. It seems one advantage of the organizational page mode is that you can split the "page wall" from "fan wall" so the promotional entries can remain as default, if desired.

Ananda, yes, I agree, the intention is not to create a "Yogani fan club." An "Advanced Yoga Practices (AYP)" fan club would be more appropriate. To change it will require deletion and restart. But before restarting, better decide whether to stay with the present mode or go to individual member and/or group mode.

I find Facebook to be pretty user unfriendly for newcomers, especially when it comes to setting things up, finding options, and even doing a simple search. I also find that the wall on the new page is not visible if not signed in. That is no good for non-member newcomers or search engines. There is probably a way to make a page public, but it isn't obvious how. We'll get there!

This Facebook page will probably be deleted soon for the reason mentioned above, so apologies to anyone who signs up there, and then finds it gone and reincarnated somewhere else with a new name. Such are the mysteries of life. That's why I do so much writing in so many places. That way, the information is less likely to get lost. :-)

Cosmic, on helping out in general, if you plant a few seeds wherever you happen to be traveling, online or offline, that will be very good. There are a lot of ways to do it. Check the border menus of this website for the many resources available to share.

Thanks!

The guru is in you.

2009/03/27 11:02:02
AYP Helpers
http://www.aypsite.org/forum/topic.asp?TOPIC_ID=3456&REPLY_ID=48040&whichpage=-1
AYP is on Facebook
PS: I am attempting to change the name of the Facebook page from "Yogani" to "Advanced Yoga Practices (AYP)." They say it takes 24 hours for a name change to take effect. It is not clear that changing the name changes the publicly displayed name. We'll see. If the public name can't be changed, the page will be removed and replaced. If anyone knows how these things work, speak up! :-)

2009/04/01 14:52:23
AYP Helpers
http://www.aypsite.org/forum/topic.asp?TOPIC_ID=3456&REPLY_ID=48227&whichpage=-1
AYP is on Facebook

quote:
_____
Originally posted by yogani

PS: I am attempting to change the name of the Facebook page from "Yogani" to "Advanced Yoga Practices (AYP)." They say it takes 24 hours for a name change to take effect. It is not clear that changing the name changes the publicly displayed name. We'll see. If the public name can't be changed, the page will be removed and replaced. If anyone knows how these things work, speak up! :-)
_____

Hi All:

The name change did not take effect, so the new AYP Facebook page was deleted yesterday. We will try again later. Thank you to those who helped test the new page by joining there.

In the meantime, we have two Facebook pages by others (linked above). The one with larger membership is linked in the left border of the website under "Communities," along with YouTube, MySpace, and other networking resources.

The guru is in you.

2009/03/23 15:14:44
AYP Helpers
http://www.aypsite.org/forum/topic.asp?TOPIC_ID=3457&REPLY_ID=47837&whichpage=-1
AYP is on MySpace

Hi All:

A few months ago, the several-year-old AYP MySpace page was accidentally deleted, and we lost the 500 members who were there. No recovery was possible.

Since then, the page has been redone, with some new features (YouTube videos!), and you are invited to take a look:

If you are a MySpace member (or would like to become one), your subscription to the Yogani/AYP page would be much appreciated. Eventually the friends there will build back up. Pass the word. :-)

Comments are always welcome, there and here.

Thanks!

The guru is in you.

2008/03/13 15:15:39
AYP Helpers
http://www.aypsite.org/forum/topic.asp?TOPIC_ID=3604&REPLY_ID=31255&whichpage=-1
AYP Meditation One Sheet

Hi Bill:

Guy's suggestion would be preferred (the small Enlightenment Series books are designed for that), but if that won't work, feel free to do a one sheet summary like you have suggested. I'll be happy to take a look at it.

If you do come up with something, we should make the end product openly available to others for similar use. It would be a toe in the water, and those with whom it resonates can move on to further reading on deep meditation and rest of the practices.

All the best!

The guru is in you.

2008/03/17 13:55:53
AYP Helpers
http://www.aypsite.org/forum/topic.asp?TOPIC_ID=3604&REPLY_ID=31415&whichpage=-1
AYP Meditation One Sheet

Hi Bill:

Looks good. Let me know when you have something.

All the best!

The guru is in you.

2008/03/17 18:02:35
AYP Helpers
http://www.aypsite.org/forum/topic.asp?TOPIC_ID=3632
StumbleUpon.com and other networks

Hi All:

Is anyone familiar with http://www.stumbleupon.com?

We are receiving a lot of new traffic from this site -- entering through the tantra lessons directory page, and on to multiple lessons from there.

Is there anyone here we should be thanking?

Suggestions on actions to take from this end, if any?

Thanks!

The guru is in you.

2008/03/17 23:33:58
AYP Helpers
http://www.aypsite.org/forum/topic.asp?TOPIC_ID=3632&REPLY_ID=31440&whichpage=-1
StumbleUpon.com and other networks

Thanks much, Jupiter and Kirtanman:

And, yes, long time no see, Kirtanman! Don't know if you saw that we finally took your advice from way back when about RSS, thanks to Jupiter resurrecting it a few days ago. Still, I have been getting emails asking what RSS is, so we added a "help" link to bring folks along.

Regarding StumbleUpon, this is all new to me, but I can't help but notice the traffic when it occurs. There has been intermittent traffic from StumbleUpon for some time, like from a lot of places. To be honest, I never gave it much thought. Then there was a spike coming from the site a few weeks ago, which simmered down after a few days. And all of a sudden today it went through the roof with well over 2000 hits on the Tantra Lessons Directory page alone.

So it has my attention, and I can see these kinds of sites have a lot of potential for sharing the AYP writings.

Unfortunately, I have no time to be playing around with it due to the writing schedule and everything else that is going on here.

Would either or both of you be willing to do some work on it? Or anyone else? I am very interested in presenting AYP in all possible locations, but not in a way that will smack of excessive promotion. What we have here is pretty unique, so no hard sell is necessary or desired. We just want to put the info in places that will make it easier for yoga practitioners to find us. Our content and wonderful community here will do the rest.

On a related subject, we are getting a lot of play on the search engines these days, having finally gotten well optimized for that last year. About 45% of all the AYP website traffic is coming from the search engines now. That is up from about 30% a few months ago. The total traffic numbers have been growing all along, so the 45% is actually a much bigger number in hits.

The website content evaluation communities you have mentioned offer a chance to kick start the whole thing to the next level. Any help with that will be much appreciated (thanks, Jupiter, for adding the AYP mainpage at StumbleUpon). If there is anything I can do that will not eat up too much time here, I am more than willing. The RSS addition was certainly worth the effort. Thanks to you both for that.

I am also open to other ways of getting the word out on the web, as long as there is help available to do it. We are never short on ideas, but always short on doers. :-)

All the best!

The guru is in you.

PS: While we have a good presence on MySpace, set up by Hunter, we are yet to get off the ground on FaceBook (nice page set up by "Nika," but no traffic). Another FaceBook page was set up by Sadhak, but I can't find a working link for that one right now. I don't think much is happening there either.

2008/03/18 14:18:57
AYP Helpers
http://www.aypsite.org/forum/topic.asp?TOPIC_ID=3632&REPLY_ID=31464&whichpage=-1
StumbleUpon.com and other networks

Hi Jupiter:

Many thanks. Go for it! :-)

Coordination can be done here in the forums, or in email as necessary. No telling who might chime in if we keep things out in the open as much as possible.

Btw, be sure to leave a space between URLs in posts here and punctuation marks, as it can kill the URL. One of those quirks in the Snitz Forum software. Parentheses are okay, but periods, commas, question marks, etc. can corrupt a URL. It is covered in a "bug note" here:
http://www.aypsite.org/forum/topic.asp?TOPIC_ID=292

Onward!

The guru is in you.

PS: Thanks, Guy! :-)

2008/03/18 14:35:51
AYP Helpers
http://www.aypsite.org/forum/topic.asp?TOPIC_ID=3632&REPLY_ID=31465&whichpage=-1
StumbleUpon.com and other networks

Hi Jupiter and All:

It should also be mentioned that we have a nice page on Zaadz, set up by Trip. Looks like Zaadz is now called "Gaia." Here it is:
http://ayp.gaia.com

We also made a few attempts to get AYP on Wikipedia a year or so ago, but it did not fly. According to the Wiki elves, "not notable enough," though there are plenty of less notable spiritual teachings with articles on Wiki. I guess they want us to go on Oprah first. Any volunteers for that? :-)

The guru is in you.

2008/03/18 19:01:02
AYP Helpers
http://www.aypsite.org/forum/topic.asp?TOPIC_ID=3632&REPLY_ID=31478&whichpage=-1
StumbleUpon.com and other networks

quote:
───────────
Originally posted by robertjames

Yes, I would love to go on Oprah to discuss AYP. Anybody have any idea how to best make contact with the Oprah people?

Guy
───────────

Hi Guy:

Kathy is in the process of contacting the Oprah people about their internet programs. As you may know, a lot has been going on there lately with Eckhart Tolle. http://www.aypsite.org/forum/topic.asp?TOPIC_ID=3504

There also could be a tie-in with the media discussion here: http://www.aypsite.org/forum/topic.asp?TOPIC_ID=3435

If anyone can do it, you can. Go for it! :-)

The guru is in you.

2008/03/30 11:09:37
AYP Helpers
http://www.aypsite.org/forum/topic.asp?TOPIC_ID=3632&REPLY_ID=31940&whichpage=-1
StumbleUpon.com and other networks

Hi Jupiter:

Thanks so much for assembling this list. I am sure it will take time for the details to get filled it by those who are willing and able, so this is a beginning. A very good one.

All the best!

The guru is in you.

2008/11/20 11:56:29
AYP Helpers
http://www.aypsite.org/forum/topic.asp?TOPIC_ID=3632&REPLY_ID=40902&whichpage=-1
StumbleUpon.com and other networks

Hi All:

A "**Share This Page**" widget has been added in the upper left corner of all pages of the AYP website and forums that enables readers to share the current page on many large bookmarking sites. I hope everyone will take advantage of this feature, as it can bring many new visitors to AYP.

Note: The "Share This Page" widget was later moved down into the "communities" section of the left border.

Due to the efforts of a few, significant influxes of new readers have come to us from these sites (hence this topic), and there is much more we can do. Tens of millions of people visit the bookmarking sites every month, so having interesting pages put there from the AYP website and forums is well worth the effort.

What is sent with the widget is the current page link (URL). If you want to share it, just use the widget while you are on the page you want to share. Simple! :-)

Note: It is even possible to zero in on a single forum post, if desired, and send it to bookmarking sites with the widget. To do this, find the post you want, copy its URL by clicking the globe icon on it, and paste that into your browser. Then go to the widget on that page and share it. The shared URL contains the information necessary open the page at that specific post.

Here is a recent ranking of the top 30 bookmarking sites: http://www.ebizmba.com/articles/social30
You will see most of them in the widget (click on "More" in the widget for the entire list)

One very popular bookmark networking site that is not available in the widget yet is "**Yahoo Buzz**." I am mulling whether or not to add it to the AYP website with its own icon. Until it is added, either in the widget or as a stand-alone, you can copy AYP page links and add "stories" to Yahoo Buzz here: http://buzz.yahoo.com/submit

----

On the subject of **video**, brought up by Jupiter in a post above, we are going to follow through on the "slideshow" idea on Youtube, though slightly in reverse. We will put the AYP audiobook previews on Youtube (and probably other sites). This possibility was pointed to by Kathy123 (thank you!). It will be audio with a cover image showing, very easy to do because we already have these audio previews in Adobe Flash on the books page. They only need to be converted to video format and they can be shared on the video sites. This can be done with the radio interviews too, though they are longer and will probably have to go on Google and other sites where there is larger video capacity. Youtube videos are limited to 10 minutes.

These initial audio/video entries are only a toe in the water, until real AYP videos happen. Not sure when that will be. It depends on when someone is willing to get in front of the camera. :-)

The guru is in you.

2008/11/30 12:16:34
AYP Helpers
http://www.aypsite.org/forum/topic.asp?TOPIC_ID=3632&REPLY_ID=41555&whichpage=-1
StumbleUpon.com and other networks

Hi All:

"Yahoo Buzz" has been added to the pull-down menu on the "Share This Page" widget. You can find it in the left border of every AYP page under "Communities."

Take a look and see how you can share any page of the AYP website or forums on the popular bookmarking services.

Thanks for helping spread the word, and all the best!

The guru is in you.

PS: Individual post URLs can be shared also by following the instructions noted in the previous post above. This is handy because posts of interest can get lost in long topics. It is possible to zero in on them with a special link by using the globe icon located on each post.

2008/12/01 10:27:46
AYP Helpers
http://www.aypsite.org/forum/topic.asp?TOPIC_ID=3632&REPLY_ID=41626&whichpage=-1
StumbleUpon.com and other networks

quote:
_____
Originally posted by krcqimpro1

Hi, Robert James/Yogani,

I think it is an excellent idea to get "experienced" members to actually "narrate" their experience in terms of when they started with AYP, what milestones they have crossed, how the advance has impacted their personal and professional lives etc. Today there are so many competing "systems" available, aggressively promoting themselves, that it is hard to decide which is genuine and which is not.

Krish

_____

Hi Krish:

Good point. Most of the bookmarking sites in the "share this page" widget provide the option for comments on the page being shared. It is an easy way to let many others know about your experiences with the whole of AYP, or any part of it.

If everyone did at least one bookmark per week, it would add up to a big network in short order.

For those who are reading the AYP books, doing book reviews and sharing personal experiences with the practices on the book seller sites is also extremely valuable for helping others find and understand what AYP is about.

Many thanks!

The guru is in you.

2009/03/27 12:39:19
AYP Helpers
http://www.aypsite.org/forum/topic.asp?TOPIC_ID=3632&REPLY_ID=48044&whichpage=-1
StumbleUpon.com and other networks

Hi All:

Over the past two days we have had over 1000 more new visitors than usual, because someone highlighted the AYP Links Section page on http://www.stumbleupon.com . Whoever did that, thank you!

We'd like to have that sort of thing happening more often on many networking sites. :-)

See the "Share This Page" gadget in the left border on any page of the AYP website.

Pass the word, and all the best!

The guru is in you.

2008/04/01 10:51:21
AYP Helpers
http://www.aypsite.org/forum/topic.asp?TOPIC_ID=3697&REPLY_ID=32023&whichpage=-1
Formatting of lessons pages

Hi Jupiter:

Tadeas is right that the <br> tags came from Yahoo Groups when the lessons were moved from there. Originally, they went to a free Yahoo Geocities website where non-widescreen formating (for 800x600) was automatically added by Yahoo Geocities website SW, so I don't believe removing the <br> tags only will remove the narrow text issue. The Geocities website has since been retired. When the content was moved to MS FrontPage and the current mirrored websites (.org and .com), the Geocities non-widescreen formatting came along with it.

Note: The right hand border is a FrontPage addition, and that is why it shows up all the way over on the right side of a widescreen page, instead of next to the text. If you view the site in 800x600 format, it looks much better. The forum does not have these format issues, because it runs on separate Snitz software.

The website will need to be upgraded to current formats and standards at some point, but not until the writing is further along here. Website upgrade will not be a small job, and help will be much appreciated.

Toward that end, feel free to take a look at the code and devise proposed solutions, but please do not engage me on it until the last two Enlightenment Series books are complete and established in distribution -- sometime this summer. Then I will be in a much better position to discuss it.

Many thanks for your interest in helping make AYP better and more visible to the world. There is lots of room for improvement. :-)

All the best!

The guru is in you.

PS: On Enlightenment Series book box sets and/or consolidation into one volume, that is for later consideration also for the same reason.

PPS: The plan is to resume online lesson posting once the E-Series books are done, so straightening out website issues in that time frame would be an appropriate move.

2008/04/01 11:21:49
AYP Helpers
http://www.aypsite.org/forum/topic.asp?TOPIC_ID=3697&REPLY_ID=32024&whichpage=-1
Formatting of lessons pages
PPPS: Wolfgang makes a good point also. I tend to get lost on those very wide text lines too. So, some sort of compromise on line length will ultimately be needed for wide screen. I am still using 800x600. Old fashioned...

2008/04/01 13:36:42
AYP Helpers
http://www.aypsite.org/forum/topic.asp?TOPIC_ID=3697&REPLY_ID=32034&whichpage=-1
Formatting of lessons pages

Thanks much, Jupiter:

Yes, very nice job, Tadeas. It looks like some words are getting split at the margin in 800x600, but I don't read Czech, so it's hard to say. But I get the idea, and clearly a site that can resize itself for the various resolutions is the way to go in this multi-formatted world. The Snitz forum software does that.

Aside from site-wide text reformatting, the top menu has to be replaced with a universal top border menu. It is currently page-by-page (the only option available in the Geocities days), which greatly limits menu changes.

Let's revisit website upgrade this summer when the E-Series books are in hand.

Between now and then, if you would like to work on the website behind the scenes, without my involvement, feel free. I can provide all the HTML, if needed. But I can't afford to get any closer to the quicksand than that right now. :-)

Many thanks!

The guru is in you.

2008/07/24 10:18:39
AYP Helpers
http://www.aypsite.org/forum/topic.asp?TOPIC_ID=3697&REPLY_ID=35727&whichpage=-1
Formatting of lessons pages

quote:

Originally posted by gray

I appreciate this has been put off as a job for later. When the time comes please bear in mind that the current formatting makes it very difficult to read on some platforms, here's how the main lessons look to me:

http://i35.tinypic.com/2h4yxr6.png

- Gray

Hi Gray:

Sorry about that. It is the line breaks that came with text copied from the original AYP Yahoo group lessons. I believe it is Apple/Safari that sees them. No known problem with that on Internet Explorer or FireFox. Not sure about Opera or other browsers.

When the website is upgraded, those hidden line breaks will be taken out (hopefully we can automate that), along with addressing the rest of the things mentioned above.

The website upgrade may be slipping into autumn, since the last Enlightenment Series book (#9 - "Eight Limbs of Yoga") will likely take most of the summer to complete and roll out into the channels. After that, it will be nice to get back to posting online lessons again, and sprucing up the website.

We'll get there. All the best!

The guru is in you.

PS: One sure way to get around the line break problem is to obtain the AYP Easy Lessons for Ecstatic Living book, which is the online lessons plus about 20% more lesson content, and no unwanted line breaks. :-)

2008/07/24 11:15:11
AYP Helpers
http://www.aypsite.org/forum/topic.asp?TOPIC_ID=3697&REPLY_ID=35729&whichpage=-1
Formatting of lessons pages
Bravo! :-)
2008/10/29 00:26:07
AYP Helpers
http://www.aypsite.org/forum/topic.asp?TOPIC_ID=3697&REPLY_ID=39600&whichpage=-1
Formatting of lessons pages

quote:

Originally posted by pahool

I would be happy to strip out the extraneous <BR> tags and could easily automate this if I can get the html for the lessons pages. Yogani, if you'd like me to, let me know. I can post up the "fixed" html on my own web server for folks to check before uploading back to the main site.

Hi Pahool:

Thank you for your kind offer.

We recently went through an effort of trying to fix all of the issues raised in the first post of this topic, and ran into difficulties having to do with the rigid table structure of the current website (can't widen the text easily), the presence of many valid <br> tags mixed in with the invalid ones (automated removal difficult), and a quirk in the editing/upload software here that overwrites changes made externally. So fixing the existing site proved to be the proverbial "can of worms," and we decided we'd rather not get caught in that quicksand.

The volunteer web developer involved is now working on redoing the entire site in CSS format (like the AYP Czech site mentioned earlier in this topic), which will solve all of the issues. But it will take time to get there -- it is a 400+ page site and a significant amount of the work will have to be done manually. In the meantime, the current website will remain intact.

If additional help is needed with the CSS project, may I contact you?

The guru is in you.

2008/11/08 18:39:25
AYP Helpers
http://www.aypsite.org/forum/topic.asp?TOPIC_ID=3697&REPLY_ID=40188&whichpage=-1
Formatting of lessons pages

Hi All:

Well, I hunkered down and did edits on the website this week. The unwanted line returns in the lessons are gone and the layout has been improved for menu editing, etc.

You will also notice a new left side border providing key lesson links and other items of interest. The plan is to add social networking and bookmarking site icons/links there as we develop them.

Jupiter, if you are still reading, any further suggestions on networking will be appreciated. We'd like to offer many more means for sharing the AYP writings around the web. Thanks for this great overview: http://www.aypsite.org/forum/topic.asp?TOPIC_ID=3632#31908

This is not a full CSS (automatic adjustable width) website redo. We looked into it, and realized it would have involved much more time than any of us have available. So this is a compromise for widescreen resolutions. Over 1024 pixels in width, there will still be a vertical gap opening up in the middle of the page, but not as much as before.

Thank you all for your suggestions and support. Further input is welcome!

The guru is in you.

2008/11/13 15:25:28
AYP Helpers
http://www.aypsite.org/forum/topic.asp?TOPIC_ID=3697&REPLY_ID=40455&whichpage=-1
Formatting of lessons pages

Hi Jupiter:

Thanks much. Looking forward to your feedback.

Unfortunately, every page on the site has its own individual text table setting, and site-wide external format edits are overwritten by the old version of Frontpage I am using. I would not mind editing the 400 pages (again) to fix the width issue, but so far the only solutions that have come to fore are adjusting the tables (and/or right border) to a fixed width, or using a % of screen width setting for the tables. There are pros and cons in these approaches, so nothing has been decided yet.

I had not considered removing the tables and copying the text between the borders with no table. The books page is done that way, though it is hard to tell, because it has a lot of formating of links that keeps it narrow also.

Another thing to consider is that any site-wide modifications will generate a certain number of "gremlims" that have to be fixed, not always easy. It takes as much time to get the gremlins out as to do the site modifications. That is what it takes to edit a 400 page website that has been through several incarnations to reach the present. Needless to say, going through such a journey is only worth it if there is a significant payoff in the end result.

In any case, expanding the sharing network to the masses is the priority now. The page width thing can be addressed when a solution become clear. It is much better than it was with the unwanted line returns gone and the left side border added -- not bad at all on 1024 pixel screen width, which is what many people are using nowadays. It is on screens wider than 1024 where the gap in the middle opens up.

I remain open to all suggestions to improve the website, and especially its ability to reach the many who are feeling the inner divine stirring these days. There has been a noticeable increase in traffic since the website upgrade was done last weekend. Something good is happening. :-)

The guru is in you.

2008/05/01 16:15:24
AYP Helpers
http://www.aypsite.org/forum/topic.asp?TOPIC_ID=3844
"Viral Marketing" of AYP Website

Hi All:

Ran across this free viral marketing service the other day. It seems harmless enough, and maybe helpful, so AYP has been signed up for it:

http://www.freeviral.com/?r=205746

That linked page has AYP in the #1 position (see near bottom of page), in what looks like a multi-level website marketing approach involving no money.

Any opinions on this are welcome. If you like it, do pass the above link on to others, as it could help increase the visibility of the AYP website.

If anyone thinks there is anything terribly wrong with this, do speak up.

AYP will not be using the unsolicited pop-up window feature of this service, or other "gimmicks" offered to get people to click over from our site to the viral marketing page. In fact, this post will likely be the only place a link to this service will appear on the AYP website.

All suggestions (and actions!) are welcome for helping make AYP more visible on the web in ethical ways.

All the best!

The guru is in you.

PS: In the end, it will not be any one thing that builds AYP website readership, but many things. Every little bit helps. :-)

2008/09/10 09:43:09
AYP Helpers
http://www.aypsite.org/forum/topic.asp?TOPIC_ID=4373&REPLY_ID=37499&whichpage=-1
Need Advice on Starting AYP Group with Addicts

Hi CarsonZi:

I agree that starting both SBP and DM on the first day is too much. 10-15 minutes of deep meditation would be a good taste, and those who connect will come back. It is best to tackle one thing at a time and let it digest.

It is a wonderful thing you are doing. Wishing you all success!

The guru is in you.

2008/09/10 10:51:46
AYP Helpers
http://www.aypsite.org/forum/topic.asp?TOPIC_ID=4373&REPLY_ID=37508&whichpage=-1
Need Advice on Starting AYP Group with Addicts

Hi CarsonZi:

I see your point, but the potential for "too much too soon" will still be there. So it is a research project to achieve the most productive impact in one session, without overdoing it.

Maybe 2-3 minutes SBP and 10 minutes DM. As you go through multiple sessions with different people, I am sure a clear path will emerge. Don't expect to hit it just right on the first attempt. Success will come with persistence and making the necessary adjustments over time. When some are coming back, you will know you are connecting.

It is new and exciting territory. Go for it!

The guru is in you.

2008/08/31 09:18:58
AYP Helpers
http://www.aypsite.org/forum/topic.asp?TOPIC_ID=4380&REPLY_ID=37032&whichpage=-1
AYP in Grade school class rooms?

Hi Anthem:

7-10 years old is a bit young to start deep meditation. Here are some AYP guidelines on teaching children: http://www.aypsite.org/256.html

Wonderful to get them started early, but careful not to overdo with those still developing nervous systems.

All the best!

The guru is in you.

2008/09/27 19:13:05
AYP Helpers
http://www.aypsite.org/forum/topic.asp?TOPIC_ID=4505&REPLY_ID=38194&whichpage=-1
Book sales

Hi Guy:

Thanks much for the feedback. That's good news. :-)

Do you think "brick and mortar" stores are ready for the AYP books? If so, that would be an indication of rising public awareness on self-directed spiritual practice, and a significant shift. So far, we have been mainly an internet phenomenon.

Sooner or later, it has to spill over into the "real world," right? Bookstores, yoga studios, meditation groups, retreats, institutional research, etc.

If anyone wants to do similar consignment set-ups with local stores, see here for the quantity discount offer:
http://www.aypsite.org/forum/topic.asp?TOPIC_ID=1248

All the best!

The guru is in you.

2008/10/16 12:32:46
AYP Helpers
http://www.aypsite.org/forum/topic.asp?TOPIC_ID=4578&REPLY_ID=38988&whichpage=-1
AYP Practice Videos

Hi VIL, and thanks for chiming in.

The subject of AYP Practice Videos has come up from time to time, and so far I have not been able to do much about it for a variety of reasons.

However, maybe we are coming into a time when AYP practice videos are becoming more viable. At this stage, we do have the beginnings of video production and distribution capability (including DVD), thanks to the extensive Enlightenment Series AudioBook work that has occurred to date. There are over 30 hours of AYP AudioBook material out there now, so I think we have the I AM mantra covered, along with many other things that can be conveyed in audio.

I agree that video would be a big boost for conveying the many physical practices included in AYP.

As you may know, the the ideas that get implemented in AYP are the ones that attract doers besides me. There is only so much one person can do, but many hands make light work.

I am willing to screen any video on AYP practices that anyone is interested in sending to me. If someone or several someones come forward with promising rough video, then we can begin to consider next steps for scripting, voice-overs by me, production, distribution and the rest.

This is a call for auditions! :-)

Is anyone interested in stepping up?

All the best!

The guru is in you.

2008/11/24 17:49:39
AYP Helpers
http://www.aypsite.org/forum/topic.asp?TOPIC_ID=4794&REPLY_ID=41165&whichpage=-1
To contribute ---An Experience of profound Joy

Hi Madhu, and welcome!

Feel free to look around the website and forums. There are plenty of places to lend a hand with spreading the word. If you have questions on helping AYP, you can contact me here: http://www.aypsite.org/contact.html

Wishing you all the best on your path. Practice wisely and enjoy!

The guru is in you.

2008/12/07 19:14:26
AYP Helpers
http://www.aypsite.org/forum/topic.asp?TOPIC_ID=4871
AYP is on YouTube!

Hi All:

All of the AYP audiobook previews and radio interviews have been put on Youtube with still cover images in place of active video. They were put on Google Video at the same time.

See here: http://www.youtube.com/user/yogani99
The link can also be found in the left border of the AYP website and forums under "Communities."

We have a new helper who is a video enthusiast, so there is more to come. The next step will be active video and/or video slide shows. But not the anonymous Yogani in front of the camera. :-)

Stay tuned...

The guru is in you.

Updates: New Enlightenment Series audiobook tracks with video that have been added to the AYP Youtube channel, with the source book/audiobook named (in parentheses):

Expansion of Divine Love in the World (Deep Meditation)
http://www.youtube.com/watch?v=pzSwM_ir0tI

Cultivating the Cosmic You (Spinal Breathing Pranayama)
http://www.youtube.com/watch?v=7hZcybFETqA

Tantra, Sex and Enlightenment (Tantra)
http://www.youtube.com/watch?v=EWWJ92T-2EY

Awakening Kundalini with Physical Practices (Asanas, Mudras & Bandhas)
http://www.youtube.com/watch?v=nUCYbvgahH0

Super-Normal Powers (Samyama)
http://www.youtube.com/watch?v=yxPDI6hdkbk

Are We What We Eat? (Diet, Shatkarmas & Amaroli)
http://www.youtube.com/watch?v=64rz_nX-kLE

A Confirmation of Unity (Self-Inquiry)
http://www.youtube.com/watch?v=75NCfAq8mVg

Dare to Dream (Bhakti & Karma Yoga)
http://www.youtube.com/watch?v=Sl10CpKkzCg

Enlightenment Milestones (Eight Limbs of Yoga)
http://www.youtube.com/watch?v=mUZZruJtIuk

Woman is Divine Goddess (Tantra)
Part 1: http://www.youtube.com/watch?v=tDLLT46qVvc
Part 2: http://www.youtube.com/watch?v=OTdK4HjvD4w

2008/12/08 19:14:00
AYP Helpers
http://www.aypsite.org/forum/topic.asp?TOPIC_ID=4871&REPLY_ID=42061&whichpage=-1
AYP is on YouTube!

quote:
_____
Originally posted by Etherfish

instead of the anonymous yogani in front of the camera, you could have yogani's voice with an animation.
See for example this video of Bjork singing "innocence". It kinda looks like her, but not really:

http://in.youtube.com/watch?v=72RFO1YtLMg

The last 15 seconds is more the kind of background effect that would go with AYP.

Hi Ether:

Thanks for the animation suggestion (and the interesting example). It is a possible direction we can go in, and has been discussed a little bit. It has implications for the Secrets of Wilder story too, much further down the road.

The next step will be a simple video slideshow for the 5 minute Deep Meditation audiobook preview. Then we will see what comes after that. We are taking it one thing at a time, depending on what happens at each step. We managed to get all the audiobook previews and interviews uploaded and organized on Youtube (44 files), no small task in itself. Now we are ready to move ahead.

Onward! :-)

The guru is in you.

2008/12/14 10:01:31
AYP Helpers
http://www.aypsite.org/forum/topic.asp?TOPIC_ID=4871&REPLY_ID=42332&whichpage=-1
AYP is on YouTube!

quote:
_____
Originally posted by YogaIsLife

Hi, I just saw this animation on meditation in youtube:

http://www.youtube.com/watch?v=inmeP8gZtrQ

I thought it was quite cool and, although it is not the same method as AYP, I think AYP could do something similar. Apparently you already have the idea of doing an animation video so I just thought of leaving here this as an example, in case you haven't seen it yet.

All the best!
_____

Hi YIL:

Thank you for that.

The quality of the animation is amazing (as is the amount of viewership), and we will continue to look into it. Of course, AYP practices are a different kettle of fish, both in practical utility and the fact that no columned temple or pedestal is required. :-)
That would be reflected in any presentations we do.

It is very helpful to see what others are doing in animation. If there are other popular examples, feel free to post them.

In particular, it would be good to know what hardware, software and artistic skills are necessary to produce such high quality animations.

All the best!

The guru is in you.

2009/01/10 12:23:02
AYP Helpers
http://www.aypsite.org/forum/topic.asp?TOPIC_ID=4871&REPLY_ID=43262&whichpage=-1
AYP is on YouTube!

Hi All:

We have been adding video uploads on YouTube, including the Jan 4th KKCR Hawaii radio interview, and new audiobook previews with real video!

http://www.youtube.com/user/yogani99

It continues to evolve...

Enjoy! :-)

The guru is in you.

2009/05/18 17:12:36
AYP Helpers
http://www.aypsite.org/forum/topic.asp?TOPIC_ID=4871&REPLY_ID=51038&whichpage=-1
AYP is on YouTube!

Hi All:

Here are the additional Enlightenment Series audiobook tracks with video that have been added to the AYP Youtube channel over the past several months:

Expansion of Divine Love in the World (DM)
http://www.youtube.com/watch?v=pzSwM_ir0tI

Cultivating the Cosmic You (SBP)
http://www.youtube.com/watch?v=7hZcybFETqA

Tantra, Sex and Enlightenment (Tantra - very popular!)
http://www.youtube.com/watch?v=EWWJ92T-2EY

Awakening Kundalini with Physical Practices (AMB)
http://www.youtube.com/watch?v=nUCYbvgahH0

Super-Normal Powers (Samyama)
http://www.youtube.com/watch?v=yxPDI6hdkbk

Are We What We Eat? (DSA)
http://www.youtube.com/watch?v=64rz_nX-kLE

A Confirmation of Unity (Self-Inquiry)
http://www.youtube.com/watch?v=75NCfAq8mVg

Our anonymous video artist is going to town with these (it's not me). Great fun! :-)

The guru is in you.

PS: See the bottom of the first post in this topic for the up to date list.

2009/06/14 12:34:54
AYP Helpers
http://www.aypsite.org/forum/topic.asp?TOPIC_ID=4871&REPLY_ID=52328&whichpage=-1
AYP is on YouTube!

Hi All:

A new audiobook preview with video has been added to the AYP Youtube Channel:

A Confirmation of Unity (Self-Inquiry)
http://www.youtube.com/watch?v=75NCfAq8mVg

It has been added to the listing above of previews with video.

Enjoy!

The guru is in you.

2009/07/23 11:30:50
AYP Helpers
http://www.aypsite.org/forum/topic.asp?TOPIC_ID=4871&REPLY_ID=53959&whichpage=-1
AYP is on YouTube!

Hi All:

A new audiobook preview with video has been added to the AYP Youtube Channel:

Dare to Dream
http://www.youtube.com/watch?v=Sl10CpKkzCg

This is is an audio/video version of a recent online lesson of the same name. Both come from the AYP Bhakti and Karma Yoga book/audiobook.

The Youtube link has also been added to the listing of previews with video in the first post of this topic.

Enjoy!

The guru is in you.

2009/08/25 13:52:47
AYP Helpers
http://www.aypsite.org/forum/topic.asp?TOPIC_ID=4871&REPLY_ID=55660&whichpage=-1
AYP is on YouTube!

Hi All:

A new audiobook preview with video has been added to the AYP Youtube Channel:

"Enlightenment Milestones"
http://www.youtube.com/watch?v=mUZZruJtIuk

This comes from the AYP Eight Limbs of Yoga book/audiobook.

The Youtube link has also been added to the listing of previews with video in the first post of this topic.

Enjoy!

The guru is in you.

2009/08/25 23:39:12
AYP Helpers
http://www.aypsite.org/forum/topic.asp?TOPIC_ID=4871&REPLY_ID=55711&whichpage=-1
AYP is on YouTube!

quote:
_____
Originally posted by Anthem11

Hi Yogani,

Fantastic video, really enjoyed it. Can I ask how the video was done, it's great!

_____

Hi Anthem:

Thank you. Glad you liked it. :-)

How the videos are put together is a mystery to me. We have an anonymous volunteer who enjoys doing them. I picked the audio tracks from the audiobooks, and the video was developed to go with them. We have now gone through all nine Enlightenment Series books for the second time with new audio tracks plus the creative video.

I'm not sure if there will be more added to Youtube beyond the three remaining KKCR interviews, which will not have custom video content (banner images only). Time will tell...

The AYP Youtube videos have been viewed/heard nearly 40,000 times since we started about 8 months ago, mostly by new visitors from all over the world. It is a nice resource for introducing folks to AYP.

The guru is in you.

2009/10/22 08:19:36
AYP Helpers
http://www.aypsite.org/forum/topic.asp?TOPIC_ID=4871&REPLY_ID=58816&whichpage=-1
AYP is on YouTube!

Hi All:

A new two part audiobook preview with video has been added to the AYP Youtube Channel:

"Woman is Divine Goddess" (...for the ladies... :-))
Part 1: http://www.youtube.com/watch?v=tDLLT46qVvc
Part 2: http://www.youtube.com/watch?v=OTdK4HjvD4w

This comes from the AYP Tantra book/audiobook.

These new Youtube links have also been added to the listing of previews with video in the first post of this topic.

Enjoy!

The guru is in you.

2009/01/02 12:52:50
AYP Helpers
http://www.aypsite.org/forum/topic.asp?TOPIC_ID=4975
AYP Website and Forum Traffic Statistics

Updated December 31, 2010

Hi All:

The AYP website and support forums have seen 351 thousand unique visitors from 213 countries and territories, and 6.2 million page views (hits) since Google record-keeping started in July 2007.

The following graph, data and map links from Google cover AYP website and forum traffic statistics. The graphs show monthly data.

All Traffic - July 2007 (when Google data started) to December 2010

Unique Visitors = 351,390
Visits (new + returning) = 910,242
Page Views (hits) = 6,173,418

Full Year 2010
Unique Visitors = 133,276
Visits (new + returning) = 330,947
Page Views (hits) = 1,983,504

Full Year 2009
Unique Visitors = 112,923
Visits (new + returning) = 280,632
Page Views (hits) = 2,020,749

Full Year 2008
Unique Visitors = 82,492
Visits (new + returning) = 218,804
Page Views (hits) = 1,604,371

6 Months 2007 (Full Year Estimates = 6 Month Stats **x 2**)
Unique Visitors = 55,894 (full year estimate)
Visits (new + returning) = 159,718 (full year estimate)
Page Views (hits) = 1,129,588 (full year estimate)

Regional Maps and Statistics

For those who are interested in regional traffic details, below are Google maps and statistics showing AYP website traffic distribution for the world, zooming in on the most active countries and regions.

World - All Countries/Territories (July 2007 - Dec 2010)
World - All Countries/Territories (12 Months Ending Dec 2010)

Most active countries/regions (July 2007 - Dec 2010):

1. United States - All
(50 states - most active first: CA, NY, PA, FL, VA, TX, MI, WI, MA, NJ, OH, IL, GA, CO, WA, AZ, MN, MD, NC, OR, CT, RI, MT, LA, KS, IN, TN, MO, DC, IA, NM, VT, UT, AR, OK, HI, AL, WV, NV, NE, KY, SC, NH, MS, ME, ID, DE, AK, SD, WY, ND)

2. United Kingdom and Ireland
3. India
4. Canada
5. Germany
6. Australia and New Zealand
7. Sweden
8. France
9. Spain
10. Czech Republic
11. Netherlands
12. Lebanon
13. Bulgaria
14. Israel
15. Norway
16. Portugal
17. Belgium
18. Singapore
19. Finland
20. Japan
21. Italy
22. Mexico
23. United Arab Emirates
24. Malaysia
25. Brazil
26. China (mainland), Hong Kong and Taiwan
27. Switzerland
28. Argentina
29. South Africa
30. Romania
31. Poland
32. Austria
33. Hungary
34. Philippines
35. Russia
36. Croatia
37. Turkey
38. Trinidad and Tobago
39. Greece
40. Thailand
41. Nepal
42. Denmark

43. Slovenia
44. Indonesia
45. Saudia Arabia
46. Pakistan
47. Iran
48. South Korea
49. Ukraine
50. Egypt

Demographics from "AYP on YouTube"

Age and Gender - Jan 2009 - Dec 2010 (based on 150,000 video views)

Note: The geographical distribution of AYP on YouTube video views is similar to the Google stats above. Since Google does not cover age and gender demographics, the YouTube stats for this are included here.

Wishing you the best on your path. Practice wisely, and enjoy!

The guru is in you.

2009/01/03 13:08:35
AYP Helpers
http://www.aypsite.org/forum/topic.asp?TOPIC_ID=4975&REPLY_ID=43018&whichpage=-1
AYP Website and Forum Traffic Statistics

quote:
_____
Originally posted by Anthem11

Hi Yogani,

As a side note, AYP also reaches a lot of people who never come to the websites.

The experience I've had with introducing AYP to people is that not more than 25% have visited the websites more than a few times, with maybe 10% visiting regularly. In my case, most that I am in contact with have learned the practices from the DM book. So AYP is far more reaching than these statistics give it credit for.
_____

Hi Anthem:

Thank you.

It is good to know there is a lot of independent study and practice going on out there, far beyond what we can see here on the internet. That is how it should be. Ultimately, I hope this will lead to many more independent meditation groups, retreats, international translations, research, etc.

Of course, anyone who visits the AYP website or forums even only once will be included in the "unique visitor" total. If they are only dropping in once or twice (pretty common, as you say), there will be less shown from them in the "page views" (hit) count. This would account for the average ratio of page views to visitors being what it is. Some make many more return visits to the website than others, and it all averages out to the stats we see here.

The reason these traffic stats have been posted publicly is not to harp on the necessity for web activity. It is more in keeping with the philosophy of openness of information in AYP. In these times, more than at any time in the past, the transmission of spiritual knowledge is part of everyone's path. So it is good for all of us to know what is going on with AYP around the world.

These stats can also be viewed as an indication of what is happening with yoga-related spiritual practices in general worldwide. The regional maps and stats are particularly revealing on this. They really show you where the action is going to be in the 21st century, and where more attention may be needed.

These stats are to remind us that AYP is a toolbox with a global reach, and that it can be a significant help to many people in many cultures.

With the evidence of steady growth, it can inspire us to do more to help increase the availability of spiritual practices to many more people around the world who may be inclined to take advantage. For those who can use the knowledge, we'd like to have it available in the most useful form possible. When we have done that, then it is up to each practitioner to take responsibility and move ahead through the process of human spiritual transformation as they are called to from within.

All the best!

The guru is in you.

2009/04/01 14:26:43
AYP Helpers
http://www.aypsite.org/forum/topic.asp?TOPIC_ID=4975&REPLY_ID=48226&whichpage=-1
AYP Website and Forum Traffic Statistics

Hi All:

The above website statistics have been updated as of March 31, 2009.

All the best!

The guru is in you.

2009/07/01 12:34:40
AYP Helpers
http://www.aypsite.org/forum/topic.asp?TOPIC_ID=4975&REPLY_ID=53098&whichpage=-1
AYP Website and Forum Traffic Statistics

Hi All:

The above website statistics have been updated as of June 30, 2009.

All the best!

The guru is in you.

2009/10/01 10:55:31
AYP Helpers
http://www.aypsite.org/forum/topic.asp?TOPIC_ID=4975&REPLY_ID=57894&whichpage=-1
AYP Website and Forum Traffic Statistics

Hi All:

The above website statistics (first post in this topic) have been updated as of September 30, 2009.

All the best!

The guru is in you.

2010/01/01 10:43:50
AYP Helpers
http://www.aypsite.org/forum/topic.asp?TOPIC_ID=4975&REPLY_ID=61990&whichpage=-1
AYP Website and Forum Traffic Statistics

Hi All:

The above website statistics (first post in this topic) have been updated as of December 31, 2009.

With it being year end, the most active countries/regions maps and statistics have been updated also.

All the best for 2010!

The guru is in you.

2010/01/01 14:27:53
AYP Helpers
http://www.aypsite.org/forum/topic.asp?TOPIC_ID=4975&REPLY_ID=61998&whichpage=-1
AYP Website and Forum Traffic Statistics

Hi Krish:

India is an interesting study. The AYP stats point to a few things.

First, as you noticed, the land of yoga is yet to catch on to the AYP approach. Perhaps because thousands of traditional gurus are available to the broad population (over 1 billion) in India. At the same time, those who have been migrating to a modern industrial lifestyle (about 300 million?) may be rejecting the old traditions, and have not yet seen AYP as part of a new way of approaching spiritual development that is compatible with the modern lifestyle, and even compatible with (supplementing) the ancient spiritual traditions.

Your comments over here provide more perspective on the situation: http://www.aypsite.org/forum/topic.asp?TOPIC_ID=3426#61841

What may not be obvious from the AYP stats is that traffic from India is accelerating. If you look at the 2.5 year country ranking, there is a significant gap in traffic between the UK and India. If you look at the country ranking in the 2009 stats (about 2/3 of the way down the PDF), you will see that in 2009 the gap between the UK and India traffic became almost nil. It is pretty clear that India is passing the UK in traffic, probably having more traffic than the UK in the second half of 2009. Let's face it, a country with 1 billion people will bring more traffic than a country with 60 million. It is only a matter of time.

The next one for India to overtake in AYP traffic is the USA. That might take a while. I'm all for it. :-)

It is interesting to look at the distribution of AYP traffic in India. The Chennai/Bangalore area (where you are) is the most active AYP region, with the Mumbai/Pune area running second, and the Delhi/New Del
Hi area running third. So the big modern cities are where AYP is finding readership. It's not surprising, considering the progressive approach we are pursuing here, geared to unfolding spiritual progress within a modern lifestyle in a self-directed fashion.

India is a sleeping giant in so many ways. It will be interesting to see how it plays out with AYP there. Your help in spreading the word is much appreciated. Not one sharing goes in vain. As you said in your other post, the potential is huge. All things in good time.

The guru is in you.

2010/01/02 07:38:12
AYP Helpers
http://www.aypsite.org/forum/topic.asp?TOPIC_ID=4975&REPLY_ID=62020&whichpage=-1
AYP Website and Forum Traffic Statistics

quote:
_____
Originally posted by krcqimpro1

Hi Yogani,
Another point of interest might be to check (if possible) how many of the visitors from countries other than India are actually of Indian origin. I expect there would be many.
Krish
_____

Hi Krish:

While I don't have statistics on that, it has been a large number (maybe 10-20%) seen here in email (and in the forums) over the years from USA, Canada, Europe, Middle East and elsewhere. These are people from India living the modern lifestyle around the world, and may well represent the path of full-scope yoga in India in coming years. So, yes, good point. India reaches far beyond her borders these days.

Some have said that the rich spiritual heritage of India is fading under the pressure of modern industrial society. I don't think this is true. It is transforming to meet the need of the times, as it always has. People everywhere have an inherent need to cultivate their infinite inner potential -- more now than ever. So adaptions and integrations of the ancient wisdom for more effective application are sure to continue in the modern age. AYP is but one example of this.

The guru is in you.

2010/01/02 08:27:39
AYP Helpers
http://www.aypsite.org/forum/topic.asp?TOPIC_ID=4975&REPLY_ID=62024&whichpage=-1
AYP Website and Forum Traffic Statistics

quote:
_____
Originally posted by krcqimpro1

Far from fading, I think there is a huge upsurge, worldwide,in (benign)spiritual activity. It is palpable in India, as I am sure it must be elsewhere, fundamentalism and fanaticism notwithstanding in some areas.
krish
_____

Definitely, but not necessarily the way traditionalists would like. Nevertheless, change is happening on the deepest levels. "The Shine" is emerging in everyone, everywhere. :-)

The guru is in you.

2010/01/08 09:48:26
AYP Helpers
http://www.aypsite.org/forum/topic.asp?TOPIC_ID=4975&REPLY_ID=62390&whichpage=-1
AYP Website and Forum Traffic Statistics

Hi All:

Because Google Analytics does not provide age and gender demographics, these have been added for 2009 from AYP on YouTube at the bottom of the above website statistics (first post in this topic).

You might find it interesting. I did. :-)

All the best!

The guru is in you.

2010/04/02 11:53:46
AYP Helpers
http://www.aypsite.org/forum/topic.asp?TOPIC_ID=4975&REPLY_ID=66799&whichpage=-1
AYP Website and Forum Traffic Statistics

Hi All:

The above website statistics (first post in this topic) have been updated as of March 31, 2010.

The most active countries/regions maps and Youtube demographics are updated annually, so those will be updated at the end of the year.

Wishing you all the best on your path!

The guru is in you.

PS: World map and stat links are now provided for both July 2007 - March 2010 and 12 Months Ending March 2010, so more recent country/territory activity can be seen in relation to the whole.

2010/07/01 14:16:55
AYP Helpers
http://www.aypsite.org/forum/topic.asp?TOPIC_ID=4975&REPLY_ID=70632&whichpage=-1
AYP Website and Forum Traffic Statistics

Hi All:

The Google website statistics and YouTube age/gender demographics (first post in this topic) have been updated as of June 30, 2010.

The world maps with ranked country statistics have also been updated through June 2010, since 2007 and for the past 12 months. The most active individual country/region maps are updated annually, so those will be updated at the end of the year.

Wishing you all the best on your path!

The guru is in you.

2010/10/01 12:26:53
AYP Helpers
http://www.aypsite.org/forum/topic.asp?TOPIC_ID=4975&REPLY_ID=73413&whichpage=-1
AYP Website and Forum Traffic Statistics

Hi All:

The Google website statistics and YouTube age/gender demographics (first post in this topic) have been updated as of September 30, 2010.

The world maps with ranked country statistics have also been updated through September 2010, since 2007 and for the past 12 months. The most active individual country/region maps are updated annually, so those will be updated at the end of the year.

Wishing you all the best on your path!

The guru is in you.

2009/04/25 14:32:30
AYP Helpers
http://www.aypsite.org/forum/topic.asp?TOPIC_ID=5521&REPLY_ID=49347&whichpage=-1
Read count suggestion

Hi ThisIsTruth:

You can get an idea about unique visitors to the AYP website and forums (the forums account for roughly 60%) by checking the website traffic statistics here: http://www.aypsite.org/forum/topic.asp?TOPIC_ID=4975

You can also get to the stats from the link in the left side border of the website, under "more resources."

All the best!

The guru is in you.

2009/04/25 15:43:57
AYP Helpers
http://www.aypsite.org/forum/topic.asp?TOPIC_ID=5521&REPLY_ID=49356&whichpage=-1
Read count suggestion

quote:

Originally posted by Etherfish

I think what he means is the read count for an individual topic.

As it is now, if a new topic is started, and the person who wrote it goes back 80 times to edit, etc. , the read count will be 80, but actually nobody read it.

Hi Ether:

Not much we can do about that without software editing. And I don't think we'd want to get into it. You can be sure the 80 returns are not in the unique visitor count for the website though. :-)

It is a matter of measuring "page hits" versus "unique visitors." On any website the page hits will be a multiple of unique visitors. The forum software measures page hits, not unique visitors, for better or worse.

The guru is in you.

PS: My visits are blocked from being counted in the website traffic stats, but they are counted here in the forums.

2009/10/19 17:35:09
AYP Helpers
http://www.aypsite.org/forum/topic.asp?TOPIC_ID=6554
All Geocities Websites Shutting Down

Hi All:

This is to let you know that the entire Yahoo Geocities free website service is shutting down on October 26th, affecting millions of internet content providers and users.

Geocities is where the first AYP website was started in 2004, at http://www.geocities.com/advancedyogapractices -- which for the past few years has had only forwarding links on it leading to our current website, http://www.aypsite.org

There are still quite a few links on the internet leading to the AYP Geocities site. If you know of any, it will be appreciated if you let the host know they will be dead links soon, and suggest that they change them to the aypsite.org address (aypsite.com links are also okay - our alternate site). The Geocities links out there contribute a tiny fraction to AYP's overall traffic, but we'd not like to lose anyone.

It has been suggested to Yahoo that many would be interested in paying a nominal fee for automatic forwarding from Geocities URLs to replacement URLs after the shutdown, but apparently they are not interested in that. The only option they are offering is to upgrade to Yahoo's paid hosting service, or be shut down. Since we are no longer using the AYP Geocities site, we will let it shut down.

For more on Geocities history and the shutdown, see here: http://en.wikipedia.org/wiki/GeoCities

The guru is in you.

2009/12/27 17:58:41
AYP Helpers
http://www.aypsite.org/forum/topic.asp?TOPIC_ID=6925&REPLY_ID=61850&whichpage=-1
State detail for Illinois?

Hi Wakeupneo, and welcome!

Here are the Illinois AYP stats for the past 2.5 years:
http://www.aypsite.org/images/AYPsite-il.pdf

All the best!

The guru is in you.

2010/04/29 14:49:10
AYP Helpers
http://www.aypsite.org/forum/topic.asp?TOPIC_ID=7692
Seeking Local AYP Contacts Around the World

Hi All:

You may have noticed that we added an "Events & Classes" heading at the top of the left border of all AYP website and forum pages. There we have provided links to the weekly global meditation and samyama healing pages, and also to a new page on the website called "Contacts - Local Meditation Groups, Classes and Retreats."

On that page, you will find the following note:

quote:
_____
We are actively seeking planning contacts and leaders for local networking, leading to AYP meditation groups, training, and retreats throughout the world. If you are interested in assisting with any of these activities, please write Yogani at yogani99@yahoo.com. We are in the early stages of creating local contact and support networks for everyone around the world. What you see below is a beginning. We'd love to hear from you.
_____

We have a number of contacts listed on the page, and we need many more around the world. I hope those of you who are using the AYP system will step up and serve as a contact for your area. It is not necessary to commit to running a meditation group or any activity other than being an email contact for coordination and planning of future activities in your area.

Once someone becomes a "planning contact," there is no telling who else might step up with an interest in starting an AYP meditation group, teach the practices, or run a retreat.

It has to begin somewhere in every community, and it can start with you.

Many thanks!

The guru is in you.

PS: And if you would like to start a meditation group or other AYP activities in your area, so much the better. Support and assistance are available for any activities you may have in mind.

2010/05/06 14:08:07
AYP Helpers
http://www.aypsite.org/forum/topic.asp?TOPIC_ID=7692&REPLY_ID=68326&whichpage=-1
Seeking Local AYP Contacts Around the World

Hi All:

This is an update on the above. A number of inquiries have been received here and we have added 6+ contacts since this was posted. Thank you to all who have responded. :-)

We are still spread pretty thin around the world. Please check the contacts/events list, and if you see a blank where you are, consider dropping me a line to be put in there. That's all it takes. No commitment required beyond being a "planning contact" for events yet to come to your area.

Don't expect a flood of email from being a contact. It isn't like that. It is a long term networking thing. Every little bit helps.

Thanks much!

The guru is in you.

Forum 23 – Yahoo AYP Forum Archive

Yahoo Groups is where the public AYP Forum first started in February 2005. In July 2005 the Yahoo forum topic threads were copied to the new
AYP Support Forums, with many new forum categories available.
http://www.aypsite.org/forum/forum.asp?FORUM_ID=13

2005/02/27
Yahoo Original Introduction
http://www.aypsite.org/forum/topic.asp?TOPIC_ID=10
Yahoo AYP Forum Introduction

Welcome to the Advanced Yoga Practices (AYP) forum. This is an open gathering where anyone can post messages. It is a place where you can share your thoughts and experiences on the AYP writings with others with similar interests. You will find practitioners at every level here that you can consult and network with.

It is hoped that this group will help facilitate the "horizontal" transmission of advanced yoga practices from person to person throughout the world. Anyone who has been around the yoga scene knows that it has become a melting pot of philosophies and practices coming from many sources and traditions. It seems no single approach holds all the keys to the vast divine kingdom that can be opened within us. These days, there are so many options for spiritual practice. How do we choose? How do we tie it all together?

The writings of AYP have aimed to collect and distill the most effective practices, from beginning to the most advanced, into a pragmatic, open system that can be flexibly applied by anyone in their daily life. With deep meditation, spinal breathing pranayama and other practices woven comfortably into our busy schedule, we find the rise of inner silence, creativity and an innate happiness gradually permeating us as we go about our daily business. This is a very practical ability we can cultivate every day within ourselves in this fast-paced world a center that does not move with the ups and downs of life. Unwavering inner peace in the midst of the constant activity of the world!

What we find is that undertaking yoga practices does not necessarily require our retreating into the forest or to the top of the mountain to achieve spiritual progress. We can be advancing steadily in our transformation to enlightenment right here where we are. If you doubt this, check out the writings of AYP, which provide effective practices, a strategy for using them and extensive feedback from real practitioners. Explore the idea of cultivating enlightenment "right where you are" with others here in the AYP forum. It can be done!

AYP started when lessons began appearing in the "main group" on Yahoo in 2003. Since then, hundreds of lessons have been posted under the Yogani name. Soon after the first group started, a second Yahoo group was opened for discussing tantric sexual practices. Then a web site was launched where all of the Yahoo lessons have been reproduced with some editorial improvements. The web site also includes additional resources: a topic index, site search, an expanded links section, a list of over 400 spiritual books, hundreds of testimonials, and so on.

In early 2005 the first AYP book came out, covering the main practices in detail, plus quite a lot of additional material beyond the online lessons. And it is continuing...

Here are links to the AYP resources just mentioned:

AYP Books (information and direct links to booksellers):
http://www.aypsite.org/books.html

AYP Web Site:
http://www.aypsite.org
or
http://www.advancedyogapractices.com

Yahoo Group - AYP Main Lessons:
http://groups.yahoo.com/group/AdvancedyogaPractices

Yahoo Group - AYP Tantra Lessons:
http://groups.yahoo.com/group/Advancedyogapractices_Tantra

AYP is not the last word on yoga. Actually it is more like some of the first words in this new era of yoga science. This is a time when the ancient methods of human spiritual transformation will be tested in the laboratories of millions of nervous systems around the planet. The methods of yoga will be blended, tested and refined. It is the technology of enlightenment that is being optimized. This is the mission of AYP to make a contribution to what will become an increasingly important branch of mainstream science in the coming decades. There is no doubt that the investigation will continue, and yoga practices will continue to be refined according to what means prove to be most effective. As the human nervous system evolves in the coming decades (and centuries), the practices will evolve to accommodate the changes. Just as we are able to achieve levels of spiritual experience with advanced yoga practices today that we could only dream of a few decades ago, so too will advances in human spiritual sensitivity be dramatic in the decades to come. Applications of yoga will evolve, just as we are evolving. But the principles will remain the same. It will be a matter of applying the most effective utilization of them.

This forum can play a role in the evolution of yoga science. We should always be asking, always testing, and always moving forward. With the essential principles of human spiritual transformation well in hand, we find that the methods of yoga can be adapted in many ways to improve the effective and safe application of the principles. Through a good knowledge of the methods of self-pacing, we are able to speed up or slow down according to the level of purification and opening occurring in our nervous system right now. This is flexible yoga based on sound principles. Let's keep up our daily practices, pace ourselves according to our experiences, and move ahead surely and safely. And, let's have fun while doing it!

The guru is in you.

2005/02/27
Yahoo Original Introduction
http://www.aypsite.org/forum/topic.asp?TOPIC_ID=11
Yahoo AYP Forum Description

Get a Link to this Message Delete Topic Description from the homepage of the original Yahoo AYP Forum, You can find it at:
http://groups.yahoo.com/group/AYPforum

****

This is an open discussion on the Advanced Yoga Practices (AYP) writings of Yogani, which include:

BOOKS

"Advanced Yoga Practices - Easy Lessons for Ecstatic Living" Easy-to-follow instructions on deep meditation, spinal breathing pranayama, tantric sexual methods, advanced mudras/bandhas and much more. The AYP lessons comprise an open, integrated system of practices that is as pragmatic as it is profound in its results.

"The Secrets of Wilder"- A powerful spiritual novel. Join John Wilder and Devi Duran and they go on a revolutionary journey of human spiritual transformation through heart, mind, body, breath and sexuality. Their discoveries are destined to change the world, but at what cost?

Both books are available in paperback and e-book format. For more information, reviews and ordering worldwide, see:
http://www.aypsite.org/books.html

FREE INTERNET LESSONS

Main AYP Website - http://www.aypsite.org
Backup Website - http://www.aypsite.com
Yahoo Main - http://groups.yahoo.com/group/AdvancedyogaPractices
Yahoo Tantra - http://groups.yahoo.com/group/Advancedyogapractices_Tantra

The focus here in the AYP Forum is on yoga practices and their effects, and developing and maintaining an effective and safe daily practice routine. AYP is a flexible, non-sectarian approach to cultivating human spiritual transformation.

While political, environmental and social causes are important, please refrain from posting messages on these, or other non-yoga practice related topics. So few forums are focused on integrated yoga practices. May this be one of them.

It is hoped you will enjoy this gathering place, and find useful knowledge and new friends.

The guru is in you.

2005/02/28
Yahoo Original Introduction
http://www.aypsite.org/forum/topic.asp?TOPIC_ID=9
A Guideline on Discussing Practices

It is hoped that those of you who have familiarity with the AYP lessons and practices will lend a hand to those who are trying to find their way.

No doubt there can be many avenues and nuances to building an effective yoga practice. The AYP practices have been used in many ways, according to the backgrounds and tendencies of the many people coming to the lessons. Whatever works for us is what we will gravitate to. It is natural, and good.

In discussing your practices with newcomers in the forum, please be sure to point out to them what is from the lessons, and what you might be doing differently. Then everyone can be working from the same basic knowledge going forward, and can make the necessary adjustments according to individual need. The lessons will always be there, and it should be clear enough to anyone who reads them what is in AYP, and what is an addition or subtraction. In the end, no matter what our practice may be, the proof of the pudding will be in the eating. It is just as it should be. It is the best pudding we are all after.

We are now at the point where the AYP lessons are sufficiently developed to support an open forum like this one. At this stage, the lessons can be a pretty good touchstone, one that will hopefully provide a sound base for stimulating and productive discussions on yoga practices and experiences.

If we keep in mind the basic principles of the rise of inner silence through deep meditation, and the cultivation of ecstatic conductivity through spinal breathing pranayama and the other advanced yoga methods discussed in the lessons, we will not wander too far from a routine of effective, safe practices that can bring us home.

So, while the discussion here will certainly be wide-ranging, as it should be, it is hoped there will be a central theme tied to the basic principles of human spiritual transformation discussed in the
lessons. If we wander off that center, let us gently ease back to the basic principles. A summary of these is given in lesson #204.

In lessons #255 and #256, on teaching yoga practices, a theme emerged that is now called the "horizontal teaching model." This is people passing on their practices and experiences to others in everyday life, as well as in the classroom and yoga studio. With so many experiencing the rise of inner silence and ecstatic conductivity around the world these days, it has become much easier to "pass it on" to those around us who are inclined to take up practices. The AYP lessons can assist with this, because they represent an integrated whole of practices that are effective, balanced and safe.

The lessons, by themselves, can inspire and empower people to take up yoga practices, and they are doing so every day. Add a few real people who are experiencing the effects of the practices, and you have all you need for "horizontal teaching."

If every candle can light a few candles, pretty soon, all the candles will be lit. This is the mathematics of spreading good in an exponentially expanding way, as discussed in lesson #166, "Pay It Forward."

May the AYP forum become a catalyst for that.

The guru is in you

2005/03/12
Yahoo AYP Forum Archive Threads
http://www.aypsite.org/forum/topic.asp?TOPIC_ID=69
Finding a Balance in the AYP Forum

Apologies to all who have been uncomfortable with the "open" posting in this new group so far. The goal is to find a balance between openness and the necessary restrictions. And we will. I think everyone should have the opportunity to share their practices and approaches to spiritual development, whatever they may be. That is what the integrative (scientific) process of yoga is about. On the other hand, if it turns to proselytizing, or outright spam, it should (and will) be stopped. The recent offender has been taken care of, as have some others who never even got posted here. Moderating at the moment is set for new members only, combined with a daily monitoring of the postings. So please know that this group is being closely watched, and adjustments will be made going forward as deemed necessary by the majority. What you say here is heard.

More than anyone, I wish to see an ongoing, productive discussion of the AYP practices here. At the same time, everyone should be able to share freely. So I am inclined to try and keep it as open as possible. Be assured that anyone who steps over the line too many times will be limited.

With so many people here, the volume of postings can be daunting. There is the option on the group home page to change your delivery preference to "daily email digest" or "no email - web viewing only." With the latter, the posts can be reviewed selectively on the web fairly quickly, focusing on those of the most interest.

In time, I am sure a balance will evolve, so those who are here can find a good experience, without having the overall discussion limited too much.

Thank you so much to those of you who have come forward and openly discussed your experiences with the AYP practices. It takes courage to do that. You are a divine blessing here, and I think many have been helped already. I encourage more of you to speak up. That is one good way to bring the discussion around more toward AYP. It is your group, and it will go where you take it -- To unshakable inner silence, ecstatic bliss and outpouring divine love, I hope!

To those arriving here who don't know about AYP, it is suggested you take a look at the lessons, starting at the beginning. The various sources are listed on the home page of this group. Most who have read the lessons agree they are pretty good food for thought on the all-important subject of spiritual practices, and the resulting inner awakenings that occur. Whether you are a beginner in yoga, or an old hand, the lessons can be a useful resource.

Best wishes as you proceed on your chosen spiritual path. Enjoy!

The guru is in you.

PS -- Due to other commitments, I am rarely able to post here. If you have a pressing question on practice that is not covered in the lessons, or by others here, please email me.

2005/06/19
Yahoo AYP Forum Archive Threads
http://www.aypsite.org/forum/topic.asp?TOPIC_ID=229
Yogani's Novel

Thanks very much for that, Jim.

The paperback ought to start showing up on the Amazon sites any time, with cover image, description, "search inside," etc. being added in the coming weeks. Here are some more links on "The Secrets of Wilder" novel (from the AYP mirror site):

Books page: http://www.aypsite.org/books.html

Press release: http://www.aypsite.org/pressrelease.html
(more on Yogani here than has been mentioned before)

Books flyer: http://www.aypsite.org/bookflyer.html

I am very interested in feedback from AYP readers on the novel, and hope everyone will do reviews on Amazon. These carry a lot of weight with visitors to the Amazon book pages.

If you like the novel, please do spread the word. The PR/advertising budget is pretty slim, so word of mouth will be important if the world is going to hear about the revealing spiritual adventures of John Wilder and Devi Duran.

A message similar to this one will be added to the main lessons group when the paperback appears on Amazon.

Wishing you all the best on your continuing journey!

The guru is in you.

2005/07/03
Yahoo AYP Forum Archive Threads
http://www.aypsite.org/forum/topic.asp?TOPIC_ID=249
I was wondering ... Yoga vs. Christianity

Thank you for bringing this up. Yes, I do have Christian roots, as do many here, I suspect.

The Secrets of Wilder novel addresses the yoga versus Christianity argument with the discovery and implementation of powerful spiritual practices (analogous with eastern methods) within a western Christian environment.

There are those who believe that the birth of Christianity was a distillation of advanced spiritual knowledge and methods from the known world at the time, including India. The Essenes hold this belief to this day, and practice according -- the so-called secret teachings of Jesus.

Over the centuries, dogmatic ideas have persisted that we must accept a particular savior or ideology or burn in hell, or that any symptom of purification in the nervous system outside the cultural norm is demonic. Interestingly, this style of belief is not unique to Christianity. It has occurred in all the religions, and has been a primary rationale for the endless persecutions and murders that have been occurring for thousands of years. Now, finally, the rise of divine
knowledge within all of us will end it.

Every person has the same doorway to the divine -- the human nervous system -- and the means for its purification and opening are universal, by whatever name these means are called. "A rose is still a rose, by any other name..."

Anyone who looks will find that the recorded experiences of saints and sages from all the religions throughout history have been essentially the same. While the cultural and religious backdrops have varied, the experience of human spiritual transformation always has the same telltale signs -- unshakable inner silence, unending ecstatic bliss and outpouring divine love. And most of all -- Joy! Joy! Joy!

While The Secrets of Wilder does not attempt to settle the arguments between the religions, or trace the cultural roots of the many spiritual techniques revealed, it does lay out a clear path of practices and experiences that are in tune with the inner spirit of Christianity, and all the religions. The means are not primarily "Hindu" or "Christian" in the Wilder story. They are human ... and that is the bottom line. Enlightenment is not mainly a religious experience, but a human one, and equally accessible to all.

The guru is in you.

2005/07/15
Yahoo AYP Forum Archive Threads
http://www.aypsite.org/forum/topic.asp?TOPIC_ID=296
New AYP Forums Launched at http://www.aypsite.org/forum

Hello All:

Since last February when this Yahoo forum was launched, a few of us have been working behind the scenes to come up with the means to implement a much broader community of forums for readers of the Advanced Yoga Practices lessons.

Thanks to inputs from a dedicated group of helpers, we now have the new "AYP Forums" being launched today at: http://www.aypsite.org/forum

You will find a wide range of forums here covering just about every aspect of spiritual practice and experience. While there is much focus on the AYP open integrated system of practices, the forums are also designed to include wide-ranging discussions on many related topics, providing opportunities for cross-pollination with systems of practice from every tradition around the globe.

There are 20 new forums on the website, plus the full Yahoo AYP forum archives have been mirrored there as well.

This Yahoo site will continue to serve as an entry point to the new AYP Forums for seekers on Yahoo looking for information and discussions on yoga practices, and as an archive backup for the many fine messages you all have posted here.

The AYP Forums are pretty much self-explanatory. Check first the "Overview and Announcements" forum, where you will find background and instructions for using the forums. Every forum has a lead-in write-up from me on the subject being covered. Many of those lead-in write-ups have new material in them, so be sure to take a look. From there, it is up to all of you. These are your forums, and they will soar as high in divine purpose as you can take them.

May you find the AYP forums to be a useful resource as you continue along your chosen path. Practice wisely, and enjoy!

The guru is in you.

2005/07/15
Yahoo AYP Forum Archive Threads
http://www.aypsite.org/forum/topic.asp?TOPIC_ID=298
New AYP Forums -- Registration Problem

Please register for the AYP Forums whether you plan on posting messages or not. It is confidential and only takes a minute. It will be very helpful for tracking reader interest and forum traffic. Just click on "Register" on the top menu of the forums.

The guru is in you

2005/07/16
Yahoo AYP Forum Archive Threads
http://www.aypsite.org/forum/topic.asp?TOPIC_ID=303
Migrating to the new AYP Forums

Hi All:

It's great that you are carrying on with the Yahoo thread discussions.

However, we are in the process of migrating to the new AYP Forums, and request that you continue your Yahoo thread discussions over there, and start new topics in the new forums.

In order to make this transition as smooth as possbile I am copying all notes posted here to the corresponding threads in the new AYP Forums Yahoo archive, so none of this will be lost.

It is time for all of you to be doing that. It will be much appreciated.

Pretty soon, the moderators here in the Yahoo forum will begin rejecting new posts (except "forum feeder" inquiries) with the note - "Please post in the AYP Forums at http://www.aypsite.org/forum"

So, kindly migrate over there with the ongoing discussions. It will be less copying and pasting for your Yogani. If others need reminders on this, feel free to drop the hint gently now and then.

The new mantra is over there, so let's just favor it easily. :-)

The guru is in you.

3194117R00442

Made in the USA
San Bernardino, CA
15 July 2013